CELL BIOLOGY

CELL BIOLOGY

THOMAS D. POLLARD, MD
Sterling Professor, Department of Molecular, Cellular, and Developmental Biology
Yale University
New Haven, Connecticut

WILLIAM C. EARNSHAW, PhD, FRSE
Professor and Wellcome Trust Principal Research Fellow
Wellcome Trust Centre for Cell Biology, ICB
University of Edinburgh
Scotland, United Kingdom

WITH JENNIFER LIPPINCOTT-SCHWARTZ, PhD
Head, Section on Organelle Biology
Cell Biology and Metabolism Branch
National Institute of Child Health and Human Development
National Institutes of Health
Bethesda, Maryland

Illustrated by Graham T. Johnson

SAUNDERS

ELSEVIER

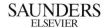

SAUNDERS
ELSEVIER

1600 John F. Kennedy Blvd.
Suite 1800
Philadelphia, PA 19103-2899

CELL BIOLOGY
SECOND EDITION
INTERNATIONAL EDITION

ISBN-13: 978-1-4160-2255-8
ISBN-10: 1-4160-2255-4
ISBN-13: 978-0-8089-2352-7
ISBN-10: 0-8089-2352-8

Notice

Knowledge and best practice in this field are constantly changing. As new research and
experience broaden our knowledge, changes in practice, treatment, and drug therapy may
become necessary or appropriate. Readers are advised to check the most current information
provided (i) on procedures featured or (ii) by the manufacturer of each product to be
administered, to verify the recommended dose or formula, the method and duration of
administration, and contraindications. It is the responsibility of the practitioners, relying on their
own experience and knowledge of the patients, to make diagnoses, to determine dosages and the
best treatment for each individual patient, and to take all appropriate safety precautions. To the
fullest extent of the law, neither the Publisher nor the Authors assume any liability for any injury
and/or damage to persons or property arising out of or related to any use of the material
contained in this book.

The Publisher

Library of Congress Cataloging-in-Publication Data
Pollard, Thomas D. (Thomas Dean), 1942–
    Cell biology / Thomas D. Pollard, William C. Earnshaw; with Jennifer Lippincott-Schwartz ;
  illustrated by Graham T. Johnson.—2nd ed.
        p. cm.
    Includes bibliographical references (p.   ).
    ISBN 1-4160-2255-4
    1. Cytology.   I. Earnshaw, William C.   II. Title.
QH581.2.P65 2008
571.6—dc22

2006048515

Publishing Director: William Schmitt
Managing Editor: Rebecca Gruliow
Senior Developmental Editor: Jacquie Mahon
Publishing Services Manager: Joan Sinclair
Senior Book Designer: Ellen Zanolle
Marketing Manager: John Gore

Printed in China

Last digit is the print number: 9 8 7 6 5 4 3 2 1

To Patty and Margarete and our families

The authors also express gratitude to their mentors, who helped to shape their views of how science should be conducted. Tom Pollard thanks Sus Ito and Ed Korn for the opportunity to learn microscopy and biochemistry under their guidance. He also thanks Hugh Huxley and Ed Taylor for their contributions as role models, his former colleagues at Johns Hopkins University for their insights regarding biophysics, and Susan Forsburg for her help in the area of yeast biology. Bill Earnshaw thanks, in particular, Jonathan King, Stephen Harrison, Aaron Klug, Tony Crowther, Ron Laskey, and Uli Laemmli, who provided a diverse range of incredibly rich environments in which to learn that science at the highest level is an adventure that lasts a lifetime.

Contributors

Jeffrey L. Corden, PhD
Professor
Department of Molecular Biology and Genetics
Johns Hopkins Medical School
Baltimore, Maryland

David Tollervey, PhD
Professor
Wellcome Trust Centre for Cell Biology
University of Edinburgh
Scotland, United Kingdom

Preface to the Second Edition

It has pleased us to know how useful the first edition of *Cell Biology* has been for both undergraduate and graduate students. We have benefited from using the book in the classroom and from helpful feedback from our students. We have also benefited from feedback from other teachers and their students, particularly Ursula Goodenough at Washington University in St. Louis. This experience validated the approach that we used for much of the material but also gave us the opportunity to identify concepts that might be presented more clearly. In response to student feedback, we reduced nonessential jargon by eliminating a number of terms that appeared only once. This helps to move the reader's focus away from nomenclature and toward an understanding of concepts. As part of our concentration on concepts and mechanisms, we moved the larger tables containing lists of specific molecules to chapter appendixes, where they can be consulted as references without disturbing the flow of the text.

We added Chapter 2, which addresses the origin of life and the evolution of the three domains of life. Evolution is not only the most important general principle in biology but also one of this text's major organizing principles.

For the second edition, we recruited a very important new member of our team. Jennifer Lippincott-Schwartz rewrote the material on membrane traffic and reorganized it into three new chapters that cover the endoplasmic reticulum (Chapter 20), the secretory pathway (Chapter 21), and the endocytic pathway (Chapter 22). Her contribution adds a new dimension that brings us up to date in one of the most dynamic areas of cell biology.

Graham Johnson, now a National Science Foundation Graduate Fellow in biophysics at the Scripps Research Institute in San Diego, remains an integral member of our team. For this edition, he added nearly 200 new figures and revised 500 figures from the first edition. His artistic gift and keen insights are evident in each of the illustrations.

Cell biology is an incredibly exciting and dynamic science. To keep our information current, we updated each chapter with the latest data about how cells work at the molecular level. Many new insights derived from real time microscopy of live cells expressing fluorescent fusion proteins. Examples include (1) the discovery that slow axonal transport is really just intermittent fast transport, (2) the discovery that many nuclear proteins are surprisingly mobile, and (3) the observation of flux of subunits within the mitotic spindle. Some particularly informative new insights came from crystal structures of a riboswitch, a new ABC translocator, several carrier proteins, several ion channels, the signal recognition particle receptor GTPase, SecYE translocon, clathrin, the EGF receptor, receptor serine/threonine kinases bound to their ligand, guanylylcyclase receptors, Toll-like receptors, the regulatory subunit bound to PKA, integrins, formins, CAD nuclease, Wee1 kinase, RFC, Mad1, Mad2, apoptosome, the Holliday junction, SCF, and other macromolecules. Careful editing allowed the inclusion of new material without significantly increasing the length of the second edition.

One reviewer of the first edition expressed concern that our coverage of cells and tissues was embedded in chapters on mechanisms. It is true that we place great emphasis on mechanisms at the cellular and molecular level, but we do so by using frequent examples from diverse experimental organisms and specialized cells and tissues of vertebrate animals to illustrate the general principles. The Guide to Figures Featuring Specific Organisms and Specialized Cells that follows the Contents lists figures by organism and cell. The relevant text accompanies the figures. The reader who wishes to assemble a unit on cellular and molecular mechanisms in the immune system, for example, will find the relevant material associated with the figures that cover lymphocytes/immune system.

Organization of the Book

We use molecular structures as the starting point for explaining how each cellular system is constructed and how it operates. Most of the ten major sections begin with one or more chapters that cover the key molecules that run the systems under consideration. For example, the section on Signaling Mechanisms begins with separate chapters on receptors, cytoplasmic signal transduction proteins, and second messengers. Noting the concentrations of key molecules and the rates of their reactions should help the student to appreciate the rapidly moving molecular environment inside cells.

We retained the general organization of the first edition, particularly the use of introductory chapters that present the machinery used in each cellular system as a precursor to the chapters that integrate concepts and describe the physiology. We moved the mechanism of the Ras GTPase from the signaling section to Chapter 4, which covers biochemical and biophysical mechanisms. This arrangement not only presents Ras as an excellent example of how to dissect an enzyme mechanism by transient kinetic analysis but also provides an early introduction of GTPases that prepares the reader for their inclusion in each subsequent section of the book. The three chapters on the central dogma of molecular biology are grouped together and include an expanded Chapter 15 that covers gene expression, contributed by Jeff Corden; a heavily reworked Chapter 16 that addresses RNA processing, contributed by David Tollervey; and a revised Chapter 17 that encompasses protein synthesis. We moved mitochondria and chloroplasts into the section on organelles, where they share a new Chapter 19 with the other organelle assembled by posttranslational import of proteins, peroxisomes. We incorporated the supplementary chapter on centrosomes included in our 2004 revised reprint edition into Chapter 34 (microtubules).

We explain the evolutionary history and molecular diversity of each class of molecules as a basis for understanding how each system works. And we ask and answer two questions: How many varieties of this type of molecule exist in animals? Where did they come from in the evolutionary process? Thus, readers have the opportunity to see the big picture rather than just a mass of details. For example, a single original figure in Chapter 10 shows the evolution of all types of membrane ion channels followed by text that spells out the properties of each of these families.

After introducing the molecular hardware, each section finishes with one or more chapters that illustrate how these molecules function together in physiological process. This organization allows for a clearer exposition regarding the general principles of each class of molecules, since they are treated as a group rather than specific examples. More important still, the operation of complex processes, such as signaling pathways, is presented as an integrated whole, without the diversions that arise when it is necessary to introduce the various components as they appear along the pathway. Teachers of short courses may choose to concentrate on a subset of the examples in these systems chapters, or

they may choose to use parts of the hardware chapters as reference material.

The seven chapters on the cell cycle that conclude the book clearly illustrate our approach. Having now covered the previous sections on nuclear structure and function, gene expression, membrane physiology, signal transduction and the cytoskeleton, and cell motility, the reader is prepared to appreciate the coordination of all cellular systems as step by step the cell transverses the cell cycle. This final section begins with a chapter that deals with general principles of cell cycle control and proceeds with chapters on each aspect of cell growth and death (including apoptosis), each integrating the contribution of all the cellular systems.

The chapters on cellular functions integrate material on specialized cells and tissues. Epithelia, for example, are covered under membrane physiology and junctions; excitable membranes of neurons and muscle under membrane physiology; connective tissues under the extracellular matrix; the immune system under connective tissue cells, apoptosis, and signal transduction; muscle under the cytoskeleton and cell motility; and cancer under the cell cycle and signal transduction. We use clinical examples to illustrate physiological functions throughout the book. This is possible, since connections have now been made between most cellular systems and disease. These medical "experiments of nature" are woven into the text along with laboratory experiments on model organisms.

Most of the experimental evidence is presented in figures that include numerous micrographs, molecular structures, and key graphs that emphasize the results rather than the experimental details. Original references are given for many of the experiments. Many of the methods used will be new to our readers. The chapter on experimental methods in cell biology introduces how and why particular approaches (such as microscopy, classical genetics, genomics and reverse genetics, and biochemical methods) are used to identify new molecules, map molecular pathways, or verify physiological functions.

In this new edition, our Student Consult site provides live links to the Protein Data Base (PDB). As in the first edition, each of the numerous structures displayed in the figures comes with a PDB accession number. With Student Consult, the reader now can access the PDB to review original data, display an animated molecule, or search links to the original literature simply by clicking on the PDB number in the on-line version of our text.

Preface to the First Edition

To understand the chain of life from molecules through cells to tissues and organisms is the ultimate goal of cell biologists. To understand how cells work, we need to know a good deal about the identities and structures of molecules, how they fit together, and what they do. It is therefore tempting to compare cells to a complex piece of machinery, like a jet airliner, whose complexity may rival certain aspects of the cell. However, cells are much more complex than jet airliners. First, cells are enormously adaptable—unlike a simple assembly of mechanical parts, they can profoundly change their structure, physiology, and functions in response to environmental changes. Second, in multicellular organisms, cells provide only an intermediate level of complexity. Groups of specialized cells organize themselves into communities called tissues, and these tissues are further organized into organs that function in coordinated ways to produce life as we experience it. Finally, cells differ from complex machines in that there exists as yet no blueprint that completely describes how cells work. However, biologists who study a wide range of different aspects of cellular structure and function are beginning to compile such a blueprint. This has elucidated not only the molecular details of fundamental processes such as oxidative phosphorylation and protein synthesis but also many ways in which defects in individual molecular components can disrupt cell function and cause diseases.

Because the blueprint does not yet exist, this book necessarily represents a collection of vignettes from the lives and functions of cells. To some extent, these stories have been selected to demonstrate the general principles that we see as important. However, to a very real extent, they have also been selected by chance. This is the nature of scientific exploration and discovery: the scientist may set out on an investigation with a particular goal in mind only to discover that he or she has landed somewhere entirely different. Ultimately, our intent is to provide the student with a working knowledge of the major macromolecular systems of the cell, together with an understanding of how these principles were discovered and how the processes are coordinated to enable cells to function both autonomously and in tissues. The latter is important because most genetic diseases result from a single mutated molecule but manifest themselves by disrupting function in tissues. Cancer, which originates as a disease of single cells and can result from many different molecular lesions, is the exception.

This book's guiding theme is that cellular structure and function ultimately result from specific macromolecular interactions. In addition to water, salts, and small metabolites, cells are composed mainly of proteins, nucleic acids, lipids, and polysaccharides. Nucleic acids store genetic information required for reproduction and specify the sequences of thousands of RNAs and proteins. Both proteins and RNA serve as enzymes for the biosynthesis of all cellular constituents. Many RNAs have structural roles, but proteins—which are able to form the specific protein-protein, protein–nucleic acid, protein-lipid, and protein-polysaccharide bonds that hold the cell together—are the predominant structural elements of cells. A remarkable feature of these vital interactions between macromolecules is that few covalent bonds are involved. The striking conclusion is that the structure and function of the cell (and therefore the existence of life on earth) depend on highly specific, but often relatively tenuous, interactions between complementary surfaces of macromolecules.

The specificity of these interactions relies to a great extent on the structure of protein molecules. Molecular biologists discovered how the information for the primary structure (the amino acid sequence) of proteins is stored in the genes, and they continue to search for the mechanisms that cells use to control the expression of the thousands of genes whose products define the properties of each cell. Biochemists and biophysicists established that the three-dimensional structure of each protein is determined solely by its amino acid sequence: once synthesized, polypeptides fold either spontaneously or with the assistance of chaperones into specific three-dimensional structures. A folded protein may be biologically active, catalyzing a reaction, binding oxygen, or carrying out a myriad of other functions. However, in many cases it is inactive, waiting for the products of other genes to convert it to an active form. The ability of cells to regulate the expression of banks of genes and to fine-tune the activities of proteins after they have been made exemplifies the plasticity that enables cells to succeed in an ever-changing world.

Seeking to take the story a step further, cell biologists ask this question: Do simple self-associations among the molecules account for the properties of the living cell? Is life merely a very complex molecular jigsaw puzzle? The answer developed in this book is both yes and no. To a large extent, cell structure and function clearly result from macromolecular interactions. However, living cells do not spontaneously self-assemble from mixtures of all their cellular constituents. The assembly reactions required for life reach completion only inside preexisting living cells; therefore, the existence of each cell depends on its historical continuity with past cells. This special historical feature sets biology apart from chemistry and physics. A cell can be viewed as the temporary repository of the genes of the species and the only microenvironment that allows macromolecular self-assembly reactions to continue the processes of life.

In our view, the field of cell biology is emerging from a Linnaean phase, where genetic and biochemical methods have been used to gather an inventory of many of the cell's molecules, into a more mechanistic phase, where new insights will come from detailed biophysical studies of these molecules at atomic resolution and of their dynamics in living cells. The molecular inventory of genes and gene products is massive, almost overwhelming, in its detail. But this genetic inventory is far from the complete story, especially at the interface of basic cell biology with medicine. On a weekly basis, investigators continue to track down the genes for defective proteins that predispose people to human disease. In addition to revealing the many genes that cause the spectrum of diseases known as cancer, this work has revealed the molecules responsible for muscular dystrophy, cystic fibrosis, hypertrophic cardiomyopathy, and blistering skin diseases, among many others, and will continue to grow as scientists seek the causes of more complex multifactorial diseases. Because virtually every gene expressed in the human body is subject to mutation, it is quite possible that eventually a great many genes will be directly or indirectly implicated in the predisposition to disease.

For both the basic scientist who seeks general principles about cellular function, often in "model" organisms, and the physician who applies knowledge of the molecular mechanisms of normal cellular function to the understanding of cellular dysfunction in human disease, the future lies in insights about how the cellular repertoire of macromolecules interact with one another. Understanding at this level requires not only the knowledge of atomic structures and rates of molecular interactions but also the development of molecular probes to follow these interactions in living cells. With respect to this area of recent explosive progress, this book presents both current technological advances and lessons already learned.

Given the complexity of the molecular inventory (about 25,000 different genes in humans), gaining an understanding of the details of molecular interactions might, in principle, be equivalent to the daunting task of learning a set of 25,000 Chinese characters and all the rules of spelling and grammar that govern their use. However, it is already clear that the origin of complex life forms by evolution has simplified the task. For example, although the genome encodes about 800 protein kinases (enzymes that transfer a phosphate from ATP to a protein), each kinase has much in common with all other kinases because of their evolution from a common ancestor. The same is true of membrane receptors with seven α-helices traversing the lipid bilayer. Detailed knowledge about any one of these kinases or receptors provides informative general principles about how the whole family of related molecules works. Thus, although there are more than a few names, structures, binding partners, and reaction rates to learn, we are confident that many general concepts have already emerged and will continue to emerge. These will enable us to develop a set of "first principles" that we can use to deduce how novel pathways are put together and function when we are confronted with new genes and structures.

Although we feel that the time is right to take a molecular approach to cellular structure and function, this is not a biochemistry book. Readers who are interested in a fuller understanding of metabolism, the biosynthesis of cellular building blocks, enzymology, and other purely biochemical topics should consult one of the many excellent biochemistry texts. Similarly, although we consider herein some of the specialized manifestations of cells found in specific tissues and how these tissues are formed, this is not a histology or developmental biology book. We focus instead on the general properties of eukaryotic cells that are common to their successful function.

We have written this book with the busy student in mind. Carefully limiting the text's size and illustrating all the main points with original drawings, we anticipate that, in a single course, an undergraduate, medical, or graduate student will be able to read through the entire book. In our effort to keep the book concise, however, we have been careful to maintain appropriate depth. Most chapters contain a few complex figures that show either how some important points were discovered or how multiple processes are integrated with one another. A few of these figures may initially present a challenge; however, an understanding of these figures will ultimately provide insight into the integrated network of cellular life. Throughout this book, we have presented the very latest discoveries in cell biology, and in each section we have defined as closely as possible the frontiers of our knowledge. We hope that upon completion of the study of this text, our readers will share not only a comprehensive, up-to-date knowledge of how cells work but also our personal excitement about these basic insights into life itself. It is our sincerest hope that the questions raised herein will inspire some of our readers to experience the challenges and rewards of cell biology research for themselves and to contribute to the ongoing challenge of completing the blueprint of the life of the cell.

We anticipate that our readers will find many ways to use this book, which covers the structure and function of all parts of the cell and all major cellular processes. We have aimed to maintain uniform depth of coverage of each topic, including up-to-date descriptions of general principles and of the structures of the major molecules and an explanation of how the system works. The emphasis is on animal cells, but we have included many examples from fungi. Our inclusion of plants and prokaryotes distinguishes their special aspects, such as rotary flagella, two-component signal transduction pathways, and photosynthesis.

We divide the material into many highly focused stories that deal with particular molecules and mechanisms. Whereas an in-depth course in cell biology might cover the whole book, a variety of shorter courses might easily be fashioned by picking a subset of topics.

Most of the papers that are cited in the chapters' Selected Readings sections are reviews of the primary literature taken from major review journals, such as the *Annual Reviews* (*of Biochemistry, Cell Biology, Biophysics*), *Trends* (*in Cell Biology, Biochemical Sciences*), and *Current Opinion* (*in Cell Biology, Structural Biology*), or from the review sections of major journals in the field, such as *Current Biology, Journal of Cell Biology, Nature, Proceedings of the National Academy of Sciences,* and *Science.* These references, although helpful to us in writing this book, will rapidly become dated. With very little effort, readers can update the reference lists on-line. PubMed (http://www.ncbi.nlm.nih.gov/entrez/query.fcgi), the wonderful tool provided by the National Institutes of Health, is an invaluable resource. Simply type in the name of the molecule or the process of interest followed by a space and the word "review" (no quotation marks). In no time, you will access an up-to-date reference list. The abstracts given in PubMed will help you choose the best articles for your purposes. Many institutions have electronic versions of the major journals in the field, so you can find and display a new review in a matter of seconds. Although the same route can be used to access the original research literature, the number of web site hits will be much greater than if the "review" restriction is used, so be prepared to spend more time searching. The PubMed site also allows searches for atomic structures, genes, genomes, and proteins. Each of the numerous molecular structures displayed in our figures comes with a Protein Data Base (PDB) accession number. Anyone with an Internet connection to PubMed or PDB can thus find the original data, display an animated molecule, and directly search links to the original literature.

Acknowledgments

Tom and Bill thank their families and their research groups for sharing so much time with "the book." Bill also owes special thanks to his long-term collaborator Scott Kaufmann. Their support and understanding made the project possible. Graham thanks his family, Margaret, Paul, and Lara Johnson. He also thanks the Benhorins for moral support; Kaitlyn Gilman and illustrator Cameron Slayden for expediting completion of various phases; and the faculty and administration of the Scripps Research Institute, especially Arthur Olson, David Goodsell, Ron Milligan, and Ian Wilson for helping him integrate the book with his evolving career goals.

Many generous individuals took their time to provide suggestions, in their areas of expertise, for revisions to chapters for the second edition. We acknowledge these individuals at the end of each chapter and here as a group: Robin Allshire, James Anderson, Michael Ashburner, Chip Asbury, William Balch, Roland Baron, Jiri Bartek, Wendy Bickmore, Susan Biggins, Julian Blow, Juan Bonifacino, Gary Brudvig, Michael Caplan, Michael Caplow, Charmaine Chan, Senyon Choe, Paula Cohen, Thomas Cremer and students, Enrique De La Cruz, Julie Donaldson, Michael Donoghue, Steve Doxsey, Mike Edidin, Barbara Ehrlich, Sharyn Endow, Don Engelman, Roland Foisner, Paul Forscher, Maurizio Gatti, Susan Gilbert, Larry Goldstein, Dan Goodenough, Ursula Goodenough, Holly Goodson, Barry Gumbiner, Kevin Hardwick, John Hartwig, Ramanujan Hegde, Phil Hieter, Kathryn Howell, Tony Hunter, Pablo Iglesias, Paul Insel, Catherine Jackson, Scott Kaufmann, Alastair Kerr, Alexey Khodjakov, Peter Kim, Nancy Kleckner, Jim Lake, Angus Lamond, Martin Latterich, Yuri Lazebnik, Dan Leahy, Robert Linhardt, Peter Maloney, Jim Manley, Suliana Manley, Ruslan Medzhitov, Andrew Miranker, David Morgan, Ciaran Morrison, Sean Munro, Ben Nichols, Bruce Nicklas, Brad Nolen, Leslie Orgel, Mike Ostap, Carolyn Ott, Aditya Paul, Jan-Michael Peters, Jonathon Pines, Helen Piwnica-Worms, Mecky Pohlschroder, Daniel Pollard, Katherine Pollard, Claude Prigent, Martin Raff, Margaret Robinson, Karin Römisch, Benoit Roux, Erich Schirmer, Sandra Schmid, Fred Sigworth, Sam Silverstein, Carl Smythe, Mitch Sogin, John Solaro, Irina Solovei, David Spector, Elke Stein, Tom Steitz, Harald Stenmark, Gail Stetten, Scott Strobel, José Suja, Richard Treisman, Bryan Turner, Martin Webb, David Wells, and Jerry Workman.

Special thanks go to our colleagues at W.B. Saunders/Elsevier, who managed the production of the book. Our editor, Bill Schmitt, provided encouragement and support; we thank him for his faith and dedication to this project for more than a decade. Our developmental editor, Jacquie Mahon, organized hundreds of documents and figures for production. Rebecca Gruliow took over the project and completed this work. Ellen Zanolle helped with the attractive new design of the second edition. Joan Sinclair coordinated the overall production process. As with the first edition, we were delighted with the editing and composition coordinated by Joan Polsky Vidal and her team. We appreciate their thoughtful attention to detail and willingness to incorporate our changes.

Contents

Guide to Figures Featuring Specific Organisms and Specialized Cells

Organism/ Specialized Cell Type	Figures
PROKARYOTES	
Archaea	1-1, 2-1, 2-4
Bacteria	1-1, 2-1, 2-4, 5-9, 12-4, 15-2, 15-5, 15-13, 17-13, 18-2, 18-9, 18-10, 19-2, 20-5, 27-11, 27-12, 27-13, 35-1, 37-12, 38-1, 38-23, 38-24, 42-3, 44-21
Viruses	5-11, 5-12, 5-13, 5-14, 5-16, 6-4, 37-12
PROTOZOA	
Amoeba	22-5, 38-1, 38-4, 38-12
Ciliates	2-8, 38-1, 38-15
Other protozoa	36-7, 38-4, 37-10, 38-6, 38-22
ALGAE AND PLANTS	
Chloroplasts	18-1, 18-2, 18-6, 19-7, 19-8, 19-9
Green algae	2-8, 37-1, 37-9, 38-19, 38-20
Plant cell wall	31-8, 32-12
Plant (general)	1-2, 2-8, 2-9, 6-4, 31-8, 33-1, 34-2, 36-7, 36-13, 38-1, 44-21, 45-8
FUNGI	
Budding yeast	1-2, 12-3, 12-4, 12-7, 12-8, 13-21, 14-10, 34-2, 34-19, 36-7, 36-13, 37-11, 42-4, 42-5, 43-9, 45-9
Fission yeast	6-3, 12-8, 33-1, 40-6, 43-2, 44-24
Other fungi	2-9, 36-13, 45-6
INVERTEBRATE ANIMALS	
Echinoderms	2-9, 36-13, 40-11, 44-22, 44-23
Nematodes	2-9, 36-7, 36-13, 38-11, 46-9
Insects	2-9, 12-4, 12-8, 12-14, 13-13, 14-12, 14-18, 36-7, 36-13, 38-5, 38-13, 44-13, 45-2, 45-10
VERTEBRATE ANIMALS	
Blood	
Granulocytes	28-3, 28-7, 28-8, 30-13, 38-1
Lymphocytes/immune system	27-8, 28-3, 28-7, 28-9, 28-10, 46-7, 46-18
Monocytes/macrophages	28-3, 28-7, 28-8, 32-11, 38-2, 46-6
Platelets	28-7, 28-10, 30-14, 32-11
Red blood cells	7-6, 7-10, 28-7, 32-11
Cancer	34-20, 38-10, 41-2, 41-9, 41-10, 42-8
Connective tissue	
Cartilage cells	28-3, 32-2, 32-3
Fibroblasts	28-2, 28-3, 28-4, 29-3, 29-4, 32-1, 32-11, 35-4, 37-1, 38-1
Mast cells	28-3, 28-5
Bone cells	28-3, 32-4, 32-5, 32-6, 32-7, 32-8, 32-9, 32-10
Fat cells	27-7, 28-3, 28-6
Epithelia	
Epidermal, stratified	29-7, 31-1, 33-2, 35-1, 35-6, 38-5, 38-7, 38-9, 40-1, 42-8
Glands, liver	21-18, 23-4, 31-4, 34-20, 41-2, 44-2
Intestine	11-2, 31-1, 32-1, 33-1, 33-2, 34-2, 46-18
Kidney	11-3, 29-18, 35-1
Respiratory system	11-4, 32-2, 34-3, 37-6, 38-17
Vascular	22-8, 29-8, 29-18, 30-13, 30-14, 31-2, 32-11
Muscle	
Cardiac muscle	11-11, 11-12, 11-13, 39-1, 39-10, 39-15, 39-18, 39-19
Skeletal muscle	11-8, 29-18, 33-3, 36-3, 36-4, 36-5, 39-1, 39-2, 39-4, 39-8, 39-9, 39-10, 39-13, 39-14, 39-15, 39-16
Smooth muscle	29-8, 33-1, 35-8, 39-1, 39-20, 39-21
Nervous system	
Central nervous system neurons	11-9, 11-10, 30-7, 34-12, 34-13, 37-7, 38-13, 39-14
Glial cells	11-8, 11-9, 29-18, 37-7
Peripheral nervous system neurons	11-8, 26-3, 26-16, 27-1, 27-2, 29-18, 33-18, 35-9, 37-1, 37-3, 37-4, 37-5, 38-1, 38-7, 39-14
Synapses	11-8, 11-9, 11-10, 39-14
Reproductive system	
Oocytes, eggs	26-15, 34-15, 40-7, 40-10, 40-12, 43-10, 45-14
Sperm	38-1, 38-3, 38-18, 45-1, 45-2, 45-4, 45-5, 45-8

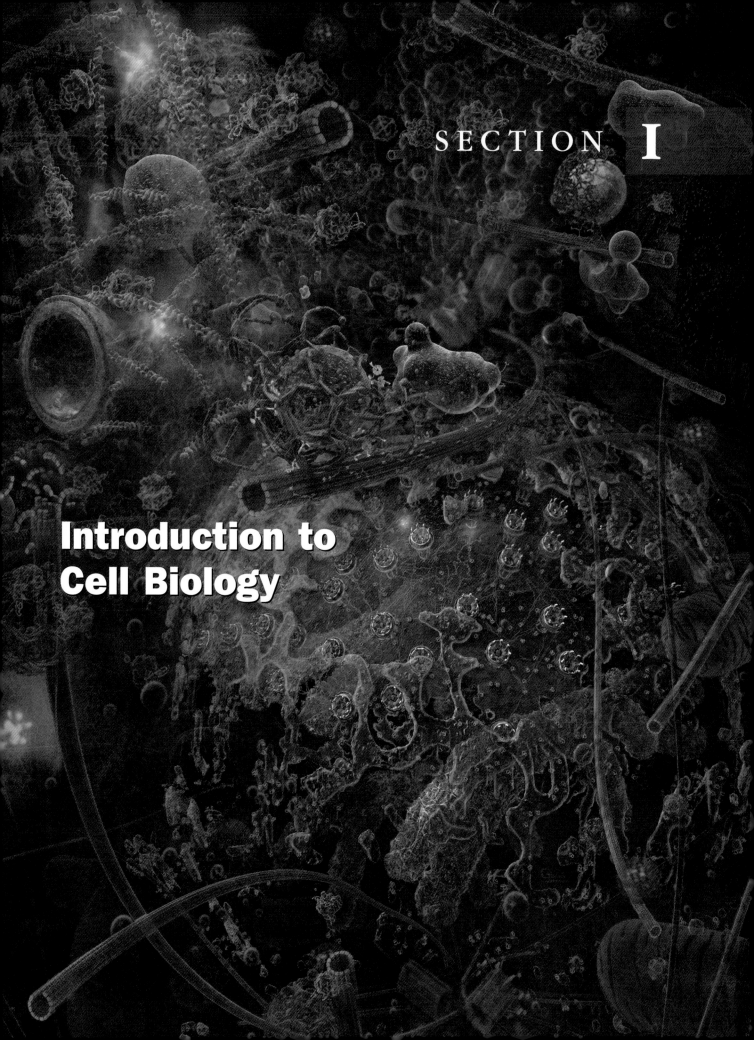

SECTION I

Introduction to Cell Biology

CHAPTER 1

Introduction to Cells

Biology is based on the fundamental laws of nature embodied in chemistry and physics, but the origin and evolution of life on earth were historical events. This makes biology more like astronomy than like chemistry and physics. Neither the organization of the universe nor life as we know it had to evolve as it did. Chance played a central role. Throughout history and continuing today, the genes of some organisms sustain chemical changes that are inherited by their progeny. Many of the changes reduce the fitness of the organism, but some changes improve fitness. Over the long term, competition between sister organisms with random differences in their genes determines which organisms survive in various environments. Although these genetic differences ensure survival, they do not necessarily optimize each chemical life process. The variants that survive merely have a selective advantage over the alternatives. Thus, the molecular strategy of life processes works well but is often illogical. Readers would likely be able to suggest simpler or more elegant mechanisms for many cellular processes described in this book.

In spite of obvious differences in size, design, and behavior, all forms of life share many molecular mechanisms because they all descended from a **common ancestor** that lived 3 or 4 billion years ago (Fig. 1-1). This founding organism no longer exists,

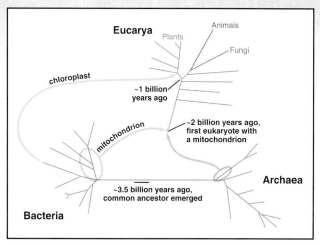

Figure 1-1 SIMPLIFIED PHYLOGENETIC TREE. This tree shows the common ancestor of all living things and the three main branches of life that diverged from this cell: Archaea, Bacteria, and Eukaryotes. Note that eukaryotic mitochondria and chloroplasts originated as symbiotic Bacteria.

but it must have utilized biochemical processes similar to the biological processes that sustain contemporary cells.

Over several billion years, living organisms diverged from each other into three great divisions: Bacteria, Archaea, and Eucarya (Fig. 1-1). Archaea and Bacteria were considered to be one kingdom until the 1970s; then ribosomal RNA sequences revealed that they were different divisions of the tree of life, having branched from each other early in evolution. The origin of eukaryotes is still uncertain, but they inherited genes from both Archaea and Bacteria. One possibility is that eukaryotes originated when an Archaea fused with a Bacterium. Note that multicellular eukaryotes (*green, blue,* and *red* in Fig. 1-1) evolved relatively recently, hundreds of millions of years after earlier, single-celled eukaryotes first appeared. Also note that algae and plants branched off before fungi, our nearest relatives on the tree of life.

Living things differ in size and complexity and are adapted to life in environments as extreme as deep-sea hydrothermal vents at temperatures of 113°C or pockets of water at 0°C in frozen Antarctic lakes. Organisms also differ in strategies to extract energy from their environments. Plants, algae, and some Bacteria derive energy from sunlight for photosynthesis. Some Bacteria and Archaea oxidize reduced inorganic compounds, such as hydrogen, hydrogen sulfide, or iron, as an energy source. Many organisms in all parts of the tree, including animals, extract energy from reduced organic compounds.

As the molecular mechanisms of life become clearer, the underlying similarities are more impressive than the external differences. Retention of common molecular mechanisms in all parts of the **phylogenetic tree** is remarkable, given that the major phylogenetic groups have been separated for vast amounts of time and subjected to different selective pressures. The biochemical mechanisms in the branches of the phylogenetic tree could have diverged radically from each other, but they did not.

All living organisms share a common genetic code, store genetic information in nucleic acids (usually **DNA**), transfer genetic information from **DNA** to **RNA** to **protein,** employ proteins (and some RNAs) to catalyze chemical reactions, synthesize proteins on **ribosomes,** derive energy by breaking down simple sugars and lipids, use adenosine triphosphate **(ATP)** as energy currency, and separate their cytoplasm from their environment by means of phospholipid **membranes** containing **pumps, carriers,** and **channels.** These ancient biochemical strategies are so well adapted for survival that they have been retained during natural selection of all surviving species.

A practical consequence of common biochemical mechanisms is that one may learn general principles of cellular function by studying any cell that is favorable for experimentation. This text cites many examples in which research on bacteria, insects, protozoa, or fungi has revealed fundamental mechanisms shared by human cells. Humans and baker's yeast have similar mechanisms to control cell cycles, to guide protein secretion, and to segregate chromosomes at mitosis. Human versions of essential proteins can often substitute for their yeast counterparts. Biologists are confident that a limited number of general principles, summarizing common molecular mechanisms, will eventually explain even the most complex life processes in terms of straightforward chemistry and physics.

Many interesting creatures have been lost to extinction during evolution. Extinction is irreversible because the cell is the only place where the entire range of life-sustaining biochemical reactions, including gene replication, molecular biosynthesis, targeting, and assembly, can go to completion. Thus, cells are such a special environment that the chain of life has required an unbroken lineage of cells stretching from each contemporary organism back to the earliest forms of life.

This book focuses on the underlying molecular mechanisms of biological function at the cellular level. Chapter 1 starts with a brief description of the main features that set eukaryotes apart from prokaryotes and then covers the general principles that apply equally to eukaryotes and prokaryotes. It closes with a preview of the major components of eukaryotic cells. Chapter 3 covers the macromolecules that form cells, while Chapters 4 and 5 introduce the chemical and physical principles required to understand how these molecules assemble and function. Armed with this introductory material, the reader will be prepared to circle back to Chapter 2 to learn what is known of the origins of life and the evolution of the forms of life that currently inhabit the earth.

Features That Distinguish Eukaryotic and Prokaryotic Cells

Although sharing a common origin and basic biochemistry, cells vary considerably in their structure and organization (Fig. 1-2). Although diverse in terms of morphology and reliance on particular energy sources, Bacteria and Archaea have much in common, including basic metabolic pathways, gene expression, lack of organelles, and motility powered by rotary flagella. All eukaryotes (protists, algae, plants, fungi, and animals) differ from the two extensive groups of prokaryotes (Bacteria and Archaea) in having a compartmentalized cytoplasm with membrane-bounded organelles including a nucleus.

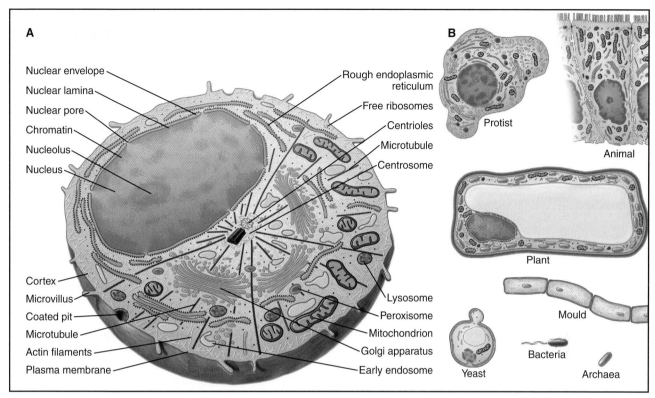

Figure 1-2 BASIC CELLULAR ARCHITECTURE. **A,** A section of a eukaryotic cell showing the internal components. **B,** Comparison of cells from the major branches of the phylogenetic tree.

A plasma membrane surrounds all cells, and additional intracellular membranes divide eukaryotes into compartments, each with a characteristic structure, biochemical composition, and function (Fig. 1-2). The basic features of eukaryotic **organelles** were refined more than 1.5 billion years ago, before the major groups of eukaryotes diverged. The **nuclear envelope** separates the two major compartments: nucleoplasm and cytoplasm. The **chromosomes** carrying the cell's **genes** and the machinery to express these genes reside inside the nucleus; they are in the cytoplasm of prokaryotes. Most eukaryotic cells have **endoplasmic reticulum** (the site of protein and phospholipid synthesis), a **Golgi apparatus** (an organelle that adds sugars to membrane proteins, lysosomal proteins, and secretory proteins), **lysosomes** (a compartment for digestive enzymes), **peroxisomes** (containers for enzymes involved in oxidative reactions), and **mitochondria** (structures that convert energy stored in the chemical bonds of nutrients into ATP in addition to other functions). **Cilia** (and flagella) are ancient eukaryotic specializations used by many cells for motility or sensing the environment. Table 1-1 lists the major cellular components and some of their functions.

Compartments give eukaryotic cells a number of advantages. Membranes provide a barrier that allows each type of organelle to maintain novel ionic and enzymatic interior environments. Each of these special environments favors a subset of the biochemical reactions required for life. The following examples demonstrate this concept:

- Segregation of digestive enzymes in lysosomes prevents them from destroying other cellular components.
- Each of the membrane-bound organelles concentrates particular proteins and small molecules in an ionic environment specialized for certain biochemical reactions.
- Special proteins in each organelle membrane contribute to the functions of the organelle.
- ATP synthesis depends on the impermeable membrane around mitochondria; energy-releasing reactions produce a proton gradient across the membrane that enzymes in the membrane use to drive ATP synthesis.
- The nuclear envelope provides a compartment where the synthesis and editing of RNA copies of the genes can be completed before the mature messenger RNAs exit to the cytoplasm where they direct protein synthesis.

Table 1-1

INVENTORY OF EUKARYOTIC CELLULAR COMPONENTS*

Cellular Component	Description
Plasma membrane	A lipid bilayer, 7 nm thick, with integral and peripheral proteins; the membrane surrounds cells and contains channels, carriers and pumps for ions and nutrients, receptors for growth factors, hormones and (in nerves and muscles) neurotransmitters, plus the molecular machinery to transduce these stimuli into intracellular signals
Adherens junction	A punctate or beltlike link between cells with actin filaments attached on the cytoplasmic surface
Desmosome	A punctate link between cells associated with intermediate filaments on the cytoplasmic surface
Gap junction	A localized region where the plasma membranes of two adjacent cells join to form minute intercellular channels for small molecules to move from the cytoplasm of one cell to the other
Tight junction	An annular junction sealing the gap between epithelial cells
Actin filament	"Microfilaments," 8 nm in diameter; form a viscoelastic network in the cytoplasm and act as tracks for movements powered by myosin motor proteins
Intermediate filament	Filaments, 10 nm in diameter, composed of keratin-like proteins that act as inextensible "tendons" in the cytoplasm
Microtubule	A cylindrical polymer of tubulin, 25 nm in diameter, that forms the main structural component of cilia, flagella, and mitotic spindles; microtubules provide tracks for organelle movements powered by the motors dynein and kinesin
Centriole	A short cylinder of nine microtubule triplets located in the cell center (centrosome) and at the base of cilia and flagella; pericentrosomal material nucleates and anchors microtubules
Microvillus (or filopodium)	A thin, cylindrical projection of the plasma membrane supported internally by a bundle of actin filaments
Cilia/flagella	Organelles formed by an axoneme of nine doublet and two singlet microtubules that project from the cell surface and are surrounded by plasma membrane; the motor protein dynein powers bending motions of the axoneme; nonmotile primary cilia have sensory functions
Glycogen particle	Storage form of polysaccharide
Ribosome	RNA/protein particle that catalyzes protein synthesis
Rough endoplasmic reticulum	Flattened, intracellular bags of membrane with associated ribosomes that synthesize secreted and integral membrane proteins
Smooth endoplasmic reticulum	Flattened, intracellular bags of membrane without ribosomes involved in lipid synthesis, drug metabolism, and sequestration of Ca^{2+}
Golgi apparatus	A stack of flattened membrane bags and vesicles that packages secretory proteins and participates in protein glycosylation
Nucleus	Membrane-bounded compartment containing the chromosomes, nucleolus and the molecular machinery that controls gene expression
Nuclear envelope	A pair of concentric membranes connected to the endoplasmic reticulum that surrounds the nucleus
Nuclear pore	Large, gated channels across the nuclear envelope that control all traffic of proteins and RNA in and out of the nucleus
Euchromatin	Dispersed, active form of interphase chromatin
Heterochromatin	Condensed, inactive chromatin
Nucleolus	Intranuclear site of ribosomal RNA synthesis and processing; ribosome assembly
Lysosome	Impermeable, membrane-bound bags of hydrolytic enzymes
Peroxisome	Membrane-bound bags containing catalase and various oxidases
Mitochondria	Organelles surrounded by a smooth outer membrane and a convoluted inner membrane folded into cristae; they contain enzymes for fatty acid oxidation and oxidative phosphorylation of ADP

*See Figure 1-2.

Some Universal Principles of Living Cells

This section summarizes the numerous features shared by all forms of life. Together with the following section on eukaryotic cells, these pages reprise the main points of the whole text.

1. *Genetic information stored in one-dimensional chemical sequences in DNA (occasionally RNA) is duplicated and passed on to daughter cells (Fig. 1-3).* The information required for cellular growth, multiplication, and function is stored in long polymers of DNA called chromosomes. Each DNA molecule is composed of a covalently linked

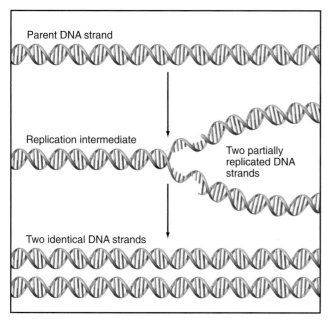

Figure 1-3 DNA STRUCTURE AND REPLICATION. The genes that are stored as the sequence of bases in DNA are replicated enzymatically, forming two identical copies from one double-stranded original.

synthesis of **polypeptides** by ribosomes. The amino acid sequence of most proteins contains sufficient information to specify how the polypeptide folds into a unique three-dimensional structure with biological activity. Two mechanisms control the production and processing of RNA and protein from tens of thousands of genes. **Genetically** encoded control circuits consisting of proteins and RNAs respond to environmental stimuli through signaling pathways. **Epigenetic** controls involve modifications of DNA or associated proteins that affect gene expression. These epigenetic modifications can be transmitted from a parent to an offspring. The basic plan for the cell contained in the genome, together with ongoing regulatory mechanisms (see points 7 and 8), works so well that each human develops with few defects from a single fertilized egg into a complicated ensemble of trillions of specialized cells that function har-

linear sequence of four different nucleotides (adenine [A], cytosine [C], guanine [G], and thymine [T]). In the double-helical DNA molecule, each nucleotide base preferentially forms a specific complex with a complementary base on the other strand. Specific noncovalent interactions stabilize the pairing between complementary nucleotide bases: A with T and C with G. During DNA replication, the two DNA strands are separated, each serving as a template for the synthesis of a new complementary strand. Enzymes that carry out DNA synthesis recognize the structure of complementary base pairs and insert only the correct complementary nucleotide at each position, thereby producing two identical copies of the DNA. Precise segregation of one newly duplicated double helix to each daughter cell then guarantees the transmission of intact genetic information to the next generation.

2. *One-dimensional chemical sequences are stored in DNA code for both the linear sequences and three-dimensional structures of RNAs and proteins (Fig. 1-4).* Enzymes called polymerases copy the information stored in genes into linear sequences of nucleotides of RNA molecules. Some genes specify RNAs with structural roles, regulatory functions, or enzymatic activity, but most genes produce **messenger RNA** (mRNA) molecules that act as templates for protein synthesis, specifying the sequence of amino acids during the

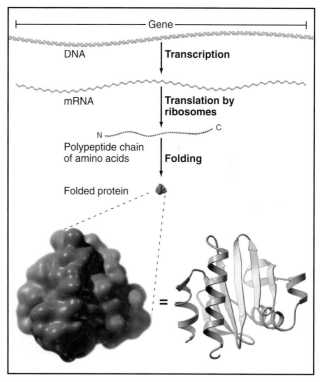

Figure 1-4 Genetic information contained in the base sequence of DNA determines the amino acid sequence of a protein and its three-dimensional structure. Enzymes copy (transcribe) the sequence of bases in a gene to make a messenger RNA (mRNA). Ribosomes use the sequence of bases in the mRNA as a template to synthesize (translate) a corresponding linear polymer of amino acids. This polypeptide folds spontaneously to form a three-dimensional protein molecule, in this example the actin-binding protein profilin. (PDB file: 1ACF.) Scale drawings of DNA, mRNA, polypeptide, and folded protein: The folded protein is enlarged at the bottom and shown in two renderings—space filling *(left)*; ribbon diagram showing the polypeptide folded into *blue* α-helices and *yellow* β-strands *(right)*.

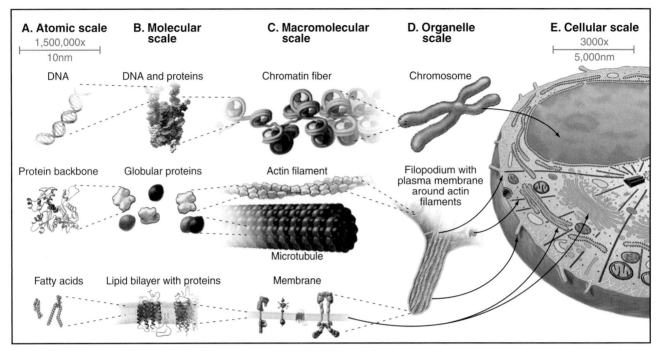

Figure 1-5 MACROMOLECULAR ASSEMBLY. Many macromolecular components of cells assemble spontaneously from constituent molecules without the guidance of templates. This figure shows the assembly of chromosomes from DNA and proteins, a bundle of actin filaments in a filopodium from proteins, and the plasma membrane from lipids and proteins. **A,** Atomic scale. **B,** Molecular scale. **C,** Macromolecular scale. **D,** Organelle scale. **E,** Cellular scale.

moniously for decades in an ever-changing environment.

3. *Macromolecular structures assemble from subunits (Fig. 1-5).* Many cellular components form by **self-assembly** of their constituent molecules without the aid of templates or enzymes. The protein, nucleic acid, and lipid molecules themselves contain the information that is required to assemble complex structures. Diffusion usually brings the molecules together during these assembly processes. Exclusion of water from their complementary surfaces ("lock and key" packing), as well as electrostatic and hydrogen bonds, provides the energy to hold the subunits together. In some cases, protein chaperones assist with assembly by preventing the precipitation of partially or incorrectly folded intermediates. Important cellular structures that are assembled in this way include **chromatin,** consisting of nuclear DNA compacted by associated proteins; **ribosomes,** assembled from RNA and proteins; cytoskeletal polymers, polymerized from protein subunits; and membranes formed from lipids and proteins.

4. *Membranes grow by expansion of preexisting membranes (Figs. 1-5 and 1-6).* Biological membranes composed of phospholipids and proteins do not form de novo in cells; instead, they grow only by expansion of preexisting lipid bilayers. As a consequence, organelles, such as mitochondria and endoplasmic reticulum, form only by growth and division of preexisting organelles and are inherited maternally starting from the egg. The endoplasmic reticulum (ER) plays a central role in membrane biogenesis as the site of phospholipid synthesis. Through a series of budding and fusion events, membrane made in the ER provides material for the Golgi apparatus, which, in turn, provides lipids and proteins for lysosomes and the plasma membrane.

5. *Signal-receptor interactions target cellular constituents to their correct locations (Fig. 1-6).* Specific recognition signals incorporated into the structures of proteins and nucleic acids route these molecules to their proper cellular compartments. Receptors recognize these signals and guide each molecule to its compartment. For example, most proteins destined for the nucleus contain short sequences of amino acids that bind receptors that facilitate their passage through nuclear pores into the nucleus. Similarly, a peptide signal sequence first targets lysosomal proteins into the lumen of the ER. Subsequently, the Golgi apparatus adds a sugar-phosphate group recognized by receptors that secondarily target these proteins to lysosomes.

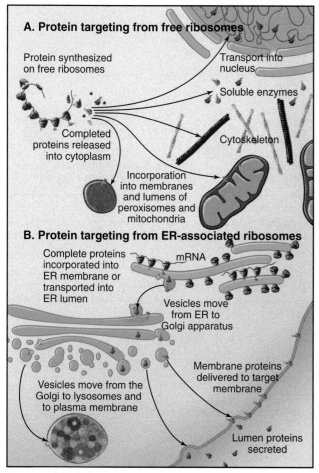

A. Protein targeting from free ribosomes

Protein synthesized on free ribosomes

Transport into nucleus

Soluble enzymes

Completed proteins released into cytoplasm

Cytoskeleton

Incorporation into membranes and lumens of peroxisomes and mitochondria

B. Protein targeting from ER-associated ribosomes

Complete proteins incorporated into ER membrane or transported into ER lumen

mRNA

Vesicles move from ER to Golgi apparatus

Membrane proteins delivered to target membrane

Vesicles move from the Golgi to lysosomes and to plasma membrane

Lumen proteins secreted

Figure 1-6 PROTEIN TARGETING. Signals built into the amino acid sequences of proteins target them to all compartments of the eukaryotic cell. **A,** Proteins synthesized on free ribosomes can be used locally in the cytoplasm or guided by different signals to the nucleus, mitochondria, or peroxisomes. **B,** Other signals target proteins for insertion into the membrane or lumen of the endoplasmic reticulum (ER). From there, a series of vesicular budding and fusion reactions carry the membrane proteins and lumen proteins to the Golgi apparatus, lysosomes, or plasma membrane.

tor. An energy-requiring reaction then transports the protein into the mitochondria.

7. *Receptors and signaling mechanisms allow cells to adapt to environmental conditions (Fig. 1-8).* Environmental stimuli modify cellular behavior and biochemistry. Faced with an unpredictable environment, cells must decide which genes to express, which way to move, and whether to proliferate, differentiate into a specialized cell, or die. Some of these choices are programmed genetically or epigenetically, but minute-to-minute decisions generally involve the reception of chemical or physical stimuli from outside the cell and processing of these stimuli to change the behavior of the cell. Cells have an elaborate repertoire of **receptors** for a multitude of stimuli, including nutrients, growth factors, hormones, neurotransmitters, and toxins. Stimulation of receptors activates diverse signal-transducing mechanisms that amplify the stimulus and also generate a wide range of cellular responses, including changes in the electrical potential of the plasma membrane, gene expression, and enzyme activity. Basic **signal transduction** mechanisms are ancient, but receptors and output systems have diversified by gene duplication and divergence during evolution. Thus, humans typically have a greater number of variations on the general themes than simpler organisms do.

8. *Molecular feedback mechanisms control molecular composition, growth, and differentiation (Fig. 1-9).* Living cells are dynamic, constantly undergoing changes in composition or activity in

6. *Cellular constituents move by diffusion, pumps, and motors (Fig. 1-7).* Most small molecules move through the cytoplasm or membrane channels by diffusion. Energy is required for movements of small molecules across membranes against concentration gradients and movements of larger objects, like organelles, through cytoplasm. Electrochemical gradients or ATP hydrolysis provides energy for molecular pumps to drive molecules across membranes against concentration gradients. ATP-burning **motor proteins** move organelles and other cargo along microtubules or actin filaments. In a more complicated example, protein molecules destined for mitochondria diffuse from their site of synthesis in the cytoplasm to a mitochondrion (Fig. 1-6), where they bind to a recep-

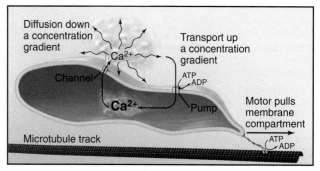

Diffusion down a concentration gradient

Transport up a concentration gradient

Ca^{2+}

Channel

ATP
ADP

Ca^{2+}

Pump

Motor pulls membrane compartment

Microtubule track

ATP
ADP

Figure 1-7 MOLECULAR MOVEMENTS BY DIFFUSION, PUMPS, AND MOTORS. Diffusion: Molecules up to the size of globular proteins diffuse in the cytoplasm. Concentration gradients can provide a direction to diffusion, such as the diffusion of Ca^{2+} from a region of high concentration inside the endoplasmic reticulum through a membrane channel to a region of low concentration in the cytoplasm. Pumps: ATP-driven protein pumps can transport ions up concentration gradients. Motors: ATP-driven motors move organelles and other large cargo along microtubules and actin filaments.

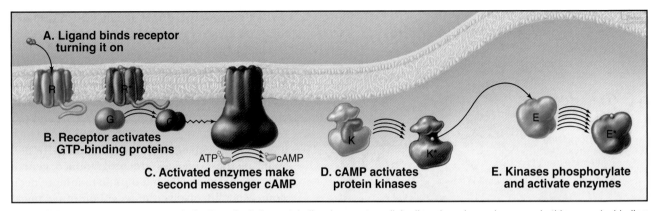

A. Ligand binds receptor turning it on

B. Receptor activates GTP-binding proteins

ATP   cAMP

C. Activated enzymes make second messenger cAMP

D. cAMP activates protein kinases

E. Kinases phosphorylate and activate enzymes

Figure 1-8 RECEPTORS AND SIGNALS. Activation of cellular metabolism by an extracellular ligand, such as a hormone. In this example, binding of the hormone **(A)** triggers a series of linked biochemical reactions **(B–E),** leading through a second messenger molecule (cyclic adenosine monophosphate, or cAMP) and a cascade of three activated proteins to a metabolic enzyme. The response to a single ligand is multiplied at steps **B, C,** and **E,** leading to thousands of activated enzymes. GTP, guanosine triphosphate.

Figure 1-9 MOLECULAR FEEDBACK LOOPS. **A,** Control of the synthesis of aromatic amino acids. An intermediate and the final products of this biochemical pathway inhibit three of nine enzymes (Enz) in a concentration-dependent fashion, automatically turning down the reactions that produced them. This maintains constant levels of the final products, two amino acids that are essential for protein synthesis. **B,** Control of the cell cycle. The cycle consists of four stages. During the G1 phase, the cell grows in size. During the S phase, the cell duplicates the DNA of its chromosomes. During the G2 phase, the cell checks for completion of DNA replication. In the M phase, chromosomes condense and attach to the mitotic spindle, which separates the duplicated pairs in preparation for the division of the cell at cytokinesis. Biochemical feedback loops called checkpoints halt the cycle (*blunt bars*) at several points until the successful completion of key preceding events.

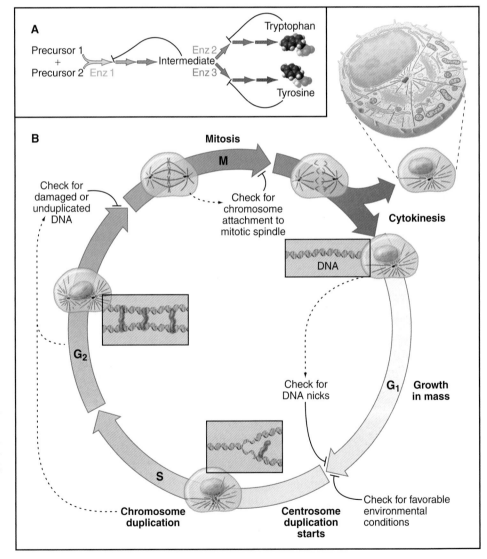

response to external stimuli, nutrient availability, and internal signals. Change is constant, but through well-orchestrated recycling and renewal, the cell and its constituents remain relatively stable. Each cell balances production and degradation of its constituent molecules to function optimally. Some "housekeeping" molecules are used by most cells for basic functions, such as intermediary metabolism. Other molecules are unique and are required for specialized functions of differentiated cells. The supply of each of thousands of proteins is controlled by a hierarchy of mechanisms: by epigenetic mechanisms that designate whether a particular region of a chromosome is active or not, by regulatory proteins that turn specific genes on and off, by the rate of translation of messenger RNAs into protein, by the rate of degradation of specific RNAs and proteins, and by regulation of the distribution of each molecule within the cell. Some proteins are enzymes that determine the rate of synthesis or degradation of other proteins, nucleic acids, sugars, and lipids. Molecular feedback loops regulate all of these processes to ensure the proper levels of each cellular constituent.

Overview of Eukaryotic Cellular Organization and Functions

This section previews the major constituents and processes of eukaryotic cells. This overview is intended to alleviate a practical problem arising in any text on cell biology—the interdependence of all parts of cells. The material must be divided into separate chapters, each on a particular topic. But to appreciate the cross-references to material in other chapters, the reader needs some basic knowledge of the whole cell.

Nucleus

The nucleus (Fig. 1-10) stores genetic information in extraordinarily long DNA molecules called chromosomes. Surprisingly, the coding portions of genes make up only a small fraction (<2%) of the 3 billion nucleotide pairs in human DNA, but more than 50% of the 97 million nucleotide pairs in a nematode worm. Regions called telomeres stabilize the ends of chromosomes, and centromeres ensure the distribution of chromosomes to daughter cells when cells divide. The functions of most of the remaining DNA are not yet known. The DNA and its associated proteins are called chromatin (Fig. 1-5). Interactions with histones and other proteins fold each chromosome compactly enough to fit inside the nucleus. During **mitosis,** chromosomes condense further into separate structural units that one can observe by light microscopy (Fig. 1-7). Between cell divisions, chromosomes are decondensed but occupy discrete territories within the nucleus.

Proteins of the transcriptional machinery turn specific genes on and off in response to genetic, developmental, and environmental signals. Enzymes called polymerases make RNA copies of active genes. Messenger RNAs specify the amino acid sequences of proteins. Other RNAs have structural, regulatory, or catalytic functions. Most newly synthesized RNAs must be processed extensively before they are ready for use. Processing involves removal of noncoding intervening sequences, alteration of bases, or addition of specific

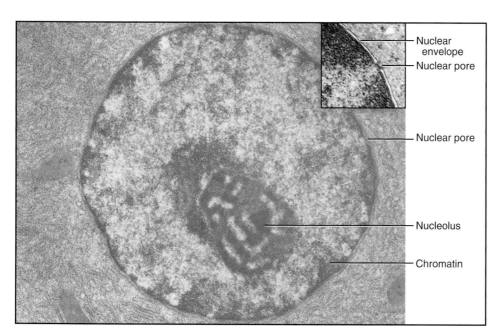

Nuclear envelope

Nuclear pore

Nuclear pore

Nucleolus

Chromatin

Figure 1-10 ELECTRON MICRO-GRAPH OF A THIN SECTION OF A NUCLEUS. (Courtesy of Don Fawcett, Harvard Medical School, Boston, Massachusetts.)

structures at either end. For cytoplasmic RNAs, this processing occurs before RNA molecules are exported from the nucleus through **nuclear pores.** The **nucleolus** assembles ribosomes from more than 50 different proteins and 3 RNA molecules. Genetic errors resulting in altered RNA and protein products cause or predispose individuals to many inherited human diseases.

The nuclear envelope is a double membrane that separates the nucleus from the cytoplasm. All traffic into and out of the nucleus passes through nuclear pores that bridge the double membranes. Inbound traffic includes all nuclear proteins, such as transcription factors and ribosomal proteins. Outbound traffic includes messenger RNAs and ribosomal subunits. Some macromolecules shuttle back and forth between the nucleus and cytoplasm.

Cell Cycle

Cellular growth and division are regulated by an integrated molecular network consisting of **protein kinases** (enzymes that add phosphate to the side chains of proteins), specific kinase inhibitors, transcription factors, and highly specific proteases. When conditions inside and outside a cell are appropriate for cell division (Fig. 1-9B), changes in the stability of key proteins allow specific protein kinases to escape from negative regulators and to trigger a chain of events leading to DNA replication and cell division. Once DNA replication is initiated, specific destruction of components of these kinases allows cells to complete the process. Once DNA replication is complete, activation of the cell cycle kinases such as Cdk1 pushes the cell into mitosis, the process that separates chromosomes into two daughter cells. Three controls sequentially activate Cdk1

through a positive feedback loop: (1) synthesis of a regulatory subunit, (2) transport into the nucleus, and (3) removal of inhibitory phosphate groups.

Phosphorylation of proteins by Cdk1 leads directly or indirectly to disassembly of the nuclear envelope (in most but not all cells), condensation of mitotic chromosomes, and assembly of the **mitotic spindle.** Selective proteolysis of Cdk1 regulatory subunits and key chromosomal proteins then allows segregation of identical copies of each chromosome and their repackaging into daughter nuclei as the nuclear envelope reassembles on the surface of the clustered chromosomes. Then daughter cells are cleaved apart by the process of **cytokinesis.**

A key feature of the cell cycle is a series of built-in quality controls, called **checkpoints** (Fig. 1-9), which ensure that each stage of the cycle is completed successfully before the process continues to the next step. These checkpoints also detect damage to cellular constituents and block cell cycle progression so that the damage may be repaired. Misregulation of checkpoints and other cell cycle controls is a common cause of cancer. Remarkably, the entire cycle of DNA replication, chromosomal condensation, nuclear envelope breakdown, and reformation, including the modulation of these events by checkpoints, can be carried out in cell-free extracts in a test tube.

Ribosomes and Protein Synthesis

Ribosomes catalyze the synthesis of proteins, using the nucleotide sequences of messenger RNA molecules to specify the sequence of amino acids (Figs. 1-4, 1-6, and 1-11). If the protein being synthesized has a signal sequence for receptors on the endoplasmic reticulum

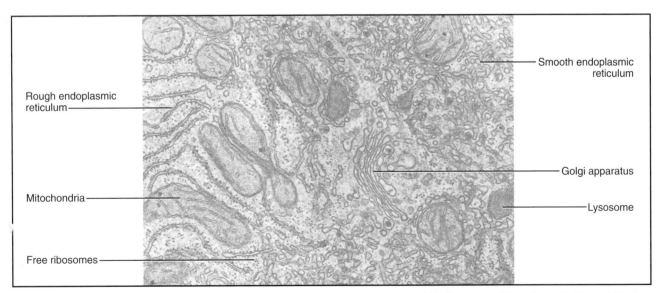

Figure 1-11   ELECTRON MICROGRAPH OF A THIN SECTION OF A LIVER CELL SHOWING ORGANELLES. (Courtesy of Don Fawcett, Harvard Medical School, Boston, Massachusetts.)

(ER), the ribosome binds to the ER, and the protein is inserted into the ER membrane bilayer or into the lumen of the ER as it is synthesized. Otherwise, ribosomes are free in the cytoplasm, and newly synthesized proteins enter the cytoplasm for routing to various destinations.

Endoplasmic Reticulum

The endoplasmic reticulum is a continuous system of flattened membrane sacks and tubules (Fig. 1-11) that is specialized for protein processing and lipid biosynthesis. Motor proteins move along microtubules to pull the ER membranes into a branching network spread throughout the cytoplasm. ER also forms the outer bilayer of the nuclear envelope. ER pumps and channels regulate the cytoplasmic Ca^{2+} concentration, and ER enzymes metabolize drugs.

Ribosomes synthesizing proteins destined for insertion into cellular membranes or for export from the cell associate with specialized regions of the ER, called rough ER owing to the attached ribosomes (Fig. 1-6). These proteins carry **signal sequences** of amino acids that guide their ribosomes to ER receptors. As a polypeptide chain grows, its sequence determines whether the protein folds up in the lipid bilayer or translocates into the lumen of the ER. Some proteins are retained in the ER, but most move on to other parts of the cell.

Endoplasmic reticulum is very dynamic. Continuous bidirectional traffic moves small vesicles between the ER and the Golgi apparatus. These vesicles carry soluble proteins in their lumens, in addition to membrane lipids and proteins. Proteins on the cytoplasmic surface of the membranes catalyze each membrane budding and fusion event. The use of specialized proteins for budding and fusion of membranes at different sites in the cell prevents the membrane components from getting mixed up.

Golgi Apparatus

The Golgi apparatus processes the sugar side chains of secreted and membrane glycoproteins and sorts the proteins for transport to other parts of the cell (Figs. 1-6 and 1-11). The Golgi apparatus is a stack of flattened, membrane-bound sacks with many associated vesicles. Membrane vesicles come from the ER and fuse with the Golgi apparatus. As a result of a series of vesicle-budding and fusion events, the membrane molecules and soluble proteins in the lumen pass through the stacks of Golgi apparatus from one side to the other. During this passage, Golgi enzymes, retained in specific layers of the Golgi apparatus by transmembrane anchors, modify the sugar side chains of secretory and membrane proteins. On the downstream side of the Golgi apparatus, processed proteins segregate into different vesicles destined for lysosomes or the plasma membrane. The Golgi apparatus is characteristically located in the middle of the cell near the nucleus and the centrosome.

Lysosomes

An impermeable membrane separates degradative enzymes inside lysosomes from other cellular components. Lysosomal proteins are synthesized by rough ER and transported to the Golgi apparatus, where enzymes recognize a three-dimensional site on the proteins' surface that targets them for addition of the modified sugar, phosphorylated mannose (Fig. 1-6). Vesicular transport, guided by phosphomannose receptors, delivers lysosomal proteins to the lumen of lysosomes.

Membrane vesicles, called **endosomes** and **phagosomes,** deliver ingested microorganisms and other materials destined for destruction to lysosomes. Fusion of these vesicles with lysosomes exposes their cargo to lysosomal enzymes in the lumen. Deficiencies of lysosomal enzymes cause many congenital diseases. In each of these diseases, a deficiency in the ability to degrade a particular biomolecule leads to its accumulation in quantities that can impair the function of the brain, liver, or other organs.

Plasma Membrane

The plasma membrane is the interface of the cell with its environment (Fig. 1-12). Owing to the hydrophobic interior of its lipid bilayer, the plasma membrane is impermeable to ions and most water-soluble molecules. Consequently, they cross the membrane only through transmembrane channels, carriers, and pumps, which provide the cell with nutrients, control internal ion concentrations, and establish a transmembrane electrical potential. A single amino acid change in one plasma membrane pump and Cl^- channel causes cystic fibrosis.

Other plasma membrane proteins mediate interactions of cells with their immediate environment. Transmembrane receptors bind extracellular signaling molecules, such as hormones and growth factors, and transduce their presence into chemical or electrical signals that influence the activity of the cell. Genetic defects in signaling proteins, which turn on signals for growth in the absence of appropriate extracellular stimuli, contribute to some human cancers.

Adhesive glycoproteins of the plasma membrane allow cells to bind specifically to each other or to the **extracellular matrix.** These selective interactions allow cells to form multicellular associations, such as epithelia. Similar interactions allow white blood cells to bind bacteria so that they can be ingested and digested in lysosomes. In cells that are subjected to mechanical forces, such as muscle and epithelia, adhesive proteins

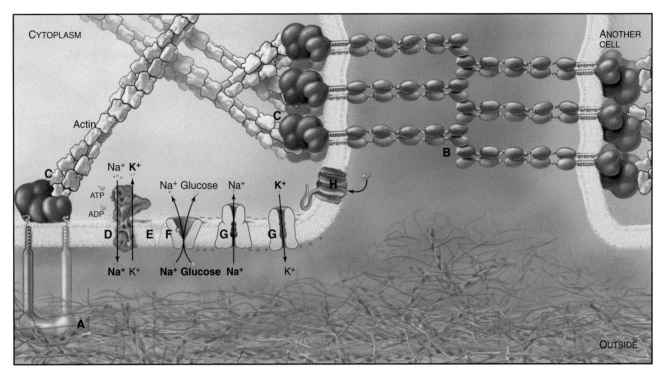

Figure 1-12   STRUCTURE AND FUNCTIONS OF AN ANIMAL CELL PLASMA MEMBRANE. The lipid bilayer forms a permeability barrier between the cytoplasm and the extracellular environment. Transmembrane adhesion proteins anchor the membrane to the extracellular matrix **(A)** or to like receptors on other cells **(B)** and transmit forces to the cytoskeleton **(C).** ATP-driven enzymes **(D)** pump Na^+ out and K^+ into the cell against concentration gradients **(E)** to establish an electrical potential across the lipid bilayer. Other transmembrane carrier proteins **(F)** use these ion concentration gradients to drive the transport of nutrients into the cell. Selective ion channels **(G)** open and shut transiently to regulate the electrical potential across the membrane. A large variety of receptors **(H)** bind specific extracellular ligands and send signals across the membrane to the cytoplasm.

of the plasma membrane are reinforced by association with cytoskeletal filaments inside the cell. In skin, defects in these attachments cause blistering diseases.

ER synthesizes phospholipids and proteins for the plasma membrane (Fig. 1-6). After insertion into the lipid bilayer of the ER, proteins move to the plasma membrane by vesicular transport through the Golgi apparatus. Many components of the plasma membrane are not permanent residents; receptors for extracellular molecules, including nutrients and some hormones, can recycle from the plasma membrane to endosomes and back to the cell surface many times before they are degraded. Defects in the receptor for low-density lipoproteins cause arteriosclerosis.

Mitochondria

Mitochondrial enzymes convert most of the energy released from the breakdown of nutrients into the synthesis of ATP, the common currency for most energy-requiring reactions in cells (Fig. 1-11). This efficient mitochondrial system uses molecular oxygen to complete the oxidation of fats, proteins, and sugars to carbon dioxide and water. A less efficient glycolytic system in the cytoplasm extracts energy from the partial break-

down of glucose to make ATP. Mitochondria cluster near sites of ATP utilization, such as sperm tails, membranes engaged in active transport, nerve terminals, and the contractile apparatus of muscle cells.

Mitochondria also have a key role in cellular responses to toxic stimuli from the environment. In response to drugs such as many that are used in cancer chemotherapy, mitochondria release into the cytoplasm a toxic cocktail of enzymes and other proteins that brings about the death of the cell. Defects in this form of cellular suicide, known as **apoptosis,** lead to autoimmune disorders, cancer, and some neurodegenerative diseases.

Mitochondria form in a fundamentally different way from the ER, Golgi apparatus, and lysosomes (Fig. 1-6). Free ribosomes synthesize most mitochondrial proteins, which are released into the cytoplasm. Receptors on the surface of mitochondria recognize and bind signal sequences on mitochondrial proteins. Energy-requiring processes transport these proteins into the lumen or insert them into the outer or inner mitochondrial membranes.

DNA, ribosomes, and messenger RNAs located inside mitochondria produce a small number of the proteins that contribute to the assembly of the organelle. This machinery is left over from an earlier stage of evolution when mitochondria arose from symbiotic Bacteria (Fig. 1-1). Defects in the maternally inherited mitochondrial genome cause several diseases, including deafness, diabetes, and ocular myopathy.

Peroxisomes

Peroxisomes are membrane-bound organelles containing enzymes that participate in oxidative reactions. Like mitochondria, peroxisomal enzymes oxidize fatty acids, but the energy is not used to synthesize ATP. Peroxisomes are particularly abundant in plants as well as some animal cells. Peroxisomal proteins are synthesized in the cytoplasm and imported into the organelle using the same strategy as mitochondria but using different targeting sequences and transport machinery (Fig. 1-6). Genetic defects in peroxisomal biogenesis cause several forms of mental retardation.

Cytoskeleton and Motility Apparatus

A cytoplasmic network of three protein polymers—actin filaments, intermediate filaments, and microtubules (Fig. 1-13)—maintains the shape of a cell. Each polymer has distinctive properties and dynamics. Actin filaments and microtubules also provide tracks for the ATP-powered motor proteins that produce most cellular movements (Fig. 1-14), including cellular locomotion, muscle contraction, transport of organelles through the cytoplasm, mitosis, and the beating of **cilia** and **flagella.** The specialized forms of motility exhibited by muscle and sperm are exaggerated, highly organized versions of the motile processes used by most other eukaryotic cells.

Networks of cross-linked actin filaments anchored to the plasma membrane (Fig. 1-12) reinforce the surface of the cell. In many cells, tightly packed bundles of actin

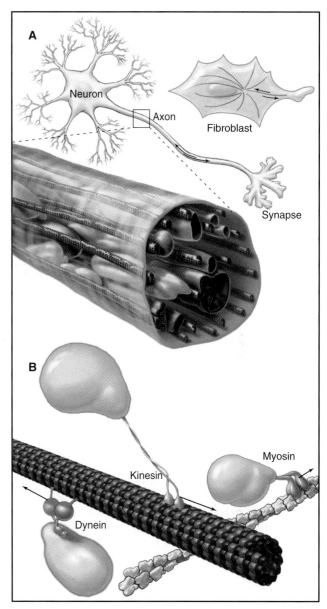

Figure 1-14 TRANSPORT OF CYTOPLASMIC PARTICLES ALONG ACTIN FILAMENTS AND MICROTUBULES BY MOTOR PROTEINS. **A,** Overview of organelle movements in a neuron and fibroblast. **B,** Details of the molecular motors. The microtubule-based motors, dynein and kinesin, move in opposite directions. The actin-based motor, myosin, moves in one direction along actin filaments. (Original drawing, adapted from Atkinson SJ, Doberstein SK, Pollard TD: Moving off the beaten track. Curr Biol 2:326–328, 1992.)

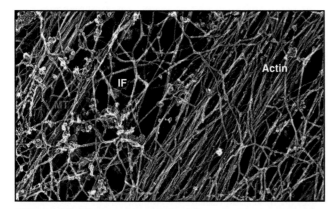

Figure 1-13 Electron micrograph of the cytoplasmic matrix of a fibroblast prepared by detergent extraction of soluble components, rapid freezing, sublimation of ice, and coating with metal. IF, intermediate filaments; MT, microtubules. (Courtesy of J. Heuser, Washington University, St. Louis, Missouri.)

filaments support finger-like projections of the plasma membrane (Fig. 1-5). These filopodia or microvilli increase the surface area of the plasma membrane for transporting nutrients and other processes, including sensory transduction in the ear. Genetic defects in a membrane-associated, actin-binding protein called dystrophin cause the most common form of muscular dystrophy.

Actin filaments participate in movements in two ways. Assembly of actin filaments produces some movements, such as the extension of pseudopods. Other movements result from force produced by the motor protein **myosin** moving along actin filaments (Fig. 1-14). A family of different types of myosin uses the energy from ATP hydrolysis to produce movements. Muscles use a highly organized assembly of actin and myosin filaments to produce forceful, rapid, one-dimensional contractions. Myosin also drives the contraction of the cleavage furrow during cell division. External signals, such as chemotactic molecules, can influence both actin filament organization and the direction of motility. Genetic defects in myosin cause enlargement of the heart and sudden death.

Intermediate filaments are flexible but strong intracellular tendons used to reinforce the epithelial cells of the skin and other cells that are subjected to substantial physical stresses. All intermediate filament proteins are related to the keratin molecules found in hair. Intermediate filaments characteristically form bundles that link the plasma membrane to the nucleus. Other intermediate filaments reinforce the nuclear envelope. Reversible phosphorylation regulates rearrangements of intermediate filaments during mitosis and cell movements. Genetic defects in keratin intermediate filaments cause blistering diseases of the skin. Defects in nuclear lamins are associated with some types of muscular dystrophy and premature aging.

Microtubules are rigid cylindrical polymers with two main functions. They serve as (1) mechanical reinforcing rods for the cytoskeleton and (2) the tracks for two classes of motor proteins. They are the only cytoskeletal polymer that can resist compression. The polymer has a molecular polarity that determines the rate of growth at the two ends and the direction of movement of motor proteins. Virtually all microtubules in cells have the same polarity relative to the organizing centers that initiate their growth (e.g., the **centrosome**) (Fig. 1-2). Their rapidly growing ends are oriented toward the periphery of the cell. Individual cytoplasmic microtubules are remarkably dynamic, growing and shrinking on a time scale of minutes.

Two classes of motor proteins use the energy liberated by ATP hydrolysis to move along the microtubules. **Kinesin** moves its associated cargo (vesicles and RNA protein particles) out along the microtubule network radiating from the centrosome, whereas **dynein** moves its cargo toward the cell center. Together, they form a two-way transport system in the cell that is particularly well developed in the axons and dendrites of nerve cells. Toxins can impair this transport system and cause nerve malfunctions.

During mitosis, the cell assembles a mitotic apparatus of highly dynamic microtubules and uses microtubule motor proteins to separate the chromosomes into the daughter cells. The motile apparatus of cilia and flagella is built from a complex array of stable microtubules that bends when dynein slides the microtubules past each other. A genetic absence of dynein immobilizes these appendages, causing male infertility and lung infections (Kartagener's syndrome).

Microtubules, intermediate filaments, and actin filaments each provide mechanical support for the cytoplasm that is enhanced by interactions between these polymers. Associations of microtubules with intermediate filaments and actin filaments unify the cytoskeleton into a continuous mechanical structure that resists forces applied to cells. These polymers also maintain the organization of the cell by providing a scaffolding for some cellular enzyme systems and a matrix between the membrane-bound organelles.

Evolution of Life on Earth

No one is certain how life began, but the **common ancestor** of all living things populated the earth over 3 billion years ago, not long (geologically speaking) after the planet formed 4.5 billion years ago (Fig. 2-1). Biochemical features shared by all existing cells suggest that this primitive microscopic cell had about 600 genes encoded in DNA, ribosomes to synthesize proteins, and a plasma membrane with pumps, carriers, and channels. Over time, mutations in the DNA created progeny that diverged genetically into numerous distinctive species, numbering about 1.7 million known to science. The total number of species living on the earth today is unknown but is estimated to be between 4 million and 100 million. On the basis of evolutionary histories preserved in their genomes, living organisms are divided into three primary domains: Bacteria, Archaea, and Eucarya.

This chapter explains our current understanding of the origin of the first self-replicating cell followed by divergence of its progeny into the two diverse groups of prokaryotes, Bacteria and Archaea. It goes on to consider theories for the origin of Eucarya and their diversification over the past 2 billion years.

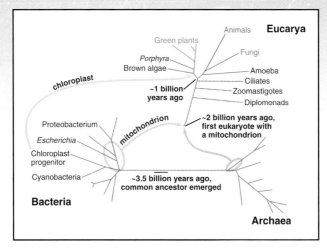

Figure 2-1 SIMPLE PHYLOGENETIC TREE WITH THE THREE DOMAINS OF LIFE—BACTERIA, ARCHAEA, AND EUCARYA (EUKARYOTES)—AND A FEW REPRESENTATIVE ORGANISMS. The origin of eukaryotes with a mitochondrion about 2 billion years ago is depicted as a fusion of an α-proteobacterium with an Archaean. An alternative explanation for the origin of eukaryotes is that the α-proteobacterium fused with a cell from a lineage that diverged directly from the common ancestor of Bacteria and Archaea. Chloroplasts arose from the fusion of a cyanobacterium with the precursor of algae and plants.

Evolution is *the* great unifying principle in biology. Research on evolution is both exciting and challenging because this ultimate detective story involves piecing together fragmentary evidence spread over 3.5 billion years. Data include fossils of ancient organisms preserved in stone, ancient DNA (going back about 45,000 years), and especially DNA of living organisms.

Prebiotic Chemistry Leading to an RNA World

But where did the common ancestor come from? A wide range of evidence supports the idea that life began with self-replicating RNA polymers sheltered inside lipid vesicles even before the invention of protein synthesis (Fig. 2-2). This hypothetical early stage of evolution is called the **RNA World.** This postulate is attractive because it solves the chicken-and-egg problem of how to build a system of self-replicating molecules without having to invent either DNA or proteins on their own. Clearly, RNA has an advantage, because it provides a way to store information in a type of molecule that can also have catalytic activity. Proteins excel in catalysis but do not store self-replicating genetic information. Today, proteins have largely superseded RNAs as cellular catalysts. DNA excels for storing genetic information, since the absence of the 2′ hydroxyl makes it less reactive and therefore more stable than RNA. Readers who are not familiar with the structure of nucleic acids should consult Chapter 3 at this point.

Experts agree that the early steps toward life involved the "prebiotic" synthesis of organic molecules that became the building blocks of macromolecules. To use RNA as an example, minerals can catalyze formation of simple sugars from formaldehyde, a chemical that is believed to have been abundant on the young earth. Such reactions could have supplied ribose for ancient RNAs. Similarly, HCN and cyanoacetylene can form nucleic acid bases, although the conditions are fairly exotic and the yields are low. On the other hand, scientists still lack plausible mechanisms to conjugate ribose with a base to make a nucleoside or add phosphate to make a nucleotide without the aid of a preexisting biochemical catalyst. Nucleotides do not spontaneously polymerize into polynucleotides in water but can do so on the surface of a clay called montmorillonite. While attached to clay, single strands of RNA can act as a template for synthesis of a complementary strand to make a double-stranded RNA.

Given a supply of nucleotides, these reactions could have created a heterogeneous pool of small RNAs, the biochemical materials required to set in motion the process of natural selection at the molecular level. The idea is that random sequences of RNA are selected for replication on the basis of useful attributes. This process of molecular evolution can now be reproduced in the laboratory by using multiple rounds of error-prone replication of RNA to produce variants from a pool of random initial sequences. Given a laboratory assay for a particular function, it is possible to use this process of directed evolution to select RNAs that are capable of catalyzing biochemical reactions (called ribozymes), including RNA-dependent synthesis of a complementary RNA strand. Although unlikely, this is presumed to have occurred in nature, creating a reliable mechanism to replicate RNAs. Subsequent errors in replication produced variant RNAs, some having desirable features such as catalytic activities that were required for a self-replicating system. Over millions of years, a ribozyme eventually evolved with the ability to catalyze the formation of peptide bonds and to synthesize pro-

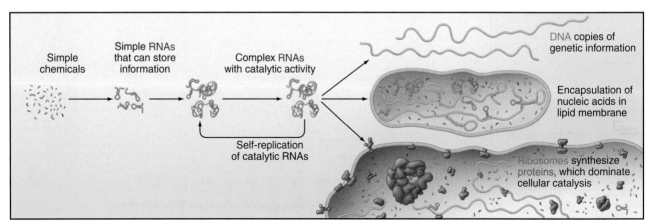

Figure 2-2 HYPOTHESIS FOR PREBIOTIC EVOLUTION TO LAST COMMON ANCESTOR. Simple chemical reactions are postulated to have given rise to ever more complicated RNA molecules to store genetic information and catalyze chemical reactions, including self-replication, in a prebiotic "RNA world." Eventually, genetic information was stored in more stable DNA molecules, and proteins replaced RNAs as the primary catalysts in primitive cells bounded by a lipid membrane.

teins. This most complicated of all known ribozymes is, of course, the ribosome (see Fig. 17-6) that catalyzes the synthesis of proteins. Proteins eventually supplanted ribozymes as catalysts for most biochemical reactions. Owing to greater chemical stability, DNA proved to be superior to RNA for storing the genetic blueprint over time.

Each of these events is improbable, and their combined probability is exceedingly remote, but given a vast number of chemical "experiments" over hundreds of millions of years, this all happened. Encapsulation of these prebiotic reactions may have enhanced their probability. In addition to catalyzing RNA synthesis, clay minerals can also promote formation of lipid vesicles, which can corral reactants to avoid dilution and loss of valuable constituents. This process might have started with fragile bilayers of fatty acids that were later supplanted by more robust phosphoglyceride bilayers (see Fig. 7-5). In laboratory experiments, RNAs inside lipid vesicles can create osmotic pressure that favors expansion of the bilayer at the expense of vesicles lacking RNAs.

No one knows where these prebiotic events took place. Some steps in prebiotic evolution might have occurred in hot springs and thermal vents deep in the ocean where conditions are favorable for some prebiotic reactions. Clay minerals are postulated to have had a role in forming both RNA and lipid vesicles. Carbon-containing meteorites contain useful molecules, including amino acids. Freezing of water can concentrate HCN in liquid droplets favorable for reactions leading to nucleic acid bases. Conditions for prebiotic synthesis were probably favorable beginning about 4 billion years ago, but the geologic record has not preserved convincing microscopic fossils or traces of biosynthesis older than 3.5 billion years.

Another mystery is how L-amino acids and D-sugars (see Chapter 3) were selected over their stereoisomers for biomacromolecules. This was a pivotal event, since racemic mixtures are not favorable for biosynthesis. For example, mixtures of nucleotides composed of L- and D-ribose cannot base-pair well enough for template-guided replication of nucleic acids. In the laboratory, particular amino acid stereoisomers (that could have come from meteorites) can bias the synthesis of D-sugars.

Divergent Evolution from the Last Universal Common Ancestor of Life

Shared biochemical features suggest that all current cells are derived from a last universal common ancestor about 3.5 billion years ago (Fig. 2-1). This primitive ancestor could, literally, have been a single cell or colony of cells, but it might have been a larger community of cells sharing a common pool of genes through interchange of their nucleic acids. The situation is obscure because no primitive organisms remain. All contemporary organisms have diverged equally far in time from their common ancestor.

Although the features of the common ancestor are lost in time, this organism is inferred to have had about 600 genes encoded in DNA. It surely had messenger RNAs, transfer RNAs, and ribosomes to synthesize proteins and a plasma membrane with all three families of pumps as well as carriers and diverse channels, since these are now universal cellular constituents. The transition from primitive, self-replicating, RNA-only particles to this complicated little cell is, in many ways, even more remarkable than the invention of the RNA World. Regrettably, few traces of these events were left behind. Bacteria and Archaea that branched nearest the base of the tree of life live at high temperatures and use hydrogen as their energy source, so the common ancestor might have shared these features.

During evolution genomes have diversified by three processes (Fig. 2-3):

- **Gene divergence:** Every gene is subject to random mutations that are inherited by succeeding generations. Some mutations change single base pairs. Other mutations add or delete larger blocks of DNA such as sequences coding a protein domain, an independently folded part of a protein (see Fig. 3-15). These events inevitably produce genetic diversity through divergence of sequences or creation of novel combinations of domains. Many mutations are neutral, but others may confer a reproductive advantage that favors persistence via natural selection. Other mutations are disadvantageous, resulting in disappearance of the lineage.

- **Gene duplication and divergence:** Rarely, a gene or part of a gene encoding a domain is duplicated during replication or cell division. This creates an opportunity for evolution. As these sister genes subsequently acquire random point mutations, insertions, or deletions, their structures inevitably diverge. Some changes may confer a selective advantage; others confer a liability. Multiple rounds of gene duplication and divergence can create huge families of genes encoding related but specialized proteins, such as membrane pumps and carrier proteins, which are found in all forms of life. Sister genes created by duplication and divergence are called **paralogs.** When species diverge, genes with common origins are called **orthologs** (Box 2-1).

- **Lateral transfer:** Another mechanism of genetic diversification involves movement of genes between organisms. How early life forms accomplished

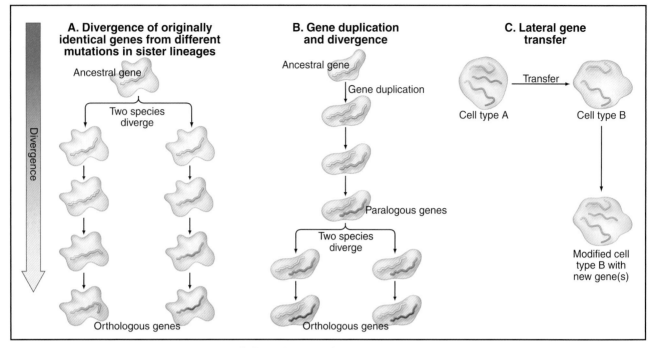

Figure 2-3   MECHANISMS OF GENE DIVERSIFICATION. **A,** Gene divergence from a common origin by random mutations in sister lineages creates orthologous genes. **B,** Gene duplication followed by divergence within and between sister lineages yields both orthologs (separated by speciation) and paralogs (separated by gene duplication). **C,** Lateral transfer can move entire genes from one species to another.

these transfers is not known. Contemporary bacteria acquire foreign genes in three ways. Pairs of bacteria exchange DNA directly during conjugation. Many bacteria take up naked DNA, as when plasmids move genes for antibiotic resistance between bacteria. Viruses also move DNA between bacteria. Such lateral transfers explain how highly

divergent prokaryotes came to share some common genes and regulatory sequences. Massive lateral transfer occurred twice in eukaryotes when they acquired symbiotic bacteria that eventually adapted to form mitochondria and chloroplasts. Lateral transfer continues to this day between pairs of prokaryotes, between pairs of protists, and even between prokaryotes and eukaryotes (such as between pathogenic bacteria and plants).

When conditions do not require the product of a gene, the gene can be lost. For example, the simple pathogenic bacteria *Mycoplasma genitalium* has but 470 genes, since it can rely on its animal host for most nutrients rather than making them de novo. Similarly, the slimmed-down genome of budding yeast, with only 6144 genes, lost nearly 400 genes found in organisms that evolved before fungi. Plants and fungi both lost about 200 genes required to assemble a eukaryotic cilium or flagellum—genes that characterized eukaryotes since their earliest days. Vertebrates also lost many genes that had been maintained for more than 2 billion years in earlier forms of life. For instance, humans lack the enzymes to synthesize certain essential amino acids, which must be supplied in our diets.

Evolution of Prokaryotes

Since the beginning of life, microorganisms dominated the earth in terms of numbers, variety of species, and

BOX 2-1
Orthologs, Paralogs, and Homologs

Genes with a common ancestor are homologs. The terms *ortholog* and *paralog* describe the relationship of homologous genes in terms of how their most recent common ancestor was separated. If a speciation event separated two genes, then they are orthologs. If a duplication event separated two genes, then they are paralogs. To illustrate this point, let us say that gene A is duplicated within a species, forming paralogous genes A1 and A2. If these genes are separated by a speciation event, so that species 1 has genes sp1A1 and sp1A2 and species 2 has genes sp2A1 and sp2A2, it is proper to say that genes sp1A1 and sp2A1 are orthologs and genes sp1A1 and sp1A2 are paralogs, but genes sp1A1 and sp2A2 are also paralogs, since their most recent common ancestor was the gene that duplicated. The situation is more complicated if one or more genes are lost. If *sp1*A2 and *sp2*A1 were lost, there would little evidence to contradict a claim that *sp1*A1 and *sp2*A2 are orthologs.

range of habitats (Fig. 2-4). Bacteria and Archaea remain the most abundant organisms in the seas and on land. They share many features, including basic metabolic enzymes and flagella powered by rotary motors embedded in the plasma membrane. Both divisions of prokaryotes are diverse with respect to size, shape, nutrient sources, and environmental tolerances, so these features cannot be used for classification, which relies instead on analysis of their genomes. For example, sequences of the genes for ribosomal RNAs cleanly separate Bacteria and Archaea (Fig. 2-4). Bacteria are also distinguished by plasma membranes of phosphoglycerides (see Fig. 7-5) with F-type adenosine triphosphatases (ATPases) that use proton gradients to synthesize adenosine triphosphate (ATP). Archaea have plasma membranes composed of isoprenyl ether lipids and V-type ATPases that can either pump protons or synthesize ATP (see Fig. 8-5).

Abetted by rapid proliferation and large populations, prokaryotes have used mutation and natural selection to explore many biochemical solutions to life on the earth. Some Bacteria and Archaea (and some eukaryotes too) thrive under inhospitable conditions such as anoxia and temperatures greater than 100°C as found in deep-sea hydrothermal vents. Other Bacteria and Archaea can use energy sources such as hydrogen, sulfate, or methane that are useless to eukaryotes. Fewer than 1% of Bacteria and Archaea have been grown successfully in the laboratory, so many varieties escaped detection by traditional means. New species are now identified by sequencing random DNA samples from ocean or soil or by amplifying and sequencing characteristic genes from minute samples. Only a very small proportion of bacterial species and no Archaea cause human disease.

Chlorophyll-based photosynthesis originated in Bacteria around 3 billion years ago. Surely, this was one of the most remarkable events during the evolution of life on the earth, because **photosynthetic reaction centers** (see Fig. 19-8) require not only genes for several transmembrane proteins but also genes for multiple enzymes to synthesize chlorophyll and other complex organic molecules associated with the proteins. Chapter 19 describes the machinery and mechanisms of photosynthesis.

Even more remarkably, photosynthesis was invented and perfected not once but twice in different bacteria. A progenitor of green sulfur bacteria and heliobacteria developed photosystem I , while a progenitor of purple bacteria and green filamentous bacteria developed photosystem II. About 2.5 billion years ago, a momentous lateral transfer event brought the genes for the two photosystems together in **cyanobacteria,** arguably the most important organisms in the history of the earth. Cyanobacteria (formerly misnamed *blue-green algae*) use an enzyme containing manganese to split water into oxygen, electrons, and protons. Sunlight energizes photosystem II and photosystem I to pump the protons out

of the cell, creating a proton gradient that is used to synthesize ATP (see Chapters 8 and 19). Using sunlight as the energy source, this form of photosynthesis is the primary source of energy to synthesize the organic compounds that many other forms of life depend on for energy. In addition, beginning about 2.4 billion years ago, cyanobacteria produced most of the oxygen in the earth's atmosphere as a by-product of photosynthesis, bioengineering the planet and radically changing the chemical environment for all other organisms as well.

Origin of Eukaryotes

Divergence from the common ancestor explains the evolution of prokaryotes but not the origin of eukaryotes. Little is known about the earliest Eucarya–neither the time of their first appearance nor much about their lifestyle–other than the fact that their genomes appear to be nearly as old (over 2 billion years) as those of Bacteria and Archaea. One problem is that early eukaryotes left no fossil record until about 1.5 billion years ago, leaving a gap of hundreds of millions of years of evolution without a physical trace except for genes that they donated to their progeny.

Therefore, researchers must analyze genome sequences to test hypotheses about the origins of eukaryotes. The mathematical methods required to analyze the genomic data are still being perfected, and the events are so ancient that their reconstruction is challenging. The bacterial ancestor donated genes for many metabolic processes carried out in the cytoplasm. The archaeal ancestor provided many distinctive genes for informational processes such as transcription of DNA into RNA and translation of RNA into protein. This explains why eukaryotes and Archaea are neighbors on molecular phylogenies based on rRNA sequences (Fig. 2-4).

Such rRNA trees imply that eukaryotes literally branched from the lineage leading to Archaea after Archaea and Bacteria diverged from each other. Such diagrams are based on the reasonable assumption of divergence from a shared ancestor. Note, however, the long line without branches diverging from the presumed ancestor of both Archaea and eukaryotes. This poorly charted territory is responsible for the uncertainty about the origins of eukaryotes.

One attractive hypothesis is that cells from the two domains of prokaryotes joined in a symbiotic relationship to form the first eukaryote (Fig. 2-5). The identities of the Bacterium and Archaean that merged to form this hybrid cell are not known, since these were cells that lived 2 billion years ago. Such a fusion with massive lateral transfer of genes into the new organism provides a simple explanation for how both types of prokaryotes contributed to eukaryotic genomes well after their forebears diverged from the common ancestor. If two

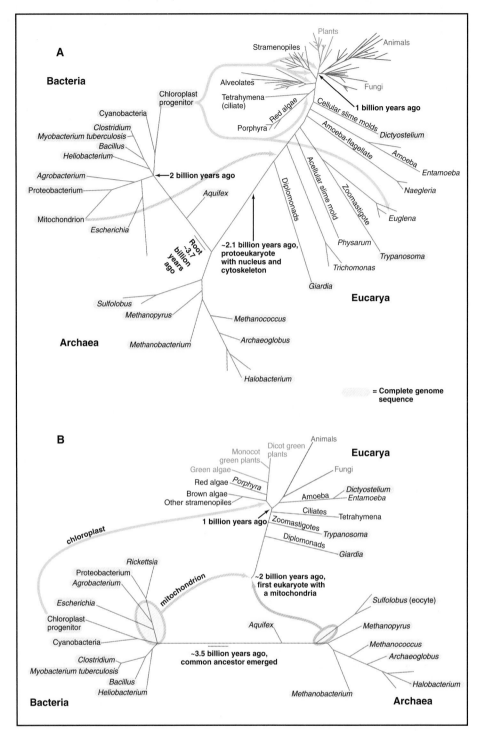

Figure 2-4 COMPARISON OF TREES OF LIFE. **A,** Universal tree based on comparisons of ribosomal RNA sequences. The rRNA tree has its root deep in the bacterial lineage 3 billion to 4 billion years ago. All current organisms, arrayed at the ends of branches, fall into three domains: Bacteria, Archaea, and Eucarya (eukaryotes). This analysis assumes that the organisms in the three domains diverged from a common ancestor. The lengths of the segments and branches are based solely on differences in RNA sequences. Because the rate of random changes in rRNA genes has not been constant, the lengths of the lines that lead to contemporary organisms are not equal. Fossil records provide estimated times of a few key events. Complete sequences of some genomes (*orange;* see http://www.tigr.org) verify most aspects of this tree but also show that genes have moved laterally between Bacteria and Archaea and within each of these domains. Multiple bacterial genes moved to Eucarya twice: First, an α-proteobacterium fused with a primitive eukaryote, giving rise to mitochondria that subsequently transferred many of their genes to the eukaryotic nucleus; and second, a cyanobacterium fused with the precursor of algae and plants to give rise to chloroplasts. Organisms formerly classified as algae, as well as organisms formerly classified elsewhere, actually belong to four large branches near the top of the tree: alveolates (including dinoflagellates, ciliates, and sporozoans), stramenopiles (including diatoms and brown algae), rhodophytes (red algae), and plants (including the green algae). **B,** Composite tree based on analysis of full genome sequences and other data. This hypothesis assumes that eukaryotes formed by fusion of an α-proteobacterium with an Archaean. Chloroplasts arose from the fusion of a cyanobacterium with the eukaryotic precursor of algae and plants. (A, Original drawing, adapted from a branching pattern from Sogin M, Marine Biological Laboratory, Woods Hole, Massachusetts. Reference: Pace N: A molecular view of microbial diversity and the biosphere. Science 276:734–740, 1997. B, Original drawing, based on multiple sources.)

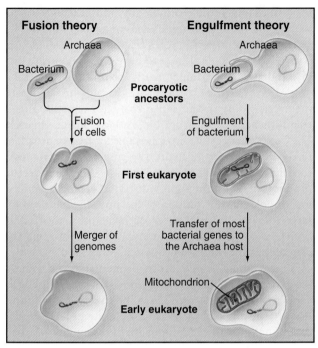

Figure 2-5 Two possible scenarios for the origin of eukaryotes.

prokaryotes literally fused, then their genomes would have been in the same cytoplasm. Later, the hybrid genome was surrounded by membranes to become the nucleus, and another proteobacterium was engulfed to form the precursor of the mitochondrion.

The more conventional view is that primitive eukaryotes first diverged from a precursor to contemporary Archaea and subsequently acquired bacterial genes by lateral transfer. One verified case of lateral transfer was the acquisition of mitochondria in the form of a symbiotic proteobacterium (see later).

Either scenario would have produced an early eukaryote endowed with a greater variety of genes than either progenitor. These single cells probably looked like prokaryotes for many millions of years before developing distinguishing features, but all traces of the original eukaryote have disappeared except for the genes that they donated to their progeny. All contemporary eukaryotes have diverged from the original eukaryote for over 2 billion years and have changed in ways that obscure the past. Although microscopic, single-celled eukaryotes called protists have been numerous and heterogeneous throughout evolution, no existing protist appears to be a good model for the ancestral eukaryote.

Origin and Evolution of Mitochondria

Overwhelming molecular evidence has established that eukaryotes acquired mitochondria when an α-**proteobacterium** became an endosymbiont. Modern-

day α-proteobacteria include pathogenic Rickettsias. When the two formerly independent cells established a stable, endosymbiotic relationship, the Bacterium contributed molecular machinery for **ATP** synthesis by oxidative phosphorylation (see Fig. 19-5). The host cell might have supplied organic substrates to fuel ATP synthesis. Together, they had a reliable energy supply for processes such as biosynthesis, regulation of the internal ionic environment, and cellular motility. Given that some primitive eukaryotes lack full-fledged mitochondria, the singular event that created mitochondria was believed to have occurred well after eukaryotes branched from prokaryotes.

An alternative idea is that the recipient of the α-proteobacterium was an archaean cell rather than a eukaryote (Fig. 2-5). If so, this union could have created not only the mitochondrion but also the first eukaryote! This parsimonious hypothesis is consistent with some but not all of the available data, so it is currently impossible to rule out other scenarios.

The mitochondrial progenitor brought along its own genome and biosynthetic machinery, but over many years of evolution, most bacterial genes either moved to the host cell nucleus or were lost. Like their bacterial ancestors, **mitochondria** are enclosed by two membranes, with the inner membrane equipped for synthesis of ATP. Mitochondria maintain a few genes for mitochondrial components and the capacity to synthesize proteins. Nuclear genes encode most mitochondrial proteins, which are synthesized in the cytoplasm and imported into the organelle (see Fig. 18-2). The transfer of bacterial genes to the nucleus sealed the dependence of the organelle on its eukaryotic host.

Even though acquisition of mitochondria might have been the earliest event in eukaryotic evolution, some eukaryotes lack fully functional mitochondria. These lineages apparently lost most mitochondrial genes and functions through "reductive evolution" in certain anaerobic environments that did not favor natural selection for respiration. The most extreme example is the anaerobic protozoan *Giardia* (the cause of "hiker's diarrhea"), which has only a remnant of a mitochondrion (used to synthesize iron-sulfur clusters for cytoplasmic ATP synthesis) and only one mitochondrial gene in the nucleus. The protist *Entamoeba histolytica* (another cause of diarrhea) is a less extreme example. It lacks mitochondria but has a remnant mitosome consisting of two concentric membranes with some rudimentary mitochondrial functions.

The First Billion Years of Eukaryotic Evolution

What is unique about eukaryotes? For years, it was believed that a membrane-bounded nucleus and a cytoskeleton set eukaryotes apart from prokaryotes. However, some Bacteria and Archaea have genes for homologs of the cytoskeletal proteins, actin, tubulin, and intermediate filaments. Although nuclei are rare in prokaryotes, a family of Bacteria called planctomycetes have rudimentary nuclei that also include all of the ribosomes. Thus, the three kingdoms of life have more in common than was appreciated in the past, as is fitting from our new appreciation for their common origins.

Molecular phylogenies (Fig. 2-4) indicate that modern eukaryotic lineages began to diverge during the period between 2 billion and 1 billion years ago. Since modern organisms from the earliest branches have nuclei, membrane-bounded organelles, and complex structures, including cilia for locomotion, much of what it takes to be a eukaryote evolved very early. These features require hundreds of genes that are absent from prokaryotes, but no fossils or other direct evidence are available about these early events. Organisms on early branches lack a few basic functions, such as the full machinery required for actin-based locomotion and cytokinesis, so the required genes likely appeared after their divergence.

Compartmentalization of the cytoplasm into membrane-bounded organelles is one feature of eukaryotes that is generally lacking in prokaryotes. Mitochondria might have created the first compartment. Endoplasmic reticulum, Golgi apparatus, lysosomes, and endocytic compartments came later by different mechanisms. Chloroplasts resulted from a late endosymbiotic event that occurred in algal cells (see later). Compartmentalization allowed ancestral eukaryotes to increase in size, to capture energy more efficiently, and to regulate gene expression in more complex ways.

Heterotrophic prokaryotes that obtain nutrients from a variety of sources appear to have carried out the first evolutionary experiment with compartmentalization (Fig. 2-6A). However, these prokaryotes are compartmentalized only in the sense that they separate digestion outside the cell from biosynthesis inside the cell. They export digestive enzymes (either free or attached to the cell surface) to hydrolyze complex organic macromolecules (see Fig. 18-10). They must then import the products of digestion to provide building blocks for new macromolecules. Evolution of the proteins required for targeting and translocation of proteins across membranes was a prokaryotic innovation that set the stage for compartmentalization in eukaryotes.

More sophisticated compartmentalization might have begun when a primitive prokaryote developed the capacity to segregate protein complexes with like functions in the plane of the plasma membrane. This created functionally distinct subdomains. Present-day Bacteria segregate their plasma membranes into domains specialized for energy production or protein translocation. Invagination of such domains might have created the endoplasmic reticulum (ER), Golgi apparatus, and lysosomes, as speculated in the following paragraphs (Fig. 2-6):

- Invagination of subdomains of the plasma membrane that synthesize membrane lipids and translocate proteins could have generated an intracellu-

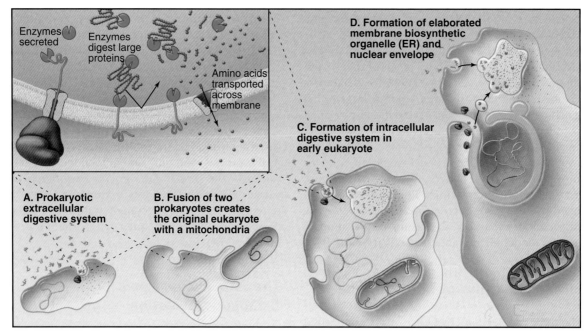

Figure 2-6   SPECULATION REGARDING THE EVOLUTION OF INTRACELLULAR COMPARTMENTS FROM PROKARYOTES TO PRIMITIVE EUKARYOTES. **A–D,** Possible stages in the evolution of intracellular compartments.

lar biosynthetic organelle that survives today as the ER.

- Translocation into the ER became coupled to cotranslational protein synthesis, particularly in later branching eukaryotes.

- The ER was refined to create the nuclear envelope housing the genome, the defining characteristic of the eukaryotic cell. This enabled cells to develop more complex genomes and to separate transcription and RNA processing from translation.

- Internalization of plasma membrane domains with secreted hydrolytic enzymes might have created a primitive lysosome. Coupling of digestion and absorption of macromolecular nutrients would increase efficiency.

This divide-and-specialize strategy might have been employed a number of times to refine the internal membrane system. Eventually, the export and digestive pathways separated from each other and from the lipid synthetic and protein translocation machinery.

As each specialized compartment became physically separated from other compartments, new mechanisms were required to allow traffic between these compartments. The solution was transport vesicles to export products to the cell surface or vacuole and to import raw materials. Transport vesicles also segregated digestive enzymes from the surrounding cytoplasm. Once multiple destinations existed, targeting instructions had to be provided to distinguish the routes and destinations.

The outcome of these events (Fig. 2-7) was a vacuolar system consisting of the ER, the center for protein translocation and lipid synthesis; the Golgi complex and secretory pathway, for posttranslational modification and distribution of biosynthetic products to different destinations; and the endosome/lysosome system, for uptake and digestion.

Production of oxygen by photosynthetic cyanobacteria raised the concentration of atmospheric oxygen about 2.2 billion years ago. This provided sufficient molecular oxygen for eukaryotic cells to synthesize cholesterol (see Fig. 20-14). Incorporation of cholesterol might have strengthened the plasma membrane without compromising fluidity and enabled early eukaryotic cells to increase in size and shed their cell walls. Having shed their cells walls, they could engulf entire prey organisms rather than relying on extracellular digestion. The increase in oxygen also precipitated most of the dissolved iron in the world's oceans, creating ore deposits that are being mined today to extract iron.

The origins of **peroxisomes** are obscure. No nucleic acids or prokaryotic remnants have been detected in peroxisomes, so it seems unlikely that peroxisomes began as prokaryotic symbionts. Peroxisomes arose as centers for oxidative degradation, particularly of products of lysosomal digestion that could not be reutilized

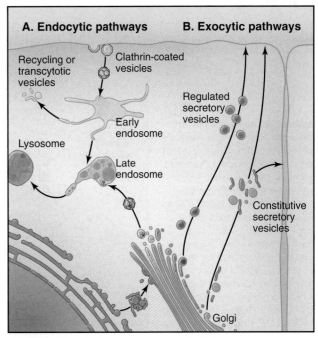

Figure 2-7 MEMBRANE-BOUNDED COMPARTMENTS OF EUKARYOTES. **A,** Pathways for endocytosis and degradation of ingested materials. **B,** Pathways for biosynthesis and distribution of proteins, lipids, and polysaccharides. Membrane and content move through these pathways by controlled budding of vesicles from donor compartments and fusion with specific acceptor compartments. Transport of membranes and content through these two pathways is balanced to establish and maintain the sizes of the compartments.

for biosynthesis (e.g., D-amino acids, uric acid, xanthine). One possibility is that they evolved as a specialization of endoplasmic reticulum.

Origins and Evolution of Chloroplasts

The acquisition of **plastids,** including chloroplasts, began when a cyanobacterial symbiont brought photosynthesis into a primitive algal cell that already had a mitochondrion (Fig. 2-8). The cyanobacterium provided both photosystem I and photosystem II, allowing the sunlight to provide energy to split water and to drive conversion of CO_2 into organic compounds with O_2 as a by-product (see Fig. 19-8). Symbiosis turned into complete interdependence when most of the genes that are required to assemble plastids moved to the nucleus of host cells that continued to rely on the plastid to capture energy from sunlight. This still-mysterious transfer of genes to the nucleus gave the host cell control over the replication of the former symbiont.

Many animals and protozoa associate with photosynthetic bacteria or algae, but the conversion of a bacterial symbiont into a plastid is believed to have been a singular event. The original photosynthetic eukaryote

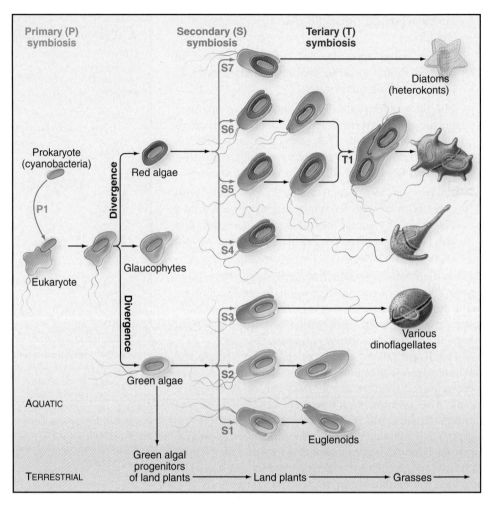

Figure 2-8 ACQUISITION OF CHLO-ROPLASTS. This is a time line from *left* to *right*. The primary event was the ingestion of a cyanobacterium by the eukaryotic cell that gave rise to red algae, glaucophytes, and green algae. Green algae gave rise through divergence to land plants. Diatoms, dinoflagellates, and euglenoids acquired chloroplasts by secondary (S1 through S7) or tertiary (T1) symbiotic events when their precursors ingested an algae with chloroplasts. (Based on Falkowski PG, Katz ME, Knoll AH, et al: Evolution of modern eukaryotic phytoplankton. Science 305:354–360, 2004.)

then diverged into three lineages: green algae, red algae, and a minor group of photosynthetic unicellular organisms called glaucophytes (Fig. 2-8). Green algae, such as the experimentally useful model organism *Chlamydomonas* (see Fig. 38-20), are still plentiful. Green algae also gave rise through divergence to about 300,000 species of land plants.

Events following the initial acquisition of chloroplasts were more complicated, since in at least seven instances, new eukaryotes acquired photosynthesis by taking in an entire green or red alga, followed by massive loss of algal genes. These secondary symbiotic events left behind chloroplasts along with the nuclear genes required for chloroplasts. For example, precursors of *Euglena* took up whole green algae, as did one family of dinoflagellates and chloroarachinophytes. Red algae participated in four secondary and one tertiary symbiotic events, giving rise to diatoms and some of the dinoflagellates. Today, photosynthesis by these marine microbes converts CO_2 into much of the oxygen and organic matter on the earth.

These secondary symbiotic events make phylogenetic relationships of nuclear genes and chloroplast

genes discordant in these organisms. For example, ribosomal RNA gene sequences show that *Euglena* diverged well before algae and later acquired a chloroplast related to those of green algae. The phylogenetic relationships of dinoflagellates are particularly complex, given that a common host cell acquired chloroplasts from three separate sources.

Evolution of Multicellular Eukaryotes

Since the origin of life on the earth, most living organisms have consisted of a single cell. Single-celled prokaryotes, protists, algae, and fungi still dominate the planet. Colonial bacteria initiated evolutionary experiments in living together over 2 billion years ago. About 1 billion years ago, the major branches of eukaryotes—fungi; cellular slime molds; red, brown, and green algae; and animals—independently evolved strategies to form multicellular organisms (Fig. 2-9).

Algae and plants separated from the cells that gave rise to fungi and animals about 1100 million years ago. This estimate is probably correct, in spite of a general

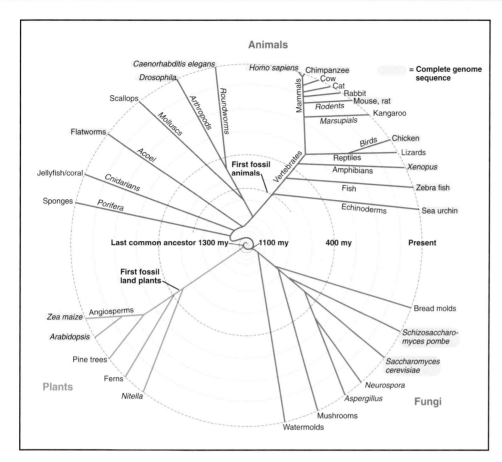

Figure 2-9 TIME LINE FOR THE DIVERGENCE OF ANIMALS, PLANTS, AND FUNGI. This tree has a radial time scale originating about 1100 million years (my) ago with the last common ancestor of plants, animals, and fungi. Contemporary organisms and time are at the circumference. Lengths of branches are arbitrary. The order of branching is established by comparisons of gene sequences. The times of the earliest branching events are only estimates, since calibration of the molecular clocks is uncertain and the early fossil records are sparse. (Original drawing, based on timing for animals, adapted from Kuman S, Hedges SB: A molecular time scale for vertebrate evolution. Nature 392:917–920, 1998; based on timing for plants, adapted from Green Plant Phylogeny Research Coordination Group at http://ucjeps.herb.berkeley.edu/bryolab/greenplantpage.html; based on timing for fungi, adapted from Tree of Life Web Project at http://tolweb.org/tree.)

lack of fossils of these lineages older than 550 million years. Early fungi may simply be difficult to distinguish from their progenitors. Molecular phylogenetics have not yet resolved unambiguously the branching of about 5000 species of red, brown, and green algae. More recent branches, such as the evolution of plants from green algae, are better established.

Fossils of early **metazoans** (multicellular animals) are difficult to find because they are so tiny. The same may be true for early plants. A few well-preserved, 600-million-year-old fossils show that animals already had complex, bilaterally symmetrical bodies at this early date. These tiny (180 μm long) animals had three tissue layers, a mouth, a gut, a coelomic cavity, and surface specializations that are speculated to be sensory structures. Formation of such tissues required membrane proteins for adhesion to the extracellular matrix and to other cells (see Chapter 30). Genes for adhesion proteins—including proteins related to cadherins, integrins, and Ig-CAMs—are found in species that branched before metazoans, so their origins are ancient. Other 570-million-year-old fossils are similar to contemporary animal embryos. These spectacular microscopic fossils support the hypothesis that early multicellular animals were small creatures similar to contemporary invertebrate larvae or embryos. Animals appear to have existed much earlier but have not yet been found in the fossil record.

The early metazoans had little in common with contemporary animals, except possibly sponges, and many were lost to extinction. As evolutionary experimentation progressed, sponges (Porifera) were the first branch of metazoans that survives today. The cells of these colonial organisms have much in common with ciliated protozoa called Chonoflagellates. Next to this branch, about 700 million years ago, were the Cnidarians: jellyfish and corals. These animals have specialized epithelial, nerve, and muscle cells in two layers.

About 540 million to 520 million years ago, conditions allowed the emergence of macroscopic multicellular animals. At the time of this "Cambrian explosion," metazoans became abundant in numbers and varieties in the fossil record. The appearance of these animals in the fossil record over a short period of time is a puzzle, since evolution of such complex body plans must actually have taken a long time. The likely explanation is that the major branches of the animal tree diverged before macroscopic animals developed, as indicated by analysis of genome sequences. Owing to their small size and lack of hard body parts, these progenitors left behind few recognizable fossils.

About 600 million years ago, all other animals branched off as three subdivisions of organisms with bilateral symmetry (at some time in their lives), three tissue layers (ectoderm, mesoderm, and endoderm), and complex organs. The three subdivisions are arthropods and nematodes; mollusks, annelid worms, brachiopods, and platyhelmiths; and echinoderms and chordata (including us).

Looking Back in Time

Viewing contemporary eukaryotic cells, one should be awed by the knowledge that they are mosaics created by historical events that occurred over a vast range of time. Roughly 3.5 billion years ago, the common ancestors of living things already stored genetic information in DNA; transcribed genes into RNA; translated mRNA into protein on ribosomes; carried out basic intermediary metabolism; and were protected by plasma membranes with carriers, pumps, and channels. More than 2.5 billion years ago, bacteria evolved the genes required for photosynthesis and eventually donated this capacity to eukaryotes via endosymbiosis about 1 billion years ago. An α-proteobacterium took up residence in an early eukaryote, giving rise to mitochondria about 2 billion years ago. Although prokaryotes have genes for homologs of all three cytoskeletal proteins, eukaryotes developed the capacity for cellular motility about 1.5 billion years ago when they shed their cell walls and evolved genes for molecular motors and many proteins that regulate the cytoskeleton. Multicellular eukaryotes with specialized cells and tissues arose only in the past 1.2 billion years after acquiring plasma membrane receptors used for cellular interactions.

It is also instructive to consider how more complex functions, such as the operation of the human nervous system, have their roots deep in time, beginning with the advent of molecules such as receptors and voltage-sensitive ion channels that originally served their unicellular inventors. At each step along the way, evolution has exploited the available materials for new functions to benefit the multitude of living organisms.

ACKNOWLEDGMENTS

Some of this chapter comes from material written by Ann L. Hubbard, J. David Castle, and Sandra Schmid for the first edition of *Cell Biology.* Thanks also go to Steve Stearns, Mike Donoghue, Mitch Sogin, Jim Lake, Daniel Pollard, Katherine Pollard, and Leslie Orgel.

SELECTED READINGS

Chen, J-Y, Bottjer DJ, Davidson EH, et al: Small bilaterian fossils from 40 to 55 million years before the Cambrian. Science 305:218-222, 2004.

Dawkins R: The Ancestor's Tale. New York, Houghton Mifflin, 2004, p 673.

Falkowski PG, Katz ME, Knoll AH, et al: Evolution of modern eukaryotic phytoplankton. Science 305:354-360, 2004.

Gerlt JA, Babbitt PC: Divergent evolution of enzymatic function: Mechanistically diverse superfamilies and functionally distinct suprafamilies. Annu Rev Biochem 70:209-246, 2001.

Harwood A, Coates JC: A prehistory of cell adhesion. Curr Opin Cell Biol 16:470-476, 2004

Joyce GF: Directed evolution of nucleic acid enzymes. Annu Rev Biochem 73:791-836, 2004.

Knoll AH: Life on a Young Planet: The First Three Billion Years of Life on Earth. Princeton, NJ, Princeton University Press, 2003, p 277.

Orgel LF: Prebiotic chemistry and the origin of the RNA world. Crit Rev Biochem Mol Biol 39:99-123, 2004.

Rivera MC, Lake JA: The ring of life provides evidence for a genome fusion origin of eukaryotes. Nature 431:152-155, 2004.

True JR, Carroll SB: Gene co-option in physiological and morphological evolution. Annu Rev Cell Dev Biol 18:53-80, 2002.

Vogel C, Bashton M, Kerrison ND, et al: Structure, function and evolution of multidomain proteins. Curr Opin Struct Biol 14:208-216, 2004.

Woese CR: A new biology for a new century. Microbiol Mol Biol Rev 68:173-186, 2004.

Internet

Deep Green Tree of Life Web Project. Available at http://tolweb.org/tree/phylogeny.html.

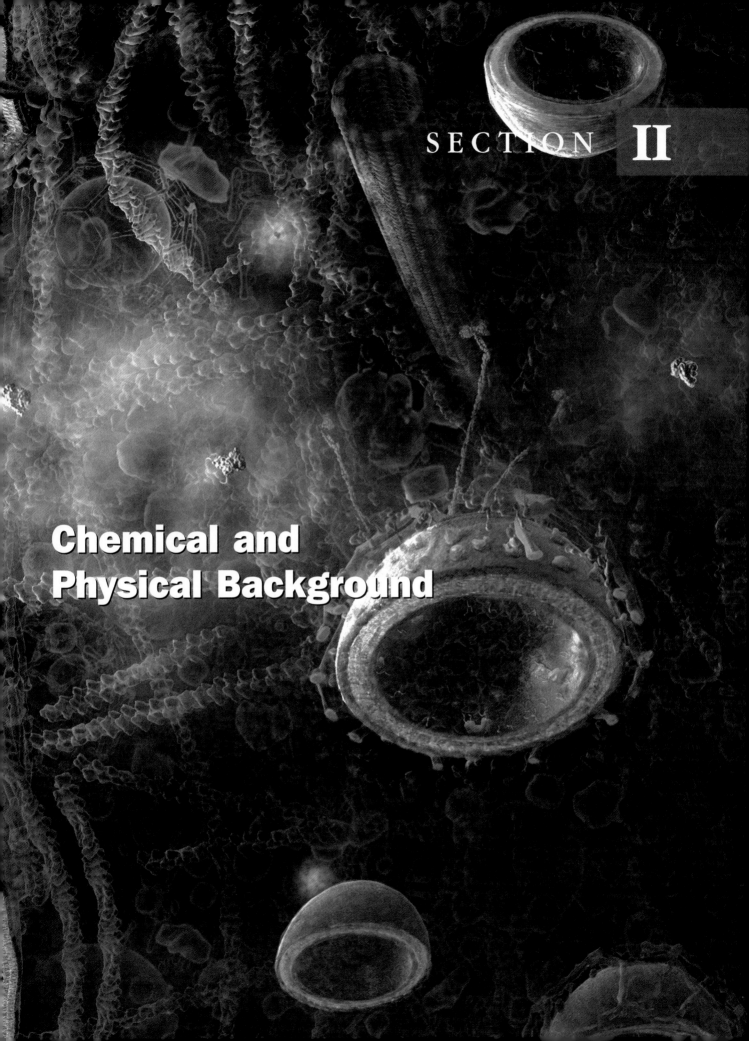

SECTION II

Chemical and Physical Background

SECTION II OVERVIEW

A primary objective of this book is to explain the molecular basis of life at the cellular level. This requires an appreciation of the structures of molecules as well as the basic principles of chemistry and physics that account for molecular interactions. The featured molecules are mostly **proteins,** but **nucleic acids, complex carbohydrates,** and **lipids** are all essential for life.

Chapter 3 explains the design principles of the major biological macromolecules in enough detail that a reader will appreciate the functions of the hundreds of proteins and nucleic acids that are considered in later chapters. Important concepts include the chemical nature of the building blocks of proteins **(amino acids),** nucleic acids **(nucleotides),** and sugar polymers **(monosaccharides);** the chemical bonds that link these units together; and the forces that drive the folding of polypeptides and nucleic acids into three-dimensional structures. Chapter 7 in the following section of the book introduces lipids in the context of the structure and function of biological membranes.

No biological macromolecule operates in isolation in cells, so Chapter 4 explains the physics and chemistry of their interactions. Many readers will never take a physical chemistry course, but they will discover in this chapter that a relatively few general principles can explain the **kinetics** and **thermodynamics** of most molecular interactions that are relevant to cells. For example, just two numbers and the concentrations of the reactants explain the forward and reverse rates of chemical reactions. Just one simple equation relates these two kinetic parameters to the key thermodynamic parameter, the **equilibrium constant**—the tendency of the reaction to go forward or backward. A second simple equation relates the equilibrium constant to the energy of the reactants and products. A third simple equation relates the change in free energy during a reaction to only two underlying parameters, the changes in heat and order in the system. These three equations explain all of the chemical reactions that make life possible. The authors hope that Chapter 4

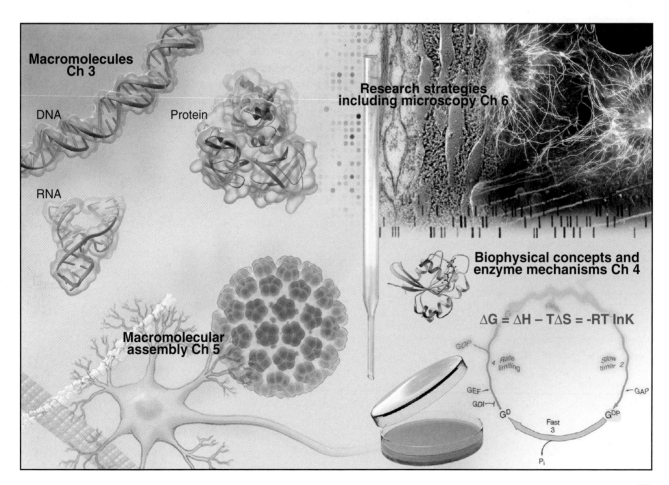

Macromolecules
Ch 3

DNA

RNA

Protein

Macromolecular
assembly Ch 5

Research strategies
including microscopy Ch 6

Biophysical concepts and
enzyme mechanisms Ch 4

$$\Delta G = \Delta H - T\Delta S = -RT \ln K$$

inspires a few readers to try a "P-chem" course to learn more.

Many cellular processes depend on macromolecular catalysts, protein enzymes, or RNA ribozymes. Chapter 4 explains how biochemists analyze enzyme mechanisms, using as the example a protein that binds and hydrolyzes a nucleotide, guanosine triphosphate (GTP). Cells use related GTPases as molecular switches for many processes, including transport of macromolecules into and out of the nucleus (see Chapter 14), protein synthesis (see Chapter 17), membrane traffic (see Chapters 20 to 22), signal transduction (see Chapters 25 and 27), regulation of the cytoskeleton (see Chapters 33 and 38) and mitosis (see Chapter 44).

Macromolecules are polymers that are held together by strong covalent bonds between the building blocks. Templates guide the synthesis of proteins (see Chapter 17) and nucleic acids (see Chapters 15 and 42), but most macromolecular structures in cells assemble spontaneously from their components without a template. These macromolecular assemblies are held together by weak, noncovalent bonds between complementary surfaces. Chapter 5 explains how simple bimolecular reactions and conformational changes guide the assembly pathways for complexes of multiple proteins and complexes of proteins with nucleic acids. Cells often use ATP hydrolysis or changes in protein conformation to control the reversible reactions required to assemble cytoskeletal polymers, signaling machines, coats around membrane vesicles, and chromosomes, among many other examples.

This book is not a manual for experimental cell biology, but to understand the experiments on which modern cell biological understanding is based, readers will want to appreciate the general strategy and the principles behind a few common methods. Chapter 6 explains that the dominant strategy in cell biology is a **reductionist approach.** Many classical questions in cell biology were defined by the behavior of cells described by early pioneers in the 19th and early 20th centuries. Subsequent microscopic analysis, genetic analysis in "model organisms," and studies of human disease have further refined these questions in a modern context. Once a cellular process of interest has been identified, biologists use genetics or biochemistry to identify the molecules that are involved. Next, chemical and physical methods are applied to learn enough about each molecule to formulate a hypothesis about mechanisms. In the best-understood situations, these hypotheses are formalized as mathematical models for rigorous comparison with biological observations.

Microscopes are the most frequently used tool in cell biology, so Chapter 6 explains how light and electron microscopes both magnify and produce contrast—the two factors that are required to image cells and molecules. Equally important are the methods that are used to prepare biological specimens for microscopy and to showcase particular molecules for microscopic observation. In particular, fusion of proteins to jellyfish fluorescent proteins has revolutionized the study of protein behavior in living cells. The chapter also explains a number of the basic genetic experiments and methods to manipulate nucleic acids in "molecular cloning" experiments. This background should help readers to understand the variety of experimental data presented in figures throughout the book.

CHAPTER 3

Molecules: Structures and Dynamics

This chapter describes the properties of water, proteins, nucleic acids, and carbohydrates as they pertain to cell biology. Chapter 7 covers lipids in the context of biological membranes.

Water

Water is so familiar that its role in cell biology and its fascinating properties tend to be neglected. Water is the most abundant and important molecule in cells and tissues. Humans are about two thirds water. Water is not only the solvent for virtually all cellular compounds but also a reactant or product in thousands of biochemical reactions catalyzed by enzymes, including the synthesis and degradation of proteins and nucleic acids and the synthesis and hydrolysis of adenosine triphosphate (ATP), to name a few examples. Water is also an important determinant of biological structure, as lipid bilayers, folded proteins, and macromolecular assemblies are all stabilized by the hydrophobic effect derived from the exclusion of water from nonpolar surfaces (see Fig. 4-5). Additionally, water forms hydrogen bonds with polar groups of many cellular constituents ranging in size from small metabolites to large proteins. It also associates with small inorganic ions.

Physical chemists are still trying to understand water, one of the most complex liquids. The molecule is roughly tetrahedral in shape (Fig. 3-1A), with two hydrogen bond donors and two hydrogen bond acceptors. The electronegative oxygen withdraws the electrons from the O—H covalent bonds, leaving a partial positive charge on the hydrogens and a partial negative charge on the oxygen. Hydrogen bonds between water molecules are partly electrostatic because of the charge separation (induced dipole) but also have some covalent character, owing to overlap of the electron orbitals. The strength of hydrogen bonds depends on their orientation, being strongest along the lines of tetrahedral orbitals. One can think of oxygens of two water molecules sharing a hydrogen-bonded hydrogen. Given two hydrogen bond donors and acceptors, water can be fully hydrogen-bonded, as it is in ice (Fig. 3-1C). Crystalline water in ice has a well-defined structure with a complete set of tetragonal hydrogen bonds and a remarkable amount (35%) of unoccupied space (Fig. 3-1D).

Neither theoretical calculations nor physical observations of liquid water have revealed a consistent picture of its organization. When ice melts, the volume decreases

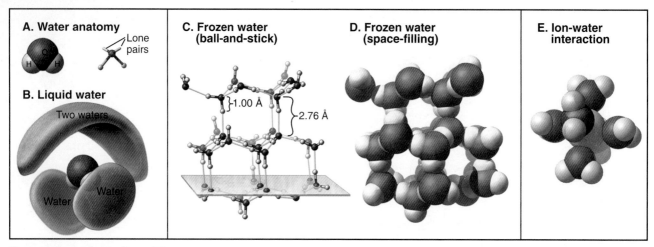

Figure 3-1 WATER. **A,** Space-filling model and orientation of the tetrahedral electron orbitals that define the directions of the hydrogen bonds. **B,** Tetrahedral local order in liquid water revealed by a theoretical calculation of a three-dimensional map of regions around the central water molecule where the local density of oxygen is at least 40% higher than average. Two adjacent water oxygens are centered near the two hydrogen bond donors, and two other waters are positioned in an elongated cap so that their protons can hydrogen-bond with the central water oxygen. **C,** Stick figure of crystallized ice showing the tetrahedral network of hydrogen bonds. **D,** A space-filling model of crystalline ice showing the large amount of unoccupied space. **E,** Shell of water molecules around a potassium ion. Small ions, such as Li^+, Na^+, and F^-, bind water more tightly than do larger ions, such as K^+, Cl^-, and I^-. (D–E, From www.nyu.edu/pages/mathmol/library/water, Project MathMol Scientific Visualization Lab, New York University. See "ice.pdb" and "waterbox.pdb.")

by only about 10%, so liquid water has considerable empty space too. The heat required to melt ice is a small fraction (15%) of the heat required to convert ice to a gas, in which all the hydrogen bonds are lost. Because the heat of melting reflects the number of bonds broken, liquid water must retain most of the hydrogen bonds that stabilize ice. These hydrogen bonds create a continuous, three-dimensional network of water molecules connected at their tetrahedral vertices, allowing water to remain a liquid at a higher temperature than is the case for a similar molecule, ammonia. On the other hand, because liquid water does not have a well-defined, long-range structure, it must be very heterogeneous and dynamic, with rapidly fluctuating regions of local order and disorder. This incomplete picture of water structure limits our ability to understand macromolecular interactions in an aqueous environment.

The properties of water have profound effects on all other molecules in the cell. For example, ions organize shells of water around themselves that compete effectively with other ions with which they might interact electrostatically (Fig. 3-1E). This shell of water travels with the ions, governing the size of pores that they can penetrate. Similarly, hydrogen bonding with water strongly competes with the hydrogen bonding that occurs between solutes, including macromolecules. By contrast, water does not interact as favorably with nonpolar molecules as it does with itself, so the solubility of nonpolar molecules in water is low, and they tend to aggregate to reduce their surface area in contact with water. Such nonpolar interactions are energetically favorable because they reduce unfavorable interactions of nonpolar groups with water and increase

favorable interactions of water molecules with each other. This is called the hydrophobic effect (see Fig. 4-5). These interactions of water dominate the behavior of solute molecules in an aqueous environment, where they influence the assembly of proteins, lipids, and nucleic acids into the structures that they assume in the cell. On the other hand, strategically placed water molecules can bridge two macromolecules in functional assemblies.

Proteins

Proteins are major components of all cellular systems. This section presents some basic concepts about protein structure that help to explain how proteins function in cells. More extensive coverage of this topic is available in biochemistry books and specialized books on protein chemistry.

Proteins consist of one or more linear polymers called **polypeptides,** which consist of various combinations of 20 different **amino acids** (Figs. 3-2 and 3-3) linked together by **peptide bonds** (Fig. 3-4). When linked in polypeptides, amino acids are referred to as residues. The sequence of amino acids in each type of polypeptide is unique. It is specified by the gene encoding the protein and is read out precisely during protein synthesis (see Fig. 18-8). The polypeptides of proteins with more than one chain are usually synthesized separately. However, in some cases, a single chain is divided into pieces by cleavage after synthesis.

Polypeptides range widely in length. Small peptide hormones, such as oxytocin, consist of as few as nine

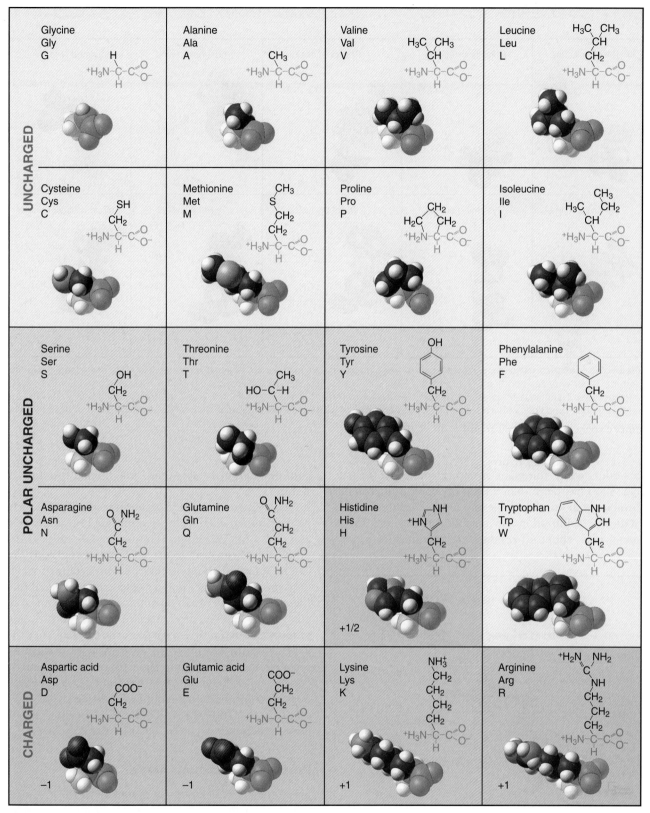

Figure 3-2 THE 20 L-AMINO ACIDS SPECIFIED BY THE GENETIC CODE. Shown for each are the full name, the three-letter abbreviation, the single-letter abbreviation, a stick figure of the atoms, and a space-filling model of the atoms in which hydrogen is *white*, carbon is *black*, oxygen is *red*, nitrogen is *blue*, and sulfur is *yellow*. For all, the amino group is protonated and carries a +1 charge, whereas the carboxyl group is ionized and carries a –1 charge. The amino acids are grouped according to the side chains attached to the α-carbon. These side chains fall into three subgroups. **Top,** The aliphatic (G, A, V, L, I, C, M, P) and aromatic (Y, F, W) side chains partition into nonpolar environments, as they interact poorly with water. **Middle,** The uncharged side chains with polar hydrogen bond donors or acceptors (S, T, N, Q, Y) can hydrogen-bond with water. **Bottom,** At neutral pH, the basic amino acids K and R are fully protonated and carry a charge of +1, the acidic amino acids (D, E) are fully ionized and carry a charge of –1, and histidine (pK: ~6.0) carries a partial positive charge. All the charged residues interact favorably with water, although the aliphatic chains of R and K also give them significant nonpolar character.

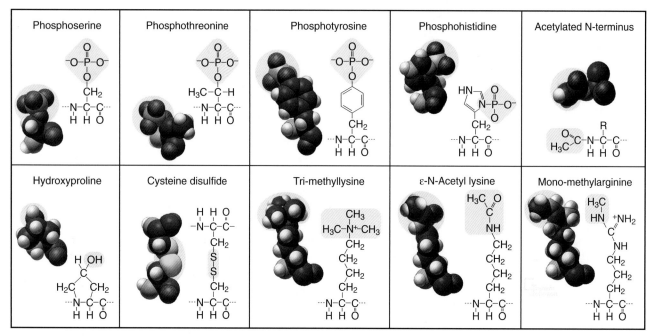

Figure 3-3 MODIFIED AMINO ACIDS. Protein kinases add a phosphate group to serine, threonine, tyrosine, histidine, and aspartic acid (not shown). Other enzymes add one or more methyl groups to lysine, arginine, or histidine (not shown); a hydroxyl group to proline; or an acetate to the N-terminus of many proteins. The reducing environment of the cytoplasm minimizes the formation of disulfide bonds, but under oxidizing conditions within the membrane compartments of the secretory pathway (see Chapter 21), intramolecular or intermolecular disulfide (S—S) bonds form between adjacent cysteine residues.

residues, while the giant structural protein titin (see Fig. 39-7) has more than 25,000 residues. Most cellular proteins fall in the range of 100 to 1000 residues. Without stabilization by disulfide bonds or bound metal ions, about 40 residues are required for a poly-

peptide to adopt a stable three-dimensional structure in water.

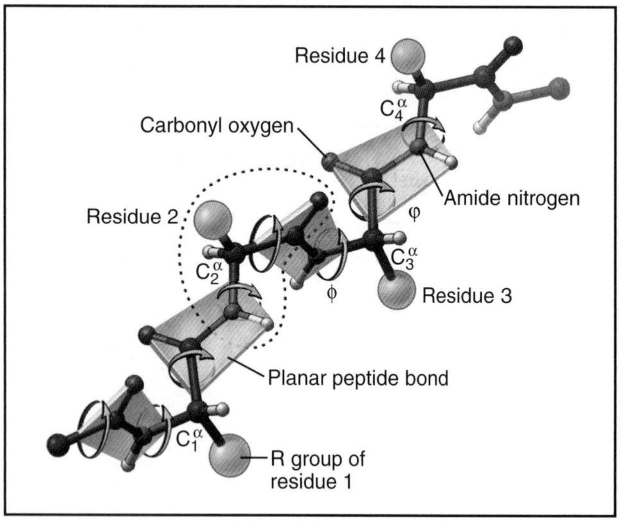

The sequence of amino acids in a polypeptide can be determined chemically by removing one amino acid at a time from the amino terminus and identifying the product. This procedure, called **Edman degradation,** can be repeated about 50 times before declining yields limit progress. Longer polypeptides can be divided into fragments of fewer than 50 amino acids by chemical or enzymatic cleavage, after which they are purified and sequenced separately. Even easier, one can sequence the gene or a complementary DNA **(cDNA)** copy of the messenger RNA for the protein (Fig. 3-16) and use the genetic code to infer the amino acid sequence. This approach misses posttranslational modifications (Fig. 3-3). Analysis of protein fragments by mass spectrometry can be used to sequence even tiny quantities of proteins.

Properties of Amino Acids

Every student of cell biology should know the chemical structures of the amino acids used in proteins (Fig. 3-2). Without these structures in mind, reading the literature and this book is like spelling without knowledge of the alphabet. In addition to their full names, amino acids are frequently designated by three-letter or single-letter abbreviations.

All but one of the 20 amino acids commonly used in proteins consist of an **amino group,** bonded to the

Figure 3-4 THE POLYPEPTIDE BACKBONE. This perspective drawing shows four planar peptide bonds, the four participating α-carbons (labeled 1 to 4), the R groups represented by the β-carbons, amide protons, carbonyl oxygens, and the two rotatable backbone bonds (φ and φ). The *dotted lines* outline one amino acid. (Adapted from Creighton TE: Proteins: Structure and Molecular Principles. New York, WH Freeman and Co, 1983.)

α-**carbon,** bonded to a **carboxyl group.** Proline is a variation on this theme with a cyclic side chain bonded back to the nitrogen to form an imino group. Both the amino group (pK > 9) and carboxyl group (pK = ~4) are partially ionized under physiological conditions. With the exception of glycine, all amino acids have a β-carbon and a proton bonded to the α-carbon. (Glycine has a second proton instead.) This makes the α-carbon an asymmetrical center with two possible configurations. The L-isomers are used almost exclusively in living systems. Compared with natural proteins, proteins constructed artificially from D-amino acids have mirror-image structures and properties.

Each amino acid has a distinctive **side chain,** or R group, that determines its chemical and physical properties. Amino acids are conveniently grouped in small families according to their R groups. Side chains are distinguished by the presence of ionized groups, polar groups capable of forming hydrogen bonds and their apolar surface areas. Glycine and proline are special cases, owing to their unique effects on the polymer backbone (see later section).

Enzymes modify many amino acids after their incorporation into polypeptides. These **posttranslational modifications** have both structural and regulatory functions (Fig. 3-3). These modifications are referred to many times in this book, especially reversible phosphorylation of amino acid side chains, the most common regulatory reaction in biochemistry (see Fig. 25-1). Methylated and acetylated lysines are important for chromatin regulation in the nucleus (see Fig. 13-3). Whole proteins such as ubiquitin or SUMO can be attached through isopeptide bonds to lysine ε-amino groups to act as signals for degradation (see Fig. 23-8) or endocytosis (see Fig. 22-16).

This repertoire of amino acids is sufficient to construct millions of different proteins, each with different capacities for interacting with other cellular constituents. This is possible because each protein has a unique three-dimensional structure (Fig. 3-5), each displaying the relatively modest variety of functional groups in a different way on its surface.

Architecture of Proteins

Our knowledge of protein structure is based largely on X-ray diffraction studies of protein crystals or nuclear magnetic resonance (NMR) spectroscopy studies of small proteins in solution. These methods provide pictures showing the arrangement of the atoms in space. X-ray diffraction requires three-dimensional crystals of the protein and yields a three-dimensional contour map showing the density of electrons in the molecule (Fig. 3-6). In favorable cases, all the atoms except hydrogens are clearly resolved, along with water molecules occupying fixed positions in and around the protein. NMR requires concentrated solutions of protein and reveals distances between particular protons. Given enough distance constraints, it is possible to calculate the unique protein fold that is consistent with these spacings. In a few cases, electron microscopy of two-dimensional crystals has revealed atomic structures (see Figs. 7-8B and 34-5).

Each amino acid residue contributes three atoms to the polypeptide backbone: the nitrogen from the amino group, the α-carbon, and the carbonyl carbon from the carboxyl group. The peptide bond linking the amino acids together is formed by dehydration synthesis (see Fig. 17-10), a common chemical reaction in biological systems. Water is removed in the form of a hydroxyl from the carboxyl group of one amino acid and a proton from the amino group of the next amino acid in the polymer. Ribosomes catalyze this reaction in cells. Chemical synthesis can achieve the same result in the laboratory. The peptide bond nitrogen has an **(amide) proton,** and the carbon has a double-bonded **(carbonyl) oxygen.** The amide proton is an excellent hydrogen bond donor, whereas the carbonyl oxygen is an excellent hydrogen bond acceptor.

The end of a polypeptide with the free amino group is called the **amino terminus** or **N-terminus.** The numbering of the residues in the polymer starts with the N-terminal amino acid, as the biosynthesis of the polymer begins there on ribosomes. The other end of a polypeptide has a free carboxyl group and is called the **carboxyl terminus** or **C-terminus.**

The peptide bond has some characteristics of a double bond, owing to resonance of the electrons, and is relatively rigid and planar. The bonds on either side of the α-carbon can rotate through 360 degrees, although a relatively narrow range of bond angles is highly favored. Steric hindrance between the β-carbon (on all the amino acids but glycine) and the α-carbon of the adjacent residue favors a *trans* configuration in which the side chains alternate from one side of the polymer to the other (Fig. 3-4). Folded proteins generally use a limited range of rotational angles to avoid steric collisions of atoms along the backbone. Glycine without a β-carbon is free to assume a wider range of configurations and is useful for making tight turns in folded proteins.

Folding of Polypeptides

The three-dimensional structure of a protein is determined solely by the sequence of amino acids in the polypeptide chain. This was established by reversibly unfolding and refolding proteins in a test tube. Many, but not all, proteins that are unfolded by harsh treatments (high concentrations of urea or extremes of pH) will refold to regain full activity when returned to physiological conditions. Although many proteins

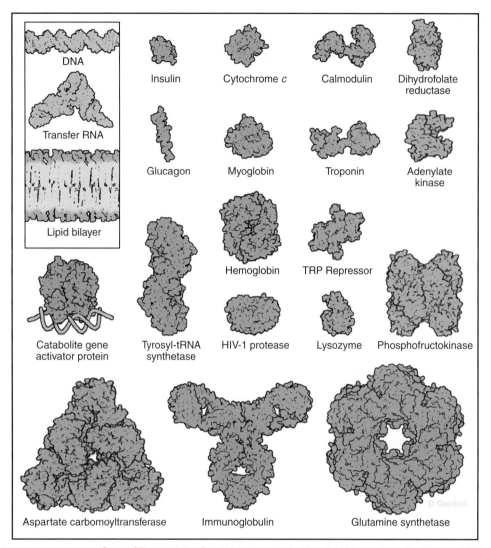

Figure 3-5   A GALLERY OF MOLECULES. Space-filling models of proteins compared with a lipid bilayer, transfer RNA, and DNA, all on the same scale. (Modified from Goodsell D, Olsen AJ: Soluble proteins: Size, shape, and function. Trends Biochem Sci 18:65–68, 1993.)

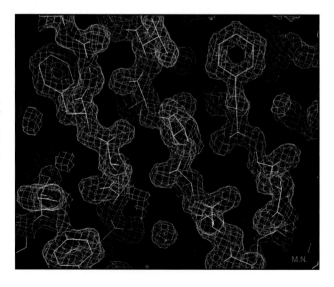

Figure 3-6   PROTEIN STRUCTURE DETERMINATION BY X-RAY CRYSTALLOG-RAPHY. A small part of an electron density map at 1.5-Å resolution of the cytoplasmic T1 domain of the shaker potassium channel from *Aplysia*. The chicken-wire map shows the electron density. The stick figure shows the superimposed atomic model. (Based on original data from M. Nanao and S. Choe, Salk Institute for Biological Studies, San Diego, California.)

are flexible enough to undergo conformational changes (see later discussion), polypeptides rarely fold into more than one final stable structure. Exceptions with medical importance are prions and amyloid (Box 3-1).

Although proteins fold spontaneously into a unique structure, it is not yet possible to predict three-dimensional structures of proteins from their amino acid sequences unless one already knows the structure of an ortholog or paralog. Then one can use the known structure and the amino acid sequence of the unknown to build a **homology model** that is often accurate enough to make reliable inferences about function. Predicting protein structures from sequence alone would have profound practical consequences, since the number of protein sequences known from genome-sequencing

projects far exceeds the number of established protein structures (about 10,000).

The following factors influence protein folding:

1. Hydrophobic side chains pack very tightly in the core of proteins to minimize their exposure to water. Little free space exists inside proteins, so the hydrophobic core resembles a hydrocarbon crystal more than an oil droplet (Fig. 3-7). Accordingly, the most conserved residues in families of proteins are found in the interior. Nevertheless, the internal packing is malleable enough to tolerate mutations that change the size of buried side chains, as the neighboring chains can rearrange without changing the overall shape of the protein. Interior charged or polar residues frequently form

---

BOX 3-1
Protein Misfolding in Amyloid Diseases

Misfolding of diverse proteins and peptides results in spontaneous assembly of insoluble **amyloid fibrils.** Such pathological misfolding is associated with Alzheimer's disease, transmissible spongiform encephalopathies (such as "mad cow disease"), and polyglutamine expansion diseases (such as Huntington's disease, in which genetic mutations encode abnormal stretches of the amino acid glutamine). Accumulation of amyloid fibrils in these diseases is associated with slow degeneration of the brain. Pathological misfolding also results in amyloid deposition in other organs such as the endocrine pancreas in Type II diabetes. The precursor of a given amyloid fiber may be the wild-type protein or a protein modified through mutation, proteolytic cleavage, posttranslational modification, or polyglutamine expansion. The pathology of amyloidosis is not well understood. Some, but not all, amyloids are intrinsically toxic to cells. Some amyloid precursors are more toxic than the fibrils themselves. In all cases, fibril initiation is very slow, but once formed, fibrils act as seeds to promote the assembly of additional protein into fibrils.

Given that many unrelated proteins and peptides form amyloid, it is remarkable that most of these twisted fibrils have similar structures: narrow sheets up to 10 μm long consisting of thousands of short β-strands that run across the width of the fibril. The β-strands can be either parallel or antiparallel, depending on the particular protein or peptide. Some amyloid fibrils consist of multiple layers of β-strands. The structures of the various parent proteins have nothing in common with each other or with amyloid cross β-sheets, so these are rare examples of polypeptides with two stable folds. To form amyloid, the native protein must either be partially unfolded or cleaved into a fragment with a tendency to aggregate.

In the common form of dementia called Alzheimer's disease, the peptide that forms amyloid is a proteolytic

fragment of a transmembrane protein of unknown function called β-amyloid precursor protein. "Infectious proteins" called **prions** cause transmissible spongiform encephalopathies. Normally, these proteins do no harm, but once misfolded, the protein can act as a seed to induce other copies of the protein to form insoluble amyloid-like assemblies that are toxic to nerve cells. Such misfolding rarely occurs under normal circumstances, but the misfolded seeds can be acquired by ingesting infected tissues.

Other proteins, including the peptide hormone insulin, the actin-binding protein gelsolin, and the blood-clotting protein fibrinogen, form amyloid in certain diseases. An inherited point mutation makes the secreted form of gelsolin susceptible to cleavage by a peptide processing protease in the trans-Golgi network. Fragments of 53 or 71 residues form extracellular amyloid fibrils in several organs.

Given that amyloid fibrils form spontaneously and are exceptionally stable, it is not surprising that functional amyloids exist in organisms ranging from bacteria to humans. For example, formation of the pigment granules responsible for skin color depends on a proteolytic fragment of a lysosomal membrane protein that forms amyloid fibrils as a scaffold from melanin pigments. Budding yeast has a number of proteins that can either assume their "native" fold or assemble into amyloid fibrils. The native fold of the protein Sup35p serves as a translation termination factor that stops protein synthesis at the stop codon (see Fig. 17-8). Rarely, Sup35p misfolds and assembles into an amyloid fibril. These fibrils sequester all the Sup35p in fibrils, where it is inactive. The faulty translation termination that occurs in its absence has diverse consequences that are inherited like prions from one generation of yeast to the next.

hydrogen bonds or salt bridges to neutralize their charge.

2. Most charged and polar side chains are exposed on the surface, where they interact favorably with water. Although many hydrophobic residues are inside, roughly half the residues that are exposed to solvent on the outer surface are also hydrophobic. Amino acid residues on the surface typically appear to play a minor role in protein folding. Experimentally, one can substitute many residues on the surface of a protein with any other residue without changing the stability or three-dimensional structure.

3. The polar amide protons and carbonyl oxygens of the polypeptide backbone maximize their poten-

tial to form hydrogen bonds with other backbone atoms, side chain atoms, or water. In the hydrophobic core of proteins, this is achieved by hydrogen bonds with other backbone atoms in two major types of **secondary structures: α-helices** and **β-sheets** (Fig. 3-8).

4. Elements of secondary structure usually extend completely across compact domains. Consequently, most loops connecting α-helices and β-strands are on the surface of proteins, not in the interior (Fig. 3-9). Exceptions are found in some integral membrane proteins (see Figs. 10-3, 10-13, 10-14, and 10-15), where α-helices can reverse in the interior of the protein.

These factors tend to maximize the stability of folded proteins in one particular "native" conformation, but the native state of folded proteins is relatively unstable. The standard free energy difference (see Chapter 4) between a folded and globally unfolded protein is only about 40 kJ mol^{-1}, much less than that of a single covalent bond! Even the substitution of a single crucial amino acid can destabilize certain proteins, causing a loss of function. In other cases, misfolding results in noncovalent polymerization of a protein into amyloid fibrils associated with serious diseases (Box 3-1).

The amino acid sequence of each polypeptide contains all the information required to specify folding into the native protein structure, just one of a near infinity of possible conformations. Chapter 17 explains how many conformations of the unfolded polypeptide are rapidly sampled through trial and error to select stable intermediates leading to the native structure. Cells use molecular chaperones to guide and control the quality of folding.

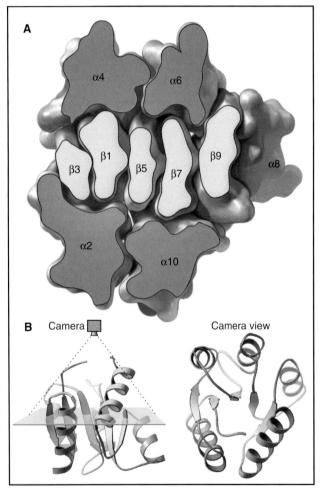

Figure 3-7 Space-filling **(A)** and ribbon **(B)** models of a cross section of the bacterial chemotaxis protein CheY illustrate some of the factors that contribute to protein folding. α-Helices pack on both sides of the central, parallel β-sheet. Most of the polar and charged residues are on the surface. The tightly packed interior of largely apolar residues excludes water. The buried backbone amides and carbonyls are fully hydrogen-bonded to other backbone atoms in both the α-helices and β-sheet. (PDB file: 2CHF.)

Secondary Structure

Much of the polypeptide backbone of proteins folds into stereotyped elements of secondary structure, especially α-helices and β-sheets (Fig. 3-8). They are shown as spirals and polarized ribbons in "ribbon diagrams" of protein organization used throughout this book. Both α-helices and β-strands are linear, so globular proteins can be thought of as compact bundles of straight or gently curving rods, laced together by surface turns.

α-Helices allow polypeptides to maximize hydrogen bonding of backbone polar groups while using highly favored rotational angles around the α-carbons and tight packing of atoms in the core of the helix (Fig. 3-8). All of these features stabilize the α-helix. Viewed with the amino terminus at the bottom, the amide protons all point downward and the carbonyl oxygens all point upward. The side chains project radially around the helix, tilted toward its N-terminus. Given 3.6 residues in each turn of the right-handed helix, the carbonyl

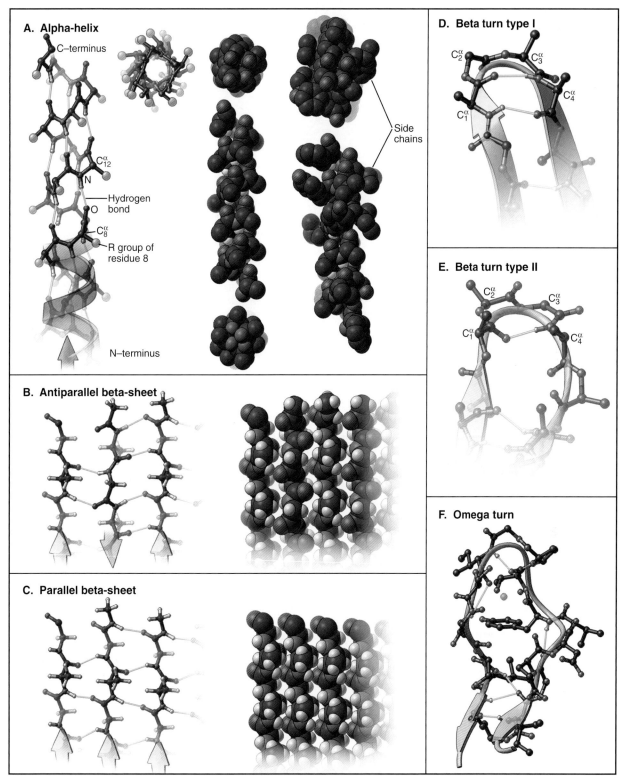

Figure 3-8 MODELS OF SECONDARY STRUCTURES AND TURNS OF PROTEINS. **A,** α-Helix. The stick figure *(left)* shows a right-handed α-helix with the N-terminus at the bottom and side chains R represented by the β-carbon. The backbone hydrogen bonds are indicated by *blue lines.* In this orientation, the carbonyl oxygens point upward, the amide protons point downward, and the R groups trail toward the N-terminus. Space-filling models *(middle)* show a polyalanine α-helix. The end-on views show how the backbone atoms fill the center of the helix. A space-filling model *(right)* of α-helix 5 from bacterial rhodopsin shows the side chains. Some key dimensions are 0.15 nm rise per residue, 0.55 nm per turn, and diameter of about 1.0 nm. (PDB file: 1BAD.) **B,** Stick figure and space-filling models of an antiparallel β-sheet. The *arrows* indicate the polarity of each chain. With the polypeptide extended in this way, the amide protons and carbonyl oxygens lie in the plane of the sheet, where they make hydrogen bonds with the neighboring strands. The amino acid side chains alternate pointing upward and downward from the plane of the sheet. Some key dimensions are 0.35 nm rise per residue in a β-strand and 0.45 nm separation between strands. (PDB file: 1SLK.) **C,** Stick figure and space-filling models of a parallel β-sheet. All strands have the same orientation *(arrows).* The orientations of the hydrogen bonds are somewhat less favorable than that in an antiparallel sheet. **D–E,** Stick figures of two types of reverse turns found between strands of antiparallel β-sheets. (PDB file: 1IMM.) **F,** Stick figure of an omega loop. (PDB file: 1LNC.)

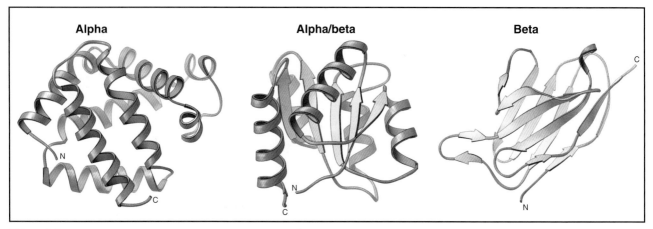

Figure 3-9 RIBBON DIAGRAMS OF PROTEIN BACKBONES SHOWING β-STRANDS AS *FLATTENED ARROWS*, α-HELICES AS COILS, AND OTHER PARTS OF THE POLYPEPTIDE CHAINS AS ROPES. **Left,** The β-subunit of hemoglobin consists entirely of tightly packed α-helices. (PDB file: 1MBA.) **Middle,** CheY is a mixed α/β structure, with a central parallel β-sheet flanked by α-helices. Note the right-handed twist of the sheet (defined by the sheet turning away from the viewer at the upper right) and right-handed pattern of helices (defined by the helices angled toward the upper right corner of the sheet) looping across the β-strands. (Compare the cross section in Figure 3-7). (PDB file: 2CHF.) **Right,** The immunoglobulin V_L domain consists of a sandwich of two antiparallel β-sheets. (PDB file: 2IMM.)

oxygen of residue 1 is positioned perfectly to form a linear hydrogen bond with the amide proton of residue 5. This *n* to *n + 4* pattern of hydrogen bonds repeats along the whole α-helix.

The orientation of backbone hydrogen bonds in α-helices has two important consequences. First, a helix has an electrical dipole moment, negative at the C-terminus. Second, the ends of helices are less stable than the middle, as four potential hydrogen bonds are not completed by backbone interactions at each end. These unmet backbone hydrogen bonds can be completed by interaction with appropriate donors or acceptors on the side chains of the terminal residues. Interactions with serine and asparagine are favored as "caps" at the N-termini of helices because their side chains can complete the hydrogen bonds of the backbone amide nitrogens. Lysine, histidine, and glutamine are favored hydrogen bonding caps for the C-termini of helices.

All amino acids are found within naturally occurring α-helices. Proline is often found at the beginning of helices and glycine at the end, because they are favored in bends. Both are underrepresented within helices. When present, proline produces bends. Glycine is more common in transmembrane helices, where it contributes to helix-helix packing.

A second strategy used to stabilize the backbone structure of polypeptides is hydrogen bonding of β-strands laterally to form β-**sheets** (Figs. 3-8 and 3-9). In individual β-strands, the peptide chain is extended in a configuration close to *all-trans* with side chains alternating top and bottom and amide protons and carbonyl oxygens alternating right and left. β-Strands can form a complete set of hydrogen bonds, with neighboring strands running in the same or opposite directions in any combination. However, the orientation of hydrogen bond donors and acceptors is more favorable in a β-sheet with antiparallel strands than in sheets with parallel strands. Largely parallel β-sheets are usually extensive and completely buried in proteins. β-Sheets have a natural right-handed twist in the direction along the strands. Antiparallel β-sheets are stable even if the strands are short and extensively distorted by twisting. Antiparallel sheets can wrap around completely to form a β-**barrel** with as few as five strands, but the natural twist of the strands and the need to fill the core of the barrel with hydrophobic residues favors barrels with eight strands.

Up to 25% of the residues in globular proteins are present in bends at the surface (Fig. 3-8D–F). Residues constituting bends are generally hydrophilic. The presence of glycine or proline in a turn allows the backbone to deviate from the usual geometry in tight turns, but the composition of bends is highly variable and not a strong determinant of folding or stability. Turns between linear elements of secondary structure are called **reverse turns,** as they reverse the direction of the polypeptide. Those between β-strands have a few characteristic conformations and are called β-bends.

Many parts of polypeptide chains in proteins do not have a regular structure. At one extreme, small segments of polypeptide, frequently at the N- or C-terminus, are truly disordered in the sense that they are mobile. Many other irregular segments of polypeptide are tightly packed into the protein structure. **Omega loops** are compact structures consisting of 6 to 16 residues, generally on the protein surface, that connect adjacent elements of secondary structure (Fig. 3-8F).

They lack regular structure but typically have the side chains packed in the middle of the loop. Some are mobile, but many are rigid. Omega loops form the antigen-binding sites of antibodies. In other proteins, they bind metal ions or participate in the active sites of enzymes.

Packing of Secondary Structure in Proteins

Elements of secondary structure can pack together in almost any way (Fig. 3-9), but a few themes are favored enough to be found in many proteins. For example, two β-sheets tend to pack face to face at an angle of about 40 degrees with nonpolar residues packed tightly, knobs into holes, in between. α-Helices tend to pack at an angle of about 30 degrees across β-sheets, always in a right-handed arrangement. Adjacent α-helices tend to pack together at an angle of either +20 degrees or −50 degrees, owing to packing of side chains from one helix into grooves between side chains on the other helix.

Coiled-coils are a common example of regular superstructure (Fig. 3-10). Two α-helices pair to form a fibrous structure that is widely used to create stable polypeptide dimers in transcription factors (see Fig. 15-18) and structural proteins (see Fig. 39-4). Typically, two identical α-helices wrap around each other in register in a left-handed super helix that is stabilized by hydrophobic interactions of leucines and valines at the interface of the two helices. Intermolecular ionic bonds between the side chains of the two polypeptides also stabilize coiled-coils. Given 3.6 residues per turn, the sequence of a coiled-coil has hydrophobic residues regularly spaced at positions 1 and 4 of a **"heptad repeat."** This pattern allows one to predict the tendency of a polypeptide to form coiled-coils from its amino acid sequence.

β-Sheets can also form extended structures. One called a **β-helix** consists of a continuous polypeptide strand folded into a series of short β-sheets that form a three-sided helix. Fig. 24-4 shows end-on and side views of two β-helices of a growth factor receptor.

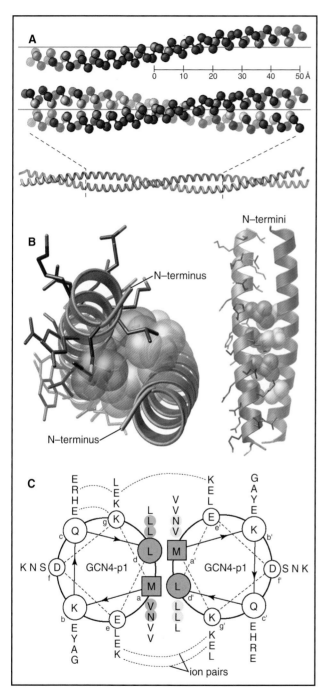

Figure 3-10 COILED-COILS. A, Comparison of a single α-helix, represented by spheres centered on the α-carbons, and a two-stranded, left-handed coiled-coil. Two identical α-helices make continuous contact along their lengths by the interaction of the first and fourth residue in every two turns (seven residues) of the helix. (PDB file: 2TMA.) **B,** Atomic structure of the GCN4 coiled-coil, viewed end-on. The coiled-coil holds together two identical peptides of this transcription factor dimer (see Fig. 15-17 for information on its function). Hydrophobic side chains fit together like knobs into holes along the interface between the two helices. (PDB file: GCN4.) **C,** Helical wheel representation of the GCN4 coiled-coil. Following the *arrows* around the backbone of the polypeptides, one can read the sequences from the single-letter code, starting with the boxed residues and proceeding to the most distal residue. Note that hydrophobic residues in the first (*a*) and fourth (*d*) positions of each two turns of the helices make hydrophobic contacts that hold the two chains together. Electrostatic interactions (*dashed lines*) between side chains at positions *e* and *g* stabilize the interaction. Other coiled-coils consist of two different polypeptides (see Fig. 15-18), and some are antiparallel (see Fig. 13-19). (C, Redrawn from O'Shea E, Klemm JD, Kim PS, Alber T: X-ray structure of the GCN4 leucine zipper, a two-stranded, parallel coiled-coil. Science 254:539–544, 1991.)

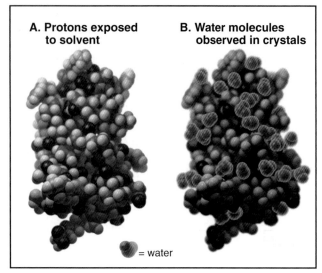

Figure 3-11 WATER ASSOCIATED WITH THE SURFACE OF A PROTEIN. **A,** Protein protons exposed to solvent *(white)* on the surface of a small protein, bovine pancreatic trypsin inhibitor. **B,** Water molecules observed on the surface of the protein in crystal structures. (PDB file: 5BTI.)

Interaction of Proteins with Solvent

The surface of proteins is almost entirely covered with protons (Fig. 3-11). Some protons are potential hydrogen bond donors, but many are inert, being bonded to backbone or side chain aliphatic carbons. Although most of the charged side chains are exposed on the surface, so are many nonpolar side chains. Many water molecules are ordered on the surface of proteins by virtue of hydrogen bonds to polar groups. These water molecules appear in electron density maps of crystalline proteins but exchange rapidly, on a picosecond (10^{-12} second) time scale. Waters that are in contact with nonpolar atoms maximize hydrogen bonding with each other, forming a dynamic layer of water with reduced translational diffusion compared with bulk water. This lowers the entropy of the water by increasing its order and provides a thermodynamic impetus to protein folding pathways that minimize the number of hydrophobic atoms displayed on the surface (see Fig. 4-5).

Protein Dynamics

Pictures of proteins tend to give the false impression that they are rigid and static. On the contrary, even when packed in crystals, the atoms of proteins vibrate around their mean positions on a picosecond time scale with amplitudes up to 0.2 nm and velocities of 200 m per second. This motion is an inevitable consequence of the kinetic energy of each atom, about 2.5 kJ mol^{-1} at 25°C. This allows the protein as a whole to explore a variety of subtly different conformations on a fast time

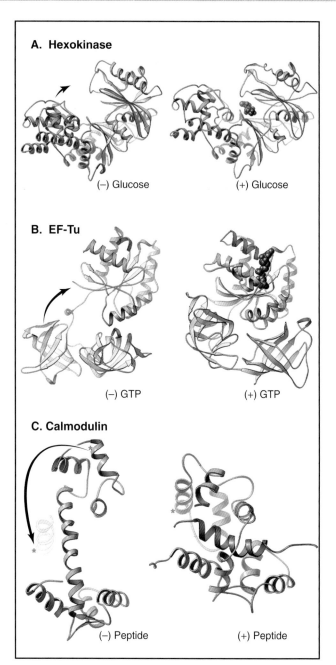

Figure 3-12 CONFORMATIONAL CHANGES OF PROTEINS. **A,** The glycolytic enzyme hexokinase. The two domains of the protein hinge together to surround the substrate, glucose. (PDB files: 2YHX and 1HKG.) **B,** EF-Tu, a cofactor in protein synthesis (see Fig. 17-10), folds more compactly when it binds guanosine triphosphate. (PDB files: 1EFU and 1EFT.) **C,** Calmodulin (see Chapter 26) binds Ca^{2+} and wraps itself around an α-helix *(red)* in target proteins. Note the large change in position of the helix marked with an *asterisk*. (PDB files: CLN and 2BBM.)

scale. Binding to a ligand or a change in conditions may favor one of these alternative conformations.

In addition to relatively small, local variations in structure, many proteins undergo large conformational changes (Fig. 3-12). These changes in structure often reflect a change of activity or physical properties. **Con-**

formational changes play roles in many biological processes ranging from opening and closing ion channels (see Fig. 10-5) to cell motility (see Fig. 36-5). Many conformational changes have been observed indirectly by spectroscopy or hydrodynamic methods or directly by crystallography or NMR. For example, when glucose binds the enzyme hexokinase, the two halves of the protein clamp around this substrate by rotating 12 degrees about a hinge consisting of two polypeptides. Guanosine triphosphate (GTP) binding to elongation factor EF-Tu causes a domain to rotate 90 degrees about two glycine residues (see Fig. 25-7)! Similarly, phosphorylation of glycogen phosphorylase causes

a local rearrangement of the N-terminus that transmits a structural change over a distance of more than 2 nm to the active site (see Fig. 27-3). The Ca^{2+} binding regulatory protein calmodulin undergoes a dramatic conformational change (Fig. 3-12) when wrapping tightly around a helical peptide of a target protein (also see Chapter 26).

Modular Domains in Proteins

Most polypeptides consist of linear arrays of multiple independently folded, globular regions, or **domains**, connected in a modular fashion (Fig. 3-13). Most domains

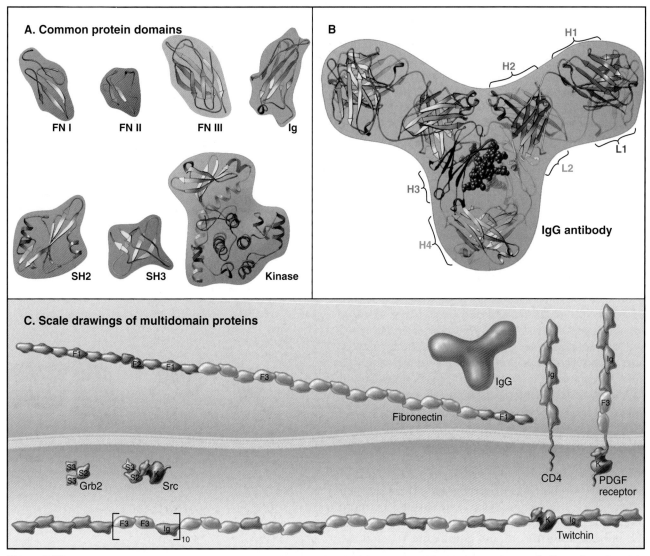

Figure 3-13 MODULAR PROTEINS CONSTRUCTED FROM EVOLUTIONARILY HOMOLOGOUS, INDEPENDENTLY FOLDED DOMAINS. **A,** Examples of protein domains used in many proteins: fibronectin 1 (FN I), fibronectin 2 (FN II), fibronectin 3 (FN III), immunoglobulin (Ig), Src homology 2 (SH2), Src homology 3 (SH3), kinase. (PDB files: FN7, 1PDC, 1FNA, 1IG2, 1HCS, 1PRM, and 1CTP.) **B,** Immunoglobulin G (IgG), a protein composed of 12 Ig domains on four polypeptide chains. Two identical heavy chains (H) consist of four Ig domains, and two identical light chains (L) consist of two Ig domains. The sequences of these six Ig domains differ, but all of the domains are folded similarly. The two antigen-binding sites are located at the ends of the two arms of the Y-shaped molecule composed of highly variable loops contributed by domains H1 and L1. (PDB file: 1IG2.) **C,** Examples of proteins constructed from the domains shown in **A:** fibronectin (see Fig. 29-15), CD4 (see Figs. 27-8 and 28-9), PDGF-receptor (see Fig. 24-4), Grb2 (see Fig. 27-6), Src (see Fig. 25-3 and Box 27-1), and twitchin (see Chapter 39). Each of the 31 FN3 domains in twitchin has a different sequence. F1 is FI, F2 is FII, and F3 is FIII.

consist of 40 to 100 residues, but kinase domains and motor domains (see Figs. 36-3 and 36-9) are much larger. Each of more than 1000 recognized families of domains is thought to have evolved from a different common ancestor. In this sense, the members of a family are said to be **homologous.** Through the processes of **gene duplication, transposition,** and **divergent evolution,** the most widely used domains (e.g., the immunoglobulin domain) have become incorporated into hundreds of different proteins, where they serve unique functions. Homologous domains in different proteins have similar folds but may differ significantly in amino acid sequences. Nevertheless, most related domains can be recognized from characteristic *patterns* of amino acids along their sequences. For example, cysteine residues of immunoglobulin G (Ig) domains are spaced in a pattern required to make intramolecular disulfide bonds (Fig. 3-3).

Rarely, protein domains with related structures may have arisen independently and converged during evolution toward a particularly favorable conformation. This is the hypothesis to explain the similar folds of immunoglobulin and fibronectin-III domains, which have unrelated amino acid sequences.

Nucleic Acids

Nucleic acids, polymers of a few simple building blocks called **nucleotides,** store and transfer all genetic information. This is not the limit of their functions. RNA enzymes, **ribozymes,** catalyze some biochemical reactions. Other RNAs are receptors **(riboswitches)** or contribute to the structures and enzyme activities of major cellular components, such as ribosomes (see Fig. 17-7) and spliceosomes (see Fig. 16-5). In addition, nucleotides themselves transfer chemical energy between cellular systems and information in signal transduction pathways. Later chapters elaborate on each of these topics.

Building Blocks of Nucleic Acids

Nucleotides consist of three parts: (1) a **base** built of one or two cyclic rings of carbon and a few nitrogen atoms, (2) a five-carbon sugar, and (3) one or more phosphate groups (Fig. 3-14). **DNA** uses four main bases: the purines **adenine** (A) and **guanosine** (G) and the pyrimidines **cytosine** (C) and **thymine** (T). In **RNA, uracil** (U) is found in place of thymine. Some RNA bases are chemically modified after synthesis of the polymer. The sugar of RNA is **ribose,** which has the aldehyde oxygen of carbon 4 cyclized to carbon 1. The DNA sugar is deoxyribose, which is similar to ribose but lacks the hydroxyl on carbon 2. In both RNA and DNA, carbon 1 of the sugar is conjugated with nitrogen

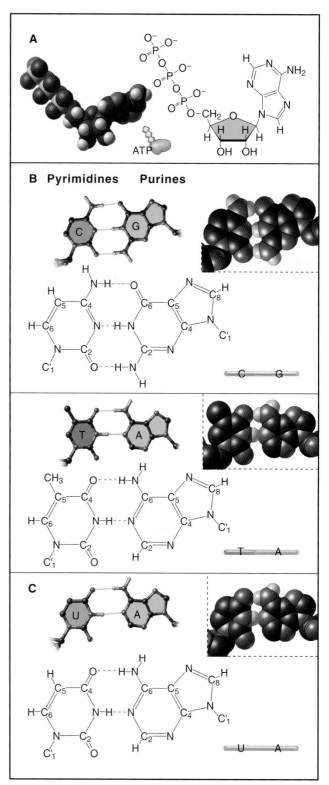

Figure 3-14   ATP AND NUCLEOTIDE BASES. **A,** Stick figure and space-filling model of ATP. **B,** Four bases used in DNA. Stick figures show the hydrogen bonds used to form base pairs between thymine (T) and adenine (A) and between cytosine (C) and guanine (G). **C,** Uracil replaces thymine in RNA. C'_1 refers to carbon 1 of ribose and deoxyribose.

1 of a pyrimidine base or with nitrogen 9 of a purine base. The hydroxyl of sugar carbon 5 can be esterified to a chain of one or more phosphates, forming **nucleotides** such as adenosine monophosphate (**AMP**), adenosine diphosphate (**ADP**), and ATP.

Covalent Structure of Nucleic Acids

DNA and RNA are polymers of nucleotides joined by **phosphodiester bonds** (Fig. 3-15). The backbone links a chain of five atoms (two oxygens and three carbons) from one phosphorous to the next—a total of six backbone atoms per nucleotide. Unlike the backbone of proteins, in which the planar peptide bond greatly limits rotation, all six bonds along a polynucleotide backbone have some freedom to rotate, even that in the sugar ring. This feature gives nucleic acids much greater conformational flexibility than polypeptides, which have only two variable torsional angles per residue. The backbone phosphate group has a single negative charge at neutral pH. The N—C bond linking the base to the sugar is also free to rotate on a picosecond time scale, but rotation away from the backbone is strongly favored. The bases have a strong tendency to stack upon each other, owing to favorable van der Waals interactions (see Chapter 4) between these planar rings.

Each type of nucleic acid has a unique sequence of nucleotides. Simple laboratory procedures employing the enzymatic synthesis of DNA allow the sequence to be determined rapidly (Fig. 3-16). All DNA and RNA

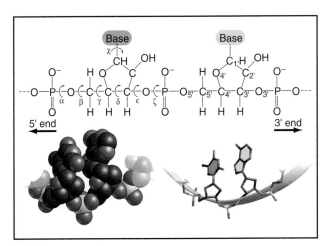

Figure 3-15 ROTATIONAL FREEDOM OF THE BACKBONE OF A POLYNUCLEO-TIDE, RNA IN THIS CASE. The stick figure of two residues shows that all six of the backbone bonds are rotatable, even the $C_{4'}$—C' bond that is constrained by the ribose ring. This gives polynucleotides more conformational freedom than polypeptides. Note the phosphodiester bonds between the residues and the definition of the 3′ and 5′ ends. Space-filling and stick figures at the bottom show a uridine (U) and adenine (A) from part of Figure 3-17. (Redrawn from Jaeger JA, SantaLucia J, Tinoco I: Determination of RNA structure and thermodynamics. Annu Rev Biochem 62:255–287, 1993.)

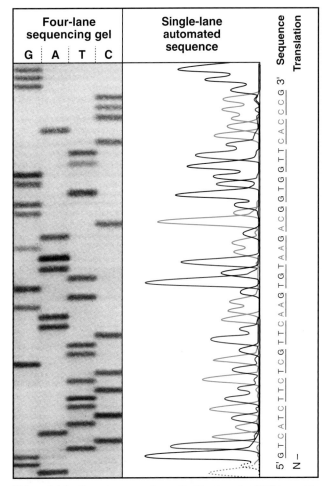

Figure 3-16   The sequence of a purified fragment of DNA is rapidly determined by in vitro synthesis (see Fig. 42-1) using the four deoxynucleoside triphosphates plus a small fraction of one dideoxynucleoside triphosphate. The random incorporation of the dideoxy residue terminates a few of the growing DNA molecules every time that base appears in the sequence. The reaction is run separately with each dideoxynucleotide, and fragments are separated according to size by gel electrophoresis (see Fig. 6-5), with the shortest fragments at the bottom. A radioactive label makes the fragments visible when exposed to an X-ray film. The sequence is read from the bottom as indicated. An automated method uses four different fluorescent dideoxynucleotides to mark the end of the fragments and electronic detectors to read the sequence. (Based on original data from W-L. Lee, Salk Institute for Biological Studies, San Diego, California.)

molecules are synthesized biologically in the same direction (see Figs. 15-11 and 42-1) by adding a nucleoside triphosphate to the 3′ sugar hydroxyl of the growing strand. Cleavage of the two terminal phosphates from the new subunit provides energy for extension of the polymer in the 5′ to 3′ direction. Newly synthesized DNA and RNA molecules have a phosphate at the 5′ end and a 3′ hydroxyl at the other end. In certain types of RNA (e.g., messenger RNA [mRNA]), the 5′ nucleotide is subsequently modified by the addition of a specialized cap structure (see Figs. 16-2 and 17-2).

Secondary Structure of DNA

A few viruses have chromosomes consisting of single-stranded DNA molecules, but most DNA molecules are paired with a complementary strand to form a right-handed **double helix,** as originally proposed by Watson and Crick (Fig. 3-17). Key features of the double helix are two strands running in opposite directions with the sugar-phosphate backbone on the outside and pairs of bases hydrogen-bonded to each other on the inside (Fig. 3-14). Pairs of bases are stacked 0.34 nm apart, nearly perpendicular to the long axis of the polymer. This regular structure is referred to as **B-form DNA,** but real

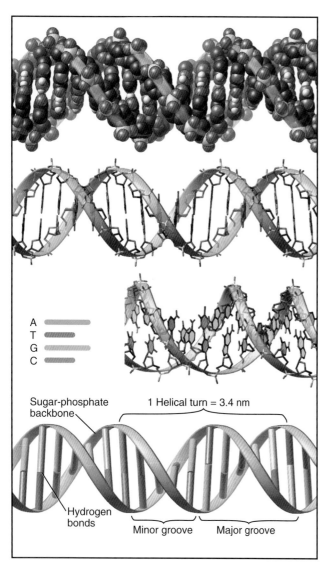

A $\rule{1.2cm}{0.4ex}$
T $\rule{1.2cm}{0.4ex}$
G $\rule{1.2cm}{0.4ex}$
C $\rule{1.2cm}{0.4ex}$

Sugar-phosphate backbone

1 Helical turn = 3.4 nm

Hydrogen bonds

Minor groove   Major groove

Figure 3-17 **MODELS OF B-FORM DNA.** The molecule consists of two complementary antiparallel strands arranged in a right-handed double helix with the backbone (Fig. 3-15) on the outside and stacked pairs of hydrogen-bonded bases (see Fig. 3-14) on the inside. **Top,** Space-filling model. **Middle,** Stick figures, with the lower figure rotated slightly to reveal the faces of the bases. **Bottom,** Ribbon representation. (Idealized 24–base pair model built by Robert Tan, University of Alabama, Birmingham.)

DNA is not completely regular. On average, in solution, B-form DNA has 10.5 base pairs per turn and a diameter of 1.9 nm. Hydrogen bonds between adenine and thymine and between guanine and cytosine span nearly the same distance between the backbones, so the helix has a regular structure that, to a first approximation, is independent of the sequence of bases. One exception is a run of As that tends to bend adjoining parts of the helix. Because the bonds between the bases and the sugars are asymmetrical, the DNA helix is asymmetrical: The major groove on one side of the helix is broader than the other, minor groove. Most cellular DNA is approximately in the B-form conformation, but proteins that regulate gene expression can distort the DNA significantly (see Fig. 15-7).

Under some laboratory conditions, DNA forms stable helical structures that differ from classic B-form DNA. All these variants have the phosphate-sugar backbone on the outside, and most have the usual complementary base pairs on the inside. A-form DNA has 11 base pairs per turn and an average diameter of 2.3 nm. DNA-RNA hybrids and double-stranded RNA also have A-form structure. Z-DNA is the most extreme variant, as it is a left-handed helix with 12 base pairs per turn. Circumstantial evidence supporting the existence of Z-DNA in cells remains controversial.

DNA molecules are either linear or circular. Human chromosomes are single linear DNA molecules (see Fig. 12-1). Many, but not all, viral and bacterial chromosomes are circular. Eukaryotic mitochondria and chloroplasts also have circular DNA molecules.

When circular DNAs or linear DNAs with both ends anchored (as in chromosomes; see Chapter 13) are twisted about their long axis, the strain is relieved by the development of long-range bends and twists called **supercoils** or **superhelices** (Fig. 3-18). Supercoiling can be either positive or negative depending on whether the DNA helix is wound more tightly or somewhat unwound. Supercoiling is biologically important, as it can influence the expression of genes. Under some circumstances, supercoiling favors unwinding of the double helix. This can promote access of proteins involved in the regulation of transcription from DNA (see Chapter 15).

The degree of supercoiling is regulated locally by enzymes called **topoisomerases.** Type I topoisomerases nick one strand of the DNA and cause the molecule to unwind by rotation about a backbone bond. Type II topoisomerases cut both strands of the DNA and use an ATP-driven conformational change (called *gating*) to pass a DNA strand through the cut prior to rejoining the ends of the DNA. To avoid free DNA ends during this reaction, cleaved DNA ends are linked covalently to tyrosine residues of the enzyme. This also conserves chemical bond energy, so ATP is not required for religation of the DNA at the end of the reaction.

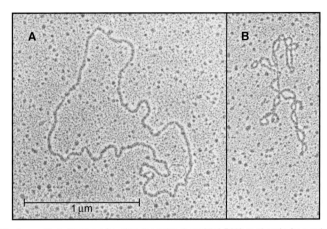

Figure 3-18 DNA SUPERCOILING. Electron micrographs of a circular mitochondrial DNA molecule in a relaxed configuration **(A)** and a super-coiled configuration **(B).** (Reproduced, with permission, from David Clayton, Stanford University, Stanford, California; originally in Stryer L: Biochemistry, 4th ed. New York, WH Freeman and Co, 1995.)

Secondary and Tertiary Structure of RNAs

RNAs range in size from micro-RNAs of 20 nucleotides (see Fig. 16-12) to messenger RNAs with more than 80,000 nucleotides. Because each nucleotide has about three times the mass of an amino acid, RNAs with a modest number of nucleotides are bigger than most proteins (see Fig. 1-4). The 16S RNA of the small ribosomal subunit of bacteria consists of 1542 nucleotides with a mass of about 460 kD, much larger than any of the 21 proteins with which it interacts (see Fig. 17-7).

Except for the RNA genomes of a few viruses, RNAs generally do not have a complementary strand to pair with each base. Instead they form specific structures by optimizing *intramolecular* base pairing (Figs. 3-19 and 3-20). Comparison of homologous RNA sequences provides much of what is known about this intramolecular base pairing. The approach is to identify pairs of nucleotides that vary together across the phylogenetic tree. For example, if an A and a U at discontinuous positions in one RNA are changed together to C and a G in homologous RNAs, it is inferred that they are hydrogen-bonded together. This **covariant method** works remarkably

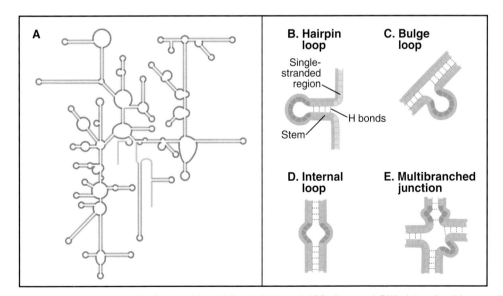

Figure 3-19 RNA SECONDARY STRUCTURES. **A,** Base pairing of *Escherichia coli* 16S ribosomal RNA determined by covariant analysis of nucleotide sequences of many different 16S ribosomal RNAs. The *line* represents the sequence of nucleotides. *Blue* sections are base-paired strands; *pink* sections are bulges and turns; *green* sections are neither base-paired nor turns. **B,** An antiparallel base-paired stem forming a hairpin loop. **C,** A bulge loop. **D,** An internal loop. **E,** A multibranched junction. (A, Redrawn from Huysmans E, DeWachter R: Compilation of small ribosomal subunit RNA sequences. Nucleic Acids Res 14(Suppl):73–118, 1987. B–E, Redrawn from Jaeger JA, SantaLucia J, Tinoco I: Determination of RNA structure and thermodynamics. Annu Rev Biochem 62:255–287, 1993.)

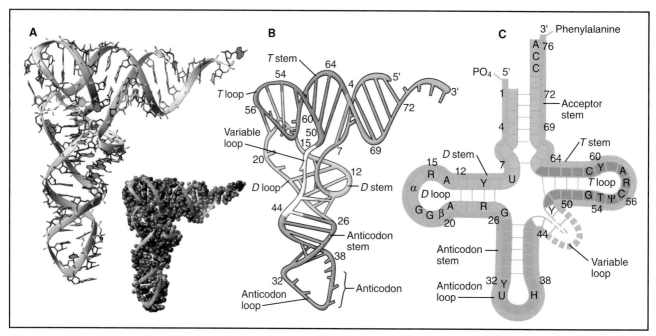

Figure 3-20   Atomic structure of phenylalanine transfer RNA (phe-tRNA) determined by X-ray crystallography. **A,** An *orange* ribbon traces the RNA backbone through a stick figure *(left)* and space filling model *(right)*. (PDB file: 6TNA.) **B,** Skeleton drawing. **C,** Two dimensional base-pairing scheme. Note that the base-paired segments are much less regular than is B-form DNA. (PDB file: 6TNA.) (B, Redrawn from an original by Alex Rich, MIT, Cambridge, Massachusetts.)

well, because hundreds to thousands of homologous sequences for the major classes of RNA are available from comparative genomics. Conclusions about base pairing from covariant analysis have been confirmed by experimental mutagenesis of RNAs and direct structure determination.

The simplest RNA secondary structure is an antiparallel double helix stabilized by hydrogen bonding of complementary bases (Figs. 3-20 and 3-21). Similarly to DNA, G pairs with C and U pairs with A. Unlike the case in DNA, G also frequently pairs with U in RNA. Helical base pairing occurs between both contiguous and dis-

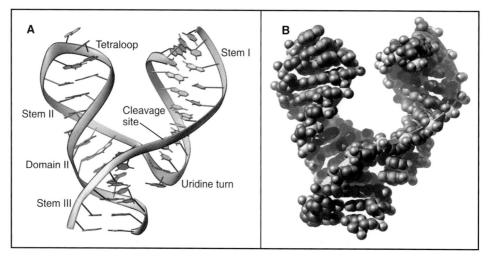

Figure 3-21   Hammerhead ribozyme, a self-cleaving RNA sequence found in plant virus RNAs. **A,** Ribbon diagram. **B,** Space-filling model. The structure consists of an RNA strand of 34 nucleotides complexed to a DNA strand of 13 nucleotides (in vivo, this is a 13-nucleotide stretch of RNA, which would be cleaved by the ribozyme). The RNA forms a central stem-loop structure (stem II) and base pairs with the substrate DNA to form stems I and III. Interactions of the substrate strand with the sharp uridine turn distort the backbone and promote its cleavage. (PDB file: 1HMH.) (A, Redrawn from Pley HW, Flaherty KM, McKay DB: Three-dimensional structure of a hammerhead ribozyme. Nature 372:68–74, 1994.)

contiguous sequences. When contiguous sequences form a helix, the strand is often reversed by a tight turn, forming an antiparallel **stem-loop** structure. These hairpin turns frequently consist of just four bases. A few sequences are highly favored for turns, owing to their compact, stable structures. Bulges due to extra bases or noncomplementary bases frequently interrupt base-paired helices of RNA.

Crystal structures of RNAs such as **tRNAs** (Fig. 3-20) and a hammerhead **ribozyme** (Fig. 3-21) established that RNAs have novel, specific, three-dimensional structures. Crystal structures of ribosomes (see Fig. 17-7) showed that larger RNAs fold into specific structures

using similar principles. Crystallization of RNAs is challenging, and NMR provides much less information on RNA than on proteins of the same size, so much is yet to be learned about RNA structures.

As in proteins, many residues in RNAs are in conventional secondary structures, especially stems consisting of base-paired double helices; however, RNA backbones make sharp turns that allow unconventional hydrogen bonds between bases, ribose hydroxyls, and backbone phosphates. Generally, the phosphodiester backbone is on the surface with most of the hydrophobic bases stacked internally. Some bases are hydrogen-bonded together in triplets (Fig. 3-22) rather than in pairs. Four

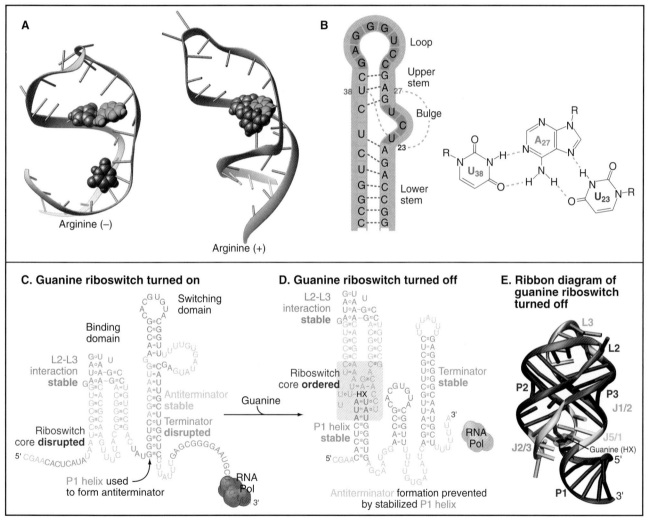

Figure 3-22 RNA CONFORMATIONAL CHANGES. A–B, Molecular models of NMR structures of TAR, a stem-loop regulator of HIV mRNA. Binding of arginine (or a protein called TAT) causes a major conformational change: Two bases twist out of the helix into the solvent (top). U23 forms a base triplet with U38 and A27 (space-filling model), and the stem straightens. This conformational change promotes transcription of the rest of the mRNA. (A, PDB files: 1ANR and 1AKX.) C–E, **Guanine-binding riboswitch from Bacillus subtilis. C,** Diagram of the mRNA showing the location of the riboswitch just upstream of the genes for the enzymes required to synthesize guanine. At low guanine concentrations, the RNA is folded in a way that allows transcription of the genes. (PDB file: 1U8D.) **D,** High guanine concentrations (the analog hypoxantine, HX, is shown here) bind to the riboswitch, causing refolding into a terminator stem loop that prevents transcription of the mRNA. **E,** Ribbon drawing of the crystal structure with bound hypoxanthine. (C, Reference: Batey RT, Gilbert SD, Montange RK: Structure of a natural guanine-responsive riboswitch complexed with the metabolite hypoxanthine. Nature 432:411–415, 2004. D, Reference: Mandal M, Boese B, Barrick JE, et al: Riboswitches control fundamental biochemical pathways in B. subtillis and other bacteria. Cell 113:577–586, 2003.)

or five Mg^{2+} ions stabilize regions of tRNA with high densities of negative charge.

Like proteins, RNAs can change conformation. The TAR RNA is a stem-loop structure with a bulge formed by three unpaired nucleotides (Fig. 3-22). TAR is located at the 5′ end of all RNA transcripts of the human immunodeficiency virus (HIV) that causes AIDS. Binding of a regulatory protein called TAT changes the conformation of TAR and promotes elongation of the RNA. Binding arginine also changes the conformation of TAR.

Like proteins, RNAs can bind ligands. About 2% of the genes in the bacterium *Bacillus subtillis* are regulated by RNA sequences located in the mRNAs. For example, mRNAs for enzymes used to synthesize purines such as guanine have a guanine-sensitive riboswitch that controls translation (Fig. 3-22C–D). At low guanine levels, the conformation allows transcription. High concentrations of guanine bind the RNA, causing a massive reorganization that blocks transcription. This negative feedback loop optimizes the cellular concentration of guanine.

Carbohydrates

Carbohydrates are a large family of biologically essential molecules made up of one or more sugar molecules. Sugar polymers differ from proteins and nucleic acids by having branches. Compared with proteins, which are generally compact, hydrophilic sugar polymers tend to spread out in aqueous solutions to maximize hydrogen bonds with water. Carbohydrates may occupy 5 to 10 times the volume of a protein of the same mass. The terms **glycoconjugate** and **complex carbohydrate** are currently preferred for sugar polymers rather than polysaccharide.

Carbohydrates serve four main functions:

1. Covalent bonds of sugar molecules are a primary source of energy for cells.

2. The most abundant structural components on earth are sugar polymers: Cellulose forms cell walls of plants; chitin forms exoskeletons of insects; and glycosaminoglycans are space-filling molecules in connective tissues of animals.

3. Sugars form part of the backbone of nucleic acids, and nucleotides participate in many metabolic reactions (see earlier discussion).

4. Single sugars and groupings of sugars form side chains on lipids (see Fig. 7-3) and proteins (see Figs. 21-26 and 29-13). These modifications provide molecular diversity beyond that inherent in proteins and lipids themselves, changing their physical properties and vastly expanding the potential of these glycoproteins and glycolipids to interact with other cellular components in specific receptor-ligand interactions (see Fig. 30-12). Conversely, other glycoconjugates block inappropriate cellular interactions.

A modest number of simple sugars (Fig. 3-23) form the vast array of different complex carbohydrates found in nature. These sugars consist of three to seven carbons with one aldehyde or ketone group and multiple hydroxyl groups. In water, the common five-carbon (**pentose**) and six-carbon (**hexose**) sugars cyclize by reaction of the aldehyde or ketone group with one of the hydroxyl carbons. This forms a compact structure that is used in all the glycoconjugates considered in this book. Given several asymmetrical carbons in each sugar, a great many **stereochemical isomers** exist. For example, the hydroxyl on carbon 1 can either be above (β-isomer) or below (α-isomer) the plane of the ring. Proteins (enzymes, lectins, and receptors) that interact with sugars distinguish these stereoisomers.

Sugars are coupled to other molecules by highly specific enzymes, using a modest repertoire of intermolecular bonds (Fig. 3-24). The common *O*-glycosidic (carbon-oxygen-carbon) bond is formed by removal of water from two hydroxyls—the hydroxyl of the carbon bonded to the ring oxygen of a sugar and a hydroxyl oxygen of another sugar or the amino acids serine and threonine. A similar reaction couples a sugar to an amine, as in the bond between a sugar and a nucleoside base. Sugar phosphates with one or more phosphates esterified to a sugar hydroxyl are components of nucleotides as well as of many intermediates in metabolic pathways.

Glycoconjugates—polymers of one or more types of sugar molecules—are present in massive amounts in nature and are used as both energy stores and structural components (Fig. 3-25). Cellulose (unbranched β-1,4 polyglucose), which forms the cell walls of plants, and chitin (unbranched β-1,4 poly *N*-acetylglucosamine), which forms the exoskeletons of many invertebrates, are the first and second most abundant biological polymers found on the earth. In animals, giant complex carbohydrates are essential components of the extracellular matrix of cartilage and other connective tissues (see Figs. 29-13 and 34-3). Glycogen, a branched α-1,4 polymer of glucose, is the major energy store in animal cells. Starch-polymers of glucose with or without a modest level of branching-performs the same function for plants.

Glycoconjugates differ from proteins and nucleic acids in that they have a broader range of conformations owing to the flexible glycosidic linkages between the sugar subunits. Although sugar polymers may be stabilized by extensive intramolecular hydrogen bonds and some glycosidic linkages are relatively rigid, NMR studies

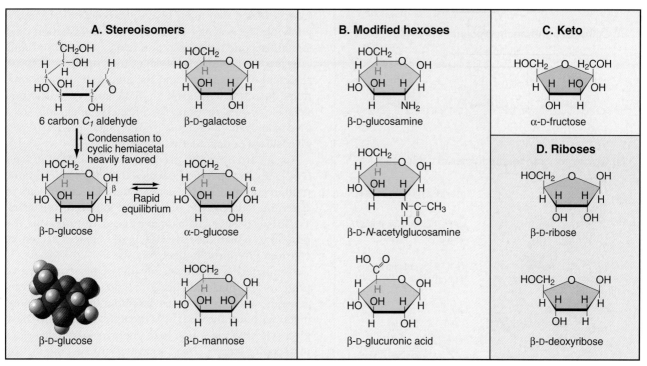

Figure 3-23   A–C, Simple sugar molecules. Stick figures and space-filling model of D-glucose showing the highly favored condensation of the carbon 5 hydroxyl with carbon 1 to form a hemiacetal. The resulting hydroxyl group on carbon 1 is in a rapid equilibrium between the α (down) or β (up) configurations. The space-filling model of β-D-glucose illustrates the stereochemistry of the ring; the stick figures are drawn as unrealistic planar rings to simplify comparisons. Stick figures show three stereoisomers of the 6-carbon glucose **(A)**, three modifications of glucose **(B)**, a 6-carbon keto sugar condensed into a five-membered ring **(C)**, and two 5-carbon riboses **(D)**.

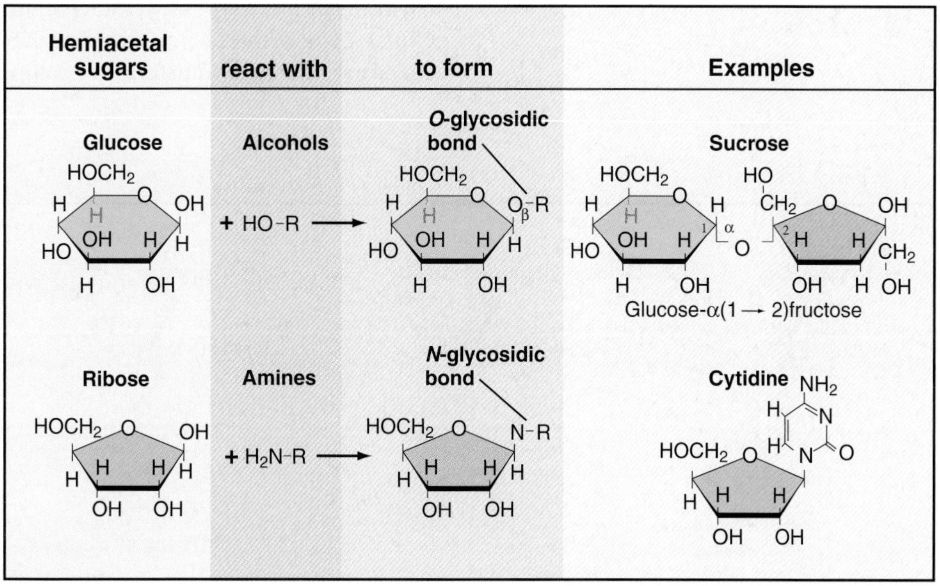

Figure 3-24   GLYCOSIDIC BONDS. Stick figures show the formation of *O*- and *N*-glycosidic bonds and a common example of each: the disaccharide sucrose and the nucleoside cytidine. Enzymes catalyze the formation of glycosidic bonds in cells. The chemical name of sucrose [glucose-α(1→2)fructose] illustrates the convention for naming the bonds of glycoconjugates.

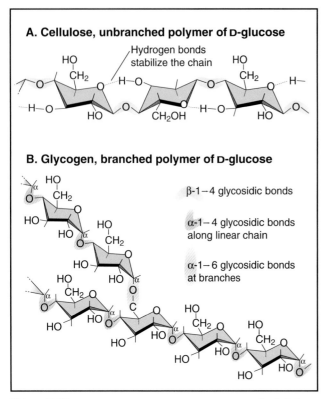

A. Cellulose, unbranched polymer of D-glucose

B. Glycogen, branched polymer of D-glucose

β-1–4 glycosidic bonds

α-1–4 glycosidic bonds along linear chain

α-1–6 glycosidic bonds at branches

Figure 3-25 EXAMPLES OF SIMPLE GLYCOCONJUGATES. **A,** Cellulose, an unbranched homopolymer of glucose used to construct plant cell walls. **B,** Glycogen, a branched homopolymer of glucose used by animal cells to store sugar. Many glycoconjugates consist of several different types of sugar subunits (see Figs. 21-26 and 29-13).

have revealed that many glycosidic bonds rotate freely, allowing the polymer to change its conformation on a submillisecond time scale. This dynamic behavior limits efforts to determine glycoconjugate structures. They are reluctant to crystallize, and the multitude of conformations does not lend itself to NMR analysis. Structural details are best revealed by X-ray crystallography of a glycoconjugate bound to a protein, such as a lectin or a glycosidase (a degradative enzyme).

Sugars are linked to proteins in three different ways (Fig. 3-26) by specific enzymes that recognize unique protein conformations. Glycoprotein side chains vary in size from one sugar to polymers of hundreds of sugars. These sugar side chains can exceed the mass of the protein to which they are attached. Chapters 21 and 29 consider glycoprotein biosynthesis.

Compared with the nearly invariant sequences of proteins and nucleic acids, glycoconjugates are heterogeneous, because enzymes assemble these sugar polymers without the aid of a genetic template. These glycosyltransferases link high-energy sugar-nucleosides to acceptor sugars. These enzymes are specific for the donor sugar-nucleoside and selective, but not completely specific, for the acceptor sugars. Thus, cells require many different glycosyltransferases to generate the hundreds of types of sugar-sugar bonds found in glycoconjugates. Particular cells consistently produce the same range of specific glycoconjugate structures. This reproducible heterogeneity arises from the repertoire of glycosyltransferases expressed, their localization in specific cellular compartments, and the availability of suitable acceptors. Glycosyltransferases compete with each

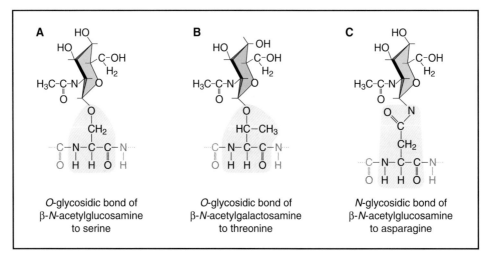

O-glycosidic bond of β-N-acetylglucosamine to serine

O-glycosidic bond of β-N-acetylgalactosamine to threonine

N-glycosidic bond of β-N-acetylglucosamine to asparagine

Figure 3-26 THREE TYPES OF GLYCOSIDIC BONDS LINK GLYCOCONJUGATES TO PROTEINS. **A,** An O-glycosidic bond links N-acetylglucosamine to serine residues of many intracellular proteins. **B,** An O-glycosidic bond links N-acetylgalactosamine to serine or threonine residues of core proteins, initiating long glycoconjugate polymers called glycosaminoglycans on extracellular proteoglycans (see Fig. 29-13). **C,** An N-glycosidic bond links N-acetylglucosamine to asparagine residues of secreted and membrane glycoproteins (see Fig. 21-26). A wide variety of glycoconjugates extend the sugar polymer from the N-acetylglucosamine. These stick figures illustrate the conformations of the sugar rings.

other for acceptors, yielding a variety of products at many steps in the synthesis of glycoconjugates. For example, the probability of encountering a particular glycosyltransferase depends upon the part of the Golgi apparatus (see Fig. 21-14) in which a particular acceptor finds itself.

The Aqueous Phase of Cytoplasm

The aqueous phase of cells contains a wide variety of solutes, including inorganic ions, building blocks of major organic constituents, intermediates in metabolic pathways, carbohydrate and lipid energy stores, and high concentrations of proteins and RNA. In addition, eukaryotic cells have a dense network of cytoskeletal fibers (Fig. 3-27). Cells control the concentrations of solutes in each cellular compartment, because many (e.g., pH, Na^+, K^+, Ca^{2+}, and cyclic AMP) have essential regulatory or functional significance in particular compartments.

The high concentration of macromolecules and the network of cytoskeletal polymers make the cytoplasm a very different environment from the dilute salt solutions that are usually employed in biochemical experiments on cellular constituents. The presence of 300 mg/mL of protein and RNA causes the cytoplasm to be crowded. The concentration of bulk water in cytoplasm is less than the 55 M in dilute solutions, but the microscopic viscosity of the aqueous phase in live cells is remarkably close to that of pure water. Crowding lowers the diffusion coefficient of the molecules by a factor of about 3, but it also enhances macromolecular associations by raising the chemical potential of the diffusing molecules through an "excluded volume" effect. Macromolecules take up space in the solvent, so the concentration of each molecule is higher in relation to the available solvent. At cellular concentrations of macromolecules, the chemical potential of a molecule (see Chapter 4) may be one or more orders of magnitude higher than its concentration. (The chemical potential, rather than the concentration, determines the rate of reactions.) Therefore, crowding favors protein-protein, protein–nucleic acid, and other macromolecular assembly reactions that depend on the chemical potential of the reactants. Crowding also changes the rates and equilibria of enzymatic reactions, usually increasing the activity as compared with values in dilute solutions.

ACKNOWLEDGMENTS

Thanks go to Tom Steitz and Andrew Miranker for their suggestions on revisions to this chapter.

SELECTED READINGS

Brandon C, Tooze J: Introduction to Protein Structure. New York, Garland Publishing, 1999, p 350.

Bryant RG: The dynamics of water-protein interactions. Annu Rev Biophys Biomol Struct 25:29-53, 1996.

Chothia C, Hubbard T, Brenner S, et al: Protein folds in the all-β and all-α classes. Annu Rev Biophys Biomol Struct 26:597-627, 1997.

Creighton TE: Proteins: Structure and Molecular Principles, 2nd ed. New York, WH Freeman, 1993, p 507.

Daggett V, Fersht AR: Is there a unifying mechanism for protein folding? Trends Biochem Sci 28:18-25, 2003.

Dobson CM: Protein folding and misfolding. Nature 426:884-890, 2003.

Doherty EA, Doudna JA: Ribozyme structures and mechanisms. Annu Rev Biophys Biomolec Struct 30: 457-475, 2001.

Feizi T, Mulloy B: Carbohydrates and glycoconjugates: Glycomics: The new era of carbohydrate biology. Curr Opin Struct Biol 13:602-604, 2003.

Huff ME, Balch WE, Kelly JW: Pathological and functional amyloid formation orchestrated by the secretory pathway. Curr Opin Struct Biol 13:674-682, 2003.

Johnson ES: Protein modification by SUMO. Annu Rev Biochem 73:355-382, 2004.

Kubelka J, James Hofrichter J, Eaton WA: The protein folding "speed limit." Curr Opin Struct Biol 14:76-88, 2004

Kuhlman B, Baker D: Exploring folding free energy landscapes using computational protein design. Curr Opin Struct Biol 14:89-95, 2004.

Lilley DMJ: The origins of RNA catalysis in ribozymes. Trends Biochem Sci 28:495-501, 2003.

Lupas A: Coiled-coils: New structures and new functions. Trends Biochem Sci 21:375-382, 1996.

Murthy VL, Srinivasan R, Draper DE, Rose GD: A complete conformational map for RNA. J Mol Biol 291:313-327, 1999.

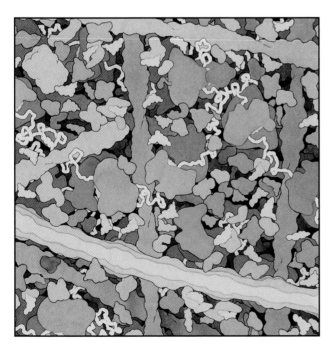

Figure 3-27 **CROWDED CYTOPLASM.** Scale drawing of eukaryotic cell cytoplasm emphasizing the high concentrations of ribosomes *(shades of red)*, proteins *(shades of tan, blue, and green),* and nucleic acids *(gray)* among cytoskeletal polymers. (Original drawing from D. Goodsell, Scripps Research Institute, La Jolla, California.)

Narlikar GJ, Hershlag D: Mechanistic aspects of enzyme catalysis: Lessons from comparisons of RNA and protein enzymes. Annu Rev Biochem 66:19-60, 1997.

Onoa B, Tinoco I: RNA folding and unfolding. Curr Opin Struct Biol 14:374-379, 2004.

Parak FG: Proteins in action: The physics of structural fluctuations and conformational changes. Curr Opin Struct Biol 13:552-557, 2003.

Pickart CM: Mechanisms underlying ubiquitination. Annu Rev Biochem 70:503-533, 2001.

Ponting CP, Russell RR: The natural history of protein domains. Annu Rev Biophys Biomolec Struct 31:45-71, 2002.

Soukup JK, Soukup GA: Riboswitches exert genetic control through metabolite-induced conformational change. Curr Opin Struct Biol 14:344-349, 2004.

Tycko R: Progress towards a molecular-level structural understanding of amyloid fibrils. Curr Opin Struct Biol 14:96-103, 2004.

Vogel C, Bashton M, Kerrison ND, et al: Structure, function and evolution of multi-domain proteins. Curr Opin Struct Biol 14:208-216, 2004.

Wedekind JE, McKay DR: Crystallographic structures of the hammerhead ribozyme: Relationship to ribozyme folding and catalysis. Annu Rev Biophys Biomol Struct 27:475-502, 1998.

CHAPTER 4

Biophysical Principles

The concepts in this chapter form the basis for understanding all the molecular interactions in chemistry and biology. To illustrate some of these concepts with a practical example, the chapter concludes with a section on an exceptionally important family of enzymes that bind and hydrolyze the nucleotide GTP. This example provides the background knowledge to understand how GTPases participate in numerous processes covered in later chapters.

Most molecular interactions are driven by diffusion of reactants that simply collide with each other on a random basis. Similarly, dissociation of molecular complexes is a random process that occurs with a probability determined by the strength of the chemical bonds holding the molecules together. Many other reactions occur within molecules or molecular complexes. The aim of biophysical chemistry is to explain life processes in terms of such molecular interactions.

The extent of chemical reactions is characterized by the **equilibrium constant;** the rates of these reactions are described by **rate constants.** This chapter reviews the physical basis for rate constants and how they are related to the thermodynamic parameter, the equilibrium constant. These simple but powerful principles permit a deeper appreciation of molecular interactions in cells. On the basis of many examples presented in this book, it will become clear to the reader that rate constants are at least as important as equilibrium constants, since the rates of reactions govern the dynamics of the cell. The chapter includes discussion of the chemical bonds important in biochemistry. Box 4-1 lists key terms used in this chapter.

First-Order Reactions

First-order reactions have one reactant (R) and produce a product (P). The general case is simply

$$R \rightarrow P$$

Some common examples of first-order reactions (Fig. 4-1) include conformational changes, such as a change in shape of protein A to shape A*:

$$A \rightarrow A^*$$

This chapter is adapted in part from Wachsstock DH, Pollard TD: Transient state kinetics tutorial using KINSIM. Biophys J 67:1260–1273, 1994.

and the dissociation of complexes, such as

$$AB \rightarrow A + B$$

The rate of a first-order reaction is directly proportional to the concentration of the reactant (R, A, or AB in these examples). The rate of a first-order reaction,

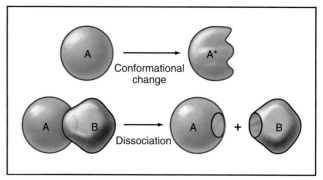

Figure 4-1 FIRST-ORDER REACTIONS. In first-order reactions, a single reactant undergoes a change. In these examples, molecule A changes conformation to A* and the bimolecular complex AB dissociates to A and B. The rate constant for a first-order reaction *(arrows)* is a simple probability.

BOX 4-1
Key Biophysical Terms

Rate constants, designated by lowercase *k*s, relate the concentrations of reactants to the rate of a reaction.

Equilibrium constants are designated by uppercase *K*s. One important and useful concept to remember is that the *equilibrium constant for a reaction is related directly to the rate constants for the forward and reverse reactions, as well as the equilibrium concentrations of reactants and products.*

The **rate of a reaction** is usually measured as the rate of change of **concentration** of a reactant (R) or product (P). As reactants disappear, products are formed, so the rate of reactant loss is directly related to the rate of product formation in a manner determined by the stoichiometry of the mechanism. In all the reaction mechanisms in this book, the arrows indicate the direction of a reaction. In the general case, the reaction mechanism is expressed as

$$R \rightleftharpoons P$$

Reaction rates are expressed as follows:

Forward rate $= k_+[R]$
Reverse rate $= k_-[P]$
Net rate $= k_+[R] - k_-[P]$

At equilibrium, the forward rate equals the reverse rate:

$$k_+[R_{eq}] = k_-[P_{eq}]$$

and concentrations of reactants R_{eq} and products P_{eq} do not change with time.

The equilibrium constant K is defined as the ratio of the concentrations of products and reactants at equilibrium:

$$K_{eq} = \frac{P_{eq}}{R_{eq}}$$

so it follows that

$$K_{eq} = \frac{k_+}{k_-}$$

In specific cases, these relationships depend on the reaction mechanism, particularly on whether one or more than one chemical species constitute the reactants and products. The equilibrium constant will be derived from a consideration of the reaction rates, beginning with the simplest case in which there is one reactant.

---

expressed as a differential equation (rate of change of reactant or product as a function of time *[t]*), is simply the concentration of the reactant times a constant, the rate constant *k,* with units of s^{-1} (pronounced "per second"):

$$\text{Rate} = -d[R]/dt = d[P]/dt = k[R]$$

The rate of the reaction has units of M s^{-1}, where M is moles per liter and s is seconds (pronounced "molar per second"). As the reactant is depleted, the rate slows proportionally.

A first-order rate constant can be viewed as a **probability** per unit of time. For a conformational change, it is the probability that any A will change to A* in a unit of time. For dissociation of complex AB, the first-order rate constant is determined by the strength of the bonds holding the complex together. This "dissociation rate constant" can be viewed as the probability that the complex will fall apart in a unit of time. The probability of the conformational change of any particular A to A* or of the dissociation of any particular AB is independent of its concentration. *The concentrations of A and AB are important only in determining the rate of the reaction observed in a bulk sample* (Box 4-2).

To review, the rate of a first-order reaction is simply the product of a constant that is characteristic of the reaction and the concentration of the single reactant. The constant can be calculated from the half-time of a reaction (Box 4-2).

Second-Order Reactions

Second-order reactions have two reactants (Fig. 4-2). The general case is

$$R_1 + R_2 \rightarrow \text{product}$$

BOX 4-2
Relationship of the Half-Time to a First-Order Rate Constant

In thinking about a first-order reaction, it is sometimes useful to refer to the half-time of the reaction. The half-time, $t_{1/2}$, is the time required for half of the existing reactant to be converted to product. For a first-order reaction, this time depends *only on the rate constant* and therefore is the same regardless of the starting concentration of the reactant. The relationship is derived as follows:

$$\frac{d[R]}{dt} = -k[R]$$

so

$$\frac{d[R]}{[R]} = -k\,dt$$

Thus, integrating, we have

$$\ln[R_t] - \ln[R_o] = -kt$$

where R_o is the initial concentration and R_t is the concentration at time t. Rearranging, we have

$$\ln[R_t] = \ln[R_o] - kt$$

or

$$[R_t] = [R_o]e^{-kt}$$

When the initial concentration R_o is reduced by half,

$$[R_t] = \tfrac{1}{2}[R_o]$$

so

$$\tfrac{1}{2}[R_o] = [R_o]e^{-kt_{1/2}}$$
$$\tfrac{1}{2} = e^{-kt_{1/2}}$$

or

$$2 = e^{kt_{1/2}}$$

Thus,

$$\ln 2 = kt_{1/2}$$

so, rearranging, we have

$$t_{1/2} = 0.693/k$$

or

$$k = 0.693/t_{1/2}$$

Therefore, a first-order rate constant can be estimated simply by dividing 0.7 by the half-time. Clearly, an analogous calculation yields the half-time from a first-order rate constant. This relationship is handy, as one frequently can estimate the extent of a reaction without knowing the absolute concentrations, and this relationship is independent of the extent of the reaction at the outset of the observations.

A common example in biology is a bimolecular association reaction, such as

$$A + B \rightarrow AB$$

where A and B are two molecules that bind together. Some examples are binding of substrates to enzymes, binding of ligands to receptors, and binding of proteins to other proteins or nucleic acids.

The rate of a second-order reaction is the product of the concentrations of the two reactants, R_1 and R_2, and the second-order rate constant, k:

$$\text{Reaction rate} = d[P]/dt = k[R_1][R_2]$$

The second-order rate constant, k, has units of $M^{-1}\,s^{-1}$ (pronounced "per molar per second"). The units for the reaction rate are

$$[R_1] \cdot [R_2] \cdot k = M \cdot M \cdot M^{-1}\,s^{-1} \text{ or } M\,s^{-1}$$

the same as a first-order reaction.

The value of a second-order "association" rate constant, k_+, is determined mainly by the rate at which the molecules collide. This collision rate depends on the rate of diffusion of the molecules (Fig. 4-2), which is

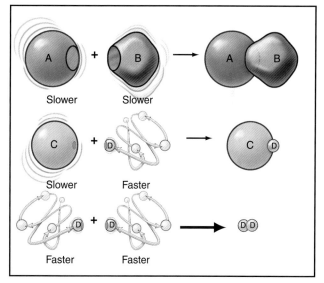

Figure 4-2 SECOND-ORDER REACTIONS. In second-order reactions, two molecules must collide with each other. The rate of these collisions is determined by their concentrations and by a collision rate constant *(arrows)*. The collision rate constant depends on the sum of the diffusion coefficients of the reactants and the size of their interaction sites. The rate of diffusion in a given medium depends on the size and shape of the molecule. Large molecules, such as proteins, move more slowly than small molecules, such as adenosine triphosphate (ATP). A protein with a diffusion coefficient of $10^{-11}\,m^2\,s^{-1}$ diffuses about 10 µm in a second in water, while a small molecule such as ATP diffuses 100 times faster. The rate constants *(arrows)* are about the same for A + B and C + D because the large diffusion coefficient of D offsets the small size of its interaction site on C. Despite the small interaction size, D + D is faster because both reactants diffuse rapidly.

determined by the size and shape of the molecule, the viscosity of the medium, and the temperature. These factors are summarized in a parameter called the **diffusion coefficient,** D, with units of $m^2 s^{-1}$. D is a measure of how fast a molecule moves in a given medium. The rate constant for collisions is described by the Debye-Smoluchowski equation, a relationship that depends only on the diffusion coefficients and the area of interaction between the molecules:

$$k = 4\pi b (D_A + D_B) N_o 10^3$$

where b is the interaction radius of the two particles (in meters), the Ds are the diffusion coefficients of the reactants, and N_o is Avogadro's number. The factor of 10^3 converts the value into units of $M^{-1} s^{-1}$.

For particles the size of proteins, D is approximately $10^{-11} m^2 s^{-1}$ and b is approximately 2×10^{-9} m, so the rate constants for collisions of two proteins are in the range of $3 \times 10^8 M^{-1} s^{-1}$. For small molecules such as sugars, D is approximately $10^{-9} m^2 s^{-1}$ and b is approximately 10^{-9} m, so the rate constants for collisions of a protein and a small molecule are about 20 times larger than collisions of two proteins, in the range of $7 \times 10^9 M^{-1} s^{-1}$. On the other hand, experimentally observed rate constants for the association of proteins are 20 to 1000 times smaller than the collision rate constant, on the order of 10^6 to $10^7 M^{-1} s^{-1}$. The difference is attributed to a steric factor that accounts for the fact that macromolecules must be correctly oriented relative to each other to bind together when they collide. Thus, the complementary binding sites are aligned correctly only 0.1% to 5% of the times that the molecules collide.

Many binding reactions between two proteins, between enzymes and substrates, and between proteins and larger molecules (e.g., DNA) are said to be "diffusion limited" in the sense that the rate constant is determined by diffusion-driven collisions between the reactants. Thus, many association rate constants are in the range of 10^6 to $10^7 M^{-1} s^{-1}$.

To review, the rate of a second-order reaction is simply the product of a constant that is characteristic of the reaction and the concentrations of the two reactants. In biology, the rates of many bimolecular association reactions are determined by the rates of diffusion-limited collisions between the reactants.

Reversible Reactions

Most reactions are reversible, so the net rate of a reaction is equal to the difference between the forward and reverse reaction rates. The forward and reverse reactions can be any combination of first- or second-order reactions. A reversible conformational change of a protein from A to A* is an example of a pair of simple first-order reactions:

$$A \rightleftharpoons A^*$$

The forward reaction rate is k_+A with units of $M s^{-1}$, and the reverse reaction rate is k_-A^* with the same units. At equilibrium, when the net concentrations of A and A* no longer change,

$$k_+[A] = k_-[A^*]$$

and

$$K_{eq} = k_+/k_- = [A^*]/[A]$$

This equilibrium constant is unitless, since the units of concentration and the rate constants cancel out.

The same reasoning with respect to the equilibrium constant applies to a simple bimolecular binding reaction:

$$A + B \rightleftharpoons AB$$

where A and B are any molecule (e.g., enzyme, receptor, substrate, cofactor, or drug). The forward (binding) reaction is a second-order reaction, whereas the reverse (dissociation) reaction is first-order. The opposing reactions are

$$\text{Rate of association} = k_+[A][B]$$
$$\text{units: } M s^{-1}$$
$$\text{Rate of dissociation} = k_-[AB]$$
$$\text{units: } M s^{-1}$$

The overall rate of the reaction is the forward rate minus the reverse rate:

$$\text{Net rate} = \text{association rate} - \text{dissociation rate}$$
$$= k_+[A][B] - k_-[AB]$$

Depending on the values of the rate constants and the concentrations of A, B, and AB, the reaction can go forward, backward, or nowhere.

At equilibrium, the forward and reverse rates are (by definition) the same:

$$k_+[A][B] = k_-[AB]$$

The equilibrium constant for such a bimolecular reaction can be written in two ways:

$$\text{Association equilibrium constant:}$$
$$K_a = [AB]/[A][B] = k_+/k_-$$
$$\text{units: } M^{-1} = M/M \times M$$

This is the classical equilibrium constant used in chemistry, where the strength of the reaction is proportional to the numerical value. For bimolecular reactions, the units of reciprocal molar are difficult to relate to, so biochemists frequently use the reciprocal relationship:

$$\text{Disassociation equilibrium constant:}$$
$$K_d = [A][B]/[AB] = k_-/k_+$$
$$\text{units: } M = M \times M/M$$

When half of the total A is bound to B, the concentration of free B is simply equal to the dissociation equilibrium constant.

Thermodynamic Considerations

The driving force for chemical reactions is the lowering of the free energy of the system when reactants are converted into products. The larger the reduction in free energy, the more completely reactants will be converted to products at equilibrium. A thorough consideration of thermodynamics is beyond the scope of this text, but an overview of this subject is presented to allow the reader to gain a basic understanding of its power and simplicity.

The change in Gibbs free energy, ΔG, is simply the difference in the chemical potential, μ, of the reactants (R) and products (P):

$$\Delta G = \mu^P - \mu^R$$

The chemical potential of a particular chemical species depends on its intrinsic properties and its concentration, expressed as the equation

$$\mu = \mu^0 + RT \ln C$$

where μ^0 is the chemical potential in the standard state (1 M in biochemistry), R is the gas constant (8.3 J mol^{-1} degree^{-1}), T is the absolute temperature in degrees Kelvin, and C is the ratio of the concentration of the chemical species to the standard concentration. Because the standard state is defined as 1 M, the parameter C has the same numerical value as the molar concentration, but is, in fact, unitless. The term $RT \ln C$ adjusts for the concentration. When $C = 1$, $\mu = \mu^0$.

Under standard conditions in which one mole of reactant is converted to one mole of product, the standard free energy change, ΔG^0, is

$$\Delta G^0 = \mu^{0P} - \mu^{0R}$$

However, because most reactions do not take place under these standard conditions, the chemical potential must be adjusted for the actual concentrations. This can be done by including the concentration term from the definition of the chemical potential. An equation for the free energy change that takes concentrations into account is

$$\Delta G = \mu^{0P} + RT \ln[P] - \mu^{0R} - RT \ln[R]$$

Substituting the definition of ΔG^0, we have

$$\Delta G = \Delta G^0 + RT \ln[P] - RT \ln[R] = \Delta G^0 + RT \ln[P]/[R]$$

This relationship tells us that the free energy change for the conversion of reactants to products is simply the free energy change under standard conditions corrected for the actual concentrations of reactant and products.

At equilibrium, the concentrations of reactants and products do not change and the free energy change is zero, so

$$0 = \Delta G^0 + RT \ln[P_{eq}]/[R_{eq}]$$

or

$$\Delta G^0 = -RT \ln[P_{eq}]/[R_{eq}]$$

The reader is already familiar with the fact that the equilibrium constant for a reaction is the ratio of the equilibrium concentrations of products and reactants. Thus, that relationship can be substituted in this thermodynamic equation:

$$\Delta G^0 = -RT \ln K$$

or

$$K = e^{-\Delta G^0/RT} = k_+/k_- = [P_{eq}]/[R_{eq}]$$

This profound relationship shows how the free energy change is related to the equilibrium constant. The change in the standard Gibbs free energy, ΔG^0, specifies the ratio of products and reactants when the reaction reaches equilibrium, *regardless of the rate or path of the reaction*. The free energy change provides no information about whether or not a given reaction will proceed on a time scale relevant to cellular activities. Nevertheless, because the equilibrium constant depends on the ratio of the rate constants, knowledge of the rate constants reveals the equilibrium constant and the free energy change for a reaction. Consider the consequences of various values of ΔG^0:

- If ΔG^0 equals 0, $e^{-\Delta G^0/RT}$ equals 1, and at equilibrium, the concentration of products will equal the concentration of reactants (or in the case of a bimolecular reaction, the product of the concentrations of the reactants).

- If ΔG^0 is less than 0, $e^{-\Delta G^0/RT}$ is greater than 1, and at equilibrium, the concentration of products will be greater than the concentration of reactants. Larger, negative, free energy changes will drive the reaction farther toward products. Favorable reactions have large negative ΔG^0 values.

- If ΔG^0 is greater than 0, $e^{-\Delta G^0/RT}$ is less than 1, and at equilibrium, the concentrations of reactants will exceed the concentration of products.

It is sometimes said that a reaction with a positive ΔG^0 will not proceed spontaneously. This is not strictly true. Reactants will still be converted to products, although relative to the concentration of reactants, the concentration of products will be small. The size and sign of the free energy change tell nothing about the rate of a reaction. For example, the oxidation of sucrose by oxygen is highly favored with a ΔG^0 of −5693 kJ/mol, but "a flash fire in a sugar bowl is an event rarely, if ever, seen."*

The free energy change is additionally related to two thermodynamic parameters that are important to the subsequent discussion of molecular interactions. The Gibbs-Helmholtz equation is the key relationship:

$$\Delta G = \Delta H - T\Delta S$$

where ΔH is the change in **enthalpy,** an approximation (with a small correction for pressure-volume work) of the bond energies of the molecules. Thus, ΔH is the heat given off when a bond is made or the heat taken up when a bond is broken. The change in enthalpy is simply the difference in enthalpy of reactants and products. In biochemical reactions, the enthalpy term principally reflects energies of the strong covalent bonds and of the weaker hydrogen and electrostatic bonds. If no covalent bonds change, as in a binding reaction or a conformational change, ΔH is determined by the difference in the energy of the weak bonds of the products and reactants.

The change in **entropy,** expressed as ΔS, is a measure of the change in the order of the products and reactants. The value of the entropy is a function of the number of microscopic arrangements of the system, including the solvent molecules. Note the minus sign in front of the $T\Delta S$ term. Reactions are favored if the change in entropy is positive, that is, if the products are less well ordered than the reactants. Increases in entropy drive reactions by increasing the negative free energy change. For example, the hydrophobic effect, which is discussed later in this chapter, depends on an increase in entropy. Increases in entropy provide the free energy change for many biologic reactions, especially macromolecular folding (see Chapters 3 and 17) and assembly (see Chapter 5).

As was emphasized in the case of ΔG, neither the rate of the reaction nor the path between reactants and products is relevant to the difference in enthalpy or entropy of reactants and products. The reader may consult a physical chemistry book for a fuller explanation of these basic principles of thermodynamics.

Linked Reactions

Many important processes in the cell consist of a single reaction, but most of cellular biochemistry involves a series of linked reactions (Fig. 4-3). For example, when two macromolecules bind together, the complex often undergoes some type of internal rearrangement or con-

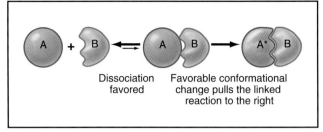

Figure 4-3 LINKED REACTIONS. Two molecules, A and B, bind together weakly and then undergo a favorable conformational change. The binding reaction is unfavorable, owing to the high rate of dissociation of AB, but the favorable conformational change pulls the overall reaction far to the right.

formational change, linking a first-order reaction to a second-order reaction.

$$A + B \rightleftharpoons AB \quad AB \rightleftharpoons AB^*$$

One of thousands of such examples is GTP binding to a G protein, causing it to undergo a conformational change from the inactive to the active state (Figs. 4-6 and 4-7 ahead).

Similarly, the basic enzyme reaction considered in most biochemistry books is simply a series of reversible second- and first-order reactions:

$$E + S \rightleftharpoons ES \quad ES \rightleftharpoons EP \quad EP \rightleftharpoons E + P$$

where E is enzyme, S is substrate, and P is product. These and more complicated reactions can be described rigorously by a series of rate equations like those explained previously. For example, enzyme reactions nearly always involve one or more additional intermediates between ES and EP, coupled by first-order reactions, in which the molecules undergo conformational changes.

Linking reactions together is the secret of how the cell carries out unfavorable reactions. All that matters is that the total free energy change for all coupled reactions is negative. An unfavorable reaction is driven forward by a favorable reaction upstream or downstream. For example, the unfavorable reaction producing adenosine triphosphate (ATP) from adenosine diphosphate (ADP) and inorganic phosphate is driven by being coupled to an energy source in the form of a proton gradient across the mitochondrial membrane (see Fig. 8-5). This proton gradient is derived, in turn, from the oxidation of chemical bonds of nutrients. To use a macroscopic analogy, a siphon can initially move a liquid uphill against gravity provided that the outflow is placed below the inflow, so that the overall change in energy is favorable.

An appreciation of linked reactions makes it possible to understand how catalysts, including biochemical catalysts—protein enzymes and ribozymes—influence

*Eisenberg D, Crothers D: Physical Chemistry with Applications to the Life Sciences. Menlo Park, Calif: Benjamin Cummings Publishing, 1979.

reactions. They do not alter the free energy change for reactions, but they enhance the rates of reactions by speeding up the forward and reverse rates of unfavorable intermediate reactions along pathways of coupled reactions. Given that the rates of both first- and second-order reactions depend on the concentrations of the reactants, the overall reaction is commonly limited by the concentration of the least favored, highest-energy intermediate, called a transition state. This might be a strained conformation of substrate in a biochemical pathway. Interaction of this transition state with an enzyme can lower its free energy, increasing its probability (concentration) and thus the rate of the limiting reaction. Acceleration of biochemical reactions by enzymes is impressive. Enhancement of reaction rates by 10 orders of magnitude is common.

Chemical Bonds

Covalent bonds are responsible for the stable architecture of the organic molecules in cells (Fig. 4-4). They are very strong. C—C and C—H bonds have energies of about 400 kJ mol^{-1}. Bonds this strong do not dissociate spontaneously at body temperatures and pressures, nor are the reactive intermediates required to form these bonds present in finite concentrations in cells. To overcome this problem, living systems use enzymes, which stabilize high-energy transition states, to catalyze formation and dissolution of covalent bonds. Energy for making strong covalent bonds is obtained indirectly by coupling to energy-yielding reactions. For example, metabolic enzymes convert energy released by breaking covalent bonds of nutrients, such as carbohydrates, lipids, and proteins, into ATP (see Fig. 19-4), which supplies energy required to form new covalent bonds during the synthesis of polypeptides. Metabolic pathways relating the covalent chemistry of the molecules of life are covered in depth in many excellent biochemistry books.

For cell biologists, four types of relatively weak interactions (Fig. 4-5) are as important as covalent bonds because they are responsible for folding macromolecules into their active conformations and for holding molecules together in the structures of the cell. These

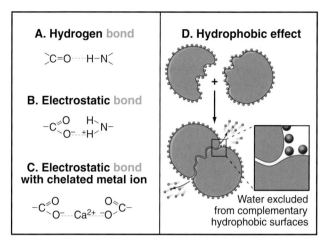

Figure 4-5 WEAK INTERACTIONS. A, Hydrogen bond. Opposite partial charges in the oxygen and hydrogen provide the attractive force. **B,** Electrostatic bond. Atoms with opposite charges are attracted to each other. **C,** Ca^{2+} chelated between two negatively charged oxygens. **D,** The hydrophobic effect arises when two complementary, apolar surfaces make contact, excluding water molecules that formerly were associated with the surfaces. The increased disorder of the water increases the entropy and provides the decrease in free energy to drive the association. Van der Waals interactions between closely packed atoms on complementary surfaces also stabilize interactions.

weak interactions are (1) **hydrogen bonds,** (2) **electrostatic interactions,** (3) the **hydrophobic effect,** and (4) **van der Waals interactions.** None of these interactions is particularly strong on its own. Stable bonding between subunits of many macromolecular structures, between ligands and receptors, and between substrates and enzymes is a result of the additive effect of many weak interactions working in concert.

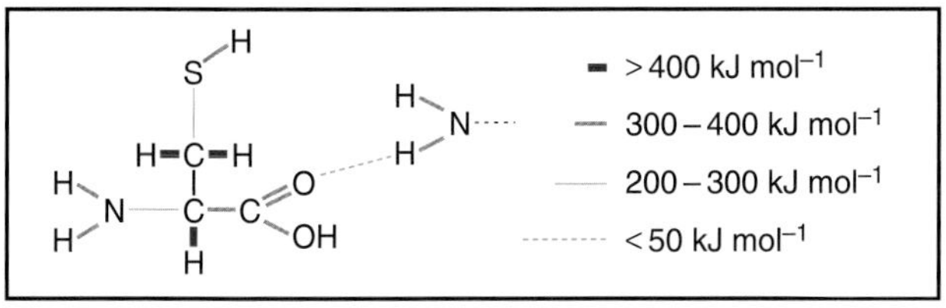

Hydrogen and Electrostatic Bonds

Hydrogen bonds (Fig. 4-5) occur between a covalently bound donor H atom with a partial positive charge, Δ+ (due to electron withdrawal by a covalently bonded O or N), and an acceptor atom (usually O or N) with a partial negative charge, Δ−. These bonds are highly directional, with optimal bond energy (12 to 29 kJ mol^{-1}) when the H atom points directly at the acceptor atom. Hydrogen bonds are extremely important in the stabilization of secondary structures of proteins, such as α-helices and β-sheets (see Fig. 3-8) and in the base pairing of DNA and RNA (see Fig. 3-14).

Electrostatic (or ionic) bonds occur between charged groups that have either lost or gained a proton (e.g., —COO$^-$ and —NH$_3^+$). Although these bonds are potentially about as strong as an average hydrogen bond (20 kJ mol^{-1}), it has been argued that they contribute little to biological structure. This is because a charged group is usually neutralized by an inorganic counterion

Figure 4-4 COVALENT BONDS. Bond energies for the amino acid cysteine.

> — >400 kJ mol^{-1}
> — 300–400 kJ mol^{-1}
> — 200–300 kJ mol^{-1}
> ····· <50 kJ mol^{-1}

(such as Na^+ or Cl^-) that is itself surrounded by a cloud of water molecules. The effect of having the cloud of water molecules is that the counterion does not occupy a single position with respect to the charged group on the macromolecule; so these interactions lack structural specificity.

The Hydrophobic Effect

Self-assembly and other association reactions that involve the joining together of separate molecules to form more ordered structures might seem unlikely when examined from the point of view of thermodynamics. Nonetheless, many binding reactions are highly favored, and when such processes are monitored in the laboratory, it can be shown that ΔS actually increases.

How can association of molecules lead to increased disorder? The answer is that the entropy of the system—including macromolecules and solvent—increases owing to the loss of order in the *water* surrounding the macromolecules (Fig. 4-5). This increase in the entropy of the water more than offsets the increased order and decreased entropy of the associated macromolecules. Bulk water is a semistructured solvent maintained by a loose network of hydrogen bonds (see Fig. 3-1). Water cannot form hydrogen bonds with nonpolar (hydrophobic) parts of lipids and proteins. Instead, water molecules form "cages" or "clathrates" of extensively H-bonded water molecules near these hydrophobic surfaces. These clathrates are more ordered than is bulk water or water interacting with charged or polar amino acids.

When proteins fold (see Fig. 17-12), macromolecules bind together (see Chapter 5), and phospholipids associate to form bilayers (see Fig. 7-5), hydrophobic groups are buried in pockets or between interfaces that exclude water. The highly ordered water formerly associated with these surfaces disperses into the less ordered bulk phase, and the entropy of the system increases.

The increase in the disorder of water that results when hydrophobic regions of macromolecules are buried is called the **hydrophobic effect.** Hydrophobic interactions are a major driving force, but they would not confer specificity on an intermolecular interaction except for the fact that the molecular surfaces must be complementary to exclude water. The hydrophobic effect is not a bond per se, but a thermodynamic factor that favors macromolecular interactions.

van der Waals Interactions

van der Waals interactions occur when adjacent atoms come close enough that their outer electron clouds barely touch. This action induces charge fluctuations that result in a nonspecific, nondirectional attraction. These interactions are highly distance dependent, decreasing in proportion to the sixth power of the separation. The energy of each interaction is only about 4 kJ mol⁻¹ (very weak when compared with the average kinetic energy of a molecule in solution, which is approximately 2.5 kJ mol⁻¹) and is significant only when many interactions are combined (as in interactions of complementary surfaces). Under optimal circumstances, van der Waals interactions can achieve bonding energies as high as 40 kJ mol⁻¹.

When two atoms get too close, they strongly repel each other. Consequently, imperfect fits between interacting molecules are energetically very expensive, preventing association if surface groups interfere sterically with each other. As a determinant of specificity of macromolecular interactions, this van der Waals repulsion is even more important than the favorable bonds discussed earlier, because it precludes many nonspecific interactions.

A Strategy for Understanding Cellular Functions

One strategy for understanding the mechanism of any molecular process—including binding reactions, self-assembly reactions, and enzyme reactions—is to determine the existence of the various reactants, intermediates, and products along the reaction pathway and then to measure the rate constants for each step. Such an analysis yields additional information about the thermodynamics of each step, as the ratio of the rate constants reveals the equilibrium constant and the free energy change, even for transient intermediates that may be difficult or impossible to analyze separately.

In earlier times, biochemists lacked methods to evaluate the internal reactions along most pathways, but they could measure the overall rate of reactions, such as the steady-state rate of conversion of reactants to products by an enzyme. To analyze these data, they simplified complex mechanisms using relationships such as the Michaelis-Menten equation (described in biochemistry textbooks). Now, abundant supplies of proteins, convenient methods for measuring rapid reaction rates, and computer programs that can be used to analyze complex reaction mechanisms generally make such simplifications unnecessary.

Analysis of an Enzyme Mechanism: The Ras GTPase

This section uses a vitally important family of enzymes called **GTPases** to illustrate how enzymes work. The example is **Ras,** a small GTPase that serves as part of a biochemical pathway linking growth factor receptors in the plasma membrane of animal cells to regulation of the cell cycle. The example shows how to dissect an enzyme reaction by kinetic analysis and how crystal structures can reveal conformational changes related to function. GTPases related to Ras regulate a host of systems (see Table 25-3) including nuclear transport (see Fig. 14-17), protein synthesis (see Figs. 17-9 and 17-10), vesicular trafficking (see Fig. 21-6), signaling pathways coupled to seven-helix receptors including vision and olfaction (see Figs. 25-8 and 25-9), the actin cytoskeleton (see Figs. 33-17 and 33-20), and assembly of the mitotic spindle (see Fig. 44-8). This section gives the reader the background required to understand the contributions of GTPases to all of these processes as they are presented in the following sections of the book.

Having evolved from a common ancestor, Ras and its related GTPases share a homologous core domain that binds a guanine nucleotide and use a common enzymatic cycle of GTP binding, hydrolysis, and product dissociation to switch the protein on and off (Fig. 4-6). The GTP-binding domain consists of about 200 residues folded into a six-stranded β-sheet sandwiched between five α-helices. GTP binds in a shallow groove formed largely by loops at the ends of elements of secondary structure. A network of hydrogen bonds between the protein and guanine base, ribose, triphosphate, and Mg^{2+} anchor the nucleotide. Larger GTPases have a core GTPase domain plus domains required for coupling to seven-helix receptors (see Fig. 25-9) or regulating protein synthesis (see Figs. 17-10 and 25-7).

The bound nucleotide determines the conformation and activity of each GTPase. The GTP-bound conformation is active, as it interacts with and stimulates effector proteins. In the example considered here, the Ras-GTP binds and stimulates a protein kinase, Raf, which relays signals from growth factor receptors to the nucleus (see Fig. 27-6). The GDP-bound conformation of Ras is inactive because it does not bind effectors. Thus, GTP hydrolysis and phosphate dissociation switch Ras and related GTPases from the active to the inactive state.

All GTPases use the same enzyme cycle, which involves four simple steps (Fig. 4-6). GTP binding favors the active conformation that binds effector proteins. GTPases remain active until they hydrolyze the bound GTP. Hydrolysis is intrinsically slow, but binding to effector proteins or regulatory proteins can accelerate this inactivation step. GTPases tend to accumulate in the inactive GDP state, because GDP dissociation is very slow. Specific proteins catalyze dissociation of GDP, making it possible for GTP to rebind and activate the GTPase. Seven-helix receptors activate their associated G-proteins. Guanine nucleotide exchange proteins (GEFs) activate small GTPases.

Figure 4-7 illustrates the experimental strategy used to establish the mechanism of the Ras GTPase cycle.

Step 1: GTP binding. GTP binds rapidly to nucleotide-free Ras in two linked reactions (Fig. 4-7A). The first is rapid but reversible association of GTP with Ras. Second is a slower but highly favorable first-

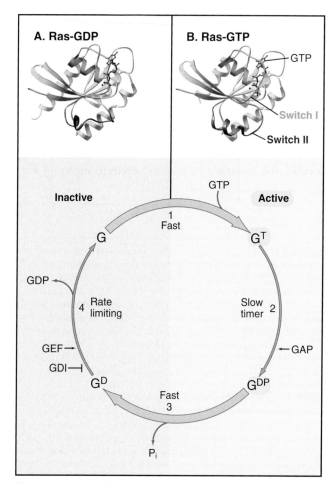

Figure 4-6 **Top (A–B),** Atomic structures of the small GTPase Ras. GTP hydrolysis and phosphate dissociation cause major changes in the conformations of the switch loops. (A, PDB file: 1Q21. B, PDB file: 121P.) **Bottom,** Generic GTPase cycle. The size of the *arrows* indicates the relative rates of the reactions. GAP, GTPase activating protein; G^D, GTPase with bound GDP; GDI, guanine nucleotide dissociation inhibitor; G^{DP}, GTPase with bound GDP and inorganic phosphate; GEF, guanine nucleotide exchange factor; G^T, GTPase with bound GTP; F_i, phosphate.

order conformational change, which produces the fluorescence signal in the experiment and accounts for the high affinity (K_d typically in the range of 10^{-11} M). The conformation change involves three segments of the polypeptide chain called switch I, switch II, and switch III. Folding of these three loops around the γ-phosphate of GTP traps the nucleotide and creates a binding site for the Raf kinase, the downstream effector (see Fig. 29-6).

Step 2: GTP hydrolysis. Hydrolysis is essentially irreversible and slow with a half-time of about 4 hours (Fig. 4-7B). Although slow, GTP hydrolysis on the enzyme is many orders of magnitude faster than in solution. Like other enzymes, interactions of the protein with the substrate stabilizes the "transition state," a high-energy chemical intermediate between GTP and GDP. In this transition state, the

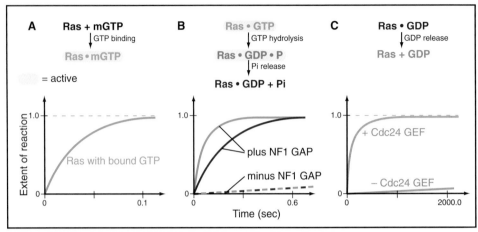

Figure 4-7   Kinetic dissection of the Ras GTPase cycle using a series of "single turnover" experiments, in which each enzyme molecule carries out a reaction only once. **A,** GTP binding. Nucleotide-free Ras is mixed rapidly with a fluorescent derivative of GTP (mGTP), and fluorescence is followed on a millisecond time scale. With 100 μM mGTP (approximately 10% of the cellular concentration), binding is fast (half-time less than 5 ms), but the change in fluorescence is slower, about 30 s^{-1}, since it depends on a subsequent, slower conformational change. Linking the association reaction to this highly favorable ($K = 10^6$) first-order conformational change accounts for the exceedingly high affinity ($K_d = \sim 10^{-11}$ M) of Ras for GTP. Binding and dissociation of GDP are similar. **B,** GTP hydrolysis and γ-phosphate dissociation. GTP is mixed with Ras, and hydrolysis is followed by collecting samples on a millisecond time scale with a "quench-flow" device, dissociating the products from the enzyme and measuring the fraction of GTP converted to GDP. The Ras-GDP-P intermediate releases γ-phosphate spontaneously in a first-order reaction. A fluorescent phosphate-binding protein is used to measure free phosphate. On this time scale in this figure, Ras alone does not hydrolyze GTP or dissociated phosphate, since the hydrolysis rate constant is 5×10^{-5} s^{-1}, corresponding to a half-time of 1400 seconds. The GTPase activating protein (GAP) neurofibromin 1 (NF1) at a concentration of 10 μM increases the rate of hydrolysis to 20 s^{-1} and allows observation of the time course of phosphate dissociation at 8 s^{-1}. **C,** GDP dissociation. Ras with bound fluorescent mGDP is mixed with GTP, which replaces the mGDP as it dissociates. The loss of fluorescence over time gives a rate constant for mGDP dissociation of 0.00002 s^{-1}. The guanine nucleotide exchange factor Cdc24^{Mn} at a concentration of 1 μM increases the rate of mGDP dissociation 500-fold to 0.01 s^{-1}. (Compiled from experiments reported by Lenzen C, Cool RH, Prinz H, et al: Kinetic analysis by fluorescence of the interaction between Ras and the catalytic domain of the guanine nucleotide exchange factor Cdc24^{Mn}. Biochemistry 37:7420–7430, 1998; and by Phillips RA, Hunter JL, Eccleston JF, Webb MR: Mechanism of Ras GTPase activation by neurofibromin. Biochemistry 42:3956–3965, 2003.)

γ-phosphate is partially bonded to both the β-phosphate and an attacking water. Hydrogen bonds between protein backbone amides and oxygens bridging the β- and γ-phosphates and on the γ- and β-phosphates stabilize negative charges that build up on these atoms in the transition state. Hydrolysis is slow in comparison with most enzyme reactions, because none of these hydrogen bonds is particularly strong. Another hydrogen bond from a glutamine side chain helps to position a water for nucleophilic attack on the γ-phosphate. The importance of this interaction is illustrated by mutations that replace glutamine 61 with leucine. This mutation reduces the rate of hydrolysis by orders of magnitude and predisposes to the development of many human cancers by prolonging the active state and thus amplifying growth-promoting signals from growth factor receptors.

Step 3: Dissociation of inorganic phosphate. After hydrolysis, the γ-phosphate dissociates rapidly. This reverses the conformational change of the three switch loops, dismantling the binding site for effector proteins.

Step 4: Dissociation of GDP. On its own, Ras accumulates in the inactive GDP state, because GDP dissociates extremely slowly with a half-time of 10 hours (Fig. 4-7C). GTP cannot bind and activate Ras until GDP dissociates.

Ras and most other small GTPases depend on regulatory proteins to stimulate the two slow steps in the GTPase cycle: GDP dissociation and GTP hydrolysis. For example, when growth factors stimulate their receptors, a series of reactions (see Fig. 27-6) brings a **guanine nucleotide exchange factor (GEF)** to the plasma membrane to activate Ras by accelerating dissociation of GDP. First the GEF binds Ras-GDP and then favors a slow conformational change that distorts a part of Ras that interacts with the β-phosphate. This allows GDP to dissociate on a time scale of seconds to minutes rather than 10 hours (Fig. 4-7C). Once GDP has dissociated, nucleotide-free Ras can bind either GDP or GTP. Binding GTP is more likely in cells, because the cytoplasmic concentration of GTP (about 1 mM) is 10 times that of GDP. GTP binding activates Ras, allowing transmission of the signal to the nucleus.

GTPase-activating proteins (GAPs) turn off Ras and related GTPases, by binding Ras-GTP and stimulating GTP hydrolysis, thereby terminating GTPase activation (Fig. 4-7B). Ras GAPs stabilize the transition state, by contributing a positively charged arginine side chain that stabilizes the negative charges on the oxygen bridging the β- and γ-phosphates and on the γ-phosphate. GAPs also help to position Gln61 and its attacking water. In the experiment in the figure, a GAP called neurofibromin (NF1) binds Ras with a half-time of 3 ms (not illustrated) and stimulates rapid hydrolysis of GTP at $20\ s^{-1}$. This is followed by rate-limiting dissociation of γ-phosphate from the Ras-GDP-P intermediate at $8\ s^{-1}$ and rapid dissociation of NF1 from Ras at $50\ s^{-1}$. NF1 is the product of a human gene that is inactivated in the disease called neurofibromatosis. Lacking the NF1 GAP activity to keep Ras in check, affected individuals develop numerous neural tumors that disfigure the skin and may compromise the function of the nervous system.

ACKNOWLEDGMENT

Thanks go to Martin Webb for his help with GTPase kinetics.

SELECTED READINGS

Berg OG, von Hippel PH: Diffusion controlled macromolecular interactions. Annu Rev Biophys 14:131-160, 1985.

Eisenberg D, Crothers D: Physical Chemistry with Applications to the Life Sciences. Menlo Park, Calif: Benjamin Cummings Publishing, 1979.

Garcia-Viloca M, Gao J, Karplus M, Truhlar DG: How enzymes work: Analysis by modern rate theory and computer simulations. Science 303:186-194, 2004.

Herrmann C: Ras-effector interactions: After one decade. Curr Opin Struct Biol 13:122-129, 2003.

Johnson KA: Transient-state kinetic analysis of enzyme reaction pathways. Enzymes 20:1-61, 1992.

Lenzen C, Cool RH, Prinz H, et al: Kinetic analysis by fluorescence of the interaction between Ras and the catalytic domain of the guanine nucleotide exchange factor Cdc^{Mn}. Biochemistry 37:7420-7430, 1998.

Northrup SH, Erickson HP: Kinetics of protein-protein association explained by Brownian dynamics computer simulation. Proc Natl Acad Sci U S A 89:3338-3342, 1992.

Phillips RA, Hunter JL, Eccleston JF, Webb, MR: Mechanism of Ras GTPase activation by neurofibromin. Biochemistry 42:3956-3965, 2003.

Wachsstock DH, Pollard TD: Transient state kinetics tutorial using KINSIM. Biophys J 67:1260-1273, 1994.

CHAPTER 5

Macromolecular Assembly

The discovery that dissociated parts of viruses can reassemble in a test tube led to the concept of **self-assembly,** one of the central principles in biology. In vitro analysis of true self-assembly from purified components of viruses, bacterial flagella, ribosomes, and cytoskeletal filaments has revealed the general properties of these processes. For example, large biological structures, such as the mitotic spindle (Fig. 5-1), are constructed from molecules that assemble by defined pathways without the aid of templates. Even large cellular components, such as chromosomes, nuclear pores, transcription initiation complexes, vesicle fusion machinery, and intercellular junctions, assemble by the same strategy. The properties of the constituents determine the assembly mechanism and architecture of the final structure. Weak but highly specific noncovalent interactions hold together the building blocks, which include proteins, nucleic acids, and lipids.

The ability of **subunit molecules** to assemble spontaneously into the complicated structures required for cellular function greatly increases the power of the information stored in the genome. The primary structure of a protein or nucleic acid specifies not only the folding of the individual protein or nucleic acid subunit but also the bonds that it can make in a larger assembly.

Assembly of macromolecular structures differs fundamentally from the template-specified, enzymatic mechanisms with which cells replicate genes (see Chapter 42) and translate genes into RNAs and proteins (see Chapters 15 and 17). Macromolecular assembly does not require templates and rarely involves enzymatic formation or

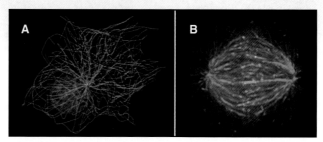

Figure 5-1 MICROTUBULES USE RECYCLED SUBUNITS TO REORGANIZE COMPLETELY DURING THE CELL CYCLE. **A,** Interphase. Microtubules *(green)* form a cytoplasmic network radiating from the microtubule organizing center at the centrosome, stained *red.* The nuclear DNA is *blue.* **B,** Mitosis. Duplicated centrosomes become the poles of the bipolar mitotic apparatus. Microtubules *(green)* radiate from the poles to contact chromosomes *(blue)* at centromeres *(red),* pulling the chromosomes to the poles. After mitosis, the interphase arrangement of microtubules reassembles. (A, Courtesy of A. Khodjakov, Wadsworth Center, Albany, New York. B, Courtesy of D. Cleveland, University of California, San Diego.)

dissolution of covalent bonds. When enzymatic processing occurs during the assembly of some viruses (see Example 7 later in the chapter, in the section titled "Regulation by Accessory Proteins"), collagen (see Fig. 29-6), and elastin (see Fig. 29-11), it usually precludes reassembly of the dissociated parts.

This chapter presents five concepts that explain most assembly processes. Also included are descriptions of a series of model systems that illustrate these principles. Subsequent chapters return repeatedly to these ideas, as they help to explain the structure, biogenesis, and function of most cellular components.

Assembly of Macromolecular Structures from Subunits

The use of subunits provides multiple advantages for assembly processes, as was originally pointed out by Crane (Box 5-1). These advantages include the following:

Assembly of large structures from subunits conserves the genome. The assembly of macromolecular structures from identical subunits, like bricks in a wall, obviates the need to specify separate parts. For example, a plant virus, the **tobacco mosaic virus** (TMV; see Example 4 in this chapter), consists of 2130 protein subunits of 158 amino acids and a single-stranded RNA molecule of 6390 nucleotides. Having a separate gene for each viral coat protein would require 1,009,620 nucleotides of RNA, which would be about 160-fold longer than the entire viral RNA! The virus conserves its genome by using a single copy of the coat protein gene (474 nucleotides—7.4% of the genome) to make 2130 identical copies of protein that assemble into the virus coat.

Using small subunits improves the chance of synthesizing error-free building blocks. All biological processes are susceptible to error, and protein synthesis by ribosomes is no exception (see Chapter 17). The error rate of translation is about 1 in 3000 amino acid residues. Therefore, the odds that any given amino acid residue is correct are 0.99967. With these odds, the chance that a TMV subunit will be translated correctly is 0.99967^{158}, or 0.949. Thus, about 95% of all TMV coat proteins in an infected cell are perfect, providing an ample supply of subunits with which to construct an infectious virus. Of the 5% of subunits with a mistake, some will be functional and others will not, depending on the nature and position of the amino acid substitution. Some amino acid substitutions pass unnoticed, whereas others result in loss of function. By contrast, the chance of correctly synthesizing the viral coat, if TMV coated its RNA with one huge polypeptide with 336,540 residues, would be only 0.99967^{336540}, or 1.87×10^{-49}.

Construction from subunits provides a mechanism for eliminating faulty components. Given that a signifi-

BOX 5-1
Crane's Hypothesis

In 1950, the physicist H. R. Crane predicted in *Scientific Monthly* that all macromolecular structures in biology are assembled from multiple subunits and according to the laws of **symmetry.** A symmetric structure is composed of numerous identical **subunits,** all in equivalent environments (i.e., making identical contacts with their neighbors). For example, Figure 5-2A shows a plane hexagonal array, with each subunit making identical contacts with the six surrounding subunits. This is the most efficient way to fill a flat surface with globular subunits.

Crane also predicted that elongated tubular structures are assembled with symmetry. This type of symmetry is known as a **helix.** One way of constructing a helix is to take a plane hexagonal array, cut it along one of its lattice lines, and roll it up into a tube (Fig. 5-2B). The bonds between adjacent subunits are nearly identical in the plane array and the helical tube, except for

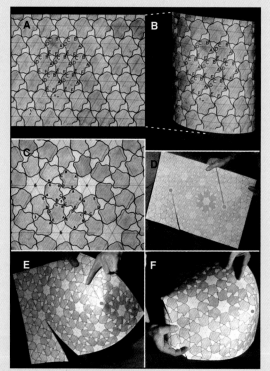

Figure 5-2 FOLDING OF PAPER MODELS OF HEXAGONAL ARRAYS OF IDENTICAL PARTICLES INTO A HELIX OR A CLOSED POLYGON. **A,** A hexagonal array of particles similar to the arrangement of subunits in the tobacco mosaic virus. **B,** The sheet is rolled around onto itself to make a helix similar to the virus. **C,** A hexagonal array of particles with three identical subunits in each triangular unit. The subunits around one sixfold axis are colored pink. **D–F,** The sheet is cut along two lattice lines and folded, creating two fivefold vertices *(green dot)*. Introduction of 12 such fivefold vertices creates an icosahedron. (From Caspar D, Klug A: Physical principles in the construction of regular viruses. Cold Spring Harbor Symp Quant Biol 27:1–24, 1962.)

the fact that each bond is distorted just enough to roll the sheet into a tube. Introduction of fivefold vertices into a hexagonal array allows it to fold up into a closed polygon (Fig. 5-2D–F).

Crane argued further that biological structures could avoid the problem of poisoning by defective subunits if such subunits were recognized and discarded. Crane's thinking about this problem was stimulated by a visit to a factory producing complex parts for vacuum tubes during World War II. When he asked the factory manager how much training the workers needed to assemble such a complex product, he was surprised to learn that the average was only 4 hours. The supervisor explained that they worked on an assembly line where each worker made only one small component (a subunit). If that component was defective, it was simply discarded, so the final product was built only from perfect components. Crane suggested that cells use the same strategy.

Crane's theories led to the hypothesis that cellular structures "build" themselves by self-assembly. Thus, the design of the final structure is somehow incorporated into the shape of the individual subunits. Remarkably, all of Crane's predictions about subunits and assembly turned out to be correct.

cant fraction of all proteins have minor errors, good and bad subunits can be segregated on the basis of their ability to form correct bonds with their neighbors at the time of assembly. Many faulty subunits will not bond and thus are simply excluded from the final structure.

Subunits can be recycled. Many macromolecular structures assemble reversibly, and because they are built of subunits, the subunits can be reused later. For example, the subunits of the mitotic spindle microtubules reassemble into the interphase array of microtubules (Fig. 5-1; see also Chapter 44). Subunits in actin (see Example 1) and myosin (see Example 2) filaments are also recycled.

Assembly from subunits provides multiple opportunities for regulation. Simple modifications of subunits can regulate the state of assembly. For example, many intermediate filaments disassemble during mitosis when their subunits are phosphorylated by protein kinases (see Figs. 35-4 and 44-6).

Specificity by Multiple Weak Bonds on Complementary Surfaces

Stable macromolecular assemblies require intermolecular interactions stronger than the forces tending to dissociate the subunits. Subunits diffusing independently in an aqueous milieu have a kinetic energy of about

$2.5 \, kJ \, mol^{-1}$ at 25°C. Interactions in macromolecular assemblies must be strong enough to overcome this thermal energy, which tends to pull them apart. Forces holding subunits together can be estimated from analysis of atomic structures (see Examples 1, 5, and 6) and the effects of solution conditions on the stability of assemblies (see Example 2).

Subunits of macromolecular assemblies are usually held together by the same four weak interactions (see Fig. 4-5) that stabilize folded proteins: the hydrophobic effect, hydrogen bonds, electrostatic interactions, and van der Waals interactions. Although none of these interactions is particularly strong on its own, stable association of macromolecular subunits is achieved by combining the effects of multiple weak interactions. This is possible because the free energy changes contributed by each weak interaction are added together. With a small correction for entropy changes, the overall binding constant for the association of subunits is the product of the equilibrium constants for each weak interaction $[K_A = (K_1)(K_2)(K_3)(. . .)(K_n)]$.

Far from being a liability, multiple weak interactions provide assembly systems with the ability to achieve exquisite specificity that is derived from the "fit" between **complementary surfaces** of interacting molecules (see Examples 4 and 5). Complementary surfaces are important for three reasons. First, atoms that have the potential to form hydrogen bonds or electrostatic bonds must be placed in a complementary arrangement for the bonds to form. Second, complementary surfaces can exclude water between subunits, as required for the hydrophobic effect. Third and most important, repulsive forces arising from collisions between even a few atoms on imperfectly matching surfaces are strong enough to effectively cancel interactions between two potential bonding partners.

To use a macroscopic analogy, the interactions between subunits of macromolecular assemblies have much more in common with Velcro fasteners than with snaps. Snaps provide an easy way to attach components to one another, and they can attach components whose surfaces touch only at the snaps. A single snap is often enough to hold two items together. By contrast, Velcro fasteners work because many tiny hooks become entrapped in a mesh of fibrous loops. The strength provided by each hook is minuscule, but when hundreds or thousands of hooks work together, bonding is strong. Velcro works best when the two bonding surfaces are smoothed against one another; in the case of rigid objects, a Velcro-like bond is tightest when the surfaces have complementary shapes. In molecular assemblies, tens of thousands of specific macromolecular associations are achieved by combining a small repertoire of weak bonds on complex, three-dimensional surfaces.

Many assembly reactions take advantage of flexibility in the protein subunits. In viral capsids (see Examples

5 and 6), hinges between the domains of the protein subunits provide the necessary flexibility to allow them to fit into more than one geometrical position. In some assemblies, flexible polypeptide strands knit subunits together (see Examples 1, 5, and 6). In other cases, assembly is coupled to the folding of the subunit proteins (see Examples 3, 4, and 6).

Symmetrical Structures Constructed from Identical Subunits with Equivalent (or Quasi-equivalent) Bonds

Studies of relatively simple systems composed of identical subunits, such as viruses and bacterial flagella, have provided most of what is known about assembly processes. The symmetry of these structures makes them ideal for analysis by X-ray crystallography and electron microscopy, and their biochemical simplicity facilitates analysis of assembly mechanisms. Subunits in asymmetric assemblies, such as transcription factor complexes (see Fig. 15-8), are likely to interact in the same way.

The subunits in a symmetrical macromolecular structure make identical bonds with one another. In practice, biological assemblies use only three fundamental types of symmetry. Proteins that assemble into flat structures, such as membranes, typically have plane hexagonal symmetry; filaments have helical symmetry; and closed structures have polygonal symmetry.

Subunits Arranged in Hexagonal Arrays in Plane Sheets

The simplest way to pack globular subunits in a plane is to form a hexagonal array with each subunit surrounded by six neighbors. This happens if one puts a layer of marbles in the bottom of a box and then tilts the box. A hexagonal array maximizes contacts between the surfaces of adjacent subunits. Membranes are the only flat surfaces in cells, and a number of membrane proteins crowd together in hexagonal arrays on or within the lipid bilayers. Connexons of gap junctions (Fig. 5-3), bacteriorhodopsin of purple membranes (see Fig. 7-8), and porin channels of bacterial membranes (see Fig. 7-8) all form regular hexagonal arrays in the plane of the lipid bilayer. Clathrin coats form hexagonal nets on the surface of membranes (Fig. 5-3).

Helical Filaments Produced by Polymerization of Identical Subunits with Like Bonds

Helical arrays of identical subunits form cytoskeletal filaments (see Examples 1 and 2), bacterial flagella (see Example 3), and some viruses (see Example 4). In helice

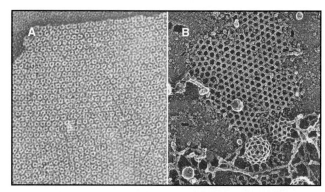

Figure 5-3   ELECTRON MICROGRAPHS SHOWING HEXAGONAL NETWORKS OF MEMBRANE PROTEINS. **A,** Integral membrane protein. Gap junction subunits called connexons span the lipid bilayer. An isolated junction was prepared by negative staining. **B,** Peripheral membrane proteins. Clathrin coats on the surface of a membrane in a hexagonal array. Introduction of fivefold vertices allows this sheet to fold up around a coated vesicle, shown at the bottom of the figure. This is a replica of the inner surface of the plasma membrane. (A, Courtesy of N. B. Gilula, Scripps Research Institute, La Jolla, California. B, Courtesy of J. Heuser, Washington University, St. Louis, Missouri.)

subunits are positioned like steps of a spiral staircase. Each subunit is located a fixed distance along the axis and rotated by a fixed angle relative to the previous subunit. Helices can have one or more strands. TMV has one strand of subunits (see Example 4), whereas bacterial flagella have 11 strands (see Example 3). Helices can be either solid, like actin filaments (see Example 1), or hollow, like bacterial flagella (see Example 3) and TMV (see Example 4).

The asymmetry of protein subunits gives most helical polymers in biology a polarity (see Examples 1, 3, and 4). Different bonding properties at the two ends of the polymer have important consequences for their assembly and functions. Myosin filaments (see Example 2) have a bipolar helix, a rare form of symmetry. (The DNA double helix [see Fig. 3-17] is geometrically symmetric, with one strand running in each direction, but the order of its nucleotide subunits gives each strand a polarity.)

Spherical Assemblies Formed by Regular Polygons of Subunits

Geometric constraints limit the ways that identical subunits can be arranged on a closed spherical surface with equivalent or nearly equivalent contacts between the subunits. By far, the most favored arrangement is based on a net of equilateral triangles. On a plane surface, these triangles will pack hexagonally with sixfold vertices (Fig. 5-2). Since the time of Plato, it has been appreciated that introducing vertices surrounded by three, four, or five triangles will cause such a network of triangles to pucker and, given an appropriate number of puckers, to close up into a complete shell (Fig. 5-4). Four

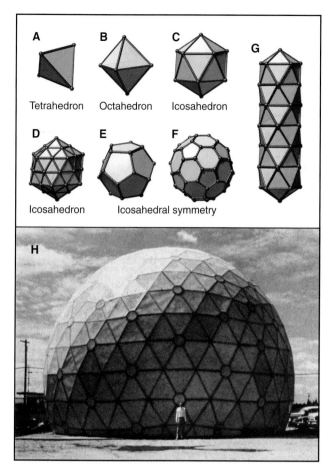

Figure 5-4 MODELS OF GEOMETRIC SOLIDS. **A,** A tetrahedron with four threefold vertices and four triangular faces. **B,** An octahedron with six fourfold vertices and eight triangular faces. **C–H, Various icosahedral solids with 12 fivefold vertices.** Many other arrangements of subunits are possible. **C,** One triangle on each face. **D,** Four triangles on each face. **E,** A dodecahedron with 20 vertices and 12 faces. **F,** An intermediate polyhedron with 60 vertices and 32 faces (12 pentagons and 20 hexagons). **G,** An extended structure made by including rings of hexagons between two icosahedral hemispheres. **H,** R. Buckminster Fuller standing in front of one of his geodesic domes. (From Caspar D, Klug A: Physical principles in the construction of regular viruses. Cold Spring Harbor Symp Quant Biol 27:1–24, 1962.)

threefold vertices make a tetrahedron, six fourfold vertices make an octahedron, and 12 fivefold vertices make an **icosahedron.** Remarkably, no other ways of arranging triangles will complete a shell. In addition to threefold, fourfold, or fivefold vertices that introduce puckers, a closed polygon can contain additional triangular faces and sixfold vertices to expand the volume. The sixfold vertices can be placed symmetrically with respect to the fivefold vertices to produce a spherical shell or asymmetrically to form an elongated structure (Fig. 5-4G).

Most closed macromolecular assemblies in biology are polygons with fivefold vertices (see Examples 5 to 7). (The cubic iron-carrying protein ferritin is an exception.) An important reason for this is that most struc-

tures require some sixfold vertices to provide sufficient internal volume. This favors fivefold vertices for the puckers, as they require much less distortion of the subunits located on the triangular faces of the hexagonal plane sheet than do threefold or fourfold vertices. Further, the distortion in the contacts between the triangles is minimized if the fivefold vertices are in equivalent positions. Closed icosahedral shells can be assembled from any type of asymmetrical subunit given two provisions: (1) The subunit must be able to form bonds with like subunits in a triangular network; and (2) these subunits must be able to accommodate the distortion required to form both fivefold and sixfold vertices. Both fibrous (Fig. 5-3B) and globular subunits (see Examples 5 to 7) can fulfill these criteria.

These considerations indicate that subunits in a closed macromolecular assembly must be arranged in rings of five or six. A simple variation has three like protein subunits on each face, but three different protein subunits, or more than three like subunits, can be used on each face to construct icosahedrons. The closest packing is achieved if the protein subunits form pentamers and hexamers, but other arrangements on the 20 faces of an icosahedron are possible (see Example 6).

New Properties from Sequential Assembly Pathways

To fully understand any assembly mechanism, it is necessary to determine the order in which the subunits bind together and the rates of these reactions. For most assembly reactions, more is known about the pathways from genetic or biochemical identification of intermediates than about the reaction rates. The following section describes some general principles about pathways.

All self-assembly processes depend on diffusion-driven, random, reversible collisions between the subunits. As is described in Chapter 4, the rate equation for such a second-order bimolecular reaction is

$$\text{Rate} = k_+(A)(B) - k_-(AB)$$

where k_+ is the association rate constant; k_- is the dissociation rate constant; and (A), (B), and (AB) are the concentrations of the reactants and products. Elongation of actin filaments (see Example 1) illustrates this mechanism.

The association rate is directly proportional to the concentration of subunits and a rate constant (k_+). This rate constant takes into account the rates of **diffusion** of the subunits, the size of their complementary surfaces, and the degree of tolerance in orientation permitted for binding. In general, association rate constants are limited by diffusion and are in the range of 10^5 to 10^7 $M^{-1} s^{-1}$ for most protein association reactions.

The rate of dissociation (k_) determines which complexes formed by random collisions are stable enough to participate in an assembly pathway. Specificity is achieved by rapid dissociation of nonspecific complexes. The sequence of random collisions, each followed by separation or bonding, can be viewed as a scanning process that allows each molecule to sample a variety of interactions. At cellular concentrations (see Fig. 3-27), intermolecular collisions between macromolecules are extremely frequent but usually involve irrelevant molecules or molecules that could assemble but that collide in the wrong orientation. Given these frequent random collisions, it is extremely important that proteins not be intrinsically "sticky." Dissociation of unrelated molecules that have collided by chance is just as important as is the formation of specific associations. Because interactions of individual atoms on the surfaces of proteins are relatively weak, random collisions are very brief unless two complementary surfaces collide in an orientation that is close enough to allow a large number of simultaneous weak interactions or to allow flexible strands to intertwine two subunits. Molecules with poorly aligned or uncomplementary surfaces rapidly dissociate by diffusing away from each other. This is how specific associations are achieved by random collisions.

The stability of macromolecular complexes varies considerably owing to two factors. First, collision complexes have a wide spectrum of dissociation rate constants ranging from greater than $1000 \, s^{-1}$ for very unstable complexes to less than $0.00001 \, s^{-1}$ for very stable complexes. (The former complexes have a half-life of 0.7 ms, whereas the half-life of the latter is 16 h. See Box 4-2 for an explanation of half-times.) Second, conformational changes often follow formation of a collision complex between subunits. These reactions are difficult to observe, but assembly of bacterial flagella provides one clear example (see Example 3). Because the equilibrium constants for all of the coupled reactions are multiplied, such conformational changes can provide the major change in free energy holding a structure together (see Fig. 4-3). The weakly associated conformation characteristic of a free subunit can be thought of as an *unsociable* state, whereas the strongly associated conformation found in a completed structure is considered an *associable* state.

Although all assembly reactions occur by chance encounters, large structures usually assemble by specific pathways in which new properties emerge at most steps. A new binding site for the next subunit may emerge from a conformational change in a newly incorporated subunit or by juxtaposition of two parts of a binding site on adjacent subunits. Such emergent properties favor addition of subunits in an orderly fashion until the process is completed. The assembly of myosin (see Example 2), tomato bushy stunt virus (see Example

5), and bacteriophage T4 (see Example 7) illustrates control of assembly by emergent properties.

Initiation of assembly is frequently much less favorable than its propagation. Free subunits associating randomly cannot participate in all the stabilizing interactions enjoyed by a subunit joining a preexisting structure. Consequently, assembly of the first few subunits to form a "nucleus" for further growth may be thousands of times less favorable than the steps that follow during the growth of the assembly (see Example 1). The chance of dissociation from the assembly is reduced once subunits can engage in the full complement of bonds made possible by conformational changes that stabilize the structure. Cells often solve the **nucleation** problem by constructing specialized structures to nucleate the formation of macromolecular assemblies (see Examples 3 and 6; also see Figs. 33-12, 33-13, and 34-16). Nucleation is not always the slowest step; in the case of myosin minifilaments, the initial step is the fastest (see Example 2).

Regulation at Multiple Steps on Sequential Assembly Pathways

Many assembly reactions proceed spontaneously in vitro, but all seem to be tightly regulated in vivo. For example, at the time of mitosis, cells disassemble their entire microtubule network and reassemble the mitotic spindle with the same subunits (Fig. 5-1). The following are some examples of the mechanisms that cells use to control assembly processes.

Regulation by Subunit Biosynthesis and Degradation

Cells regulate the supply of building blocks for assembly reactions. For example, a feedback mechanism controls the concentration of tubulin subunits available to form microtubules. The concentration of unpolymerized tubulin regulates the stability of tubulin mRNA. Experimental release of tubulin subunits in the cytoplasm results in degradation of tubulin mRNA and a decline in the rate of tubulin synthesis. On the other hand, red blood cells regulate the assembly of their membrane skeleton (see Fig. 7-10) by synthesizing a limiting amount of one subunit of the spectrin heterodimer. Following assembly of the membrane skeleton, proteolysis destroys the excess of the other subunit.

Regulation of Nucleation

Regulation of a rate-limiting nucleation step is particularly striking in the case of microtubules. Microtubule nucleation from subunits is so unfavorable that it rarely, if ever, occurs in a cell. Instead, all the microtubules grow from a discrete microtubule organizing center (Fig. 5-1). In animal cells, the principal microtubule organizing center is the centrosome, a cloud of amorphous material surrounding the centrioles (see Fig. 34-16). Varying the number, position, and activity of microtubule organizing centers helps cells to produce completely different microtubule arrays during interphase and mitosis.

Regulation by Changes in Environmental Conditions

Weak bonds between subunits allow cells to regulate assembly processes with relatively mild changes in conditions, such as in pH or ion concentrations. For example, when TMV infects a plant cell, the low concentration of Ca^{2+} in cytoplasm promotes disassembly of the virus because Ca^{2+} links the protein subunits together (see Example 4). Uncoating the RNA genome begins a new cycle of replication.

Regulation by Covalent Modification of Subunits

Phosphorylation of specific serine, threonine, or tyrosine residues (see Fig. 25-1) can regulate interactions of protein subunits in macromolecular assemblies. This is an excellent strategy because cell cycle and extracellular signals can control the activities of the kinases that add phosphate and the enzymes, called protein phosphatases, that reverse the modification. Given the uniform bonding between subunits of symmetrical macromolecular structures, phosphorylation of the same amino acid residue on each subunit can cause the whole structure to disassemble.

Reversible phosphorylation regulates the assembly of the nuclear lamina, the filamentous network that supports the nuclear envelope (see Fig. 14-8). At the onset of mitosis, a protein kinase adds several phosphate groups to the lamina subunits (see Fig. 44-6). The network of filaments falls apart when negatively charged phosphate groups overcome the weak interactions between the protein subunits. Removing these phosphates at the end of mitosis is one step in the reassembly of the nucleus. Similarly, phosphorylation of centrosomal proteins may be responsible for changes in their microtubule nucleation properties during mitosis (Fig. 5-1).

Several other chemical modifications regulate assembly reactions. Proteolysis is a drastic and irreversible modification used in the assembly of the bacteriophage T4 head (see Example 7) and collagen (see Fig. 29-4). Collagen is an extreme example, since its assembly also requires hydroxylation of prolines and lysines, glycosylation, disulfide bond formation, oxidation of lysines, and chemical cross-linking. Subunits in other assemblies are modified by methylation, acetylation, glycosylation, fatty acylation, tyrosination, polyglutamylation, or linkage to ubiquitin (or related proteins).

Regulation by Accessory Proteins

Self-assembly processes were originally thought to require only the components found in the final structure, but many assembly reactions either require or are facilitated by auxiliary factors. The **molecular chaperones** that promote protein folding (see Fig. 17-13) also promote assembly reactions. In fact, bacterial mutations that compromised assembly of bacteriophages led to the discovery of the original chaperonin-60, GroEL (see Fig. 17-16). This class of chaperones also facilitates assembly of oligomeric proteins, such as the chloroplast enzyme RUBISCO. These effects of chaperones may simply be due to their role in preventing aggregation during the folding of subunit proteins prior to their assembly. They may also participate directly in macromolecular assembly reactions, but this has not been proven.

Bacteriophage assembly also requires accessory proteins coded by the virus. T4 uses accessory proteins to assemble its head. Often, proteolysis destroys these accessory proteins prior to insertion of the viral DNA (see Example 7). Bacteriophage P22 uses an accessory **"scaffolding protein"** to guide assembly of its icosahedral capsid protein. The building blocks are apparently heterodimers or small oligomers of the two proteins. Scaffolding protein forms an internal shell inside the capsid. Before the DNA is inserted, the scaffolding proteins exit intact from the head (by an unknown mechanism) and recycle to promote the assembly of another virus.

Accessory molecules can specify the size of assemblies. The length of the RNA genome precisely regulates the size of TMV (see Example 4). A giant α-helical polypeptide called nebulin runs from end to end of skeletal muscle actin filaments, determining their length (see Chapter 39). By contrast, a kinetic mechanism determines the length of skeletal muscle myosin filaments (see Example 2).

Numerous proteins regulate assembly of the cytoskeleton, and some are incorporated into the polymer network. Taking actin as an example, different classes of proteins regulate nucleotide exchange, determine the concentration of monomers available for assembly, nucleate and cap the ends of filaments, sever filaments, and cross-link filaments into bundles or random networks (see Fig. 33-10). Similar regulatory proteins likely are involved in other macromolecular assemblies, such as microtubules, intermediate filaments, myosin filaments, and coated vesicles.

The following examples demonstrate how the principles that were discussed previously govern the assembly of real biological structures.

EXAMPLE 1

Actin Filaments: Rate-Limiting Nucleation and the Concept of Critical Concentration

Actin filaments consist of two strands of subunits wound helically around one another (Fig. 5-5). (The structure can also be described as a single short-pitch helix with all of the subunits repeating every 5.5 nm.) Each subunit contacts two subunits laterally and two other subunits longitudinally. Hydrogen bonds, electrostatic bonds, and hydrophobic interactions stabilize contacts between subunits. Subunits all point in the same direction, so the polymer is polar. The appearance of actin filaments with bound myosin (see Fig. 33-8) originally revealed the **polarity** now seen directly at atomic resolution. The decorated filament looks like a line of arrowheads with a point at one end and a barb at the other.

Actin binds adenosine diphosphate (ADP) or adenosine triphosphate (ATP) in a deep cleft. Irreversible hydrolysis of bound ATP during polymerization complicates the assembly process in a number of important ways (see Fig. 33-8). Here, assembly of ADP-actin, a relatively simple, reversible reaction, illustrates the concepts of nucleation and critical concentration.

Initiation of polymerization by pure actin monomers, also called **nucleation,** is so unfavorable that polymer accumulates only after a lag (Fig. 5-6C). This time is required to nucleate enough filaments to yield

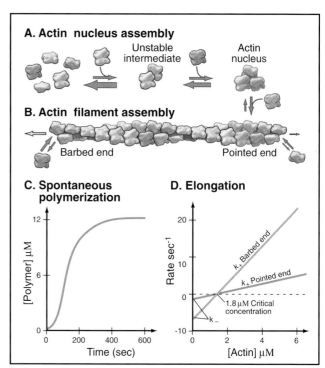

Figure 5-6 ACTIN FILAMENT ASSEMBLY. **A,** Formation of a trimeric nucleus from monomers. **B,** Elongation of the two ends of a filament by association and dissociation of monomers. **C,** Time course of spontaneous polymerization of purified ADP-actin under physiological conditions. **D,** Dependence of the rates of elongation at the two ends of actin filaments on the concentration of ADP-actin monomers. (Reference: Pollard TD: Rate constants for the reactions of ATP- and ADP-actin with the ends of actin filaments. J Cell Biol 103:2747–2754, 1986.)

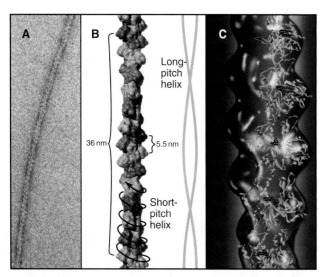

Figure 5-5 ACTIN FILAMENT STRUCTURE. **A,** Electron micrograph of a negatively stained actin filament. **B,** Atomic model showing two ways to describe the helix: (1) two long-pitch helices (*orange/yellow* and *blue/green*) or (2) a one start short-pitch helix including all of the subunits (*yellow* to *green* to *orange* to *blue*). **C,** Ribbon model of actin, including a space-filling model of ADP superimposed on a reconstruction of the filament from electron micrographs. (Courtesy of U. Aebi, University of Basel, Switzerland.)

a detectable rate of polymerization. Initiation of each new filament is slow because small actin oligomers are exceedingly unstable. Actin dimers dissociate on a microsecond time scale, so their concentration is low, making addition of a third subunit rare. Actin trimers are the nucleus for filament growth (Fig. 5-6A) because they are more stable than dimers and can add further monomers rapidly. A trimer is a reasonable nucleus, since it is the smallest oligomer with a complete set of intermolecular bonds. Unfavorable nucleation reduces the chance that new filaments form spontaneously. This enables the cell to control this reaction with specific nucleating proteins (see Figs. 33-12 and 33-13).

Elongation of actin filaments is a bimolecular reaction between monomers and a single site on each end of the filament (Fig. 5-6B–D). The growth rate of each filament is directly proportional to the concentration of subunits. (In a bulk sample, the rate of change in polymer concentration by elongation is proportional to both the concentrations of filament ends and subunits.) If the rate of assembly is graphed as a function of the concentration of actin monomer, the slope is the association rate constant, k_+. The y-intercept is the dissociation rate constant, k_-. The elongation rate is zero where the plot crosses the x-axis. This monomer concentration is called the **critical concentration.** Above this concentration, polymers grow longer. Below this concentration, polymers shrink. Polymers grow until the monomer concentration falls to the critical concentration. At the critical concentration, subunits bind and dissociate at the same rate. The rates of association and dissociation are somewhat different at the two ends of the polar filament. The rapidly growing end is called the barbed end, and the slowly growing end is called the pointed end.

EXAMPLE 2

Myosin Filaments: New Properties Emerge as the Filaments Grow

Myosin-II forms bipolar filaments held together by interactions of the α-helical, coiled-coil tails of the molecules (Fig. 5-7). Antiparallel overlap of tails forms a central bare zone flanked by filaments with protruding heads. On either side of the bare zone, parallel interactions extend the filament. The simplest myosin-II minifilaments from nonmuscle cells consist of just eight molecules (Fig. 5-7B). Muscle myosin filaments are much larger but are built on the same plan (Fig. 5-7A). Molecules are staggered at 14.3-nm intervals in these filaments. This arrangement maximizes the ionic bonds between zones of positive and negative charge that alternate along the tail. Hydrophobic interactions are also important; 170 water molecules dissociate from every molecule incorporated into a muscle myosin filament.

Myosin-II minifilaments form in milliseconds by three successive dimerization reactions (Fig. 5-8). Under experimental conditions in which filaments are partially assembled, antiparallel dimer and antiparallel tetramer intermediates can be detected. Computer modeling of the time course of assembly provides limits on the rate constants for each transition. The association rate constants for formation of dimers and tetramers are larger than those predicted by diffusional collisions. Perhaps the long tails of the subunits form a variety of weakly bound complexes that rearrange rapidly to form stable intermediates without dissociating.

This simple mechanism shows how new properties can emerge during an assembly process. The parallel interactions of tails seen in tetramers and octamers are not favored until the myosin has formed antiparallel dimers in the first step.

The elongation of muscle myosin filaments from the central bare zone provides a second example of how assembly properties can change as a structure forms. Muscle myosin forms stable dimers by side-by-side association of the tails. These are called parallel dimers because both pairs of heads are at the same end. Parallel dimers add to the ends of filaments in a diffusion-limited, bimolecular reaction. The reaction is unusual in that the dissociation rate constant increases with the length of the filament, eventually limiting the length of the polymer at the point where the dissociation rate equals the association rate.

EXAMPLE 3

Bacterial Flagella: Assembly with a Rate-Limiting Folding Reaction

Bacterial flagella are helical polymers of a protein called flagellin (Fig. 5-9). Eleven strands of subunits surround a narrow central channel.

Nucleation of a flagellar filament is even less favorable than for an actin filament, so assembly from purified flagellin depends absolutely on the presence of preexisting flagellar ends. Bacteria use structures called the base plate and hook assembly to initiate flagellar growth and to anchor the flagellum to the rotary motor that turns it (see Fig. 38-24).

Amazingly, flagella grow only at the end located farthest from the cell. Flagellin subunits synthesized in the cytoplasm diffuse through the narrow central channel of the flagellum (Fig. 5-9) out to the distal tip, where a cap consisting of an accessory protein prevents their escape before assembly.

Elongation of a filament by addition of purified flagellin is expected to be a bimolecular reaction dependent on the concentrations of flagellin monomers and polymer ends. This behavior is observed at

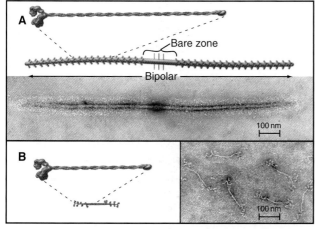

Figure 5-7 STRUCTURE OF MYOSIN FILAMENTS. **A,** Skeletal muscle myosin filament. Drawing and electron micrograph of a negatively stained filament. **B,** *Acanthamoeba* myosin-II minifilament. Drawing and electron micrograph of a negatively stained filament. (A, Courtesy of J. Trinick, Bristol University, England.)

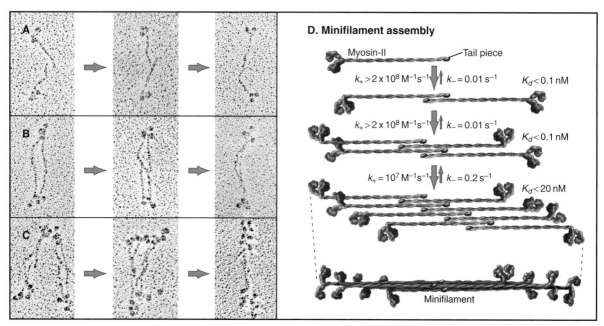

Figure 5-8 **ASSEMBLY OF AMOEBA MYOSIN-II MINIFILAMENTS. A–C,** Electron micrographs showing the successive assembly of dimers, tetramers, and octamers. **D,** Diagram of the assembly pathway with rate and equilibrium constants. A nonhelical tailpiece at the tip of the tail engages another myosin tail to form an antiparallel dimer with a 15-nm overlap. Two dimers form a tetramer, and two tetramers form an octamer. The second and third steps depend on completion of the first step. (A–C, Courtesy of J. Sinard, Yale Medical School, New Haven, Connecticut. D, Reference: Sinard JH, Pollard TD: *Acanthamoeba* myosin-II minifilaments assemble on a millisecond time scale. J Biol Chem 265:3654–3660, 1990.)

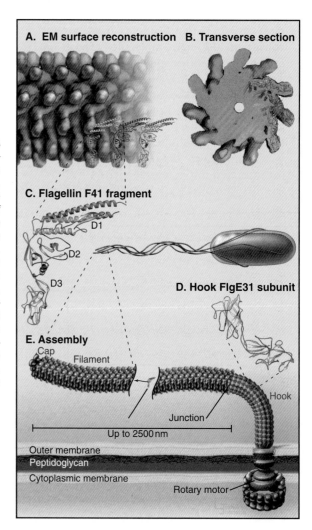

Figure 5-9 **STRUCTURE OF THE FLAGELLA FROM THE BACTERIUM *SALMONELLA TYPHIMURIUM*. A,** Surface rendering from reconstructions of electron micrographs with superimposed ribbon diagrams of the structure of the flagellin subunit. **B,** Cross section from image processing of electron micrographs, showing the central channel and superimposed ribbon diagrams of the structure of the flagellin subunit. (PDB file: 1IO1.) **C,** Ribbon diagram of part of the flagellin subunit. (PDB file: 1WLG.) **D,** Ribbon diagram of the hook subunit, FlgE31. **E,** Drawing of a flagellar filament attached via the hook segment to the basal body, the rotary motor that turns the flagellum. The cap structure is found at the distal end of the filament. A flagellin subunit in transit through the central channel from its site of synthesis in the cytoplasm to the distal tip is shown in the break in the filament. (A–B, From Mimori-Kiyosue Y, Yamashita I, Fujiyoshi Y, et al: Role of the outermost subdomain of *Salmonella* flagellin in the filament structure revealed by electron cryomicroscopy. J Mol Biol 284:521–530, 1998. B, Reference: Samatey FA, Imada K, Nagashima S, et al: Structure of the bacterial flagellar protofilament and implications for a switch for supercoiling. Nature 410:331–337, 2001. C, Reference: Samatey FA, Matsunami H, Imada K, et al: Structure of the bacterial flagellar hook and implication for the molecular universal joint mechanism. Nature 431:1062–1068, 2004.)

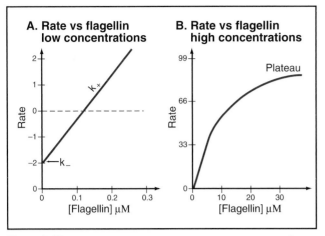

A. Rate vs flagellin low concentrations

B. Rate vs flagellin high concentrations

Figure 5-10 ELONGATION OF FLAGELLAR FILAMENTS FROM SEEDS (FRAGMENTS OF FLAGELLA) IN VITRO. The plots show the dependence of the elongation rate on subunit concentration. **A,** Low concentrations. **B,** High concentrations. (Redrawn from Asakura S: A kinetic study of in vitro polymerization of flagellin. J Mol Biol 35:237–239, 1968.)

low concentrations of flagellin, where the rate of elongation is proportional to the concentrations of flagellin and nuclei (Fig. 5-10A). Unexpectedly, the rate of elongation plateaus at a maximum of about three monomers per second at high subunit concentrations (Fig. 5-10B). This rate-limiting step is thought to be a relatively slow conformational change that is required before the next subunit can bind. The parts of the flagellin monomer that form the core of the

polymer are disordered in solution, so the slow step may involve folding of these disordered peptides into α-helices that interact to form the two concentric cylinders inside the flagellum. Slow folding converts an unsociable monomer into an associable subunit of the flagella and allows further growth.

EXAMPLE 4

Tobacco Mosaic Virus: A Helical Polymer Assembled with a Molecular Ruler of RNA

Tobacco mosaic virus (TMV) was the first biological structure recognized to be a helical array of identical subunits, and it was the first helical protein structure to be determined at atomic resolution (Fig. 5-11). The virus is a cylindrical copolymer of one RNA molecule (the viral genome) and 2130 protein subunits. The protein subunits are constructed from a bundle of four α-helices, shaped somewhat like a bowling pin. These subunits pack tightly in the virus and are held together by hydrophobic interactions, hydrogen bonds, and salt bridges. The RNA follows the protein helix in a spiral from one end of the virus to the other, nestling in a groove in the protein subunits. This groove is lined with arginine residues to neutralize the negative charges along the RNA backbone (Fig. 5-11C–D). Each protein subunit also makes hydrophobic and electrostatic interactions with three of the RNA bases.

Production of infectious TMV from RNA and protein subunits was the first self-assembly reaction

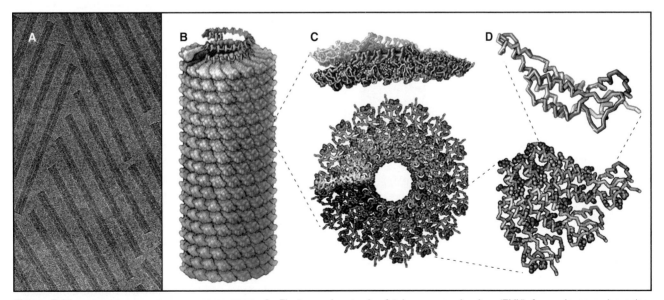

Figure 5-11 STRUCTURE OF TOBACCO MOSAIC VIRUS. **A,** Electron micrograph of tobacco mosaic virus (TMV) frozen in amorphous ice. **B,** Atomic structure showing the protein subunits in *gray* and the individual nucleotides of RNA in *red*. **C–D,** Details of the atomic structure of one turn of the helix and of subunits. Basic residues are *blue;* note the basic residues in the groove that binds the RNA. Acidic residues are *red*. (PDB file: 2TMV. A, Courtesy of R. Milligan, Scripps Research Institute, La Jolla, California. B–D, Courtesy of D. Caspar, Florida State University, Tallahassee, Florida; Reference: Namba K, Caspar D, Stubbs G: Enhancement and simplification of macromolecular images. Biophysical J 53:469–475, 1988.)

reproduced from purified components. At the time, during the 1950s, newspapers proclaimed, "Scientists create life in a test tube!"

RNA regulates assembly of the protein subunits in two ways. First, RNA allows the protein to polymerize at a physiological pH. Protein alone forms helical polymers of varying lengths at nonphysiological acidic pH; but at neutral pH, it forms only unstable oligomers of 30 to 40 protein subunits, slightly more than two turns of the helix (Fig. 5-12). Monomers and small oligomers of coat protein exchange rapidly with these oligomers, but disorder in the polypeptide loops lining the central channel limits growth beyond 40 subunits. RNA promotes folding of these disor-

dered loops, acting as a switch to drive propagation of the helix by the incorporation of additional protein subunits. Second, RNA is the molecular ruler that determines the precise length of the assembled virus. Only after interacting with RNA at the growing end of the polymer can subunits fold into a structure compatible with a stable virus.

EXAMPLE 5

Tomato Bushy Stunt Virus: Flexibility within Protein Subunits Accommodates Quasi-equivalent Bonding

The first atomic structure of a virus (tomato bushy stunt virus, TBSV) revealed that the flexibility required to form both fivefold and sixfold icosahedral vertices lies within the protein subunit rather than in the bonds between subunits. The 180 identical subunits associate in pairs in two different ways, distinguished in Figure 5-13 by the green-blue and red colors. The blue subunit of the green-blue pairs is used exclusively for fivefold vertices. Three red subunits and three green subunits form six-fold vertices. External contacts of both green-blue and red pairs with their neighbors are similar, but the contacts between pairs of red subunits differ from pairs of green-blue subunits. The difference is achieved by changing the position of the amino-terminal portion of the coat protein polypeptide chain. Two subunits in green-blue pairs pack tightly against each other, providing the sharp curvature required at fivefold vertices. In red dimers, the amino-terminal peptide acts as a wedge to pry the inner domains of the subunits apart and flatten the surface, as is appropriate for sixfold vertices. Thus, the flexible arm acts like a switch to determine the local curvature. This subunit flexibility accommodates the 12-degree difference in packing at fivefold and sixfold vertices. Other spherical viruses use a similar strategy to achieve **quasi-equivalent** packing of identical subunits.

TBSV provided the first of many examples of flexible arms that lace subunits together. Amino-terminal extensions of three red subunits intertwine at sixfold vertices. As if holding hands, these arms form a continuous network on the inner surface, reinforcing the coat.

Icosahedral plant viruses like TBSV assemble from pure protein and RNA. An attractive hypothesis is that local information built into the growing shell specifies the pathway, as follows. Building blocks are dimers of coat protein. To initiate assembly, three dimers in the red conformation bind a specific viral RNA sequence, forming a structure similar to a sixfold vertex. Folding of the arms in this nucleus forces the next three dimers to take the green-blue conforma-

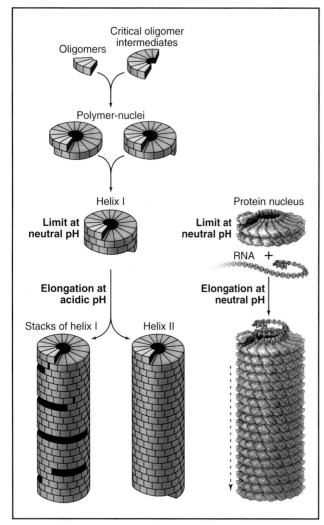

Figure 5-12 ASSEMBLY PATHWAY OF TOBACCO MOSAIC VIRUS. The subunit protein forms small oligomers of two plus turns at neutral pH that can elongate in the presence of RNA. On their own, the protein oligomers can form imperfect protein helices at acid pH. (Redrawn from Potschka M, Koch M, Adams M, Schuster T: Time resolved solution X-ray scattering of tobacco mosaic virus coat protein, kinetics, and structure of intermediates. Biochemistry 27:8481–8491, 1988.)

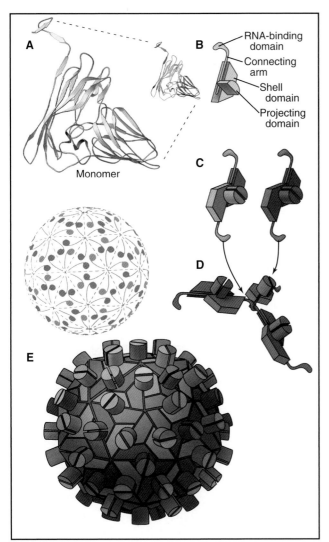

Figure 5-13 TOMATO BUSHY STUNT VIRUS STRUCTURE AND ASSEMBLY
PATHWAY. **A,** Ribbon diagram of a coat protein subunit. (PDB file:
2TBV.) **B,** Block diagram of one subunit. **C,** Block diagrams of
dimers of coat protein subunits. **D,** Proposed nucleus for a sixfold
vertex with three dimers (*red*). Three additional dimers (*green-blue*)
are proposed to add to complete a sixfold vertex. Five *blue* subunits
associate to make a fivefold vertex. **E,** Two different surface repre-
sentations of the viral capsid showing the quasi-equivalent positions occupied by *red, blue,* and *green* subunits. (C–D, Redrawn
from Olsen A, Bricogne G, Harrison S: Structure of tomato bushy
stunt virus IV. The virus particle at 2.9 Å resolution. J Mol Biol
171:61–93, 1983.)

tion, since no intermolecular binding sites are available for their arms. The greater curvature of the
green-blue dimers dictates that fivefold vertices form
at regular positions around the nucleating sixfold
vertex. Additional fivefold vertices form appropriately as positions for this more favored association
become available around the growing shell. The
beauty of this idea is that local information (the availability of intermolecular binding sites for strands)

automatically favors the insertion of green-blue or
red dimers, as appropriate, to complete the icosahedral shell.

EXAMPLE 6

Simian Virus 40: Quasi-equivalent Bonding of Protein Subunits with a Flexible Adapter

Flexible polypeptide strands, even more extensive
than those of plant viruses, lace together the icosahedral capsid of DNA tumor viruses of animal cells,
such as polyomavirus (Fig. 5-14A) and simian virus
40 (SV40) (Fig. 5-14B–E). The geometry is more complicated than that of TBSV, since all 360 subunits are
clustered in groups of five, called pentamers. Bonds
between subunits within these pentamers are all
identical. Icosahedral geometry is achieved by surrounding 12 pentamers with 5 other pentamers, and
surrounding the remaining 60 pentamers with 6
pentamers.

Connections that accommodate both fivefold and
sixfold packing link pentamers together. Each subunit
has three parts: (1) a rigid structural unit that makes
up one-fifth of the wall of a pentamer, (2) a "hook"
that interacts with a subunit in an adjacent pentamer,
and (3) a flexible connector between the structural
unit and the hook. The hook attaches firmly to its
neighbor by being incorporated into a β-sheet, formed
mainly by the other polypeptide chain. The flexible
connector deforms to accommodate different angles
in groups of five and six. These helical bundles,
together with connectors from adjacent subunits,
reinforce the connections made by the hook. Little is
known about the assembly pathways for DNA viruses,
such as SV40, but it is safe to predict that lacing
together the helical bundles and the β-sheets from
two different protein subunits requires careful
control of protein folding.

With its surface lattice composed entirely of pentamers, SV40 is an extreme example of how large
viruses have departed from true icosahedral symmetry to assemble shells with sufficient carrying
capacity to enclose the viral chromosome. Adenovirus solves the problem by using 60 copies of one
protein for its fivefold vertices and 720 copies of a
second protein organized into 240 units of three
subunits each.

EXAMPLE 7

Bacteriophage T4: Three Irreversible Assembly Pathways Form a Metastable Structure

Bacteriophage T4 is a virus of the bacterium *Escherichia coli* (Fig. 5-15). Genetic analysis established
that more than 49 distinct gene products contribute to assembly of this virus. Three separate,

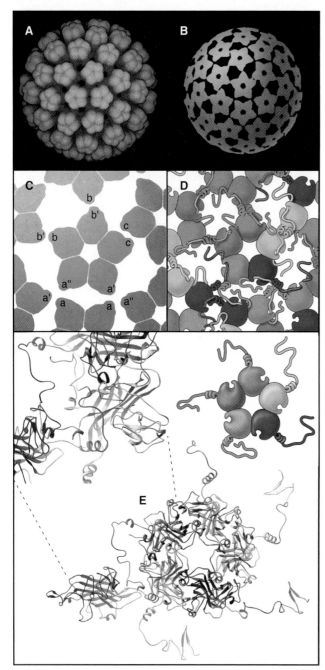

Figure 5-14 STRUCTURE AND ASSEMBLY OF DNA TUMOR VIRUSES. **A,** Surface view of a polyomavirus capsid shell. **B–E, Simian virus 40 structure.** (PDB file: 1SID.) **B–C,** Packing of capsid subunits. **D,** Diagrammatic representation of capsid subunits and their extended C-terminal tails that knit the capsid together by engaging neighboring subunits. **E,** Ribbon diagram of the pentamer of subunits with details of the C-terminal tails. Note the association of the *red* tail with the *blue* subunit and the association of the *blue* tail with the *gold* subunit. (A, Courtesy of D. Caspar, Florida State University, Tallahassee. Reference: Namba K, Caspar D, Stubbs G: Enhancement and simplification of macromolecular images. Biophysical J 53:469–475, 1988. B–D, Redrawn from Caspar DLD: Virus structure puzzle solved. Curr Biol 2:169–171, 1992. B–E, Reference: Liddington R, Yan Y, Moulai J, et al: Structure of simian virus 40 at 3.8 Å resolution. Nature 354:278–284, 1991.)

multicomponent substructures—heads, tails, and tail fibers—assemble along independent pathways and combine to form the virus (Fig. 5-16). Emergence of new properties automatically orders the steps along each pathway, so assembly occurs sequentially even in the presence of reactive pools of all of the subunits. A good product is ensured because defective subassemblies fail to attach and are rejected.

A protein complex nucleates the growth of a preliminary version of the icosahedral head and later attaches one vertex of the head to the tail. A complex of the major head protein with several accessory proteins adds to the growing head. The accessory proteins end up inside the precursor head. After proteolysis cleaves 20% of the peptide from the N-terminus of the major head protein and degrades the accessory proteins, a major conformational change shifts part of the head protein from inside to outside and expands the volume of the head

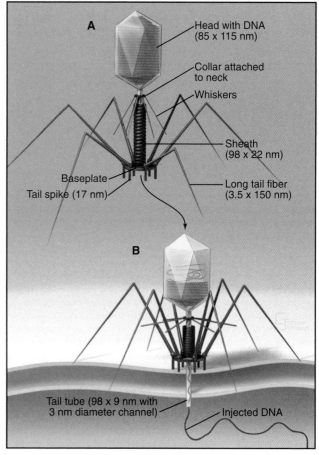

Figure 5-15 STRUCTURE OF BACTERIOPHAGE T4. **A,** Infectious phage particle. **B,** Association with *Escherichia coli* and injection of DNA by contraction of the sheath. (Reference: Leiman PG, Chipman PR, Kostyuchenko VA, et al: Three-dimensional rearrangement of proteins in the tail of bacteriophage T4 on infection of its host. Cell 118:419–429, 2004. Also see the movie on the journal web site: http://download.cell.com/supplementarydata/cell/118/4/419/DC1/leiman-et-al.movie-2.)

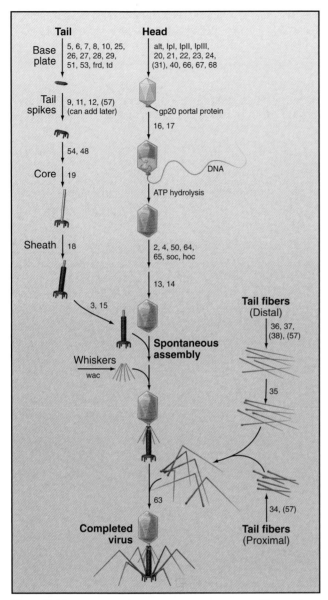

Figure 5-16 ASSEMBLY PATHWAY OF BACTERIOPHAGE T4. The numbers refer to genes required at each step. (Redrawn from Wood WB, Edgar RS, King J, et al: Bacteriophage assembly. Fed Proc 27:1160–1166, 1968.)

by 16%. Then, an ATP-driven rotary motor inserts the 166,000-base-pair DNA molecule into the head through a hole in a vertex. This motor, one of the strongest in nature, can produce a force of 70 pN, enough to compress the DNA inside the head to a pressure of 60 atmospheres. Within the head, the pressurized DNA is restrained in a near-crystalline, metastable state until it is released during infection of the *E. coli* host.

The tail is a double cylinder of a rod-like, helical core and a loosely fitting helical sheath, both attached to a base plate. A complicated pathway involving at least 15 gene products and 13 steps assembles the hexagonal base plate. One of these proteins, acting

like a "safety" on a gun, stabilizes its shape. A plug in the middle of the hexagonal base plate nucleates the polymerization of core subunits. Next, the sheath subunits polymerize into a helical lattice that mimics the underlying core. In mutants that lack base plates, sheath subunits assemble inefficiently into a shorter and fatter helix.

The three assembly lines converge, joining heads to tails and then adding the six long, independently assembled tail fibers that give the completed virus its spider-like appearance. Attachment of tail fibers to the base plate somehow removes the "safety" that held the base plate in its hexagonal form. The finished bacteriophage is hardy enough to survive for 20 years at 4°C in a metastable state, poised to infect its bacterial host.

When tail fibers contact a susceptible bacterium, dramatic structural changes in the sheath force the tail core through both bacterial membranes in a syringe-like fashion (Fig. 5-15B). The base plate changes from a hexagon into a six-pointed star that cuts loose the central plug with its attached tail core. The weakness of the contacts between sheath and core allows the sheath to "recrystallize" into its preferred short, fat, helical form. Because the sheath is firmly attached at both the base plate and the top of the tail core, this spring-like contraction drives the core through the base plate into the bacterium. This action also unplugs the head, allowing the pressurized DNA to extrude through the channel in the core into the bacterium. Thus, the linear assembly reactions and an ATPase motor produce a machine that can, when triggered, do physical work.

SELECTED READINGS

Caspar DLD: Virus structure puzzle solved. Curr Biol 2:169–171, 1992.

Caspar DLD, Klug A: Physical principles in the construction of regular viruses. Cold Spring Harbor Symp Quant Biol 27:1–24, 1962.

Harrison SC: What do viruses look like? Harvey Lect 85:127–152, 1991.

Leiman PG, Chipman PR, Kostyuchenko VA, et al: Three-dimensional rearrangement of proteins in the tail of bacteriophage T4 on infection of its host. Cell 118:419–429, 2004. [Also see movie on the journal web site: http://download.cell.com/supplementarydata/cell/118/4/419/DC1/leiman-et-al.movie-2.]

Liddington RC, Yan Y, Moulai J, et al.: Structure of simian virus 40 at 3.8 A resolution. Nature 354:278–284, 1991.

Namba K, Stubbs G: Structure of tobacco mosaic virus at 3.6 A resolution: Implications for assembly. Science 231:1401–1406, 1986.

Oosawa F, Asakura S: Thermodynamics of the Polymerization of Protein. New York, Academic Press, 1975.

Pollard TD, Blanchoin L, Mullins RD: Biophysics of actin filament dynamics in nonmuscle cells. Ann Rev Biophys Biomolec Struct 29:545–576, 2000.

Rossmann MG, Mesyanzhinov VV, Fumio Arisaka F, Leiman PG: The bacteriophage T4 DNA injection machine. Curr Opin Struct Biol 14:171–180, 2004.

Simpson AA, Tao Y, Leiman PG, et al: Structure of the bacteriophage phi29 DNA packaging motor. Nature 408:745-750, 2000.

Sinard JH, Pollard TD: *Acanthamoeba* myosin-II minifilaments assemble on a millisecond time scale with rate constants greater than those expected for a diffusion limited reaction. J Biol Chem 265:3654-3660, 1990.

Smith DE, Tans SJ, Smith SB, et al: The bacteriophage straight phi29 portal motor can package DNA against a large internal force. Nature 413:748-752, 2001.

Wood WB: Genetic control of bacteriophage T4 morphogenesis. Symp Soc Dev Biol 31:29-46, 1973.

Research Strategies

Research in cell biology aims to discover how cells work at the molecular level. Powerful tools are now available to achieve this goal. To understand how these methods contribute to the broad effort to explain cellular function, this chapter begins with a brief account of the synthetic approach used in cell biology. This strategy is based on the premise that one can understand a complex cellular process by reducing the system to its constituent parts and characterizing their properties. This approach, also called **reductionism**, has dominated cell biology research since the middle of the 20th century and has succeeded time after time. For example, most of what is understood about protein synthesis has come from isolating and characterizing ribosomes, messenger RNAs (mRNAs), transfer RNAs (tRNAs), and accessory factors. In this and many other cases, proof of function has been established by reconstituting a process from isolated parts of the molecular machine and verifying these conclusions with genetic experiments.

This reductionist approach involves much more than simply identifying the molecular parts of a cellular machine. Essential tasks include the following:

1. Defining a biological question
2. Making a complete inventory of molecular constituents
3. Localizing these molecules in cells
4. Measuring the cellular concentrations of these molecules
5. Determining atomic structures of these molecules
6. Identifying molecular partners (and pathways)
7. Measuring rate and equilibrium constants
8. Reconstituting the biological process from purified molecules
9. Testing for physiological function
10. Formulating a mathematical model of system behavior

This agenda is complete for remarkably few biological processes. Bacterial chemotaxis is one example (see Figs. 27-12 and 27-13). Often, much is known about some aspects of a process, such as a partial list of participating molecules, the localization of these molecules in a cell, or a test for function by removing the genes for one or more molecules from an experimental organism. Rarely is enough information available about molecular concentrations and reaction rates to formulate a mathematical model of the process to verify that the system actually works as anticipated. Thus, much work remains to be done.

Box 6-1 is a guide for locating descriptions of methods used throughout this book. This chapter begins with imaging, one extremely valuable method for studying cells. Microscopy of live and fixed cells often provides initial hypotheses about the mechanisms of cellular process. It is also a valuable adjunct to genetic analysis and testing mechanisms. The chapter then covers a selection of other methods that are used for cell biology research.

Imaging

Microscopy is useful for cell biologists, owing to fortunate coincidences within the electromagnetic spectrum. First, the wavelength of visible light is suitable for imaging whole cells, and the wavelength of electrons is right for imaging macromolecular assemblies and cellular organelles. Second, glass lenses may be used to focus visible light, and electromagnetic lenses can focus electrons. Resolution, the ability to discriminate two points, is directly related to the wavelength of the light. The equation is

$$D = 0.61\lambda/N\sin\alpha$$

where D is the resolution, λ is the wavelength of light, N is the refractive index of the medium between speci-

mens, and $\sin\alpha$ is the numerical aperture of the lens. The limit of resolution with visible light and glass lenses is normally about 0.2 μm. Although short-wavelength X-rays are not useful for imaging because there is no convenient way to focus them, analysis of their diffraction by molecular crystals is still the chief method for determining structures of cellular macromolecules at atomic resolution.

Microscopes carry out two functions. The first is to enlarge an image of the specimen so that it can be seen with the eye or a camera. Everyone is familiar with the concept that a magnifying lens can enlarge an image. Just as important, but less appreciated, microscopes must produce **contrast** so that details of the enlarged image stand out from each other.

Light Microscopy

A half dozen optical tricks are used to produce contrast in light micrographs of biological specimens (Table 6-1 and Fig. 6-1). These are called wide-field methods, as a broad beam of illuminating light is focused on the specimen by a condenser lens.

The classic light microscopic method is **bright field,** whereby the specimen is illuminated with pure white light. Most cells absorb very little visible light and thus show little contrast with bright-field illumination (Fig. 6-2A). For this reason, staining is used to increase light absorption and contrast. Because staining makes it difficult to see through thick tissues, specimens must also be relatively thin, about 1 μm for critical work. Slides for histologic and pathological study are produced by fixing cells with cross-linking chemicals, embedding them in paraffin or plastic, making sections with a microtome (a device that cuts a series of thin slices from the surface of a specimen), and staining with a variety of dyes (for examples, see Figs. 28-2, 28-5, 28-6, 28-7, 29-3, 29-8, 32-1, and 32-2). Alternatively, thin slices may be taken from frozen tissue and then stained. In either case, the cells are killed by fixation or sectioning prior to observation.

Observations of live cells require other methods to produce contrast. In every case, these methods are also useful for fixed cells. **Phase-contrast** microscopy generates contrast by interference between light scattered by the specimen and a slightly delayed reference beam of light. Small variations in either thickness or refractive index (speed of light) can be detected, even within specimens that absorb little or no light (Fig. 6-2B). **Differential interference contrast** (DIC) produces an image that looks as though it is illuminated by an oblique shaft of light (Fig. 6-2C). What actually happens is that two nearby beams interfere with each other, producing contrast in proportion to local differences (gradient) in the refractive index across the specimen. Thus, a vesicle with a high refractive index (slow speed of light) in

Table 6-1

METHODS FOR PRODUCING CONTRAST IN LIGHT MICROSCOPY

Type	Principle	Requirements	Live Cells	Fixed Cells
Bright field	Absorption of visible light	Light-absorbing stains on a thin specimen	No	Yes
Fluorescence	Emission of light by fluorescent molecule	Cellular molecules labeled with fluorescent dyes or expression of fluorescent proteins	Yes	Yes
Phase contrast	Variations in thickness and refractive index within specimen	Relatively flat cells	Yes	Yes
Differential interference contrast (DIC)	Gradient of refractive index across the specimen	None; may be used on thick, unstained specimens	Yes	Yes
Dark field	Scattering of light	Relatively thin, simple specimen	Yes	Yes
Polarization	Differences in refractive index for perpendicular beams of polarized light	Birefringent (highly ordered along a linear axis) elements in specimen	Yes	Yes

cytoplasm will appear light on one side (where the refractive index is increasing with respect to the cytoplasm) and dark on the other (where the refractive index is decreasing).

Fluorescence microscopy requires a fluorescent dye or protein in the specimen. Remarkable sensitivity makes fluorescence microscopy a powerful tool. Under favorable conditions, single fluorescent dyes or fluorescent protein molecules can be imaged. When a fluorescent molecule absorbs a photon of light, an electron is excited into a higher state. Nanoseconds later, a longer-wavelength (lower-energy) photon is emitted when the

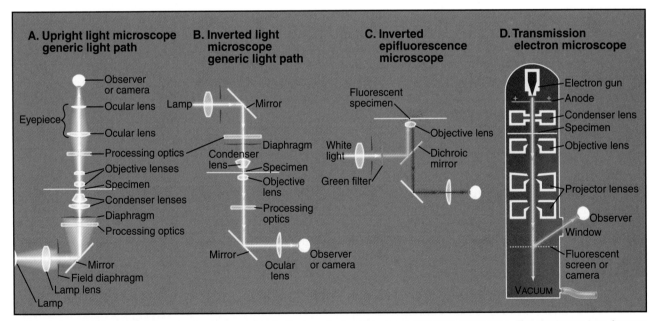

Figure 6-1 **LIGHT PATHS THROUGH VARIOUS MICROSCOPES. A,** Basic optical path in an upright light microscope. The condenser lens focuses light on the specimen. Light interacts with the specimen. The objective lens collects and recombines the altered beam. An ocular lens projects the enlarged image onto the eye or a camera. Processing optics produce contrast by phase contrast, differential interference, or polarization. **B,** Optical path in an inverted light microscope. **C,** Epi-illumination for fluorescence microscopy. The objective lens acts as the condenser to focus the exciting, short-wavelength light (*green,* in this example) on the specimen. Fluorescent molecules in the specimen absorb exciting light and emit longer-wavelength light (*red,* in this example). The same objective lens collects emitted long-wavelength light. A dichroic mirror in the light path reflects exciting light and transmits emitted light. An additional filter (not shown) blocks any short-wavelength light from reaching the viewer. **D,** Optical path in a transmission electron microscope. Electromagnetic lenses carry out the same functions as glass lenses in a light microscope. For visual observations, the electrons produce visible light from a fluorescent screen.

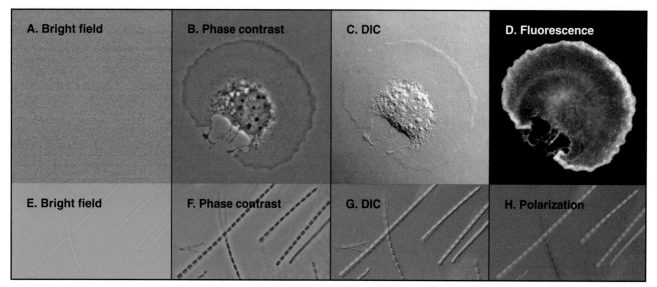

Figure 6-2 COMPARISON OF METHODS TO PRODUCE CONTRAST. **A–D,** Micrographs of a spread mouse 3T3 cell grown in tissue culture on a microscope slide, then fixed and stained with rhodamine-phalloidin, a fluorescent peptide that binds actin filaments. Contrast methods include bright field **(A)**, phase contrast **(B)**, differential interference contrast **(C)**, and fluorescence **(D)**. **E–H,** Micrographs of myofibrils isolated from skeletal muscle. Contrast methods include bright field **(E)**, phase contrast **(F)**, differential interference contrast **(G)**, and polarization **(H)**. The A-bands, consisting of parallel thick filaments of myosin (see Fig. 39-3), appear as dark bands with phase contrast and are birefringent (either bright or dark, depending on the orientation) with polarization. (A–D, Courtesy of R. Mahaffy, Yale University, New Haven, Connecticut.)

electron falls back to its ground state. For example, the fluorescent dye rhodamine absorbs green light (shorter wavelength) and emits red light (longer wavelength). Fluorescence microscopes use filters and special dichroic mirrors that reflect short wavelengths of light used to illuminate and excite fluorescent specimens but transmit the longer-wavelength emitted fluorescent light into the imaging system (camera). Strategically placed emission filters remove the exciting light reflected by the specimen so that only the fluorescent regions of the specimen appear bright. To provide fluorescence, a purified lipid, protein, or nucleic acid can be labeled with a fluorescent dye and injected into a live cell, where it will seek its natural location (see Figs. 37-6 and 38-9). Molecules labeled with a fluorescent dye can also be used to locate a target in a fixed and permeabilized cell. A powerful version of this strategy uses antibodies, proteins produced by the immune system (see Fig. 28-9), to react with specific molecular targets. Antibodies are tagged with fluorescent dyes and used to localize molecules in fixed cells by fluorescence microscopy (Fig. 6-3E). This is called immunofluorescence. Another strategy is to label an oligonucleotide with a fluorescent dye to probe for nucleic acids with complementary sequences in fixed cells (see Fig. 13-15). Yet another approach is to localize individual structures, such as actin filaments, with a fluorescent dye attached to a small peptide that binds tightly to these filaments (Fig. 6-2D).

The discovery of proteins whose amino acid sequence renders them naturally fluorescent, such as **green fluorescent protein** (GFP) from jellyfish, made fluorescence microscopy immensely valuable for observation of individual proteins in live cells. Typically, DNA-encoding GFP is joined to one end of the coding sequence for a cellular protein and introduced into cells, which then synthesize a fusion protein consisting of GFP linked to the protein of interest. GFP fluorescence marks the fusion protein wherever it goes in the cell and can be quantified to determine how many labeled molecules reside in a particular cellular location (Fig. 6-3). Ideally, the coding sequence for GFP fusion protein is inserted into the genome of the test cell in place of the wild type gene, and the fusion protein is shown to function normally by genetic or biochemical experiments. Where this is difficult or impossible (e.g., in most studies of metazoan cells), the GFP fusion protein can be produced from exogenous DNA or RNA introduced into the cell. Mutations in GFP can change its fluorescence properties, providing probes in a range of colors and with differing sensitivities to distinct biochemical parameters in the cell, such as pH, Ca^{2+} concentration, and kinase activity. When attached to different protein types, these probes allow two or more protein species to be visualized simultaneously in the same cell and can serve as "biosensors" to measure changes in the intracellular environment and in a protein's behavior/interactions.

Dark-field microscopy and **polarization microscopy** have specialized uses in biology. In dark-field microscopy, the specimen is illuminated at an oblique angle so that only light scattered by the specimen is

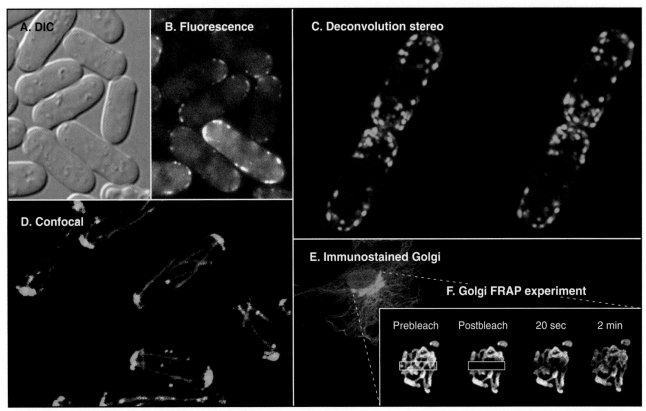

Figure 6-3 FLUORESCENCE MICROSCOPY METHODS. **A–C, Light micrographs of live fission yeast expressing GFP fused to myosin-I. A,** Differential interference contrast (DIC). **B,** Standard wide-field fluorescence of the same cells. **C,** Stereo pair of a three-dimensional reconstruction of a stack of optical sections made by deconvolution of wide-field images. Removal of out-of-focus blur improves the resolution and contrast of small patches enriched in myosin-I. A stereo view is obtained by focusing your left eye on the left image and right eye on the right image. This can be achieved by holding the micrographs close to your eyes and then gradually withdrawing the page about 12 inches. **D,** Confocal fluorescence micrograph of fission yeast cells showing *red* microtubules and *green* Tea 1 protein (a protein involved in determining cell shape). This thin optical section eliminates the blur from fluorescence in other planes of focus. **E–F, Fluorescence recovery after photobleaching. E,** A fibroblast cell in tissue culture stained with fluorescent antibodies for the Golgi apparatus *(yellow)* and microtubules *(green)* and with the fluorescent dye DAPI for DNA *(blue)*. **F,** A series of fluorescence micrographs of a fibroblast cell expressing GFP-galactosyltransferase, which concentrates in the Golgi apparatus. The GFP in a bar-shaped zone is bleached with a strong pulse of light, and the fluorescence is followed over time. After 2 minutes GFP-galactosyltransferase redistributes by lateral diffusion in the membranes to fill in the bleached zone. (A–C, From Lee W-L, Bezanilla M, Pollard TD: Fission yeast myosin-I, Myo1p, stimulates actin assembly by Arp2/3 complex and shares functions with WASp. J Cell Biol 151:789–800, 2000. D, Courtesy of Hilary Snaith and Kenneth Sawin, University of Edinburgh, Scotland. E–F, Courtesy of J. Lippincott-Schwartz, N. Altan, and K. Hirschberg, National Institutes of Health, Bethesda, Maryland.)

collected by the objective lens. Recall how easy it is to detect tiny dust particles in a beam of light in a dark room. The contrast is so great that single microtubules stand out brightly from the dark background. However, for the images to be interpretable, the specimen must be very simple, much simpler than a cell. A dark-field image of something as complicated as cytoplasm is very confusing, owing to multiple overlapping objects that scatter light.

Like dark-field microscopy, polarization microscopy produces a bright image on a dark background. When a specimen is viewed between two crossed polarizing filters, only light whose polarization state is modified by the specimen will pass through the second polarizer to the image. Polarization microscopy relies on a specimen's crystalline order, or birefringence, to provide con-

trast. Birefringent specimens, such as filaments in striated muscle (Fig. 6-2H) or microtubules in a mitotic spindle, are aligned enough that polarized light, oriented so that it vibrates along the length of the polymers, passes through more slowly than does light vibrating perpendicular to the polymers (much as a knife cuts through meat faster with the grain than across it). Most cells do not have sufficient birefringence to produce a useful image with a conventional polarization microscope. New methods are making this approach more applicable for future work.

Computer processing can greatly enhance contrast and remove optical artifacts from images. For example, computer-enhanced DIC can image single microtubules (see Fig. 34-7). New methods of **image processing** can even improve detection beyond the classic limit determined by the wavelength of light (about 0.2 μm with green light). A processing method called **deconvolution** produces clear fluorescence images of thick specimens by using an iterative computer process to restore light that is blurred out of focus to its proper focal plane. Starting with a stack of blurry images taken at different focal planes all the way through the specimen using a traditional wide-field microscope, this method produces a remarkably detailed three-dimensional image in sharp focus throughout (Fig. 6-3C).

Confocal microscopy also produces thin optical sections of fluorescent specimens. Rather than illuminating with a wide beam of light, this method uses a point of laser light sharply focused in all three directions: *x, y,* and *z.* The point of light is scanned across the specimen in a raster pattern (checkerboard pattern, like the electron beam in a TV) to excite fluorescent molecules. Light emitted at each consecutive point in the specimen passes through a pinhole placed next to the detector to remove any light that does not come directly from each focal point. A computer reassembles the image from the fluorescence at each point in this checkerboard of fluorescence signals (Fig. 6-3D; see also Figs. 13-12, 14-2, and 44-23). A series of confocal images taken at different planes of focus can be used for three-dimensional reconstructions.

Electron Microscopy

A **transmission electron microscope** (Fig. 6-1D) can resolve points below 0.3 nm, but the practical resolution is usually limited by damage to the specimens from the electron beam and the methods used to prepare specimens. Historically, the most common method used to prepare cells for electron microscopy was to fix the specimen with chemicals, embed it in plastic, cut the specimen into **thin sections,** and stain the sections with heavy metals (Fig. 6-4F). With this technique, the resolution is limited to about 3 nm, but that is sufficient to bridge the gap between light microscopy and molecular structures. During the heyday of electron microscopy in cell biology, between 1950 and 1970, thin sections revealed most of what is known about the organization of organelles in cells.

The highest resolution is attained with regular specimens, such as two-dimensional protein crystals rapidly frozen and viewed while embedded in a thin film of vitreous (i.e., amorphous, noncrystalline) ice (see Fig. 5-11A). This is called **cryoelectron microscopy** because the stage holding the frozen specimen is cooled to liquid nitrogen temperature. Electron micrographs and electron diffraction of frozen crystals have produced structures of bacteriorhodopsin (see Fig. 7-8), aquaporin water channels (see Fig. 10-15), and tubulin (see Fig. 34-4) at resolutions of 3 to 4 nm. Computational image processing methods are used to calculate the three-dimensional structure of proteins in these regular specimens. These methods are similar to those used to calculate electron density maps from X-ray diffraction patterns (see Fig. 3-10). Although the resolution is limited and data collection is tedious in electron crystallography, electron microscopic images have the advantage of containing the phase information that is often difficult to ascertain with X-ray diffraction.

Electron microscopy is valuable for studying protein polymers and other large macromolecular specimens at less-than-atomic resolution. Diverse methods are used to prepare specimens and impart contrast. One way is to freeze filaments or macromolecular assemblies in vitreous ice, as described earlier (see Figs. 34-7 and 36-4A). A second is negative staining, whereby specimens are dried from aqueous solutions of heavy metal salts (Fig. 6-4B). A shell of dense stain encases particles on the surface of a thin film of carbon and can preserve structural details at a resolution of about 1 nm. Alternatively, macromolecules dried on a smooth surface can be shadowed with a thin coat of metal evaporated from an electrode (Fig. 6-4C). A variation of this approach that improves preservation is to freeze specimens rapidly, evaporate the ice surrounding the molecules, and then apply a coat of platinum (see Figs. 30-4 and 34-11).

Computer image processing of micrographs of certain types of structures can yield an average three-dimensional reconstruction of a molecular structure. Particles with helical symmetry, such as actin filaments (see Fig. 33-7) and microtubules (see Fig. 34-5), are analyzed by an image-processing method called deconvolution to reconstruct the three-dimensional structure. Single particles may also be reconstructed by first classifying images of thousands of randomly oriented particles into categories corresponding to different views. Then, an average three-dimensional structure is calculated computationally from this ensemble. One example is the Sec61p translocon associated with a ribosome (see Fig. 20-6). More recently, computing advances have led to the development of electron microscope tomography, in which many pictures are taken of a relatively thick specimen from different angles (by tilting the specimen inside the microscope). Superimposition blurs each picture, but when they are merged together into a three-dimensional map, structures as complex as entire cells can be visualized at a resolution of a few nanometers.

Cells and tissues can also be frozen rapidly and prepared for electron microscopy without chemical fixation. In the **freeze-fracture method,** the frozen specimen is cleaved to expose the inside of the cells, and exposed surfaces are rotary-shadowed with a thin coat of platinum. This surface coat is then viewed by using a transmission electron microscope (Fig. 6-4D). Frequently, the cleavage plane splits lipid bilayers in half to reveal proteins embedded in the plane of the mem-

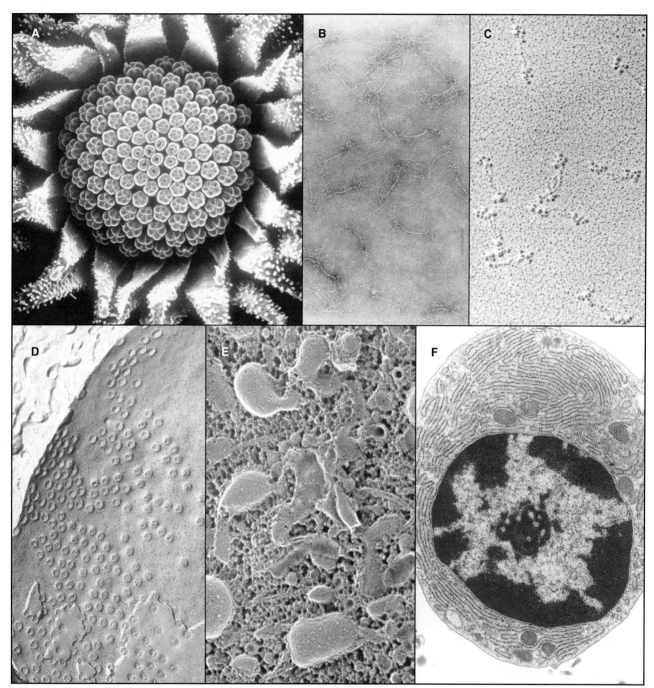

Figure 6-4 ELECTRON MICROGRAPHS. **A,** Scanning electron micrograph of developing flowers of the Western mountain aster. **B–F,** Transmission electron micrographs. **B,** Myosin-II minifilaments on a thin carbon film prepared by negative staining with uranyl acetate. **C,** Myosin-II minifilaments on a mica surface prepared by rotary shadowing with platinum. **D,** Freeze-fracturing. The cleavage plane passed through the cytoplasm and then split apart the two halves of the bilayer of the nuclear envelope. This fractured surface was then shadowed with platinum. The cytoplasm is in the upper left. Nuclear pores are prominent in the nuclear envelope. **E,** A cultured cell prepared by rapid freezing, fracturing, deep etching, and rotary shadowing with platinum. Membranes of the endoplasmic reticulum stand out against the porous cytoplasmic matrix. **F,** Thin section of a plasma cell, an immune cell specialized to synthesize and secrete antibodies. (A, Courtesy of J. L. Bowman, University of California, Davis. C, Courtesy of J. Sinard, Yale University, New Haven, Connecticut. E, Courtesy of John Heuser, Washington University, St. Louis, Missouri. D–F, Courtesy of Don W. Fawcett, Harvard Medical School, Boston, Massachusetts.)

brane. If some of the frozen water in a fractured speci-men is evaporated from the surface before shadowing, three-dimensional details of deeper parts of the cyto-plasm can be revealed. A variation of this method involves extracting soluble molecules and membranes with mild detergents before freezing, fracturing, evapo-rating frozen water, and rotary-shadowing (Fig. 6-4E; see also Fig. 1-13).

A **scanning electron microscope** (SEM) can be used on thicker specimens, such as whole cells or tissues that have been fixed, dried, and coated with a thin metal film. Here, an electron beam scans a raster pattern over the surface of specimens, and secondary electrons emitted from the surface at each point are collected and used to reconstruct an image (Fig. 6-4A). The resolution of conventional SEM is limited, but nonetheless valu-able, for studying surface features of cells and their three-dimensional relationships in tissues. SEMs that use special high-energy (field emission) guns to produce the electron beam have greatly improved resolution, and these have been very useful for studying cellular sub-structures, such as nuclear pores (see Fig. 14-6B).

Choice of Organisms for Biological Research

Given the origin of life from a common ancestor (see Fig. 2-1), one can learn about basic cellular processes in any organism that has the molecules of interest. It is useful to select an organism that specializes in the

process, such as skeletal muscle to study contractile proteins (see Chapter 39) or Chlamydomonas to study flagella (see Fig. 38-20). Some organisms are much more amenable to investigation because communities of sci-entists have invested years of hard work to develop genetic, molecular genetic, and biochemical methods for experimentation. These valuable experimental tools have attracted investigators to a growing number of "model" organisms (Table 6-2).

Model Organisms

Ideal model organisms have completely sequenced genomes and facile methods to manipulate the genes, including replacement of a gene with a modified gene, by the process of homologous recombination. Haploid organisms with one copy of each chromosome after mitotic division are particularly favorable for detecting the effects of changes in genes, called mutations (Box 6-2). It is useful for a haploid organism to have a diploid stage with two copies of each chromosome and a sexual phase, during which meiotic recombination occurs between the chromosomes from the two parents. (See Fig. 45-7 for details on recombination.) This allows one to construct strains with a variety of mutations and facilitates mapping mutations to a particular gene. In addition, diploids carrying a lethal mutation of a gene that is essential for life can be propagated, provided that the mutation is recessive.

Budding yeast and fission yeast meet all of these criteria, so they are widely used to study basic cellular

Table 6-2

MODEL GENETIC ORGANISMS

Organism	Genome Size and Ploidy	Genome Sequenced	Number of Genes	Homologous Recombination	Meiotic Recombination	Biochemistry
Gram-negative bacterium, *Escherichia coli*	4.6 Mb, haploid	Yes	4288	Yes	No	Excellent
Cellular slime mold, *Dictyostelium discoideum*	34 Mb, haploid	Yes	~12,000	Yes	No	Excellent
Budding yeast, *Saccharomyces cerevisiae*	12.1 Mb, haploid	Yes	~6604	Yes	Yes	Good
Fission yeast, *Schizosaccharomyces pombe*	14 Mb, haploid	Yes	~4900	Yes	Yes	Good
Nematode worm, *Caenorhabditis elegans*	97 Mb, diploid	Yes	~18,266	Difficult	Yes	Poor
Fruit fly, *Drosophila melanogaster*	180 Mb, diploid	Yes	~13,338	Difficult	Yes	Fair
Mustard weed, *Arabidopsis thaliana*	100 Mb, diploid	Yes	~25,706	No	Yes	Poor
Mouse, *Mus musculus*	3000 Mb, diploid	Yes	~25,000	Yes	Yes	Good
Human, *Homo sapiens*	3000 Mb, diploid	Yes	~25,000	Yes, cultured cells	Yes	Good

Allele. A version of a gene

Complementation. Providing gene function in *trans* (i.e., by another copy of a gene)

Conditional Mutation. A mutation that gives an altered phenotype only under certain conditions, such as temperature, medium composition, and so on.

Diploid. A genome with two copies of each chromosome, one from each parent

Dominant Mutation. A mutation that gives an altered phenotype, even in the presence of a copy of the wild-type gene

Essential Gene. A gene whose function is required for viability

Gene. The nucleotide sequence required to make a protein or RNA product, including the coding sequence, flanking regulatory sequences, and introns, if present

Genome. The entire genetic endowment of an organism

Genotype. The genetic complement, including particular mutations

Haploid. A genome with single copies of each chromosome

Mutant. An organism that contains a mutation of interest

Mutation. A change in the chemical composition of a gene, including changes in nucleotide sequence, insertion, deletions, and so on.

Pedigree. Family history of a genetic trait

Phenotype. (From the Greek term for "shining" or "showing") Appearance of the organism as dictated by its genotype

Plasmid. A circular DNA molecule that self-replicates in the cytoplasm of a bacterium or nucleus of a eukaryote

Recessive Mutation. A mutation that gives an altered phenotype only when no wild-type version is present

Recombination. Physical exchange of regions of the genome between homologous chromosomes or between a plasmid and a chromosome

Wild Type. The naturally occurring allele of a gene; the phenotype of the naturally occurring organism

biochemical, and microscopic analysis revolutionized research in cell biology. However, yeast are solitary cells with specialized lifestyles.

Multicellular organisms are required to study the development and function of tissues and organs. Flies, nematode worms, mice, and humans share many ancient, conserved genes that control their cellular and developmental systems, so flies and worms are popular for basic studies of animal development and tissue function. However, vertebrates have evolved a substantial number of new gene families (roughly 7% of total genes) and a large number of new proteins by rearranging ancient domains in new ways. Therefore, mice are used for experiments on specialized vertebrate functions, especially those of the nervous system, despite being more difficult to work with than flies and worms are. Although not an experimental organism, humans are included on this list because much can be learned by analysis of human genetic variation and its relationship to disease. Humans are, of course, much more eloquent than the model organisms when it comes to describing their medical problems, many of which have a genetic basis that can be documented by analysis of pedigrees and DNA samples. Arabidopsis is the most popular plant for genetics because its genome is small, reproduction is relatively rapid, and methods for genetic analysis are well developed. Its genome was the first of a plant to be completely sequenced. One drawback is the lack of methods to replace genes by homologous recombination (see later section).

By focusing on a limited number of easy-to-use model organisms, biological research raced forward in the last quarter of the 20th century. This focus does have liabilities. For one, these organisms represent a very limited range of lifestyles. Thousands of other solutions to survival exist in nature, and they tend to be ignored. At the cellular level, these liabilities are less severe, since most cellular adaptations are ancient and shared by most organisms.

Cell Culture

Regardless of the species to be studied, growing large populations of isolated cells for biochemical analysis and microscopic observation is helpful. This is straightforward for the unicellular organisms such as fungi or bacteria, which can be grown suspended in a nutrient medium. These organisms can also be grown on the surface of gelled agar in a petri dish. When single cells are dispersed widely on an agar surface, each multiplies to form a macroscopic colony, all descendents of a single cell. This family of cells is called a clone.

For multicellular organisms, it is often possible to isolate single live cells by dissociating a tissue with proteolytic enzymes and media that weaken adhesions between the cells. Many but not all isolated cells can be

functions. These free-living haploid organisms have a tractable diploid stage in their life cycles. Moving between haploid and diploid stages greatly simplifies the process of creating and analyzing recessive mutations. This is important because most loss-of-function mutations are recessive. Even before their genomes were sequenced, the availability of yeast for genetic,

grown in sterile media, a method called tissue culture or cell culture. Terminally differentiated cells such as muscle or nerve cells do not reenter the cell cycle and grow. Cells that are predisposed to grow in the body including fibroblasts (see Fig. 28-4) and endothelial cells from blood vessels (see Fig. 30-13) will grow if the nutrient medium is supplemented with growth factors to drive the cell cycle (see Fig. 41-7). This is accomplished by adding fetal calf serum, which contains a particularly rich mixture of growth factors. Some cultured cells grow in suspension, but most prefer to grow on a surface of plastic or glass (Fig. 6-2), often coated with extracellular matrix molecules for adhesion (see Fig. 30-11). This is the origin of the term *in vitro,* meaning "in glass," used to describe cell culture. Normal cells grow until they cover the artificial surface, when contacts with other cells arrest further growth. Dissociation and dilution of the cells onto a fresh surface allow growth to resume. Most "primary cells" isolated directly from tissues divide a limited number of times (see Fig. 12-15). Primary cells can become immortal, either through mutations or transformation by a tumor virus that overcomes cell cycle controls. Such immortal cells are called cell lines. Similar changes allow cancer cells to grow indefinitely. HeLa cells are a famous cell line derived from Henrietta Lax, an African-American patient with cervical cancer. HeLa cells have been growing in laboratories for more than half a century.

A variation on cell culture is to grow a whole organ or part of an organ in vitro. The requirements for organ culture are often more stringent than those for growing individual cells, but the method is used routinely for experiments on slices of brain tissue and for studying the development of embryonic organs.

Inventory: Gene and Protein Discovery

Classical Genetics: Identification of Genes through Mutations

The approach in classical genetics is to identify mutations that compromise a particular cellular function and then to find the responsible gene(s). This approach is extremely powerful, especially when little or nothing is known about a process or when the gene product (usually a protein) is present at low concentrations. Yeast genetic studies have been spectacularly successful in mapping out complex pathways, including identification of the proteins that regulate the cell cycle (see Chapters 40 to 44) and the proteins that operate the secretory pathway (see Chapter 21).

Because one generally does not know the relevant genes in advance, it is important that mutations are introduced randomly into the genome and, ideally, limited to one mutation in each organism tested. A prerequisite for such a genetic screen is a good assay for the biological function of interest. Simplicity and specificity are essential, as interesting mutations may be rare, and much effort may be expended characterizing each mutation. The assay may test the ability to grow under certain conditions, drug resistance, morphologic changes, cell cycle arrest, or abnormal behavior. Mutations arise spontaneously at low rates, so often a chemical (e.g., ethyl methyl sulfonate or nitrosoguanidine) or radiation is used to increase the frequency of damage. Another approach is to insert an identifiable segment of DNA randomly into the genome. This simultaneously disrupts genes and marks them for subsequent analysis. Because the damage is random, the trick is to find the particular damage that changes the physiology of the organism in an informative way.

Haploid organisms are favorable for detecting mutations because damage to the single copy of a relevant gene will alter function, and either a loss of function or a gain of function can be detected with suitable test conditions (i.e., the ability to grow under certain conditions), biochemical assay, or morphologic assay. A disadvantage is that haploid organisms are not viable following the loss of function of an essential gene. Selecting for **conditional mutant** alleles allows the haploid organism to survive mutation of an essential gene under **permissive conditions** (e.g., low temperatures) but not under **restrictive conditions** (e.g., high temperatures). A further advantage of haploid organisms is that one can usually identify the mutated gene by a **complementation** experiment. Mutant cells are induced to take up a plasmid library containing fragments of the wild-type genome or cDNAs. **Plasmids** are circular DNA molecules that can be propagated readily in bacteria and, if suitably designed, in eukaryotes as well. Plasmids carrying the wild-type gene will correct loss-of-function mutations, allowing colonies of cells to grow normally. Plasmids complementing the mutation are isolated and sequenced. Additional tests are required to confirm that the wild-type gene in the plasmid corresponds to the mutant gene, as in some cases, raising the level of an unrelated gene can rescue a mutant phenotype. However, once this is done, the mutant gene can be isolated and sequenced to determine the nature of the damage. This complementation test can also be used to discover genes from other species that correct the mutation in the model organism. For example, genes for human cell cycle proteins can complement many cell cycle mutations in yeast (see Chapter 40). For gain-of-function mutations, a gene library from the mutant cell is inserted into plasmids, which are then tested for their ability to cause the altered phenotype in wild-type cells.

Genetics in obligate diploid organisms is more complicated. Many mutations will appear to have no effect, provided that the corresponding gene on the other chromosome functions normally. These **recessive mutations** produce a phenotype only after crossing two mutant organisms, yielding 25% of offspring with two copies of the mutant gene. (Consult a genetics textbook for details on Mendelian segregation.) Other mutations will yield an altered phenotype even when only one of the two genes is affected. These **dominant mutations** include simple loss of function when two wild-type genes are required to make sufficient product for normal function (called **haplo-insufficiency**); production of an altered protein that compromises the formation of a large assembly by normal protein subunits produced by the wild-type gene (called **dominant negative**); and production of an unregulated protein that cannot be controlled by partners in the cell (another type of dominant negative).

The classic method for identifying a mutated gene is **genetic mapping.** One observes the frequency of recombination between known markers and the mutation of interest in genetic crosses. This is usually sufficient to map a gene to a broad region of a particular chromosome. If a complete genome sequence is available, the database of sequenced genes in the area highlighted by mapping is examined to look for sensible candidate genes. These candidates can then be studied to establish which one carries the mutation. Another approach is to make the mutation by inserting a piece of DNA (called a transposable element) randomly into the genome. If one of these insertions causes a mutant phenotype, the transposable element may be recovered together with some of the surrounding chromosome, which is sequenced to identify the disrupted gene.

Once a gene required for the function of interest is sequenced (see Fig. 3-16), the primary structure of the protein (or RNA) is deduced from translating the coding sequence with a computer. Much can be learned by identifying RNAs or proteins with similar sequences or domains in the same or other species, particularly if something is known about the function of the corresponding gene product. Protein can often be expressed from a cDNA copy of the mRNA, tested for activity and binding partners, and (when fused to GFP or when used to make an antibody) localized in cells.

Further insights regarding function are often obtained by disruption of a gene. Genomic DNA can be used to construct a plasmid that contains two substantial regions of the chromosome (usually several thousand base pairs) flanking either the entire gene to be targeted or a significant portion thereof. In the plasmid, these "targeting" regions flank a selectable marker, for example, a gene encoding resistance to a particular drug that would normally kill the cells. If introduced into cells capable of homologous recombination, the targeting regions can recombine into the chromosome, thereby replacing the DNA between the targeting sequences with the selectable marker and disrupting the gene, ideally creating a **null mutation.** The selectable marker is used to enrich for cells with the disrupted gene. Gene disruption is readily accomplished in yeast and, with somewhat more difficulty, in vertebrate cells but is more complicated in flies, in which this gene-targeting technology is less well developed. Fortunately, an alternative method called RNAi (for **RNA interference**) can lower the levels of particular mRNAs from many cells, including those in worms and cultured cells of flies and humans (discussed later, and see Fig. 16-12 for details).

Genomics and Reverse Genetics

Thanks to large-scale DNA sequencing projects, nearly complete sequences of the coding regions of the most popular experimental organism are now available (see Figs. 2-4 and 2-9). When fully annotated (i.e., all sequences coding for genes have been identified and catalogued), these genome sequences will be the definitive inventory of genes. This is easier said than done, as accurate and complete identification of genes in raw sequence data is still challenging (see Chapter 12). The task has been aided by constructing databases containing millions of sequence fragments derived from cDNA copies of expressed genes (**expressed sequence tags,** or ESTs), which help to document the diversity of products created by transcription and RNA processing (see Chapter 15).

Nevertheless, even before genome annotation is complete, these sequences make possible a new approach for relating genes to biological function. Given the sequence of a gene of interest, the initial strategy is to search computer databases for proteins with similar sequences and known functions to try to predict what the protein might do. This is surprisingly fruitful, as many genes occur as extended families. First, one scans the protein sequence for conserved **sequence motifs** (regions of a few to several hundred amino acid residues). To accomplish particular tasks, for example, to be a protein kinase, proteins use motifs that arose early in evolution and are now widely scattered throughout the genome (see Fig. 25-4). Dozens of motifs are now known (and more are discovered daily), so finding such a motif in your protein can reveal that it binds to phosphorylated tyrosine, is an enzyme that methylates other proteins, or has one of the dozens of functions that are ascribed to particular motifs. Once predicted sequences have been analyzed, one can check when and where the gene is expressed in the organism, test the consequences of deleting the gene, or test for interactions of the protein with other proteins (see later section). These tests can be done one gene at a time or on a genome-wide scale. For example, investigators created strains of budding yeast lacking each of the 6000 genes and tested for interaction of the products of each of these genes with the products of all other genes. These preliminary screening tests often yield some clues about function. Ultimately, however, function is understood only when representatives of each protein family are studied in detail by the biophysical, biochemical, and cellular methods described in the following sections.

Reverse genetics refers to the process of starting with a known gene and selectively disrupting its function. One common approach used in yeasts is gene disruption, described previously. For metazoans, gene disruption is also used, but the most widely used method of reverse genetics is RNAi (discussed later in the chapter in the section titled "Physiological Testing").

Biochemical Fractionation

The biochemical approach (to the inventory) is to purify active molecules for analysis of structure and function. This requires a sensitive, quantitative assay to detect the component of interest in crude fractions, an assay to assess purity, and a battery of methods to separate the molecule from the rest of the cellular constituents. Assays are as diverse as the processes of life. Enzymes are often easy to measure. Many molecules are detected by binding a partner molecule. For example, nucleic acids bind complementary nucleotide sequences and sequence-specific regulatory proteins; receptors bind ligands; antibodies bind their antigens; and particular proteins bind partner proteins. More difficult assays reconstitute a cellular process, such as membrane vesicle fusion, nuclear transport, or molecular motility. Devising a sensitive and specific assay is one of the most creative parts of this approach. A second prerequisite for purification is a simple method for assessing purity. Various types of **gel electrophoresis** often work brilliantly (Box 6-3 and Fig. 6-5).

With a functional assay and a method to assess purity, one sets about purifying the molecule of interest. Highly abundant constituents, such as actin or tubulin, may require purification of only 20- to 100-fold, but many important molecules, such as signaling proteins and transcription factors, constitute less than 0.1% of the cell protein, so extensive purification is required.

First, the cell is disrupted gently to avoid damage to the molecule of interest. This may be accomplished physically by mechanical shearing with various types of **homogenizers** or, where appropriate, chemically, with mild detergents that extract lipids from cellular membranes. Next, the homogenate is **centrifuged** to separate particulate and soluble constituents. If the molecule of interest is soluble, it can be purified by sophisticated **chromatography** methods (Box 6-4 and Fig. 6-6) given sufficient starting material.

If a cDNA copy of the mRNA for a protein of interest is available, rare proteins or modified proteins can often be expressed in large quantities in bacteria, yeast, or insect cells. An advantage of this approach is that mutations can be made at will, including substitution of one or more amino acids or deletion of parts of the protein. Addition of domains can be useful for characterizing the protein such as the following:

- **GFP:** Addition of a fluorescent protein, such as GFP (described earlier) allows localization in cells.
- **Epitope tag:** Addition of short amino acid sequences corresponding to the binding site (epitope) for particular antibodies can be used to purify the protein or to localize the protein on gel blots or in cells.
- **GST:** Fusions with the enzyme glutathione S-transferase (GST) are widely used for affinity chromatography and binding assays. GST binds tightly to glutathione, which can be immobilized on beads.

If the molecule of interest is part of an organelle, centrifugation can be used to isolate the organelle. Typically, the crude cellular homogenate is centrifuged multiple times at a succession of higher speeds (and therefore forces). Particles move in a centrifugal field according to their mass and shape. Large particles such as nuclei pack into a pellet at the bottom of the centrifuge tube at low speeds, whereas high speeds are required to pellet small vesicles. These pellets may be enriched in particular organelles but are never pure. Next, the impure pellet is centrifuged for many hours in a tube containing a concentration gradient of sucrose. In **sedimentation velocity** gradients, particles are centrifuged in a gradient of sucrose (e.g., 5% sucrose in buffer at the top of the tube, increasing to 20% sucrose at the bottom). Because the motion of particles in a centrifugal field depends on the square of the distance from the center of the rotor (think of a spinning ice skater), the farther down the tube the particle travels, the faster it will go. However, the motion of particles in a centrifugal force field also depends on the difference between their density and that of the surrounding medium. Thus, the increasing density of sucrose gradient tends to slow the particle down. Ideally, the two factors counteract one another so that the particle moves at a constant rate, yielding the best separation. In **sedimentation equilibrium** gradients, particles move until their density equals that of the gradient, at which point they move no farther, regardless of how long or hard they are spun. Membrane-containing organelles can be isolated in this way in sucrose gradients. The small differences in size and buoyant density among many of the membrane-bound organelles limit the resolution of subcellular fractionation by sedimentation velocity and sedimentation equilibrium, so additional methods are useful in purifying preparations of organelles. For example, antibodies

BOX 6-3
Gel Electrophoresis

An electrical field draws molecules in a sample through a gel matrix. **Agarose gels** (Fig. 6-5A) are used commonly for nucleic acids, whereas **polyacrylamide gels** are used for both nucleic acids (see Fig. 3-16) and proteins (Fig. 6-5B). Most often, buffers are employed to dissociate the components of the sample and to make their rate of migration through the gel depend on their size. The ionic detergent sodium dodecylsulfate **(SDS)** serves this purpose for proteins. SDS binding unfolds polypeptide chains and gives them a uniform negative charge per unit length. Small molecules move rapidly and separate from slowly moving large molecules, which are more impeded by the matrix. By the time small molecules reach the end of the gel, all of the components in the sample are spread out according to size. Buffers containing the nonionic, denaturing agent urea also dissociate and unfold protein molecules. Electrophoresis in urea separates the proteins depending on both their charge *and* size. Negatively charged proteins move toward the positive electrode, whereas positively charged proteins move in the other direction. Another approach, called **isoelectric focusing,** uses a buffer that contains molecules called ampholines, which have both positive and negative charges. In an electrical field across a gel, ampholines set up a pH gradient. Proteins (usually dissociated in urea) migrate to the pH where they have a net charge of zero, their isoelectric point. This is a sensitive approach to detect charge differences in proteins, such as those introduced by phosphorylation. Isoelectric focusing in one gel followed by SDS-gel electrophoresis in a second dimension can resolve hundreds of individual proteins in complex samples (see Fig. 38-16A).

Many methods are available to detect molecules separated by gel electrophoresis. Proteins are detected by binding colored dyes or more sensitive metal reduction techniques. Obtaining a single stained band on a heavily loaded SDS gel is the goal of those purifying proteins. Of course, some pure proteins consist of multiple polypeptide chains (Fig. 6-5C); in such cases, multiple bands in characteristic ratios are seen. Specific proteins are often detected with antibodies. Typically, proteins are transferred electrophoretically from the polyacrylamide gel to a sheet of nitrocellulose or nylon before reaction with antibodies. This transfer step is called **blotting.** Antibodies labeled with radioactivity are detected by exposing a sheet of X-ray film. Antibodies are also detected by reaction with a second antibody conjugated to an enzyme that catalyzes a light-emitting reaction **(chemiluminescence),** which exposes a sheet of X-ray film. Some proteins can be detected by reaction with naturally occurring binding partners. Fluorescent dyes, such as ethidium bromide, bind nucleic acids (Fig. 6-5A). Following blotting of separated nucleic acids from the gel onto nitrocellulose or nylon films, specific sequences can be detected with complementary oligonucleotides or longer sequences of cloned DNA (probes) labeled with radioactivity or fluorescent dyes.

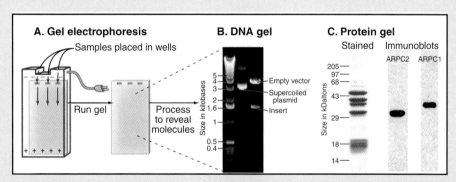

Figure 6-5 GEL ELECTROPHORESIS. **A,** Schematic diagram showing a (generic) gel with three sample wells and an electric field. **B,** Agarose gel electrophoresis of DNA samples stained with ethidium bromide. The lane on the left shows size standards. The middle lane has a bacterial plasmid, a supercoiled (see Fig. 3-18) circular DNA molecule carrying an insert (Fig. 6-8 provides details). The right lane has the same plasmid digested with a restriction enzyme that cleaves the DNA twice, releasing the insert. Although smaller than the circular plasmid, the empty vector runs more slowly on the gel because the linear DNA offers more resistance to movement than the supercoiled circular plasmid. **C,** Polyacrylamide gel electrophoresis of the Arp2/3 complex, an assembly of seven protein subunits involved with actin polymerization (see Fig. 33-13). All three samples are identical. In the left lane, the proteins are stained with the nonspecific protein dye Coomassie blue. The proteins in the other two lanes were transferred to nitrocellulose paper; each reacted with an antibody to one of the subunit proteins (ARPC2 and ARPC1). The position of the bound antibody is determined with a second antibody coupled to an enzyme that produces light and exposes a piece of film black. This method is called chemiluminescence. (B, Courtesy of V. Sirotkin, Yale University, New Haven, Connecticut. C, Courtesy of H. Higgs, Dartmouth Medical School, Hanover, New Hampshire.)

BOX 6-4
Chromatography

Affinity chromatography (Fig. 6-6) is the most selective purification method. A ligand that binds the target molecule is attached covalently to a solid matrix. When a complex mixture of molecules passes through the column, the target molecule binds, whereas most of the other molecules flow through. After the column is washed, the target protein is eluted by competition with free ligand or changing conditions, such as changes in pH or salt concentration. The ligand and target in Fig. 6-6 are both nucleic acids, but they can be any molecules that bind together, including pairs of proteins, drugs and proteins, proteins and nucleic acids, and so on.

Gel filtration separates molecules on the basis of size. Inert beads of agarose, polyacrylamide, or other polymers are manufactured with pores of a particular size. Large

molecules are excluded from the pores and elute first from the column in a volume (void volume) equal to the volume of buffer outside the beads in the column. Small molecules, such as salt, penetrate throughout the beads and elute much later in a volume equal to the total volume of the column. Molecules of intermediate size penetrate the beads to an extent that depends on their molecular radius. This parameter, called the **Stokes radius,** can be measured quantitatively if the column is calibrated with standards of known size. Such molecules elute between the void volume and the total volume.

Ion exchange chromatography utilizes charged groups attached covalently to inert beads. These charged groups may be positive (e.g., the tertiary amine diethylaminoethyl [DEAE]) or negative (e.g., carboxylate or phos-

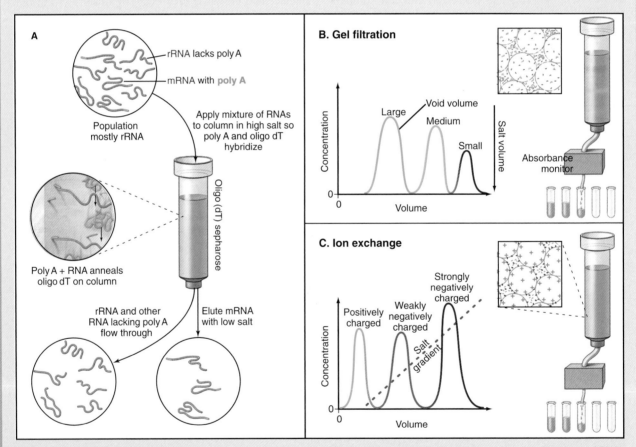

Figure 6-6 CHROMATOGRAPHY. **A,** Affinity chromatography to purify poly A mRNAs with poly dT attached to beads. A mixture of RNAs is extracted from cells and applied to the column in a buffer containing a high concentration of salt. Only poly (A)⁺ mRNA binds and is then eluted with buffer containing a low concentration of salt. (rRNA, ribosomal RNA.) **B,** Gel filtration chromatography separates molecules on the basis of size. Large molecules *(blue)* are excluded from the beads and travel through the column in the void volume outside the beads. Smaller molecules *(green)* penetrate the beads depending on their size. Tiny molecules *(red),* such as salt, completely penetrate the beads and elute in a volume (the salt volume) equal to the size of the bed of beads. Material eluting from the column is monitored for absorbance of ultraviolet light (260 nm for nucleic acids, 280 nm for proteins) to measure concentration and then collected in tubes in a fraction collector. **C,** Anion exchange chromatography. The beads in the column have a positively charged group that binds negatively charged molecules. A gradient of salt elutes bound molecules depending on their affinity for the beads. For cation exchange chromatography, the beads carry a negative charge.

phate). Ionic interactions retain oppositely charged solutes on the surface of the column particles, provided that the ionic strength of the buffer is low. Typically, a gradient of salt is used to elute bound solutes.

Other types of chromatography media are widely used. Crystals of calcium phosphate, called hydroxyapatite, bind both proteins and nucleic acids, which can be eluted selectively by a gradient of phosphate buffer. Beads with hydrophobic groups, such as aromatic rings, absorb many proteins in concentrated salt solutions. They can be eluted selectively by a declining gradient of salt.

The resolution of all chromatography methods depends on the size of the particles (usually beads) that form the immobile phase in the column. Resolution improves with small particles, but so does the resistance to flow. Therefore, high pressures are used to maintain good flow rates in the most high-resolution systems (e.g., high-pressure liquid chromatography [HPLC]).

specific for a molecule on the surface of an organelle can be attached to a solid support and used to bind the organelle. Contaminating material can then be washed away. Certain particles, such as DNA or RNA molecules, are denser than sucrose. They can be centrifuged to equilibrium in gradients of dense salts, such as cesium chloride.

Once a protein of interest has been purified, the path to its gene(s) is relatively direct. Traditionally, each constituent polypeptide was cut into fragments by proteolytic enzymes, after which these fragments were isolated by chromatography and their amino acid sequence determined by Edman degradation (see Chapter 3). Given part of the amino acid sequence, the corresponding gene can then be identified in a genomic data base or isolated by using oligonucleotide probes as the assay (see next section).

Increasingly, proteins are identified by **mass spectrometry.** Proteins are fragmented by cleavage at specific sites with a proteolytic enzyme, such as trypsin, and the masses of the fragments produced are measured exactly with a mass spectrometer. If the protein comes from an organism with a sequenced genome, the gene encoding the protein can be identified by matching the experimental masses of the tryptic fragments with masses of all the peptides predicted from the genome sequence. The sensitivity of these methods has been improved to the point where a stained protein band on a gel suffices to identify the corresponding gene. Alternatively, fragments of known weight are bombarded inside the mass spectrometer under conditions that break the peptide backbone. Analysis of the masses obtained by fragmenting a particular peptide can be used to deduce the sequence of that fragment. Another method starts with isolation of cellular components composed of a complex mixture of proteins such as the nuclear envelope. The sample is digested with the proteolytic enzyme trypsin, fractionated by chromatography, and analyzed by mass spectrometry. Routinely, hundreds of proteins can now be identified in complex cellular structures.

Isolation of Genes and cDNAs

A variety of methods make isolation of specific nucleic acids relatively routine. Genomic DNA is isolated from whole cells by selective extraction. mRNAs are purified by affinity chromatography, taking advantage of their polyadenylate (poly A) tails (see Fig. 16-3), which bind by base pairing to poly dT attached to an insoluble matrix (Fig. 6-6A). Because DNA is easier to work with than RNA (e.g., it can be cleaved by restriction endonucleases and cloned), RNAs are usually converted to **complementary DNA (cDNA)** by reverse transcriptase, a viral DNA polymerase that uses RNA as a template.

Several options exist to purify a particular DNA from a complex mixture:

1. The **polymerase chain reaction (PCR)** uses a heat-stable DNA polymerase and two primers (oligonucleotides, each complementary to one of the ends of a DNA sequence of interest) to synthesize a strand of DNA complementary to another DNA strand (Fig. 6-7A). This reaction is repeated to double the number of copies. Because the DNA duplex product must be dissociated at high temperature before each round of duplication, this method was facilitated by isolation of DNA polymerases from bacteria that live at high temperatures. Repeated steps of synthesis and denaturation allow an exponential amplification in the amount of the chosen DNA sequence. Designing the primers requires knowledge of the sequence of the gene of interest, which may be available from databases or which may be guessed from the sequence of the same gene in a related species or a similar gene in the same species. If the reaction is successful, a single sequence is amplified in quantities sufficient for cloning, sequencing, or large-scale biological production by expression in a bacterium (see later discussion). At its best, PCR is so sensitive that DNA sequences from a single cell can be cloned and characterized.

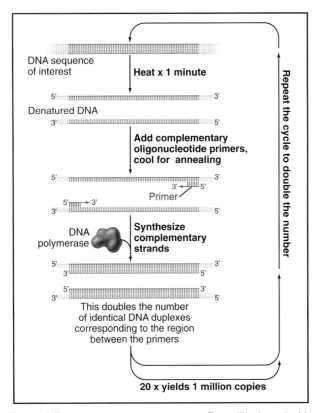

Figure 6-7 POLYMERASE CHAIN REACTION. **From the top,** double-stranded DNA with a sequence of interest is denatured by heating to separate the two strands. An excess of oligonucleotide primers complementary to the ends of the sequence of interest are added and allowed to bind by base pairing. DNA polymerase synthesizes complementary strands, starting from the primers. This cycle is repeated many times to amplify the sequence of interest. Use of a DNA polymerase from a thermophilic bacterium allows many cycles at high temperature without losing activity.

2. A DNA segment of interest can be isolated by **cloning** in a bacterial virus or plasmid (Fig. 6-8A). Such cloning strategies use **"libraries"** of DNA sequences, highly complex mixtures that often have more than 10^6 different cDNAs or genomic DNA fragments. These DNA molecules are transferred into the genome of a virus (usually a bacteriophage) or into a plasmid, a circular DNA molecule that is capable of replication in a host bacterium. The viruses or plasmids are introduced into susceptible bacteria, which grow on agar in petri dishes. In the case of viral vectors, cycles of virus infection and cell lysis in a continuous layer of bacteria produce small clear spots devoid of bacteria, called plaques. For plasmids, conditions are chosen in which only those bacteria carrying a plasmid will grow to form a colony. To clone the DNA sequence of interest, the virus (or cells with plasmid library) are plated at very high density on a petri dish. Next, some of the virus or cells are picked up with a nylon membrane, and the DNA they carry is tested for hybridization to a DNA probe complementary to the sequence of interest. This probe may be a

chemically synthesized oligonucleotide based on a sequence in a database or may be inferred from the amino acid sequence of the protein of interest. Commonly, the probe is a small piece of cloned DNA generated by PCR or obtained from an EST repository. Plaques or colonies that react with the probe are recovered from the petri dish. Initially, these isolates are complex mixtures of viruses or cells bearing plasmids. A uniform population (clone) is obtained by successive rounds of dilution, recovery, and replating until all of the DNA corresponds to the sequence of interest.

3. An alternative approach, called **"expression cloning,"** typically uses a cDNA library inserted into a viral vector or plasmid next to a bacterial promoter and translational start codon (see Fig. 17-9) so that the host bacterium will copy the DNA, starting at the 5′ end of the clone, into mRNA and synthesize the protein. Viral plaques or bacterial colonies on a petri dish are transferred to a membrane and probed with a specific antibody that recognizes the protein of interest. If the bacterium makes the protein, this cloning method is easy. However, there are pitfalls, particularly in cloning genes from organisms whose preference for the use of particular codons differs from the bacterial host or if the protein of interest is not soluble. In such cases, cDNA libraries can be introduced into yeasts or even vertebrate cells, which are tested for expression of a particular trait, such as a membrane channel.

4. If the desired sequence is known in part, it can often be obtained directly from a repository of ESTs. However, because ESTs are only DNA sequence fragments, some of the coding region of the gene is often missing. The rest of the coding sequence can be isolated from cellular RNA or DNA by PCR or cloning.

Once a gene or cDNA has been cloned, it is sequenced and used to deduce the sequence of the encoded protein. Of course, analysis of a DNA sequence cannot reveal posttranslational modifications of a protein, such as phosphorylation, glycosylation, or proteolytic processing. Such modifications, which are often critical for function, can be identified only by analysis of proteins isolated from cells. This analysis entails mass spectrometry or amino acid sequencing.

Cloned cDNAs are used to express native or modified proteins in bacteria or other cells for biochemical analysis or antibody production. This approach has two advantages. First, the quantity of protein produced is often far greater than that from the natural source. Second, cloned DNA can readily be modified by **site-directed mutagenesis** to make predetermined amino acid substitutions and other alterations that are useful for studying protein function (Fig. 6-9). The behavior of

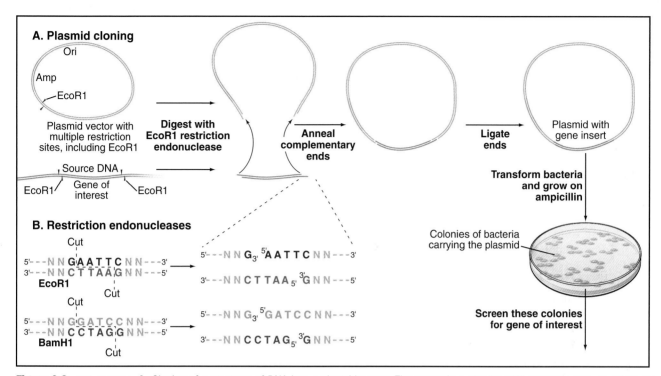

Figure 6-8 DNA CLONING. **A,** Cloning of a segment of DNA into a plasmid vector. The vector is a circular DNA molecule with an origin of replication (Ori) that allows it to replicate in a host bacterium. Most vectors also include one or more genes conferring antibiotic resistance—in this example, resistance to ampicillin (Amp). This enables one to select only those bacteria carrying a plasmid by the ability to grow in the presence of ampicillin. Vectors also contain a sequence of DNA with multiple restriction enzyme digestion sites (see part **B**) for the insertion of foreign DNA molecules. In this example, a single restriction enzyme, EcoR1, is used to cut both the source DNA and the plasmid vector, leaving both with identical single-strand overhangs. The ends of the insert and the cut vector anneal together by base pairing and are then covalently linked together by a ligase enzyme, forming a complete circle of DNA. Plasmids are introduced into bacteria, which are then grown on ampicillin to select those with plasmids. Colonies of bacteria are screened for those containing the desired insert using, for example, DNA probes for sequences specific to the gene of interest. Figure 6-5B shows gel electrophoresis of a plasmid carrying an insert before and after digestion with a restriction enzyme to liberate the insert from the vector. **B,** Sequence-specific cutting of DNA with restriction enzymes. EcoR1 and BamH1 are two of the hundreds of different restriction enzymes that recognize and cleave specific DNA sequences. Both of these restriction enzymes recognize a palindrome of six symmetrical bases. Note that these enzymes leave overhangs with identical sequences on both cut ends that are useful for base pairing with DNA having the same cut. Other restriction enzymes recognize and cut from 4 to 10 bases.

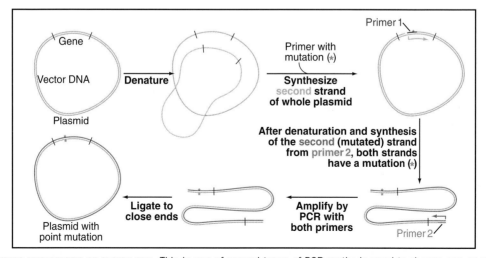

Figure 6-9 IN VITRO MUTAGENESIS OF CLONED DNA. This is one of several types of PCR methods used to change one or more nucleotides (the symbol * in this example) in a cloned gene using a primer with altered bases. In this particular method, primer 1 has the altered base and is used to duplicate the entire plasmid. Primer 2 is used to synthesize the whole plasmid from the other end. After amplification with both primers, the two ends are ligated together, and the plasmid is produced in quantity by growth in bacteria.

mutant proteins in cells can provide evidence for the role of a given protein in particular cellular functions. Thus, biochemical, genetic, and molecular cloning approaches may be applied collectively to reveal the function of proteins.

Molecular Structure

Primary Structure

DNA sequences are now determined by automated dye-termination methods (see Fig. 3-16). The same automated dye-termination methods, when applied to cDNAs, are used to deduce the sequence of proteins and structural RNAs. Protein sequencing by Edman degradation is still occasionally used to detect modified amino acids (see Fig. 3-3); however, mass spectrometry is faster and more sensitive.

Subunit Composition

Gel electrophoresis of many isolated proteins has revealed that they consist of more than one polypeptide chain. Their stoichiometry can be determined from the size and intensity of the stained bands on the gel, but the only way to determine the total number of subunits is to measure the molecular weight of the native protein or protein assembly. The definitive method is a sedimentation equilibrium experiment carried out in an analytical ultracentrifuge. A sample of purified material is centrifuged in a physiological salt solution at relatively low speed in a rotor that allows the measurement of the mass concentration from the top to bottom of the sample cell. At equilibrium, the sedimentation of the material toward the bottom of the tube is balanced by diffusion from the region of high concentration at the bottom of the tube. This balance between sedimentation and diffusion uniquely defines the molecular weight of the particle. A less direct approach to measuring the molecular weight of the native protein or protein assembly is to measure the **sedimentation coefficient** (the parameter relating the rate of sedimentation to the centrifugal force) during centrifugation at high speed and to measure the diffusion coefficient separately, most often by analytical gel filtration (Fig. 6-6B). These two parameters are used to calculate the molecular weight. (Note that neither measurement separately is sufficient to measure molecular weights, despite numerous assertions in the literature that they are sufficient!) An advantage of the latter approach is that it can be used with impure material, provided that an assay is available that is applicable to the two types of measurements. Light scattering can also be used to estimate molecular weights.

Atomic Structure

X-ray crystallography and **nuclear magnetic resonance (NMR)** spectroscopy are used to determine the structure of proteins and nucleic acids at atomic resolution (see Fig. 3-8). Although X-ray crystallography has determined structures as large as the ribosome (see Fig. 17-7) and viruses (see Figs. 5-11 and 5-14), some large structures are currently outside the size range of this high-resolution method. Alternatively, large structures can be studied by electron microscopy of single particles or regular assemblies. If available from crystallography or NMR, atomic structures of subunits can be fit into lower-resolution reconstructions of large assemblies made by electron microscopy (see Figs. 36-4 and 36-10). NMR avoids the requirement to crystallize the protein to be studied, but the protein must be soluble at high concentrations, and NMR is difficult for proteins larger than 20 kD.

Partners and Pathways

It is hard to think of a cellular molecule that functions in isolation, as virtually all cellular components are parts of assemblies, networks, or pathways. Thus, a major challenge in defining biological function is to place each molecule in its physiological context with all of its molecular partners. The classic example of such an endeavor is the biochemical mapping of major metabolic pathways (see Fig. 19-4 or a biochemistry textbook). Genetics played a prominent role in the discovery of the network of proteins that control the cell cycle (see Fig. 40-2). Currently, signaling, regulation of gene expression, membrane trafficking, and the control of development are pathways of particular interest.

Biochemical Methods

Once a molecule of interest has been purified, finding partners with which it functions in the cell is often the next step. This requires a method to separate the macromolecular complex containing the molecule being studied away from other cellular proteins. One approach is **affinity chromatography** with the probe molecule attached by a chemical crosslink to an insoluble support, such as small beads. A popular variation is to express a probe protein fused to GST that can be bound with high affinity to a small molecule attached to beads. A crude cellular extract is run through the column with immobilized probe molecules and washed. Then molecules bound to the probe are eluted with high salt, extremes of pH, specific ligands, or, if necessary, with denaturing agents, such as urea. Eluted proteins are analyzed by gel electrophoresis and identified with antibodies, sequencing, or mass spectrometry. Eluted nucleic acids are cloned and sequenced.

An alternative to column chromatography is to mix beads with attached probe molecules with a crude cellular extract and then isolate the beads with

bound molecules by centrifugation into a pellet. Bound molecules are eluted for analysis. Varying the concentration of such beads is a simple way to measure the affinity of the probe for its various partners. Antibodies are frequently used to separate a protein and its partners from crude extracts. An antibody specific for the probe molecule can be attached directly or indirectly to a bead and used to bind the protein of interest along with any associated molecules. This is called **immunoprecipitation.**

Proteins tagged with combinations of peptides can be purified by affinity methods along with tightly associated proteins. A popular method called **TAP (tandem affinity purification) tagging** adds to any protein of interest DNA sequences encoding two different peptide epitopes separated by a cleavage site for a highly specific viral protease. The cell makes the doubly tagged protein. The tagged protein, together with associated proteins, is purified from a cellular extract using immobilized antibodies to the outermost tag. The TEV protease, which has no natural targets in the cell, cleaves the tagged protein from the immobilized antibody. Then an entirely different set of reagents permits a second round of purification using the remaining tag. Two successive affinity steps remove most proteins that bind nonspecifically to the protein of interest or the affinity reagents. This is a quick method to purify stable protein complexes from crude whole-cell lysates.

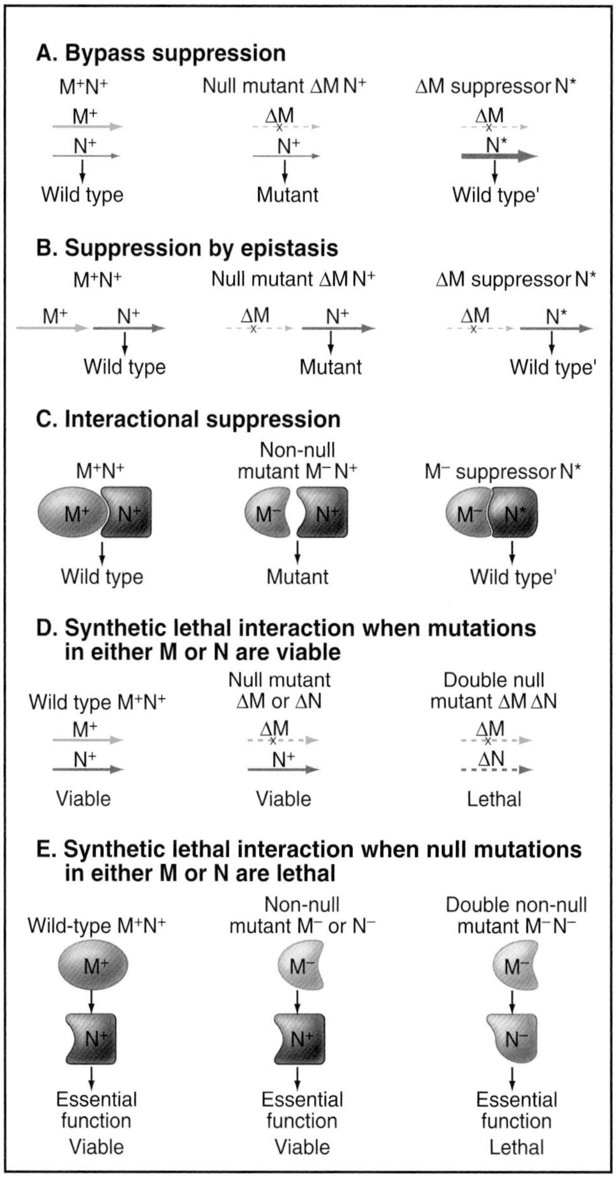

Genetics

Given a mutation in a gene of interest, two genetic tests are used to search for partners: (1) identification of a second mutation that ameliorates the effects of the primary mutation (a **suppressor mutation,** Fig. 6-10A–B) and (2) identification of a second mutation that makes the phenotype more severe, often lethal (an **enhancer mutation** [Fig. 6-10C–E]). A specialized class of enhancer mutations, called **synthetic lethal mutations,** is particularly useful in the analysis of genetic

Figure 6-10 ANALYSIS OF GENETIC INTERACTIONS BETWEEN TWO GENES, M AND N. The sizes of the *arrows* indicate the level of function of the gene product, usually a protein. The phenotype is indicated for each example. Mutant phenotype means an altered function dependent on gene products M and N. In the diagram, the symbol $^+$ indicates a wild-type allele, the symbol * indicates a suppressor allele, and the symbol Δ indicates a null mutation. **A,** Bypass suppression. Gene products M and N operate in parallel, with M making the larger contribution. Loss of M yields a mutant phenotype because N alone does not provide sufficient function. Mutation N* enhances the function of N, allowing it to provide function on its own. **B,** Suppression by epistasis. Products M and N act in series on the same pathway. Loss of M function blocks the pathway. Mutation N* allows N to function without stimulation by product M. **C,** Interactional suppression. Function requires interaction of gene products M and N. Mutation M$^-$ interferes with the interaction. Suppressor mutation N* allows product N* to interact with M$^-$. **D,** Synthetic lethal interaction when null mutations in either M or N are viable. The products of genes M and N operate in parallel to provide function. N provides sufficient function in the absence of M (ΔM) and vice versa. Loss of both M and N is lethal. **E,** Synthetic lethal interaction when null mutations in either M or N are lethal. Products M and N function in series. N can provide residual function even when M is compromised by mutation M$^-$, and vice versa. When both M and N are compromised (M$^-$, N$^-$), the pathway provides insufficient function for viability. (Redrawn from Guarente L: Synthetic enhancement in gene interaction: A genetic tool comes of age. Trends Genet 9:362–366, 1993.)

pathways in yeast. In this case, mutations in two genes in the same pathway, if present in the same cell, even as heterozygotes (i.e., each cell having one good and one mutant copy of each gene), cannot be tolerated, so the cell dies. It is thought that each mutation lowers the level of production of some critical factor just a bit and that the combination of the two effectively means that the output of the pathway is insufficient for survival. These tests can be made with existing collections of mutations by genetically crossing mutant organisms. Alternatively, one can seek new mutations created by a second round of mutagenesis. The results depend on the architecture of the particular pathway. If the products of the genes in question operate in a sequence, analysis of single and double mutants can often reveal their order in the pathway. For essential genes in haploid organisms, a conditional allele of the primary mutation simplifies the experiment. Synthetic interactions (suppression or lethality) may also be discovered by overproduction of wild-type genes on a plasmid. Caution is required in interpreting suppressor and enhancer mutations, given the complexity of cellular systems and the possibility of unanticipated consequences of the mutations.

Another approach to find protein partners is called a **two-hybrid assay** (Fig. 6-11). This assay depends on the observation that some activators of transcription have two modular domains with discrete functions: One domain binds target sites on DNA, and the other recruits the transcriptional apparatus (see Fig. 15-19). The target gene is expressed if both activities are present at the transcription start site, even if the activities are on two different proteins. For the two-hybrid assay, the coding sequence of the protein whose partners are to be identified is fused to the coding sequence of a yeast protein that recognizes a target DNA sequence upstream of a gene that provides the readout of the assay. This so-called bait protein is expressed constitutively in yeast cells. A plasmid library is constructed consisting of cDNA sequences of all possible interaction partners ("prey"), each fused to the coding sequence of an "activator domain" and a nuclear localization sequence. This library of "prey" proteins is introduced into the "bait" yeast strain. The readout gene is expressed if a "prey" protein binds the "bait" protein and recruits the transcriptional apparatus. Many variations of this assay exist. One produces an enzyme that makes a colored product, so colonies of yeast with interacting proteins can be identified visually. In another version, the target gene encodes a gene essential for production of a particular amino acid, so only cells with a bait-prey interaction will grow on agar plates lacking that amino acid. Putative interactions must subsequently be tested carefully to define specificity, as false-positive results are common. Moreover, some valid interactions are missed owing to false-negative results.

Large-Scale Screening with Microarrays

Microarrays display thousands of tiny spots on a glass slide, each with a particular DNA sequence or protein (Fig. 6-12). This allows many reactions to be monitored in parallel. One type of microarray has cDNAs or oligonucleotides for thousands of genes. Probing such an array with complementary copies of mRNAs from a test sample reveals which genes are expressed. This can be used to find partners, because expression of genes

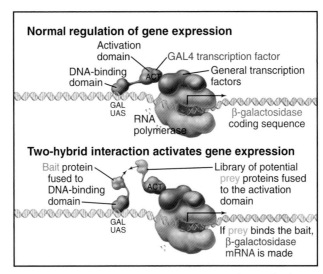

Figure 6-11 ONE VERSION OF THE YEAST TWO-HYBRID ASSAY FOR INTERACTING PROTEINS. Interaction between "bait" protein and "prey" protein *(bottom)* brings together the two halves of a transcription factor required to turn on the expression of β-galactosidase. The DNA-binding domain of the GAL4 transcription factor binds a specific DNA sequence: GAL UAS. Generally, a library of random cDNAs or gene fragments is used to express test prey proteins as fusions with the activation domain.

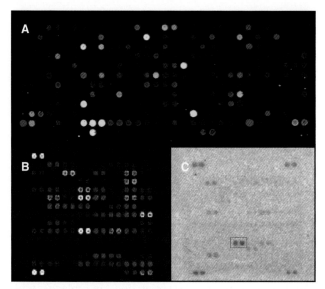

Figure 6-12 LARGE-SCALE ANALYSIS OF GENE EXPRESSION AND KINASE ACTIVITY WITH MICROARRAYS. **A,** Gene expression. PCR was used to make cDNA copies of mRNAs from two parts of the human brain. The cDNAs from cerebral cortex mRNAs were labeled with a *red* fluorescent dye, whereas those from the cerebellum were labeled with a *green* fluorescent dye. A mixture of equal proportions of the two fluorescent cDNA preparations was reacted with 384 different known cDNAs arrayed in tiny spots on a glass slide. The fluorescence-bound cDNAs were imaged with a microscopic fluorescent scanner similar to a confocal microscope. *Yellow* spots bound equal quantities of cDNAs from the two sources. *Red* spots bound more cDNA from the cortex, indicating a higher concentration of those mRNAs. *Green* spots bound more cDNA from the cerebellum, indicating a higher concentration of those mRNAs. **B–C,** Large-scale identification of substrates for a protein kinase. Thousands of different budding yeast proteins tagged with GST- and 6 histidines were overexpressed in yeast and purified by affinity chromatography. Each protein was spotted in duplicate on a glass slide, a small portion of which is shown here. **B,** The amount of bound protein in each spot was detected with a fluorescent antibody to GST (indicated by varying intensity of fluorescence from *dark red* to *white*). **C,** The slide was incubated with a yeast kinase in the presence of ^{33}P-ATP. Radioactive phosphorylated proteins were detected as pairs of dark spots by autoradiography. One pair is boxed. (A, Courtesy of C. Barlow and M. Zapala, Salk Institute, La Jolla, California. B–C, Courtesy of Geeta Devgan and Michael Snyder, Yale University, New Haven, Connecticut. Reference: Zhu H, Bilgin M, Bangham R, et al: Global analysis of protein activities using proteome chips. Science 293:2101–2105, 2001.)

contributing proteins to a particular pathway is often coordinated as conditions change. For example, unfolded proteins in the lumen of the endoplasmic reticulum trigger the expression of nearly 300 genes for proteins of the endoplasmic reticulum (see Fig. 20-11). Microarrays of thousands of different proteins can be used to test for interactions. For example, reaction of protein arrays with each yeast protein kinase, one kinase per slide, identified the substrates phosphorylated by each kinase (Fig. 6-12B).

Rates and Affinities

Information about reaction rates is important for two reasons. First, reaction rates are required to account for the dynamic aspects of any biological system. Second, although the methods in the previous section usually provide initial clues about the integration of proteins into pathways, knowledge of reactant concentrations and **rate constants** is the only way to fully understand biochemical pathways. Fortunately, just two types of reactions occur in biology: first-order reactions, such as conformational changes and dissociation of molecular complexes, and second-order reactions between two molecules. Chapter 4 explains the rate constants for such reactions, the relationship of rate constants to the equilibrium constant for a reaction, and the relationship of the equilibrium constant to thermodynamics. Figure 4-7 illustrates how transient kinetics experiments were used to determine the mechanism of the Ras GTPase (see Fig. 4-6).

Despite their importance, rate constants and the physiological concentrations of the molecules in a pathway are usually the least understood aspects of most biological systems. A common impediment is the lack of an assay with sufficient sensitivity and time resolution to measure reaction rates. Optical methods, such as those using fluorescence, are usually the best and can be devised for most processes.

Tests of Physiological Function

Reconstitution of Function from Isolated Components

The classic biochemical test of function is **reconstitution** of a biological process from purified components. This involves creating conditions in the test tube in which isolated molecules can perform a complex process normally carried out by a cell. The difficulty of the task depends on the complexity of the function. Successful reconstitution experiments reveal the molecular requirements and mechanisms involved in a process. Examples of successful tests include reconstitution of ion channel function in pure lipid membranes (see Chapter 10), protein synthesis and translocation of proteins into the endoplasmic reticulum (see Fig. 20-7), and motility of bacteria powered by assembly of actin filaments (see Fig. 37-12).

Anatomic Tests

No biological process can be understood without knowledge of where the components are located in the cell. Often, cellular **localization** of a newly discovered molecule provides the first clue about its function. This accounts for why cell biologists put so much effort into localizing molecules in cells. Cell fractionation, fluorescent antibody staining, and expression of GFP fusion proteins are all valuable approaches, illustrated by numerous examples in this book. For more detailed localization, antibodies can be adsorbed to small gold beads and used to label fixed specimens for electron microscopy (see Fig. 29-7).

GFP fusion proteins are particularly valuable because of the ease of their construction and expression and because they can be used to monitor both the behavior and dynamics of molecules within living cells. However, it should always be kept in mind that attaching GFP may affect either the localization or function of the protein being tested. Demonstration that a GFP fusion protein is fully functional, that is, that it can replicate the parent protein's biochemical and biophysical properties, can be done only by genetic replacement of the native protein with the GFP fusion protein. This is routinely done in yeast but rarely for vertebrate proteins, as the required genetics are difficult or impossible. Instead, correct function is inferred from the fusion protein exhibiting morphologic, biochemical, and biophysical properties similar to those of the native protein. This is better than nothing but incorporates an element of wishful thinking.

The use of GFP fusions to study cellular dynamics has yielded many surprises, as structures that were thought to be inert have turned out to be remarkably dynamic. One powerful technique is to photobleach the GFP fusion protein in one part of the cell and to observe how the fluorescent proteins in other parts of the cell redistribute with time (fluorescence recovery after photobleaching, or FRAP; see Fig. 6-3E). The speed of fluorescence recovery into the photobleached area provides information on the mobility of the fusion protein (i.e., whether it diffuses freely, is immobilized on a scaffold, or is actively transported) and its interaction properties within the cell (see Figs. 7-11 and 14-4). These properties play important roles in how a protein functions within a cell, which cannot be determined by merely observing the protein's steady-state distribution.

Proteins and other cellular components, including DNA, RNA, and lipids, can be labeled with fluorescent dyes to study their intracellular localization and dynamics. Fluorescent RNAs and proteins can be microinjected into cells. Fluorescent lipids can be inserted into the outer leaflet of the plasma membrane in living cells; from there, they move to appropriate membranes and then mimic rather faithfully the behavior of their natural lipid counterpart.

Physiological Tests

Although often obscured by technical jargon, just three methods are available to test for physiological function:

(1) reducing the concentration of active protein (or other molecule), (2) increasing the concentration of active molecule, and (3) replacing a native protein with a protein that has altered biochemical properties. Biochemical, pharmacological, and genetic methods are available for each test, the genetic methods often yielding the cleanest results. These experiments are most revealing when robust assays are available to measure quantitatively how the cellular process under investigation functions when the concentration of native molecule is varied or an altered molecule replaces the native molecule. When done well, these experiments provide valuable constraints for quantitative models of biological systems, as described in the next section.

The definitive way to reduce the concentration of active protein or RNA is to prevent its expression. This option is available if the molecule is not required for viability. If a protein is essential, one can replace it with an altered version that is fully active under a certain set of conditions and completely inactive under other conditions (a **conditional** mutant). Proteins that are active at one temperature and inactive at another are widely used. Even then, it is difficult to control for the effects of temperature on all of the other processes in the cell. A second option is to put the expression of the protein or RNA under the control of regulatory proteins that are sensitive to the presence of a small molecule, such as a vitamin or hormone. Then, expression of the molecule can be turned on and off at will. This is commonly done for vertebrate cells by using promoters of gene expression engineered so that they can be turned on or off by the antibiotic tetracycline, which alters the ability of a bacterial protein (the tetracycline repressor) to bind particular regulatory sequences on DNA. A limitation of this technology is that some proteins are so stable that days are required to reduce their concentrations. During this time, cells may be able to compensate for the loss of the protein of interest.

RNA interference (RNAi) is a powerful method to reduce the concentration of a particular RNA, especially mRNAs (see Fig. 16-12). Introducing a double-stranded RNA copy of part of an RNA sequence into the cytoplasm generates a response that results in the degradation of the target RNA. Animals, fungi, and plants use this process to suppress expression of foreign RNAs, such as those introduced by viruses. If double-stranded RNA is introduced into cells, it is fragmented into pieces of about 21 nucleotides (see Fig. 16-12). Base pairing of these fragments with cellular RNAs having the complementary sequence (usually an exact match is required) targets the RNA for cleavage. To suppress a particular RNA in human cells experimentally, one synthesizes a double-stranded RNA including a sequence of 21 nucleotides matching the target cellular RNA. Introduction of this oligonucleotide into cells often (not always) results in destruction of the target RNA. If successful, the level of the targeted protein falls 5- to 10-fold as it is degraded naturally over the next several days. Loss of the protein may produce a cellular phenotype. RNAs and proteins can be depleted from *Drosophila* and *Caenorhabditis elegans* by using slightly different procedures. The simplicity of this approach makes RNAi very powerful and suitable for scaling up to study thousands of genes. However, false-negative results are common because some targeted protein usually remains. If the protein is an enzyme, a few protein molecules can turn over numerous substrate molecules and maintain function. One must also be cautious regarding other unanticipated consequences.

Another strategy is to inhibit a particular protein with a drug, inhibitory peptide, antibody, or inactive partner protein. Drugs as probes for function have a long and distinguished history in biology, but their use is hampered by the difficulty of ruling out side effects, including action on other unknown targets. One wag even asserted that "drugs are only specific for about a year," roughly the time it takes someone to find an unexpected second target. Nevertheless, many drugs have the advantages that the onset of their action is rapid and their effects are reversible, so one can follow the process of recovery when they are removed. The use of libraries of small molecules to probe biological processes has been given the name *chemical genetics.*

If microinjected into cells, antibodies can be very specific, but the effects on their target must be fully characterized, and sufficient antibody must be introduced into the target cell to inactivate the target molecule. Some arginine-rich peptides, such as one from the HIV Tat protein, can also be used to carry inhibitory peptides across the plasma membrane into the cytoplasm. Other peptides can guide experimental peptides into various cellular compartments. It is also possible to inactivate pathways by the introduction of dominant negative mutants that can do part, but not all, of the job of a given protein. Dominant negative mutants of protein kinases are particularly effective. The active site is modified to eliminate enzymatic activity, but the modified protein can still bind to its regulatory proteins and substrates. This can interfere with signal transduction pathways very effectively by competing with functional endogenous kinases for regulatory factors and substrates. Dominant negative mutants offer the advantage that they can be expressed in many types of cells. However, all too often, little is known about the concentrations of these dominant negative agents or the full range of their targets.

The concentration of active protein can be increased by **overexpression,** for example, driving the expression of a cDNA from a very active viral promoter. Some expression systems are conditional, being turned on, for example, by an insect hormone that does not activate endogenous genes. Interpreting the consequences of overexpression tends to be more problematic than other approaches, as specificity of interactions with other cellular components can be lost at high concentrations.

Genetics is the best way to replace a native protein with a protein that has altered biochemical properties. Such **gene replacement** requires homologous recombination in the genome, which is not readily available in all experimental systems (Table 6-2). Examples of altered proteins include an enzyme with an altered catalytic function or a protein with altered affinity for a particular cellular partner. In the best cases, the altered protein is fully characterized before its coding sequence is used to replace that of the wild-type protein, and the cellular concentration of the altered protein is confirmed to be the same as the wild-type protein. On the relatively long time scale of such experiments (up to a year in vertebrates), interpreting the outcome may be compromised by the ability of cells to adapt to the change imposed by the gene substitution in unknown ways.

Mathematical Models of Systems

Even with an inventory of molecular components; their structures, concentrations, molecular partners, and reaction rates; and genetic tests for their contributions to a physiological process, one really does not know whether a system operates according to one's expectations unless a mathematical model can match the performance of the cellular system over a range of conditions and, when challenged, with mutations in one or more component. In the best cases (bacterial metabolic pathways, bacterial chemotaxis, yeast cell cycle, muscle calcium transients, and muscle cross-bridges), the mathematical models usually have fallen short of duplicating the physiological process. This means that some aspect of the process is incompletely understood or that assumptions in the mathematical model are incorrect. In either case, these failures offer important clues about the shortcomings of current knowledge and point the way toward improvements in underlying assumptions, experimental parameters, or mathematical models.

SELECTED READINGS

Altieri AS, Byrd TA: Automation of NMR structure determination of proteins. Curr Opin Struct Biol 14:547–553, 2004.

Bader GD, Heilbut A, Andrews B, et al: Functional genomics and proteomics: Charting a multidimensional map of the yeast cell. Trends Cell Biol 13:344–356, 2003.

Brent R, Finley RLJ: Understanding gene and allele function with two-hybrid methods. Ann Rev Genet 31:663–704, 1997.

Carthew RW: Gene silencing by double-stranded RNA. Curr Opin Cell Biol 13:244–248, 2001.

Celis J (ed): Cell Biology: A Laboratory Handbook, vols 1–3. New York: Academic Press, 1994.

Danuser G, Waterman-Storer CM: Quantitative fluorescent speckle microscopy of cytoskeleton dynamics. Annu Rev Biophys Biomol Struct 35:361–387, 2006.

Falk MM: Genetic tags for labelling live cells: Gap junctions and beyond. Trends Cell Biol 12:399–404, 2002.

Frank J: Single-particle imaging of macromolecules by cryo-electron microscopy. Annu Rev Biophys Biomol Struct 31:303–319, 2002.

Frey TG, Perkins GA, Ellisman MH: Electron tomography of membrane-bound cellular organelles. Annu Rev Biophys Biomol Struct 35:199–224, 2006.

Gariepy J, Kawamura K: Vectorial delivery of macromolecules into cells using peptide-based vehicles. Trends Biotechnol 19:21–28, 2001.

Guarente L: Strategies for the identification of interacting proteins. Proc Natl Acad Sci U S A 90:1639–1641, 1993.

Guarente L: Synthetic enhancement in gene interaction: A genetic tool come of age. Trends Genet 9:362–366, 1993.

Hahn K, Toutchkine A: Live-cell fluorescent biosensors for activated signaling proteins. Curr Opin Cell Biol 14:167–172, 2002.

Inoué S: Video Microscopy. New York: Plenum Press, 1986.

Inoué S, Oldenbourg R: Microscopes. In Bass M, Van Stryland EW, Williams DR, Wolf WL (eds): Handbook of Optics, vol 2. New York: McGraw-Hill, 1995, pp 17.1–17.52.

International Human Genome Sequencing Consortium: Initial sequencing and analysis of the human genome. Nature 409:860–921, 2001. [Also see related articles in the same issue.]

Mayer TU: Chemical genetics: Tailoring tools for cell biology. Trends Cell Biol 13:270–277, 2003.

McIntosh JR, Nicastro D, Mastronarde D: New views of cells in 3D: An introduction to electron tomography. Trends Cell Biol 15:43–51, 2005.

Mogilner A, Wollman R, Marshall WF: Quantitative modeling in cell biology: What good is it? Dev Cell 11:1–9, 2006.

Murphy DB: Fundamentals of Light Microscopy and Electronic Imaging. New York: Wiley-Liss, 2001.

Panda S, Sato TK, Hampton GM, Hogenesch JB: An array of insights: Application of DNA chip technology in the study of cell biology. Trends Cell Biol 13:151–156, 2003.

Papin JA, Price ND, Wiback SJ, et al: Metabolic pathways in the post-genome era. Trends Biochem Sci 28:250–258, 2003.

Sambrook J, Russell D: Molecular Cloning, 3rd ed. Plainview, NY: Cold Spring Harbor Laboratory, 2001.

Slayter EM: Optical Methods in Biology. New York: Wiley-Interscience, 1970.

Slepchenko BM, Schaff JC, Carson JH, Loew LM: Computational cell biology: Spatiotemporal simulation of cellular events. Annu Rev Biophys Biomolec Struct 31:423–441, 2002.

Steven AC, Aebi U: The next ice age: Cryo-electron tomography of intact cells. Trends Cell Biol 13:107–110, 2003.

Subramaniam S, Milne JLS: Three-dimensional electron microscopy at molecular resolution. Annu Rev Biophys Biomolec Struct 33:141–155, 2004.

Wu RZ, Bailey SN, Sabatini DM: Cell-biological applications of trans-fected-cell microarrays. Trends Cell Biol 12:485–488, 2002.

Xia Y, Yu H, Jansen R, et al: Analyzing cellular biochemistry in terms of molecular networks. Annu Rev Biochem 73:1051–1087, 2004.

Yates JR III: Mass spectral analysis in proteomics. Annu Rev Biophys Biomolec Struct 33:297–316, 2004.

Zhu H, Bilgin M, Snyder M: Proteomics. Annu Rev Biochem 72:783–812, 2003.

Internet

Web site for biophysical methods. Available at http://www.biophysics.org/education/resources.htm.

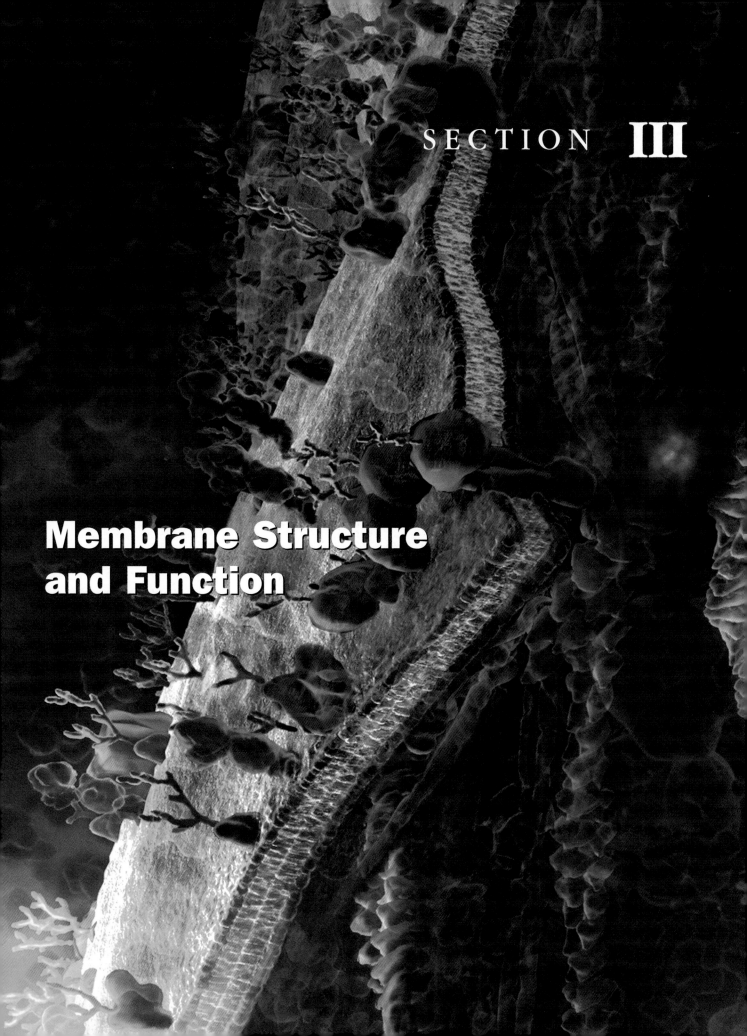

SECTION **III**

Membrane Structure and Function

SECTION III OVERVIEW

Life, as we know it, depends on a fragile lipid membrane that separates each cell from the surrounding world. These membranes, composed of two layers of lipids, are generally impermeable to ions and macromolecules. Proteins embedded in the lipid membrane facilitate the movement of ions, allowing cells to create an internal environment different from that outside. Membranes also subdivide the cytoplasm of eukaryotic cells into compartments called organelles. Chapter 7 introduces the features that are shared by all biological membranes: a **bilayer** of lipids, **integral proteins** that cross the bilayer, and **peripheral proteins** associated with the surfaces.

Membranes are a planar sandwich of two layers of lipids that act as two-dimensional fluids. Each lipid has a polar group from which extend hydrocarbon tails that are insoluble in water. The hydrocarbon tails are in the middle of the membrane bilayer with polar head groups exposed to water on both surfaces. In spite of the rapid, lateral diffusion of these lipids in the plane of the membrane, the hydrophobic interior of the bilayer is poorly permeable to ions and macromolecules. This impermeability makes it possible for cellular membranes to form barriers between the external environment, cytoplasm, and organelles. The selectively permeable membrane around each organelle allows the creation of a unique interior space for specialized biochemical reactions that contribute to the life process. Chapters 18 to 23 consider in detail all of the organelles, including mitochondria, chloroplasts, peroxisomes, endoplasmic reticulum, Golgi apparatus, lysosomes, and the vesicles of the secretory pathway.

Peripheral membrane proteins that are found on the surfaces of the bilayer often participate in enzyme and signaling reactions. Others form a membrane skeleton on the cytoplasmic surface that reinforces the fragile lipid bilayer and attaches it to cytoskeletal filaments.

Integral membrane proteins that cross lipid bilayers feature prominently in all aspects of cell biology. Some are enzymes that synthesize lipids for biological membranes (see Chapter 20). Others serve as adhesion proteins that allow cells to interact with each other or extracellular substrates (see Chapter 30). Cells need to sense hormones and many other molecules that cannot penetrate a lipid bilayer. Therefore, they have evolved thousands of protein receptors that span the lipid bilayer (see Chapter 24). Hormones or other extracellular signaling molecules bind selectively to receptors exposed on the cell surface. The energy from binding is used to transmit a signal across the membrane and turn on biochemical reactions in the cytoplasm (see Chapters 25 to 27).

A large fraction of the energy that is consumed by organs such as our brains is used to create ion gradients across membranes. Several large families of integral membrane proteins control the movement of ions and other solutes across membranes. Chapter 8 introduces

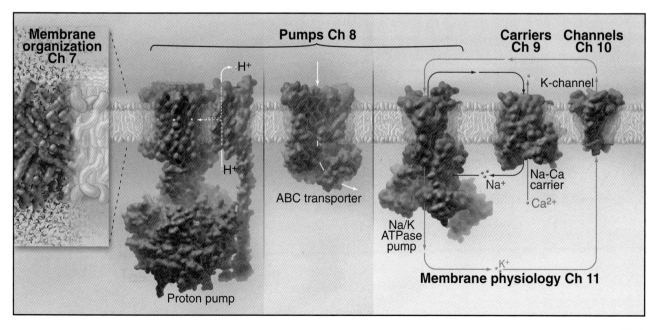

three families of **pumps** that use adenosine triphosphate (ATP) hydrolysis as the source of energy to transport ions or solutes up concentration gradients across membranes. For example, pumps in the plasma membranes of animal cells use ATP hydrolysis to expel Na^+ and concentrate K^+ in the cytoplasm. Another type of pump creates the acid environment inside lysosomes. A related pump in mitochondria runs backward, taking advantage of a proton gradient across the membrane to synthesize ATP. A third family, called ABC transporters, use ATP hydrolysis to move a wide variety of solutes across plasma membranes.

Carrier proteins (Chapter 9) facilitate the movement of ions and nutrients across membranes, allowing them to move down concentration gradients much faster than they can penetrate the lipid bilayer. Some carriers couple movement of an ion such as Na^+ down its concentration gradient to the movement of a solute such as glucose up a concentration gradient into the cell. Carriers generally change their shape reversibly to transport their cargo across the membrane one molecule at a time.

Channels are transmembrane proteins with selective pores that allow ions, water, glycerol, or ammonia to move very rapidly down concentration gradients across membranes (Chapter 10). Taking advantage of ion gradients created by pumps and carriers, cells selectively open ion channels to create electrical potentials across the plasma membrane and some organelle membranes. Many channels open and close their pores in response to local conditions. The electrical potential across the membrane regulates voltage-gated cation channels. Binding of a chemical ligand opens other channels. For instance, nerve cells secrete small organic ions (called neurotransmitters) to stimulate other nerve cells and muscles by binding to an extracellular domain of cation channels. The bound neurotransmitter opens the pore in the channel. In the cytoplasm, other organic ions and Ca^{2+} can also regulate channels. Cyclic nucleotides open plasma membrane channels in cells that respond to light and aromas. Inositol triphosphate and Ca^{2+} control channels that release Ca^{2+} from the endoplasmic reticulum.

All living organisms depend on combinations of pumps, carriers, and channels for many physiological functions (Chapter 11). Cells use ion concentration gradients produced by pumps as a source of potential energy to drive the uptake of nutrients through plasma membrane carriers. Epithelial cells lining our intestines combine different carriers and channels in their plasma membranes to transport sugars, amino acids, and other nutrients from the lumen of the gut into the blood. Many organelles use carriers driven by ion gradients for transport. Most cells use ion channels and transmembrane ion gradients to create an electrical potential across their plasma membranes. Nerve and muscle cells create fast-moving fluctuations in the plasma membrane potential for high-speed communication; operating on a millisecond time scale, voltage-gated ion channels produce waves of membrane depolarization and repolarization called action potentials.

Our abilities to perceive our environment, think, and move depend on transmission of electrical impulses between nerve cells and between nerves and muscles at specialized structures called synapses. When an action potential arrives at a synapse, voltage-gated Ca^{2+} channels trigger the secretion of neurotransmitters. In less than a millisecond, the neurotransmitter stimulates ligand-gated cation channels to depolarize the plasma membrane of the receiving cell. Muscle cells respond with an action potential that sets off contraction. Nerve cells in the central nervous system integrate inputs from many synapses before producing an action potential. Pumps and carriers cooperate to reset conditions after each round of synaptic transmission.

Membrane Structure and Dynamics

Membranes composed of lipids and proteins form the barrier between each cell and its environment. Membranes also partition the cytoplasm of eukaryotes into compartments, including the nucleus and membrane-bounded organelles. Each type of membrane is specialized for its various functions, but all biological membranes have much in common: a planar fluid **bilayer** of lipid molecules, **integral membrane proteins** that cross the lipid bilayer, and **peripheral membrane proteins** on both surfaces.

This chapter opens with a discussion of the lipid bilayer. It then considers examples of integral and peripheral membrane proteins before concluding with a discussion of the dynamics of both lipids and proteins. The following three chapters introduce three large families of membrane proteins: pumps, carriers, and channels. Chapter 11 explains how pumps, carriers, and channels cooperate in a variety of physiological processes. Chapters 24 and 30 cover plasma membrane receptor proteins.

Development of Ideas about Membrane Structure

Our current understanding of membrane structure began with E. Overton's proposal in 1895 that cellular membranes consist of lipid bilayers (Fig. 7-1A). Biochemical experiments in the 1920s supported the bilayer hypothesis. It was found that the lipids extracted from the plasma membrane of red blood cells spread out in a monolayer on the surface of a tray of water to cover an area sufficient to surround the cell twice. (Actually, offsetting errors—incomplete lipid extraction and an underestimation of the membrane area—led to the correct answer!) X-ray diffraction experiments in the early 1970s established definitely that membrane lipids are arranged in a bilayer.

During the 1930s, cell physiologists realized that a simple lipid bilayer could not explain the mechanical properties of the plasma membrane, so they postulated a surface coating of proteins to reinforce the bilayer (Fig. 7-1B). Early electron micrographs strengthened this view, since when viewed in cross sections, all membranes appeared as a pair of dark lines (interpreted as surface proteins and carbohydrates) separated by a lucent area (interpreted as the lipid bilayer). By the early 1970s, two complementary approaches showed that proteins cross the lipid bilayer. First, electron micrographs of membranes that are split in two while frozen (a technique called freeze-fracturing; see Fig. 6-4D) revealed protein particles embedded in the lipid bilayer. Later, chemical labeling showed that many membrane proteins traverse the

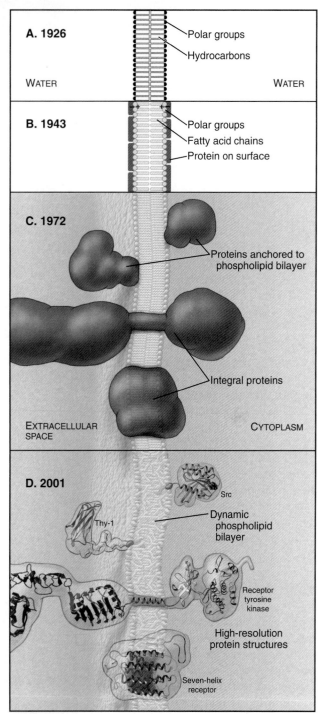

A. 1926

WATER   WATER

Polar groups
Hydrocarbons

B. 1943

Polar groups
Fatty acid chains
Protein on surface

C. 1972

Proteins anchored to
phospholipid bilayer

Integral proteins

EXTRACELLULAR
SPACE   CYTOPLASM

D. 2001

Src
Thy-1
Dynamic
phospholipid
bilayer

Receptor
tyrosine
kinase

High-resolution
protein structures

Seven-helix
receptor

Figure 7-1 DEVELOPMENT OF CONCEPTS IN MEMBRANE STRUCTURE. **A,** Gorder and Grendel model from 1926. **B,** Davson and Danielli model from 1943. **C,** Singer and Nicholson fluid mosaic model from 1972. **D,** Contemporary model with peripheral and integral membrane proteins. The lipid bilayer shown here and used throughout the book is based on an atomic model (Fig. 7-5).

bilayer, exposing different regions of the polypeptide to the aqueous phase on the two sides. Light microscopy with fluorescent tags demonstrated that membrane lipids and some membrane proteins diffuse in the plane of the membrane. Quantitative spectroscopic studies

showed that lateral diffusion of lipids is a rapid process but that flipping from one side of a bilayer to the other is a slow one. The fluid mosaic model of membranes (Fig. 7-1C) incorporated this information, showing transmembrane proteins floating in a fluid lipid bilayer. Subsequent work revealed structures of many proteins that span the lipid bilayer, the existence of lipid anchors on some membrane proteins, and a network of cytoplasmic proteins that restricts the motion of many integral membrane proteins (Fig. 7-1D).

Lipids

Lipids form the framework of biological membranes, anchor soluble proteins to the surfaces of membranes, store energy, and carry information as extracellular hormones and as intracellular second messengers. Lipids are organic molecules generally less than 1000 D in size that are much more soluble in organic solvents than in water. They consist predominantly of aliphatic or aromatic hydrocarbons.

This chapter concentrates on major lipids found in biological membranes. After an introduction to their structures, the following section explains how the hydrophobic effect drives lipids to self-assemble stable bilayers. Membranes also contain hundreds of minor lipids, some of which might have important biological functions that are not yet appreciated. For example, during the 1980s, a minor class of lipids with phosphorylated inositol head groups first attracted attention when investigators found that they had a major role in signaling (see Fig. 26-7).

Phosphoglycerides

Phosphoglycerides (also called glycerolphospholipids) are the main constituents of membrane bilayers (Fig. 7-2). (These lipids are often called phospholipids, an imprecise term, as other lipids contain phosphate.) Phosphoglycerides have three parts: a three-carbon backbone of glycerol, two long-chain fatty acids esterified to carbons 1 and 2 (C_1 and C_2) of the glycerol, and phosphoric acid esterified to C_3 of the glycerol. Fatty acids have a carboxyl group at one end of an aliphatic chain of 13 to 19 additional carbons (Table 7-1). More than half of the fatty acids in membranes have one or more double bonds, which create a bend in the aliphatic chain. These bends contribute to the fluidity of the bilayer. Fatty acids and phosphoglycerides are **amphiphilic,** since they have both **hydrophobic** (fears water) and **hydrophilic** (loves water) parts. The aliphatic chains of fatty acids are hydrophobic. The carboxyl groups of fatty acids and the head groups of phosphoglycerides are hydrophilic.

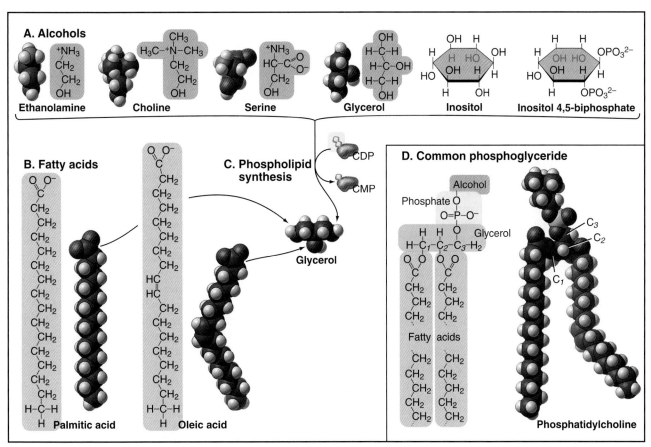

Figure 7-2 STRUCTURE AND SYNTHESIS OF PHOSPHOGLYCERIDES. **A,** Stick figures and space-filling models of the alcohol head groups. **B,** Stick figures and space-filling models of a saturated and an unsaturated fatty acid. **C,** Combination of an alcohol, a glycerol, and two fatty acids to make a phosphoglyceride. In some cases CDP provides the phosphate linking glycerol to the alcohol. **D,** Diagram of the parts of a phosphoglyceride and a space-filling model of phosphatidylcholine.

The cross-sectional areas of the head groups and the aliphatic tails are similar, so a phosphoglyceride is shaped approximately like a cylinder—an important factor in membrane structure. The hydrophobic effect (see Fig. 4-5) drives amphiphilic phosphoglycerides to assemble bilayers (see later).

Cells make more than 100 major phosphoglycerides by using several different fatty acids and by esterifying one of five different alcohols to the phosphate. In general, the fatty acids on C_1 have no or one double bond, whereas the fatty acids on C_2 have two or more double bonds. Each double bond creates a permanent bend in the hydrocarbon chain. The alcohol head groups, rather than the fatty acids, give phosphoglycerides their names:

phosphatidic acid [PA] (no head group)

phosphatidylglycerol [PG] (glycerol head group)

phosphatidylethanolamine [PE] (ethanolamine head group)

phosphatidylcholine [PC] (choline head group)

phosphatidylserine [PS] (serine head group)

phosphatidylinositol [PI] (inositol head group)

The several head groups confer distinctive properties to the various phosphoglycerides. All have a negative charge on the phosphate esterified to glycerol. Neutral phosphoglycerides—PE and PC—have a positive charge

Table 7-1

COMMON FATTY ACIDS OF MEMBRANE LIPIDS

Name	Carbons	Double Bonds (Positions)
Myristate	14	0
Palmitate	16	0
Palmitoleate	16	1 (Δ9)
Stearate	18	0
Oleate	18	1 (Δ9)
Linoleate	18	2 (Δ9, Δ12)
Linolenate	18	3 (Δ9, Δ12, Δ15)
Arachidonate	20	4 (Δ5, Δ8, Δ11, Δ14)

on their nitrogens, giving them a net charge of zero. PS has extra positive and negative charges, giving it a net negative charge like the other acidic phosphoglycerides (PA, PG, and PI). PI can be modified by esterifying one to five phosphates to the hexane ring hydroxyls. These **polyphosphoinositides** are highly negatively charged.

The complicated metabolism of phosphoglycerides can be simplified as follows: Enzymes can interconvert all phosphoglyceride head groups and remodel fatty acid chains. For example, three successive enzymatic methylation reactions convert PE to PC, whereas another enzyme exchanges serine for ethanolamine, converting PS to PE. Other enzymes exchange fatty acid chains after the initial synthesis of a phosphoglyceride. These enzymes are located on the cytoplasmic surface of the smooth endoplasmic reticulum. Biochemistry texts provide more details of these pathways.

Several minor membrane phospholipids are variations on this general theme. Plasmalogens have a fatty acid linked to carbon 1 of glycerol by an ether bond rather than an ester bond. They serve as sources of arachidonic acid for signaling reactions (see Fig. 26-9). Cardiolipin has two glycerols esterified to the phosphate of PA.

Sphingolipids

Most sugar-containing lipids of biological membranes are sphingolipids. Sphingolipids get their name from **sphingosine,** a nitrogen-containing base (Fig. 7-3) that is the structural counterpart of glycerol and one fatty acid of phosphoglycerides. Sphingosine carbons 1 to 3 have polar substituents. A double bond between C_4 and C_5 begins the hydrocarbon tail. Two variable features distinguish the various sphingolipids: the fatty acid (often lacking double bonds) attached by an amide bond to C_2 and the nature of the polar head groups esterified to the hydroxyl on C_1.

The head groups of **glycosphingolipids** consist of one or more sugars. Some are neutral; others are negatively charged. Note the absence of phosphate. Sugar head groups of some glycosphingolipids serve as receptors for viruses. Alternatively, a phosphate ester can link a base to C_1. These so-called **sphingomyelins** have phosphorylcholine or phosphoethanolamine head groups just like PC and PE. Receptor-activated enzymes remove phosphorylcholine from sphingomyelin to produce the second messenger ceramide (see Fig. 26-11). Sphingolipids are much more abundant in the plasma membrane than in membranes inside cells. The hydrocarbon tails of sphingosine and the fatty acid contribute to the hydrophobic bilayer, and polar head groups are on the surface.

Sterols

Sterols are the third major class of membrane lipids. **Cholesterol** (Fig. 7-4) is the major sterol in animal plasma membranes, with lower concentrations in internal membranes. Plants, lower eukaryotes, and bacteria have other sterols in their membranes. The rigid four-ring structure of cholesterol is apolar, so it inserts into

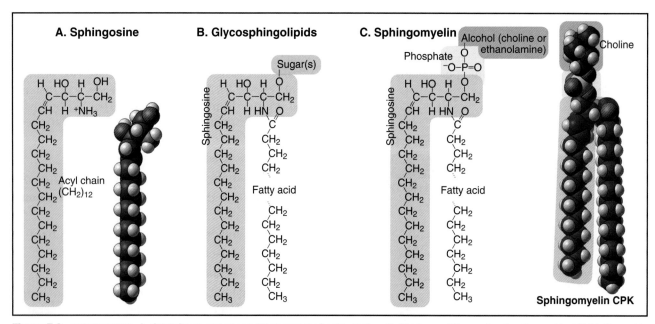

Figure 7-3   SPHINGOLIPIDS. **A,** Stick figure and space-filling model of sphingosine. **B,** Diagram of the parts of a glycosphingolipid. Ceramide has a fatty acid but no sugar. **C,** Stick figure and space-filling model of sphingomyelin.

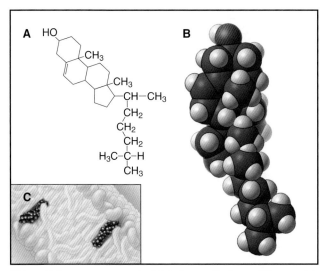

Figure 7-4 **CHOLESTEROL. A,** Stick figure. **B,** Space-filling model. **C,** Disposition of cholesterol in a lipid bilayer with the hydroxyl oriented toward the surface. The rigid sterol nucleus tends to order fluid bilayers in the region between C_1 and C_{10} of the fatty acids but promotes motion of the fatty acyl chains deeper in the bilayer owing to its wedge shape.

the core of bilayers with the hydroxyl on C_3 oriented toward the surface.

Cholesterol is vital to metabolism, being situated at the crossroads of several metabolic pathways, including those that synthesize steroid hormones (such as estrogen, testosterone, and cortisol), vitamin D, and bile salts secreted by the liver. Cholesterol itself is synthesized (see Fig. 20-13) from **isopentyl** (5-carbon) building blocks that form 10-carbon **(geranyl),** 15-carbon **(farnesyl),** and 20-carbon **(geranylgeranyl) isoprenoids.** As is described later, these isoprenoids are used as hydrocarbon anchors for many important membrane-associated proteins. Isoprenoids are also precursors of natural rubber and of cofactors present in visual pigments.

Glycolipids

Cells have three types of glycolipids: (1) sphingolipids (the predominant form), (2) glycerol glycolipids with sugar chains attached to the hydroxyl on C_3 of diglycerides, and (3) **glycosylphosphatidylinositols (GPI).** Some glycosylphosphatidylinositols simply have a short carbohydrate chain on the hydroxyl of inositol C_2. Others use a short sugar chain to link C_6 of phosphatidylinositol to the C-terminus of a protein (Fig. 7-9C).

Triglycerides

Triglycerides are simply glycerol with fatty acids esterified to all three carbons. Lacking a polar head group, they are not incorporated into membrane bilayers.

Instead, triglycerides form large, oily droplets in the cytoplasm that are a convenient way to store fatty acids as reserves of metabolic energy. In white adipose cells, specialized for lipid storage, the triglyceride droplet occupies most of the cytoplasm (see Fig. 28-6). Mitochondria oxidize fatty acids and convert the energy in their covalent bonds into ATP (see Fig. 19-4).

Physical Structure of the Fluid Membrane Bilayer

In an aqueous environment, amphiphilic lipids spontaneously self-assemble into ordered structures in microseconds. The cylindrical shapes and amphiphilic nature of phosphoglycerides and sphingolipids favor formation of lamellar bilayers, planar structures with fatty acid chains lined up more or less normal to the surface and polar head groups on the surfaces exposed to water (Fig. 7-1D). Bilayer formation is energetically favorable, owing to the increase in entropy when the hydrophobic acyl chains interact with each other and exclude water from the core of the bilayer. This hydrophobic effect increases the entropy of the system and drives the assembly process.

An atomic model of a phosphoglyceride bilayer (Fig. 7-5) has the hydrocarbon chains on the inside and polar head groups facing the surrounding water. The model accounts for the physical properties of biological membranes. It emphasizes the tremendous disorder of the lipid molecules, as expected for a liquid. Polar head groups vary widely in their orientation, and some protrude far into water. This makes the bilayer surface very rough at the nanometer level. The phosphorylcholine head groups are oriented nearly parallel to the bilayer rather than sticking out into water. Fatty acid chains undergo internal motions on a picosecond time scale, making them highly irregular, with about 25% of the bonds in the bent (gauche) configuration. The molecular density is lowest in the middle of the bilayer.

In the model, water penetrates the bilayer only to the level of the deepest carbonyl oxygens, leaving a dehydrated layer about 1.5 nm thick in the center of the bilayer. Nevertheless, a few water molecules move across the bilayer. Water molecules near the bilayer tend to orient with their negative dipole toward the hydrocarbon interior. This generates an electrical potential (positive inside) between the hydrocarbon and the aqueous phase despite an oppositely oriented potential arising from the electrical dipole between the P and N atoms of the head groups. This inside positive potential may contribute to the barrier to the transfer of positively charged polypeptides across membranes.

The model also accounts for the mechanical properties of membranes. Although bilayers neither stretch nor compress readily, they are very flexible, owing to rapid

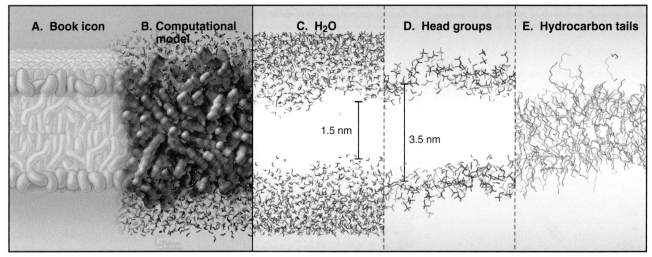

Figure 7-5 ATOMIC MODEL OF A HYDRATED PHOSPHATIDYLCHOLINE BILAYER DETERMINED BY SIMULATION ON A SUPERCOMPUTER. **A,** Lipid bilayer–based icon used throughout this book based on the model of a phosphatidylcholine bilayer shown in **B**. **B,** Space-filling model with all the lipid atoms in the simulation. Stick figures of the water molecules are *red*. The polar regions of phosphatidylcholine (PC) from the carbonyl oxygen to the choline nitrogen are *blue*. Hydrocarbon tails are *yellow*. **C,** Water molecules only. **D,** Polar regions of PC from the carbonyl oxygen to the choline nitrogen only. **E,** Hydrocarbon tails only. This model was calculated from first principles rather than experimental data, such as X-ray diffraction or NMR. This computational approach is both necessary and appropriate, as a lipid bilayer is a fluid without a regular structure. Such models account for virtually all molecular parameters (electron density, surface roughness, distance between phosphates of the two halves, area per lipid [0.6 nm²], and depth of water penetration) of similar bilayers obtained by averaging techniques, including NMR, X-ray diffraction, and neutron diffraction. The simulation started with 100 PC molecules (based on an X-ray diffraction structure of PC crystals) in a regular bilayer with 1050 molecules of bulk phase water on each side. Taking into account surface tension and distribution of charge on lipid and water, the computer simulated the molecular motion of all atoms on a picosecond time scale using simple Newtonian mechanics. After less than 100 picoseconds of simulated time (taking weeks of computation), the liquid phase of the lipids appeared. The model shown here is after 300 picoseconds of simulated time. (Courtesy of E. Jakobsson, University of Illinois, Urbana. Redrawn from Chiu S-W, Clark M, Balaji V, et al: Incorporation of surface tension into molecular dynamics simulation of an interface: A fluid phase lipid bilayer membrane. Biophys J 69:1230–1245, 1995.)

fluctuations in the arrangement of the lipids. Thus, one can also draw out a narrow tube of membrane by sucking gently on the surface of a cell. Little force is required to deform bilayers into the complex shapes observed for cell membranes. Both these features are illustrated by the response of a red blood cell plasma membrane to changes in volume (Fig. 7-6). Because the membrane area is constant, a reduction in volume throws the membrane into folds, whereas swelling distends it to a spherical shape until it eventually bursts. If osmotic forces rupture a lipid bilayer, it will reseal.

A variety of biophysical methods, including fluorescence recovery after photobleaching (Fig. 7-11), have shown that lipid molecules diffuse rapidly in the plane of a bilayer. A typical lateral diffusion coefficient (D) for a membrane lipid is approximately 1 $\mu m^2\ s^{-1}$. Given that the rate of diffusion is $2(Dt)^{1/2}$ (t = time), a lipid molecule moves laterally about 1 $\mu m/s$ in the plane of the membrane. Thus, a diffusing lipid circumnavigates the membrane of a bacterium in a few seconds. Cholesterol flips between the two side of a bilayer on a second time scale. Rarely (about $10^{-5}\ s^{-1}$), a neutral phosphoglyceride, such as PC, flips unassisted from one side of a bilayer to the other. Charged phosphoglycerides are slower. Proteins can facilitate this flipping in cellular membranes (see Fig. 20-12).

Despite all the lateral movement of the molecules, phospholipid bilayers are stable and impermeable to polar or charged compounds, even those as small as Na^+ or Cl^-. This poor electrical conductivity is essential for many biological processes (see Fig. 11-6). Small, uncharged molecules, such as water and glycerol, pass slowly across lipid bilayers and more rapidly through channels (see Figs. 10-14 and 10-15).

Biological membranes vary considerably in their lipid composition. In addition to phosphoglycerides, plasma membranes are about 35% cholesterol and over 10% sphingolipids (Fig. 7-7), while internal membranes have little of these lipids. Like bilayers of pure phosphatidylcholine cellular membranes have limited permeability to ions, high electrical resistance, and the ability to self-seal. The length of fatty acids and the presence of unsaturated bonds strongly influence the physical properties of membranes. Fatty acids with 18 or more carbons are solid at physiological temperatures unless they contain double bonds. Hence, phosphoglycerides in biological membranes usually contain C16 saturated fatty acids and longer-chain fatty acids with double bonds (C18 with one to three double bonds and C20 with four double bonds [Table 7-1]). Permanent bends created by double bonds contribute to bilayer fluidity by preventing tight packing of fatty acid tails in the middle of the

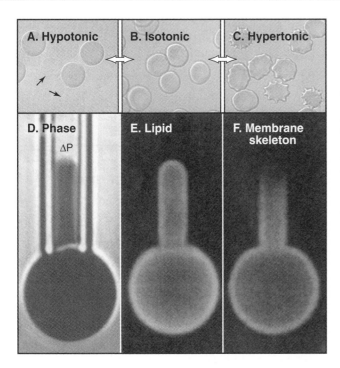

Figure 7-6 MEMBRANE DEFORMABILITY ILLUSTRATED BY THE PLASMA MEMBRANE OF HUMAN RED BLOOD CELLS. **A–C,** Differential interference contrast light micrographs. In an isotonic medium, the cell is a biconcave disk. In a hypotonic medium, water enters the cytoplasm, and the cell rounds up. The cell will burst *(arrows)* when the area of the membrane cannot accommodate the volume. In a hypertonic medium, water leaves the cell, and the membrane is thrown into spikes and folds. **D,** Phase contrast micrograph showing that the plasma membrane is flexible enough to be drawn by suction into a capillary tube. **E,** Fluorescence micrograph showing that membrane lipids, marked with a fluorescent dye, evenly surround the membrane extension. **F,** The elastic membrane skeleton, marked with another fluorescent dye, stretches into the capillary but not to the tip of the extension. (D–F, Courtesy of N. Mohandas, Lawrence Berkeley Laboratory, Berkeley, California. Reference: Discher D, Mohandas N, Evans E: Molecular maps of red cell deformation. Science 266:1032–1035, 1994.)

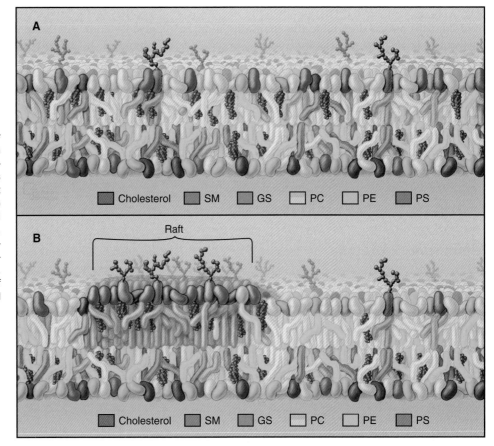

Figure 7-7 LIPID COMPOSITION OF A PLASMA MEMBRANE ILLUSTRATING THE HETEROGENEITY AND ASYMMETRICAL DISTRIBUTION OF THE LIPIDS BETWEEN THE TWO HALVES OF THE BILAYER. **A,** Sphingomyelin (SM) and cholesterol form a small cluster in the external leaflet. GS, glycosphingolipid; PC, phosphatidylcholine; PE, phosphatidylethanolamine; PS, phosphatidylserine. **B,** Lipid raft in the outer leaflet of the plasma membrane enriched in cholesterol and sphingolipids.

bilayer. The presence of cholesterol in a bilayer makes the acyl chains pack more compactly. This allows lateral mobility of the lipids but restricts movement of small molecules across the bilayer.

With the exception of cholesterol, most lipids distribute asymmetrically between the two halves of biological membranes. In plasma membranes, glycosphingolipids are outside, while phosphatidylserine and phosphatidylinositol face the cytoplasm (Fig. 7-7). Phosphatidylserine asymmetry gives the cytoplasmic surface of the plasma membrane a net negative charge. **Lipid asymmetry** established during biosynthesis of membranes (see Chapter 20) is maintained, owing to the low rate of flipping of charged lipids from one side of a bilayer to the other. The lipid composition of prokaryotic membranes differs from that of eukaryotes. Bacterial membranes consist of phosphatidylethanolamine, phosphatidylglycerol, cardiolipin, and other lipids. Archaeal membranes have a mixture of glycolipids, neutral lipids, and ether-linked lipids, and some include single fatty acids.

Since cholesterol interacts favorably with sphingolipids, they have been proposed to form a separate phase in the outer leaflet of plasma membranes named **rafts** (Fig. 7-7B). It has been hard to pin down the size of such lipid domains and to determine the composition of the adjacent inner leaflet. A variety of indirect evidence is consistent with this idea, but these lipids might actually be dispersed in the outer leaflet of the plasma membrane (Fig. 7-7A), except for special invaginations called caveolae (see Fig. 22-6). Some transmembrane proteins, GPI-anchored proteins, and fatty acid–anchored proteins (Figs. 7-8 and 7-9) associate with sphingolipids and cholesterol in membrane extracts and in artificial bilayers. Consequently, establishing the degree of segregation of these lipids in membranes will also shed light on many membrane functions including signaling.

Membrane Proteins

Proteins are responsible for most membrane functions. The variety of membrane proteins is great, comprising about one third of proteins in sequenced genomes. Integral membrane proteins cross the lipid bilayer, and peripheral membrane proteins associate with the inside or outside surfaces of the bilayer. Transmembrane segments of integral membrane proteins interact with hydrocarbon chains of the lipid bilayer and have few hydrophilic residues on these surfaces. Like other soluble proteins, peripheral membrane proteins have hydrophilic residues exposed on their surfaces and a core of hydrophobic residues. Chemical extraction experiments distinguish these two classes of membrane proteins. Alkaline solvents (e.g., 0.1 M carbonate at pH 11.3) solubilize most peripheral proteins, leaving behind the lipid bilayer and integral membrane proteins. Detergents, which interact with hydrophobic transmembrane segments, solubilize integral membrane proteins.

Integral Membrane Proteins

Atomic structures of a growing number of integral membrane proteins and primary structures of thousands of others show how proteins associate with lipid bilayers (Fig. 7-8). Many integral membrane proteins have a single peptide segment that fulfills the energetic criteria (Box 7-1) for a membrane-spanning α-helix. Glycophorin from the red blood cell membrane was the first of these proteins to be characterized (Fig. 7-8A). Nuclear magnetic resonance experiments established that the single **transmembrane segment** of glycophorin is an α-helix. This helix interacts more favorably with lipid acyl chains than with water. By analogy with glycophorin, it is generally accepted that single, 25-residue hydrophobic segments of other transmembrane proteins fold into α-helices. In many cases, independent evidence has confirmed that the single segment crosses the bilayer. For example, proteolytic enzymes might cleave the peptide at the predicted membrane interface. Potential glycosylation sites might be located outside the cell. Chemical or antibody labeling might identify parts of the protein inside or outside the cells.

Transmembrane segments of integral membrane proteins that cross the bilayer more than once are folded into α-helices or β-strands. Hydrogen bonding of all backbone amides and carbonyls in the secondary structure minimizes the energy required to bury the backbone in the hydrophobic lipid bilayer. For the same reason, most amino acid side chains in contact with fatty acyl chains in the bilayer are hydrophobic. Chapter 21 considers how transmembrane proteins fold during their biosynthesis.

Integral membrane proteins with all α-helical transmembrane segments are the most common. Examples are bacteriorhodopsin (Fig. 7-8B; see also Fig. 24-2), pumps (see Figs. 8-3, 8-5, 8-7, and 8-9), carriers (see Fig. 9-3), channels (see Fig. 10-3), cytochrome oxidase (see Fig. 19-5), and photosynthetic reaction centers (see Fig. 19-9). All of these proteins have polar and charged residues in the plane of the bilayer, generally facing away from the lipid toward the interior of the protein, in contrast to the opposite arrangement in water-soluble proteins.

Many transmembrane proteins consist of multiple subunits that associate in the plane of the bilayer (Fig. 7-8). The transmembrane helix of glycophorin A has a strong tendency to form homodimers in the plane of the membrane. Dimers are favored because complementary surfaces on a pair of helices interact more precisely with each other than with lipids. The positive entropy change

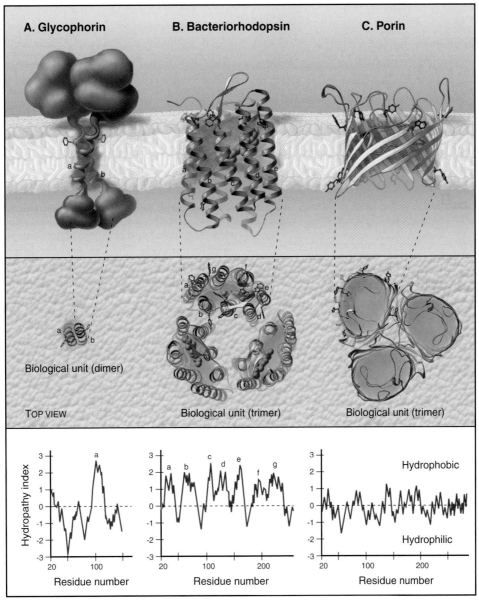

A. Glycophorin **B. Bacteriorhodopsin** **C. Porin**

Biological unit (dimer)

TOP VIEW   Biological unit (trimer)   Biological unit (trimer)

Hydropathy index

Hydrophobic

Hydrophilic

Residue number   Residue number   Residue number

Figure 7-8 STRUCTURES OF REPRESENTATIVE INTEGRAL MEMBRANE PROTEINS. **Top row,** Views across the lipid bilayer. **Middle row,** Views in the plane of the lipid bilayer. **Bottom row,** Hydrophobicity analysis. **A,** Glycophorin, a human red blood cell protein, has a single transmembrane α-helix. The extracellular and cytoplasmic domains are artistic conceptions. The transmembrane helices have a strong tendency to form homodimers in the plane of the membrane. (PDB file: 1MSR.) **B,** Bacteriorhodopsin, a light-driven proton pump from the plasma membrane of a halophilic bacterium, has seven transmembrane helices. The green space-filling structure is retinal, the covalently bound, light-absorbing "chromophore." This structure was first determined by electron microscopy of two-dimensional crystals and extended to higher resolution by X-ray diffraction. (PDB file: 1AT9.) **C,** Porin, a nonselective channel protein from the outer membrane of a bacterium, is composed largely of transmembrane β-strands. This structure was determined by X-ray crystallography of three-dimensional crystals. (PDB file: 1PRN.) Hydropathy plots are calculated from the energy required to transfer an amino acid from an organic solvent to water. One sums the transfer free energy for segments of 20 residues. Segments with large, positive (unfavorable) transfer free energies (around 1.5 on this scale) are more soluble in the hydrophobic interior of a membrane bilayer than in water and thus are candidates for membrane-spanning segments.

associated with dissociation of lipids from interacting protein surfaces (comparable to the hydrophobic effect in water) drives the reaction. Unconventional hydrogen bonds between backbone carbonyl oxygens and C-α hydrogens also stabilize dimers. Bacteriorhodopsin molecules self-associate in the plane of the membrane to

form extended two-dimensional crystals. Many membrane channels form by association of four similar or identical subunits with a pore at their central interface (see Fig. 10-1). Acetylcholine receptors are pentamers of identical or related subunits. Together, they form a cation channel that opens transiently when the

Amino Acid Sequences Identify
Candidate Transmembrane Segments

Amino acid sequences of integral membrane proteins frequently provide important clues about segments of the polypeptide that cross the lipid bilayer. Each crossing segment must be long enough to span the bilayer with a minimum of charged or polar groups in contact with the lipid (Fig. 7-8). Polar backbone amide and carbonyl atoms are buried in α-helices or β-sheets to avoid contact with lipid. In many transmembrane segments, aromatic residues project into the lipid near the level where acyl chains are bonded to the lipid head groups (red side chains in Fig. 7-8). A helix of 20 to 25 residues or a β-strand of 10 residues is long enough (3.0 to 3.8 nm) to span a lipid bilayer.

Quantitative analysis of the side chain and backbone **hydropathy** (aversion to water) of the sequence of an integral membrane protein usually identifies one or more hydrophobic sequences long enough to cross a bilayer (see the legend for Fig. 7-8 for details). The approach works best for helices that are inserted directly in the lipid, like the single transmembrane helix of glycophorin A, which has mostly apolar side chains. If a protein has multiple transmembrane helices, some may escape detection by hydrophobicity analysis, because the helices may group together to surround a hydrophilic channel lined with charged and polar side chains. For example, two of seven transmembrane helices of bacteriorhodopsin contain charged residues facing the interior of the protein, so they are less hydrophobic than the other transmembrane helices. Transmembrane β-strands are more challenging, since only half of the side chains face the membrane lipids. None of the transmembrane strands of porin qualify in terms of hydrophobicity criteria. They are short, and many contain polar residues. Independent biochemical or structural data are required to confirm the identity of transmembrane polypeptides.

neurotransmitter acetylcholine binds to the two α-subunits (see Fig. 10-12). Bacterial cytochrome oxidase is an assembly of four different subunits with a total of 22 transmembrane helices (see Fig. 19-5). The purple bacterium photosynthetic reaction center consists of three unique helical subunits plus a peripheral cytochrome protein (see Fig. 19-9).

A minority of integral membrane proteins use β-strands to cross the lipid bilayer. Porins form channels for many substances, up to the size of proteins, to cross the outer membranes of gram-positive bacteria and their eukaryotic descendents, mitochondria and chloroplasts. Porins consist of an extended β-strand barrel with a hydrophobic exterior surrounding an aqueous pore

(Fig. 7-8C). These subunits associate as trimers in the lipid bilayer.

In addition to transmembrane helices or strands, many integral membrane proteins have structural elements that pass partway across the bilayer. Porins have extended polypeptide loops inside the β-barrel. Many channel proteins have a short helices and loops that reverse in the middle of the membrane bilayer. These structural elements help to form pores specific for potassium (see Fig. 10-3), chloride (see Fig. 10-13), and water (see Fig. 10-15).

Peripheral Membrane Proteins

Six strategies bind peripheral proteins to the surfaces of membranes (Fig. 7-9). One of three different types of acyl chains can anchor a protein to a membrane by inserting into the lipid bilayer. Other proteins bind electrostatically to membrane lipids, and some insert partially into the lipid bilayer. Many peripheral proteins bind directly or indirectly to integral membrane proteins.

Isoprenoid Tails

A 15-carbon isoprenoid (farnesyl) tail (see Fig. 20-13) is added posttranslationally to the side chain of a cysteine residue near the C-terminus of the guanosine triphosphatase (GTPase) Ras (see Fig. 4-6) and many other proteins. The enzyme making this modification recognizes the target cysteine followed by two aliphatic amino acids plus any other amino acid (a CAAX recognition site). Membrane attachment by this farnesyl chain is required for Ras to participate in growth factor signaling (see Fig. 27-6).

Myristoyl Tails

Myristate, a 14-carbon saturated fatty acid, anchors the tyrosine kinase Src (see Box 27-1) and other proteins involved in cellular signaling to the cytoplasmic face of the plasma membrane. Myristate is added to the amino group of an N-terminal glycine during the biosynthesis of these proteins. Insertion of this single fatty acyl chain into a lipid bilayer is so weak (K_d: ~10^{-4} M) that additional electrostatic interactions between basic side chains of the protein and head groups of acidic phosphoglycerides are required to maintain attachment to the membrane. As a consequence, phosphorylation can dissociate some myristoylated proteins from membranes by competing with these secondary electrostatic interactions.

Glycosylphosphatidylinositol Tails

A short oligosaccharide-phosphoglyceride tail links a variety of proteins to the outer surface of the plasma

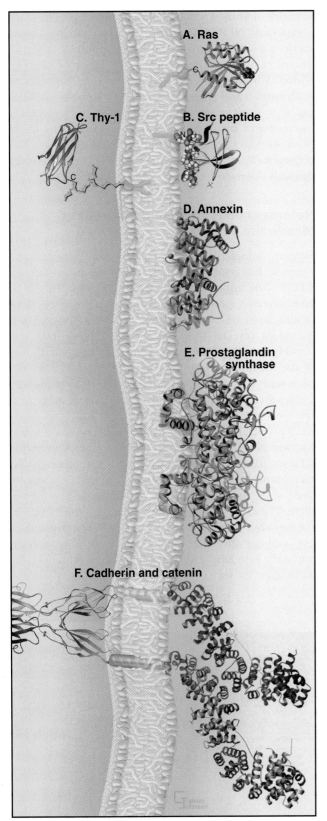

membrane. The C-terminus of these proteins is attached covalently to the oligosaccharide, and the two fatty acyl chains of phosphatidylinositol anchor the link to the lipid bilayer. In animal cells, this glycosylphosphatidylinositol (GPI) anchors important plasma membrane proteins, including enzymes (acetylcholine esterase; see Fig. 11-8), adhesion proteins (T-cadherin; see Fig. 30-5), and cell surface antigens (Thy-1). The protozoan parasite *Trypanosoma brucei* covers itself with a high concentration of a GPI-anchored protein. If challenged by an antibody response from the host, the parasite sheds the protein by hydrolysis of the lipid anchor and expresses a variant protein to evade the immune system.

Electrostatic Interaction with Phospholipids

As was postulated in the 1930s (Fig. 7-1), a number of soluble cytoplasmic proteins bind the head groups of membrane lipids. The full range of these electrostatic interactions has yet to be explored, as the concept was largely neglected for two decades after the recognition of transmembrane proteins and the emergence of the fluid mosaic model of membranes. Annexins, a family of calcium-binding proteins implicated in membrane fusion reactions, bind tightly to phosphatidylserine. Myosin-I motor proteins (see Fig. 36-7) also bind strongly to acidic phosphoglycerides, a possible step in targeting to cellular membranes.

Partial Penetration of the Lipid Bilayer

For years, it was believed that no proteins penetrate the lipid bilayer only partially. It was thought that they either traverse the membrane fully one or more times or bind to the surface. However, some peptide venoms (such as bee venom mellitin) intercalate into half of a lipid bilayer. Hydrophobic α-helices of prostaglandin H_2 synthase (see Fig. 26-9) are also postulated to anchor the enzyme to membranes by partially penetrating the lipid bilayer.

Association with Integral Proteins

Many peripheral proteins bind cytoplasmic domains of integral membrane proteins. For example, catenins bind

Figure 7-9 SIX DIFFERENT WAYS FOR PERIPHERAL MEMBRANE PROTEINS TO ASSOCIATE WITH THE LIPID BILAYER. **A,** A C-terminal isoprenoid tail attaches Ras to the bilayer. (PDB file: 121P.) **B,** An N-terminal myristoyl tail binds Src weakly to the bilayer. Electrostatic interactions between acidic lipids and basic amino acids stabilize the interaction. **C,** A C-terminal GPI tail anchors Thy-1 (similar to an immunoglobulin variable domain) to the bilayer. **D,** Electrostatic interactions with phospholipids bind annexin to the bilayer. (PDB file: 1A8A.) **E,** Hydrophobic helices of prostaglandin H_2 synthase are postulated to penetrate the lipid bilayer partially. (PDB file: 1CQE.) **F,** The peripheral protein β-catenin (*blue* [PDB file: 1I7W]) associates with the cytoplasmic portion of the transmembrane adhesion protein cadherin (*red* and *green* [PDB file: 1FF5]).

transmembrane cell adhesion proteins called cadherins. These protein–protein interactions may provide more specificity and higher affinity than do the interactions of peripheral proteins with membrane lipids. Such protein–protein interactions anchor the cytoskeleton to transmembrane adhesion proteins (see Fig. 31-7) and guide the assembly of coated vesicles during endocytosis (see Fig. 22-11). Protein–protein interactions also provide a way to transmit information across a membrane. Ligand binding to the extracellular domain of a transmembrane receptor can change the conformation of its cytoplasmic domain, promoting interactions with cytoplasmic, signal-transducing proteins (see Chapter 24 and Fig. 46-17).

The **membrane skeleton** on the cytoplasmic surface of the plasma membrane of human red blood cells (Fig. 7-10) provided the first insights regarding interaction of peripheral and integral membrane proteins. Two types of integral membrane proteins—an anion carrier called Band 3 and glycophorin—anchor a two-dimensional network of fibrous proteins to the membrane. The main component of this network is a long, flexible, tetrameric, actin-binding protein called **spectrin** (after its discovery in lysed red blood cells, "ghosts"; see Fig. 33-16). A linker protein called ankyrin binds tightly to both Band 3 and spectrin. About 35,000 nodes consisting of a short actin filament and associated proteins interconnect the elastic spectrin network. This membrane skeleton reinforces the bilayer, allowing a cell to recover its shape elastically after it is distorted by passage through the narrow lumen of blood capillaries.

Heterogeneous, Dynamic Behavior of Membrane Proteins

Several complementary methods can monitor the dynamic behavior of plasma membrane proteins (Fig. 7-11A). One approach—the one used originally—is to label proteins with a fluorescent dye, either by covalent modification or by attachment of an antibody with a bound fluorescent dye. After a spot of intense light irreversibly bleaches the fluorescent dyes in a small area of the membrane, one observes the fluorescence over time with a microscope. If the test protein is mobile, unbleached proteins from surrounding areas move into the bleached area. The rate and extent of fluorescence recovery after **photobleaching** (FRAP) revealed that a fraction of the population of most membrane proteins diffuses freely in two dimensions in the plane of the membrane but that a substantial fraction is immobilized, since the recovery from photobleaching is incomplete. The same photobleaching method is used to study the mobility of fluorescent fusion proteins targeted to any cellular membrane (see Fig. 6-3). The second approach is to label individual membrane proteins with antibodies or lectins (carbohydrate-binding proteins)

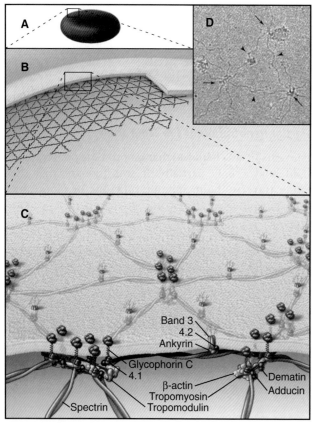

Figure 7-10 THE MEMBRANE SKELETON ON THE CYTOPLASMIC SURFACE OF THE RED BLOOD CELL PLASMA MEMBRANE. **A,** Whole cell. **B,** Cut-away drawing. **C,** Detailed drawing. Nodes consisting of a short actin filament and associated proteins interact with multiple spectrin molecules, which, in turn, bind to two transmembrane proteins: glycophorin and (via ankyrin) Band 3. **D,** An electron micrograph of the actin-spectrin network. (D, Courtesy of R. Josephs, University of Chicago, Illinois.)

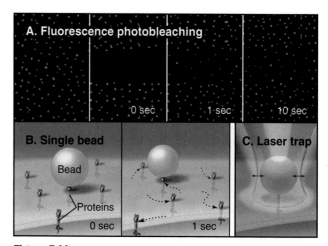

Figure 7-11 METHODS USED TO DOCUMENT THE MOVEMENTS OF MEMBRANE PROTEINS. **A,** Fluorescence recovery after photobleaching. **B,** Single-particle tracking. **C,** Optical trapping.

attached to small particles of gold or plastic beads (Fig. 7-11B). High-contrast light microscopy can follow the motion of a particle attached to a membrane protein. Despite their size, the particles have minimal effects on diffusion of membrane proteins. The third method is an extension of single-particle tracking. Instead of merely watching spontaneous movements, the investigator can grab a particle in an **optical trap** created by focusing an infrared laser beam through the microscope objective (Fig. 7-11C). Manipulation of particles with an optical trap reveals what happens when force is applied to a membrane protein.

Membrane proteins exhibit a wide range of dynamic behaviors (Fig. 7-12). Some molecules diffuse freely. Others diffuse intermittently, alternating with periods of restricted movement. A substantial number of membrane proteins are immobilized, presumably by direct or indirect associations with the membrane skeleton or cytoskeleton. Others exhibit long-distance directed movements, presumably powered by motor proteins in the cytoplasm.

The population of a given type of membrane protein (e.g., a cell adhesion protein) may exhibit more than one class of dynamic behavior. For example, most proteins with GPI anchors diffuse freely, as is expected from their association with the lipid bilayer, but a fraction of any GPI-anchored protein has restricted mobility. Some transmembrane proteins also diffuse freely, but a fraction may become trapped or immobilized at any time. Diffusing proteins must be free of interactions with the membrane skeleton and with anchored membrane proteins. Cell adhesion proteins (cadherins; see Fig. 30-5) and nutrient receptors (transferrin receptors; see Fig. 22-14) are examples of transmembrane proteins that diffuse intermittently. They alternate between free diffusion and temporary trapping for 3 to 30 seconds in local domains measuring less than 0.5 μm in diameter. In some cases, trapping depends on the cytoplasmic tails of transmembrane proteins, which are thought to interact reversibly with the cytoskeleton or with immobilized membrane proteins. Tugs with an optical trap

show that the cages that confine these particles are elastic, as expected for cytoskeletal networks. Extracellular domains of these proteins may also interact with adjacent immobilized proteins. Immobilized proteins do not diffuse freely, and particles attached to them resist displacement by optical traps. Remarkably, the lipid bilayer can flow past immobilized transmembrane elements without disrupting the membrane. If the plasma membrane of a red blood cell is sucked into a narrow pipette (Fig. 7-6), lipids of the fluid membrane bilayer extend uniformly over the protrusion, leaving behind the immobilized membrane proteins and the membrane skeleton.

Some membrane proteins undergo long-distance translational movements in relatively straight lines. Diffusion cannot account for these linear movements, so they must be powered by motor proteins attached to cytoplasmic domains. Because disruption of cytoplasmic actin filaments by drugs impedes these movements, myosins (see Fig. 36-7) are the most likely, but still unproved, motors for these movements. In some instances, members of the integrin family of adhesion proteins (see Fig. 30-9) use this transport system.

Movement of membrane proteins in the plane of the membrane is essential for many cellular functions. During receptor-mediated endocytosis, receptors are concentrated in coated pits before internalization (see Fig. 22-11). Similarly, transduction of many signals from outside the cell depends on the formation of receptor dimers or trimers (see Figs. 24-5, 24-7, 24-8, 24-9, 24-10, 24-11, and 46-17). Some freely diffusing receptor subunits may be brought together by binding extracellular ligands. In other cases, ligand binding changes the conformation of preexisting dimers in the membrane. In both cases, juxtaposition of the cytoplasmic domains of receptor subunits activates downstream signaling mechanisms, such as protein kinases. Similarly, clustering of adhesion receptors, allowed by movements in the plane of the plasma membrane, enhances binding of cells to their neighbors or to the extracellular matrix (see Figs. 30-6 and 30-11).

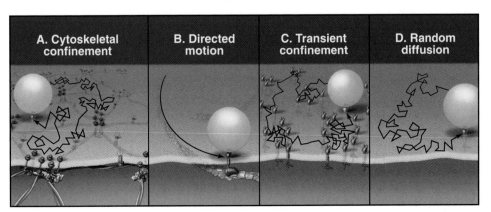

| A. Cytoskeletal confinement | B. Directed motion | C. Transient confinement | D. Random diffusion |

Figure 7-12 MOVEMENTS OF PROTEINS IN THE PLANE OF MEMBRANES. **A,** Transient confinement by obstacle clusters. **B,** Directed movements. **C,** Transient confinement by the membrane skeleton. **D,** Free diffusion. (Reference: Jacobson K, Sheets ED, Simson R: Revisiting the fluid mosaic model of membranes. Science 268:1441–1442, 1995.)

ACKNOWLEDGMENTS

Thanks go to Michael Edidin and Donald Engelman for their suggestions on this chapter.

SELECTED READINGS

Bijlmakers M-J, Marsh M: The on-off story of protein palmitoylation. Trends Cell Biol 13:32–42, 2003.

Casey PJ, Seabra MC: Protein prenyltransferases. J Biol Chem 271:5289–5292, 1996.

Curran AR, Engelman DM: Sequence motifs, polar interactions and conformational changes in helical membrane proteins. Curr Opin Struct Biol 13:412–417, 2003.

Dowhan W: Molecular basis for membrane phospholipid diversity: Why are there so many lipids? Annu Rev Biochem 66:199–232, 1997.

Edidin M: The state of lipid rafts: From model membranes to cells. Annu Rev Biophys Biomol Struct 32:257–283, 2003.

Edwards PA, Ericsson J: Sterols and isoprenoids: Signaling molecules derived from the cholesterol biosynthesis pathway. Annu Rev Biochem 68:157–186, 1999.

Engelman DM: Lipid bilayer structure in the membrane of Mycoplasma laidlawii. [Bilayer structure established by x-ray diffraction.] J Mol Biol 58:153–165, 1971.

Gahmberg GG, Tolvanen M: Why mammalian surface proteins are glycoproteins. Trends Biochem Sci 21:308–311, 1996.

Jakobsson E: Computer simulation studies of biological membranes: Progress, promise and pitfalls. Trends Biochem Sci 22:339–344, 1997.

Jayasinghe S, Hristova K, White SH: Energetics, stability, and prediction of transmembrane helices. J Mol Biol 312:927–934, 2001.

McNeil PL, Steinhardt RA: Plasma membrane disruption: Repair, prevention, adaptation. Annu Rev Cell Devel Biol 19:697–731, 2003.

Munro S: Lipid rafts: Elusive or illusive? Cell 115:377–388, 2003.

Robertson JD: Membrane structure. [Historical perspective.] J Cell Biol 91:1895–2045, 1981.

Sachs JN, Engelman DM: Introduction to the membrane protein reviews: The interplay of structure, dynamics, and environment in membrane protein function. Annu Rev Biophys Biomol Struct 35:707–712, 2006.

Senes A, Engel DE, DeGrado WF: Folding of helical membrane proteins: The role of polar, GxxxG-like and proline motifs. Curr Opin Struct Biol 14:465–479, 2004.

Simons K, Vaz WLC: Model systems, lipid rafts and cell membranes. Annu Rev Biophys Biomol Struct 33:269–295, 2004.

Stoeckenius W, Engelman DM: Current models for the structure of biological membranes. [Historical perspective.] J Cell Biol 42:613–646, 1969.

Torres J, Stevens TJ, Samsó M: Membrane proteins: The "Wild West" of structural biology. Trends Biochem Sci 28:137–144, 2003.

White SH: The progress of membrane protein structure determination. Protein Sci 13:1948–1949, 2004.

White SH, Wimley WC: Membrane protein folding and stability: Physical principles. Annu Rev Biophys Biomol Struct 28:319–365, 1999.

Zhang FL, Casey PJ: Protein prenylation: Molecular mechanisms and functional consequences. Annu Rev Biochem 65:241–270, 1996.

Membrane Pumps

Membrane Permeability: An Introduction

Although lipid bilayers provide a barrier to diffusion of ions and polar molecules larger than about 150 D, protein pores provide selective passages for ions, and other larger molecules across membranes. Integral proteins that control membrane permeability fall into three broad classes—pumps, carriers, and channels—each with distinct properties (Fig. 8-1). These proteins allow cells to control solute traffic across membranes, an essential feature of many physiological processes.

- **Pumps** are enzymes that utilize energy from adenosine triphosphate (ATP), light, or (rarely) other sources to move ions (generally, cations) and other solutes across membranes at relatively modest rates. They establish concentration gradients between membrane-bound compartments.

- **Carriers** are enzyme-like proteins that provide passive pathways for solutes to move across membranes down their concentration gradients from a region of higher concentration to one of lower concentration. Each conformational change in a carrier protein translocates a limited number of solutes across the membrane. Carriers use ion gradients as a source of energy to perform a remarkable variety of work. Some carriers use translocation of an ion down its concentration gradient to drive another ion or solute up a concentration gradient.

- **Channels** are ion-specific pores that typically open and close transiently in a regulated manner. When a channel is open, a flood of ions passes quickly across the membrane through the channel, driven by electrical and concentration gradients. The movement of ions through open channels controls the electrical potential across membranes, so that changes in channel activity produce rapid electrical signals in excitable membranes of nerves, muscles, and other cells.

This chapter and Chapters 9, 10, and 11 consider, in turn, the three classes of proteins that control membrane permeability. Pumps are discussed first because they create the solute gradients required for the function of carriers and channels. The concluding chapter in this section, Chapter 11, illustrates how pumps, carriers, and channels work together to perform a remarkable variety of functions. An important point is that differential expression of a subset of isoforms of these proteins in specific membranes allows differentiated cells to perform a wide range of complex functions.

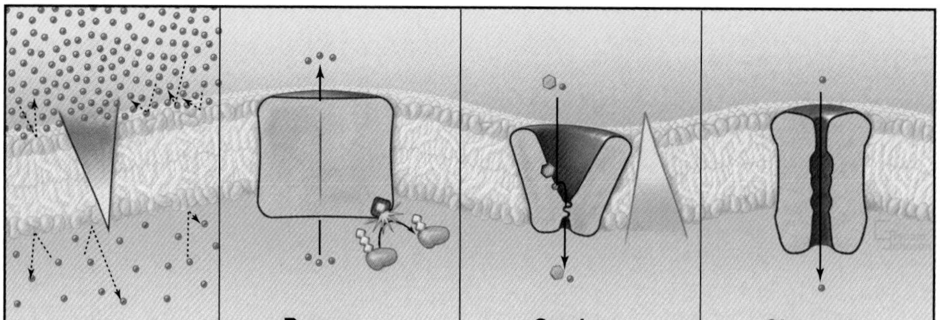

Figure 8-1 PROPERTIES OF THE THREE TYPES OF PROTEINS THAT TRANSPORT IONS AND OTHER SOLUTES ACROSS MEMBRANES. The triangle represents the concentration gradients of Na^+ *(blue)* and glucose *(green)* across the membrane.

	Pump	Carrier	Channel
Specificity	Absolute	Intermediate	Only 10–20×
Rate (ions/s)	100	<1000	10^6
Gradient	Uphill	Downhill*	Downhill
Energy input	Required	No	No
Ions/conformational change	~1	~1	Many
		*May pull another solute uphill	

Membrane Pumps

Protein pumps transport ions and other solutes across membranes up concentration gradients as great as 1 million-fold. Energy for this task can come from a variety of sources: light, oxidation-reduction reactions, or, most commonly, hydrolysis of ATP (Table 8-1). Energy is conserved in the form of transmembrane electrical or chemical gradients of the transported ion or solute. The potential energy in these ion gradients drives a variety of energy-requiring processes (Fig. 8-2). Most known biological pumps translocate cations. Although they could just as well move anions, cations were selected during the evolution of early life forms 3 billion years ago.

Pumps are also called **primary active transporters** because they transduce electromagnetic or chemical energy directly into transmembrane concentration gradients. Some carriers use ion gradients created by pumps to drive the uphill movement of other ions or solutes, so these are called **secondary transporters** (see Chapter 9). Channels are **passive transporters**, allowing net diffusion of ions and water only down their concentration gradients (see Chapter 10).

Diversity of Membrane Pumps

A vast array of integral membrane proteins can capture energy from an external source to pump ions and other solutes across biological membranes (Table 8-1). The protein families differ in their energy sources and transported materials. Fortunately, these pumps had a limited number of common ancestors, providing a relatively simple classification and generalizations about their structures and mechanisms. Given the importance of pumps in establishing transmembrane electrochemical gradients, the simplicity of this list is remarkable. Its brevity may be attributable to the fact that a single pump can drive a whole host of secondary reactions mediated by different carriers.

Table 8-1

DIVERSITY OF MEMBRANE PUMPS*

Energy Source	Pump	Driven Substance	Distribution
Light	Bacteriorhodopsin	H^+	Halobacteria
	Halorhodopsin	Cl^-	Halobacteria
Light	Photoredox	H^+	Photosynthetic organisms
Redox potential	Electron transport chain NADH oxidase	H^+	Mitochondria, bacteria
		Na^+	Alkalophilic bacteria
Decarboxylation	Ion-transporting decarboxylases	Na^+	Bacteria
Pyrophosphate	H^+-pyrophosphatase	H^+	Plant vacuoles, fungi, bacteria
ATP	Transport ATPases	Various ions and solutes	Universal

*Each class of pumps has a different evolutionary origin and structure.

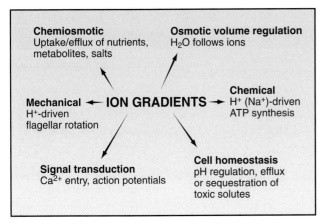

Figure 8-2 CELLULAR PROCESSES DRIVEN BY THE ENERGY STORED IN ION GRADIENTS.

This chapter considers four representative pumps, emphasizing examples in which both high-resolution structures and detailed biochemical analysis of pathways are available. Chapter 19 provides additional details on H^+ translocation by redox-driven cytochrome c oxidase and the role of F-type pumps in ATP synthesis by mitochondria and chloroplasts. Microbiology texts provide more information on pumps driven by decarboxylases and pyrophosphatases.

Light-Driven Proton Pumping by Bacteriorhodopsin

Owing to its simplicity, its small size, and the availability of a high-resolution structure (Fig. 8-3), more is known about light-driven transport of protons by **bacteriorhodopsin** than about any other pump. This pump allows the halophilic (salt-loving) Archaea *Halobacterium halobium* to convert light energy into a proton gradient across its plasma membrane. The 26-kD pump packs into two-dimensional crystalline arrays in the plasma membrane. The polypeptide is folded into seven α-helices that cross the lipid bilayer. The light-absorbing chromophore retinal (vitamin A aldehyde) is bound covalently to the side chain of lysine 216 (Lys216) via a Schiff base. This chromophore makes the protein and the membrane purple.

Bacteriorhodopsin absorbs light and uses the energy to pump protons out of the cell. A proton-driven ATP synthase uses this proton gradient to make ATP (Fig. 8-5). The proton pathway includes the side chains of aspartate 96 (Asp96), aspartate 85 (Asp85), glutamate 204 (Glu204), and the Schiff base. Local environments give the two aspartates remarkably different ionization constant (pK_a) values. Asp96 has a very high pK_a of about 10, so it can serve as a proton donor. Asp85 has a low pK_a of about 2, so it serves as a proton acceptor.

Absorption of a photon changes the conformation of the retinal and the pK_a of the Schiff base. These four groups work together to transfer a single proton from the cytoplasm to the extracellular space.

1. The mechanism starts with retinal in the all-*trans* configuration and protons bound to the Schiff base and Asp96 at the hydrophobic, cytoplasmic end of the proton pathway.

2. Absorption of a photon isomerizes retinal to the 13-*cis* configuration and changes the conformation of the protein, favoring transfer of the Schiff base proton to Asp85.

3. Asp85 transfers the proton to Glu204, which releases the proton outside the cell.

4. A further conformational change reorients the Schiff base toward Asp96. The pK_a of Asp96 is lower in this conformation, so a proton transfers from Asp96 to the Schiff base.

5. Asp96 is reprotonated from the cytoplasm.

6. The retinal reisomerizes to the all-*trans* configuration in preparation for another cycle.

The net result of this cycle is rapid vectorial transport of a proton from the cytoplasm out of the cell. Steps 4 to 6 are rate limiting, occurring at a rate of about 100 s^{-1}. The other reactions are fast, provided that there is an adequate flux of light. Retinal not only captures energy by absorbing a photon but also acts as a switch that

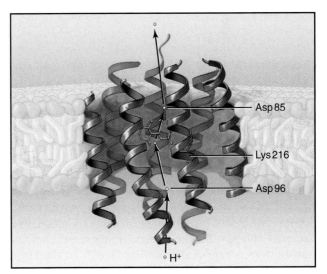

Figure 8-3 PROTON PATHWAY ACROSS THE MEMBRANE THROUGH BACTERIORHODOPSIN. The atomic structure, together with analysis of a wide array of mutations, reveals the pathway for protons through the middle of the bundle of helices. Further insights come from analysis of reaction intermediates, which differ in light absorption. A cytoplasmic proton binds successively to Asp96, the Schiff base linking retinal to lysine 216 (Lys216) and Asp85 before release outside the cell. Absorption of light by retinal drives conformational changes in the protein that favor the transfer of the proton across the membrane up its concentration gradient.

Table 8-2

ATP-DRIVEN TRANSPORT ATPASE PUMPS

Pump	Subunits	Distribution	Substrate	Function
F_0F_1 Family				
F_0F_1	8 or more	Mitochondria, chloroplasts, bacterial, plasma membranes	H^+ (rarely Na^+)	ATP synthesis or ATP-driven H^+ pumping
V_0V_1	8 or more	Eukaryotic endomembranes, Archaea	H^+ (rarely, Na^+)	ATP-driven H^+ (or rarely, Na^+) pumping
P-type ATPase Family				
Na^+K^+-ATPase	2	Plasma membrane	3 Na^+ for 2 K^+	Generation of Na^+, K^+ gradient
H^+K^+-ATPase	2	Stomach and kidney plasma membranes	1 H^+ for 1 K^+	Gastric and renal H^+ secretion
SERCA Ca-ATPase	1	Sarcoplasmic reticulum, endoplasmic reticulum	2 Ca^{2+} for 2 H^+	Lowering of cytoplasmic Ca^{2+}
PMCA Ca-ATPase	1	Plasma membrane	1 Ca^{2+} for 1 H^+	Lowering of cytoplasmic Ca^{2+}
H^+-ATPase	1	Plasma membrane in yeast, plants, protozoa	1 H^+	Generation of proton gradient
ABC Transporters				
MDR1 P-glycoprotein	1	Plasma membrane	Drugs	Drug secretion
CFTR	1	Respiratory tract and pancreatic epithelial plasma membranes	ATP, Cl^-	Cl^- secretion
TAP1, 2	2	Endoplasmic reticulum	Antigenic peptides	Transport of antigenic peptides from cytoplasm into ER
MDR2	1	Liver cell apical plasma membrane	Phosphatidylcholine	Phosphoglyceride flippase, bile secretion?
STE6	1	Yeast plasma membrane	Mating pheromone peptide	Signaling for mating
HisQMP	4 + pp	Bacteria plasma membrane	Histidine	Histidine uptake
PstSCAB	4 + pp	Bacteria plasma membrane	Phosphate	Phosphate uptake
OppDFBCA	4 + pp	Bacteria plasma membrane	Oligopeptides	Peptide uptake
HlyB	2	*Escherichia coli* plasma membrane	Hemolysin A (107-kD protein)	Hemolysin A uptake

pp, periplasmic protein.

changes both the accessibility and affinities of the proton-binding groups in a sequential fashion.

In addition to bacteriorhodopsin, halobacterial plasma membranes contain two related proteins: halorhodopsin and sensory rhodopsin. Halorhodopsin absorbs light and pumps chloride into the cell. Interestingly, a single amino acid substitution can reverse the direction of pumping. Sensory rhodopsin couples light absorption by its bound retinal to phototaxis (swimming toward light) with a tightly coupled transducer protein. In the absence of this transducer, sensory rhodopsin transports protons out of the cell much like bacterial rhodopsin. The design of these seven-helix transporters is remarkably similar to that of the large family of seven-helix receptors, especially the photoreceptor proteins that vertebrates use for vision (see Fig. 24-2).

ATP-Driven Pumps

Three families of transport ATPases (Table 8-2) are essential for the physiology of all forms of life. F_0F_1-ATPases and P-type ATPases differ in structure, but both generate electrical and/or chemical gradients across membranes. ABC transporters not only produce ion gradients but also transport a much wider range of solutes across membranes. Chemical inhibitors have been useful in characterizing these pumps, and some are also used therapeutically (Table 8-3).

Free energy released by ATP hydrolysis puts a limit on the concentration gradient that these pumps can produce. If transport is electrically neutral (i.e., if it does not produce a membrane potential; see Fig. 10-17), the

Table 8-3

TOOLS FOR STUDYING PUMPS

Agent	Target
Cardiac glycosides* (e.g., ouabain, digitalis)	Na^+K^+-ATPase
Omeprazole*	H^+K^+-ATPase (parietal cell)
Oligomycin	F_0F_1-ATP synthase

*Used clinically as drugs.

maximum gradient is about 1 million-fold. Such an extraordinary gradient is actually created by the P-type, electrically neutral H^+K^+-ATPase of gastric epithelial cells, which acidifies the stomach down to a pH of 1.

F_0F_1-ATPase Family

The two major subdivisions of this family are called F_0F_1-ATPases (or F-type ATPases) and V_0V_1-ATPases (or V-type ATPases) (Figs. 8-4 and 8-5). V_0V_1-ATPases, named for their location in the vacuolar system of eukaryotes, pump protons into organelles and out of Archaea. F_0F_1-ATPases of Bacteria, mitochondria, and chloroplasts generally run in the opposite direction, using proton gradients generated by other membrane proteins to drive ATP synthesis. However, purified F_0F_1-ATPases are freely reversible, using ATP hydrolysis to pump protons or alternatively proton gradients to synthesize ATP. Hence, these enzymes are called both ATP-synthases and F-type ATPases.

Phylogenetic analysis of the subunit polypeptides traces the origin of V-type ATPases to the precursor of all contemporary life forms (see Fig. 1-1). The genes for F-type ATPase subunits arose by divergence in Bacteria after they separated from Archaea. Eukaryotes came to have both F-type ATPases and V-type ATPases when symbiotic Bacteria gave rise to mitochondria and chloroplasts. Two subtle points are of interest here. First, a few Bacteria still have a V-type ATPase. Second, in contrast to the situation in eukaryotes, archaeal V-type ATPases function as ATP synthases similar to mitochondrial and bacterial F-type ATP synthases.

F-type ATPases (ATP Synthases)

F-type ATPases of mitochondria, chloroplasts, and bacterial plasma membranes produce most of the world's ATP during aerobic metabolism (see Chapter 19). Redox-driven and light-driven pumps create proton gradients to drive ATP synthesis by F-type ATPases. When required by circumstances, many Bacteria use their F-type ATPase to produce a proton gradient at the expense of ATP hydrolysis. Eukaryotes have elaborate mechanisms to inactivate the ATPase and prevent futile cycles of ATP synthesis and hydrolysis. For example, in mitochondria, an inhibitory protein binds the F_1-ATPase if the oxygen supply required to generate the proton gradient is compromised.

F_0F_1-ATPase has two parts (Fig. 8-5). Water-soluble, globular F_1 catalyzes ATP hydrolysis or synthesis. F_0 is embedded in the membrane and passively conducts protons across the lipid bilayer. A stalk connects F_1 to F_0, providing a way to couple proton translocation to ATP synthesis. Given a higher concentration of protons outside a Bacterium or mitochondrion than inside, protons pass through F_0 and drive the synthesis of ATP by F_1. Conversely, in bacteria, ATP hydrolysis by F_1 can drive protons out of the cell.

Pioneering biochemical studies and the crystal structure of F_1 (Fig. 8-4) suggested that rotation of a protein

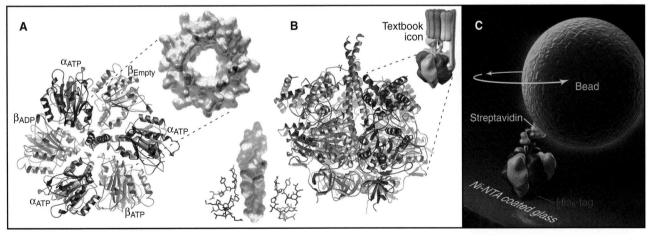

Figure 8-4 CRYSTAL STRUCTURE AND MECHANICS OF MITOCHONDRIAL F_1. **A,** A ribbon diagram viewed from the membrane *(bottom)* side with α-subunits *(red)*, β-subunits *(yellow),* and the γ-subunit *(blue).* All three α-subunits have a bound ATP. The β-subunits are empty or bind ATP or ADP. At the *upper right* is a space-filling bottom view of the parts of the α- and β-subunits forming the asymmetrical central channel for the γ-subunit (not shown). The electrostatic potential is *blue* for positive, *red* for negative, and *gray* for neutral. **B,** Oblique view of a ribbon diagram. The γ-subunit forms an antiparallel coiled-coil. At the bottom left is a space-filling model of the γ-subunit. Parts of the surrounding α- and β-subunits are shown as stick diagrams. Note that the surfaces of both the γ-subunit and the channel formed by the α- and β-subunits are hydrophobic and suitable to act as a molecular bearing. **C,** Drawing of the experimental set-up to show ATP-driven rotation of the γ-subunit relative to the α- and β-subunits. Streptavidin and biotin link the γ-subunit to a bead, which is observed to rotate by light microscopy. (PDB file: 1BMF. Reference: Abrahams JP, Leslie AGW, Lutter R, Walker JE: Structure at 2.8 Å resolution of F_1-ATPase from bovine heart mitochondria. Nature 370:621–628, 1994.)

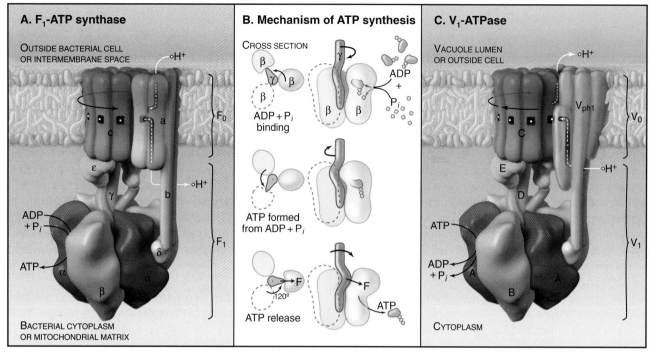

| A. F₁-ATP synthase | B. Mechanism of ATP synthesis | C. V₁-ATPase |

Figure 8-5   A–C, Models of the mitochondrial F_0F_1–ATP synthase and the V_0V_1 pump based on the atomic structure of F_1-ATPase and electron micrographs of the whole enzyme. Colors code the homologous subunits. F_0 is the oligomycin-sensitive factor. F_1 is the ATPase. Proton transfer across the membrane can drive ATP synthesis, or ATP hydrolysis can pump protons across the membrane. The text explains the reversible ATPase reaction. (Based on Elston T, Wang H, Oster G: Energy transduction in ATP synthesis. Nature 391:510–513, 1998.)

shaft couples proton fluxes in F_0 to ATP synthesis or, alternatively, couples ATP hydrolysis in F_1 to proton pumping by F_0. In the simplest case, bacterial F_1 consists of five different types of polypeptides in the ratio $\alpha_3\beta_3\gamma\Delta\epsilon$. Mitochondrial F_1 has additional subunits. The α- and β-subunits are folded similarly and arranged alternately like segments of a orange. The γ-subunit is folded into a long, antiparallel, α-helical coiled-coil that forms a shaft. This hydrophobic shaft fits tightly in a hydrophobic sleeve in the middle of the hexamer of α- and β-subunits. To accommodate the asymmetrical shaft, each of the surrounding α- and β-subunits has a slightly different conformation. Each α- and β-subunit has an adenine nucleotide-binding site at the interface with its neighbor. ATP bound stably to α-subunits does not participate in catalysis. Nucleotide-binding sites on β-subunits catalyze ATP synthesis and hydrolysis.

Mechanical rotation of the γ-subunit inside F_1 is tightly coupled to ATP synthesis or hydrolysis. A proton gradient across the membrane can drive a flux of protons through the F_0 complex. This drives clockwise (when viewed from F_0) rotation of the γ-subunit inside the $\alpha\beta$ hexamer, like the camshaft in a motor. The mechanical force produced by the asymmetric camshaft drives conformational changes in β-subunits that synthesize ATP (Figs. 8-5 and 8-6). When the machine operates in the other direction, ATP hydrolysis drives counterclockwise rotation of the shaft, which can pump protons through F_0.

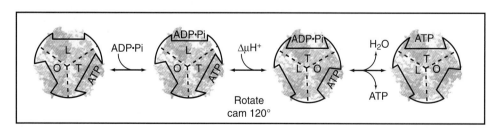

Figure 8-6   THE BINDING CHANGE MODEL FOR ATP SYNTHESIS BY F₁. Each of the three β-subunits differs in conformation and affinity for nucleotides. The three subunits cycle in succession from the loose (L) state (that binds ADP and P_i), to the tight (T) state (that favors ATP synthesis) to the open (O) state (that releases ATP). Energy provided by the electrochemical gradient of protons ($\Delta\mu H^+$) is required for the γ-subunit to drive each successive transition from loose to tight. (Reference: Boyer PD: The ATP synthase: A splendid molecular machine. Annu Rev Biochem 66:717–749, 1997.)

Light microscopy is used to observe rotation directly (Fig. 8-4C). F_1 is attached to a glass coverslip, and a tiny bead or actin filament is attached to the free end of the γ-subunit. ATP hydrolysis by the β-subunits drives the rotation of the bead or filament on the γ-subunit. If the bead is magnetic, a rotating magnet field can be used to drive the shaft and synthesize ATP from ADP and phosphate. The γ-subunit rotates at a maximum rate of about 130 times per second (8000 rpm) in mitochondria and twice as fast in chloroplasts.

During ATP hydrolysis or synthesis, the catalytic sites on the β-subunits participate cooperatively, in a sequence of steps coupled to rotation of the shaft. The β-subunits can be in one of three conformations—open, loose, and tight—designating their increasing affinities for adenine nucleotides. At any time in an F_1 molecule, one β-subunit is open, one is loose, and one is tight. All three subunits pass in lock step through the sequence of three states.

In hydrolyzing ATP, the rate-limiting step is ATP binding to the open β-subunit. The energy from ATP binding causes a conformational change that drives an 80° counterclockwise rotation of γ-subunit in less than a millisecond and favors hydrolysis of ATP on the β-subunit that just previously bound ATP. After about 2 milliseconds, another reaction, possibly ADP dissociation from the third β-subunit, rapidly rotates the γ-subunit another 40°, completing a 120° step of the motor.

In synthesizing ATP, the β-subunit in the loose conformation binds ADP and inorganic phosphate (P_i). Energy provided by a 120° rotation of the γ-subunit converts this site to the tight conformation. In the environment created by the active site, ADP and P_i spontaneously form ATP. Energy from a subsequent 120° of the shaft drives the tight state to the open state, which allows ATP to dissociate.

The membrane-embedded F_o complex is a second rotary motor consisting of 12 to 15 protein subunits in the ratio ab_2c_{9-12}. The c-subunits are simple hairpins of two α-helices. A ring of c-subunits is attached to γ-subunit. The single a-subunit provides a channel for protons to move across the lipid bilayer. This proton channel is thought to be divided into two physically separated parts. To cross the membrane, a proton enters one side of the channel, transfers to aspartate 61 (Asp61) of a c-subunit. Rotation of the ring of c-subunits relative to the a-subunit aligns a protonated Asp61 with the second half of the channel in the a-subunit, allowing the proton to escape on the opposite side from the membrane from which it came. Each ATP synthesized or hydrolyzed is coupled to the transport of three or four protons. Given three ATPs synthesized/hydrolyzed per complete F_1 cycle, 9 to 12 copies of c-subunits in various types of F_o provide the correct stoichiometry if each transports a single proton.

All of these transitions are reversible in bacterial F_0F_1. With input of energy from proton translocations, F_1 moves through this cycle of states and produces ATP. Alternatively, these reactions can pump protons at the expense of ATP hydrolysis. Reaction of the chemical DCCD with Asp61 on a single c-subunit blocks H^+ conduction and ATP hydrolysis or synthesis. This inhibition emphasizes the tight coupling of all the subunits of F_0F_1.

V-Type ATPases

Vacuolar ATPases (Fig. 8-5) are found in the membranes bounding acidic compartments in eukaryotic cells, including clathrin-coated vesicles, endosomes, lysosomes (see Chapter 22), Golgi apparatus (see Chapter 21), secretory vesicles (including synaptic vesicles), and plant vacuoles. V-type pumps are also present in the plasma membranes of cells specialized to secrete protons, such as osteoclasts (see Fig. 32-6), macrophages, and kidney tubule intercalated cells.

V-type pumps have two functions. First, they acidify all the compartments listed here using rotation of the c-subunits to drive proton translocation. The acidic pH promotes ligand dissociation from receptors in endosomes and activates lysosomal hydrolases, as well as many other reactions (see Chapter 22). Second, proton gradients across these membranes provide the energy source to drive H^+-coupled transport of other solutes by carriers, such as the uptake of neurotransmitters by synaptic vesicles (see Figs. 11-8 and 11-9).

Like F-type pumps, V-type ATPases are rotary motors. Most protein subunits of V-type pumps are homologs of their counterparts from F-type pumps. An ancient gene duplication made the c-subunits of eukaryotic V-type pumps twice as large as those in F-type pumps. Six copies of V-type c-subunits provide the same total number of membrane-spanning helices as the 12 F-type c-subunits, but each has only one glutamate equivalent to Asp61. Accordingly, V-type pumps transport only 1 to 2 H^+ per ATP hydrolyzed.

P-Type Cation Pumps: E_1E_2-ATPases

All living organisms depend on P-type ATPases (Table 8-2) to pump cations across membranes. Their name comes from the fact that they utilize a high-energy covalent β-**aspartyl phosphate intermediate.** They are also called E_1E_2-ATPases from a description of the conformational changes that they undergo during the course of their mechanism.

Eukaryotic P-type ATPases generate primary ion gradients across the plasma membrane that are required for the function of ion channels (see Chapter 10) and most cation-coupled transport mediated by carrier proteins (see Chapter 9). In animal cells, **Na^+K^+-ATPase** produces the primary gradients of Na^+ and K^+. In plants and fungi, the functional homolog H^+-ATPase generates a proton gradient. Production of these primary ion gradients is expensive, consuming up to 25% of total cellular ATP. Other eukaryotic P-type ATPases acidify the stomach and clear cytoplasm of the second messenger, Ca^{2+} (see Fig. 26-12). Bacterial P-type ATPases scavenge K^+ and Mg^{2+} from the medium and export Ca^{2+}, Cu^{2+}, and toxic heavy metals.

The P-type ATPase that is best understood is the sarco(endo)plasmic reticulum **Ca^{2+}-ATPase** (SERCA1), which pumps Ca^{2+} out of the cytoplasm into the endoplasmic reticulum (Fig. 8-7). ATP hydrolysis provides energy to move Ca^{2+} across the membrane up a steep concentration gradient. The mechanism is understood in detail, thanks to extensive biochemical analysis and crystal structures of five of the chemical intermediates along the pathway (Fig. 8-8). This analysis was possible because the enzyme is abundant in the sarcoplasmic reticulum of skeletal muscle (see Fig. 39-10), allowing it to be purified in large quantities.

The 100-kD Ca^{2+}-ATPase consists of two regions. Ten α-helices cross the membrane bilayer and bind two Ca^{2+} ions side by side in the middle of the membrane. The globular region in the cytoplasm consists of three domains. The N-domain binds ATP and transfers its γ-phosphate to aspartic acid 351 (Asp351) in the P-domain. The A-domain transmits large conformational changes in the cytoplasmic domains to the transmembrane helices, which (6 of 10 helices) alternate between two conformations. The E_1 conformation allows access to the Ca^{2+} binding sites from the cytoplasm (Fig. 8-8A). The E_2 conformation allows access from the lumen of the endoplasmic reticulum (Fig. 8-8B). Each step along the pathway—Ca^{2+} binding, ATP binding, phosphorylation of the enzyme, dissociation of ADP, and hydrolysis of the β-aspartyl phosphate intermediate—causes linked conformational changes in both the cytoplasmic domains and six of the transmembrane helices. The changes in the transmembrane domain alters the affinity of the protein for Ca^{2+} and the exposure of Ca-binding sites on the two sides of the membrane. Figure 8-8 describes the cycle of ATP hydrolysis and Ca^{2+} transport in detail. Note that the transition between the E_1 and E_2 conformations involves an "occluded" state in which the bound Ca^{2+} is not accessible on either side of the membrane. This occluded state allows the pump to transport against a large concentration gradient without a leak.

Because the cycle transfers two Ca^{2+} into the lumen and two H^+ out, it generates an electrical potential (see Chapter 10). In the steady state, the Ca^{2+} gradient is maintained, but the H^+ gradient dissipates, owing to H^+ permeability across the membrane and to the buffering capacity of the lumen. All reactions in the pathway are reversible, so a large gradient of Ca^{2+} across the membrane can drive the synthesis of ATP.

All P-type ATPases consist of homologous α-subunits with large cytoplasmic domains and a minimum of six transmembrane helices. Eukaryotic P-type ATPases,

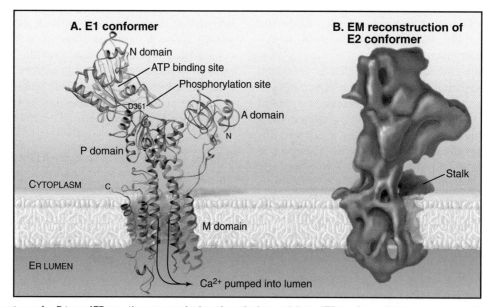

Figure 8-7 Structure of a P-type ATPase, the sarcoendoplasmic reticulum calcium–ATPase from skeletal muscle. **A,** The structure of the 2Ca-E1 conformation was determined by X-ray diffraction of crystals formed in the presence of Ca^{2+}. Two Ca^{2+} ions bind among four of the ten transmembrane helices near the middle of the membrane bilayer. In the cytoplasm, the N-domain binds nucleotide (ATP) and transfers the γ-phosphate to Asp351 (D351) in the P-domain. (PDB file: 1EUL.) **B,** Reconstruction of the E2 conformation of the pump from electron micrographs. (A, Reference: Toyoshima C, Nakasako M, Nomura H, Ogawa H: Crystal structure of the calcium pump of sarcoplasmic reticulum at 2.6 Å resolution. Nature 405:647–655, 2000. B, From Toyoshima CH, Sasabe H, Stokes DL: Three-dimensional cryoelectron microscopy of the calcium ion pump in the sarcoplasmic reticulum membrane. Nature 362:467–471, 1993.)

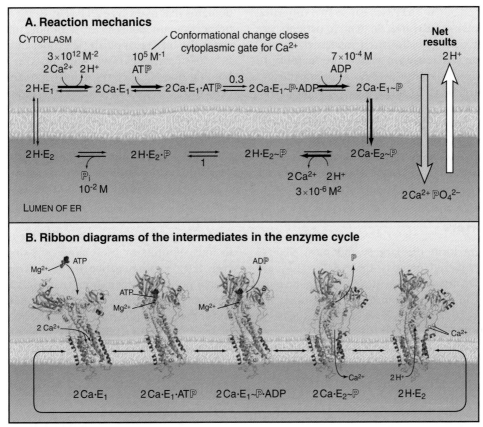

Figure 8-8 Reaction mechanism of the sarcoendoplasmic reticulum calcium–ATPase. **A,** Biochemical pathway. The E stands for enzyme, having two conformations: E_1 and E_2. E_1 has the Ca^{2+}-binding site oriented toward the cytoplasm. E_2 has the Ca^{2+}-binding site oriented toward the lumen of the endoplasmic reticulum. Ca^{2+} binds E_1 on the cytoplasmic side. Subsequent binding of ATP and phosphorylation of the enzyme drive the enzyme toward the E_2 state and transport Ca^{2+} up a steep concentration gradient into the lumen of the endoplasmic reticulum. Dephosphorylation of the enzyme favors a return to the E_1 state. **B,** Ribbon diagrams of structures along the biochemical pathway. Conformational changes are coupled to ATP hydrolysis and transport of Ca^{2+}. Starting on the left side of part A, the pump without bound Ca^{2+} or ATP vacillates between the E_2 and E_1 conformations, alternatively exposing the Ca^{2+}-binding sites on the two sides of the membrane. If Ca^{2+} ions are available in the cytoplasm, such as after activation of muscle (see Fig. 39-16), they bind cooperatively to the E_1 conformation with micromolar affinity. Ca^{2+} binding strongly stimulates enzyme activity by favoring Mg-ATP binding to the N-domain. Mg-ATP can bind simultaneously to both the N- and the P-domains, so its presence favors a striking change in conformation that requires the N-domain to rotate and the A-domain to pull on a transmembrane helix that closes a gate between the bound Ca^{2+} and the cytoplasm. This conformation brings the γ-phosphate of ATP into proximity with the side chain of Asp351 and allows formation of the phosphoenzyme intermediate. The equilibrium constant for phosphorylation is near unity, so most of the energy from ATP hydrolysis is stored in a high-energy conformation of the protein. After transfer of γ-phosphate to the enzyme, ADP dissociates. This results in a rotation of the A-domain that moves several transmembrane helices to expose the Ca^{2+}-binding sites to the lumen of the endoplasmic reticulum and reduces the affinity for Ca^{2+} by several orders of magnitude. Thus Ca^{2+} dissociates into the lumen, completing its uphill transfer from the cytoplasm. Hydrolysis of the phosphorylated intermediate and dissociation of phosphate reverse the conformational changes in both the cytoplasmic and transmembrane domains, completing the cycle. (References: Toyoshima C, Nomura H, Tsuda T: Lumenal gating mechanism revealed in calcium pump crystal structures with phosphate analogues. Nature 432:361–368, 2004; and Soerensen T, Moeller JV, Nissen P: Phosphoryl transfer and calcium ion occlusion in the calcium pump. Science 304:1672–1675, 2004. PDB files: 1EUL, 1T5S, 1T5T, IWPG, IIWO.)

such as the Na^+K^+- and Ca^{2+}-ATPases have 10 transmembrane helices. Many P-type ATPase are about 110 kD, like the Ca-ATPase, but some are larger or smaller, owing to variable features. Na^+K^+-ATPase and H^+K^+-ATPase require a 50-kD glycosylated β-subunit with a single transmembrane segment for both transport and intracellular trafficking.

Other P-type ATPases work the same way as the Ca^{2+}-ATPase, but with adaptations to pump other ions. For example, the E_1 conformation of the Na^+K^+-ATPase of eukaryotic plasma membranes picks up three Na^+ from the cytoplasm. The P-E_2 conformation releases these Na^+ one after another outside the cell and then binds two K^+. Binding of extracellular K^+ leads to dephosphorylation of the enzyme and results in the occlusion of K^+ in the KE_2 conformation. ATP binding leads to the release of this K^+ on the cytoplasmic side and regenerates the E_1 conformation so that the cycle can start over again.

Some P-type ATPases are involved in human diseases. Mutations in Ca^{2+}-ATPase cause muscle stiffness and cramps. Mutations in Cu^{2+}-ATPases cause two inherited diseases: **Menkes' syndrome,** in which patients are copper-deficient owing to impaired intestinal absorption, and **Wilson's disease,** in which the inability to remove copper from the liver is toxic. Omeprazole and related drugs are used to treat ulcers by inhibiting gastric H^+K^+-ATPase. Drugs called **cardiac glycosides** strengthen the heartbeat by inhibiting the cardiac isoform of Na^+K^+-ATPase (see Fig. 11-13 for details). These drugs, which derive originally from the foxglove plant, were among the first used to treat congestive heart failure.

ABC Transporters

ABC transporters form the largest and most diverse family of ATP-powered pumps (Table 8-2). They are found in all known organisms, so the founding gene must have originated in the common ancestor of all living things. The genome of baker's yeast encodes at least 30 ABC transporters, compared with 16 P-type ATPases, one F-type ATPase, and one V-type ATPase. ABC transporters are the largest gene family in the colon bacterium *Escherichia coli*. In eukaryotes particular family members are located in the plasma membrane, endoplasmic reticulum, and, most likely, other membranes.

Each ABC transporter is specific for one or a few related substrates, but the family as a whole has an enormous range of substrates, including inorganic ions, sugars, amino acids, complex polysaccharides, peptides, and even proteins. Given diverse substrates, the sequences of the transmembrane domains of ABC transporters have diverged much more than their cytoplasmic domains. Specialized members of the family act as ion channels (e.g., the **cystic fibrosis transmembrane regulator, CFTR**) or regulate other membrane proteins, such as the sulfonylurea receptor.

ABC transporters have a modular design that includes two transmembrane domains and two cytoplasmic domains that hydrolyze ATP (Fig. 8-9A). Each transmembrane domain consists of a bundle of α-helices that spans the bilayer: typically six times but up to ten times in some examples. Two sequences in the nucleotide-binding domain give the family its name (ATP-binding cassette). The Walker A motif (GXXGXGKS/T, where X is any residue) is also called a P loop, since it binds the γ-phosphate of ATP in ABC transporters and other ATP-binding proteins. The Walker B motif ($RX_{6-8}F_4D$, where F is any hydrophobic residue) interacts with the Mg^{2+} bound to ATP. Motif B is typically separated from motif A by 100 to 150 residues along the sequence.

Various "experiments" of nature during evolution show that the four independently folded domains of an ABC transporter can be assembled by association of up to four subunits or by folding of a single polypeptide (Fig. 8-9). Gram-negative bacterial transporters often utilize periplasmic subunits that bind and concentrate transported substrates in the vicinity of the pump. Some vertebrate ABC transporters include an additional cytoplasmic R-domain in the single polypeptide for regulation by phosphorylation.

The crystal structure of the *E. coli* BtuCD vitamin B_{12} transporter (Fig. 8-10) suggests how ABC transporters might work. The molecule consists of four subunits: two copies of the transmembrane BtuC subunit and two copies of the nucleotide-binding BtuD subunit. Each transmembrane subunit consists of ten transmembrane helices. The interface between the BtuC subunits forms a large chamber open outside the cell (the periplasmic space in this case). The chamber is lined by hydrophobic side chains that are expected to interact with vitamin B_{12}. The chamber penetrates more than halfway across the lipid bilayer but is blocked on the cytoplasmic side by residues that form a gate. The nucleotide-binding cytoplasmic subunits form large interfaces with their partner transmembrane subunits and have a small but highly conserved interface with the other nucleotide-binding subunit. This small interface positions ATP-

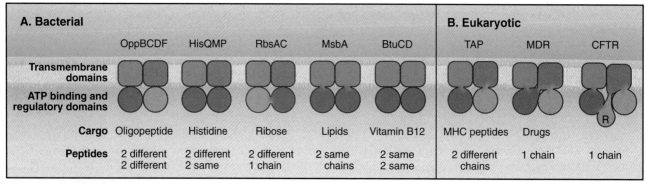

Figure 8-9 DOMAIN ARCHITECTURE OF ABC TRANSPORTERS. **A,** Bacterial transporters. **B,** Eukaryotic transporters. Each transporter has two ATP-binding domains in the cytoplasm (*purple circles*) and two transmembrane domains, each consisting of 6 to 10 α-helices (*blue* or *pink squares*). CFTR has an additional regulatory (R) domain in the cytoplasm. The four domains required for activity may be four separate polypeptides or may be incorporated in several ways into polypeptides with two or four domains.

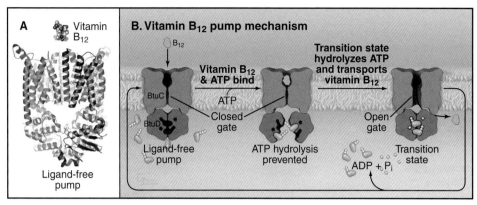

Figure 8-10 Structure and proposed mechanism of the *E. coli* BtuCD vitamin B_{12} transporter. **A,** Ribbon diagram of the crystal structure of BtuCD. Two identical BtuC subunits *(blue)* traverse the membrane. Two identical BtuD subunits *(red)* bind and hydrolyze ATP. A periplasmic protein BtuF binds vitamin B_{12} and delivers it to BtuCD. (PDB file: 1L7V.) **B,** A hypothesis for the mechanism of vitamin B_{12} transport: BtuCD begins free of both vitamin B_{12} and ATP; vitamin B_{12} binding to BtuC promotes ATP binding to BtuD; during a transition state, ATP hydrolysis is coupled to conformational changes that open the gate of BtuC, admitting vitamin B_{12} into the cytoplasm. Release of ADP and phosphate returns the transporter to its initial state. (Reference: Locher K, Lee A, Rees D: The *E. coli* BtuCD structure: A framework for ABC transporter architecture and mechanism. Science 296:1091–1098, 2002.)

binding sites of the two subunits next to each other. A periplasmic protein binds vitamin B_{12} and presents it to the transporter.

It is postulated that ATP binding and hydrolysis drive a cycle of conformational changes that opens the gate, allowing vitamin B_{12} to escape into the cytoplasm. Binding of substrate to the chamber is expected to increase the affinity of the ABC cassettes for ATP. What happens next is less clear, but an attractive hypothesis is that ATP binding and hydrolysis at the two opposed BtuD active sites transiently open the gate and release B_{12} in the cytoplasm. Release of ADP and phosphate are presumed to be coupled to closure of the gate. Structures of additional intermediates and more biochemical parameters are required to clarify the mechanism.

ABC transporters with similar mechanisms include bacterial permeases that pump nutrients into the cell, and **TAP1** and **TAP2** that pump peptide fragments of antigenic proteins into the lumen of the endoplasmic reticulum. Some substrates are membrane bound. ABC transporters such as the *E. coli* "flippase" MsbA move phospholipids from one leaflet of the bilayer to the other, while yeast STE6 transports a small, prenylated pheromone peptide out of the cell.

Other family members are more problematic. The vertebrate cystic fibrosis transmembrane conductance regulator (CFTR [Fig. 8-9B]) looks like a pump but acts like a channel. It allows Cl^- to move down its concentration gradient out of the cell. ATP binding and hydrolysis by the nucleotide-binding domains may open and shut this channel. Mutations in CFTR are responsible for cystic fibrosis (see Fig. 11-4). Of more than 1000 CFTR mutations known to cause cystic fibrosis, by far the most common mutation is deletion of phenylalanine 508.

This position corresponds to a highly conserved hydrophobic residue in the vitamin B_{12} transporter that is important for the interaction of BtuD with BtuC. Mutant $\Delta F508$ CFTR misfolds and is retained in the ER and destroyed, depriving the plasma membrane of chloride channel activity. Depleting Ca^{2+} from the ER by inhibiting the SERCA Ca^{2+} ATPase can apparently allow $\Delta F508$ CFTR to escape from calcium-dependent chaperones (see Fig. 20-10) and function on the cell surface.

The **multiple drug resistance** proteins (**MDR1** and **MDR2**) are ABC transporters that provide a challenge for cancer chemotherapy (Fig. 8-11). In about half of the cases in which chemotherapy fails to cure cancer in humans, the cause is the emergence of clones of tumor cells that overexpress an MDR. Normal cells use a low level of MDR1 to export unknown substrates, perhaps a steroid, a phospholipid, or another hydrophobic molecule. MDR can also transport many hydrophobic compounds, including some chemotherapeutic drugs. These drugs enter cells by dissolving in the membrane, and they subsequently poison vital cellular processes. Cells that overexpress MDR survive by pumping the drug out of the cell.

The multiple drug resistance protein 2 (MDR2) is another unconventional pump located in the apical plasma membrane of liver cells. It is a flippase that moves phosphatidylcholine from the inner to the outer half of the lipid bilayer, perhaps in preparation for secretion in bile.

Some even less conventional ABC transporters appear to regulate ion channels. The sulfonylurea receptor (SUR) is an ABC transporter required for the function of an ATP-sensitive potassium channel (K_{ATP}) that regulates insulin secretion. SUR binds drugs called sulfonylureas that are used to treat forms of diabetes involving

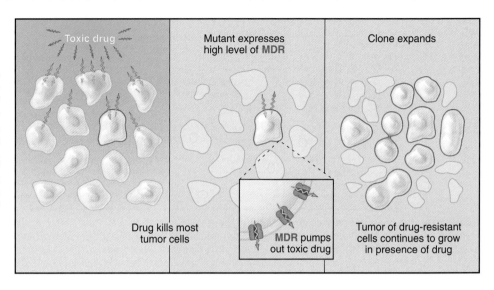

Figure 8-11 MULTIPLE DRUG RESISTANCE IN CANCER CHEMOTHERAPY. In a population of tumor cells, most are sensitive to killing by a chemotherapeutic drug. However, variants that express high levels of the ABC transporter, MDR, can clear the cytoplasm of the drug. A clone of these variant cells may expand, allowing the tumor to grow in the presence of the drug.

inadequate insulin secretion. These drugs activate secretion by inhibiting the K_{ATP} channel (see Chapter 10).

ACKNOWLEDGMENT

Thanks go to Michael Caplan for suggestions on revisions to this chapter.

SELECTED READINGS

Abrahams JP, Leslie AGW, Lutter R, Walker JE: Structure at 2.8 Å resolution of F_1-ATPase from bovine heart mitochondria. Nature 370: 621-628, 1994.

Borst P, Oude Elferink R: Mammalian ABC transporters in health and disease. Annu Rev Biochem 71:537-592, 2002.

Cross RL: Turning the ATP motor. Nature 427:407-408, 2004.

Davidson A: Not just another ABC transporter. Science 296:1038-1040, 2002.

Davidson AL, Chen J: ATP-binding cassette transporters in bacteria. Annu Rev Biochem 73:241-268, 2004.

Facciotti MT, Rouhani-Manshadi S, Glaeser RM: Energy transduction in transmembrane ion pumps. Trends Biochem Sci 29:445-451, 2004.

Kaplan JH: Biochemistry of the Na,K-ATPase. Annu Rev Biochem 71: 511-535, 2002.

Kinosita K, Jr, Adachi K, Itoh H: Rotation of F_1-ATPase: How an ATP-driven molecular machine may work. Annu Rev Biophys Biomol Struct 32:245-268, 2004.

Kuhlbrandt W: Biology, structure and mechanism of P-type ATPases. Nat Rev Mol Cell Biol 5:282-295, 2004.

Lancaster CRD: Ion pumps in the movies. Nature 432:286-287, 2004.

Lanyi JK: Bacteriorhodopsin. Annu Rev Physiol 66:665-688, 2004.

Locher KP: Structure and mechanism of ABC transporters. Curr Opin Struct Biol 14:426-431, 2004.

Locher K, Lee A, Rees D: The *E. coli* BtuCD structure: A framework for ABC transporter architecture and mechanism. Science 296:1091-1098, 2002.

Nishizaka T, Oiwa K, Noji H, et al: Chemomechanical coupling in F_1-ATPase revealed by simultaneous observation of nucleotide kinetics and rotation. Nat Struct Mol Biol 11:142-148, 2004.

Oster G, Wang H: Rotary protein motors. Trends Cell Biol 13:114-121, 2003.

Soerensen T, Moeller JV, Nissen P: Phosphoryl transfer and calcium ion occlusion in the calcium pump. Science 304:1672-1675, 2004.

Subramaniam S, Hirai T, Henderson R: From structure to mechanism: Electron crystallographic studies of bacteriorhodopsin. Phil Trans A Math Phys Eng Sci 360:859-874, 2002.

Toyoshima C, Inesi G: Structural basis of ion pumping by Ca^{2+}-ATPase of the sarcoplasmic reticulum. Annu Rev Biochem 73:269-292, 2004.

Toyoshima C, Nomura H: Structural changes in the calcium pump accompanying the dissociation of calcium. Nature 418:605-611, 2002.

Toyoshima C, Nomura H, Tsuda T: Lumenal gating mechanism revealed in calcium pump crystal structures with phosphate analogues. Nature 432:361-368, 2004. (The journal web site associated with this paper has a movie of the structural changes during the ATPase cycle: http://www.nature.com/nature/journal/v432/ n7015/suppinfo/nature02981.html.)

Membrane Carriers

Carriers are integral membrane proteins that use electrochemical gradients to move select chemical substrates across lipid bilayers (Fig. 9-1). Transport by well-characterized carriers depends on a conformational change to move each substrate. Typically, the carriers work step by step, more like enzymes than channels. Channels simply provide a selective pore for transport, and they generally transport at much higher rates (see Chapter 10). Common substrates for carriers are ions and small soluble organic molecules, but in some cases, substrates are lipid soluble.

Like pumps and channels, carriers are found in all membranes, wherever cells need to exchange molecules for metabolism or extrude wastes. Carriers are also known as facilitators or porters.

Carriers that transport a single substrate across a membrane down its concentration gradient are called **uniporters.** Remarkably, many carriers also transport substrates up concentration gradients, provided that their passage through the carrier and across the membrane is coupled to the transport of another substrate down its electrochemical gradient. Glucose provides good examples of both downhill and uphill movement through different carriers. The GLUT1 uniporter allows glucose to move down its concentration gradient from plasma into red blood cells. On the other hand, the SGLT1 carrier uses a gradient of Na^+ established by the Na^+K^+-ATPase pump to move glucose up its concentration gradient into intestinal cells. It is called a **symporter,** since glucose and Na^+ move in the same direction. Another class of carriers called **antiporters** move a substrate in the opposite direction to the ion gradient driving the reaction. All carrier-mediated reactions are reversible, so substrates can move in either direction across the membrane, depending on the polarity of the driving forces.

When a carrier uses an ion gradient to provide the energy to transport a substrate, it is said to catalyze a secondary reaction. In this sense, pumps catalyze primary transport reactions, using energy from ATP hydrolysis, electron transport, or absorption of light to create ion gradients (see Chapter 8). Coupling an ion gradient created by pumps to drive transport by a carrier is called a chemiosmotic cycle (see Fig. 11-1).

Diversity of Carrier Proteins

Biological experimentation and exploration of genomes have revealed more than a hundred families of carriers, many of which can be grouped into superfamilies. The **major facilitator superfamily** (MFS) is the focus of this chapter, since it includes about one third of all known carrier proteins, including many of the best-characterized

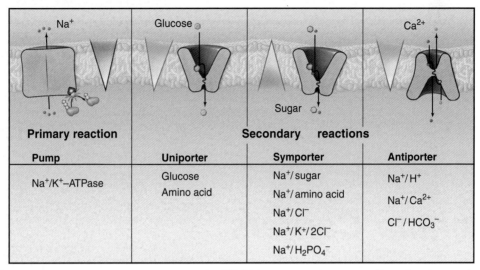

Figure 9-1 PRIMARY AND SECONDARY TRANSPORT REACTIONS. An ATP-driven pump produces a gradient of an ion, such as Na⁺, across a membrane. The triangles represent gradients of Na⁺ *(purple)*, glucose *(green)*, sugar *(blue)*, and Ca²⁺ *(light blue)* across the membrane. This ion gradient drives secondary transport reactions mediated by carriers. Uniporters allow an ion or other solute to move across the membrane down its concentration gradient. Symporters and antiporters couple transport of an ion (Na⁺ in this example) down its concentration gradient with the transport of a solute (glucose or Ca²⁺ in these examples) up its concentration gradient. Antiporters carry out these reactions in succession, picking up Na⁺ outside, reorienting, dissociating Na⁺ inside, picking up Ca²⁺ inside, reorienting, and releasing Ca²⁺ outside.

carriers. Thousands of MFS genes in all branches of the phylogenetic tree are likely to have arisen from a common ancestor. Two thirds of known carriers have other origins and structures but have converged on mechanical solutions for solute transport similar to MFS carriers. No one knows how many structurally distinct groups exist in nature. Box 9-1 illustrates a small selection of carrier families with different evolutionary origins and structures.

Structure of MFS Carrier Proteins

Crystal structures of two MFS carrier proteins from *Escherichia coli* (Fig. 9-3A–B) confirmed much of what had been learned about their organization from less direct methods. GlpT is a glycerol-3-phosphate–phosphate antiporter. LacY, the lactose permease, is a lactose-proton symporter. Both proteins consist of 12 transmembrane α-helices. The sequences and structures of the two halves of each protein are homologous, so it is believed that the original gene was created by duplication of an ancestral gene, which coded for a six-helix protein that formed functional dimers. As the MFS gene family grew during evolution, the ancient gene duplication and fusion process had two advantages. First, it allowed the two halves of each gene to diversify separately to increase specificity for a wide variety of substrates. Second, a single polypeptide simplifies assembly of a functional carrier, as two half-sized subunits do not have to find each other. If the two halves of a 12-helix

MFS carrier are expressed in the same cell, they can assemble functional carriers, but less efficiently than the intact protein.

Both carriers bind substrates in the center of a cluster of transmembrane helices. LacY achieves specificity for lactose by providing geometrically favorable hydrogen bonds and hydrophobic interactions for the substrate. GlpT has a pair of conserved arginines near the middle of the bilayer that are required to bind phosphate.

MFS carriers are believed to alternate between two conformations: one with the substrate-binding site(s) open to the cytoplasmic side of the membrane, as in the crystals, and another with the substrate-binding site(s) exposed on the opposite side of the membrane. The architecture of both proteins is compatible with the proposed conformational change, but structures of the proteins in the alternate conformation must be understood before the mechanism can be established. When open to the periplasmic side of the membrane, GlpT binds glycerol-3-phosphate preferentially, since its affinity is higher than that of phosphate. Bound substrates may facilitate interconversion of the two conformations. When exposed to the cytoplasm, glycerol-3-phosphate dissociates and is replaced by phosphate, which is present at a higher concentration in the cytoplasm. Transport of lactose by LacY is coupled to transport of a proton. A glutamic acid is a likely candidate for proton binding, but it is not yet clear why the conformation of the protein that is open on the periplasmic side of the membrane favors binding of lactose plus a proton.

BOX 9-1
Crystal Structures of Diverse Carrier Proteins

Four crystal structures (Fig. 9-2) illustrate the diversity of carrier proteins. They differ in evolutionary origins and structures, but all function as carriers. They converged toward common mechanisms implemented by different structures. Conformational changes are believed to contribute to transport in all cases, so their mechanisms will be better understood when structures of additional conformations of each protein are available.

- MFS carriers consist of single polypeptides that form 10 to 14 (usually 12) transmembrane helices (Fig. 9-2B). Substrates bind in a pocket among these helices. A conformational change exposes this binding site on either side of the membrane so that substrates can bind and dissociate. These carriers are active as monomers.

- Mitochondrial adenine nucleotide carriers transport ATP and ADP across the membranes of mitochondria and chloroplasts. Their genes were formed by a threefold duplication and divergence of a sequence that encodes a pair of transmembrane helices. These six transmembrane helices form a cup exposing a nucleotide binding site near the middle of the membrane bilayer. These carriers are believed to operate in pairs to enable cooperative binding of ATP and ADP on opposite sides of the inner mitochondrial membrane. Once bound, the nucleotides are transported down their concentration gradients.

- Multidrug transporters help bacteria to live in hostile environments by extruding a wide variety of toxic hydrophobic chemicals. Substrates include bile salts,

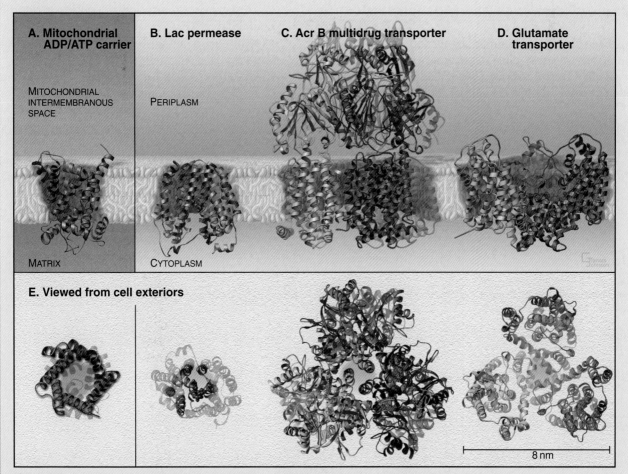

Figure 9-2 **STRUCTURES OF MEMBRANE CARRIER PROTEINS.** Ribbon diagrams illustrate their diversity. **A,** Bovine mitochondrial ADP/ATP transporter. (PDB file: 1OKC.) **B,** *E. coli* Lac Y. (PDB file: 1PV7.) **C,** *E. coli* AcrB multidrug transporter. The three identical subunits are shown in different colors. (PDB file: 1OY8.) **D,** *Pyrococcus horikoshii* glutamate transporter. The three identical subunits are shown in different colors. (PDB file: 1XFH.) **E,** Views of the exterior of the cell or mitochondrion with the presumed transport pathway shaded tan. (References: Pebay-Peyroula E, Dahout-Gonzalez C, Kahn R, et al: Structure of mitochondrial ADP/ATP carrier in complex with carboxyatrachtyloside. Nature 426:39–44, 2003; Abramson J, Smirnova I, Kasho V, et al: Structure and mechanism of the lactose permease of *E. coli*. Science 301:610–615, 2003; Muakami S, Nakashima R, Yamashita E, Yamaguchi A: Crystal structure of bacterial multidrug efflux transporter AcrB. Nature 419:587–593, 2002; Yernool D, Boudker O, Jin Y, Gouaux E: Structure of a glutamate transporter homologue from *Pyrococcus horikoshii*. Nature 431:811–818, 2004.)

Continued

dyes, detergents, and lipid-soluble antibiotics. When overexpressed these carriers can make bacteria resistant to antibiotics. The protein is a homotrimer of huge subunits, each with 12 transmembrane helices. Large domains above the membrane help to span the periplasmic space. Substrates that are soluble in the membrane diffuse into a hydrophobic binding site in the center of the carrier and are transported out of the cell by a mechanism that depends on a proton gradient across the plasma membrane.

- Glutamate transporters remove the excitatory neurotransmitter glutamate from the synaptic cleft after a nerve impulse and transport glutamate into bacteria. The protein is a trimer of identical subunits, each composed of eight complex transmembrane helices. Each subunit has two α-helical hairpin loops that partially cross the bilayer and bind a glutamate. Each glutamate transported across the membrane is accompanied by three Na^+ and one H^+ moving in the same direction and one K^+ moving in the opposite direction. Transport may involve transient fluctuations that open and close a gate near the bound glutamate, but the details are not known.

Carrier Physiology and Mechanisms

Investigators have identified about 500 different reactions that are attributable to secondary transporters and have characterized about a dozen carriers well enough to understand their mechanisms. These model systems (Table 9-1) provide a framework to divide carriers into three broad classes (Fig. 9-4) based on mechanism:

- **Uniporters** transport a single substrate that moves alone down its concentration gradient. This reaction is also called **facilitated diffusion**—facilitated in the sense that the carrier provides a low-resistance pathway across a poorly permeable lipid bilayer. GLUT carriers for glucose are an example of a uniporter found in mammalian tissues.

- **Antiporters** exchange substrates in opposite directions across a membrane. The driving ion moves in one direction, the driven substance in the other. The mitochondrial ANC exchanger for ADP and ATP is an antiporter (Fig. 9-2A).

- **Symporters** allow two or more substrates to move together in the same direction across a membrane. The driving ion and the driven substance move

Figure 9-3 STRUCTURES AND TRANSPORT REACTIONS OF TWO MFS CARRIER PROTEINS FROM *E. COLI*. A, LacY, a proton-lactose symporter. The *red* space-filling model is bound lactose. (PDB file: 1PV7.) **B,** GlpT, a glycerol-3-phosphate (G_3P)–phosphate antiporter. **Bottom,** Transport reactions carried out by postulated reorientation of transmembrane helices. Only 6 of the 12 transmembrane helices of each carrier are shown. (References: Abramson J, Smirnova I, Kasho V, et al: Structure and mechanism of the lactose permease of *E. coli*. Science 301:610–615, 2003; Huang Y, Lemieux MJ, Song J, et al: Structure and mechanism of the glycerol-3-phosphate transporter from *E. coli*. Science 301:616–620, 2003.)

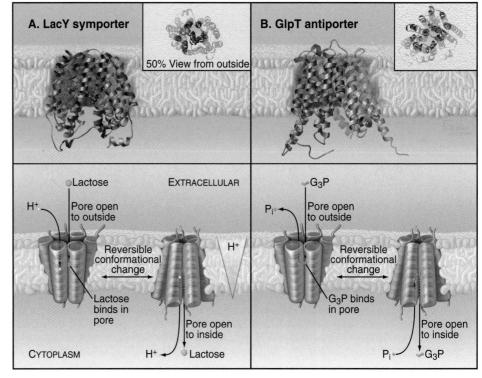

Table 9-1

EXAMPLES OF CARRIER PROTEINS

Carrier	Subunits	Distribution	Substrate	Function
Uniporters				
GLUT1	1×12 helix	Red blood cells	Glucose	Glucose uptake
GLUT4	1×12 helix	Fat, muscle	Glucose	Insulin-responsive glucose uptake
UCP	2×6 helix	Mitochondria	H^+	Uncoupling protein, thermal regulation
Antiporters				
NHE-1	1 or 2×12 helix	Kidney, gut	Na^+/H^+	Acid-base balance
Band 3	1×14 helix	Red blood cells	HCO_3^-/Cl^-	Acid-base balance
UhpT	1×12 helix	*E. coli*	P_i/glucose 6-phosphate	Glucose 6-phosphate uptake
NCE	1×12 helix	Muscle	$3\ Na^+/Ca^{2+}$	Ca^{2+} homeostasis; regulation of heart contractility
ANC	2×6 helix	Mitochondria	ADP/ATP	ATP, ADP exchange
TPE	2×7 helix	Chloroplast	P_i/2 PGA	ATP generation
Symporters				
LacY	1×12 helix	*E. coli*	H^+/lactose	Lactose uptake
NKC1	1×12 helix	Kidney, gut, lung	Na^+/K^+/2 Cl^-	NaCl regulation, fluid secretion
SGLT1	1×12 helix	Gut	Na^+/glucose	Glucose uptake
Various	1×12 helix	Central nervous system neurons	Na^+/Cl^-/γ-gamma-aminobutyric acid (GABA)	Neurotransmitter reuptake

together across the membrane. This is also known as **cotransport.** Examples are the *E. coli* LacY protein (Fig. 9-3A) and the mammalian Na^+-coupled glucose transporters.

Dividing carriers into these three classes should not obscure the important point that these proteins are remarkably similar. In fact, relatively simple mutations can convert a carrier from one class to another.

A few carriers are more complicated than is indicated by this classification. For example, neurotransmitter carriers catalyze both antiporter and symporter reactions, with Na^+ and Cl^- going in one direction and a neurotransmitter in the opposite direction. This example also makes the important general point that the stoichiometry of antiporter and symporter reactions need not be one-to-one. Table 9-1 provides other examples.

All three classes of MFS carriers use similar mechanisms to transfer bound substrates across membranes. This follows naturally from having a common evolutionary ancestor and similar architectures. They work like enzymes, binding substrates on one side of membranes, undergoing a conformational change that reorients this binding site, and releasing substrate on the opposite side of the membrane. Substrate concentrations on the two sides determine the direction of net transfer across the membrane. Whether a carrier is a uniporter, antiporter, or symporter depends simply on the number of substrate-binding sites and the rate and equilibrium constants for the various species to reorient across the membrane. The actual rate of transfer depends on the concentrations of substrates. A limited number of specific inhibitors (Table 9-2) have been useful in establishing physiological functions of carriers.

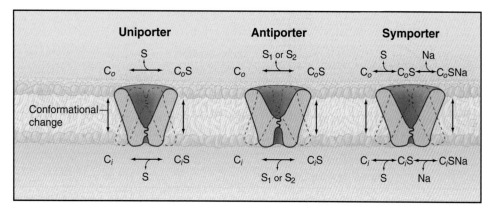

Figure 9-4   CARRIER HYPOTHESIS WITH KINETIC INTERMEDIATES OF THREE CLASSES OF CARRIER. C_o has the substrate-binding site oriented toward the outside of the cell. C_i has the substrate-binding site oriented inside. S, S_1, S_2, and Na are substrates. The *arrows* indicate transitions among the intermediates. Transport occurs when a substrate binds on one side of the membrane and is released on the opposite side after the carrier changes conformation.

Table 9-2

TOOLS FOR STUDYING CARRIERS

Agent	Target
Furosemide*	$Na^+/K^+/2\ Cl^-$ symporter
Amiloride*	Na^+/H^+ antiporter
SITZ, DITZ	HCO_3^-/Cl^- antiporter
Cytochalasin B	GLUT isoforms
Phloretin	GLUT isoforms
Phlorizin	SGLT isoforms

*Used clinically as a drug.

Uniporters

The prefix "uni-" indicates that a single substrate moves across the membrane along its own electrochemical gradient. Nonelectrolytes, such as glucose, use uniporters simply to move across membranes down a chemical gradient. Movement of charged substrates is influenced by the membrane potential and by pH gradients in the case of weak acids or bases.

Classic experiments with **GLUT1** in the plasma membrane of red blood cells led to the carrier concept in the 1950s. Human red blood cells are convenient to use because they express high concentrations of GLUT carriers and because blood banks can provide large quantities of cells. The time course of radioactive glucose accumulation (Fig. 9-5A) shows that transport is stereospecific for D-glucose and that net transport stops when the concentrations of D-glucose are equal inside and out. Slow equilibration of L-glucose across the membrane probably represents passive diffusion across the lipid bilayer, as this rate can be predicted from the solubility of glucose in membrane lipids. This experiment showed that something in the membrane causes an acceleration

in the rate of glucose entry, giving rise to the concept of facilitated diffusion.

The dependence of the initial rate of D-glucose entry on its concentration (Fig. 9-5B) provided evidence for a specific, saturable, carrier molecule in the membrane. Because the rate of D-glucose entry includes both diffusion across the bilayer and movement through a carrier, the L-glucose rate must be used to correct for the rate of diffusion. Once this has been done, the rate of facilitated D-glucose entry has a hyperbolic dependence on the concentration of D-glucose (Fig. 9-5C). This concentration dependence is just like a bimolecular binding reaction (see Fig. 4-2) or the rate of a simple enzyme mechanism that depends on the rate of substrate binding to the enzyme. Thus, the substrate concentration at the half-maximal velocity provides an estimate of the affinity of the carrier for the substrate. At high substrate concentrations, the substrate-binding sites on the carrier are saturated, and the rate plateaus at a maximal velocity owing to rate-limiting conformational changes. These enzyme-like properties, along with the ability to stop facilitated transport with protein inhibitors, suggest that carriers are proteins with specific binding sites for their substrates.

The carrier hypothesis is now understood in terms of carrier proteins embedded in the lipid bilayer; these proteins bind substrate and undergo readily reversible first-order transitions between at least two different conformations (Fig. 9-3). One conformation exposes a substrate-binding site on one side of the membrane. Another conformation exposes a binding site on the other side. Thus, a single substrate molecule can bind on one side of the membrane and be released on the other, thus moving across the membrane. (The carrier does not physically diffuse across the membrane, as was formerly believed.)

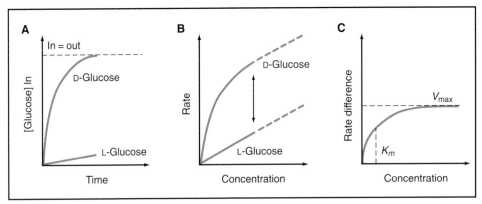

Figure 9-5   EXPERIMENTS ON TRANSPORT OF RADIOACTIVE GLUCOSE INTO RED BLOOD CELLS ESTABLISHING THE EXISTENCE OF MEMBRANE CARRIERS.
A, Time course of the uptake of D- and L-glucose. **B,** Rate of uptake of D- and L-glucose as a function of extracellular concentration. Uptake of L-glucose is by diffusion across the lipid bilayer. **C,** Rate of uptake of D-glucose corrected for diffusion as a function of extracellular concentration. The curve is similar to the dependence of an enzyme on substrate concentration, yielding the maximum rate (V_{max}) at high substrate concentration and the apparent affinity of the carrier (K_m) for the substrate at half the maximal rate.

Net transport requires a concentration gradient, as the conformational change that reorients substrate-binding sites is reversible, and substrate can move either way. The rates of substrate movement depend on the rates of formation of substrate-carrier complex on the two sides of the membrane. The rates of these second-order reactions depend directly on the substrate concentrations, so the binding sites of the carrier are more fully occupied on the uphill side, and the net movement of substrate is therefore in the downhill direction. When substrate concentrations are the same on the two sides, exchange continues without net movement because the carrier is equally saturated on both sides of the membrane.

This simple carrier model clarified a large body of confusing information and clearly distinguished carriers from channels for the first time. The original carrier model for the GLUT1 uniporter also led directly to kinetic schemes for antiporters and symporters (Fig. 9-4).

Carrier mechanisms involve a series of reversible reactions, including rate-limiting conformational changes in the carrier that move substrates across the membrane. Carriers generally translocate substrates at rates of 10^{-1} to 10^3 s^{-1}, similar to the rates of enzyme reactions, whereas channels transfer ions at rates of 10^6 to 10^9 s^{-1} during the brief times that they open (see Chapter 10).

See Figure 11-2 for a depiction of epithelial cells using glucose symporters and uniporters to take up glucose from the intestine after a meal. See Figure 28-6 for an illustration of brown fat cells using uncoupling protein, a proton uniporter in mitochondria, to generate heat when animals arise from hibernation and mammalian infants are born.

Antiporters

Antiporters translocate two different substrates and use a concentration gradient of one substrate to drive another substrate up its concentration gradient. Like uniporters, these carriers undergo reversible, conformational changes that expose substrate-binding sites on one or the other side of a membrane. Two modifications of the uniporter mechanism provide a model for antiporters (Fig. 9-4). First, two substrates, S_1 and S_2, compete for binding antiporters. Second, a substrate-free carrier cannot undergo the conformational changes required to change the orientation of its binding sites. These differences make transport of two substrates dependent on each other in an obligate fashion.

For example, the heart 3Na$^+$/Ca^{2+} exchanger binds either Na$^+$ or Ca^{2+} and uses the large Na$^+$ gradient across the plasma membrane to drive the transport of Ca^{2+} out of the cytoplasm up a concentration gradient (see Fig. 11-13). On the outer surface of the cell, the carrier binds three Na$^+$. After the conformational change that reorients the binding site, the three Na$^+$ dissociate inside and one Ca^{2+} binds. Reorientation of the binding site carries this Ca^{2+} to the outer surface of the cell, where it dissociates. (In addition to the substrate concentrations, the membrane potential must also be taken into account, as this exchange is not electrically neutral, and the potential may affect the binding of one or both substrates to the carrier.)

Antiporters generally exchange like substrates: cations for cations, anions for anions, sugars for sugars, and so on. The Na$^+$/H$^+$ antiporter of kidney, gut, and most other cells allows cells to manipulate their internal pH. Band 3 antiporter of red blood cells exchanges Cl$^-$ for HCO$_3^-$. Carbon dioxide produced in tissues by oxidative reactions diffuses into red blood cells, where a cytoplasmic enzyme—carbonic anhydrase—transforms carbon dioxide into HCO$_3^-$. The antiporter provides a way for the HCO$_3^-$ to return to the plasma, where it is carried to the lungs as the bicarbonate anion. UhpT antiporter (uptake of hexose phosphate transporter) allows *E. coli* to scavenge glucose 6-phosphate from the medium in exchange for inorganic phosphate. Antiporters in mitochondria, consisting of dimers (each with six helices like the presumed ancestor of MFS carriers), exchange cytoplasmic ADP for ATP synthesized by these organelles.

Symporters

The prefix "sym-" indicates that two substrates are transported in the same direction. A simple extension of the uniporter mechanism provides a model for symporters (Fig. 9-4). Like uniporters, the carrier has two conformations with substrate-binding sites open to either side of the membrane. The binding site may be free or occupied by a single substrate, like a uniporter, but in addition, two substrates can bind together. A second difference is that transmembrane reorientation of substrate-binding sites is much more favorable for free carrier and carrier with two bound substrates than for carrier with only one bound substrate. This feature of symporters minimizes leaks of one substrate across the membrane.

E. coli LacY symporter uses a proton gradient across the plasma membrane to drive accumulation of lactose (Fig. 9-3A). The proton gradient is created by the respiratory chain under aerobic conditions or by the F-type ATPase pump under anaerobic conditions (see Fig. 8-5). Protons move down their concentration gradient as lactose moves up its concentration gradient into the cell. Mutations in LacY can cause internal leaks that uncouple sugar transport from proton movements. Vertebrate SGLT1 symporter carries out a comparable reaction for intestinal epithelial cells using the Na$^+$ gradient to take up glucose from the lumen of the gut (see Fig. 11-2).

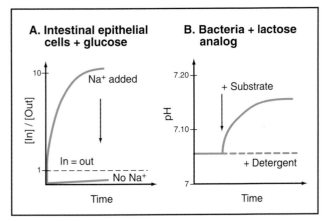

Figure 9-6 EXPERIMENTAL EVIDENCE FOR THE EXISTENCE OF SYMPORT-ERS. **A,** The effect of Na$^+$ on the uptake of radioactive glucose by apical plasma membrane vesicles isolated from intestinal epithelial cells containing the Na$^+$/glucose symporter SGLT1. The addition of Na$^+$ to the external buffer strongly favors glucose uptake against its concentration gradient. **B,** Cotransport of protons and lactose by bacteria expressing LacY H/lactose symporter. Bacteria are suspended in a weakly buffered medium. Lactose added to the medium moves into the cells and down its concentration gradient. Protons accompany the lactose through the symporter, raising the pH of the medium. If detergent makes the membrane permeable, the pH does not change.

Two key experiments (Fig. 9-6) established the symporter concept. The first demonstrated that extracellular Na$^+$ was required for intestinal cells with the SGLT1 transporter to accumulate D-glucose against a concentration gradient. This experiment left open the possibility that Na$^+$ simply activates the carrier in some way without being used directly to drive glucose accumulation. Second, an experiment with LacY demonstrated that sugar and cation move across the membrane together. Not only was a proton gradient required for sugar transport but also a high concentration of another sugar (a nonmetabolizable lactose analog) in the medium could drive H$^+$ into the cell along with the sugar. Additional experiments confirmed that the stoichiometry of the reaction was one lactose transported in for every H$^+$ transported in. (Because this transport reaction is not electrically neutral, the membrane potential is a factor, and another pathway must be available to balance the charge—e.g., by carrying K$^+$ in the opposite direction.) These experiments established that both substrates move together across the membrane with a fixed stoi-chiometry and that a concentration gradient of either can drive the other. Parallel experiments on plasma membrane vesicles isolated from vertebrate kidney cells showed that Na$^+$ moving inward down its electrochemical gradient can drag glucose in with it. When the Na$^+$ concentration is equal on the two sides, the carrier facilitates the movement of glucose across the membrane but not its net accumulation.

ACKNOWLEDGMENT

Thanks go to Peter Maloney for material used in the first edition and for his suggestions on revisions to this chapter.

SELECTED READINGS

Abramson J, Kaback HR, Iwata S: Structural comparison of lactose permease and the glycerol-3-phosphate antiporter: Members of the major facilitator superfamily. Curr Opin Struct Biol 14:413–419, 2004.

Abramson J, Smirnova I, Kasho V, et al: Structure and mechanism of the lactose permease of E. coli. Science 301:610–615, 2003.

Guan L, Kaback HR: Lessons from lactose permease. Annu Rev Biophys Biomol Struct 35:67–91, 2006.

Huang Y, Lemieux MJ, Song J, et al: Structure and mechanism of the glycerol-3-phosphate transporter from E. coli. Science 301:616–620, 2003.

Malandro MS, Kilberg MS: Molecular biology of mammalian amino acid transporters. Annu Rev Biochem 65:305–336, 1996.

Maloney PC: Bacterial transporters. Curr Opin Cell Biol 6:571–582, 1994.

Muakami S, Nakashima R, Yamashita E, Yamaguchi A: Crystal structure of bacterial multidrug efflux transporter AcrB. Nature 419:587–593, 2002.

Nury H, Dahout-Gonzalez C, Trézéguet V, et al: Relations between structure and function of the mitochondrial ADP/ATP carrier. Annu Rev Biochem 75:713–741, 2006.

Orlowski J, Grinstein S: Na$^+$/H$^+$ exchangers of mammalian cells. J Biol Chem 272:22373–22376, 1997.

Pebay-Peyroula E, Dahout-Gonzalez C, Kahn R, et al: Structure of mitochondrial ADP/ATP carrier in complex with carboxyatrachty-loside. Nature 426:39–44, 2003.

Walmsley AR, Barrett MP, Bringaud F, Gould GW: Sugar transporters from bacteria, parasites and mammals: Structure-activity relationships. Trends Biochem Sci 23:476–480, 1998.

Wright EM, Loo DDF, Turk E, Hirayama BA: Sodium cotransporters. Curr Opin Cell Biol 8:468–473, 1996.

Yernool D, Boudker O, Jin Y, Gouaux E: Structure of a glutamate transporter homologue from Pyrococcus horikoshii. Nature 431:811–818, 2004.

Yu EW, McDermott G, Zgurskaya HI, et al: Structural basis of multiple drug-binding capicity of the AcrB multidrug efflux pump. Science 300:976–980, 2003.

Membrane Channels

Channels are integral membrane proteins with transmembrane pores that allow particular ions or small molecules to cross a lipid bilayer. Some channels are open constitutively, but most open just part time. Each time a channel opens, thousands to millions of ions diffuse down their electrochemical gradient across the membrane. Carriers and pumps are orders of magnitude slower, since they use rate-limiting conformational changes to transport each ion (see Chapters 8 and 9).

The ability to control diffusion across membranes allows channels to perform three essential functions (Fig. 10-1). First, certain channels cooperate with pumps and carriers to transport water and ions across cell membranes. This is required to regulate cellular volume and for secretion and absorption of fluid, as in salivary glands, kidney, inner ear, and plant guard cells. Second, ion channels regulate the **electrical potential** across membranes. The sign and magnitude of the membrane potential depend on ion gradients created by pumps and carriers and the relative permeabilities of various channels (Appendix 10-2). Open channels allow unpaired ions to diffuse down concentration gradients across a membrane, separating electrical charges and producing a **membrane potential.** Coordinated opening and closing of channels change the membrane potential and produce an electrical signal that spreads rapidly over the surface of a cell. Nerve and muscle cells use these **action potentials** (see Fig. 11-6) for high-speed communication. Third, other channels admit Ca^{2+} from outside the cell or from the endoplasmic reticulum into the cytoplasm, where it triggers a variety of processes (see Fig. 26-12), including secretion (see Fig. 21-19) and muscle contraction (see Fig. 39-16).

Cells control channel activity in two ways. In the long term, each cell type expresses a unique repertoire of channels from among hundreds of channel genes. **Excitable cells,** such as nerve and muscle, express plasma membrane voltage-gated channels to produce action potentials. Epithelial cells express Na^+ channels, Cl^- channels, K^+ channels, and water channels to produce the salt and water fluxes required for secretion and reabsorption of fluids in glands and the kidney. In the short term, cells open and shut specific types of channels in response to physiological or environmental stimuli. Some channels respond to changes in membrane potential. Others respond to intracellular or extracellular ligands or to mechanical forces. Still others, such as kidney water channels, are shifted from one membrane compartment to another to mediate physiological functions.

Channels are important in medicine. Ion channels are targets of powerful drugs and toxins, including curare, tetrodotoxin ("voodoo toxin"), paralytic shellfish toxins, cobra toxin, local anesthetics, antiarrhythmic agents, and probably general anesthetics (Table 10-1). Defects in ion channel genes cause many inherited disorders, including

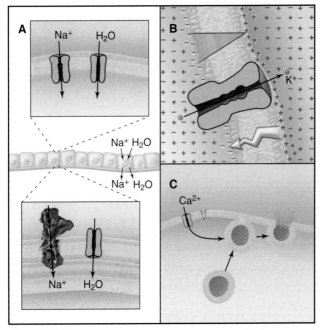

Figure 10-1 FUNCTIONS OF MEMBRANE CHANNELS. **A,** Transport of salt and water across an epithelium by water channels in both the apical and basolateral membranes, a Na^+ channel in the apical membrane, and a Na^+ pump in the basolateral membrane. **B,** Regulation of membrane potential. The triangle represents the concentration difference of K^+ across the membrane. The *zigzag arrow* represents the membrane potential, negative inside. **C,** Ca^{2+} signaling in secretion.

some cardiac arrhythmias and kidney stones. In the human autoimmune disorder myasthenia gravis antibodies target ion channels.

This chapter covers 12 large families of plasma membrane channels. Other chapters discuss cystic fibrosis transmembrane regulator Cl^- channels (see Fig. 11-4), gap junction channels used for communication between adjacent cells (see Fig. 31-6), and intracellular Ca^{2+} release channels that participate in signal transduction (see Figs. 26-13 and 39-15). Understanding channels requires not only information about their structure and activity but also some knowledge of electrical phenomena. Appendixes 10-1 to 10-3 contain essential material about electrophysiology.

Physiologists introduced the concept of channels in the 1950s to explain ion currents during action potentials. Proof that channels are integral membrane proteins followed in the 1970s with isolation of the nicotinic acetylcholine receptor channel and the voltage-gated Na^+ channel. The great diversity of channels was revealed initially by cloning complementary DNAs (cDNAs) using functional assays and homology with known channels. Ultimately, the full repertoire of channels emerged from sequenced genomes.

A new channel can be characterized by expressing its cDNA in a test cell and then making electrical recordings of ion currents from the cell or patches of its membrane (Appendix 10-1). If expression of a single-channel protein fails to reproduce the channel activity observed in the cell of origin, auxiliary subunits are probably

Table 10-1

EXAMPLES OF CHANNEL-BLOCKING AGENTS

Compound (Chemical Class)	Source	Physiological Effect
Sodium Channel Blockers		
Tetrodotoxin (alkaloid)	Japanese puffer fish	Paralyzes skeletal muscle
Saxitoxin (alkaloid)	Dinoflagellates	Paralyzes skeletal muscle
μ-Conotoxins (peptide)	Maine snails	Paralyzes skeletal muscle
Batrachotoxin (alkaloid)	Arrow poison frogs	Opens Na-channels, paralyzes skeletal muscle
Lidocaine	Chemical synthesis	Reduces cardiac and nerve excitability
Potassium Channel Blockers		
Quaternary amino alkanes	Chemical synthesis	Blocks K-currents, increases nerve excitability
Scorpion toxin	Scorpions	Blocks K-currents, increases nerve excitability
Calcium Channel Blockers		
Dihydropyridines	Chemical synthesis	Reduces excitability of L-type channels of striated muscles
ω-conotoxin (peptide)	Pacific cone snail	Inhibits nervous system N-type channels; blocks synaptic transmission
Nicotinic Acetylcholine Receptor		
α-Bungarotoxin (peptide)	Snake, Bungaris multicinctus	Blocks neuromuscular transmission; paralyzes skeletal muscle
α-Cobra toxin	Cobra	Blocks neuromuscular transmission; paralyzes skeletal muscle
Curare	Plant, strychnos toxifera	Blocks neuromuscular transmission; paralyzes skeletal muscle

required. Historically, investigation of channel functions has relied on toxins and drugs that inhibit particular channels more or less specifically (Table 10-1). This approach is often limited by a lack of specificity. Mutations, including those in human disease, provide definitive tests for physiological functions and have yielded some surprising results.

Channel Diversity and Evolution

Humans have about 400 genes that encode channel proteins. The historical channel nomenclature based variously on the ion transported, mode of regulation, physiological role, or drug sensitivity is often ambiguous. Fortunately, knowledge of channel protein structures clarified evolutionary relationships and provided a framework to classify most plasma membrane channels into a few large families (Fig. 10-2).

Channels are integral membrane proteins, usually with two or more α-helices crossing the lipid bilayer. Porins are an exception; they are built from transmembrane β-strands (see Fig. 7-8C). Channels generally consist of two to six subunits, but some are single, large polypeptides. The transmembrane pores for conducting ions or other substrates are often located in the middle of a group of subunits or subunit-like domains, but the pores of chloride, water, and ammonia channels are located within single subunits.

A limited number of genes in early forms of life appear to have given rise to most channel genes. For example, the gene for a simple prokaryotic channel with just two transmembrane segments (called S5 and S6) was the progenitor of a huge family of channels with 2 to 24 transmembrane segments. Some channels with two transmembrane segments acquired features to produce rectified ion fluxes (see later section), extracellular ligand binding (neuropeptides and ATP), and intracellular ligand binding (cyclic adenosine monophosphate [cAMP], G proteins). A simple duplication of one of these genes yielded channels with four segments. Even before the emergence of eukaryotes, the addition of four segments (S1 to S4) yielded channels with six transmembrane segments. Acquisition of positive charges by S4 provided for voltage sensitivity. Two rounds of gene duplication and divergence produced voltage-gated channels consisting of four domains, each with six transmembrane segments, such as voltage-gated Na^+ channels. Water channels originated in prokaryotes by duplication of a gene that encoded three hydrophobic transmembrane segments. The extracellular domain of glutamate-gated channels originated as a bacterial glutamate-binding protein. Ammonia channels and double-barreled Cl^- channels also had bacterial ancestors. The origins of ligand-gated neurotransmitter receptors related to the nicotinic acetylcholine receptor, gap junction connexins, and calcium release channels are still obscure.

Channels in higher eukaryotes are products of multigene families that arose from multiple rounds of gene duplication and divergence. Alternative splicing also enriches the variety of channels. Combining different subunit isoforms in one channel creates increased specialization. All of this diversity suggests a sophistication of function that is difficult to demonstrate with current assays. For example, it is not known why the sodium channels that produce action potentials in neurons cannot substitute for their counterparts in skeletal muscle.

Channel Structure

The K^+ channel **KcsA** from the Bacterium *Streptomyces lividans* serves the model for channels in general and the whole family of **S5/S6 channels** in particular (Fig. 10-3). Four identical subunits are composed of two transmembrane helices connected by a **P loop** (for pore)—a short third helix and a crucial strand that makes the **selectivity filter.** The transmembrane helices are packed close together on the cytoplasmic side of the bilayer but splay apart on the extracellular side to make room for the **pore helices** and selectivity filter.

The selectivity filter is a centrally located pore where the four identical subunits meet, each subunit contributing a quarter of the wall. Highly conserved residues (GYG) in an unusual linear conformation line the pore. The backbone carbonyl oxygens (C=O) of four successive residues all point toward the pore. The pore is 1.2 nm long and about 0.2 nm in diameter, just wide enough to accommodate a dehydrated K^+ ion. This passage distinguishes between K^+ and Na^+ with a fidelity of 1000 to 1 even though Na^+ (with a diameter of 0.095 nm) is smaller than K^+ (0.133 nm in diameter). A simple explanation is that K^+ fits so perfectly into the pore that the carbonyl oxygens replace the water shell of K^+ without an energy penalty, whereas the smaller Na^+ binds more strongly to its hydration shell than to the pore. However, the protein is not sufficiently rigid to discriminate a difference of 0.38 Å, so local electrostatic interactions between ions and carbonyl oxygens and between carbonyl oxygens themselves contribute to selectivity. Carbonyl oxygens carry the optimal electric dipole to favorably counterbalance the hydration free energy of K^+ over that of Na^+, thereby giving robust selectivity despite thermal fluctuations of the protein.

The selectivity filter accommodates two K^+ ions, a local concentration exceeding that inside or outside the cell by more than 10-fold, so it actually concentrates K^+. However, it does not impede diffusion through the pore, since electrostatic repulsion between these closely spaced ions forces them apart. Outside the filter, the pore is lined with hydrophobic groups, but a cavity in

Postulated Primordial Channel	Known Prokaryote Channels	Postulated Primitive Eukaryote Channels	Known Eukaryote Channels	Predicted Membrane Topology	Likely Subunit Composition
S5-S6	S5-S6	S5-S6	Neuropeptide ⮜ Isoforms ENaC ⮜ Isoforms XC-ATP Isoforms	S5 S6 N C	
	S5-P-S6 (KscA)	S5-P-S6	Kir ⮜ Isoforms	N C	
		Duplication	TWIK ⮜ Isoforms	N C	
	S1–S5-P-S6 (KCh)	S1–S5-P-S6	IC ligand-gated ⮜ Isoforms	S1 S6 N C	
	S1–S5-P-S6	S1–S5-P-S6	TRP ⮜ Isoforms		
	S1–S4-S5-P-S6	S1–S4-S5-P-S6	VG-K-Ch ⮜ Isoforms	N C	
		Duplication Duplication 4×[S1–S4-S5-P-S6]	VG-NaCh ⮜ Isoforms VG-CaCh ⮜ Isoforms	N C	
Glutamate-binding protein	Glutamate R M1–P–M2	Glutamate R	Glutamate R ⮜ Isoforms	N C	
	?	?	5HT3R ⮜ Isoforms nAChR ⮜ Isoforms GABA·R ⮜ Isoforms	N C	
?	S1–S12 (eeClC)	S1–S12	ClC ⮜ Isoforms	S1 S14 N C	
3-segment ↓ Duplication 6-segment	Aquaporin	Aquaporin	Aquaporin ⮜ Isoforms	N C	
11 helix	Ammonia ch	Ammonia ch	Ammonia ch ⮜ Isoforms	N C	
		?	Connexins ⮜ Isoforms	N C	
		?	IP₃-R Ryanodine-R	N C N C	

Figure 10-2 CLASSIFICATION OF CHANNEL PROTEINS. This scheme is based on primary structure, atomic structures (where known), and postulated evolutionary origins. The predicted transmembrane topology has the extracellular side at the top and uses rectangles to indicate helices labeled "S." P loops are shown as a short helix and loop between two transmembrane helices. S4 voltage-sensing helices are *pink;* pore positions are *yellow.* The *last column* shows the known (or likely) subunit compositions. In many cases, it is possible to trace the origins of a channel family back to prokaryotes. In other cases, family members are known only in vertebrate organisms. In most families, relatively recent gene duplications and divergence have given rise to multiple isoforms of each type of channel. Channel nomenclature is not uniform. Some names indicate the transported ion (Na+, K+, Ca2+, Cl−), whereas others signify the regulatory modality (i.e., voltage-gated [VG] or neurotransmitter-gated), a physiologic role (intracellular calcium release), drug binding (ryanodine receptor), or some other feature. ClC, chloride channel; ENaC, epithelial sodium channel; GABA, γ-amino butyric acid; 5-HT, 5-hydroxytryptamine; IC, intracellular ligand; IP$_3$, inositol triphosphate; Kir, potassium inward rectifier; nAch, nicotinic acetylcholine; R, receptor; Ryanodine, a chemical that binds calcium-release channels; TRP, transient receptor potential; VG, voltage-gated; XC-ATP, extracellular ATP-gated channel.

the middle of this passage accommodates a hydrated K+ in an environment with a negative electrostatic potential that is thought to reduce the electrostatic barrier to the ion as it crosses the membrane, as predicted by earlier physiological studies.

Channel Activity

Single-channel electrical recordings show that channel pores are either open or closed (Figs. 10-4 and 10-5). Open channels, also called the **active state,** pass selected ions across the membrane at rates approaching their diffusion in water. Closed channels have a different conformation that does not pass ions, small solutes, or water. Many channels also have an **inactivated state** in which part of the channel protein or an impermeant ion blocks the pore of an otherwise open channel, preventing diffusion of ions through the pore. Inactivation makes a channel unresponsive to conditions that favor the active state. Voltage-gated Na+ channels provide a good example; they cycle from closed to open and then inactivate before returning to the closed state.

Selectivity in the Open State

Open channels vary widely in their ability to discriminate among ions. Highly selective channels, such as voltage-gated K+ channels, pass ions without bound water. Less selective channels, such as the nicotinic acetylcholine receptor, are equally permeable to Na+ and K+, which probably pass through as hydrated ions.

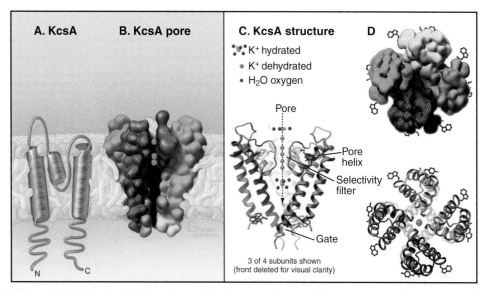

Figure 10-3 Atomic structure of KcsA, a K+ channel from *Streptomyces lividans.* **A,** Transmembrane topology. The short helix and loop between the two transmembrane helices are called a P loop because they form the pore. **B,** Space-filling model with each subunit shaded a different color and with a cutaway view to expose the central pore, which contains three K+ ions *(blue).* **C,** Ribbon model of KcsA with the front subunit removed to reveal the central pore. Starting on the extracellular side, the 4.5-nm-long pore consists of a negatively charged vestibule; the 1.2-nm-long selectivity filter with binding sites for four dehydrated K+ ions (each site is partially occupied at any time); a central cavity with space for a single hydrated K+; a gate (closed here); and a negatively charged cytoplasmic vestibule. **D,** Views from outside the cell. Aromatic side chains (shown as stick figures) at both ends of the transmembrane helices of each subunit project radially into the lipid. (PDB file: 1BL8. References: Doyle DA, Morais-Cabral J, Pfuetzner RA: The structure of the potassium channel: Molecular basis of K+ conduction and selectivity. Science 280:69–77, 1998; Zhou Y, Morais-Cabral JH, MacKinnon R: Chemistry of ion coordination and hydration revealed by a K+-channel-Fab complex at 2.0 Å resolution. Nature 414:43–48, 2001.)

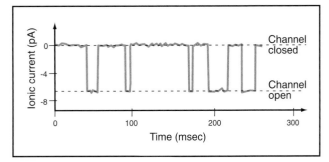

Figure 10-4 PATCH RECORDING OF A SINGLE-CATION CHANNEL MOLE-CULE. This time course shows the current that results when a single channel opens and closes at random. When open, it conducts Na^+ ions at a rate of about 36×10^6 per second, yielding a current of -6 pA. The transitions between open and closed are so fast that they appear instantaneous on this time scale.

Gap junction channels pass most molecules smaller than 800 D without discrimination (see Fig. 31-4).

Extensive physiological data and the structure of KcsA suggest that channels achieve their selectivity by virtue of the fact that particular dehydrated ions bind the channel filter as well as their water shell does (Fig. 10-3). Ions that fit poorly in the pore are rejected, as it is energetically unfavorable to shed their hydration shell. The **ion flux** through an open channel (at a fixed membrane potential) is approximately proportionate to the ion concentration on the side from which the ions migrate. The maximum rate of ion flux—10^6 to 10^8 ions/second—is limited by the time required for binding

and dissociation at specific sites as an ion traverses the pore. At this high rate, channels discriminate between selected ions that bind and rejected ions that do not during an interaction lasting only 10 to 100 nanoseconds! Ions may move in single file through the pore, driven in part by electrostatic repulsion between the ions.

Transition between the Closed, Open, and Inactivated States

Switching between conducting and nonconducting states is called **gating.** Gating determines channel activity because channels generally do not open partway or change their ion selectivity. Transitions between closed and open states are so fast that channels are effectively either fully open or fully closed (Fig. 10-4). The steady-state **probability of being open** (P_o) is simply the fraction of the total time that the channel is open. For a given channel, the fraction of time in the open state determines the ion flux. Because channels act independently, the total flux across a membrane depends on the number of channels that are open at a given time.

Comparison of two K^+ channel structures shows how a conformational change physically opens and closes a gate (Fig. 10-5). In the closed state (the KcsA structure), the helices at the cytoplasmic end of the pore occlude the lumen. The gate is open in the Ca-gated K^+ channel by virtue of a bend in these helices produced by force exerted by a regulatory domain. Energy from Ca^{2+}

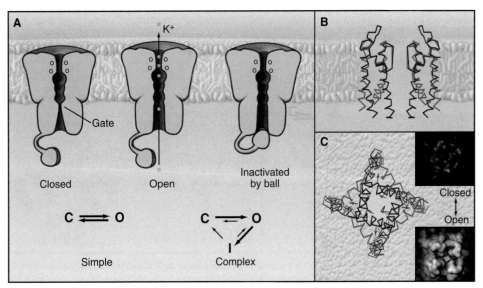

Figure 10-5 FUNCTIONAL STATES OF A TYPICAL ION CHANNEL EMBEDDED IN A LIPID BILAYER. **A,** Drawings of three functional states. Closed channels are inactive. Open channels are active, forming a selective pore for particular ions across the bilayer. The pore rejects other ions because of inappropriate size or charge. Either the channel protein itself or a large ion can inactivate channels by blocking the pore. In this example, an inactivation ball blocks the pore to inactivate the channel. Simple channels switch between two conformations: open and closed. Complex channels switch from closed to open to inactivated and then back to closed without returning to the open state. **B–C,** Drawings of side and top views of the polypeptide backbones of two potassium channels. *Red* is KcsA from *Streptomyces lividans* with the gate closed. *Blue* is a calcium-gated MthK K-channel from *Methanobacterium autotrophicum* with the gate open. The selectivity filters are identical in the closed and open states. (Reference: Jiang Y, Lee A, Chen J, et al: Crystal structure and mechanism of a calcium-gated potassium channel. Nature 417:515–522, 2002.)

binding to the regulatory domain is converted into mechanical work to pull open the gate. Other gating mechanisms are likely to use this principle.

Some channels fluctuate spontaneously between open and closed, but in most cases, local physiological conditions, which are considered in detail in the following sections, control gating from moment to moment. External or internal ligands open some channels. The membrane potential opens and closes other channels without affecting the conductance of the open channels. Mechanical force gates some channels. Cells also use the full range of signaling mechanisms (see Chapters 24 to 26) from phosphorylation to second messengers to guanosine-triphosphate (GTP)–binding proteins to influence the probability that particular channels open or close. By modulating the sensitivity of various channels, cells modify the behavior of their membranes and their responses to external conditions. This modulation makes channels in general, and membrane excitability in particular, highly adaptable. Chapter 11 illustrates how channel modulation regulates the heart rate, changes the efficiency of communication between nerve cells, and adapts cells to some stresses.

In some cases, a process called **inactivation** stops the flux of ions through active channels. The pore of an inactivated channel remains in the open conformation, so it admits ions, but a part of the channel itself or an ion blocks the pore and prevents ions from crossing the membrane (Fig. 10-5). Flexible cytoplasmic domains inactivate voltage-gated channels (see later discussion) by plugging the open pore. Large organic or inorganic ions, such as polyamines and Mg^{2+}, block other open channels simply by binding within and occluding the pore. The membrane potential influences ion blocking because it drives ions into or out of channels. A blocking ion that binds an open channel and dissociates slowly turns off the channel for a long time. Blockers that dissociate on a millisecond time scale cause the current through the channel to flicker on and off multiple times every time the channel opens. Even faster blocking events cannot be resolved but reduce the rate at which ions move through active channels. Local anesthetics such as lidocaine are pharmacological channel blockers. Binding sites for blocking ions can be found on the outside, the inside, or both sides of the membrane, depending on the channel.

Opening a channel for a few milliseconds can change the membrane potential but not the cytoplasmic ion composition, because only a few ions must cross the membrane to produce a large change in membrane potential (Appendixes 10-2 and 10-3). This conserves energy because ion gradients created by energy-requiring pumps are not dissipated. Longer openings of tens of milliseconds can alter the ion composition of the cell. For example, voltage-gated Ca^{2+} channels remain open long enough to change the intracellular Ca^{2+} concentration and trigger cellular events (see Fig. 39-15B). In this way, they convert an electrical signal to a chemical signal.

Channels with One Transmembrane Segment

The simplest known channel is found in the membrane envelope of influenza virus. This **M_2 channel** consists of four small subunits, each with but one transmembrane helix. After an infected cell takes the virus into an endosome (see Chapter 22), the acidic environment opens the channel, allowing protons to enter the virus and to begin to disassemble the protein shell that surrounds the genome. The antiviral drug amantadine blocks these channels. Bacteria secrete peptides (gramicidin, alamethicin, and colicins) that are designed to kill other species by forming highly selective and conductive channels. Only 13 amino acids are required for gramicidin A to form β-helical homodimers that function as K^+-selective channels.

Vertebrates also have simple channel proteins of about 130 residues with a single transmembrane segment and no sequence homology with other known channels. These **minK** molecules do not form channels on their own but are accessory subunits for a conventional P loop, voltage-gated, K^+-specific channel. Both subunits contribute to the pore of the channel. Mice that lack the minK gene have defects in hearing and balance. Epithelial cells in the inner ear fail to secrete the K^+-rich fluid required for the function and viability of hair cells that transduce sound waves.

Channels with Two Transmembrane Segments

Mechanosensitive Channels

MscL from *Mycobacterium tuberculosis* (Fig. 10-6) is a simple channel of five subunits. One of the two transmembrane helices forms the wall of the pore. A third C-terminal helix extends the pore 4 nm into the cytoplasm. The central pore is lined with polar residues except for a gate at its narrowest constriction, where an isoleucine and a value reduce the diameter to about 0.2 nm. Tension in the plane of the membrane created by osmotic stress is believed to rearrange these helices and open the channel. Cations pass through the open channels indiscriminately at high rates, since they lack a selectivity filter like that of KcsA. This response avoids osmotic lysis of the cell. Such channels are widespread in prokaryotes and are also found in eukaryotes.

Inward Rectifier Potassium Channels

The Kir family of channels has the same evolutionary origin as KcsA (S5-P-S6 [Fig. 10-2]). Like KcsA (Fig. 10-3), Kir channels consist of two transmembrane helices with a P loop in between. The P loop and helix S6 line the K^+-selective pore. In spite of these common features, these channels vary in many respects.

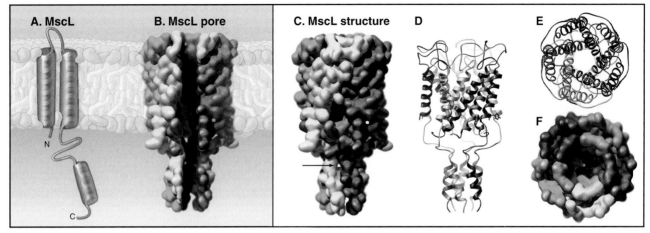

Figure 10-6   Atomic structure of MscL, a mechanosensitive channel from *Mycobacterium tuberculosis*. **A,** Subunit topology. Ribbon model with each subunit shaded a different color. **B,** Space-filling model with each subunit shaded a different color and a cutaway view to expose the central pore, which is 8 nm long. **C–F,** Space-filling and ribbon models. The *arrow* indicates the probable ion entry site on the cytoplasmic side of the pore. (PDB file: 1MSL. Reference: Chang G, Spencer RH, Lee AT, et al: Structure of the MscL homolog from *Mycobacterium tuberculosis:* A gated mechanosensitive ion channel. Science 282:2220–2226, 1998.)

Several channels in this family (Kir2.1, Kir2.3, Kir3 family, and Kir4.1) are **inward rectifiers.** A rectifier is an electronic component that passes current preferentially in one direction. Inward rectifier K^+ channels pass K^+ into the cell when the membrane potential is below E_K (Appendix 10-2), a membrane potential that is not achieved physiologically. Above the resting potential, these K^+ channels pass only a small K^+ current out of the cell when they open. The reason is that impermeant cytoplasmic cations, Mg^{2+}, and polyamines (ornithine metabolites having net positive charges of 2+ to 4+) bind to negatively charged residues on the cytoplasmic end of the S6 segment of open channels and block the passage of K^+. Despite their low permeability, these channels help to maintain the resting membrane potential in many cells and to repolarize excitable cells during an action potential.

Divergence from a common ancestor created a number of channels with differing physiological properties:

- Kidney Kir1.1 channels provide a pathway for K^+ to leave renal conducting duct cells for the urine. Accordingly, they are constitutively open and not blocked by cytoplasmic ions.

- Kir2 channels in the heart and brain contribute to maintaining the resting membrane potential by keeping it from being hyperpolarized. They are constitutively active with inward rectification sensitive to membrane potential.

- Kir3 or Kir3.1 and Kir3.4 channels in the pacemaker cells of the heart regulate heart rate under the control of trimeric GTP–binding proteins (see Fig. 11-12).

- *Cytoplasmic* ATP regulates Kir6.2 channels. These channels, also called K_{ATP} channels, have a novel

function in the pancreas requiring interaction with a member of the ABC transporter family, the **sulfonylurea receptor (SUR).** High blood glucose levels raise *intracellular* ATP concentrations, which closes Kir6.2 channels. This pushes the membrane potential toward threshold for opening a Ca^{2+} channel, which triggers insulin secretion. Sulfonylurea drugs used to treat diabetes mellitus promote insulin secretion by inhibiting these ATP-sensitive channels.

Epithelial Sodium Channels

Epithelial Na^+ channels accelerate the rate-limiting step in Na^+ transport, an essential process that moves salt and water across epithelia in a number of organs (Fig. 10-1A). Typically, epithelial Na^+ channels in the apical plasma membrane provide pores for Na^+ to diffuse down its concentration gradient into the cytoplasm, and Na^+/K^+-ATPases in the basolateral plasma membrane pump Na^+ out of the cell into the underlying extracellular space. Water follows Na^+ through water channels. Renal collecting tubules use this strategy to resorb salt and water. Lung epithelial cells do the same to clear fluid from air spaces. Mice with knockout mutations in the lung epithelial Na^+ channel gene die at birth with fluid in their lungs.

Epithelial Na^+ channels consist of multiple α-, β-, and γ-subunits, but their stoichiometry is not known. All have two hydrophobic segments that are thought to be transmembrane helices but no verified P loops. The second putative helix probably lines a pore that is 10 times more permeable to Na^+ than to K^+. The channel opens and closes randomly for relatively long periods, between 0.5 and 5 seconds, unaffected by the membrane potential or any known natural ligand. The drug

amiloride blocks epithelial Na$^+$ channels, so they are called amiloride-sensitive Na$^+$ channels to distinguish them from voltage-gated Na$^+$ channels. The steroid hormone **aldosterone,** produced in response to salt loss, increases the plasma membrane content of Na$^+$ channels and the rate of Na$^+$ resorption by the kidney.

Liddle's syndrome illustrates the importance of epithelial Na$^+$ channels. Mutations in the C-terminal tails of the β- or γ-subunits of epithelial Na$^+$ channels increase the open time of the channels, leading to excess salt and water resorption by the kidney. Humans with these mutations develop severe high blood pressure at a young age. Hypersecretion of aldosterone by adrenal tumors has similar effects. One type of epithelial sodium channel expressed in brain is activated by the acidic environment when the blood supply is compromised in a stroke. They admit not only Na$^+$ but also Ca^{2+}, which is responsible for much of the damage in stroke patients.

ATP-Gated Channels

Vertebrates express subunits for at least seven cation channels with two transmembrane segments that open in response to *extracellular* ATP. This might be surprising, as ATP is an intracellular energy carrier. However, ATP is stored along with neurotransmitters in many synaptic vesicles, so it is released at such synapses, including sympathetic nerves that innervate blood vessels and transmit pain perception. The subunit composition and stoichiometry are unknown. No ATP-binding site is obvious in the primary structure. These ATP-gated "purinergic" channels are called P2X receptors to distinguish them from P2Y ATP receptors, members of the seven-helix family that are coupled to GTP-binding proteins.

Peptide-Gated Channels

The discovery of channels gated by small peptides in the nervous systems of invertebrates was unanticipated, as all previously known channels gated by extracellular ligands bound small amines or amino acids. These channels are also unusual because they are selective for Na$^+$ and sensitive to amiloride. They are related to epithelial Na$^+$ channels. The human brain expresses related proteins, but little is known about their functions.

Channels with Four Transmembrane Helices

K$^+$ channels with four transmembrane segments and two P loops (Fig. 10-2, TWIK) are abundant in animal genomes, with 40 to 50 genes in *C. elegans*. Two of these subunits form a channel with four domains similar to KcsA. They help to establish the resting potential of the plasma membrane by allowing K$^+$ to leak out of the cell, independent of the membrane potential. These leak channels are activated by volatile anesthetics, leading to hyperpolarization of the membrane and reduced excitability.

Voltage-Gated Cation Channels

Voltage-gated channels have two main functions. First, voltage-gated K$^+$ and Na$^+$ channels produce action potentials in excitable cells (see Fig. 11-6). Depolarization of the membrane opens these channels transiently, driving the membrane potential first toward the Na$^+$ equilibrium potential (Appendix 10-2) and then back toward the K$^+$ equilibrium potential. Second, voltage-gated Ca^{2+} channels convert electrical signals into chemical signals when they admit Ca^{2+} to the cytoplasm, where it acts as a second messenger (see Figs. 11-8, 11-9, and 26-12) to stimulate secretion, activate protein kinases, trigger muscle contraction, or influence gene expression.

Voltage-gated channels share a common domain organization (Fig. 10-2). Crystal structures of voltage-gated K$^+$ channels from a thermophilic Archaea and rat brain (Fig. 10-7) confirmed that hydrophobic segments S5 and S6 are transmembrane helices with a P loop just like KcsA. The P loop is the selectivity filter, since transplantation of the P loop from one channel to another can yield a chimeric channel with the ion conductance of the foreign P loop. Hydrophobic segments S1 to S4 form a separate domain lateral to the central pore.

In voltage-gated K$^+$ channels, the domains consisting of S1 to S6 are four separate polypeptides that associate noncovalently as homo-oligomers or hetero-oligomers. Animal voltage-gated Na$^+$ and Ca^{2+} channels consist of four similar but nonidentical domains (each with S1 to S6) linked in a single polypeptide (Fig. 10-2). Voltage-gated channels have additional specialized domains and/or subunits, but the four main domains carry out the basic functions.

The probability that a voltage-sensitive channel is open depends on the membrane potential (Fig. 10-8). The transition is sharp, likely because all four domains respond cooperatively. A negative internal membrane potential stabilizes the closed state. A **voltage sensor** couples membrane depolarization to channel opening, physically moving charged residues a small distance across the lipid bilayer. Helix S4 is a key part of the sensor. One side of this helix has a spiral of positively charged lysines or arginines. Spectroscopic measurements suggest that the S4 helix makes a subtle motion such as a rotation in response to membrane depolarization. This movement would bring positive charges on

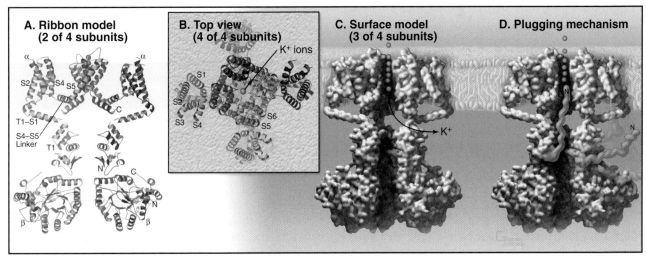

Figure 10-7 VOLTAGE-GATED POTASSIUM CHANNEL. Crystal structure of the Kv1.2 K⁺ channel with β2-subunits from rat brain. **A,** Ribbon diagram of two of the four α-subunits and two of the four β-subunits viewed from the side. Each of the four α-subunits contributes an S5 helix, P loop, and S6 helix to form a channel similar to KcsA. Helices S1 through S4 form a separate domain connected to the channel domain by the S4–S5 linker helix. Movements of the S4 helix in response to the membrane potential pull the channel gate open and closed. The N-terminal T1 domains of each α-polypeptide are located in the cytoplasm, interacting with the tetrameric β-subunit. **B,** Ribbon diagram viewed from outside the cell, illustrating the central channel domains and the peripheral voltage-sensing domains. **C,** Side view of a space-filling model of three of the four subunits, showing K⁺ ions *(blue),* one above the membrane, four in the selectivity pore, and one in the vestibule. **D,** Space-filling model with an artist's conception of the N-terminal "ball and chain" plugging the open gate of an inactivated channel. (PDB file: 2A79. Reference: Long SB, Campbell EB, MacKinnon R: Crystal structure of a mammalian voltage-dependent Shaker Family K⁺ channel. Science 309:897–902, 2005.)

S4 closer to the external side of the membrane, accounting for the charge movement that is detected as a **"gating current."** Movement of S4 pulls on the helix connecting S4 and S5 (Fig. 10-7A), producing force to open the gate of the channel.

Inactivation is accomplished by flexible parts of these channels, either a ball and chain at the N-terminus of some K⁺ channels (Fig. 10-7D) or a loop between the domains of Na⁺ channels. Inactivation depends on membrane depolarization in the sense that the channel must first open to expose a binding site for the **inactivation peptide,** which then occludes the pore and blocks conduction. As a result, the channel opens only transiently. Less is known about the transition from the inactivated state to the closed state, but a conformational change must occlude the pore before the ball dissociates from the cytoplasmic side of the pore.

Potassium Channels

All known voltage-gated K⁺ channels assemble from four α-subunits. Each subunit forms a voltage-gated channel domain with helices S1 to S6 and a P loop forming a central pore. Sequencing of the *Drosophila shaker* gene first revealed the architecture of these α-subunits.

Vertebrates and invertebrates use three strategies to produce voltage-gated K⁺ channels with diverse physiological properties. First, they express many different K⁺ channel proteins from about 20 genes (in *Caenorhabditis elegans*), augmented by alternate splicing of messenger RNAs. Metazoons appear to have four subfamilies of voltage-sensitive K⁺ channels. T1 domains near the N-termini of these subunits (Fig. 10-7A) restrict formation of tetramers to subunits from the same subfamily. Second, some K⁺ channels are heterotetramers, providing a combinatorial strategy with the potential to

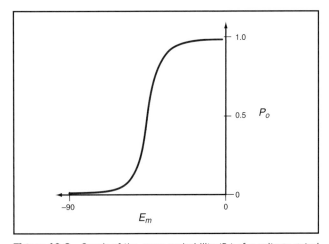

Figure 10-8 Graph of the open probability *(Pₒ)* of a voltage-gated Na⁺ channel as a function of membrane potential *(Eₘ)*. Essentially, all channels are closed at the resting potential of −70 mV, and all are open above a threshold potential of about −40 mV.

produce thousands of different tetramers. Third, soluble β-subunits associate with the cytoplasmic side of some α-subunits (Fig. 10-7A) and modify the behavior of the K$^+$ channel tetramer. One type of voltage-gated K$^+$ channel has a Ca^{2+} binding site at the C-terminus. Signaling events that raise cytoplasmic Ca^{2+} make these channels more sensitive to membrane depolarization, reducing the excitability of the membrane.

Shaker K$^+$ channels are voltage-gated and rapidly inactivated by a globular "ball" on a flexible polypeptide "chain" at the N-termini of either α- or β-subunits (Fig. 10-7D). After a channel opens, a ball from any α- or β-subunit may inactivate the channel by binding in the open pore. Amputation of the ball residues eliminates inactivation, but a soluble peptide consisting of residues number 6 to 46 can rescue inactivation by binding open channels in reconstitution experiments.

Mutations in the gene for the cardiac K$^+$ channel, called HERG, cause an autosomal-dominant human disease called **long QT syndrome.** The QT interval is the time between depolarization and repolarization of the heart muscle on electrocardiograms. HERG codes for a heart K$^+$ channel of the delayed-rectifier type, which is responsible for repolarizing the membrane during action potentials (see Fig. 11-11). Mutant channels open more slowly in response to depolarization of the membrane. Affected patients have a mixture of normal and defective K$^+$ channels, which prolongs the action potential and predisposes to abnormal cardiac rhythms and sudden death. Some HERG mutations also cause deafness.

Na$^+$ Channels

Voltage-gated Na$^+$ channels consist of one large α-subunit of four domains linked in series, each with S1 to S6 helices and a P loop (VG-NaCh [Fig. 10-2]). The 260-kD protein is 25% to 30% carbohydrate. These α-subunits alone form voltage-gated Na$^+$ channels in vertebrate hearts and other organs. In some tissues, one or more small β-subunits help to target α-subunits to their proper places in the cell or modify channel behavior.

Vertebrates express more than 10 Na$^+$ channel isoforms that share many common features: transient activation by membrane depolarization, selectivity for Na$^+$ over K$^+$ and other monovalent ions, and the capacity to propagate action potentials. They differ slightly in their sensitivity to local anesthetics and neurotoxins. Neurons, cardiac muscle, and neonatal skeletal muscle express isoforms with a polypeptide insert between domains I and II containing five to seven phosphorylation sites that modulate channel activity.

Voltage-gated Na$^+$ channels depolarize the plasma membrane during action potentials (see Fig. 11-6), so their distribution effectively defines the excitable regions of nerve cell membranes (see Fig. 11-9A). When activated by membrane depolarization, Na$^+$ channels cycle from closed to open to inactivated in 1 to 2 msec. At the threshold voltage, most Na$^+$ channels open synchronously over a narrow range of membrane potential (Fig. 10-8). Open channels are selectively permeable to Na$^+$ (P_{Na}/P_K = 12 to 45). In 1 to 2 msec after opening, the channel inactivates when a short cytoplasmic segment between domains III and IV binds to and blocks the open pore. The channel remains inactivated until the membrane repolarizes. Then the channel rearranges to the closed state without reopening. Inactivation does not depend on membrane potential, but because it rarely occurs unless the channel is open, inactivation appears to be voltage dependent.

Local anesthetics and a variety of neurotoxins block Na$^+$ channels, inhibiting generation of action potentials. Several of these agents are specific for Na$^+$ channels in particular tissues. For example, Na$^+$ channels of sensory nerves and cardiac muscle cells are sensitive to local anesthetics, such as lidocaine and procaine. They bind to Na$^+$ channels in the open state and block passage of Na$^+$. Because they reduce the excitability of cardiac muscle, local anesthetics are used to treat potentially fatal disorders of cardiac rhythm. Anyone who has had dental work knows that local anesthetics also block the perception of painful stimuli. Snails use paralytic toxins to paralyze their prey, and puffer fish toxins are a health hazard for those who eat this fish.

Mutations in the gene for a heart Na$^+$ channel are another cause of long QT syndrome in humans. Patients have a mixture of normal and defective Na$^+$ channels. Most of the time, the mutant channels open and close normally, but occasionally, they fail to inactivate, sustaining the inward Na$^+$ current that depolarizes the membrane. These rare abnormal events in a large population of Na$^+$ channels delay the repolarization of the membrane, prolong the action potential, and predispose the patient to abnormal cardiac rhythms and sudden death.

Calcium Channels

Ca^{2+} channels are structurally the most complex voltage-gated ion channels (VG-CaCh [Fig. 10-2]). Heart Ca^{2+} channels were purified by using their affinity for dihydropyridine drugs, so they are also called **dihydropyridine receptors.** The α$_1$-subunit has four internally homologous domains with sequence features similar to a Na$^+$ channel. It forms voltage-gated, Ca^{2+}-selective channels. The α$_2$-subunit is a glycoprotein with no homology to other channel subunits. Its role is uncertain, but coexpression of α$_2$ appears to be essential for assembly and normal gating kinetics of α$_1$. The roles of the other, smaller peptide subunits designated β, γ, and Δ are less well characterized.

Like voltage-gated Na^+ channels, Ca^{2+} channels are activated by membrane depolarization, inactivated by a first-order process, and returned to the resting state when the membrane repolarizes. Inactivation is generally slower than that for Na^+ channels.

Ca^{2+} channels have numerous functions. First, in some cells, Ca^{2+} channels contribute to membrane depolarization during action potentials. Given the very low Ca^{2+} concentration inside cells (see Fig. 26-12), open Ca^{2+} channels have a powerful effect on membrane potential. During an action potential, Ca^{2+} currents supplement Na^+ currents in vertebrate heart cells and replace Na^+ currents in heart pacemaker cells (see Fig. 11-11) and some invertebrate neurons.

Second, given their long activity cycles, Ca^{2+} channels can convert electrical signals (membrane depolarization) into chemical signals by raising the cytoplasmic Ca^{2+} concentration. In cardiac muscle, Ca^{2+} triggers the release of Ca^{2+} from internal stores to stimulate contraction (see Fig. 39-15). In nerve terminals, an influx of Ca^{2+} triggers the secretion of neurotransmitters (see Figs. 11-8 and 11-9). In some neurons, changes in postsynaptic Ca^{2+} levels are associated with changes in the strength of synaptic signals. These changes constitute one level of synaptic learning (see Fig. 11-10).

Third, plasma membrane Ca^{2+} channels act as voltage sensors in skeletal muscle. Action potentials stimulate Ca^{2+} channels, which use direct physical contact to activate **Ca^{2+} release channels** located in the endoplasmic reticulum (see Fig. 39-15). The released Ca^{2+} stimulates contraction.

To carry out these diverse physiological functions, vertebrate cells express a variety of Ca^{2+} channel proteins with different physiological properties. Traditionally, Ca^{2+} channels have been divided into several classes, termed N, T, L, and P/Q, based on their sites of expression, voltage required for activation, open channel currents, inactivation kinetics, and sensitivity to drugs (Table 10-2). For example, only L-type calcium channels are sensitive to dihydropyridines, which are used therapeutically to dilate blood vessels by relaxing smooth muscle. N-type Ca^{2+} channels resist dihydropyridines but are blocked selectively and nearly irreversibly by ω-conotoxin, which prevents neurotransmitter release at some synapses. Although this classification is still useful, the continued discovery of channels with novel properties has blurred these distinctions. Now cDNA cloning, expression, and characterization of single molecules provide more discrimination.

TRP Channels

Organisms from most parts of the phylogenetic tree use the TRP family of channels for sensation of diverse stimuli, including chemicals, osmolarity of their environment, and temperature. TRP channels enable humans to sense bitter and sweet tastes, high temperature (and hot spices), and cool temperatures (and cooling chemicals). Mutations that cause defects in fly photoreception led to the first known TRP (transient receptor potential) channel. Some of the large family of nearly 30 mammalian TRP genes were subsequently discovered by sequence homology and assigned function by physiological tests. Other TRP channels were found by expression cloning of cDNAs that allowed test cells to respond to hot spices or cooling chemicals by admitting Ca^{+2}.

No high-resolution structures are available, but the sequences of TRP channels indicate six transmembrane helices and a possible P-loop (Fig. 10-9). These subunits form tetrameric channels that are thought to be similar in architecture to voltage-sensitive K-channels, including a gate on the cytoplasmic side of the ion-conducting pore.

All TRP family members are cation channels, admitting modest amounts of both extracellular Na^+ and Ca^{+2} when active. Diverse stimuli activate the various TRP channels, but the mechanisms are still poorly understood and subject to controversy. In the simplest case, extracellular ligands such as hot spices or cooling chemicals open particular channels. High temperature also activates the hot spice channels, accounting for the perception of such spices as being "hot." The brain cannot discern whether the TRP channels in a sensory nerve are activated by heat or a spice. Similarly, cold temperatures activate another TRP channel that responds also to cooling chemicals such as menthol. Signaling mechanisms downstream from seven-helix receptors and

Table 10-2			
CALCIUM CHANNEL CLASSIFICATION			
Type	**Distribution**	**Functions**	**Blockers**
L-type	Heart; skeletal muscle	Excitation-contraction coupling	Dihydropyridines
N-type	Heart; sympathetic neurons; CNS presynaptic terminals	Neurotransmitter secretion	ω-conotoxin
P/Q-type	Synapses	Neurotransmitter secretion	
T-type	Neurons	Neuron excitation	Ni^{2+}

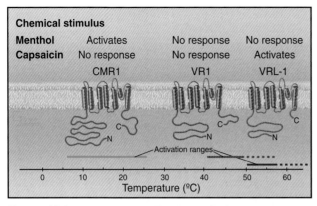

Figure 10-9 TRP CHANNELS. Topology of three temperature-sensitive TRP channel subunits. Note the similar transmembrane segments coupled to cytoplasmic domains that vary in size. The *blue* to *red* shading indicates the range of temperatures that activates each of these channels. The cooling chemical menthol activates CMR1. Capsaicin, the active ingredient of hot chili peppers, activates VRL-1. (Reference: McKemy DD, Neuhausser WM, Julius D: Identification of a cold receptor reveals a general role for TRP channels in thermosensation. Nature 416:52–58, 2002.)

receptors tyrosine kinases (see Chapter 24) activate other TRP channels, in some cases by producing a second messenger (see Chapter 26) such as the membrane lipids PIP₂ and diacylglycerol.

Channels Gated by Intracellular Ligands

Genes for families of channels gated by cytoplasmic Ca^{2+}, cyclic nucleotides, or β/γ-subunits of trimeric G-proteins (see Fig. 25-9) diverged from K^+ channels relatively recently in evolution, about the time when animals diverged from fungi. Their sequences are similar to each other (LC ligand-gated [Fig. 10-2]).

Ca^{2+}-activated K^+ channels are first cousins of voltage-gated K^+ channels. They have six transmembrane segments and a P loop. The Ca^{2+}-binding protein, **calmodulin** (see Fig. 3-12C), binds constitutively to the cytoplasmic tail following S6. Ca^{2+}, entering the cytoplasm through the plasma membrane or released from intracellular stores (see Fig. 26-12), binds this associated calmodulin and activates the channel by making it more sensitive to membrane depolarization. Expression from different genes and alternative splicing produce a variety of these channels with different physiological properties.

Cyclic nucleotide–gated ion channels have six membrane-spanning segments with a P loop and a C-terminal cyclic nucleotide–binding domain homologous with bacterial cyclic nucleotide–binding proteins (Fig. 10-10). Four of these subunits, some of which may be

different isoforms, form a functional channel. Binding of cyclic adenosine monophosphate (cAMP) to the cytoplasmic receptor domain opens a pore for Na^+ and Ca^{2+} and depolarizes the membrane. Changes in cyclic nucleotide concentration provide a sharp on/off switch, as ligand must occupy at least three of the four subunits to open the channel. Ca^{2+} entering the cytoplasm binds to calmodulin associated with the N-terminal cytoplasmic part of the protein. This provides negative feedback to the channel.

Ion channels gated by intracellular cyclic nucleotides are particularly important in sensory systems, including olfaction (see Fig. 27-1) and vision (see Fig. 27-2). Odorant molecules stimulate olfactory sensory neurons by binding seven-helix receptors in the plasma membrane. These receptors work through trimeric G-proteins to increase the cytoplasmic concentration of cAMP. cAMP opens cAMP-gated cation channels, depolarizes the membrane, and activates voltage-gated Na^+ channels to fire an action potential. Visual transduction also uses a cyclic nucleotide–gated channel. Light activates a seven-helix receptor, leading to a decline in cytoplasmic cyclic guanosine monophosphate (cGMP). This closes cGMP-gated channels, hyperpolarizing the photoreceptor plasma membrane and reducing the secretion of neurotransmitter (see the next section).

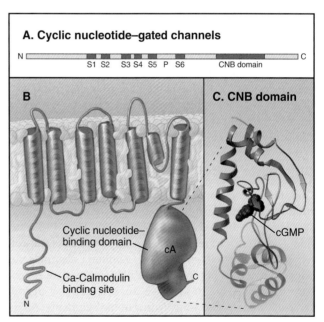

Figure 10-10 CYCLIC NUCLEOTIDE–GATED CATION CHANNELS. **A,** Domain architecture with six predicted transmembrane helices (S1 to S6), a P loop, and a C-terminal cyclic nucleotide–binding domain. **B,** Predicted transmembrane topology of each of the four identical subunits. The N-terminal cytoplasmic domain has a binding site for calcium-calmodulin. **C,** Atomic structure of the bacterial cyclic nucleotide–binding protein, CAP, which is homologous to the ligand-binding domains of these channels. cGMP, cyclic guanosine monophosphate. (PDB file: 3GAP.)

Ion Channels Gated by Extracellular Ligands

Channels that are gated by chemicals mediate communication between nerve terminals and other nerves or muscles. This communication takes place at specializations called synapses, which facilitate chemical transmission (see Figs. 11-8 and 11-9). On the sending side, presynaptic terminals are specialized for exocytosis of chemicals called neurotransmitters, which they package in small synaptic vesicles. Neurotransmitters include acetylcholine, serotonin, glutamic acid, glycine, and γ-aminobutyric acid (GABA) (see Fig. 11-7). When an action potential arrives at a nerve terminal, voltage-gated Ca^{2+} channels admit Ca^{2+} to the cytoplasm, causing synaptic vesicles to fuse with the plasma membrane, releasing transmitter outside the cell. Transmitters diffuse to the postsynaptic membrane in microseconds.

On the receiving side, the transmitter activates ligand-gated ion channels in the postsynaptic membrane. Many of these receptor-channels appear to have diverged from a still mysterious common ancestor, but glutamate receptors had a separate origin in bacteria. Some ligand-gated channels trigger action potentials in the postsynaptic membrane by admitting cations, which drive the membrane potential toward threshold. Others inhibit action potentials by admitting Cl^-, which hyperpolarizes the postsynaptic membrane.

Stimulation of ligand-gated channels is transient because of an inactivating conformational change called desensitization and because neurotransmitters are rapidly removed from the synaptic cleft between the cells (see Figs. 11-8 and 11-9). An extracellular enzyme degrades acetylcholine. Carriers (see Chapter 9) remove all other neurotransmitters by pumping them back into the presynaptic cell.

Glutamate Receptors

Glutamate receptors depolarize the postsynaptic membrane when glutamate binding opens a cation channel that is permeable to both Na^+ and K^+ (see Fig. 11-9). This depolarization of the plasma membrane excites the cell by activating voltage-sensitive sodium channels to trigger an action potential. Eukaryotic glutamate receptor channels (Fig. 10-11) have an extracellular ligand-binding domain and four hydrophobic segments: M2 is a P loop between transmembrane helices M1 and M3. Four subunits form a channel with their P loops on the cytoplasmic side of the plasma membrane rather than outside, like KcsA and its many relatives. A change in the conformation of the extracellular domain induced by glutamate binding opens a pore through the middle of the channel. Successive binding of glutamate to each of the four subunits opens the pore in steps (although

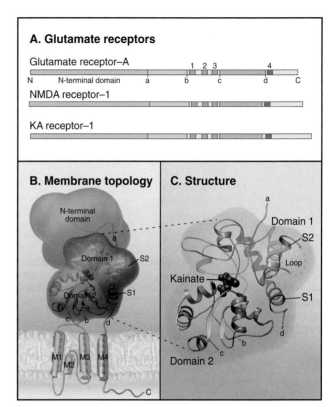

Figure 10-11　GLUTAMATE-GATED ION CHANNELS. A, Domain organization with the glutamate-binding domain between a and b and four predicted transmembrane segments, M1 to M4. M2 is probably a cytoplasmically oriented P loop. **B,** Transmembrane topology and orientation of the atomic structure of the glutamate-binding domain. The N-terminal domain is shown approximately to scale. Four of these subunits are thought to constitute a channel similar to an inverted K^+ channel. **C,** Atomic structure of the ligand-binding extracellular domain from the vertebrate kainate (KA) receptor. (PDB file: 1GR2. From Armstrong N, Sun Y, Chen G-Q, Gouaux E: Structure of a glutamate-receptor ligand-binding core in complex with kainate. Nature 395:913–917, 1998.)

binding is usually too fast to resolve these partially open states).

Multiple genes, alternative splicing, and RNA editing (see Fig. 16-7) all provide a diversity of glutamate receptor subunits, which assemble into homomeric and heteromeric channels used in different parts of the nervous system. Three families of isoforms are sensitive to different pharmacologic agonists in addition to glutamate: *N*-methyl-D-aspartate **(NMDA),** α-amino-3-hydroxy-5-methyl-4-isoxazole propionate **(AMPA),** or **kainate.** NMDA receptors are more permeable to Ca^{2+} than to Na^+ and K^+. Because excess intracellular Ca^{2+} can be damaging, overstimulation of NMDA receptors by glutamate released from cells during strokes or constitutive activation of NMDA receptors by point mutations can kill nerve cells.

Eukaryotic glutamate receptor channels apparently originated in Bacteria by fusion of genes for a periplasmic amino acid–binding protein (similar to *Escherichia coli* glutamine-binding protein) and an S5/P/S6 potassium channel similar to KcsA. The domain organization of plant glutamate receptors is similar to that of animal brain glutamate receptors. Glutamate receptors participate in the response of developing plants to light.

Nicotinic Acetylcholine Receptor

The best-characterized ligand-gated channel is an excitatory cation channel—the nicotinic acetylcholine receptor from the plasma membrane of skeletal muscle cells. This receptor triggers action potentials that stimulate muscle contraction (see Figs. 11-8 and 39-14). It is called the nicotinic acetylcholine receptor because it also

binds the tobacco alkaloid **nicotine.** Related nicotinic acetylcholine receptors in the central nervous system are the targets in tobacco addiction.

The muscle nicotinic acetylcholine receptor is a pentamer of four different, but homologous, subunits with the composition $\alpha_2\beta\gamma\epsilon$ (Fig. 10-12). Each subunit has a large N-terminal extracellular segment, four transmembrane α-helices (M1 to M4), and a large cytoplasmic segment between M3 and M4. M2 α-helices from the five subunits line a central transmembrane pore like staves of a barrel. Hydrophobic side chains line this pore except for a few negative charges that may contribute to cation selectivity. Three other α-helices of each subunit separate the M2 helices from the surrounding lipid. The N-terminal segments of each subunit form massive extracellular domains, each folded into similar,

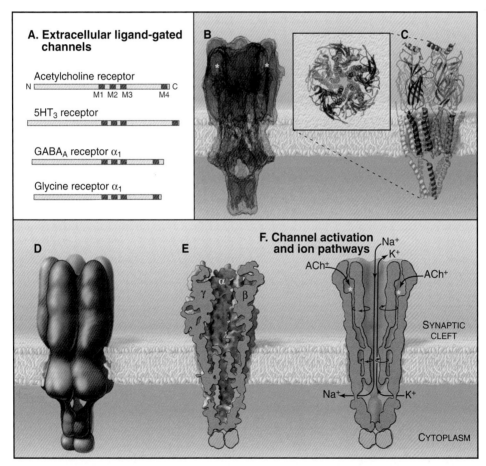

Figure 10-12 **NICOTINIC ACETYLCHOLINE RECEPTOR. A,** Domain organization of the acetylcholine receptor and related receptors gated by neurotransmitters. All four hydrophobic segments, M1 to M4, form transmembrane helices. **B–C,** Structure of the pentameric nicotinic acetylcholine receptor from the electric organ of the electric ray determined by electron microscopy. **B,** Reconstruction at a resolution of 0.46 nm. **C,** Ribbon diagrams of the nicotinic acetylcholine receptor from a structure at a resolution of 0.40 nm. **Left,** View from the extracellular side, showing five M2 helices lining the central pore. **Right,** Side view of model. The extracellular domains of two *red* α-subunits bind acetylcholine. **D,** Space-filling surface representation. **E,** Central section through the pore. **F,** Diagram showing the acetylcholine-binding sites, the proposed conformational changes following activation, and the passages for Na$^+$ into the cell and K$^+$ out of the cell. A 43-kD protein called rapsyn *(blue)* binds on the cytoplasmic side. (PDB file: 1OED. Reference: Miyazawa A, Fujiyoshi Y, Unwin N: Structure and gating mechanism of the acetylcholine receptor pore. Nature 423:949–955, 2003.)

highly twisted β-sandwiches. The α-subunits have deep cavities that bind acetylcholine.

Gating and ion selectivity of acetylcholine receptors differ in concept from the P-loop family of channels. In closed channels, the narrowest part of the closed pore is less than 7 Å in diameter, too small for hydrated K^+ and Na^+ ions, and the hydrophobic pore does not provide a passage for unhydrated ions. Acetylcholine binding to the two α-subunits changes the conformations of the extracellular domains, which rotate the M2 helices and open a channel that is more permeable to K^+ and Na^+ than to Ca^{2+}. The resulting permeability to all three ions causes the membrane potential to collapse toward a reversal potential (see the section titled "Net Current through Ion-Selective Channels") around 0 mV. This triggers voltage-gated Na^+ channels to initiate a self-propagating action potential in the muscle plasma membrane with nearly 100% efficiency (see Fig. 11-8).

Muscle cells and some central nervous system neurons express more than two dozen different isoforms of nicotinic acetylcholine receptors, most with a mixture of subunits but some with five identical subunits.

Many toxins bind nicotinic acetylcholine receptors, blocking transmission of impulses between motor nerves and skeletal muscle (Table 10-1). α-**Bungarotoxin** has been used to characterize the receptor. **Curare** is a powerful muscle relaxant that is used during surgery because it blocks acetylcholine-binding sites without opening the channel. Local anesthetics, such as procaine, bind within the channel and block ion conductance.

Some people produce autoimmune antibodies to nicotinic acetylcholine receptors, resulting in a disease called **myasthenia gravis.** When antibody binds to the receptor, the skeletal muscle internalizes the receptor, reducing its response to acetylcholine and causing weakness.

Other Neurotransmitter Receptors

Receptors activated by the neurotransmitters GABA or glycine consist of five subunits with sequences similar to those of nicotinic acetylcholine receptors. They are Cl^- channels that hyperpolarize the postsynaptic membrane. Several isoforms of GABA receptors bind **benzodiazepines,** drugs used to treat depression. They increase the probability that the channel will open. **Strychnine** inhibits glycine receptors, making neural circuits oversensitive to stimulation. Channels opened by 5-hydroxytryptamine (serotonin) consist of five similar subunits.

ClC Chloride Channels

Organisms ranging from bacteria to yeast and animals have genes for members of a large family of ClC chloride channels. ClCs control membrane excitability and contribute to volume regulation and epithelial transport. Like P-loop cation channels, ClCs are selective for a particular ion, Cl^- in this case, and are gated by the membrane potential. Nevertheless, P-loop cation channels and ClCs differ in evolutionary origins and structure.

ClC subunits are triangular transmembrane proteins formed from 18 α-helices (Fig. 10-13). These helices surround a pore that passes through the middle of each subunit, like the pores of ammonia channels (Fig. 10-14), aquaporins (Fig. 10-15), and porins (see Fig. 7-8C). Several helices around the pore extend only part way across the lipid bilayer. Highly conserved residues in the loops between these helices form the selectivity filter for Cl^- in the middle of the protein and the membrane bilayer. Two subunits associate tightly in the lipid bilayer, so each channel has two pores.

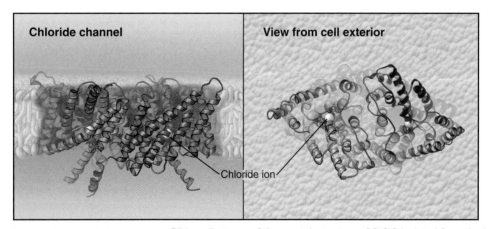

Figure 10-13 STRUCTURE OF CLC CHLORIDE CHANNEL. Ribbon diagrams of the crystal structure of StClC isolated from the bacterium *Salmonella typhimurium*. One subunit is *red;* the other is *blue.* The *white* sphere shows the position of a Cl^- ion in the selectivity filter. This structure is the model for other chloride channels, but it actually works more like a carrier than a channel. (PDB file: 1KPK. Reference: Dutzler R, Campbell EB, Cadene M, et al: X-ray structure of a ClC chloride channel at 3.0 Å reveals the molecular basis of anion selectivity. Nature 415:287–294, 2002.)

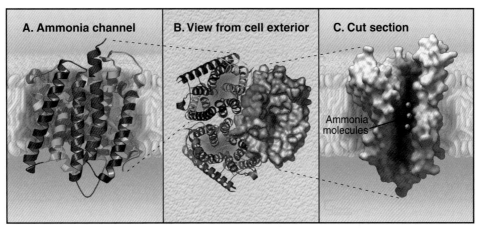

Figure 10-14   AMMONIA CHANNELS. **A,** Ribbon diagram of one subunit of the trimeric AmtB ammonia channel from *E. coli* with the extracellular side at the top. **B,** Ribbon and space-filling diagram of the channel viewed from outside the cell. Each of the three identical subunits has a pore for ammonia to cross the lipid bilayer. **C,** Space-filling cutaway drawing of one subunit exposing the channel for passage of ammonia *(blue)*. In the vestibule facing outside the cell, an ammonium ion gives up a proton to an amino acid side chain before passing through the hydrophobic pore through the core of the protein as uncharged ammonia. At the narrowest point of the pore, hydrogen bonds between the ammonia and two histidines contribute to the specificity. (PDB file: 1U77. Reference: Khademi S, O'Connell J, Remis J, et al: Mechanism of ammonia transport by Amt/MEP/Rh: Structure of AmtB at 1.35 Å. Science 305:1587–1594, 2004.)

The best-known member of the family is ClC0 from skeletal muscle. Like voltage-gated cation channels, ClC0 channels open when the membrane depolarizes and subsequently inactivate. In contrast to cation channels, which have a single conductance state, active Cl⁻ channels conduct at two levels: 10 or 20 pS (picosiemens; see the section titled "Net Current through Ion-Selective Channels"). The pairing of two subunits, each with a pore capable of conducting at 10 pS, explains this behavior. When active, either one or both subunits conduct Cl⁻. A negatively charged glutamate side chain is believed to block the pore of inactive channels and to swing out of the way in active channels. In an unexpected turn of events, physiological analysis of the bacterial ClC channel used for structural studies revealed many features of a carrier that exchanges Cl⁻ for H⁺ rather than features of a typical ion channel behavior like other members of this family. This is one of several examples of blurred distinctions among channels, carriers, and pumps.

Mutations in Cl⁻ channel genes cause several human diseases. Defective skeletal muscle ClC1 channels cause recessive and dominant myotonias. Mutations in kidney ClC5 channels predispose individuals to the formation of kidney stones.

Ammonia Channels

One ancient channel family evolved in early prokaryotes to conduct ammonia across the cell membrane. Ammonia can directly penetrate lipid bilayers, but these channels allow low concentrations of ammonia to serve as a source of nitrogen that prokaryotes use to synthesize proteins and nucleic acids. Bacteria, Archaea, and eukaryotes still depend on these channels. In humans, these channels conduct both ammonia and carbon dioxide across the plasma membranes of red blood cells, where they are known as **Rh antigens** (Box 10-1). These channels are also important for ammonia transport in the human kidney and liver.

Ammonia channels consist of three identical subunits, each composed of 11 transmembrane helices and having its own conducting pore (Fig. 10-14). These are the only known trimeric channels (Fig. 10-2). The interfaces between these subunits are tightly sealed, but each subunit has a narrow internal pore that is highly selective for ammonia and methylammonium. Chloride channels (Fig. 10-13) and aquaporins (Fig. 10-15) also have conducting pores through subunits rather than the more common strategy of forming pores at a central interface among subunits. Both

---

BOX 10-1
Rh Antigens

Before anything was known about membrane proteins or ammonia transport, immunologists discovered that injection of rhesus monkey red blood cells into rabbits produced antibodies that reacted with most but not all human red blood cells. This Rh antigen, now known to be the most common isoform of the human ammonia channel, is clinically relevant because the red blood cells of an "Rh-positive" fetus inheriting this isoform from the father can provoke an immunologic response from the mother if she lacks this isoform and is "Rh negative." During subsequent pregnancies, these maternal antibodies can attack the red blood cells of an Rh-positive fetus.

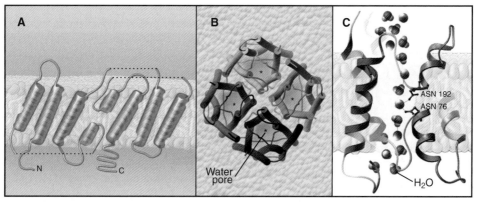

Figure 10-15   WATER CHANNELS. **A,** Membrane topology of aquaporin-1 deduced from the primary structure. The two halves of the polypeptide have similar sequences but are inverted relative to each other. **B,** Structure determined by electron crystallography, showing four identical units, each with a pore *(red asterisk)*. Helices are depicted as cylinders. **C,** Detail of the water pore, with a chain of water molecules crossing the membrane. Two asparagines in the middle of the pore hydrogen bond one water. (PDB file: 1FQY. Courtesy of P. Agre, Johns Hopkins Medical School, Baltimore, Maryland. Reference: Murata K, Mitsuoka K, Hirai T, et al: Structural determinants of water permeation through aquaporin-1. Nature 407:599–605, 2000.)

substrates (ammonium NH_4^+ and methylammonium $CH_3NH_3^+$) are charged in aqueous solution and must leave behind a proton to pass through the pore as uncharged species (NH_3, CH_3NH_2). They pick up a replacement proton on the other side of the membrane as they exit the channel. Selectivity is achieved by the tight fit of the substrates in the hydrophobic pore and by transient formation of an unusual hydrogen bond within the pore. With millimolar ammonium on one side of a membrane, these channels conduct hundreds of ammonia molecules per second without leaking water, protons, or other charged species.

Water Channels

Water diffuses relatively slowly across lipid bilayers, so membranes are barriers to water movement unless the membranes contain water channels. Such channels were postulated years ago to explain the water permeability of certain cell membranes, but they eluded identification until investigators tested a small hydrophobic protein from red blood cells for water channel activity. When expressed in frog eggs, this protein made the eggs permeable to water, so they swelled and burst when placed in hypotonic media. Knowledge of this **aquaporin** rapidly led to the characterization of a family of related water channels from many species, including bacteria, fungi, and plants. A related channel transports glycerol across bacterial membranes.

Aquaporins provide highly permeable pores for water to cross membranes. Four identical subunits form a stable tetramer in the plane of the membrane (Fig. 10-15). Each subunit has a narrow pore that is selective for water passing through the middle of a bundle of

α-helices. About 10 water molecules line up in a pore about 0.3 nm in diameter. Hydrogen bonding of waters with a pair of asparagine residues at a narrow point in the pore allows the channel to be selective for water. The two halves of the protein arose by a gene duplication, since their sequences are remarkably similar.

Osmotic pressure created by pumps, carriers, and the macromolecular composition of the cytoplasm drives water through aquaporins at rates exceeding 10^9 molecules per second. This explains why red blood cells rapidly swell and shrink passively, depending on the osmolarity of the surrounding fluid (see Fig. 7-6). Water channels have no gates, so they are open constitutively.

Various human tissues express 12 different aquaporin isoforms. Aquaporin-1 is found in red blood cells, renal proximal tubules, blood vessel endothelial cells, and the choroid plexus (which makes spinal fluid in the brain). A few humans carry mutations that inactivate aquaporin-1; remarkably, homozygotes have no symptoms, despite the low water permeability of their red blood cells (and presumably other tissues that depend on this isoform). Aquaporin-2 is required for renal collecting ducts to reabsorb water. A patient with inactivating mutations in both aquaporin-2 genes suffered from severe water loss, called nephrogenic diabetes insipidus. **Antidiuretic hormone** (vasopressin) controls the placement of aquaporin-2 in the collecting duct membrane. It activates a seven-helix receptor, causing cytoplasmic vesicles storing aquaporin-2 to fuse with the plasma membrane. This increases the permeability of apical plasma membranes to water, allowing it to move from the urine into the hypertonic extracellular space of the renal medulla. Reaction of sensitive cysteine residues with mercuric chloride closes the water pores of aquaporins. This explains how mercurials, used therapeutically as diuretics in the past, inhibit the reabsorption of water filtered by the kidney. The reversible inhibition of aquaporins with mercurials provides a test for their participation in physiological processes.

Aquaporins are also important in plants, which depend on water to maintain turgor and to expand cells in growing tissues. When the stomata in leaves open, water moves continuously from roots through xylem vessels and cells in tissues to exit from leaves as vapor. The movement across cell and tonoplast membranes depends on aquaporins. Water deprivation induces expression of tonoplast aquaporins in some plants and may provide a mechanism for plants to compete for water when it is scarce.

Porins

Porins are channels with wide, water-filled pores found in the outer membranes of gram-negative bacteria and mitochondria. The subunits are composed of an anti-parallel barrel of 16 or 18 β-strands that cross the membrane (see Fig. 6-8C). One to three of the loops connecting the strands extend into the center of the barrel and line the pore. The functional molecule consists of three identical subunits.

Most porins are relatively nonselective pores for small, water-soluble molecules, although some are specific for certain solutes, such as sugars. *E. coli* uses a related protein with 22 transmembrane β-strands to transport iron complexes across the outer membrane. A central "cork" domain occludes the lumen of this β-barrel. Interactions across the periplasmic space with plasma membrane proteins open and close the pore. A variety of viruses use bacterial porins as receptors.

ACKNOWLEDGMENTS

Thanks go to Fred Sigworth for material used in the first edition and to Fred Sigworth and Benoit Roux for their suggestions on revisions to this chapter.

SELECTED READINGS

Armstrong CM: Voltage-gated K channels. Sci STKE 188:re10, 2003. Available at http://stke.sciencemag.org/cgi/content/gloss/sigtrans;2003/188/re10.

Bichet D, Haass FA, Jan LY: Merging functional studies with structures of inward-rectifier K(+) channels. Nat Rev Neurosci 4:957–967, 2003.

Birnbaum SG, Varga AW, Yuan LL, et al: Structure and function of Kv4-family transient potassium channels. Physiol Rev 84:803–833, 2004.

Catterall WA, Goldin AL, Waxman SG: International Union of Pharmacology. XXXIX. Compendium of voltage-gated ion channels: Sodium channels. Pharmacol Rev 55:575–578, 2003.

Catterall WA, Striessnig J, Snutch TP, Perez-Reyes E: International Union of Pharmacology. XL. Compendium of voltage-gated ion channels: Calcium channels. Pharmacol Rev 55:579–581, 2003.

Clapham DE: TRP channels as cellular sensors. Nature 426:517–524, 2003.

Dolphin AC: G protein modulation of voltage-gated calcium channels. Pharmacol Rev 55:607–627, 2003.

Dutzler R: The structural basis of ClC chloride channel function. Trends Neurosci 27:315–320, 2004.

Gulbis JM, Doyle DA: Potassium channel structures: Do they conform? Curr Opin Struct Biol 14:440–446, 2004.

Hille B: Ion Channels of Excitable Membranes, 3rd ed. Sunderland, Mass, Sinauer Associates, 2001.

Hulme JT, Scheuer T, Catterall WA: Regulation of cardiac ion channels by signaling complexes: Role of modified leucine zipper motifs. J Mol Cell Cardiol 37:625–631, 2004.

Jiang Y, Lee A, Chen J, et al: Crystal structure and mechanism of a calcium-gated potassium channel. Nature 417:515–522, 2002.

Jiang Y, Lee A, Chen J, et al: X-ray structure of a voltage-dependent K+ channel. Nature 423:33–41, 2003.

Khademi S, O'Connell J, Remis J, et al: Mechanism of ammonia transport by Amt/MEP/Rh: Structure of AmtB at 1.35 Å. Science 305:1587–1594, 2004.

King LS, Kozono D, Agre P: From structure to disease: The evolving tale of aquaporin biology. Nat Rev Mol Cell Biol 5:687–698, 2004.

Li B, Gallin WJ: VKCDB: Voltage-gated potassium channel database. BMC Bioinformatics 5:3, 2004.

Lu Z: Mechanism of rectification in inward-rectifier K+ channels. Annu Rev Physiol 66:103–129, 2004.

Matulef K, Zagotta WN: Cyclic nucleotide-gated ion channels. Annu Rev Cell Devel Biol 19: 23–44, 2003.

Miyazawa A, Fujiyoshi Y, Unwin N: Structure and gating mechanism of the acetylcholine receptor pore. Nature 423:949–955, 2003.

Noskov SY, Berneche S, Roux B: Control of ion selectivity in potassium channels by electrostatic and dynamic properties of carbonyl ligands. Nature 431:830–834, 2004.

Perozo E, Rees DC: Structure and mechanism in prokaryotic mechanosensitive channels. Curr Opin Struct Biol 13:432–442, 2003.

Roosild TP, Lê K-T, Choe S: Cytoplasmic gatekeepers of K+-channel flux: A structural perspective. Trends Biochem Sci 29:39–45, 2004.

Schild L: The epithelial sodium channel: From molecule to disease. Rev Physiol Biochem Pharmacol 151:93–107, 2004.

Sigworth F: Life's transitors. Nature 423:21–22, 2003.

Stocker M: Ca(2+)-activated K+ channels: Molecular determinants and function of the SK family. Nat Rev Neurosci 5:758–770, 2004.

Stroud, RM, Miercke LJW, O'Connell J, et al: Glycerol facilitator GlpF and the associated aquaporin family of channels. Curr Opin Struct Biol 13:424–431, 2003.

Viswanathan PC, Balser JR: Inherited sodium channelopathies: A continuum of channel dysfunction. Trends Cardiovasc Med 14:28–35, 2004.

Yu FH, Catterall WA: The VGL-chanome: A protein superfamily specialized for electrical signaling and ionic homeostasis. Sci STKE 253:re15, 2004.

APPENDIX 10-1

Electrical Recordings in Biology

Analysis of electrical activity across biological membranes requires sensitive methods to detect electrical potential differences and the flow of current on a rapid time scale. Physiologists and clinicians use four general methods, with different sensitivities, to detect electrical activity of single channels (patch electrodes), cell membranes (microelectrodes and fluorescent dyes), and whole tissues (extracellular electrodes).

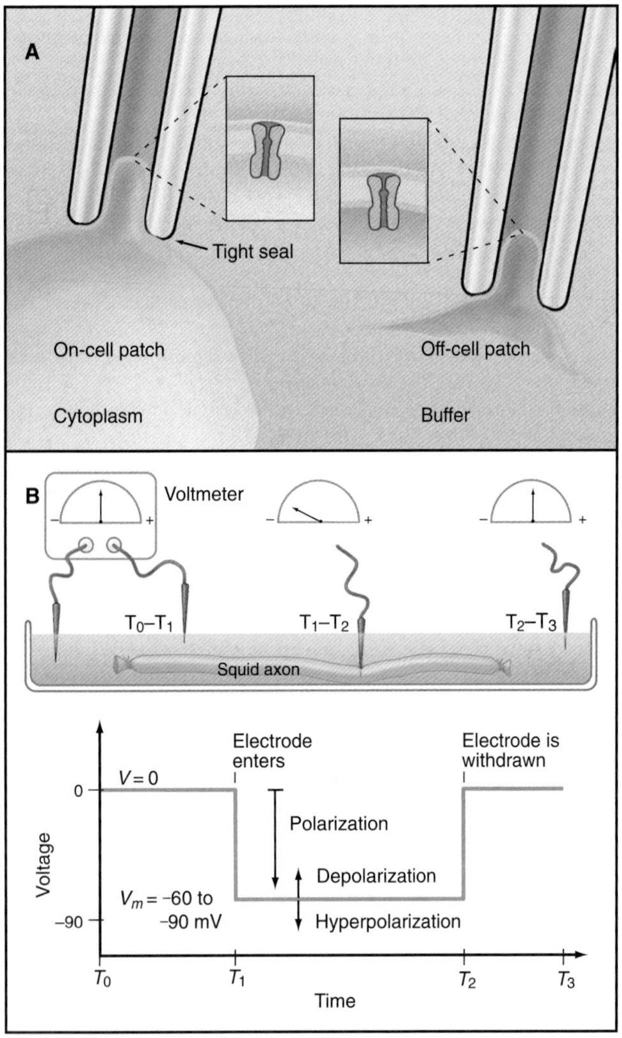

Single-Channel Recordings with Patch Electrodes

Patch-clamp microelectrodes (Fig. 10-16A) provide the best way to characterize the behavior of individual channels. A small-diameter, fire-polished glass capillary is pressed onto the surface of a cell and suction is used to form a high-resistance seal (10 to −50 gigaohms). The membrane patch is small enough to contain just a few ion channels. The electrode becomes part of an electric circuit that can measure current or voltage across the membrane. The high-resistance seal between micropipette and membrane ensures that more electrical current (composed of ions) flows through a single open channel than leaks in around the side of the electrode. When a channel opens, a sensitive ammeter connected to the micropipette records the direction and magnitude of ion flow through the channel as an electrical current. Patch electrodes give direct information about both current and the time that individual channels spend open or closed.

Variations of the patch-clamp technique provide access to channel properties. Leaving the membrane patch on the cell (cell-attached configuration) reveals properties of the channels in their cellular context. Lifting the membrane patch off the cell (excised-patch configuration) exposes the cytoplasmic surface of the membrane to ions, enzymes, or second messengers that

Figure 10-16 ELECTROPHYSIOLOGICAL MEASUREMENTS. **A,** Patch electrode. Fine-tipped glass micropipettes form a tight seal with a small patch of plasma membrane. The salt solution inside the pipette conducts current flowing through an open channel in the patch for recording. Lifting the patch of membrane off the cell exposes the cytoplasmic surface of the membrane to experimental manipulation from the bath. Solutes in the micropipette can stimulate the extracellular face of the membrane. **B,** Measurement of membrane potentials and currents with microelectrodes. A fine-tipped micropipette penetrates the plasma membrane of a cell and is part of a circuit that can record either membrane potential or current flowing across the membrane. *To measure membrane potential,* a voltmeter in the circuit records the voltage inside the cell relative to the bath and follows any changes that occur when ion channels open and close. *To measure current,* an electronic feedback device is placed in the circuit to hold the membrane potential at a constant value. Under these "voltage-clamped" conditions, the feedback device provides current to balance any current that results from opening of membrane channels. The current from the feedback device is a record of current across the membrane channels. The membrane potential is an ensemble property of a large number of individual molecules. Microelectrodes can measure the membrane potential on a submillisecond time scale.

the investigator adds to the bath. Similarly, the investigator can test the effects of potential ligands, drugs, and ions in the micropipette.

Measurement of Membrane Potentials with Intracellular Microelectrodes and Fluorescent Dyes

A glass capillary is drawn to a fine tip (~0.5 μm), filled with a conducting solution (3 *M* KCl), and inserted through the plasma membrane. The tip penetrates the cell with minimal damage, and the membrane seals tightly around it. The microelectrode is connected to a meter to record current and voltage (Fig. 10-16B). Alternatively, the investigator can apply a patch electrode to the cell surface and suck forcefully to breach the membrane, putting the micropipette in continuity with the cytoplasm for recordings from the rest of the membrane.

Two microelectrodes inserted into a beaker of saline register no potential difference. If one electrode is inserted into a cell, the meter registers a potential difference of −60 to −90 mV inside the cell relative to the bath. This **membrane potential** arises from the combined action of many membrane pumps, carriers, and channels.

New fluorescent dyes provide an optical signal that is sensitive to membrane potential. This is the only convenient approach for acquiring information about the spatial distribution of potential charges within cells.

Extracellular Electrical Measurements

Synchronous electrical activity of thousands of cells produces small electrical currents outside the cells, which can be recorded with extracellular electrodes or even with electrodes on the surface of the body. Physicians take advantage of this phenomenon to record the ensemble electrical activity of the heart (**electrocardiogram** [ECG]), brain (**electroencephalogram** [EEG]), and muscle (**electromyogram** [EMG]). These recordings reflect the behavior of thousands of cells, so they provide little information about events at molecular or cellular levels.

APPENDIX 10-2

The Biophysical Basis of Membrane Potentials

The membrane potential arises from separation of charges across an insulating surface (Fig. 10-17). The lipid bilayer provides the insulation required to separate charges. Either pumps or channels can produce unpaired charges. Pumps that transport unpaired ions generate membrane potentials directly. Channels that pass unpaired ions can use ion concentration gradients across membranes to generate membrane potentials. The concentration gradient provides a diffusional force to drive ions through channels. Because channels are ion specific, an excess of charge builds up after very few ions cross a membrane. This excess charge creates a membrane potential and stops the net movement of additional ions across the membrane.

This discussion starts with a qualitative description of forces behind membrane potentials and then develops a quantitative account of membrane potentials with single or multiple types of ion channels.

Diffusion Potentials

An impermeable membrane enclosing concentrated potassium chloride is suspended in a bath of more dilute potassium chloride (Fig. 10-17). If the membrane contains a pore that is *selectively permeable* for bidirectional diffusion of K^+, the concentration gradient drives K^+ out of the membrane compartment. Because Cl^- cannot pass through this selective pore or the membrane bilayer, the inside compartment loses positive charge. Charge imbalance creates an electrical field, negative inside, called the **membrane**

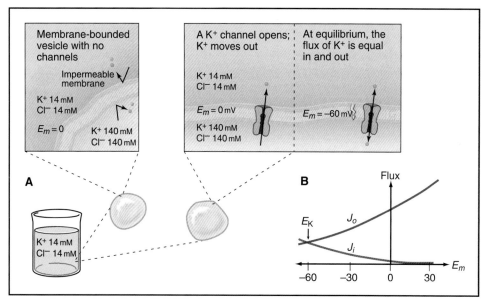

Figure 10-17 MEMBRANE POTENTIAL. **A,** Production of a membrane potential, E_m, by a K^+-selective ion channel and a 10-fold potassium chloride concentration gradient across a membrane. The three panels illustrate the situations without a channel, when a channel first opens, and at equilibrium. **B,** Dependence of K^+ fluxes out of the vesicle (J_o) and into the vesicle (J_i) as a function of membrane potential (E_m). K^+ passes into the vesicle (driven by the concentration gradient) and out of the vesicle (driven by the voltage across the membrane). At a potential of −60 mV, these fluxes are balanced. This is called the resting potential, or E_K. If the membrane potential is greater than −60 mV, the flux of K^+ into the vesicle (driven by the concentration gradient) exceeds the flux out of the vesicle (driven by the voltage across the membrane). This pushes the potential toward E_K.

potential. By convention, extracellular voltage is defined as zero.

Force provided by the membrane potential influences the diffusion of ions through the pore in both directions. The positive potential outside opposes the diffusion of K^+ out of the vesicle and drives K^+ into the vesicle, up its concentration gradient. Net K^+ efflux continues until a charge imbalance builds up a membrane potential large enough to drive K^+ influx at the same rate that the concentration gradient drives K^+ efflux. The electrical potential required to stop net ion movement is called the **equilibrium potential** for K^+, or **Nernst potential**, E_K.

Quantitative Relationships

The quantitative description of membrane potentials by the Nernst equation is *the* central concept of electrophysiology. This relationship between an ion concentration gradient and a balancing membrane potential is derived as follows, using K^+ as an example.

The concentration gradient provides the first force. J_o is the rate (expressed in ions per second) of efflux through the K^+-selective pore. J_i is the rate of influx. The fluxes are proportionate to the concentrations on the side from which the ions come. The ratio of these rates is equal to the ratio of the inside and outside K^+ concentrations, K_i and K_o:

$$\frac{J_o}{J_i} = \frac{K_i}{K_o}$$

A typical cell has a $K_i : K_o$ ratio of about 35.

The membrane potential provides a second force. A positive potential gives a positive ion a higher energy, driving it down the electrical gradient. A negative potential has the opposite effect. The difference in electrical energy per mole of ions is equal to zFE, where z is the valence (+1 for K^+), F is the faraday constant (10^5 coulombs/mol), and E is the potential in volts. This difference in energy enters the equation for the flux ratio as an exponential term (the "Boltzmann factor"), with the electrical energy difference divided by the thermal energy:

$$\frac{J_o}{J_i} = \frac{K_i e^{zFE/RT}}{K_o}$$

where R is the gas constant and T is the absolute temperature.

The K^+ fluxes in and out are equal when

$$\frac{K_i e^{zFE/RT}}{K_o} = 1$$

This famous Nernst equation can be rearranged to give the equilibrium (Nernst) potential in terms of the ion concentrations.

$$E_K = \frac{RT}{zF} \ln K_o/K_i$$

RT is the thermal energy of a mole of particles. The ratio *RT/zF* has the dimensions of voltage and provides the electrical potential that gives a mole of charged particles with valence *z* an electrical energy *(zFE)* equal to the thermal energy *(RT)*. At physiological temperatures, its value is about 25 mV for univalent ions where *z* = 1. The ratio of *RT/zF* establishes the range of potentials (tens of millivolts) that occur in cells.

Another form of the Nernst equation is more convenient. Since ln*(x)* = 2.3 log*(x)* and 2.3 *RT/F* = 60 mV at 30°C, the Nernst equation can be rewritten as

$$E_K = \frac{60 \text{ mV}}{z} \log K_o / K_i$$

Thus, the membrane potential is −60 mV when the K^+ concentration inside is 10 times the concentration outside.

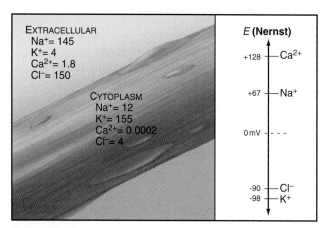

Figure 10-18 PHYSIOLOGICAL ION CONCENTRATIONS AND MEMBRANE POTENTIALS. Ion concentrations in the cytoplasm and outside a vertebrate muscle cell. The scale on the right shows the corresponding equilibrium membrane potentials (Nernst potentials) that would result if channels for each one of these ions opened.

Nernst Potential for Various Ions

The Nernst potential can be calculated for each ion known to have a selective channel in cell membranes: Na^+, K^+, Ca^{2+}, and Cl^- (Fig. 10-18). Given physiological gradients of these ions across the plasma membrane, the membrane potential could range from −98 to +128 mV, depending on which channels are open. In resting cells, only K^+ channels are open, so the resting membrane potential is close to E_K. Thus, variation of extracellular K^+ concentration changes the membrane potential. In vertebrates, the normal extracellular K^+ concentration is about 4 mM, but it varies from 2 mM to >8 mM in disease states. This fourfold variation in K_o changes the membrane potential by 30 to 37 mV, enough to affect cellular processes that are sensitive to the membrane potential. Other channels open and close selectively in response to extracellular or intracellular ligands, membrane potential, physical forces, or other factors (see text). Selective activation of channels is responsible for action potentials and other behavior of excitable membranes (see Fig. 11-6).

APPENDIX 10-3

Charging and Discharging the Membrane

Opening or closing ion channels influences the membrane potential and the flux of ions across the membrane. This discussion explains how movement of just a few ions allows cells to change their membrane potential without dissipating ion gradients across the membrane. Consequently, flux through a few ion channels rapidly changes the membrane potential during action potentials. The result of opening multiple channels with different ion selectivities and concentration gradients is also explained.

Membrane Capacitance

The membrane potential *(E)* produced by a given net charge inside the cell *(Q)* depends on the physical properties of the membrane, summarized in a constant called **capacitance** *(C)*:

$$E = \frac{Q}{C}$$

Capacitance depends on membrane area, thickness (physical separation between internal and external charges), and dielectric constant. If the capacitance is large, many ions must move to change the membrane potential. For cell membranes, the capacitance is approximately $1 \, \mu F/cm^2$. One farad is 6×10^{18} charges per volt.

Charge Movement for a Small Cell

The following calculation shows why *ion concentration gradients change little during most electrical events in cells.* This is important to obviate the requirement for excessive energy to restore ion gradients. A cell that is $18 \, \mu m$ in diameter might have a capacitance of 10^{-11} F, or 6×10^7 charges per volt of membrane potential. Thus, movement of 6 million positive charges out of the cell produces a membrane potential of -0.1 V, or -100 mV. A cell of this size with an internal concentration of 150 mM K^+ contains about 2.7×10^{11} K^+, so movement of fewer than one out of 40,000 K ions from inside to outside creates a large membrane potential. This fraction of ions is far less for large cells, owing to their smaller ratio of surface area to volume. Thus, little energy is required for a large change in membrane potential, such as an action potential. When ion channels open, few ions cross the membrane before an opposing electrical field develops and retards further flux.

In Chapters 8 and 9, pumps and carriers were also noted to produce opposing membrane potentials when moving ions across membranes. This can be avoided by opening ion channels that short-circuit the change in membrane potential by providing pathways for counterions to move in the same direction or similar ions to move in the opposite direction across the membrane.

Rate of Charge Movement through Channels

A current is the rate of movement of charge. The ionic current *(I)* across a membrane is taken as *positive* when charges move *outward*. According to this definition, the equation for conservation of charge in a cell is

$$\frac{dQ}{dt} = -I$$

A positive current reduces the net charge inside the cell, and vice versa. Including the relationship for capacitance $(E = Q/C)$, the equation relates the current to the rate of change of membrane potential:

$$\frac{dE}{dt} = \frac{-I}{C}$$

Because channels conduct about 6×10^6 charges per second, a single open channel changes E at a rate of -100 mV/sec on this 18-μm cell.

Because most channels occur at densities of 50–200/μm^2, an 18-μm cell will have 50,000 to 200,000 channels. If a few channels open together, the membrane potential rapidly approaches the Nernst potential for the selected ion. This explains why most electrical events in cells transpire in a millisecond time frame. Because the rate of current flow through ion channels is not limiting, the time course of electrical events depends on the kinetics of channel opening and closing. This focuses attention on factors that control whether channels are open or closed, also known as **gating.**

Net Current through Ion-Selective Channels

Another way to describe ionic current across a membrane is

$$I = ze_o (J_o - J_i)$$

where e_o is the elementary charge. The dependence of current on membrane potential for real channels is complicated (Fig. 10-17B), so electrophysiologists approximate this current-voltage relationship of channels by a linear relationship, such as Ohm's law $(E = IR)$:

$$I = g(E - E_{ion})$$

where g is **conductance** (inverse of resistance) and E_{ion} is the **reversal potential** of a particular ion channel (the potential at which current reverses from out to in). For perfectly selective pores, the reversal potential for each ion equals its Nernst potential, even in the face of other ionic gradients. The unit used for current is siemens (equivalent to 1 ampere per volt). Most channels have currents in the picosiemens range $(10^{-12}$ S).

For a simple pore, a plot of current versus membrane potential is linear, with no current at E_{ion}; real channels are more complicated. Typical plots of current versus voltage deviate from a straight line. This is called **rectification.** Deviation may be attributable to voltage-dependent conformational changes in the channel protein or to nonpermeant ions blocking the pore.

Each channel contributes independently to the total current, so given *n* channels on a cell membrane, the total current is

$$I = ng(E - E_{ion})$$

Opening Na^+ and K^+ channels has opposite effects because the ion concentration gradients are reversed. The Nernst potential for Na^+ is about +65 mV in a typical cell, given a 10-fold excess of Na^+ outside the cell. Current through an Na^+ channel is negative (i.e., inward) at membrane potentials below E_{Na}. Thus, if a Na^+ channel opens on a cell in which E equals 0, the membrane potential rises toward E_{Na}.

Consequence of Multiple Channel Types Opening Simultaneously

More than one type of open channel creates a situation more complicated than the *equilibrium* described by the Nernst potential for a single-ion species (Figs. 10-18 and 10-19). Consider a cell with physiological ion gradients and two channels—one open K^+ channel and one open Na^+ channel—having conductances of g_K and g_{Na}. The total current through these two channels is the sum of the individual currents:

$$I_{total} = g_K(E - E_K) + g_{Na}(E - E_{Na})$$

Note from this relationship that current is zero at the midpoint between E_K and E_{Na}, and the line has twice the slope of a single channel (i.e., twice the conductance).

Which channel predominates? The equation for I_{total} can also be written as

$$I_{total} = g_{eff}(E - E_{eff})$$

where the effective conductance g_{eff} and reversal potential E_{eff} are given by

$$g_{eff} = g_K + g_{Na}$$

and

$$E_{eff} = \frac{g_K E_K}{g_K + g_{Na}} + \frac{g_{Na} E_{Na}}{g_K + g_{Na}}$$

The two channels together act like a single channel with an effective conductance equal to the sum of their conductances and a reversal potential that is the weighted average of their reversal potentials, that is, weighted by their relative conductances (Fig. 10-19A).

Goldman, Hodgkin, and Katz formulated another equation for E. It uses permeability (P, in units of cm/sec) to describe the membrane potential:

$$E = \frac{RT}{F} \ln \frac{P_{Na}[Na]_o + P_K[K]_o + P_{Cl}[Cl]_o + \cdots}{P_{Na}[Na]_i + P_K[K]_i + P_{Cl}[Cl]_i + \cdots}$$

This equation summarizes the concepts presented here about membrane potentials. Just *two factors* determine the membrane potential: (1) the **concentration gradients** of different ions (e.g., the Nernst potentials for

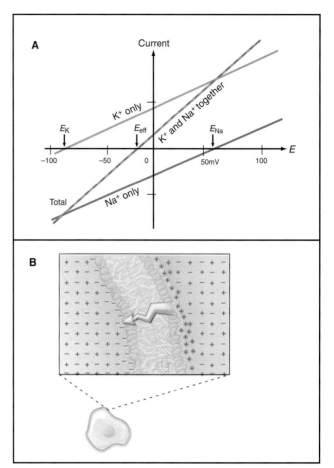

Figure 10-19 MEMBRANE POTENTIAL AND CURRENTS ACROSS A MEMBRANE WITH TWO TYPES OF CHANNELS. **A,** Dependence of currents on membrane potential resulting from opening either K^+ channels or Na^+ channels individually or together. In contrast to Figure 10-17, which shows ion fluxes in each direction, this is a plot of net current. E_K and E_{Na} are the equilibrium potentials (zero current) when only potassium or sodium channels are open. When both types of channels are open, the equilibrium potential (E_{eff}) is midway between the equilibrium potentials of the two types of channels. **B,** Distribution of positive (red) and negative (blue) ions across the plasma membrane and around a cell having a negative membrane potential. Excess negative charge builds up near the inside of the membrane, with the excess positive charge near the outside.

each ion) and (2) the relative permeabilities of the membrane to these ions. When all Na^+ and Cl^- channels are closed ($P_{Na}, P_{Cl} = 0$), the equation reduces to the Nernst relationship for K. When all K^+ and Cl^- channels are closed ($P_K, P_{Cl} = 0$), the equation collapses to the Nernst relationship for Na^+.

In nerve cells, the resting membrane is most permeable to K^+ but also slightly permeable to Na^+, so the resting potential is near E_K. Opening more K^+ channels or lowering extracellular K^+ makes the resting potential more negative. Opening more Na^+ channels or raising extracellular Na^+ makes the resting potential more positive.

Charge Redistribution by Electrical Conduction

Most cellular ions have balancing counterions, whereas unpaired ions contributing to membrane potentials are confined to boundary layers near the membrane (Fig. 10-19B). Like-charged ions repel one another, so unpaired ions tend to accumulate at boundaries where they can move no farther.

During electrical events, unpaired ions redistribute over membrane surfaces by electrical conduction at rates much faster than diffusion. This works as follows: Ions are always in motion, exchanging places. Introduction of extra ions sets off a chain of movements as neighbors repel each other, resulting in rapid spread of unbalanced charge near the membrane. Diffusion of the entering ions over to the membrane would take much longer than this electrical wave. Thus, electrical signaling is the fastest signaling process in cells.

CHAPTER

Membrane Physiology

This chapter describes how pumps, carriers, and channels cooperate in living systems. These three components often work together in circuits or cycles. Pumps establish gradients of ions across membranes (see Chapter 8). Channels regulate membrane permeability to these ions to maintain the electrical potential (see Chapter 10) required for membrane excitability. Carriers use ion gradients as a source of energy to drive transport as well as to do other work (see Chapter 9). Coupling ion fluxes through pumps and carriers to do work is called a **chemiosmotic cycle.**

Selective expression of a repertoire of pumps, carriers, and channels in specific membrane compartments enables cells to build sophisticated machines from a stockpile of standard components. If the pumps, carriers, and channels produced by a cell are known, it is relatively easy to explain complicated physiological processes by applying general principles for the operation of these membrane proteins. The examples in this chapter also show how defects in pumps and channels cause disease and how pharmacological manipulations can alleviate symptoms of disease.

Chemiosmotic Cycles

A simple chemiosmotic cycle couples a cation transporting pump to solute transport by a carrier (Fig. 11-1). The membrane could be a plasma membrane or an organelle

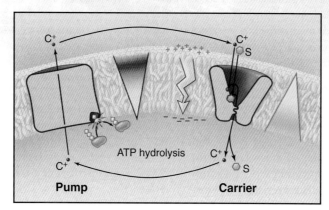

Figure 11-1 A MODEL CHEMIOSMOTIC CYCLE IN A MEMBRANE SURROUNDING A CLOSED SPACE. An ATP-driven pump transports a cation C⁺ out of the compartment. The energy derived from ATP is stored as a concentration gradient of C⁺ *(red triangle)* and a membrane potential *(yellow arrow)* across the membrane. The carrier uses the electrochemical gradient of C⁺ to drive the transport of both C⁺ and a solute up a concentration gradient *(green triangle)* across the membrane.

membrane. The driving reaction is called the primary transport step, indicating an input of energy and, in most cases, some chemical reaction. Other reactions are called secondary transport reactions, indicating that they depend on ion gradients. The transported substrate is the same chemically on both sides of the membrane. Although they are simple in concept, the importance and power of chemiosmotic cycles should not be underestimated. They operate in every membrane of every cell.

Pumps use energy derived from ATP hydrolysis, light absorption, or another chemical reaction (see Table 8-1) to move ions in one direction across a membrane. This raises the concentration of a cation (C^+) on one side and depletes it on the other side of a membrane-bounded compartment. An ion gradient is characterized by both a chemical term, the concentration gradient, and an electrical gradient (the membrane potential explained in Fig. 10-17). The electrochemical potential across a membrane represents a reservoir of power and a capacity to do work, also known as an ion-motive force. A mechanical analog would be using a pump to fill an elevated reservoir with fluid.

Carriers and other membrane proteins use the potential energy of ion gradients to drive other processes. This is analogous to using fluid flow out of a reservoir to drive a turbine, which puts the energy to use for other types of work. Many carriers use energy derived from the downhill passage of one substrate to transport one or more other substances up their concentration gradients across the same membrane barrier. In Figure 11-1, the carrier links the transport of solute S to the movement of cation C^+ down its gradient. Recirculation of cations allows a cell to accumulate solute against its concentration gradient. In addition to the osmotic work illustrated in the figure, chemiosmotic cycles can do chemical work. During both oxidative and photosynthetic phosphorylation, proton cycles drive ATP synthesis by F_0F_1-ATP synthases (see Fig. 19-5). Chemiosmotic cycles can also perform mechanical work. The electrochemical gradient of protons across the plasma membrane drives rotation of bacterial flagella (see Fig. 38-24).

Chemiosmotic cycles using protons dominate the biological world. Most bacterial cycles involve proton pumps, proton-linked carriers, or other proton-linked events. The same is true of lower eukaryotes, fungi, and plants. Plasma membranes of plant cells have a powerful proton pump and a collection of proton carriers. Proton chemiosmotic cycles are also characteristic of most eukaryotic organelles, including the Golgi apparatus, endosomes, lysosomes, mitochondria, and chloroplasts. Animal cell plasma membranes are a major exception, because they use predominantly sodium ions for their chemiosmotic cycles.

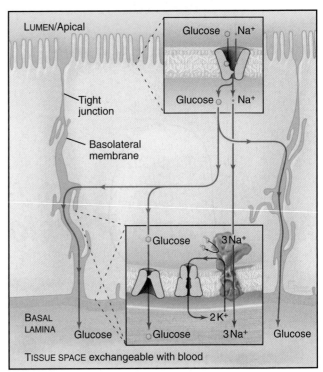

Figure 11-2 GLUCOSE TRANSPORT BY THE INTESTINAL EPITHELIUM. Tight junctions seal the epithelium of polarized epithelial cells. Na^+K^+-ATPase pumps (space-filling model) in the basolateral plasma membrane drive Na^+/glucose symporters in the apical plasma membrane *(upper inset)* and glucose uniporters in the basolateral plasma membrane *(left icon in lower inset)* to move glucose from the lumen of the intestine to the blood. Basolateral K^+ channels *(middle icon)* recycle K^+ pumped into the cell.

Epithelial Transport

Net transport across an epithelium depends on tight junctions (see Fig. 31-2) that seal the extracellular space between the cells (Fig. 11-2). These junctions separate two extracellular compartments. The **apical compartment** is the free surface (e.g., the skin) or the lumen of the organ (e.g., the intestine, respiratory tract, or kidney tubules). The **basolateral compartment** lies between epithelial cells and is continuous with the underlying connective tissue and its blood vessels. Tight junctions seal the extracellular space, inhibiting diffusion of solutes, between the apical and basolateral compartments of the extracellular space. The extent of this seal varies from very tight to leaky. Tight junctions also separate the plasma membrane into apical and basolateral domains, restricting the movement of integral membrane proteins between these domains.

Glucose Transport in the Intestine, Kidney, Fat, and Muscle

A chemiosmotic cycle transports glucose uphill from the lumen of the intestine to the blood (Fig. 11-2). Tight junctions restrict movement of glucose between the epithelial cells, so all of the glucose must move through the cytoplasm. Glucose transport across the epithelial cells requires the following components:

- Na^+K^+-ATPase, located in the basolateral plasma membrane
- SGLT1 Na^+/glucose symporter, restricted to the apical plasma membrane
- GLUT5 glucose uniporter, restricted to the basolateral plasma membrane

The molecular composition of the membrane domains explains the mechanism of glucose transport. Na^+K^+-ATPases use ATP hydrolysis to produce Na^+ and K^+ gradients across the plasma membrane by continuously pumping Na^+ out of and K^+ into the cell. SGLT Na^+/glucose symporters use Na^+ moving inward down its electrochemical gradient to accumulate high internal concentrations of glucose from the lumen. In this step, energy is expended (dissipation of the Na^+ gradient) to move glucose uphill. GLUT uniporters in the basolateral membrane simply facilitate movement of cytoplasmic glucose down its concentration gradient out of the cell. In the gut, this process provides for the uptake of glucose from food. Renal proximal tubule cells use a similar strategy to recapture glucose filtered from blood, transporting it across the tubule cell and back into the blood.

Glucose uptake by fat and muscle cells offers a different perspective. These tissues are designed to take up glucose from the blood when it is plentiful following a meal. Mammals have genes for six isoforms of the classical D-glucose uniporter. Insulin in the blood regulates the availability of the GLUT4 isoform in the plasma membrane. Muscle and fat express GLUT4 but store it internally in membrane vesicles. After a meal, high blood glucose stimulates secretion of insulin into blood. Signal transduction mechanisms (see Fig. 27-7) lead to fusion of these GLUT4 vesicles with the plasma membrane. That increases the rate of glucose transport into fat and muscle by 5-fold to 20-fold, lowering the blood glucose concentration and providing these cells with glucose, which they then convert to glycogen and triglycerides for storage.

Salt and Water Transport in the Kidney

In a section of the kidney tubule called the loop of Henle, the epithelium uses Na^+K^+-ATPase pumps and $Na^+/K^+/2Cl^-$ symporters to reabsorb NaCl that is filtered from blood into the excretory pathway (Fig. 11-3). Without this provision, salt would be lost in urine. Tight junctions seal this epithelium, so that salt must pass through the cells to return to the blood. $Na^+/K^+/2Cl^-$ symporters in the apical plasma membrane provide a way for NaCl to enter the cell down its concentration

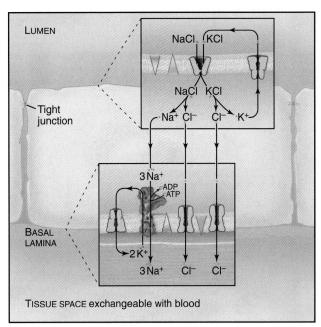

Figure 11-3 **SODIUM CHLORIDE TRANSPORT BY THE EPITHELIUM OF THE KIDNEY TUBULE.** Tight junctions seal the space between these polarized epithelial cells of the thick ascending limb of the loop of Henle. Na^+K^+-ATPase pumps (space-filling model) in the basolateral plasma membrane drive $Na^+/K^+/2Cl^-$ symporters in the apical plasma membrane. K^+ channels in the apical plasma membrane and K^+ channels and Cl^- channels in the basolateral plasma membrane provide paths for K^+ to circulate and for Cl^- to follow Na^+ across the cell from the lumen of the tubule to the blood compartment.

gradient. Abundant Na^+K^+-ATPases in the basolateral plasma membrane ($5000/\mu m^2$) create a Na^+ gradient to drive the symporter and to clear the cytoplasm of Na^+ accumulated from the tubule lumen. KCl that enters with Na^+ through the $Na^+/K^+/2Cl^-$ symporter leaves the cell through channels: K^+ channels in apical and basolateral membranes and Cl^- channels in basolateral membranes.

A drug that is used to treat congestive heart failure—furosemide—inhibits the $Na^+/K^+/2Cl^-$ symporter in the loop of Henle. A weak heart leads to accumulation of fluid in the lungs (causing shortness of breath) and other tissues (causing swelling of the ankles). Inhibition of the $Na^+/K^+/2Cl^-$ symporter reduces NaCl reabsorption, so the kidney produces large quantities of urine, clearing excess fluid from the body and relieving symptoms.

Cystic Fibrosis as a Transporter Disease

Normally, cells in the lung and gastrointestinal tract use a complicated selection of familiar pumps and carriers to secrete salt and water at their apical surfaces (Fig. 11-4). Na^+K^+-ATPases in the basolateral membrane set up an electrochemical gradient of Na^+, which is exploited by basolateral membrane $Na^+/K^+/2Cl^-$ sym-

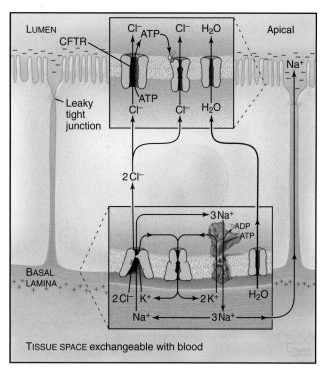

Figure 11-4 SALT AND WATER TRANSPORT ACROSS THE EPITHELIUM LINING THE RESPIRATORY TRACT. Leaky tight junctions partially seal the space between these polarized epithelial cells. Na^+K^+-ATPase pumps in the basolateral plasma membrane drive $Na^+/K^+/2Cl^-$ symporters in the basolateral plasma membrane. CFTR Cl^- channels in the apical plasma membrane allow Cl^- to move into the lumen, creating a negative electrical potential that pulls Na^+ between the cells into the lumen. CFTR also releases ATP, which activates additional Cl^- channels. Water follows sodium chloride into the lumen through water channels and between the cells. Basolateral K^+ channels allow K^+ to circulate.

porters to take in Na^+, along with K^+ and Cl^- anions. The inward movement of Na^+ down its electrochemical gradient drives the entry of K^+ and Cl^- up their gradients. This brings excess potassium chloride into the cell. (The K^+ brought in by both the Na^+K^+-ATPase and the $Na^+/K^+/2Cl^-$ symporter recycles after exiting from the cell by way of channels in the basolateral plasma membrane. Thus, K^+ is merely catalytic.) Excess Cl^- is left inside the cell. The cystic fibrosis transmembrane regulator (CFTR) protein, an ABC pump, in the apical plasma membrane acts as a Cl^- channel. When protein kinase phosphorylates the regulatory domain and ATP binds to the cytoplasmic domains, a conformational change opens a Cl^- channel across the membrane. Cl^- moves down its electrochemical gradient out of the cell, carrying charge to the outside. The whole epithelium becomes polarized, with the lumen electrically negative relative to the extracellular fluid compartment. This electrical driving force allows Na^+ to move between cells, from the extracellular fluid compartment through leaky tight junctions to the surface of the epithelium. Sodium chloride on the apical surface creates an osmotic force that draws water down its concentration gradient across the

cells to the outside through water channels (see Fig. 10-15). CFTR also appears to inhibit the transport mechanisms that reabsorb fluid from the lumen of the epithelium. A balance between this fluid secretion and fluid reabsorption normally keeps the surface of the epithelium properly hydrated, allowing the cilia to clear the lung of bacteria and secretions and the ducts of the pancreas to secrete digestive enzymes.

Patients with cystic fibrosis have mutations in CFTR that result in defects in apical Cl^- transport and secretion. Their lungs are too dry as a result of this imbalance in fluid secretion and reabsorption on the surface of epithelia. This situation is life-threatening because cilia in the respiratory tract cannot move sticky, dry, mucus containing bacteria and viruses out of the lungs, thereby predisposing to respiratory infections. Sticky secretions in the pancreatic ducts also interfere with the secretion of digestive enzymes by the pancreas. Many different mutations in the CFTR gene cause the disease. The most common mutation (67% of cases) deletes the codon for phenylalanine 508 (F508). The resulting protein is temperature-sensitive, not folding properly at 37°C and failing to negotiate the secretory pathway to the plasma membrane. Patients with two copies of this mutation on chromosome 7 have classic cystic fibrosis. Heterozygotes with one normal gene (about 5% of the population) have no symptoms. Patients who have a combination of this ΔF508 mutation with a number of other mutations in the other copy of the gene vary in the severity of their pancreatic problems but still have typical lung disease.

Cellular Volume Regulation

Cells employ both short- and long-term strategies involving pumps, carriers, and channels to maintain a constant volume (Fig. 11-5). These compensatory mechanisms are required because water moves across the plasma membrane through water channels and slowly through lipid bilayers if the osmotic strength of the environment differs even slightly from that inside the cell. Water moves to maintain an osmotic equilibrium, as is illustrated for red blood cells in Figure 7-6. In a hypotonic medium, water moves into a cell to dilute the cytoplasm. In a hypertonic medium, water moves out to concentrate the cytoplasm. Mechanisms that are employed to compensate for these volume changes are well defined, but the mechanisms that sense volume changes and trigger these responses are still being investigated.

Animal cells respond acutely to loss of water by activating Na^+/H^+ antiporters, Cl^-/HCO_3^- antiporters, and/or $Na^+/K^+/2Cl^-$ symporters that bring potassium chloride and sodium chloride into the cell. Water follows, returning the cell to its original volume in minutes. The acute response to swelling activates K^+ channels, Cl^-

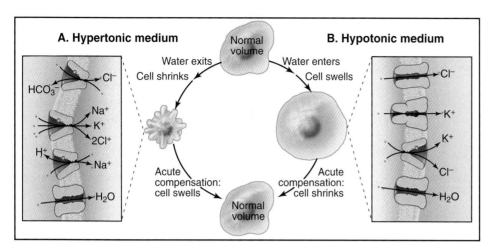

Figure 11-5 ACUTE CELLULAR VOLUME CONTROL. A, Cell is placed in hypertonic medium. **B,** Cell is placed in hypotonic medium. Cells compensate for volume changes by activating channels and carriers to move inorganic ions into or out of the cell. Water follows passively through channels and across the lipid bilayer.

channels (ClC-3), and/or a K^+/Cl^- symporter, taking potassium chloride and water out of the cell. Compensation by moving inorganic ions works in the short run but is not an acceptable long-term solution because changes in the internal concentrations of K^+, Na^+, and Cl^- affect the membrane potential and other physiological processes.

In the long term, cells use small organic molecules called osmolytes to adjust the osmotic strength of cytoplasm and to maintain their volume. Osmolytes include amino acids, polyalcohols (sorbitol and inositol), and methylamines that do not interfere with cellular biochemistry or membrane excitability. Adjustment of osmolyte concentrations takes longer than that for ions, as it requires synthesis or degradation of transport proteins. In response to swelling, cells immediately activate channels that allow osmolytes and Cl^- to escape from cytoplasm; this is followed later by a reduction in the number of plasma membrane Na^+/osmolyte symporters. In response to shrinking, cells close the osmolyte channels and synthesize additional Na^+/osmolyte symporters.

Excitable Membranes

Regulation of membrane potential is particularly important in higher organisms, which use electrical signals generated by membrane channels for communication in their nervous and muscular systems. For example, reading and understanding this page depend on rapid creation and processing of electrical and chemical signals by cells in the visual system and brain. Ion channels produce the key event, a transient change in electrical potential of the plasma membrane, called an action potential. These energy-efficient electrical signals are the fastest means of communication in the body, spreading over the plasma membrane at tens of meters per second. Similarly, action potentials trigger skeletal

muscle contraction, control the timing of the heartbeat, and coordinate the peristaltic motions of the gut and contractions of the uterus.

Electrical excitability is not limited to nerves and muscles. Eggs use a form of action potential as an early step in blocking fertilization by more than one sperm. Chemotaxis by macrophages and secretion of insulin and other hormones both depend on electrical excitability. The reader should be familiar with the appendixes in Chapter 10 to appreciate the following material.

Description of an Action Potential

If a microelectrode (see Fig. 10-16A) drives a small positive or negative current into a cell, a second microelectrode a short distance away detects a small voltage response. These electrotonic potentials decline rapidly with distance if the cell in nonexcitable.

In striking contrast to these small local currents, when the plasma membrane of an excitable cell, such as **neuron** or **muscle,** is depolarized beyond a certain level, called a **threshold,** the membrane responds over a few milliseconds with a large, stereotyped change in membrane potential, called an **action potential** (Fig. 11-6). Voltage-gated ion channels (see Fig. 10-7) generate this powerful electrical signal that spreads rapidly (10 m/sec) over the entire plasma membrane. During an action potential, the membrane potential can reach a peak of +40 to 50 mV before repolarizing to the resting potential. Because action potentials are self-triggering, they travel without dissipation over long distances. This high-speed transmission is very efficient, requiring movement of very few ions across the membrane.

The molecular events during an action potential were first characterized around 1950 in squid giant axons using microelectrodes coupled to an electronic feedback circuit. This clever "voltage clamp" holds the membrane potential constant by providing the cell with electrical current to compensate for changes in ion

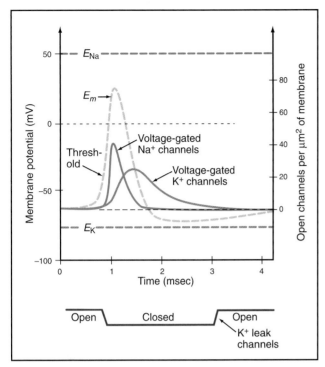

Figure 11-6 THE TIME COURSE OF AN ACTION POTENTIAL PASSING A MEASURING ELECTRODE INSERTED THROUGH THE PLASMA MEMBRANE OF A SQUID GIANT AXON. Spread of an action potential from an adjacent area of the membrane brings the membrane potential E_m, to threshold, triggering the action potential at this point on the membrane. The other curves show the conductance of the membrane at this point for Na^+ and K^+ expressed as the concentration of open channels. The lower trace shows the times during which K^+ leak channels open and close at this point. E_{Na} is the Na^+ equilibrium potential, and E_K is the K^+ equilibrium potential.

currents. Investigators discovered that changes in permeability to Na^+ and K^+ ions produced action potentials. Changing one variable at a time, they determined the time and voltage dependence of ion-specific conductance. They also determined the relationship between conductance and voltage. From these relationships, measured under controlled conditions, they could calculate the membrane response to virtually any experimental condition. To explain these changes in permeability, they postulated the existence of ion channels. The voltage clamp provided a direct measure of this channel activity. This approach also revealed the behavior of channels held at a potential more positive than their resting potential.

Three Channels Generating Action Potentials

Voltage-gated Na^+ and K^+ channels open and close in sequence to produce action potentials. Depending on the type of open channel, the membrane potential varies in time between the K^+ equilibrium potential (E_K) and the Na^+ equilibrium potential (E_{Na}) (see Fig. 10-18).

Because membrane depolarization activates these ion channels, and because the response spreads this depolarization, triggering an action potential initiates a cascade of reactions that moves over the membrane, first to depolarize and then to repolarize the membrane. In nerves, just three types of voltage-gated channels are required to generate action potentials:

- K^+-selective leak channels of the Kir family and the TWIK family (see Fig. 10-2) are open at resting potentials. Cytoplasmic Mg^{2+} blocks Kir channels when the membrane depolarizes.

- Voltage-gated Na^+ channels are closed at the resting potential but open if the membrane depolarizes to about −40 mV. They open only transiently because a first-order inactivation reaction closes the pore, even if the membrane potential is at or above zero. These channels return to the closed state without passing again through the open state.

- Delayed-rectifier voltage-gated K^+ channels have a low probability of being open at the resting potential. They respond to membrane depolarization by opening, but more slowly than Na^+ channels do. They stay open long enough to allow the repolarizing membrane potential to approach E_K.

The properties of these channels explain the time course of an action potential as follows:

Stage 1: At rest, the membrane is slightly permeable to K^+ but not to other ions, so the resting potential is near E_K, about −70 mV. K^+-selective leak channels and a few open voltage-gated K^+ channels contribute to this basal K^+ permeability.

Stage 2: If the membrane is depolarized by an oncoming action potential and reaches the threshold potential, K^+-selective leak channels *close* and voltage-gated Na^+ channels *open*. Because the membrane is permeable only to Na^+ and because many Na^+ channels open, Na^+ moves into the cell and the membrane potential rapidly approaches E_{Na}, about +45 mV.

Stage 3: After 1 to 2 msec, Na^+ channels spontaneously *inactivate* and slowly responding delayed-rectifier K^+ channels *open*. Now the membrane is strongly and selectively permeable to K^+, so K^+ moves out of the cell, and the membrane potential reverses all the way to E_K, about −80 mV. K^+ channels are less synchronized than Na^+ channels, so the membrane potential falls more slowly than it rises.

Stage 4: Delayed-rectifier K^+ channels close progressively as the membrane repolarizes, and K^+-selective leak channels open, returning the membrane potential to the resting voltage, just above E_K.

During an action potential, the membrane voltage changes by 100 to 150 mV in 1 to 2 msec. The membrane bilayer is approximately 7 nm thick, so this voltage corresponds to a field variation on the order of 150,000 volts/cm in 1 to 2 msec. Such strong forces elicit conformational changes in membrane proteins, such as voltage-gated ion channels.

Membrane Depolarization: The Stimulus for Action Potentials

The initial depolarization of the plasma membrane that triggers an action potential can arise from activation by a neurotransmitter (see the section that follows) or spread of an action potential from an adjacent membrane or from an adjacent cell through a gap junction. Membrane depolarization must exceed a certain threshold to trigger an action potential. The threshold arises directly from the properties of the ion channels. Depolarization less than threshold activates a few Na^+ channels, producing a small inward Na^+ current, but it also activates some delayed-rectifier K^+ channels, resulting in K^+ efflux. If the Na^+ conductance is small in relation to the K^+ conductance, outward currents predominate and the membrane repolarizes. Depolarization greater than threshold activates additional Na^+ channels, yielding inward Na^+ currents greater than outward K^+ currents, at least briefly. This positive feedback loop further depolarizes the membrane, amplifying activation of Na^+ channels and producing the cascade of channel activation that makes action potentials an all-or-nothing event.

Synaptic Transmission

Most neurons use chemical messengers called **neurotransmitters** (Fig. 11-7) to communicate rapidly with each other and with effector cells, such as skeletal muscle and glands. This chemical communication occurs at sites called **synapses** (Figs. 11-8 and 11-9), where the sending cell is specialized to secrete a particular neurotransmitter and the receiving cell is specialized to respond to that neurotransmitter. The sending side of a synapse is referred to as **presynaptic,** whereas the receiving side is designated **postsynaptic.** Small vesicles containing neurotransmitter pack the presynaptic nerve terminal. **Neurotransmitter receptors** concentrate in the postsynaptic plasma membrane. Modest changes in either the presynaptic release of neurotransmitter or postsynaptic receptor activation can profoundly influence how a neuron processes this information. Analysis of synaptic transmission has revealed much about the mechanisms of secretion (see Chapter 22), signal transduction, and psychoactive drugs that affect behavior. Not all synapses use chemical transmitters. In special cases, gap junctions (see Fig. 31-6) connect neurons at "electrical synapses," where current moves directly between the two cells.

Neurotransmitters are generally small organic molecules with an amino group. These include acetylcholine, norepinephrine, 5-hydroxytryptamine (serotonin), and the amino acids glycine and glutamic acid (Fig. 11-7). Secretory mechanisms are similar at all synapses, but each neurotransmitter requires its own biochemical machinery for synthesis, packaging in synaptic vesicles, and reception by postsynaptic cells. Such distinctive features of synapses using a particular transmitter make it possible to modify synaptic transmission selectively, such as in treatment with psychoactive drugs.

This section compares two types of synapses that use extracellular ligand-gated ion channels: the neuromuscular junction and central nervous system (CNS) synapses. These examples also show how pumps, carriers, and channels work together during synaptic transmission.

In addition to activating ligand-gated ion channels, most neurotransmitters also stimulate particular seven-helix receptors (Fig. 11-7; see also Fig. 24-3). For example, acetylcholine stimulates the seven-helix **muscarinic acetylcholine receptor,** which uses a trimeric G-protein intermediary to activate Kir3.1 K^+ channels (Fig. 11-12). Glutamate stimulates seven-helix "**metabo-**

Transmitter	Acetylcholine	Dopamine	γ-Aminobutyric acid (GABA)	Glutamate	Glycine	Norepinephrine	Serotonin
Structure	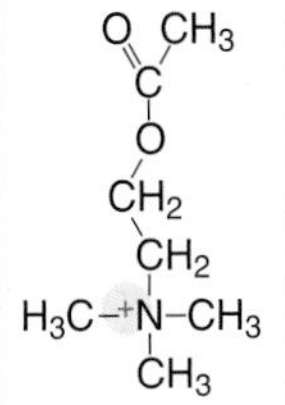 (structure)	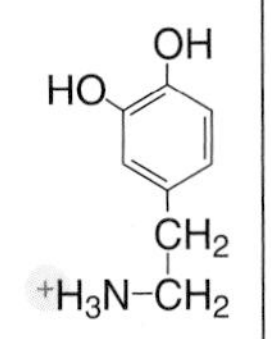 (structure)	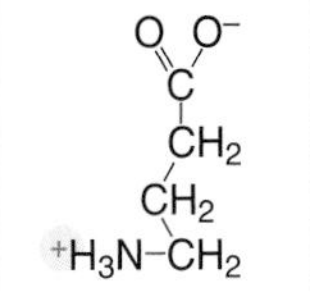 (structure)	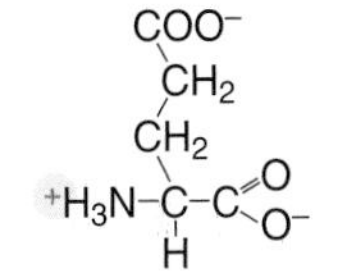 (structure)	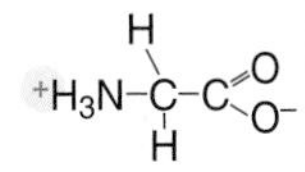 (structure)	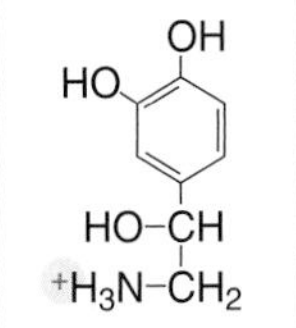 (structure)	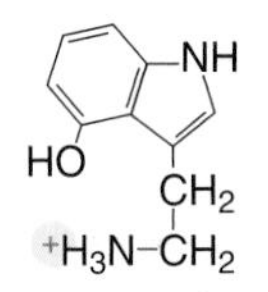 (structure)
Receptors — Channels	Excitatory (nicotinic) Na^+/K^+ channel	—	Inhibitory Cl^- channel	Excitatory Na^+/K^+ channel or $Na^+/K^+/Ca^{2+}$ channel	Inhibitory Cl^- channel	—	Excitatory Na^+/K^+ channel
Receptors — Seven-helix	Muscarinic receptor	Dopamine receptor	β-type GABA receptor	Metabotropic glutamate receptor	—	Adrenergic receptor	Serotonin receptor

Figure 11-7   NEUROTRANSMITTERS AND THEIR LIGAND-GATED ION CHANNELS AND SEVEN-HELIX RECEPTORS.

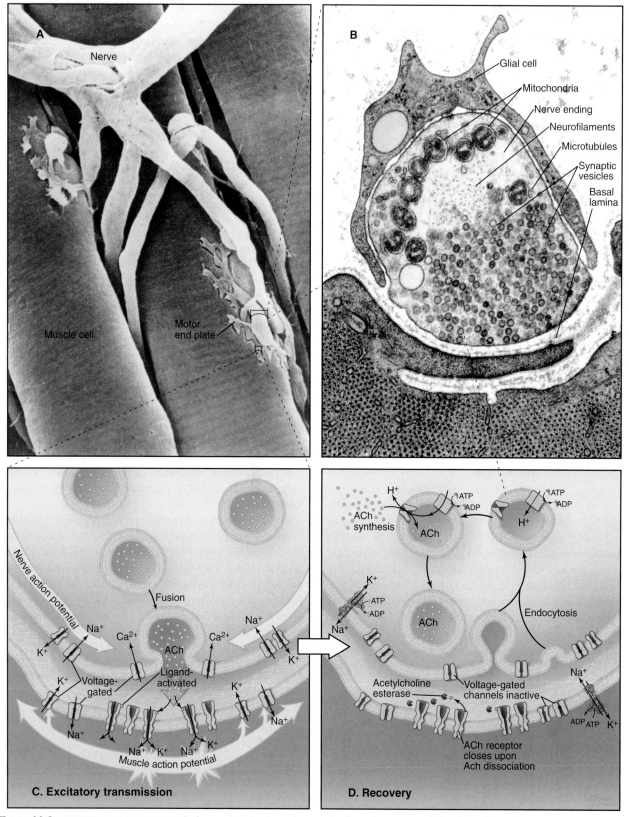

Figure 11-8   NEUROMUSCULAR JUNCTION. A, A scanning electron micrograph of a motor nerve and the skeletal muscle cells that it innervates. **B,** An electron micrograph of a thin section of a frog neuromuscular junction. **C,** Excitatory synaptic transmission. The nerve action potential opens voltage-gated calcium channels. Entry of Ca^{2+} triggers fusion of a synaptic vesicle containing acetylcholine (ACh) with the plasma membrane. Acetylcholine binds and opens postsynaptic channels on the muscle cell, which trigger an action potential. **D,** Recovery includes acetylcholine hydrolysis, recycling of synaptic vesicle membranes, and loading of synaptic vesicles with new acetylcholine. (A, Courtesy of Don Fawcett, Harvard Medical School, Boston, Massachusetts. B, Courtesy of J. E. Heuser, Washington University, St. Louis, Missouri.)

tropic" receptors, which also act through trimeric G proteins. Disruption of the gene for metabotropic glutamate receptors leaves mice with defects in coordination and learning, and overstimulation of these receptors might contribute to some forms of mental retardation in humans.

Neuromuscular Junction

Motor neurons in the spinal cord and brainstem control contraction of skeletal muscle cells (see Fig. 39-14). Long axons from these neurons terminate in synapses on skeletal muscle cells, called **neuromuscular junctions** (Fig. 11-8A–B). Every neuronal action potential that reaches a neuromuscular junction evokes an action potential that spreads over the postsynaptic surface of the muscle cell and initiates contraction. This highly reliable, one-to-one communication depends on chemical transmission by **acetylcholine** between the nerve and muscle. Highly concentrated nicotinic acetylcholine receptors in the postsynaptic membrane (~20,000/μm^2) transduce the arrival of extracellular acetylcholine into membrane depolarization.

Figure 11-8C illustrates the membrane proteins required for neuromuscular transmission. Both the nerve terminal and muscle depend on Na$^+$K$^+$-ATPase and Ca^{2+}-ATPase pumps to maintain gradients of Na$^+$, K$^+$, and Ca^{2+} across their plasma membranes. Both presynaptic and postsynaptic cells need voltage-gated Na$^+$ channels and K$^+$ channels for action potentials. Additionally, the presynaptic membrane requires voltage-gated Ca^{2+} channels to trigger secretion of acetylcholine.

A neuronal action potential initiates synaptic transmission by admitting Ca^{2+} into the presynaptic terminal through voltage-gated Ca^{2+} channels. Within less than 1 msec, Ca^{2+} triggers fusion of **synaptic vesicles** containing acetylcholine with the plasma membrane. Within microseconds, acetylcholine released into the synaptic cleft between the cells reaches millimolar concentrations and binds postsynaptic acetylcholine receptors.

Weak but cooperative binding of acetylcholine to two subunits of the **acetylcholine receptor** (see Fig. 10-12) opens a nonselective cation channel. The open pore is about equally permeable to K$^+$ and Na$^+$ and less permeable to Ca^{2+}, so the membrane potential collapses toward a reversal potential (see the section titled "Consequence of Multiple Channel Types Opening Simultaneously") of about 0 mV. This is above threshold for triggering a self-propagating action potential in the muscle plasma membrane, which occurs with nearly 100% efficiency. The action potential traveling over the muscle plasma membrane activates voltage-sensitive Ca^{2+} channels that trigger Ca^{2+} release from smooth endoplasmic reticulum, resulting in contraction (see Fig. 39-15).

Two different mechanisms terminate activation of acetylcholine receptors. First, an extracellular enzyme, **acetylcholinesterase,** rapidly degrades free acetylcholine, usually depleting acetylcholine from the synaptic cleft in a few milliseconds. Acetylcholine then dissociates from the receptor, closing the channel. Second, during prolonged exposure to acetylcholine, a conformational change in the acetylcholine receptor increases its affinity for bound acetylcholine and *closes* the channel. In this **desensitized state,** acetylcholine dissociates only when its extracellular concentration is very low. Once acetylcholine dissociates, the receptor slowly returns to rest.

Nerve terminals retrieve synaptic vesicle membrane by endocytosis (see Chapter 22). Cytoplasmic enzymes synthesize new acetylcholine. A V-type ATPase proton pump (see Fig. 8-5C) acidifies the lumen of synaptic vesicles, providing an electrochemical potential to drive an acetylcholine/H$^+$ antiporter, which concentrates acetylcholine in vesicles.

Central Nervous System Synapses

Synaptic transmission between neurons in the CNS (Fig. 11-9) differs fundamentally from the efficient, one-to-one coupling at neuromuscular junctions, where every presynaptic action potential triggers a postsynaptic action potential. The approximately 100 billion (10^{11}) neurons in the human brain receive synaptic inputs from many neurons, forming about 10^{15} synapses. Synapses cover the surface of dendrites and the cell body (Fig. 11-9A). Some synapses excite the postsynaptic cell by opening ligand-gated cation channels that depolarize the membrane locally. Such small, local changes tend to push the membrane toward threshold for an action potential. Other synapses are inhibitory, hyperpolarizing the postsynaptic membrane locally by opening ligand-gated Cl$^-$ channels. These changes are inhibitory, since they drive the membrane potential away from threshold (see Fig. 10-18). From moment to moment, neurons spatially average excitatory and inhibitory stimuli and fire action potentials when the combined effects of these opposing stimuli exceed threshold potential in the proximal part of the axon, called the **axon hillock.** Both the pattern and frequency of action potentials carry information in the brain.

Transmission at chemical synapses in the CNS depends on cooperation of pumps, carriers, and channels (Fig. 11-9C–D). ATPase pumps maintain concentration gradients of Na$^+$, K$^+$, and Ca^{2+} across both presynaptic and postsynaptic plasma membranes. Potassium channels establish the resting membrane potential, and voltage-gated K$^+$ and Na$^+$ channels fire action potentials. Neurotransmitters secreted by the presynaptic cell activate ligand-gated channels that control the postsynaptic membrane potential. Carriers in the presynaptic membrane and adjacent supporting cells termi-

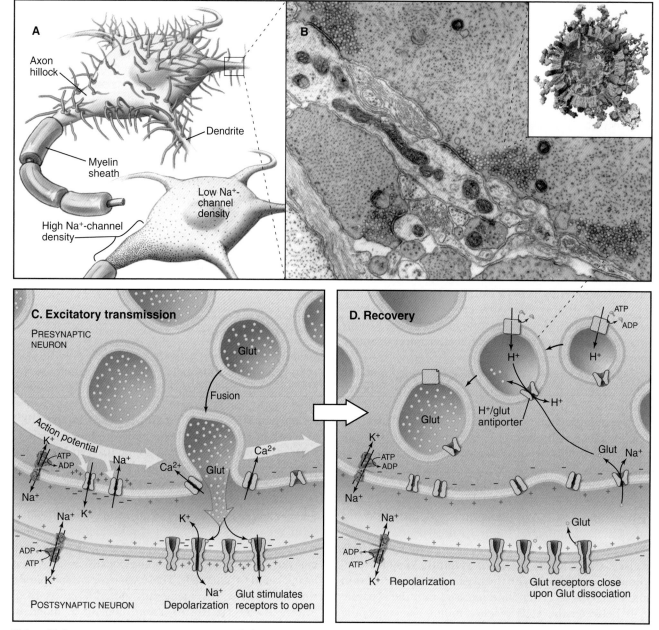

Figure 11-9 **CENTRAL NERVOUS SYSTEM SYNAPSES. A,** A neuron with its cell body and dendrites covered with a mixture of excitatory and inhibitory synapses. A high density of voltage-gated Na^+ channels in the proximal part of the axon, called the axon hillock, favors the generation of an action potential when the sum of postsynaptic potentials brings the axon hillock to threshold. **B,** An electron micrograph of a thin section of brain showing synapses with vesicles *(green)* clustered in the presynaptic axon. The *inset* shows an anatomically correct molecular model of a synaptic vesicle. **C,** Synaptic transmission at a CNS excitatory synapse. A presynaptic action potential opens voltage-gated Ca^{2+} channels. Entry of Ca^{2+} stimulates fusion of synaptic vesicles filled with glutamate (Glut) with the plasma membrane. Glutamate binds and opens postsynaptic AMPA receptors that generate a local postsynaptic potential change. **D,** Recovery from excitatory stimulation includes retrieval of glutamate by a presynaptic Na^+/glutamate symporter and concentration of glutamate in synaptic vesicles by a H^+/glutamate antiporter. (B, Courtesy of Don Fawcett, Harvard Medical School, Boston, Massachusetts. Inset, Adapted from Takamori S, Holt M, Stenius K, et al.: Molecular anatomy of a trafficking organelle. Cell 127:831–846, 2006. Copyright 2006, with permission from Elsevier.)

nate transmission by removing neurotransmitter from the synaptic cleft.

Incoming information takes the form of action potentials that arrive at synapses. As in the neuromuscular junction, action potentials open voltage-gated Ca^{2+} channels in the presynaptic membrane. This transient rise in

cytoplasmic Ca^{2+} can trigger the fusion of synaptic vesicles with the presynaptic plasma membrane, releasing transmitter, but the probability of successful fusion is lower than at neuromuscular junctions. After vesicle fusion transmitter diffuses rapidly to its receptors in the postsynaptic membrane.

Transmitters activate ligand-gated channels that cause a local, short-lived change in membrane potential, called a **postsynaptic potential** (PSP). At **excitatory synapses,** the neurotransmitter **glutamate** activates receptors (see Fig. 10-11) that open **cation channels** that depolarize the membrane. However, in contrast to the neuromuscular junction, individual PSPs do not fire action potentials. First, individual PSPs raise the membrane potential only a few millivolts, so they do not bring the postsynaptic membrane to threshold. Second, dendritic and cell body plasma membranes contain few voltage-gated Na^+ channels. Furthermore, **inhibitory synapses** on the same cell counteract excitatory synapses by secreting **glycine** or γ-**aminobutyric acid** (GABA) to activate Cl^- **channels** that hyperpolarize the membrane, taking it farther from threshold.

Excitatory and inhibitory PSPs spread passively over the postsynaptic membrane and generate an action potential only when their sum at a particular time brings the membrane potential at the axon hillock to threshold (Fig. 11-9A). The axon hillock is located at the base of each axon. This part of the plasma membrane is particularly sensitive to voltage, owing to a high concentration of voltage-gated Na^+ channels. At threshold, they open, depolarizing the membrane (Fig. 11-6). Delayed-rectifier K^+ channels then repolarize the membrane in preparation for subsequent action potentials. Each action potential is identical and propagates down the axon.

Because bringing the axon hillock to threshold in the CNS typically requires multiple excitatory postsynaptic potentials, the frequency of the postsynaptic output depends on the intensity of the presynaptic input. In fact, the frequency of postsynaptic action potentials is proportional to the intensity of the presynaptic input above a threshold. This threshold depends on additional voltage-gated K^+ channels that suppress the firing rate at low levels of stimulation.

Removal of neurotransmitters from the synaptic cleft terminates activation of postsynaptic receptors (Fig. 11-8D). Na^+K^+-ATPase pumps provide a Na^+ gradient to drive symporters that return neurotransmitters to their presynaptic cells. Within the presynaptic cell, a second proton-driven chemiosmotic cycle concentrates transmitter in synaptic vesicles. A V-type, proton-translocating ATPase acidifies the lumen of the synaptic vesicle and establishes the proton electrochemical gradient across the vesicle membrane to drive the antiporter.

Modification of CNS Synapses by Drugs and Disease

The transport systems that retrieve CNS neurotransmitters from the synaptic cleft and repackage them in vesicles determine the duration of synaptic stimulation, so inhibiting these transport processes with drugs pro-longs stimulation at particular classes of CNS synapses, with profound effects on brain function and behavior. A plasma membrane dopamine transporter is the main target of **cocaine.** Cocaine also inhibits transporters for serotonin and norepinephrine. Tricyclic **antidepressants** inhibit norepinephrine uptake, and other drugs inhibit serotonin uptake. These drugs have dramatic effects on the symptoms of depression as well as a range of milder psychiatric disorders. Millions of people take these drugs, even though the physiological consequences of transporter inhibition are incompletely understood.

Excess stimulation of N-methyl-D-aspartate (NMDA) receptors rapidly kills postsynaptic neurons, most likely owing to the deleterious effects of excess cytoplasmic Ca^{2+}. This occurs when glutamate is released from ischemic brain tissue during a stroke caused by compromising the blood supply to a region of the brain. Such damage might also contribute to neuron death in degenerative diseases of the nervous system, such as amyotrophic lateral sclerosis and Alzheimer's disease.

Acetylcholine secreted by neurons and **nicotine** from tobacco modulate synaptic transmission in the CNS by activating the same neurotransmitter receptor. In the CNS, acetylcholine acts on *presynaptic* terminals rather than participating directly in fast synaptic transmission as it does at the neuromuscular junction. Nicotinic acetylcholine receptors in the *presynaptic* plasma membrane are highly permeable to Ca^{2+}, so their stimulation admits Ca^{2+} into the presynaptic terminal. This enhances both the spontaneous release of neurotransmitter and release in response to action potentials. The isoform composition of CNS acetylcholine receptors differs from that of muscles (see Fig. 10-12). Some are homopentamers of α-subunits. Others are heteropentamers of α- and β-subunits. Activation of these ligand-gated channels in different regions of the brain may account for the enhancing effects of nicotine on learning and memory but also for tobacco addiction. Loss of CNS neurons that secrete acetylcholine might contribute to dementia in Alzheimer's disease.

Modification of CNS Synapses by Use

Memories are thought to be laid down in structural changes that modify the strength or numbers of synapses between neurons in the brain. Particular patterns of stimulation can produce long-term changes that enhance or reduce the efficiency of transmission of various glutamate-mediated synapses (Fig. 11-10). The **hippocampus,** a region of the vertebrate cerebral cortex that is known to participate in some forms of learning and memory, is favorable for observing a simple form of cellular learning. Intense stimulation of excitatory glutamate synapses (20 pulses over a period of 200 msec) can increase synaptic strength for days or weeks. This is called **long-term potentiation (LTP).**

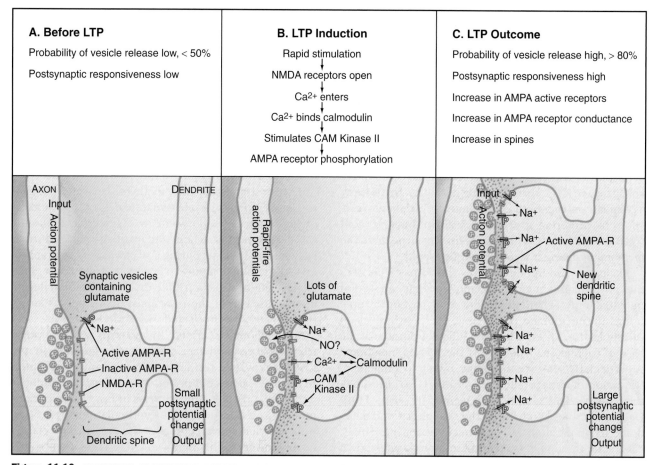

A. Before LTP	B. LTP Induction	C. LTP Outcome
Probability of vesicle release low, < 50%	Rapid stimulation	Probability of vesicle release high, > 80%
Postsynaptic responsiveness low	NMDA receptors open	Postsynaptic responsiveness high
	Ca^{2+} enters	Increase in AMPA active receptors
	Ca^{2+} binds calmodulin	Increase in AMPA receptor conductance
	Stimulates CAM Kinase II	Increase in spines
	AMPA receptor phosphorylation	

Figure 11-10 MECHANISM OF LONG-TERM POTENTIATION OF SYNAPTIC TRANSMISSION AT EXCITATORY SYNAPSES IN THE HIPPOCAMPUS. **A,** Prior to long-term potential (LTP), postsynaptic responses to presynaptic action potentials are unreliable and small. **B,** Some acute responses to vigorous stimulation. **C,** After induction of LTP, postsynaptic responses are more reliable and larger. AMPA-R and NMDA-R are two classes of glutamate receptors; NO is nitric oxide, a candidate for the retrograde signaling molecule; CAM Kinase II is calcium-calmodulin Kinase II.

Conversely, slow, prolonged stimulation of glutamate synapses reduces the response for hours. This is called **long-term depression (LTD).** The mechanisms of LTP and LTD are under intense investigation, because high-order brain functions, such as learning and memory, depend on changes in the flow of impulses through neural circuits, and the changes in transmission during LTP and LTD occur on an appropriate time scale.

Induction of LTP typically involves two types of glutamate receptors (see Fig. 10-11): **AMPA receptors** and **NMDA receptors** found in postsynaptic specializations called dendritic spines (Fig. 11-10). AMPA receptors open and close rapidly in response to glutamate. When open, AMPA receptors admit Na^+ and NMDA receptors admit Ca^{2+} to depolarize the postsynaptic plasma membrane. The slow response of NMDA receptors to glutamate depends on the membrane potential, as partial depolarization is required to displace an extracellular Mg^{2+} ion blocking the channel. This dual dependence on glutamate and membrane potential makes NMDA receptors coincidence detectors, responsive to rapid stimulation or stimulation at nearby excitatory synapses. A synapse with only NMDA receptors is functionally "silent." Such silent synapses can be aroused when presynaptic release of glutamate is coordinated with sufficient membrane depolarization from neighboring synaptic activation. This results in the insertion of AMPA receptors, waking up the synapse.

In principle, LTP and LTD might alter the efficiency of synaptic transmission by changing glutamate release from the presynaptic cell or responsiveness of the postsynaptic cell to glutamate. In fact, a wide range of experiments suggests that both presynaptic and postsynaptic processes contribute. The best-documented presynaptic change is an increase in the probability that an action potential will stimulate the fusion of a glutamate-containing synaptic vesicle with the plasma membrane. In the resting state, exocytosis of these vesicles is unreliable. LTP increases the probability of exocytosis from less than 0.5 to greater than 0.8. In addition, the postsynaptic side responds more robustly to glutamate for two reasons: a higher concentration of active AMPA receptors with enhanced conductance when open and formation of additional synapses with the stimulating axon.

The mechanisms that bring about these changes are incompletely understood, but the following is well established. LTP depends on stimulation of NMDA receptors and Ca^{2+} entry. Within the postsynaptic dendritic spine, Ca^{2+} activates processes that initiate and maintain LTP. Within seconds, Ca^{2+} binds calmodulin (see Fig. 3-12C) and triggers events that depend on calcium-calmodulin, including activation of protein kinases, such as CAM-kinase II (see Fig. 25-4A). Phosphorylation of AMPA receptors by CAM-kinase II increases their responsiveness to glutamate, perhaps "waking up silent synapses." AMPA receptors divide their time between the postsynaptic membrane and intracellular recycling endosomes. LTP shifts more AMPA receptors from endosomes to the postsynaptic membrane. No consensus has been reached on the nature of the extracellular messengers that provide feedback to the presynaptic terminal to modify its exocytosis efficiency.

Within minutes, induction of LTP triggers signaling cascades that maintain the increased efficacy, leading to structural changes and increased protein synthesis. These changes may induce dendrites to stabilized existing spines or sprout new filopodia and spines; these are presumed to account for the increased number of synapses observed after an hour or so. Extension of these processes and remodeling of the shape of dendritic spines depend on actin filament assembly (see Fig. 38-8). Growth of axons and formation of new synapses provide mechanisms to generate novel connections in response to use. Over the longer term, the postsynaptic cell initiates gene transcription and protein synthesis, bringing about further changes that stabilize enhanced synaptic transmission.

LTD appears, in many ways, to be the reverse of LTP, with less reliable presynaptic exocytosis and less responsive postsynaptic AMPA receptors. It, too, depends on NMDA receptors, but the biochemical basis for the synaptic changes is even less well understood.

Cardiac Membrane Physiology

Spontaneous Action Potentials of Pacemaker Cells

Intrinsically excitable **pacemaker cells** in the **sinoatrial node** drive rhythmic contractions of the heart (see Fig. 39-19). The membrane potential of these cells drifts spontaneously toward threshold, setting off action potentials about once each second (Fig. 11-11). Cardiac action potentials spread via **gap junctions** (see Fig. 31-6) from cell to cell throughout the heart, activating contraction in a reproducible pattern.

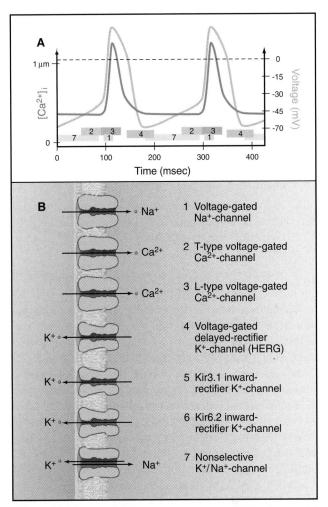

Figure 11-11 MECHANISM OF SPONTANEOUS CARDIAC PACEMAKER ACTION POTENTIALS. Sequential activation and inactivation of seven different plasma membrane channels account for the time course of action potentials and cytoplasmic Ca^{2+} transients in pacemaker cells of the sinoatrial node. **A,** Time courses of the fluctuations in membrane potential (orange) and cytoplasmic Ca^{2+} concentration (blue). Colored boxes indicate when the various channels enumerated in part B are open. Kir3.1 and Kir6.2 are inactive under these conditions. **B,** Channels contributing to pacemaker activity.

Spontaneous action potentials of cardiac pacemaker cells are more complicated than those of nerves. Seven different plasma membrane channels determine their frequency:

1. *Voltage-gated Na^+ channels.* As in nerves, these channels rapidly activate at membrane potentials above threshold and then rapidly inactivate.

2. *T-type, voltage-gated Ca^{2+} channels.* These low-conductance channels activate transiently at membrane potentials more negative than Na^+ channels, about −70 mV.

3. *L-type, voltage-gated Ca^{2+} channels.* These high-conductance channels slowly activate and inactivate when the membrane depolarizes to about −40 mV. Sympathetic nerve stimulation sensitizes

these channels to membrane depolarization. Drugs called dihydropyridines block these channels.

4. *Delayed-rectifier, voltage-gated K⁺ channels.* As in nerves, these HERG channels activate and inactivate slowly in response to membrane depolarization. Sympathetic nerves stimulate these channels.

5. *Kir3.1 inward-rectifier K⁺ channels.* These channels conduct K⁺ over a limited range of membrane potential, between about −30 and −80 mV. Parasympathetic nerve stimulation activates these channels.

6. *Kir6.2 inward-rectifier K⁺ channels.* Normal levels of cytoplasmic ATP inhibit these channels. Depletion of cytoplasmic ATP activates these channels.

7. *Nonselective K⁺/Na⁺ channels.* Repolarization of the membrane activates these channels.

Acting together, these channels produce a spontaneous cycle of pacemaker action potentials. At the threshold potential (about −40 mV), voltage-gated Na⁺ channels open synchronously and rapidly depolarize the membrane. As they inactivate, L-type Ca^{2+} channels open, prolonging the depolarization and admitting Ca^{2+}; this, in turn, triggers contraction by releasing more Ca^{2+} from internal stores (see Fig. 39-15B). As these Ca^{2+} channels slowly inactivate, delayed-rectifier K⁺ channels open and drive the membrane potential toward E_K, the K⁺ equilibrium potential. As the membrane potential reaches a minimum, delayed-rectifier K⁺ channels inactivate, but the two Kir channels open. In the absence of other channel activity, the membrane potential would remain near E_K, but the nonselective Na⁺/K⁺ channels open and the membrane slowly depolarizes, drifting toward threshold. T-type Ca^{2+} channels contribute to the slow, spontaneous depolarization. At threshold, the cycle repeats.

Mutations in six different human ion channel genes are linked to disorders of cardiac muscle electrophysiol-ogy. These inherited diseases are called *long-QT syndrome* because the interval between the initial depolarization of the muscle cells and their relaxation is prolonged. This change predisposes the person to abnormal cardiac rhythms that might be fatal.

Regulation of Heart Rate by G Proteins and Phosphorylation

Regulation of pacemaker cells by neurotransmitters secreted by autonomic nerves is an example of the widespread regulation of channels by G proteins and phosphorylation (Fig. 11-12). Neurotransmitters from the two parts of the autonomic nervous system have opposite effects on the frequency of cardiac contraction. The resting rate reflects a compromise in the competition between these two inputs. Acetylcholine from **parasympathetic nerves** slows the heartbeat, whereas norepinephrine from **sympathetic nerves** speeds the rate and increases the strength of contraction. These neurotransmitters modify their target channels indirectly by activating two different seven-helix receptors and their associated trimeric G-proteins (see Fig. 25-9).

Norepinephrine increases the heart rate by modulating L-type Ca^{2+} channels. Norepinephrine that binds to plasma membrane β-adrenergic receptors activates trimeric G proteins, which stimulate **adenylyl cyclase,** the enzyme that makes cyclic adenosine monophosphate (cAMP) (see Fig. 26-2). This second messenger stimulates cyclic **AMP**–dependent protein kinase (see Fig. 25-3) to phosphorylate cytoplasmic residues of L-type, voltage-gated Ca^{2+} channels in the plasma membrane. Phosphorylated Ca^{2+} channels are more likely to open in response to membrane depolarization than are unphosphorylated channels. Phosphorylation increases the rate at which the membrane potential drifts toward threshold. This increases the frequency of action potentials of pacemaker cells and the heart rate. In a parallel pathway, cAMP stimulates HCN cation channels, which

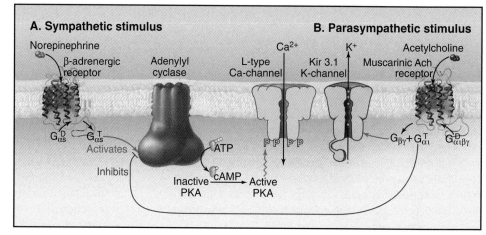

Figure 11-12 Regulation of the rate of cardiac pacemaker cells by sympathetic **(A)** and parasympathetic **(B)** nerves. GTP-Gα$_s$ stimulates adenylyl cyclase. GTP-Gα$_i$ inhibits adenylyl cyclase. D is GDP associated with G protein α-subunits; T is GTP. cAMP, cyclic adenosine monophosphate; PKA, protein kinase A.

push the membrane potential toward threshold and increase the heart rate.

Acetylcholine released by parasympathetic nerves activates Kir3.1 inward-rectifier K$^+$ channels that slow the heartbeat. Acetylcholine binds to different seven-helix receptors, called muscarinic acetylcholine receptors (because they bind muscarine), to distinguish them from the nicotinic acetylcholine receptors. Acetylcholine binding to muscarinic receptors activates a trimeric G protein, different from that activated by norepinephrine. Two G-protein subunits, which make up the G$\beta\gamma$ complex, dissociate from the Gα_i subunit and activate Kir3.1/3.4 channels. When open, these channels reduce the rate at which the membrane potential drifts toward threshold. In addition the Gα_i subunit inhibits cyclic AMP production and reduces Ca^{2+} channel phosphorylation. This decreases the probability that Ca^{2+} channels are open, contributing to a lowering of the heart rate. If the energy supply of the heart is compromised, ATP levels fall. This activates Kir6.2 channels, which reduce the rate of spontaneous depolarization and the heart rate until ATP levels are restored.

Regulation of Cardiac Contractility

A set of channels similar to those in the sinoatrial node generate action potentials in cardiac muscle cells and stimulate contraction. Cardiac muscle cells can generate spontaneous action potentials, but they have fewer T-type Ca^{2+} channels and more Kir K$^+$ channels, so the rate of spontaneous action potentials is lower than that of pacemaker cells. Except in disease, pacemaker cells drive action potentials throughout the rest of the heart. Sympathetic nervous stimulation, acting through cyclic AMP–dependent protein kinase, strengthens cardiac contraction. Phosphorylated L-type Ca^{2+} channels admit more Ca^{2+} to activate the contractile machinery more fully. The same kinase activates delayed-rectifier K$^+$ channels, which prevent activated Ca^{2+} channels from prolonging the action potential. This allows heart muscle cells to keep up with stimuli generated at a higher rate from pacemaker cells. Cyclic AMP–dependent protein kinase also enhances contractility by phosphorylating proteins of the contractile apparatus and smooth endoplasmic reticulum (see Chapter 39).

Therapeutic Effect of Digitalis in Congestive Heart Failure

In congestive heart failure, cardiac contraction fails to produce enough force to maintain adequate circulation of blood. **Cardiac glycosides,** such as digitalis (from the foxglove plant), ameliorate this common human condition by inhibiting an isoform of Na$^+$K$^+$ATPase in the plasma membrane of heart cells (Fig. 11-13). Plasma membrane L-type Ca^{2+} channels and endoplasmic retic-

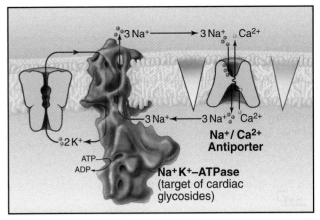

Figure 11-13 The chemiosmotic cycle that helps to clear Ca^{2+} from the cytoplasm of cardiac muscle cells. Na$^+$K$^+$-ATPase pumps create a Na$^+$ gradient *(purple triangle)* to drive the Na$^+$/Ca^{2+} antiporter to transport Ca^{2+} up its concentration gradient *(blue triangle)* out of the cell. Cardiac glycosides inhibit the cardiac isoform of Na$^+$K$^+$-ATPase, raising the concentration of cytoplasmic Ca^{2+} and strengthening cardiac contraction. K$^+$ channels *(left)* allow K$^+$ to circulate.

ulum Ca^{2+} release channels activate contraction by transiently increasing cytoplasmic Ca^{2+}. Calcium ATPase pumps (see Fig. 8-8) in smooth endoplasmic reticulum clear most of this Ca^{2+} from cytoplasm, but plasma membrane Na$^+$/Ca^{2+} antiporters, driven by the plasma membrane Na$^+$ gradient, contribute as well.

Digitalis and related compounds, such as ouabain, strengthen cardiac contraction indirectly by inhibiting an isoform of Na$^+$K$^+$-ATPase found in the cardiac plasma membrane. Reduced sodium pump activity lowers the electrochemical gradient of Na$^+$ across the plasma membrane and provides less driving force for Na$^+$ to exchange for Ca^{2+}. The result is a slightly higher steady-state concentration of Ca^{2+} in cytoplasm, which strengthens contraction. A drug that targets Ca^{2+} export directly would be desirable, but thus far, researchers have failed to find a satisfactory inhibitor.

The success of cardiac glycosides depends on their selectivity for the α_2 isoform of the α-subunit of the Na$^+$K$^+$-ATPase, which is expressed in heart, skeletal muscle, and fat. This α_2 isoform is much more sensitive to cardiac glycosides than is the α_1 isoform. Although the α_2 isoform represents a minority of cardiac sodium pumps, its inhibition lowers the Na$^+$ gradient across the heart cell plasma membrane without deleterious effects on other tissues. One reason might be that the Na$^+$/Ca^{2+} symporter that works with the sodium pump in the heart is not expressed in skeletal muscle or fat.

ACKNOWLEDGMENTS

Thanks go to Michael Caplan, Paul Forscher, John Solaro, and David Wells for their suggestions on revisions to this chapter.

SELECTED READINGS

Chklovskii DB, Mel BW, Svoboda K: Cortical rewiring and information storage. Nature 431:782-788, 2004.

Cohen-Cory S: The developing synapse: Construction and modulation of synaptic structures and circuits. Science 298:770-776, 2002.

Danbolt NC: Glutamate uptake. Prog Neurobiol 65:1-105, 2001.

Dorwart M, Thibodeau P, Thomas P: Cystic fibrosis: Recent structural insights. J Cystic Fibrosis 3:91-94, 2004.

Fernández-Alfonso T, Ryan TA: The efficiency of the synaptic vesicle cycle at central nervous system synapses. Trends Cell Biol 16:413-420, 2006.

Hogg RC, Bertrand D: What genes tell us about nicotine addiction. Science 306:983-984, 2004.

Keating MT, Sanguinetti MC: Molecular and cellular mechanisms of cardiac arrhythmias. Cell 104:569-580, 2001.

Malenka RC, Bear MF: LTP and LDP: An embarrassment of riches. Neuron 44:5-21, 2004.

Malinow R, Malenka RC: AMPA receptor trafficking and synaptic plasticity. Annu Rev Neurosci 25:103-126, 2002.

Record MT, Courtenay ES, Cayley DS, Guttman HJ: Responses of *E. coli* to osmotic stress: Large changes in amounts of cytoplasmic solutes and water. Trends Biochem Sci 23:143-150, 1998.

Schuske K, Jorgensen EM: Vesicular glutamate transporter: Shooting blanks. Science 304:1750-1752, 2004.

Severs NJ: The cardiac muscle cell. Bioessays 22:188-199, 2000.

Strange K: Cellular volume homeostasis. Adv Physiol Educ 28:155-159, 2004.

Vankeerberghen A, Cuppens H, Cassiman J-J: The cystic fibrosis transmembrane conductance regulator: An intriguing protein with pleiotropic functions. J Cystic Fibrosis 1:13-29, 2002.

Vincent GM: The long QT syndrome: Bedside to bench to bedside. New Engl J Med 348:1837-1838, 2003.

Zagotta WN, Olivier NB, Black KD, et al: Structural basis of modulation and agonist specificity of HCN pacemaker channels. Nature 425:200-205, 2003.

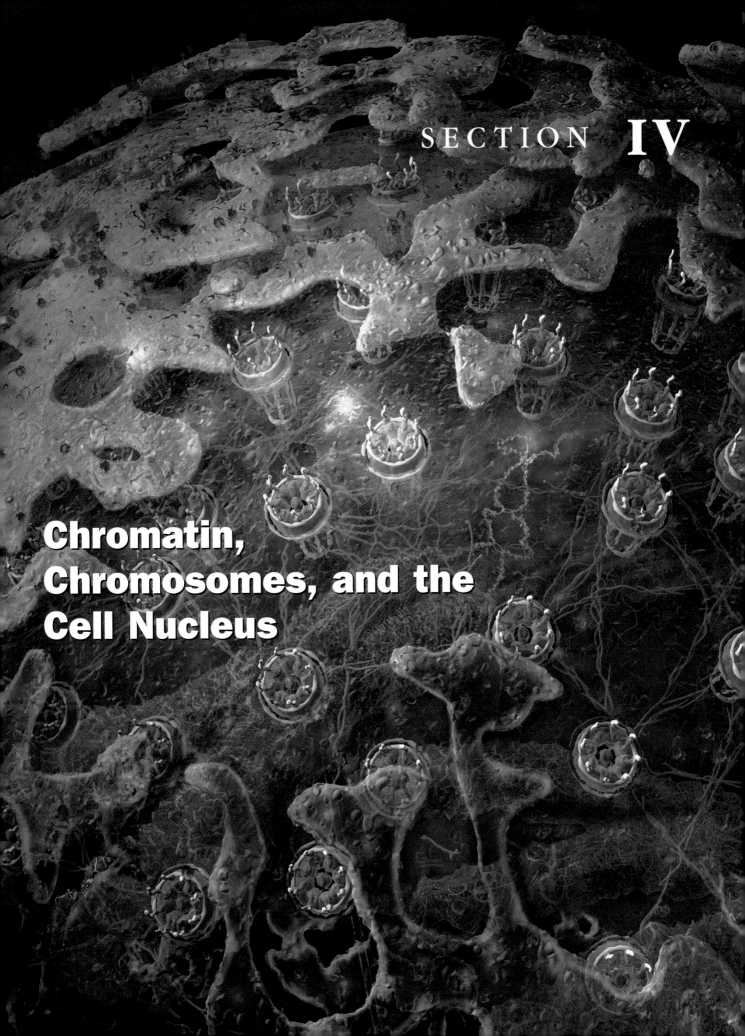

Chromatin, Chromosomes, and the Cell Nucleus

SECTION **IV** OVERVIEW

Every organism is defined by a blueprint consisting of information stored in its **chromosomes.** With the exception of a few viruses, these chromosomes are composed of enormously long circular or linear molecules of DNA. (Those few viruses use RNA instead.) Chromosomes have fascinated biologists ever since it was realized that they contain the genetic information that defines each organism—its **genome.** After Watson and Crick's proposal of a structure for DNA in 1953, it was realized that the DNA is a linear sequence of A, T, G, and C bases that can be thought of as a code to describe the physical attributes for every organism.

Originally, this code was thought to be impossibly complex, but recent technological advances have permitted scientists to determine the complete sequence of large DNA molecules. Between 1996 and 2006, investigators determined the sequences of the DNA molecules that make up the genomes of over 300 prokaryotes and 20 eukaryotes, including several fungi, the nematode worm *Caenorhabditis elegans,* 12 species of fruit flies (including *Drosophila melanogaster*), the plant *Arabidopsis thaliana,* chickens, mice, rats, and humans. These genome sequences not only reveal much about the biology of living organisms but also are the most important source of information about the evolution of life on earth (see Chapter 2).

This does not mean that we understand everything about chromosomes, however. Far from it. We still know very little about how chromosomal DNA molecules are packaged so that they not only fit into cells but also allow access to the library of genetic information that they contain. In prokaryotes, the single chromosome is concentrated in a specialized region of the cytoplasm called the nucleoid. In eukaryotes, the chromosomes are packaged in a specialized membrane-bounded compartment known as the **nucleus.** This difference in organization has important consequences for the regulation of gene expression.

Chapter 12 describes the organization of chromosomal DNA molecules. Every species has a characteristic number of chromosomes that occupy distinct territories within the nucleus and can be visualized as separate entities only during cell division. For example, humans have 46 chromosomes that contain, in total, about 6.2 $\times 10^9$ base pairs of DNA.

Analysis of the human genome sequence revealed that the genes that encode proteins and RNAs are often surrounded by huge noncoding deserts. In fact, the vast majority of the chromosomal DNA in humans has no coding function and might instead serve a structural role. Two specific DNA structures are essential for the maintenance of a constant chromosome complement in a given species: **centromeres** and **telomeres.** Centromeres consist of DNA sequences that, together with 60 or more proteins (Chapter 13), direct the segregation of chromosomes during cell division. Telomeres are spe-

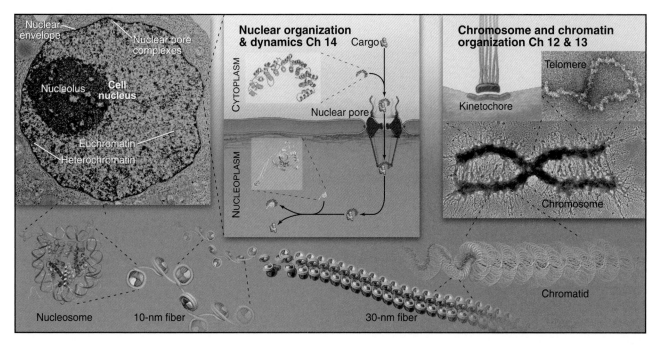

Nuclear envelope · Nuclear pore complexes · Nucleolus · **Cell nucleus** · Euchromatin · Heterochromatin

Nuclear organization & dynamics Ch 14 · Cargo · CYTOPLASM · Nuclear pore · NUCLEOPLASM

Chromosome and chromatin organization Ch 12 & 13 · Telomere · Kinetochore · Chromosome · Chromatid

Nucleosome · 10-nm fiber · 30-nm fiber

cialized structures that protect the ends of chromosomes and permit complete replication of the chromosomal DNA.

Given the spacing of 3.4 Å per base pair in B-form DNA, each human cell contains more than 2 m of DNA packaged into a nucleus only 5 to 20×10^{-6} m in diameter! Chapter 13 explains how DNA is extensively folded to fit into the nucleus. The first levels of packaging shorten the DNA about 40-fold by wrapping it around histone proteins to form nucleosomes and then twisting the nucleosomes into 30-nm fibers. Higher levels of packaging of the chromatin fiber are still poorly understood.

The complex of DNA with its packaging proteins is called **chromatin.** Nuclei contain two broad classes of chromatin: **heterochromatin,** which is highly condensed throughout the cell cycle and is generally inactive in transcription, and **euchromatin,** which is less condensed and contains actively transcribed genes. Different types of chromatin are defined by complex patterns of posttranslational modifications of the histone proteins. This "histone code" directs the binding of other proteins that induce the chromatin to adopt either a more compact or more open and active structure.

Chapter 14 discusses the structure and physiology of the nucleus. The boundary of the nucleus is a **nuclear envelope** composed of inner and outer nuclear membranes, separated by a perinuclear space that is continuous with the lumen of the endoplasmic reticulum. The inner nuclear membrane is supported by a protein layer called the **nuclear lamina.** Mutations in the lamina and other nuclear envelope proteins cause a wide spectrum of inherited human diseases, with mutations in the lamin A gene alone causing over a dozen different diseases.

Traffic into and out of the nucleus moves through **nuclear pore complexes** that span the two membrane bilayers of the nuclear envelope. Newly processed RNAs head out to the cytoplasm. So do the ribosomal subunits that will translate them into proteins, some of which then wend their way back into the nucleus. Proteins that are destined for transport across the nuclear envelope (either alone or associated with RNA molecules) typically contain short stretches of amino acids, called **nuclear localization sequences** or **nuclear export sequences,** that bind to specific adapter and receptor proteins to facilitate transport across the nuclear pore. A small guanosine triphosphatase (GTPase) called **Ran** regulates the directionality of this transport, because it is present primarily in its GTP-bound form in the nucleus and its GDP-bound form in the cytoplasm. Ran-GTP in the nucleus causes imported cargos to fall off their transporters and cargos destined for export to bind to their carriers.

The nucleus contains a number of substructures. The most prominent of these is the **nucleolus,** a versatile factory for transcription of ribosomal RNA (rRNA) from a tandem array of genes and processing of rRNA and other noncoding RNAs, as well as ribosome assembly. Nuclei also contain several other specialized regions. Although in many cases, their functions are not known, the presence of these specialized subdomains suggests that compartmentalization of the nucleus contributes to the regulation of nuclear functions.

Chromosome Organization

Chromosomes are enormous DNA molecules that can be propagated stably through countless generations of dividing cells (Fig. 12-1). Genes are the reason for the existence of the chromosomes, but in higher eukaryotes, they actually make up only a small fraction of the chromosomal DNA, much of which does not encode proteins or other known functional RNAs. Cells package chromosomal DNA with roughly twice its weight of protein. This DNA-protein complex, called chromatin, is discussed in Chapter 13.

In addition to the genes, only three classes of specialized DNA sequences are needed to make a fully functional chromosome: (1) a centromere, (2) two telomeres, and (3) an origin of DNA replication for approximately every 100,000 base pairs (bp). Centromeres regulate the partitioning of chromosomes during mitosis and meiosis. Telomeres protect the ends of the chromosomal DNA molecules and ensure their complete replication. DNA replication is discussed in Chapter 42. Chapter 15 considers the structure of genes. Box 12-1 lists a number of key terms presented in this chapter.

Chromosome Morphology and Nomenclature

With few specialized exceptions, chromosomes from somatic cells of higher eukaryotes are visualized directly only during mitosis. Each mitotic chromosome consists of two **sister chromatids** that are held together at a waist-like constriction called the **centromere.** The portions of the chromosomes that are not in the centromere itself are called chromosome "arms" (Fig. 12-2).

One DNA Molecule per Chromosome

Each eukaryotic chromosome contains one DNA molecule that stretches between the **telomeres** at either end. Most prokaryotic and mitochondrial chromosomes are circular DNA molecules that lack telomeres, but naturally occurring eukaryotic nuclear chromosomes are generally linear DNA molecules with two telomeres. The clearest proof that each chromosome is composed of a single DNA molecule has been obtained for budding and fission yeasts, where intact chromosomal DNA molecules may be visualized by pulsed-field gel electrophoresis as a characteristic series of bands (Fig. 12-3). This technique can display the largest chromosome of fission yeast at 5,598,923 bp, but even the smallest human chromosome, which is about 40 million bp long, is too large to resolve in this way.

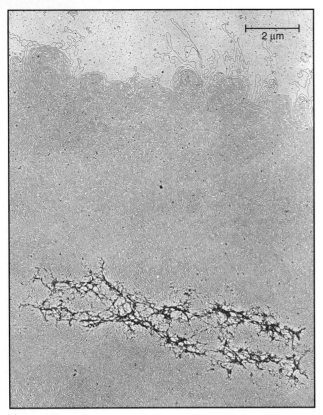

Figure 12-1 ELECTRON MICROGRAPH OF A CHROMOSOME FROM WHICH MOST PROTEINS WERE EXTRACTED, ALLOWING DNA *(THIN LINES)* TO SPREAD OUT FROM THE RESIDUAL SCAFFOLD. Enormous amounts of DNA are packaged in each chromosome. This image shows less than 30% of the DNA of this chromosome. (From Paulson JR, Laemmli UK: The structure of histone-depleted chromosomes. Cell 12:817–828, 1977.)

BOX 12-1
Key Terms

Centromere: The chromosomal locus that regulates the movements of the chromosomes during mitosis and meiosis. The centromere is defined by specific DNA sequences plus proteins that bind to them. In higher eukaryotes, the centromere of mitotic chromosomes can be visualized as a constricted region where sister chromatids are held together most closely.

Chromatin: DNA plus the proteins that package it within the cell nucleus.

Chromosome: A DNA molecule with its attendant proteins that moves as an independent unit during mitosis and meiosis. Before DNA replication, each chromosome consists of a single DNA molecule plus proteins and is called a *chromatid.* After replication, each chromosome consists of two identical DNA molecules plus proteins. These are called *sister chromatids.* Chromosomal DNA molecules are usually linear but can be circular in organelles, bacteria, and viruses.

Kinetochore: The centromeric substructure that binds microtubules and directs the movements of chromosomes in mitosis.

Telomere: The specialized structure at either end of the chromosomal DNA molecule that ensures the complete replication of the chromosomal ends and protects the ends within the cell.

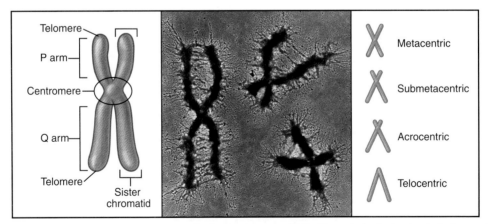

Figure 12-2 ANATOMY OF MITOTIC CHROMOSOMES FROM HIGHER EUKARYOTES. **Left,** The principal structural features of chromosomes. **Center,** An electron micrograph of human mitotic chromosomes. **Right,** A diagram of the various classes of chromosomes. At mitosis, chromosomes of higher eukaryotes consist of sister chromatids held together at the centromeric region. Chromosomes are classified on the basis of the position of the centromere relative to the arms. In *metacentric* chromosomes, the centromere is located midway along the chromatid. In *submetacentric* chromosomes, the centromere is located asymmetrically so that each chromatid can be divided into short (P) and long (Q) arms. In *acrocentric* chromosomes, the centromere is located near the end of the arms. In *telocentric* chromosomes, the centromere appears to be located very near the end of the cell chromatid. (Micrograph courtesy of William C. Earnshaw.)

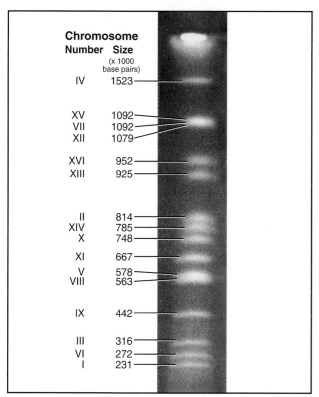

Figure 12-3 PULSED-FIELD GEL ELECTROPHORESIS OF BUDDING YEAST CHROMOSOMES. Intact cells embedded in a block of agarose are treated under very gentle conditions with proteases and detergents to free the chromosomal DNA from other cellular constituents. The DNA is then moved under the influence of an electrical field out of the agarose block and directly into an agarose gel. The technique uses a specialized gel apparatus in which the direction and strength of the electrophoretic field is varied periodically. This technique permits the separation of very long DNA molecules (of up to several million bp). (Courtesy of P. Hieter, University of British Columbia, Vancouver, Canada.)

The Organization of Genes on Chromosomes

The first chromosome to be completely sequenced (in 1977) was that of the bacterial virus φx174 (Table 12-1). Starting in the 1990s much effort worldwide has been devoted to determining the complete sequences of the chromosomes of a wide variety of organisms (see Fig. 2-4). Sequencing efforts that have been completed to date have generated an enormous bank of data on the genetic composition of simple and complex organisms. For example, over 100 microbial genomes have been sequenced. One major goal of this effort—the sequence of the human genome—is now essentially complete.

Complex genomes that have been sequenced thus far range in size from 580,000 bp for *Mycoplasma genitalium,* which causes urinary tract infections in humans to 2,863,476,365 bp for humans themselves. Numbers of protein-coding genes identified range from 480 in *M. genitalium* to 20,000 to 25,000 for humans (Table 12-1).

However, because gene prediction algorithms are still being perfected, only rough estimates of gene number are available, even for completely sequenced genomes.

As a rule of thumb, the bacterial genomes tend to make very efficient use of space, about 90% of the genome being devoted to coding sequences. The remaining 10% is mostly taken up by sequences involved in gene regulation. One notable exception to this is *Rickettsia prowazekii,* for which only 76% of the genome is devoted to coding sequences. Because this intracellular parasite derives many of its metabolic functions from the host cell, much of its noncoding DNA may be remnants of unneeded genes undergoing various stages of gradual loss from the genome.

The first eukaryote whose genome was entirely sequenced was the budding yeast *Saccharomyces cerevisiae.* The 14 million bp yeast genome is subdivided into 16 chromosomes ranging in size from 230,000 bp to over 1 million bp (Fig. 12-3). This genome has a dramatic history. Ancestral budding yeast apparently had eight chromosomes but at one point underwent a duplication of the entire genome. This event was followed by numerous small deletions that resulted in the subsequent loss of most of the duplicated genes, with about 10% remaining. As a result, the modern budding yeast genome contains about 5700 predicted genes, many of which are paralogs (genes produced by duplication that have evolved to take on distinct functions; see Box 2-1). As a result, only about 1000 of these genes are indispensable for life. About 5% of yeast genes are segmented, containing regions that appear in mature RNA molecules **(exons)** and regions that are removed by splicing **(introns)** (discussed in detail in Chapter 16). Exons occupy approximately 75% of the budding yeast genome, with the remainder in regulatory regions, repeated DNAs, and introns (Fig. 12-4).

Subsequent analysis of the fission yeast genome yielded some surprises. First, many more (43%) of the genes have introns. Second, despite the fact that the genome is about 15% larger than that of budding yeast, the number of genes is substantially less. People were very surprised to learn that a free-living eukaryote could "get by" with fewer than 5000 genes. An important point here is that this genome was not duplicated and later pared down, so it does not have so many sister (paralogous) genes. Although it has fewer genes than budding yeast, the variety of genes is actually greater. The biggest difference between the fission and budding yeast chromosomes is in the structure of their centromere regions (see later).

The next genome sequences to be completed were those of two very important "model" organisms that have been widely used by cell and developmental biologists: the nematode worm *Caenorhabditis elegans* and the fruit fly *Drosophila melanogaster.* These sequences revealed a number of important organiza-

Table 12-1

DNA CONTENT OF VARIOUS GENOMES

Organism	Haploid Genome Size (bp)	Predicted Number of Protein-Coding Genes
$\phi X174$ (bacterial virus)	5386	11
Mycoplasma genitalium (pathogenic bacterium)	580,070	480*
Rickettsia prowazekii (endoparasitic bacterium)	1,111,523	834
Escherichia coli (free-living bacterium)	4,639,221	4288
Bacillus subtilis (free-living bacterium)	4,214,810	4100
Saccharomyces cerevisiae (budding yeast)	14,000,000	6604
Schizosaccharomyces pombe (fission yeast)	13,800,000	4824
Caenorhabditis elegans (nematode worm)	9.7×10^7	19,100
Drosophila melanogaster (fruit fly)	1.4×10^8	13,525
Arabadopsis thaliana (plant)	1.25×10^8	25,498
Anopheles gambiae (malaria mosquito)	2.78×10^8	14,000
Oryza sativa japonica (rice)	4.2×10^8	32,000–50,000
Mus musculus (house mouse)	2.6×10^9	~30,000
Rattus norvegicus (Brown Norway rat)	2.75×10^9	~21,000–46,000
Xenopus laevis (South African clawed frog)	3.1×10^9	?
Homo sapiens (human)	3.1×10^9	20,000–25,000
Triturus cristatus (salamander)	2.2×10^{10}	?

*It appears that only 265 to 350 of these genes are essential for life.

Note: In most higher eukaryotes, with the exception of some plants, the huge tracts of repeated DNA sequences in and around centromeres are poor in genes and beyond the limits of present technology to sequence. Thus, when statistics are given on chromosome sizes in descriptions of genome sequencing projects, these portions are generally omitted. Where possible, the genome size figures given here reflect the entire genome (sequenced and unsequenced).

tional differences from budding yeast. Although its genome is eight times larger than that of budding yeast (97 million bp distributed in six chromosomes), the nematode has only about three times more genes. Surprisingly, the fly, despite its even larger genome and more complex body plan and life cycle, has about one third fewer genes than the worm. In fact, only about 27% of the *C. elegans* genome and 13% of the *Drosophila* genomic DNA code for proteins. Instead, the fly has much more noncoding repetitive DNA than the worm.

The "finished" sequence of the human genome, published in 2004, revealed an even lower density of genes.

Figure 12-4 COMPARISON OF THE DISTRIBUTION OF GENES OVER 90,000 BP OF THE CHROMOSOME OF A TYPICAL BACTERIUM (*B. SUBTILIS*), THE BUDDING YEAST *S. CEREVISIAE*, THE FRUIT FLY *D. MELANOGASTER*, AND HUMANS. To give a more accurate representation of the distribution of human genes, we also show a stretch of chromosome 21 spanning 500,000 bp. *Arrows* show the direction of transcription. Regions of genes encoding a product are shown as *thick orange arrows*. Intervening sequences (introns) are shown as *thin lines*. (Courtesy of A. Kerr, University of Edinburgh, Scotland.)

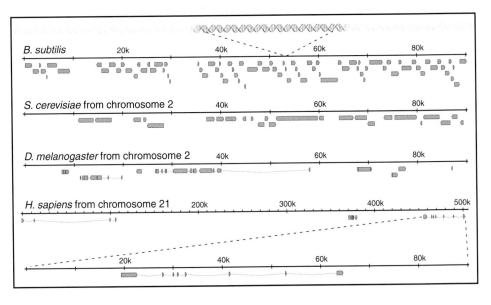

Humans have far fewer genes than had been predicted: about 20,000 to 25,000, in contrast to some earlier predictions of up to 100,000 (Table 12-1). Protein-coding regions occupy only about 1.2% of the chromosomes. In contrast, various repeated-sequence elements and pseudogenes appear to occupy about 50% of the genome, as is discussed in a later section. To put this all in perspective, every million bp of DNA sequenced yielded 483 genes in *S. cerevisiae*, 197 genes in *C. elegans*, 117 genes in *D. melanogaster*, and only 7 to 9 genes in humans. If the *Escherichia coli* chromosome were the size of chromosome 21, the smallest human chromosome at ~40×10^6 bp, it would have nearly 37,000 genes—more than the entire human complement! In fact, chromosome 21 is predicted to have only 225 genes.

Human genes range in size from a few hundred bp to well over 10^6 bp, the average being about 28,000 bp. Most human protein-coding genes have introns separating an average of 9 exons averaging only 145 bp each. The average intron is a bit over 3000 bp in length, but the variability is enormous. Genes can have over 100 exons or only 1, and introns can be over 500,000 bp long. It is therefore not surprising that the discovery of new genes using the genomic DNA sequence is a complex art that is still in its infancy.

The distribution of protein-coding genes along chromosomes is also highly variable. For example, on chromosome 9, gene density ranges from 3 to 22 genes per 10^6 bp. On chromosome 21 one region of 7×10^6 bp, encompassing nearly 20% of the whole chromosome, has no identified genes at all. This region is almost twice the size of the entire *E. coli* chromosome! Approximately 25% of the genome is made up of regions of greater than 5×10^5 bp that are devoid of genes and are termed *gene deserts*.

Much of this "noncoding DNA"—up to 40% to 50% in humans—is actually transcribed into RNA. The functions of these RNAs are unknown, but they could have important roles in chromosome structure and function.

Transposons Make Up Much of the Human Genome

Eukaryotic genomes contain large amounts of **repetitive DNA** sequences that are present in many copies (thousands, in some cases). By contrast, coding regions of genes (which are typically present in a single copy per haploid genome) are referred to as **unique-sequence DNA.**

Repetitive DNA shows two patterns of distribution in the chromosomes. **Satellite DNAs** are clustered in discrete areas, such as the centromeres. They are discussed in the next section. Other types of repetitive DNA are dispersed throughout the genome. In humans, most of this dispersed repetitive DNA is composed of **transposable elements**—small, discrete DNA elements dispersed throughout the genome—that either are now or were formerly capable of moving from place to place within the DNA. There are many types of these elements, but for purposes of simplicity, they are divided here into two overall classes. **Transposons** move via DNA intermediates, and **retrotransposons** move via RNA intermediates. Transposons generally move by a cut-and-paste mechanism, that is, the starting element cuts itself out of its location within the genome and inserts itself somewhere else. There is currently no evidence for active transposons in humans, but in *Drosophila*, transposition by transposons such as the **P element** accounts for at least half of spontaneous mutations.

Even though humans no longer have active transposons, we still use at least two functional vestiges of these elements. It has been known for years that one of the ways in which the diversity of the immune system is generated is by cutting and pasting portions of the genes that encode the variable regions of the immunoglobulin chains (see Fig. 28-10). This process involves moving bits of DNA around, and it now appears that the enzymes that accomplish this process were originally encoded by ancient transposons. In addition, CENP-B (centromere protein B; see Fig. 13-23), an abundant protein that binds to the α-satellite DNA repeats in primate centromeres, is closely related to a transposase enzyme encoded by one family of transposons.

Retrotransposons transcribe themselves into RNA, then convert this RNA into DNA as it is being inserted at another site in the genome. Retrotransposons move (transpose) from one place in the DNA to another through production of an RNA intermediate. Therefore, on completion of a transposition event, the original retrotransposon remains in its original chromosomal location, and a newly generated element (which may be either full-length or partial) is inserted at a new site in the genome. The copying of RNA into DNA is carried out by a specialized type of DNA polymerase called a **reverse transcriptase.** These enzymes were discovered in tumor viruses with RNA chromosomes, but human cells also have a number of genes encoding reverse transcriptases.

The best-known retrotransposons are **LINES** (long interspersed nuclear elements) and **SINES** (short interspersed nuclear elements). Reverse transcriptases encoded by LINES are responsible for movements of both LINES and SINES. The L1 class of LINES encodes two proteins, one of which has reverse transcriptase activity (Fig. 12-5). All DNA polymerases, including reverse transcriptases, work by elongating a preexisting stretch of double-stranded nucleic acid (see Chapter 42 for a discussion of the mechanism of DNA synthesis). L1

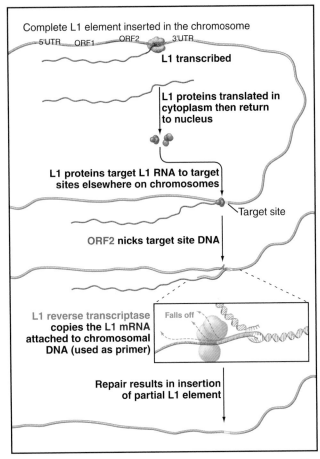

Complete L1 element inserted in the chromosome
5'UTR   ORF1   ORF2   3'UTR

L1 transcribed

L1 proteins translated in cytoplasm then return to nucleus

L1 proteins target L1 RNA to target sites elsewhere on chromosomes

Target site

ORF2 nicks target site DNA

L1 reverse transcriptase copies the L1 mRNA attached to chromosomal DNA (used as primer)

Falls off

Repair results in insertion of partial L1 element

Figure 12-5 MECHANISM OF TRANSPOSITION OF AN L1 ELEMENT. The element is transcribed by RNA polymerase II (see Fig. 15-4). Proteins encoded by the element nick the chromosome, promote base pairing of the L1 transcript with the target site, and reverse transcribe the RNA into DNA. The L1 DNA is synthesized as an extension of the chromosome. The mechanism of final closing up of the nicks and gaps is not yet fully understood.

elements insert themselves into the chromosome by first nicking the chromosomal DNA, then using the newly created end as a primer for synthesis of a new DNA strand (Fig. 12-5). The template for this DNA synthesis by the reverse transcriptase is the LINE RNA, and the newly synthesized DNA is made as a direct extension of the chromosomal DNA molecule. Most LINES are only partial copies of the full-length element. Apparently, the reverse transcriptase is not very efficient (processive): It usually falls off before it completes copying the entire element.

Interestingly, the key enzyme responsible for maintaining DNA sequences at telomeres, **telomerase** (see later), is a specialized form of reverse transcriptase, and its mechanism is closely related to that of the L1 reverse transcriptase.

LINES and SINES plus other remnants of transposable elements account for up to 45% of the human genome. LINES, with a consensus sequence of 6 to 8 kb, make up about 20% of the genome. (A consensus sequence is the average arrived at by comparing a number of different sequenced DNA clones.) About 79% of human genes have at least one segment of L1 sequence inserted, typically in an intron. The Alu class of SINES, with a consensus sequence of about 300 bp, constitutes about 13% of the total DNA—almost a million copies scattered throughout the genome. Alu elements are derived from the 7SL RNA gene, which encodes the RNA component of signal recognition particle (see Fig. 20-5). They are actively transcribed by RNA polymerase III (see Fig. 15-10) but are short and do not have enough coding capacity to encode for complex proteins. They therefore rely on the L1 machinery to move around. It is therefore somewhat paradoxical that SINES and LINES have quite different distributions along the chromosomes. LINES are concentrated in gene-poor regions of the chromosomes with a relatively higher content of A + T base pairs. In contrast, the Alu SINES are concentrated in gene-rich regions with a relatively higher content of G + C base pairs.

Transposition can be harmful, as along the way, genes can be disrupted, deleted, or rearranged. Because of their tendency to insert into gene-rich regions of chromosomes, Alu elements are one of the most potent endogenous human mutagens, with a new Alu insertion occurring once in every 100 births. In contrast, although LINES can cause genome instability when they move, several factors appear to minimize the damage that they cause. Despite the large fraction of the human genome that is derived from LINES, they cause only 0.07% of spontaneous mutations seen in humans, owing to several mitigating features: (1) Only about 60 to 100 L1 elements are active, and these appear to be active only in the germ line (i.e., during production of gametes). (2) LINE elements prefer to move into gene-poor areas of chromosomes. (3) Most LINE sequences are only fragments of the complete element. In contrast, mice apparently have many more active L1 elements (~3000), and L1 transposition causes about 2.5% of spontaneous mutations in mice. One of the ancestral roles of the RNAi machinery (see Fig. 16-12) might have been to suppress the deleterious activity of transposable elements.

The physiological role, if any, of these elements is much debated. One long-favored possibility is that they do nothing advantageous and are analogous to an infection of the DNA that is tolerated as long as it does not move into genes that are essential for life. This is called the "**selfish DNA**" hypothesis. This notion has been challenged for Alu sequences, which are efficiently transcribed into RNA. Alu transcripts accumulate under conditions of cellular stress such as viral infection. This is interesting, because Alu transcripts can bind very efficiently to a protein kinase called **PKR**, which is induced by interferon as part of the cell's antiviral protection pathways. The best-known function of PKR is phosphorylation of eukaryotic initiation factor 2α-subunit (eIF-2α; see Fig. 17-9). This profoundly inhibits protein synthesis. PKR is generally activated by dsRNAs, and this is presumably important for its antiviral role, as many viruses have RNA chromosomes. Alu transcripts at low levels activate PKR (i.e., suppress protein synthesis), but at higher levels, they inactivate the enzyme (i.e., promote protein synthesis). Thus, it has been suggested that Alu transcripts might be natural regulators of protein synthesis under conditions of cellular stress.

LINES can also modulate transcription of genes by influencing the behavior of RNA polymerase as it passes through them. Thus, they might have a role in the control of gene expression. As discussed at the end of this chapter, the structure of telomeres (the ends of chromosomes) is in part maintained by telomerase, a reverse transcriptase that is likely have originated as part of a retrotransposon.

Pseudogenes

One surprise that emerged from analysis of the human genome sequence was the number of pseudogenes, which may exceed the number of genes. **Pseudogenes** are derived from genes but are no longer functional. They arise in two ways, both involving transposable elements. **Processed pseudogenes,** the more common variety, are created by reverse transcription of mature mRNA sequences into DNA apparently by a LINE reverse transcriptase that then inserts the copy back into the genome. Because these sequences come from mature mRNA, they lack introns. They also lack sequences that regulate transcription initiation and termination (Chapter 15), so they are not expressed. **Unprocessed pseudogenes** are created either by reverse transcription of unspliced precursor mRNAs or by local duplications of the chromosome that generally occur as a result of recombination between transposable elements. Such duplications initially create bona fide functional gene copies that become pseudogenes as they accumulate mutations that render their transcripts nonfunctional. Because pseudogenes are not functional, mutation of their DNA is not selected against during evolution, as are harmful mutations in the coding sequences of genes. Thus, over time, pseudogenes become less and less recognizable, and they eventually are lost from recognition in the sea of noncoding DNA.

Segmental Duplications in the Human Genome

About 5% of the human genome is composed of regions of **segmental duplication** that have formed relatively recently in evolutionary time. Segmental duplications are regions of 1000 or more bp with a DNA sequence identity of 90% or more that are present in more than one copy but are not transposons. They are of considerable interest because they can have a significant impact on human health. Regions of highly related DNA sequence are able to base-pair with one another and can consequently undergo recombination with one another. Depending on how these regions are distributed on the chromosomes, this recombination can eliminate intervening regions of nonduplicated DNA. If the deleted region contains genes important for human health, then the end result can be human disease.

One example of this is found on chromosome 7, where deletion of a portion of the long arm is associated with Williams-Beuren syndrome, a complex developmental disorder associated with a highly variable range of symptoms that can include elfin-like facial features, defects in certain mental skills, and a wide range of physical problems (Fig. 12-6). These deletions, which typically remove about 1.6×10^6 bp, occur because of large segmental duplications of blocks of >140,000 bp distributed across a region of 2×10^6 bp. These duplications flank a unique sequence region of 1.15×10^6 bp that is lost when recombination occurs between the regions of segmental duplication. Because of the highly complex organization of this region and the large size of the duplications, this turned out to be the most

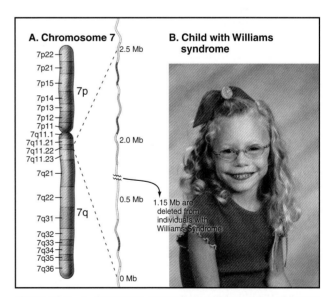

Figure 12-6 A, Segmental duplications within a region of human chromosome 7 give rise to Williams-Beuren syndrome. Inappropriate recombination between duplicated sequences causes the deletion of a region of the chromosome. **B,** Williams-Beuren syndrome is a rare congenital disorder that is characterized by an outgoing personality, a characteristic elfin-like facial appearance, moderate to mild mental retardation, and a range of physical problems. (Courtesy of the Williams Syndrome Association. To learn more, visit the association's website at http://www.williams-syndrome.org/.)

difficult region of chromosome 7 to sequence, and in fact, some ambiguities still remain.

The Centromere: Overview

The **centromere** is at the heart of all chromosomal movements in mitosis and meiosis, as it is the region where the chromosome becomes attached to the mitotic spindle (the microtubule-based apparatus upon which chromosomes move; see Chapter 44). The centromere also has an important role in monitoring the attachment of the chromosomes to the spindle and controlling the progress of cells through mitosis. The centromere is a nucleoprotein structure, and both DNA and proteins are essential to its function.

In chromosomes of most higher eukaryotes, the centromere may be visualized directly as a waist-like stricture or **primary constriction** where the two sister chromatids are most intimately paired. Several abundant families of repetitive DNAs are concentrated in the centromeres of human chromosomes. The chromatin of human centromeres is entirely embedded within **constitutive heterochromatin,** a form of chromatin characterized by the presence of special proteins and special modifications of the histone proteins, that is generally nonpermissive for gene transcription and that remains condensed throughout the cell cycle (see Fig. 13-9). At least some of the repeated DNA elements are transcribed into dsRNA, and the cellular RNAi machinery is required for the assembly of heterochromatin. (For a discussion of heterochromatin, see Chapter 13.) At the surface of the centromeric heterochromatin is a button-like structure called the **kinetochore,** which directs chromosomal movements in mitosis (see Fig. 13-20). Kinetochores are packaged into a specialized form of chromatin called centrochromatin.

Variations in Centromere Organization among Species

Each chromosome has particular DNA sequences, called **CEN** sequences, that specify protein-binding sites required for assembly of the kinetochore. In budding yeast, CEN sequences are autonomous; if inserted into circular DNA molecules (plasmids), they can render them capable of interacting with the mitotic spindle and segregating during mitosis (Fig. 12-7). In other organisms, including the fission yeast *Schizosaccharomyces pombe,* CEN sequences appear to require an activation event in order to nucleate kinetochore formation. This event appears to involve some sort of modification of the DNA and/or chromatin (discussed later).

CEN sequences from all 16 chromosomes of budding yeast have a common organization based around three

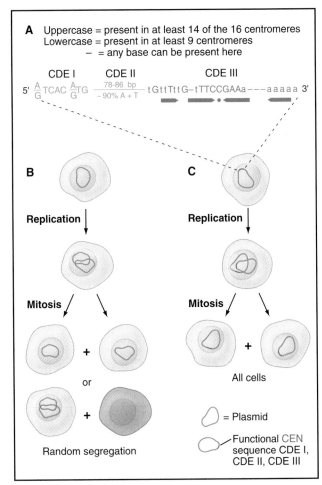

Figure 12-7   A, The budding yeast centromere is specified by a 125-bp sequence, with three conserved DNA elements (CDE I to CDE III). CDE I and CDE III bind proteins in a sequence-specific manner. CDE III has mirror symmetry: a central C *(dot)* is flanked by two regions of complementary DNA sequence *(arrows).* All that seems to be important about CDE II is its abundance of A and T nucleotides and its overall length. **B–C,** The assay for mitotic stability of a plasmid used to clone CEN DNA from most budding yeast chromosomes. The plasmid carries a gene encoding an enzyme involved in adenine metabolism. When the plasmid is present, colonies are white. If the plasmid is lost, the colonies become red as a result of the accumulation of a metabolic by-product. If the plasmid is capable of replication but lacks a centromere, the colonies will be mostly red, reflecting the inefficient segregation of the plasmid at mitosis **(B).** If the plasmid carries a functional centromere, the colonies will be white, as the plasmid will be successfully transmitted at nearly every division **(C).**

conserved sequence elements (Fig. 12-7). These are designated (in the 5′ to 3′ direction) **CDE I** (centromere DNA element I, 8 bp), **CDE II** (78 to 86 bp), and **CDE III** (25 bp). A 125-bp region spanning CDE I to CDE III is sufficient to direct the efficient segregation of a yeast chromosome, which can reach a size of more than 1 million bp. This type of centromere, in which the kinetochore is assembled as a result of protein recognition of specific DNA sequences, is known as a **point cen-**

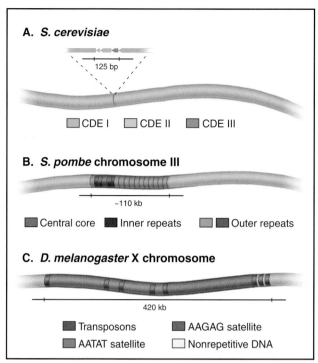

Figure 12-8 Organization of the centromeric DNAs of budding yeast, fission yeast, and fruit fly. **A,** The budding yeast **point centromere** is specified by a 125-bp sequence. **B,** The fission yeast **regional centromeres** all contain central core DNA flanked by complex arrays of repeated sequences. Embedded within these repeated sequences are a number of genes encoding transfer RNAs, not shown here. The minimum region required to construct a functional centromere in fission yeast artificial chromosomes is about 10 kb in length and includes the central core DNA plus a portion of the flanking repeated DNA. **C,** The fruit fly also has a regional centromere encompassing 420 kb. This is rich in satellite DNA and contains a number of transposable elements. Interestingly, the same satellite DNAs and transposons are also found at other, noncentromeric, regions of the chromosomes.

tromere. Kinetochores assembled on point centromeres bind a single microtubule.

Even though the average size of *S. pombe* chromosomes is only fivefold larger than their counterparts in *S. cerevisiae* (4.6 Mb versus 0.87 Mb), fission yeast centromeres are 300- to 600-fold larger (Fig. 12-8). The smallest *S. pombe* centromere consists of 35,000 bp, whereas the largest spans 110,000 bp. Fission yeast centromeres are also much more complex than are their counterparts from budding yeast, containing a central core of unique-sequence DNA that is 4 to 7 kb long, flanked by complex arrays of repeated sequences. This type of centromere, where the kinetochore is assembled on a variable array of repeated DNA sequences, is known as a **regional centromere.** Kinetochores assembled on regional centromeres bind multiple microtubules (2 to 4 in the case of *S. pombe*).

Studies of *S. pombe* centromeres revealed an additional level in the regulation of centromere function. *S.*

pombe CEN DNA apparently must undergo an **epigenetic** activation event to function as a centromere. Epigenetic events are inheritable properties of chromosomes that are not directly encoded in the nucleotide sequence. They are thought to be explained either by enzymatic modification of the DNA (e.g., methylation of cytosine) or by modification of proteins that are stably associated with the DNA. There is increasing evidence that epigenetic mechanisms play an essential role in the assembly of centromeres in higher eukaryotes, including humans. What this means in practice is that (with the exception of budding yeast), no single DNA sequence can be put into cells and function directly as a centromere. If a piece of *S. pombe* centromeric DNA is introduced into cells, it must undergo a series of packaging events and modifications that turn it into a functional centromere. These events are so rare that when candidate DNA molecules with CEN sequences are introduced into *S. pombe* cells, only about one in 10^5 assembles into a functional centromere.

In both *S. pombe* and metazoans, these epigenetic changes involve the construction of a special chromatin environment. *S. pombe* kinetochores assemble into a specialized form of chromatin containing the kinetochore-specific histone variant CENP-A (see Fig. 13-23). This flanking heterochromatin is important because it is required for binding a protein complex that regulates the pairing of replicated chromosomal DNA molecules during mitosis. Mutations in *S. pombe* that impair formation of heterochromatin also impair centromere function.

The best-characterized centromere of a metazoan comes from rice, in which the centromere of chromosome 8 has been completely sequenced. This was possible because this particular centromere contains relatively limited amounts of the rice centromeric satellite DNA (CentO), and this is dispersed in a number of blocks separated by transposons, retrotransposons, and fragments. All in all, 72% of this centromere is composed of repetitive sequences. The kinetochore, as defined by sequences associated with the kinetochore-specific histone H3 variant CENP-A (see Fig. 13-23), spans 750 kb and appears to be interspersed with regions of chromatin containing normal histone H3. The state of posttranslational modifications of that H3 indicates that it is packaged heterochromatin (a "closed" state of the chromatin usually associated with the absence of active gene transcription; see Fig. 13-9). It was therefore surprising that this centromere region contains at least four genes that are actively transcribed. The structure of this centromere appears to be intermediate between that of a canonical vertebrate centromere and a neocentromere (see later); however, rice centromere 8 is not a new variant but has had this organization for at least the last 10,000 years, since the *indica* and *japonica* cultivars of rice were separated.

The centromere organization of the fruit fly *D. melanogaster* shows important similarities and differences to the plant centromeres. The centromere of the fly's X chromosome is contained within a stretch of roughly 420,000 bp (Fig. 12-8) that is composed mostly of simple-sequence satellite DNAs interspersed with transposable DNA elements. This resembles the situation in plants; however, in *Drosophila*, no sequences were found in this region that are unique to the fly centromeres; all sequences that are found at centromeres can also be found on the chromosome arms. Thus, it appears that something other than the DNA sequence alone must be responsible for conferring centromere activity on this region of the chromosome.

Most higher eukaryotes have regional centromeres, but a third variant is also observed in many insects as well as in the nematode *C. elegans*. **Holocentric** chromosomes have centromere activity distributed along the whole surface of the chromosome during mitosis. Thus, instead of having a tight bundle of 20 microtubules binding to a disk-like kinetochore at a centromeric constriction, as in humans, in *C. elegans* about 20 microtubules bind at scattered sites along the whole poleward-facing surface of the chromosome during mitosis. If a holocentric chromosome is fragmented, all the pieces have the ability to bind microtubules and segregate in mitosis. Perhaps surprisingly, the proteins of the holocentric kinetochore are the same as those found at disk-like regional kinetochores (see Chapter 13). At the moment, nothing is known about the DNA sequences, presumably interspersed throughout the genome, that direct the assembly of holocentric kinetochores. One possibility is that in these chromosomes, any chromatin can serve to nucleate kinetochore assembly—perhaps the requirement for special epigenetic marks has been relaxed.

Mammalian Centromere DNA

Vertebrate centromeres have proven extremely difficult to characterize in molecular detail, largely due to their large size and complex, highly repeated, organization. For example, the centromere of chromosome 21 (the smallest human chromosome at ~40 million bp) has been estimated to encompass more than 5 million bp. This entire region appears to be composed of many thousands of copies of short DNA sequences that are clustered together in head-to-tail arrays. Such clustered DNA repeats are known as satellite DNA.

The major human centromeric satellite DNA, α-**satellite,** is a complex family of repeated sequences that constitutes approximately 5% of the genome. Monomers averaging around 171 bp long are organized into higher-order repeats (Fig. 12-9). Some of the monomers have a conserved 17-bp sequence (the CENP-B

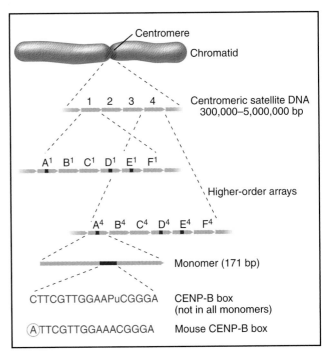

Figure 12-9 HIERARCHICAL ORGANIZATION OF α-SATELLITE DNA AT HUMAN CENTROMERES. The numbers (1 to 4) indicate higher-order repeats of α-satellite DNA. These may contain from 2 to 32 monomers (indicated by A^1, B^1, and so on). DNA sequences of adjacent monomers within a repeat (e.g., A^1, B^1, C^1) may differ by as much as 40% from one another. DNA sequences of monomers occupying identical positions within the higher-order repeats (A^1, A^4, an so on) are nearly 99% identical to one another. The *red* sequence shown at the *bottom* represents the binding site for centromeric protein CENP-B.

box), which forms the binding site for the centromeric protein CENP-B (mentioned earlier as having its origin in an ancient DNA transposon). The organization of higher-order repeats varies greatly from chromosome to chromosome, and numerous repeat patterns, comprising 2 to 32 monomers, have been described. Each chromosome has one or a few types of higher-order repeats of α-satellite DNA.

Human chromosomes also contain several other families of satellite DNA. Classical satellites I to IV, which together constitute 2% to 5% of the genome, are composed of divergent repeats of the sequence GGAAT. These satellites occur in blocks more than 20,000 bp long that are immediately adjacent to the centromeres of chromosomes 1, 9, and 16 and that may be found at much lower levels near most centromeres. The so-called pericentromeric region adjacent to the centromere of chromosome 9 apparently contains 7 to 10 million bp of satellite III sequence. The long arm of the Y chromosome also contains huge amounts of satellite III DNA (up to 40% of its total DNA).

What is human CEN DNA, that is, the DNA that nucleates kinetochore formation? The best candidate thus far is α-satellite, which occurs at all natural centromeres. The entire centromeric region of certain chromosomes may be composed of α-satellite monomers, apparently with little or no interspersed DNA of other types. The amount of α-satellite DNA at different centromeres varies widely: from as little as 300,000 bp on the Y chromosome to up to 5 million bp on chromosome 7. In addition, the α-satellite DNA content of a given chromosome can vary by more than a million bp between different individuals. Thus, whatever the function of α-satellite DNA may be, clearly, a wide variation in local organization is tolerated.

If α-satellite DNA arrays longer than about 50,000 bp are introduced into cultured human cells, they occasionally form tiny minichromosomes with functional centromeres. For this to work, the α-satellite DNA arrays must have a highly regular organization, and some of the monomers must contain binding sites for CENP-B. Formation of these mammalian artificial chromosomes is very inefficient, so it is clear that α-satellite DNA arrays cannot automatically function as CEN DNA—some type of epigenetic activation is required.

There is an interesting corollary of this role of epigenetic modifications in assembly of a functional centromere. Suppose a bit of noncentromeric DNA somehow acquired the right set of modifications. Could that now function as a centromere? The answer is yes. The formation of **neocentromeres** on noncentromeric DNA has been seen in fruit flies and humans and was first described in plants.

Rare individuals have a chromosome fragment that segregates in mitosis, despite the fact that the normal centromere has been lost. Such chromosomes have acquired a new centromere or neocentromere in a new location on one of the chromosome arms. Remarkably, neocentromeres are composed of the normal DNA that exists at that location on the chromosome arm and yet somehow has acquired centromere function. Neocentromeres are bona fide centromeres; for example, they bind all known centromeric proteins except for CENP-B, which requires specific sequences on α-satellite DNA for binding. Different neocentromeres need have no sequences in common. These observations strongly support models in which the centromere is specified by epigenetic markers rather than the exact DNA sequence per se. It could be that the linkage that is observed between α-satellite DNA and centromeres actually reflects a propensity of α-satellite DNA to acquire the epigenetic mark, rather than a sequence-specific mechanism as occurs in *S. cerevisiae*.

The epigenetic mark that defines an active centromere can be lost as well as gained. Thus, it is possible for a centromere to retain its normal DNA composition and yet lose the ability to assemble a kinetochore. This has been seen most clearly in naturally occurring human dicentric chromosomes. The example shown in Figure 12-10 arose through a breakage and fusion near the long arm of chromosome 13. Thus, it has two centromeres. As shown in the figure, one of these, even though it retains its α-satellite, has lost the ability to assemble a kinetochore.

Once a DNA sequence has acquired the proper epigenetic mark, it can assemble a functional kinetochore that can regulate chromosome behavior in mitosis. This involves the binding and function of a great many proteins, to be discussed in Chapter 13 (see Fig. 13-23).

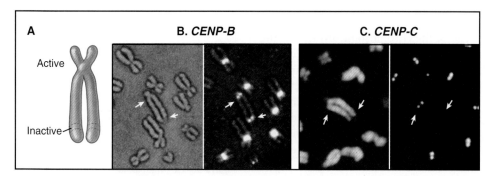

Figure 12-10 **EPIGENETIC REGULATION OF HUMAN CENTROMERE FUNCTION.** An unusual chromosome was discovered during prenatal screening of a fetus that sonography had indicated to be abnormal. This chromosome consisted of two copies of the maternal chromosome 13 linked end to end. It thus contained two centromeres and so was termed *dicentric*. Such dicentric chromosomes are normally very unstable during mitosis, as the two centromeres on one chromatid often become attached to opposite spindle poles. This causes the chromosome to be stretched between opposite spindle poles and ultimately break. In the case of this particular dicentric chromosome, one of the centromeres has been inactivated (presumably, it lost its epigenetic mark). This chromosome thus behaves perfectly normally in mitosis. When the distribution of centromere proteins at the active and inactive centromeres was compared, it was found that CENP-B was present at both but that CENP-C, a marker for kinetochores that can bind microtubules, was present only at the active centromere. **A,** Organization of the dicentric chromosome. **B,** Phase-contrast view of chromosomes from the amniocytes *(left)*. Phase-contrast view taken with superimposed antibody staining for CENP-B *(right)*. **C,** DNA stain of a different chromosome spread *(left)*. Staining with antibody specific for CENP-C *(right)*. (Micrographs courtesy of William C. Earnshaw.)

The Ends of the Chromosomes: Why Specialized Telomeres Are Needed

The ends of chromosomal DNA molecules pose at least two problems that cells solve by packaging the chromosome ends into specialized structures called **telomeres.** First, it is essential that cells distinguish the ends of a chromosome from breaks in DNA. When cells detect DNA breaks, they stop their progression through the cell cycle and repair the breaks by joining the ends together (see Box 43-1). Telomeres keep normal chromosome ends from inducing cell cycle arrest and from being joined to other DNA ends by the repair machinery. Second, telomeres permit the chromosomal DNA to be replicated out to the very end (see later discussion).

The Structure of Telomeric DNA

Telomeres in all eukaryotes tested to date (with the curious exception of flies such as *Drosophila*) are composed of many repeats of short DNA sequences. The sequence 5′ TTAGGG 3′ is found at the ends of chromosomes in organisms ranging from human to rattlesnake to the fungus *Neurospora crassa.* In the human, roughly 650 to 2500 copies of this sequence are found at the ends of each chromosome, yielding a total length of about 4000 to 15,000 bp (this varies in different tissues). Higher plant telomeres have the sequence TTTAGGG, and other variations of this repeat sequence have been noted in protozoans and yeasts.

The telomeric repeat is organized in a unique orientation with respect to the chromosome end. Thus, the end of every chromosome has one G-rich strand and one complementary C-rich strand. The G-rich strand always makes up the 3′ end of the chromosomal DNA molecule. Thus, the very 3′ end of the chromosome always has the following structure: .... (TTAGGG)-OH. Furthermore, the end of the chromosome is not a blunt structure; the G-rich strand ends in a single-stranded overhang that is approximately 200 bp long. Recent evidence suggests that this single-stranded DNA might "invade" the double helix of telomeric repeats, causing the ends of chromosomes to form large loops, called T loops (see later discussion).

How Telomeres Replicate the Ends of the Chromosomal DNA

One role of telomeres is to prevent the erosion of the end of the chromosomal DNA molecule during each round of replication (for a more extensive discussion of DNA replication, see Chapter 42). All DNA replication

proceeds with a polarity of 3′ to 5′ on the template DNA (5′ to 3′ in the newly synthesized DNA). Furthermore, all DNA polymerases (but not RNA polymerases) work by elongating a preexisting stretch of double-stranded nucleic acid. During cellular DNA replication, this is achieved by making a short RNA primer and then elongating the RNA : DNA duplex with DNA polymerase. The primer is subsequently removed, and the newly opened gap is filled by a DNA polymerase elongating from the next upstream DNA end (Fig. 12-11).

If the terminus of the chromosomal DNA is replicated from an RNA primer that sits on the very end of the DNA molecule, it follows that when this primer is removed, there is no upstream DNA on which to put a primer. How, then, is the DNA underneath the last RNA primer replicated? Years of searching for a DNA polymerase that could operate in the opposite direction

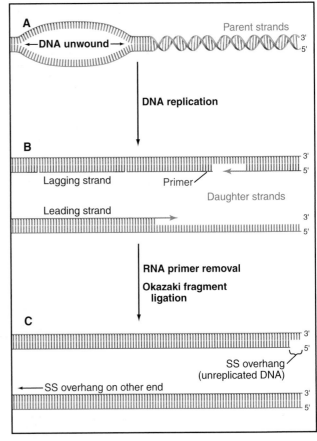

Figure 12-11 THE DNA REPLICATION PROBLEM AT CHROMOSOME ENDS. DNA polymerases cannot initiate the formation of DNA on a template de novo; they can only extend preexisting nucleotide strands (see Chapter 42). In contrast, RNA polymerases can initiate synthesis without a primer. All replicating DNA chains start from a short region of RNA, which is used to "prime" DNA polymerase. **A,** DNA strand separation. **B,** RNA primer synthesis. Replication of DNA starts with the synthesis of an RNA primer complementary to a short sequence of DNA, which is extended by DNA polymerase. **C,** The RNA primer is degraded and the gap is filled in by DNA polymerase. This being true, how is the DNA underneath the very last RNA primer replicated?

Figure 12-12 TELOMERASE PROVIDES A SPECIAL MECHANISM FOR LENGTHENING CHROMOSOMAL ENDS. **A–B,** Normal mechanisms of DNA replication are unable to replicate the very 3' end of the chromosomal DNA. **C,** Telomerase solves this problem by providing its own template in the form of an intrinsic RNA subunit. This RNA subunit contains a sequence complementary to that found at the chromosome terminus on the 3' strand. This sequence is able to base-pair with the DNA at the chromosome terminus and act as a template for DNA synthesis. In this case, the primer is the 3' end of the chromosomal DNA, and the template is the RNA of the telomerase enzyme. Thus, the process of telomere elongation is a specialized form of reverse transcription (copying RNA into DNA), a process similar to that occurring during transposition of LINE elements (see Fig. 12-5), and most well known during the life cycle of certain RNA-containing tumor viruses. The telomerase enzyme releases and rebinds its template after each 6 to 7 bp of new DNA has been synthesized. Up to several hundred bp may be added to the telomere in this way. **D,** In most cells, the cycle of telomerase activity and subsequent DNA replication leaves a single-stranded G-rich strand about 200 nucleotides long.

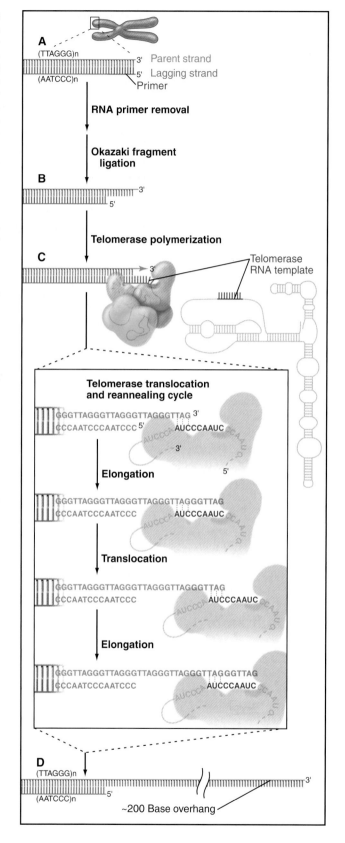

proved fruitless. The answer that ultimately emerged turned out to be both elegant and unexpected.

One solution to this problem was taken by dipterans such as *Drosophila melanogaster,* in which the ends of the chromosomes are composed of transposable elements. In the fly, a few bp are lost from the end of the chromosome at every round of replication. This erosion of the chromosome ends is remedied by the occasional transposition of a transposable element to the chromosome end. Thus, this appears to be an example of an originally "selfish DNA" that has become recruited for an essential cellular function.

Most other organisms have an enzymatic activity whose specific function is to lengthen the 3' end of the chromosomal DNA. This activity is referred to as **telomerase.** Telomerases are enzymes that contain both protein and RNA subunits. The sequences of these components provide an essential clue to how this enzyme works.

The sequence of the human telomere is TTAGGG. When the RNA component of human telomerase was characterized, it was found to contain the sequence AUCCCAAUC, which could base-pair with the TTAGGG repeat at the end of the chromosome. This observation led to a proposal for the mechanism of telomerase action (Fig. 12-12). In brief, the enzyme uses its own RNA as a template for the synthesis of DNA, which it attaches to the end of the chromosome. This hypothesis has been confirmed by studies that show that alterations in the sequence of the telomerase RNA lead to alterations in the telomere sequence at the end of the chromosome.

According to this model, the telomerase actually synthesizes DNA from an RNA template. Thus, telomerase is a reverse transcriptase similar to that involved in the movement of the LINE retrotransposons (see Fig. 12-5).

Interestingly, the L1 family of LINE retrotransposons appear to insert themselves into the chromosome by a similar mechanism, in which a DNA end created at a nick in the chromosome is used to prime synthesis of a DNA strand using the LINE RNA as template, the newly synthesized DNA being a direct extension of the chromosomal DNA molecule.

Telomerases have been characterized from budding yeast, mice, humans, and two ciliated protozoans. The enzymes consist of at least two protein subunits complexed to the RNA. The telomerase RNA varies in size and sequence between species, the human RNA, hTR, being 450 nucleotides long. hTR is complexed with two polypeptides: TP1 (a 240-kD protein that specifically binds to the RNA) and hTERT (a 127-kD protein that is the telomerase reverse transcriptase). Active human telomerase can be reconstituted in vitro from purified hTR and hTERT in the presence of a cell-free lysate from reticulocytes (which appears to provide essential protein-folding factors).

Telomerase is subject to tight biological regulation, active enzyme being detected in only a few normal tissues of adult humans. These include the intestine and testis. In addition, about 85% of cancer cells express active telomerase. In cells that lack telomerase, an alternative pathway, thought to involve DNA recombination, can help to maintain the telomeric repeats at chromosome ends. Paradoxically, hTR and TP1 are not tightly regulated. They are detected in many tissues, most of which lack telomerase activity. By contrast, the expression of hTERT correlates tightly with telomerase activity. Furthermore, introduction of a DNA-encoding hTERT into telomerase-negative cells is sufficient to convert those cells to telomerase-positive. This can have extremely important consequences for the proliferation of the cells (Fig. 12-15).

Structural Proteins of the Telomere

Telomeres provide special protected ends for the chromosomal DNA molecule, in part by coating the end of the DNA molecules with protective proteins and by adopting a specialized DNA loop structure. In organisms in which telomeric DNA sequences are relatively short, these sequences are packaged into a specialized chromatin structure. In mammals, in which the telomeric sequences are much longer, the bulk of the telomeric DNA is packaged into conventional chromatin (see Chapter 13).

Three types of proteins associate with telomeres (Fig. 12-13). The first binds in a sequence-specific manner to the double-stranded telomeric repeats. In budding yeast, the best known such protein is Rap1p. Mammals have two essential proteins of this type: TRF1 and TRF2 (telomere repeat factor). TRF1 and its associated factors regulate telomerase activity, thus helping to maintain the proper length of telomeres. A similar function has been proposed for Rap1p in budding yeast, where the telomeres appear to elongate only until they create a threshold number of binding sites for this protein. TRF2 and its associated factors protect the chromosome ends; interference with the binding of this protein to telomeres results in a loss of the G-strand overhangs and a dramatic increase in the tendency of chromosomes to fuse end to end. This may be because TRF2 can promote the formation of a special looped configuration of DNA in which the single-stranded G-strand overhang is base-paired with "upstream" DNA (Fig. 12-13B). Figure 12-14 shows the phenotype of a *Drosophila* mutant that lacks a protein essential for the assembly of the proper protective structure at telomeres and therefore undergoes extensive chromosome fusion.

Telomeric proteins of the second class bind to the single-stranded DNA of the G-strand overhang. One such protein, called Pot1, is conserved from humans to yeasts. Pot1 binds to single-stranded telomeric DNA and controls telomere length. The budding yeast homolog of Pot1 binds to the G-strand overhang and protects the end of the recessed C-rich strand at telomeres. In mutants lacking this protein, the C-rich strand is rapidly degraded, with lethal consequences for the cell.

Proteins of the third class pose a conundrum. At telomeres, they are required to protect the chromosome ends and prevent them from fusing with the ends of other chromosomes. Elsewhere on chromosomes, these same proteins function in the repair of DNA breaks by joining bits of broken DNA together, a pathway known as **nonhomologous end joining (NHEJ).** This appears to be exactly the opposite of their role at telomeres. The proteins involved are the Ku70/80 complex, which can recognize DNA ends, and a complex called MRN (MRE11, RAD50, NBS1). These proteins are highly conserved components of telomeres—from yeast to human—and if they are inactivated by mutations, telomeres frequently fuse together. It thus appears that chromosome ends are recognized by the breakage repair machinery but that some aspect of the telomeric structure changes the function of this machinery so that it assumes an end-blocking protection role rather than an end-joining role.

Telomeres may also direct chromosome ends to their proper location within the cell. In budding yeast (and many other species), telomeres prefer to cluster together at the nuclear periphery. Mutants in the telomere-binding SIR proteins, or in regions of the histones with which they intersect, disrupt this clustering in yeast. This results in activation of genes that are normally silenced when located in close proximity to telomeres. Thus, positioning of the telomere within the nucleus may be used to sequester genes into compartments where their transcriptional activity is repressed.

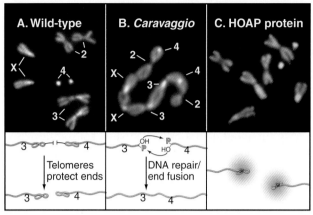

Figure 12-14 DISRUPTION OF THE PROTECTIVE COMPLEX AT TELOMERES RESULTS IN CHROMOSOME FUSION. **A,** The chromosomes of a wild-type female *Drosophila melanogaster* seen at mitotic metaphase (see Chapter 44). **B,** The *caravaggio* mutant is characterized by a "train" of chromosomes generated by telomere-telomere fusions. (Caravaggio is the name of an Italian train.) **C,** The cav gene encodes HP1/Orc2 Associated Protein (HOAP), which specifically localizes at all *Drosophila* telomeres. (Images courtesy of Gianni Cenci and Maurizio Gatti, University of Rome, Italy. B, From Cenci G, Siriaco G, Raffa GD, et al: Drosophila HOAP protein is required for telomere capping. Nat Cell Biol 5:82–84, 2003. C, Part of montage on *Nature Cell Biology* cover.)

Telomeres, Aging, and Cancer

Although the average length of telomeric repeats in humans is about 4000 bp, this length varies. Chromosomes of older individuals have shorter telomeres, and gametes have longer telomeres. This suggested the interesting possibility that chromosomes might lose telomeric sequences during the life of an individual.

The relationship between telomere length and aging can be studied in cultured cells. Normal cells in culture grow for only a limited number of generations (often called the Hayflick limit) before undergoing **senescence** (this involves cessation of growth, enlargement in size, and expression of marker enzymes, such as β-galactosidase). Because normal somatic cells lack telomerase activity, their telomeres shorten by about 50% before the cells senesce. Senescent cells stop divid-

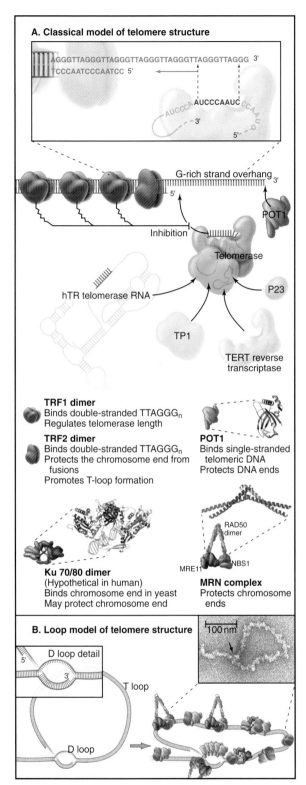

Figure 12-13 MODELS FOR TELOMERE STRUCTURE. **A,** The proposed structure of the end of a human chromosome. TRF1 and TRF2 bind to the double-stranded (TTAGGG)n repeats at telomeres. TRF1 somehow regulates the action of telomerase. TRF2 is responsible for protecting the integrity of chromosomal ends. If it is lost, chromosomes fuse with one another, and many abnormalities are seen. In yeast, a protein called Ku binds to the ends of the DNA. (Pot1: 1QZG.pdb. Ku 70/80: 1JEY.pdb. Rad 50: 1L8D.pdb.) **B,** Alternative loop model for vertebrate telomeres. Chromosomal ends may form a T-loop structure when a single-stranded G-rich 3′ end of the chromosome "invades" a double-stranded portion of the telomere, base-pairing with one strand and displacing the other strand (D loop). TRF2 can promote formation of T loops in vitro. **Inset,** A T loop excised together with its chromatin proteins from a chicken erythrocyte chromosome. (Inset, From Nikitina T, Woodcock CL: Closed chromatin loops at the ends of chromosomes. J Cell Biol 166:161–165, 2004.)

ing before their telomeres become critically short. In some cases, it is possible to force the senescent cells to resume proliferation (e.g., by expressing certain viral oncogenes). These "driven" cells continue to divide and their telomeres continue to shorten until a **crisis** point is reached. In crisis, cells suffer chromosomal instability (chromosomal fusions and breaks can occur) and cell death. In populations of human cells in crisis, very rarely (in about 1 in a million cases), cells appear that once again grow normally. These cells now express telomerase. These observations with cultured cells led to the suggestion that senescence might occur in cells when the telomeric repeats of one or more chromosomes are reduced to some critical level.

If this model is correct, it suggests very interesting (and controversial) implications for the regulation of cell life. Suppose that telomerase is active only in the germ line, so that all gametes have long telomeres. Now, if the enzyme were inactivated in somatic cells, this would effectively provide every cell lineage with a limitation on how many times it could divide before loss of telomeric sequences caused it to become senescent. Provided that the starting telomeres were sufficiently long and that telomerase was expressed in unusual tissues, like testis and intestine, in which rapid division occurs throughout the life of the individual, this would have no deleterious effect on the life span of the organism. In fact, such a mechanism might provide an important advantage by minimizing the chances that a clone of cells would escape from the normal regulation of growth control and become cancerous.

This model has been tested in two ways. First, mice were prepared in which the gene coding for the RNA component of telomerase was disrupted. These mice were healthy and fertile for six generations in the complete absence of telomerase but then abruptly became sterile as a result of cell death in the male germ line. The abrupt cell death presumably occurred when the telomeres shortened below a critical threshold. Having telomeres about three times longer than humans might have contributed to their initial survival through several generations. This experiment thus showed that telomerase is not essential for the day-to-day life of a mammal, but clearly, it is needed for the survival of the species.

In a second experiment, the hTERT reverse transcriptase subunit of telomerase was introduced into normal cells growing in culture. This caused an increase in the level of active telomerase with dramatic results. Instead of undergoing senescence, these cells kept dividing in culture, apparently indefinitely (Fig. 12-15). However, unlike cancer cells, which are also immortal, these cells did not acquire the ability to cause tumors. Thus, this experiment showed convincingly that telomeres are part of a mechanism that regulates the proliferative capacity of somatic cells.

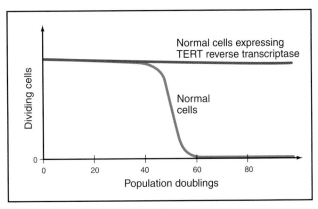

Figure 12-15   Introduction of hTERT, the human reverse transcriptase subunit of telomerase, into normal cells is sufficient to overcome the senescence limit and immortalize the cells. These cells are not transformed into invasive cancer cells; instead, they act like normal cells that can now grow indefinitely.

ACKNOWLEDGMENTS

Thanks go to Robin Allshire, Michael Ashburner, Maurizlo Gatti, Ursula Goodenough, Paul Hieter, and Alastair Kerr for their suggestions on revisions to this chapter.

SELECTED READINGS

de Lange T: T-loops and the origin of telomeres. Nat Rev Mol Cell Biol 5:323-329, 2004.

Doolittle RF: Microbial genomes opened up. Nature 392:339-342, 1998.

Dujon B: The yeast genome project: What did we learn? Trends Genet 12:263-270, 1996.

Fukagawa T: Centromere DNA, proteins and kinetochore assembly in vertebrate cells. Chromosome Res 12:557-567, 2004.

Hall AE, Keith KC, Hall SE, et al: The rapidly evolving field of plant centromeres. Curr Opin Plant Biol 7:108-114, 2004.

International Human Genome Sequencing Consortiuim: Finishing the euchromatic sequence of the human genome. Nature 431:931-945, 2004.

Kim SH, Kaminker P, Campisi J: Telomeres, aging and cancer: In search of a happy ending. Oncogene 21:503-511, 2002.

Maiato H, DeLuca J, Salmon ED, Earnshaw WC: The dynamic kinetochore-microtubule interface. J Cell Sci 117:5461-5477, 2004.

McAinsh AD, Tytell JD, Sorger PK: Structure, function, and regulation of budding yeast kinetochores. Annu Rev Cell Dev Biol 19:519-539, 2003.

McEachern MJ, Krauskopf A, Blackburn EH: Telomeres and their control. Annu Rev Genet 34:331-358, 2000.

Pidoux AL, Allshire RC: Centromeres: Getting a grip of chromosomes. Curr Opin Cell Biol 12:308-319, 2000.

Rubin GM, Yandell MD, Wartman JR, et al: Comparative genomics of the eukaryotes. Science 287:2204-2215, 2000.

Shay JW, Zou Y, Hiyama E, Wright WE: Telomerase and cancer. Hum Mol Genet 10:677-685, 2001.

Smit AF: Interspersed repeats and other mementos of transposable elements in mammalian genomes. Curr Opin Genet Dev 9:657-663, 1999.

Smogorzewska A, de Lange T: Regulation of telomerase by telomeric proteins. Annu Rev Biochem 73:177-208, 2005.

CHAPTER 13

DNA Packaging in Chromatin and Chromosomes

Chromosomal DNA molecules of eukaryotes are thousands of times longer than the diameter of the nucleus and must therefore be highly compacted throughout the cell cycle. This folding is accomplished by combining the DNA with structural proteins to make **chromatin.** A hierarchy of levels of chromatin folding compacts the DNA but permits transcriptional machinery access to those regions of the chromosome required for gene expression.

The first level of folding involves coiling DNA around a protein core to yield a **nucleosome.** This shortens DNA about sevenfold relative to naked DNA. The string of nucleosomes is next folded into a shorter, thicker filament, called a **30-nm fiber,** which is about 40-fold shorter than naked DNA. The structure of the 30-nm fiber is not yet known unambiguously, and the details of the higher-order packing of chromatin in nuclei and mitotic chromosomes remain quite controversial.

The First Level of Chromosomal DNA Packaging: The Nucleosome

The continuous DNA fiber of each chromosome links hundreds of thousands of nucleosomes in series. Individual nucleosomes can be isolated following cleavage of DNA between neighboring particles. Random digestion of chromatin by DNA-cutting enzymes called nucleases initially yields a mixture of particles consisting of one or more nucleosomes containing multiples of about 200 base pairs of DNA (Fig. 13-1). Continued nuclease cleavage yields a stable particle with 146 base pairs of DNA (1.75 turns of the DNA around the protein core). This is called a **nucleosome core particle.**

The nucleosome core particle is disk-shaped, with DNA coiled in a left-handed superhelix around an octamer of **core histones.** This octamer consists of a central tetramer composed of two closely linked **H3** : **H4** heterodimers, flanked on either side by two **H2A** : **H2B** heterodimers. High-resolution crystal structures of nucleosome core particles revealed that each core histone has a compact domain of 70 to 100 amino acid residues that adopts a characteristic Z-shaped "histone fold" consisting

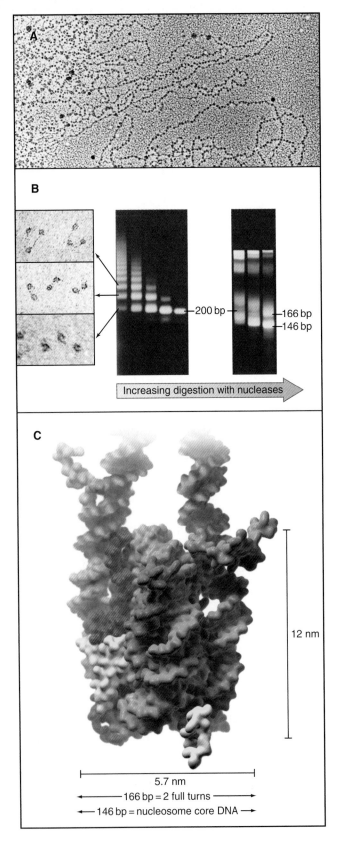

Figure 13-1 **NUCLEOSOMES. A,** Electron micrograph showing chromosomal loops covered in nucleosomes, which under these conditions look like beads on a string. **B,** Nuclease digestion of chromosomes releases fragments containing varying numbers of nucleosomes *(left),* in which the DNA fragments vary by multiples of 200 base pairs *(center).* More extensive nuclease digestion results in production of the nucleosome core particle, with 146 base pairs of DNA *(right).* **C,** The crystal structure of the nucleosome core particle. The DNA wraps around a compact core of histones. (A, Courtesy of William C. Earnshaw. B, *left panel,* Composite of excerpts from Woodcock CL, Sweetman HE, Frado LL: Structural repeating units in chromatin. II: Their isolation and partial characterization. Exp Cell Res 97:111–119, 1976. B, *center and right panels,* Excerpts from Allan J, Cowling GJ, Harborne N, et al: Regulation of the higher-order structure of chromatin by histones H1 and H5. J Cell Biol 90:279–288, 1981. C, PDB file: 1KX5.)

of a long α-helix flanked by two shorter α-helices (Fig. 13-2).

The amino-terminal approximately 30 amino acid residues of the core histones (referred to as **N-terminal tails**) are important for interactions both inside and outside the nucleosome. They project outward from the cylindrical faces of the nucleosomal core as well as between the adjacent winds of the DNA on the nucleosome surface. Although these N-terminal tails are not ordered either in crystals of nucleosome core particles or in solution, they are among the most highly conserved regions of these very highly conserved proteins, as they serve two essential functions. First, specific modifications of these N-terminal tails are used to regulate the accessibility of the DNA within the chromatin fiber to the transcription, replication, and repair machinery (see later section). The N-terminal tails also promote interactions between nucleosomes that favor formation of the compact 30-nm fiber.

Epigenetics and the Histone Code

The revolution in biology that began with the structure of DNA and the realization that the sequence of bases in DNA provides a code that specifies the structure of proteins culminated 50 years later with the near complete sequencing of all the gene-rich portions of the human genome. To take advantage of this coding information, cells must control when to use it. Initial studies of the processes controlling **gene expression** focused on regulation of transcription by proteins that bind specific DNA sequences at the 5′ end of genes (see Chapter 15), as this is the way in which bacteria regulate their genes. This is now known to be only part of the story.

Eukaryotes impose another level of regulation on the utilization of their genes. This has been referred to as a **histone code.** The histone code hypothesis proposes that combinations of **posttranslational modifications** of histones are "read" by proteins that

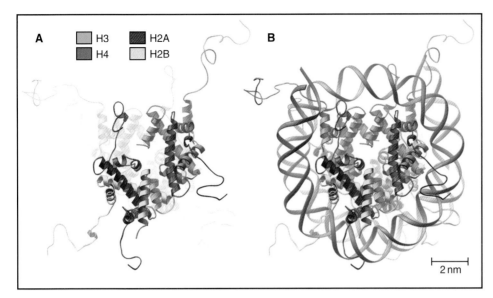

Figure 13-2 SECONDARY STRUCTURE OF THE HISTONES WITHIN THE CORE PARTICLE. **A,** A ribbon diagram shows that each histone protein in the octameric core of the nucleosome has a characteristic α-helical structure (the histone fold). Portions of the flexible N-terminal portions of the histones, which have a critical role in regulating chromatin structure, did not occupy a unique location in the crystal and do not appear in this structure. **B,** The histone octamer surrounded by one of the two turns of DNA. (PDB file: 1KX5. Modified from Luger K, Mäder AW, Richmond RK, et al: Crystal structure of the nucleosome core particle at 2.8 Å resolution. Nature 389:251–260, 1997.)

bind modified histones and then dictate whether particular regions of chromatin are transcribed by RNA polymerases or are held in an inactive state. Post-translational modifications of histones include acetylation, phosphorylation, methylation, ubiquitination, and poly(ADP)ribosylation at many sites in the N-terminal tails and elsewhere (Fig. 13-3). Chromatin states created by histone modifications can be stably inherited through many rounds of cell division. Thus, this hypothesis can explain the phenomenon of epigenetic regulation (see Fig. 12-10): the stable, heritable regulation of chromosomal functions by information that is not simply encoded in the DNA sequence.

Regulation of Chromatin Structure by the Histone N-Terminal Tails

Human nuclei contain roughly 3.3×10^7 nucleosomes distributed along the DNA. Despite the fact that more than 70% of the molecular surface of nucleosomal DNA is accessible to solvent, most nonhistone proteins involved in gene regulation bind nucleosomal DNA 10-fold to 10^4-fold less well than naked DNA. Thus, nucleosomes establish a general environment in which DNA replication and gene transcription are repressed unless signals are given to the contrary.

The N-terminal histone tails provide a molecular "handle" to manipulate DNA accessibility in chromatin (Fig. 13-3). This complex area can only be outlined here. The two key modifications contributing to the histone code are acetylation and methylation of lysine residues. Histones with acetylated lysines are generally associated with "open" chromatin that is permissive for RNA transcription, while histones with methylated lysines can be associated with either "open" or "closed" chromatin states. It should be emphasized that the histone code is complex and not fully understood. Since the histone modifications are read as combinations, individual

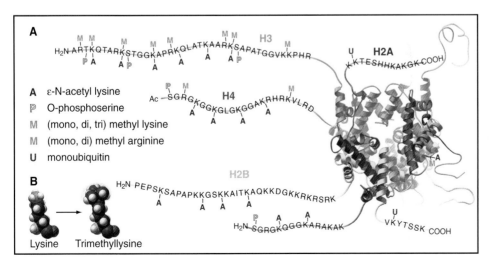

Figure 13-3 THE HISTONE CODE. **A,** Modification of the amino- and carboxy-terminal domains of the histones creates a "histone code" that regulates nucleosome assembly, transcription, and mitotic chromosome condensation. The modifications are described in the figure key. **B,** Structure of trimethyllysine. Arginine, R; lysine, K; serine, S. (PDB file: 1KX5. Adapted from Khorasanizadeh S: The nucleosome: From genomic organization to genomic regulation. Cell 116:259–272, 2004.)

modifications do not necessarily always have the same consequences. One example of this is the phosphorylation of histone H3 on serine 10 (H3-S10P). In mitotic cells, this correlates with a condensed and transcriptionally inactive chromatin structure, but when combined with acetylation of surrounding amino acid residues, it is also associated with the activation of gene transcription as nonproliferating cells reenter the cell cycle (see Chapter 41).

Acetylation reduces the net positive charge of the N-terminal domain, causing the chromatin to adopt an "open" conformation that is more favorable to transcription, as the histones bind less tightly to DNA. Acetylation also provides binding sites for a number of proteins with an approximately 100-amino-acid sequence motif called a bromodomain. Bromodomain binding to acetylated histone N-terminal tails is analogous to the binding of SH2 domains to phosphorylated tyrosine in cellular signaling pathways (see Fig. 25-10). Bromodomain-containing enzymes recruited to chromatin by acetylated histones often modify histones in other ways that promote or limit the accessibility of the DNA for transcription into RNA.

Proteins called transcription factors regulate gene expression by binding specific DNA sequences in promoter regions adjacent to the coding sequences of genes and recruiting transcriptional machinery (RNA polymerases and associated proteins) to the gene (see Fig. 15-19). Many transcription factors recruit a protein complex, called a **coactivator,** that facilitates loading of the transcriptional apparatus onto the gene. Often, coactivators are enzymes that modify N-terminal histone tails. One yeast coactivator contains over 10 proteins, including a histone acetyltransferase that transfers acetate groups from acetyl coenzyme A (CoA) to the ε-amino groups of lysine-14 and lysine-8 in the N-terminal tails of histone H3 (Fig. 13-4). Histone acetylation is crucial for life. Yeast cells die if these lysines are mutated to arginines, thus preserving their positive charge but preventing them from being acetylated.

Histone acetylation is dynamic. Just as transcriptional coactivators contain histone acetyltransferases that add acetyl groups to nucleosomes and promote gene activation, so *corepressors,* which are recruited in a similar manner, can contain histone deacetylases that remove acetyl groups from selected lysine residues. This tends to inactivate gene expression. This mechanism regulates cell cycle progression during the G_1 phase of the cell cycle (see Fig. 41-8).

In addition to marking nucleosomes by modification of their N-terminal tails, cells also use the energy provided by ATP hydrolysis to actively remodel nucleo-

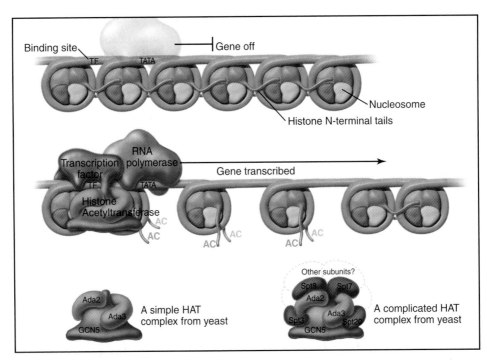

Figure 13-4   Acidic transcription factors *(purple)* bind specific DNA sequences and recruit coactivators to the 5′ ends of genes. Many of these coactivators have histone acetyltransferase activity and work by acetylating the N-terminal tails of the core histones, thereby loosening the chromatin structure and promoting the binding and activation of the RNA polymerase holoenzyme (see Chapter 15). The coactivators vary in composition and complexity from the relatively simple histone acetyltransferase complex *(bottom left)* to the huge and elaborate SAGA complex *(bottom right).* (AC, acetylation; TATA, DNA sequence in the gene promoter [see Chapter 15]). In this side view, only one of the two turns of DNA around the nucleosome is seen. GCN5, Ada2, Ada3, Spt3, Spt7, Spt8, and Spt20 are the names of budding yeast genes whose products are found in these complexes.

somes. This involves complex protein "machines" that can alter nucleosome structure, move nucleosomes around, or both. Two large "machines" in yeast—RSC (remodels the structure of chromatin) with 15 subunits and SWI/SNF (switch/sniff) with 11 subunits—each has a key subunit that utilizes ATP hydrolysis to translocate along the DNA helix. One proposal is that these "machines" use ATP hydrolysis to force an extra 40 to 60 base pairs of DNA onto the nucleosome. Since this excess DNA cannot fit smoothly against the surface of the histone octamer, it presumably bulges out in a loop from the nucleosomal surface. If the position of this loop migrates around the surface of the nucleosome, the nucleosome will "jump" 40 to 60 base pairs along the DNA. This process can uncover sequences that are important for gene regulation that had been hidden by association with a nucleosome. Alternatively, this mechanism may be used to loosen the nucleosome and allow the exchange of histone dimers in and out.

Histone Acetylation and Nucleosome Assembly

During DNA replication, existing nucleosomes are partitioned randomly between daughter DNA strands. Newly assembled nucleosomes then fill the gaps. When not associated with DNA, histones are always bound to protein chaperones. Newly translated H3 and H4, which are acetylated on lysine-9 of H3 and lysine-5 and lysine-12 of H4, associate with a chromatin assembly factor, called CAF1. One of the three subunits of CAF1 is a chaperone called retinoblastoma-associated protein of 48 kD (RbAp48). CAF1 is targeted to sites of DNA replication by interaction with proliferating cell nuclear antigen (PCNA), a doughnut-shaped protein that helps DNA polymerase to slide along the DNA during replication (see Fig. 42-11). Thus, CAF1 delivers newly synthesized histones to sites on the chromosome where new nucleosomes are required as DNA is synthesized during the S phase of the cell cycle (see Chapter 42). H3 and H4 are deposited first on the new DNA, followed by two H2A : H2B heterodimers to complete the assembly of the nascent nucleosome.

Histone Variants

About 75% of histone H3 in chromatin is deposited during DNA replication by CAF1. The remaining 25% is a special isoform of H3, called H3.3, that is encoded by a different gene and deposited on chromatin by an entirely different mechanism. Histone H3.3 is transcribed throughout the cell cycle, not coordinated with DNA synthesis. Newly synthesized H3.3 associates with the RbAp48 chaperone, but this then forms a complex with a protein called histone regulator A (HIRA) instead of the other two CAF1 subunits. Some H3.3 assembles

into nucleosomes at the time of DNA replication, just like the canonical H3. However, H3.3 can also be inserted into chromatin at other times of the cell cycle. For example, the HIRA : RbAp48 complex swaps H3.3/H4 dimers for H3/H4 dimers in chromatin during transcription, which transiently perturbs the nucleosomes on the underlying gene. Such replacement of histone H3 methylated on lysine 9 (H3-K9me) with unmethylated H3.3 is one way to convert "closed" chromatin, where transcription is disfavored, into "open" chromatin that is favorable for transcription. Alternatively, demethylases can remove the methyl groups from histone H3. H3-K9me marks inactive chromatin, while H3.3 tends to associate with actively transcribed genes.

Other specialized histone variants also contribute to the microdiversity of chromatin. For example, the H3 isoform called CENP-A is a key component of the kinetochore, the structure that assembles at centromeres to promote the segregation of chromosomes during mitosis (see later).

The largest number of variant forms has been described for H2A. Interaction between the N-terminus of H4 and a patch on the surface of H2A on the adjacent nucleosome has an important role in promoting chromatin fiber compaction. Therefore, altering the local H2A composition and consequently influencing the strength of this interaction provides an effective way to vary the accessibility of the DNA for gene expression. One variant, H2AX, which constitutes about 15% of the cellular H2A, helps to maintain genome integrity. At sites of DNA damage, H2AX is phosphorylated within a minute by protein kinases. This serves as a mark for the assembly of multiprotein complexes that repair the damage.

Linker DNA and the Linker Histone H1

When examined by electron microscopy at low ionic strength, nucleosomal chromatin resembles a string of beads with diameters of about 10 nm and **linker DNA** extended between adjacent nucleosomes (Fig. 13-1). Each nucleosome in chromosomes is typically associated with about 200 base pairs of DNA. With subtraction of 166 base pairs for two turns around the histone octamer, this leaves 34 base pairs of linker DNA between adjacent nucleosomes. Linker DNA can vary widely in length in different tissues and cell types.

A fifth histone, **H1** or **linker histone,** is thought to bind to linker DNA at the side of each nucleosome core where the DNA molecule enters and exits the structure (Fig. 13-5). H1 histones have a "winged helix" central domain flanked by unstructured basic domains at both the N- and C-termini (Fig. 13-3). Mammals have at least eight variant forms (called subtypes) of H1 histones ($H1_{a-e}$, $H1^0$, $H1_t$, and $H1_{oo}$). The amino acid sequences of these variants differ by 40% or more. Of these, $H1^0$ is

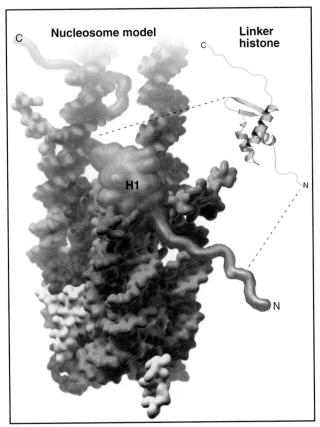

Figure 13-5   ARTIST'S RENDITION SHOWING THE BINDING SITE OF HISTONE H1 ON THE NUCLEOSOME, NEAR THE SITE WHERE DNA STRANDS ENTER AND EXIT THE CORE PARTICLE. *Orange*, DNA; *blue*, H3; *purple*, H4; *red*, H2A; *yellow*, H2B. (A, PDB file: 1KX5. B, PDB file: 1HST.)

found in cells entering the nondividing G$_o$ state (see Chapter 41), while H1$_t$ and H1$_{oo}$ are found exclusively in developing sperm and oocytes, respectively.

The role of H1 linker histone in chromatin remains enigmatic. The protein was originally assumed to have a structural role, yet it is mobile in the nucleus, spending no more than a few minutes at any given location. Deletion of the sole linker histone genes from yeast and *Tetrahymena* (a ciliated protozoan) causes no obvious ill effects, but H1 is essential in mice. Although genes that encode individual H1 isoforms can be deleted in mice, simultaneous deletion of the genes for three isoforms causes embryonic death. Death is thought to be due to alterations in chromatin structure that perturb normal patterns of gene expression.

The Second Level of Chromosomal DNA Packaging: The 30-nm Fiber

Levels of chromatin structure beyond the nucleosome are poorly understood. One job of linker histone H1 is to promote the packaging of chromatin into the **30-nm fiber,** a condensed filament of nucleosomes that can be observed by electron microscopy. Investigators now agree that the 30-nm fiber is unlikely to be a simple helix (solenoid) of nucleosomes. More complex models, similar to those shown in Figure 13-6B and D, are now favored.

Higher Levels of Chromosomal DNA Packaging in Interphase Nuclei

Dense packing of macromolecules in the nucleus makes it very difficult to observe the details of higher-level folding of chromatin fibers directly. Visualization of specific DNA loci within fixed interphase nuclei by in situ hybridization (see Fig. 13-15) can be used to estimate the degree of chromatin compaction by comparing the physical distance between two DNA sequences with a known number of base pairs between them. For regions of DNA up to about 250,000 base pairs apart, the chromatin fiber is shortened about twofold to threefold relative to the 30-nm fiber. When sequences are separated by tens of millions of base pairs, the shortening increases by another 20-fold to 30-fold. This suggests that there are at least two levels of chromatin folding beyond the 30-nm fiber.

The organization of chromatin fibers can be observed by fluorescence microscopy of living cells after labeling with a fluorescent marker, such as the jellyfish green fluorescent protein (GFP [see Fig. 6-3]) (Fig. 13-7). These labeled chromosome arms are dynamic, changing both their structure and location as cells traverse the cell cycle. At times in the cycle when a chromosome arm becomes relatively more decondensed, it is possible to observe the presence of a fiber, 100 to 300 nm in diameter, called a **chromonema fiber.** Similar fibers are seen in electron micrographs of interphase cells. It is not yet known whether the chromonema fiber is the next level of chromatin packing above the 30-nm fiber.

Functional Compartmentation of the Nucleus: Heterochromatin and Euchromatin

Chromatin has traditionally been divided into two main classes based on structural and functional criteria. **Euchromatin** contains almost all of the genes, both actively transcribed and quiescent. **Heterochromatin** is transcriptionally inert and is generally more condensed than the euchromatin; it was initially recognized because it stains more darkly with DNA-binding dyes than the remainder of the nucleus. A typical nucleus has both euchromatin and heterochromatin, the latter

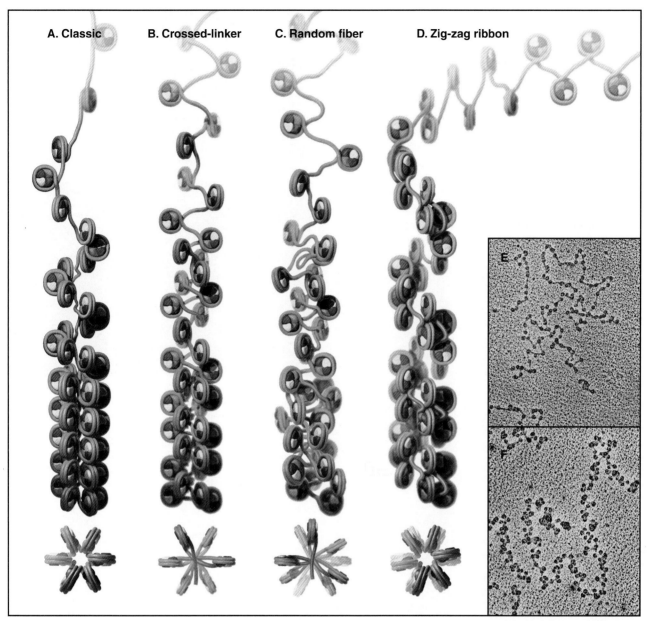

A. Classic **B. Crossed-linker** **C. Random fiber** **D. Zig-zag ribbon**

Figure 13-6 ALTHOUGH IT HAS BEEN STUDIED INTENSIVELY FOR 30 YEARS, THE STRUCTURE OF THE 30-NM CHROMATIN FIBER REMAINS CONTROVERSIAL. **A–D,** Various models of the 30-nm fiber: classic solenoid (a type of helix), crossed-linker solenoid, random fiber, and zig-zag ribbon. The classic solenoid model was originally favored, but it now appears that the crossed-linker and zig-zag ribbon are more likely. **E–F,** Histone H1 causes a compaction of the chromatin filament. **E,** Chromatin spread for electron microscopy following removal of histone H1: the 10-nm fiber or so-called beads on a string. **F,** A similar preparation with H1 present: the 30-nm fiber. (E–F, From Thoma F, Koller T: Influence of histone H1 on chromatin structure. Cell 12:101–107, 1977.)

usually being concentrated near the nuclear envelope and around nucleoli. Much of the interior of nuclei is occupied by pale-staining euchromatin rich in actively transcribing genes. Nuclei that are less active in transcription have relatively more heterochromatin (Fig. 13-8). Two types of heterochromatin are recognized.

Constitutive heterochromatin is associated with special types of DNA sequences, such as satellite DNAs (see Fig. 12-9), that are packaged into a particular type of "closed" conformation in every cell. Establishment of constitutive heterochromatin involves transcription of

these repeated DNA elements to produce double-stranded RNAs that are cleaved into short fragments by the RNAi machinery (see Fig. 16-12). The resulting short RNAs are thought to target components that promote heterochromatin formation to their sites of transcription in the chromosome (see Fig. 16-13).

Facultative heterochromatin is epigenetic: Rather than showing an invariant link with particular DNA sequences, it consists of sequences that are in heterochromatin in some cells and in euchromatin in others. X chromosome inactivation is the classic example of facultative heterochromatin in mammals. In females, one X chromosome in each cell (selected at random) is inactivated early in development prior to implantation of the embryo. The inactivated X chromosome forms a discrete patch of heterochromatin at the nuclear periphery known as the **Barr body** (Fig. 13-8). Because most genes carried on the inactivated X chromosome become transcriptionally silent, females with two X chromosomes have the same levels of gene expression as do males with a single X chromosome.

The epigenetic mark that best defines heterochromatin is methylation of histone H3 on lysine 9 (H3-K9me). This modification acts as a specific binding site for **heterochromatin protein 1 (HP1).** The amino-terminal

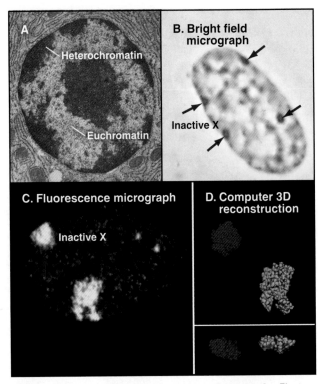

Figure 13-8 EUCHROMATIN AND HETEROCHROMATIN. **A,** Electron micrograph of a thin section of a plasma cell nucleus. Euchromatin is decondensed. Heterochromatin (mostly clumped near the nuclear envelope and nucleolus) remains condensed. **B,** Light micrograph of a female nucleus with four Barr bodies *(arrows)* (facultative heterochromatin composed of the inactive X chromosome). This woman has a highly abnormal genetic makeup, with five X chromosomes. The X chromosome inactivation system has a built-in counting mechanism that ensures that only one X chromosome remains active. **C–D,** The Barr body is structurally distinct from the active X chromosome. This figure is excerpted from a three-dimensional study in which the X chromosome was identified by in situ hybridization "painting" with probes that covered the entire chromosome. **C,** One slice through the three-dimensional data set. **D,** Two different views of the X chromosomes reconstructed in three dimensions. The inactive X chromosome is shown in red. Because of X chromosome inactivation, females are mosaic for functions encoded on the X chromosome. Each female embryo has two X chromosomes: X^{pat} and X^{mat} (for paternal and maternal). Following X chromosome inactivation, some cells will express genes from X^{pat} and others will express genes from X^{mat}. The inactivation is permanent; all progeny of a cell with X^{pat} inactivated will also have X^{pat} inactivated and vice versa. This inactivation occurs randomly in different cells of the embryo. In cats, genes responsible for coat color are encoded on the X chromosome. The patchy color pattern of calico cats reflects the underlying pattern of X chromosome inactivation. All calico cats are females. (A, From Fawcett DW: The Cell. Philadelphia, WB Saunders, 1981. B, Courtesy of Barbara Hamkalo, University of California, Irvine. C–D, From Eils R, Dietzel S, Bertin E, et al: Three-dimensional reconstruction of painted human interphase chromosomes: Active and inactive X chromosome territories have similar volumes but differ in shape and surface structure. J Cell Biol 135:1427–1440, 1996.)

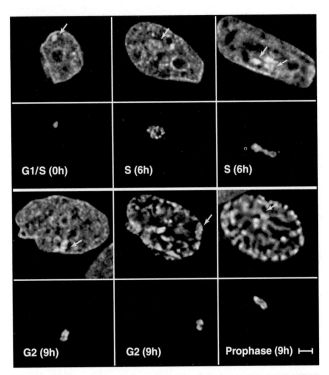

Figure 13-7 DIRECT VISUALIZATION OF CHANGES IN THE COMPACTION AND LOCATION OF A CHROMOSOME ARM IN A LIVING CELL. DNA molecules carrying the binding sites for a specific DNA-binding protein were integrated into the chromosomes of a cell at random and caused to amplify into large arrays, which, in some cases, corresponded to whole chromosome arms. These cells were then induced to express the DNA-binding protein as a fusion to jellyfish green fluorescent protein (GFP). In the lower panel at each time point, the fluorescently labeled chromosome arm can be seen to change both its degree of condensation and its position within the nucleus as a function of the cell cycle. The upper panels show total DNA stained with DAPI. DNA replication occurs in the S phase, which is separated from mitosis (cell division) by the G$_1$ and G$_2$ gap phases (see Chapter 40). These studies are potentially revealing, but they should be interpreted cautiously, as the labeled regions represent artificial arrays of DNA sequence rich in particular binding sites and may not exactly mimic the behavior of natural segments of chromosomes. (From Li G, Sudlow G, Belmont AS: Interphase cell cycle dynamics of a late-replicating, heterochromatic homogeneously staining region: Precise choreography of condensation/decondensation and nuclear positioning. J Cell Biol 140:975–989, 1998.)

region of HP1 contains a motif of 50 amino acids called a **chromodomain** (chromatin modification organizer) that binds to histone H3 methylated on lysine 9. HP1 recruits other proteins, including histone methyltransferases and deacetylases, that further adjust the array of posttranslational modifications on the amino-terminal tails of the histones in order to establish a "closed" chromatin conformation that represses transcription.

HP1 also recruits DNA methyltransferases that modify the underlying DNA by adding a methyl group to the 5′ position on cytosine in the dinucleotide CpG. If methylation occurs near the 5′ promoters of genes (see Chapter 15), in regions with an above average concentration of CpG and referred to as **CpG islands,** it can inactivate gene transcription and promote formation of heterochromatin. Several specific binding proteins recognize DNA containing 5-methyl-cytosine. One of these, methyl cytosine–binding protein (MeCP2), represses expression of nearby genes by recruiting a histone deacetylase complex that removes acetyl groups from the core histone N-terminal tails (Fig. 13-9). A second methyl-CpG-binding protein also binds to HP1, which in turn recruits histone deacetylases and enzymes that methylate histone H3 on lysine 9. This creates more HP1-binding sites and causes the heterochromatin to spread laterally along the chromosome.

Thus, both chromatin and DNA structure contribute to the assembly of heterochromatin. As a result of the interplay between these factors, heterochromatin is richer in histone H3-K9me and methyl-CpG and lower in histone acetylation than active chromatin. All of this promotes a "closed" chromatin structure that is repressive to transcription.

Not all silent chromatin is classical heterochromatin. For example, the polycomb group proteins, which help to confirm the identity of particular body segments during development by regulating the expression of a number of homeodomain transcription factors (see Fig. 15-17), do so by creating an alternative type of "closed" euchromatin environment that is unfavorable for gene transcription.

Polycomb group proteins are found in two complexes: PRC1 and PRC2 (polycomb repressive complex). Polycomb silencing starts with methylation of histone H3 lysine 27 (H3-K27me) by the PRC2 complex. The polycomb protein itself, in the PRC1 complex, has a chromodomain that binds specifically to H3-K27me. Two functions have been proposed for the PRC1 complex. First, its binding causes nucleosomes to form dense clumps that are resistant to remodeling and "opening" by ATP-dependent remodeling "machines." Second, PRC1 contains an E3 ubiquitin ligase activity (see Chapter 23) that transfers a single ubiquitin molecule to lysine119 of histone H2A. Together, these activities do not turn genes on and off; instead, they apparently lock genes that are already off in a silent epigenetic state

that is stable even through many generations of cell division.

Polycomb group proteins also have a role in X chromosome inactivation and facultative heterochromatin formation. In mammals, the *inactive* X chromosome expresses a large (15 kb) RNA called XIST, which encodes no proteins but associates with and "coats" the inactive X chromosome. Shortly after XIST RNA is produced, the PRC2 complex associates with the inactive X, producing H3-K27me and transiently recruiting PRC1, which conjugates ubiquitin to lysine119 of H2A. In addition to ubiquitinated H2A, the inactive X has low levels of histone acetylation, is highly enriched in the H2A variant macroH2A, and has high levels of CpG methylation in many CpG islands. Exactly how this extensive series of epigenetic modifications leads to X inactivation remains to be determined.

Controlling the Influence and Spread of Heterochromatin

Most HP1 is highly mobile in nuclei, moving on a time frame of seconds. Moreover, it recruits chromatin and DNA-modifying enzymes that can act on multiple substrates. As a result, heterochromatin is not a static "closed" chromatin compartment but can "invade" nearby genes along the chromosome. If an actively transcribed gene is moved into close proximity to constitutive heterochromatin by a chromosomal rearrangement, transcription from the gene is repressed as heterochromatin spreads across it (Fig. 13-9). This is called **position effect.**

Naturally occurring regions of chromosomes containing actively transcribed genes are often adjacent to inactive regions that form heterochromatin. How are these genes protected from position effect? This appears to be the role of two types of chromosomal regions: **locus control regions** and **insulators.** Both provide examples in which the epigenetic regulation of gene activity appears to involve formation of large chromatin loops.

Locus control regions (LCRs) have been identified on the basis of their ability to influence the transcriptional activity of cloned DNA sequences in transgenic animals. When genes are introduced into cells in the laboratory, they normally insert at random into the chromosomes. Such inserted test genes are known as *transgenes.* If the transgenes insert into an active chromosomal domain, they are expressed. If they insert into an inactive chromosomal domain, they are repressed. LCRs permit transgenes to be expressed no matter where they insert into the chromosomes, suggesting that these elements create functional domains independent of the surrounding chromosome.

About 20 human LCRs have been identified to date. They generally regulate the proper expression of genes that are expressed only in particular tissues and at

Figure 13-9 USE OF POSITION EFFECT TO ILLUSTRATE THE STEPS IN FORMATION OF HETEROCHROMATIN. If a transcriptionally active gene is moved next to a region of heterochromatin, it is repressed as the heterochromatin spreads. **A,** The relative position of the gene is shown on mitotic chromosomes as it would be determined by in situ hybridization (Fig. 13-15). **B–F,** Diagrammatic representation of the effects of this gene translocation on transcription of the gene during interphase. Stages in the process of heterochromatin formation involve the following: removal of acetyl groups from the histones by a histone deacetylase **(B–C);** addition of two or three methyl groups to lysine 9 of H3 **(D);** binding of HP1, which recruits a DNA methyltransferase plus other heterochromatin proteins **(E);** in heterochromatin the methylation of DNA and the subsequent binding of HP1 plus other heterochromatin proteins **(E–F).** The gene is silent. In this side view, only one of the two turns of DNA around the nucleosome is seen. AC, acetylation; Me, methylation. (Inset, From Fawcett DW: The Cell. Philadelphia, WB Saunders, 1981.)

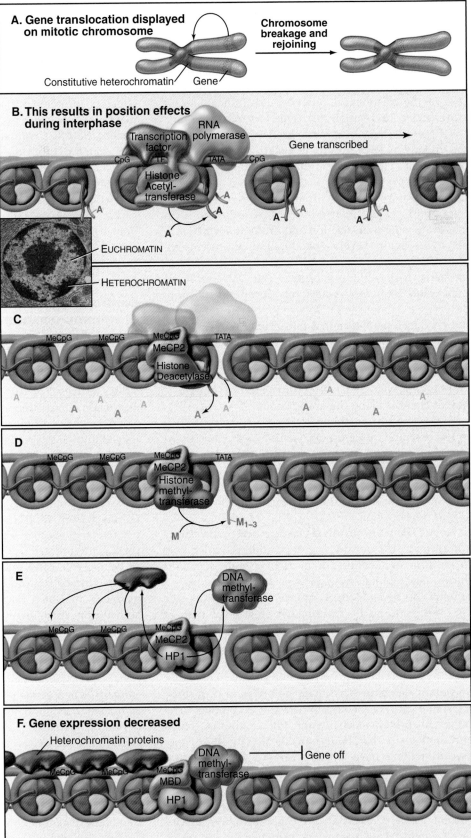

particular times. How they do this is not entirely clear. LCRs typically consist of short regions (often a 150 to 300 base pair stretch of DNA) that are rich in binding sites for transcriptional regulators (see Chapter 14). Somehow, the concerted action of these factors promotes formation of an "open" chromatin region containing acetylated histones that may stretch for thousands of base pairs away from the LCR. Experiments in which a single LCR drives the expression of a cluster of several genes reveal that the LCR stimulates the expression of only one gene at a time. Thus, LCRs appear to work by physically associating with a gene, forming a loop in the chromatin and actively turning on its expression rather than by setting up a broad domain in which gene expression is insulated from the surrounding chromosome.

Insulators are short DNA sequence elements that protect regions of a chromosome from the effects of neighboring regions. In one example in which an active gene cluster borders on a region of heterochromatin, the distribution of H3-K9me characteristic of heterochromatin ends just next to the insulator, which itself is rich in H3 acetylated on K9. Acetylation of lysine 9 blocks the methylation of this residue. Therefore, maintenance of this acetylation is an effective way for the insulator to provide a barrier to the spreading of H3-K9 methylation and thereby limit the spread of the heterochromatin. This insulator also has a number of bind-ing sites for a protein called CCCTC binding factor (CTCF). Binding CTCF to DNA can physically block the DNA from being methylated, providing another defense against the spread of heterochromatin.

In *Drosophila*, protein components of one insulator bind to about 500 sites along the chromosomes. These proteins form about 25 foci near the nuclear envelope in somatic cells. This binding and clustering process causes the DNA between binding sites to form loops. Genes within these loops are thought to be coordinately regulated and insulated from epigenetic effects that act outside the loop.

Imprinting: A Specialized Type of Gene Silencing

The factors described previously are also involved in a second, very specific type of gene silencing known as **imprinting.** An imprinted gene is stably turned off during formation of the egg or sperm. For example, if the maternal copy of a gene is imprinted, then expression can come only from the corresponding homologous chromosome contributed by the father. Currently, about 80 imprinted genes are known.

One well-studied system involves the insulin-like growth factor-2 (IGF2) and H19 genes of the mouse (H19 is an RNA that does not encode for a protein; Fig. 13-10).

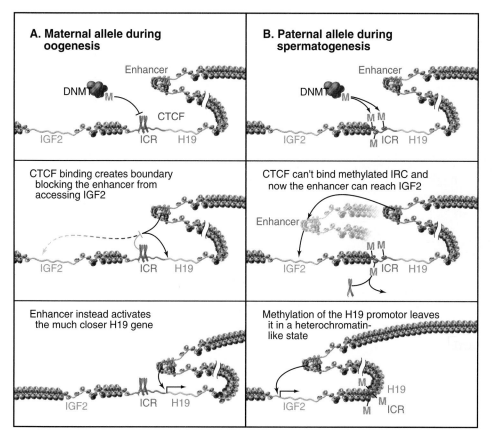

A. Maternal allele during oogenesis

DNMT M

Enhancer

CTCF

IGF2   ICR   H19

CTCF binding creates boundary blocking the enhancer from accessing IGF2

IGF2   ICR   H19

Enhancer instead activates the much closer H19 gene

IGF2   ICR   H19

B. Paternal allele during spermatogenesis

DNMT M

Enhancer

M M

M ICR   H19

IGF2

CTCF can't bind methylated IRC and now the enhancer can reach IGF2

Enhancer

M M

IGF2   M ICR   H19

Methylation of the H19 promotor leaves it in a heterochromatin-like state

H19

M

IGF2   M ICR

Figure 13-10 IMPRINTING OF THE IGF2 AND H19 LOCI. **A,** During oogenesis, CTCF binding to the imprinting control region (ICR) prevents methylation of the DNA. In the zygote, this methylated chromosome from the mother is bound by CTCF, which acts as an insulator, blocking the IGF2 gene from gaining access to its enhancer. As a result, the maternal chromosome expresses H19 and not IGF2. **B,** During spermatogenesis, the ICR is methylated. In the zygote, the ICR on the chromosome derived from the father cannot bind CTCF. As a result, the IGF2 gene gains access to its enhancer and is expressed. The H19 gene is off.

The imprinting control region (ICR) of the DNA that controls these two genes has binding sites for the CTCF protein discussed previously. When CTCF binds to the chromosome derived from the egg, it acts as an insulator element, preventing access of the IGF2 gene to a transcriptional enhancer, keeping it turned off. Under these conditions, the H19 gene is expressed. In chromosomes derived from the sperm, the control region is methylated on CpG sequences. This stops CTCF from binding, and as a result, the paternal copy of IGF2 has access to its enhancer and is expressed. Under these conditions, the H19 gene is not expressed. This simple switch ensures that only the paternal copy of the IGF2 gene and the maternal copy of H19 are expressed in the offspring.

Large-Scale Structural Compartmentation of the Nucleus

Although interphase nuclei lack a high degree of order, a number of general organizational principles are recognized. First, individual chromosomes tend to concentrate within discrete territories and intermingle with one another only to a limited extent. This is seen most clearly in human somatic cell nuclei when individual chromosomes are visualized by a special type of in situ hybridization called chromosome painting (Fig. 13-11). Actively transcribing genes are frequently located on the surface of territories occupied by individual chromosomes. However, in some cases, active genes can be located well outside of the territories, as though their activation involved looping out a much larger domain from the remainder of the chromosome. In some cases, this movement during gene activation involves relocation from regions ("compartments") of the nucleus

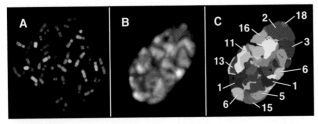

Figure 13-11 CHROMOSOMES OCCUPY DISCRETE TERRITORIES IN INTERPHASE NUCLEI. **A,** Metaphase chromosome labeled by fluorescence in situ hybridization (FISH) using chromosome paint probes (probes distributed all along the chromosome, excluding repetitive DNA). In this 24-color FISH image, every chromosome is marked with two or three fluorochromes (true color image). **B,** The same combinatorial probe was used in 24-color FISH on a fibroblast nucleus under conditions preserving the 3D architecture. Every chromosome forms distinct chromosome territory. **C,** Every chromosome territory of the same nuclear optical section as on B was identified and false-colored after classification. (Images courtesy of I. Solovei, A. Bolzer, and T. Cremer, University of Munich, LMU, Germany.)

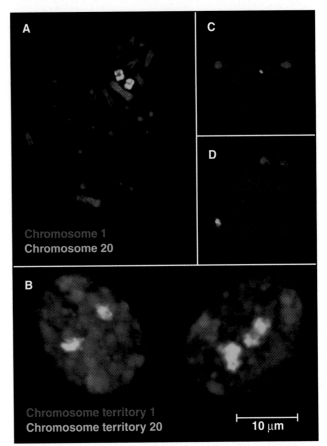

Figure 13-12 CHROMOSOME POSITION IN THE NUCLEUS CORRELATES WITH TRANSCRIPTIONAL ACTIVITY. **A,** Metaphase chromosome spread from a healthy donor with painted chromosomes 1 *(red)* and 20 *(green)*. **B,** The same paint probes were used in FISH experiments on three-dimensionally preserved fibroblast nuclei (3D-FISH): they revealed two pairs of chromosome territories. Note the more central positioning of small-size chromosome 20 territories and the more peripheral positioning of chromosome 1 territories. **C–D,** The CD4 gene *(green)* is located in the nucleoplasm in cells where it is expressed **(C)** but is associated with centromeric heterochromatin in cells where it is silent **(D).** (A and B, Courtesy of I. Solovei, A. Bolzer, and T. Cremer, University of Munich, LMU, Germany. C–D, From Lamond AI, Earnshaw WC: Structure and function in the nucleus. Science 280:547–553, 1998; and Brown KE, Guest SS, Smale ST, et al: Association of transcriptionally silent genes with Ikaros complexes at centromeric heterochromatin. Cell 91(6): 845–854, 1997.)

where transcription is relatively infrequent into areas where transcription is favored (Fig. 13-12C–D).

Second, heterochromatin tends to be concentrated near the nuclear periphery in a wide range of cell types. This was the first indication that particular chromosomal regions might have preferred locations within the nucleus. Subsequent studies confirmed that the distribution of chromosomes within interphase nuclei is not random. Rather, chromosomes that are rich in actively transcribed genes tend to be localized toward the interior of the nucleus, while chromosomes with a lower gene content tend to be found near the nuclear periphery (Fig. 13-12A).

A much less well resolved issue is whether chromosomes change their positions within nuclei as cells traverse the cell cycle or undergo more long-term developmental programs. In human lymphocytes, centromeres tend to cluster together near the periphery of the nucleus during the G_1 phase of the cell cycle. During the S phase, they tend to be more dispersed and in the nuclear interior. These movements of chromosome domains depend on actin and myosin, but the detailed mechanism is not known.

Higher-Order Structure of Chromosomes

Special Interphase Chromosomes with Clearly Resolved Structures

Studies of specialized chromosomes from organisms ranging from flies to mammals suggest that chromosomes have large-scale structural domains composed of loops containing thousands to millions of base pairs. Such loop domains are clearly seen in **lampbrush chromosomes,** found during meiotic prophase in oocytes of many species (Fig. 13-13A). Lampbrush chromosome loops are sites of intense transcriptional activity as oocytes stockpile huge stores of the components needed for rapid cell division during early development of the fertilized egg. The loops are easily seen because the DNA is coated with many RNA transcripts, together with proteins that package them.

Similar loops can be seen in the giant **polytene chromosomes** found in some tissues of *Drosophila* larvae. Each polytene chromosome consists of more than 1000 identical DNA molecules packed side by side in precise linear register. Light microscopy reveals that polytene chromosomes have a complex pattern of thousands of bands (Fig. 13-13B–D) representing

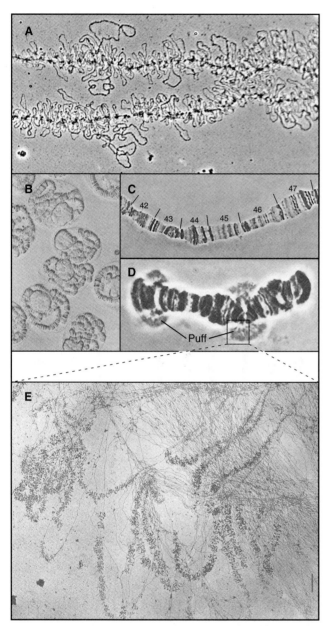

Figure 13-13 CHROMATIN LOOPS IN SPECIAL INTERPHASE CHROMOSOMES. **A,** Phase contrast view of the left end of meiotic lampbrush chromosome 6 from the newt *Notophthalmus viridescens*. **B–D,** Domain organization of polytene chromosomes. Once fly larvae achieve a certain size, most cells stop dividing, and larval growth proceeds via an increase in the size of individual cells. To keep the protein synthesis machinery of these huge cells supplied with messenger RNA, DNA replication is uncoupled from cell division so that ultimately, the cells contain many times the normal complement of cellular DNA (i.e., they are *polyploid*). In certain tissues, the numerous copies of the chromosomes are maintained in strict alignment with respect to one another, making giant *polytene* chromosomes, the best-known of which occur in the salivary gland. **B,** Giant polytene chromosomes are visible within isolated salivary gland nuclei. **C,** A portion of a high-resolution map of the *Drosophila* polytene chromosomes. **D,** Polytene chromosome showing puffs. The *inset box* shows an area analogous to that used in panel **E. E,** Electron micrograph of puff showing transcribing DNA loops. These loops are covered with a "fuzz" corresponding to growing RNA chains coated with proteins. (A, Reproduced from Roth MB, Gall JG: Monoclonal antibodies that recognize transcription unit proteins on newt lampbrush chromosomes. J Cell Biol 105:1047–1054, 1987. B, From Robert M: Isolation and manipulation of salivary gland nuclei and chromosomes. Methods Cell Biol 9:377–390, 1975. C, Courtesy of Margarete Heck, University of Edinburgh, Scotland. D, From Andersson K, Mahr R, Bjorkroth B, et al: Rapid reformation of the thick chromosome fiber upon completion of RNA synthesis at the Balbiani ring genes in Chironomus tentans. Chromosoma 87:33–48, 1982. E, From Lamb MM, Daneholt B: Characterization of active transcription units in Balbiani rings of Chironomus tentans. Cell 17:835–848, 1979.)

domains of differentially compacted chromatin. Each band contains one or several genes and potentially constitutes a domain for gene expression. Stress or stimulation of gene expression by hormones causes certain bands to lose their compact shape and puff out laterally. Such **puffs** are composed of hundreds of identical chromatin loop domains, all being actively transcribed (Fig. 13-13E).

Higher-Order Structure of Mitotic Chromosomes

Although polytene chromosomes provide the clearest demonstration of structural domains along an interphase chromosome, the arms of typical diploid mitotic chromosomes also appear to have a domain substructure. This can be seen when mammalian chromosomes are subjected to G-banding (Fig. 13-14). G-banded human chromosomes from the early (prometaphase) stage of mitosis have up to 2000 discrete bands. Although the structural basis for the bands is not known, dark G-bands tend to be relatively enriched for A : T residues, poor in genes, and rich in LINE elements (see Fig. 12-5) and tend to replicate later in S phase than light G-bands (also called R, or reverse, bands). Cytogeneticists have used these highly reproducible banding patterns for years to identify individual human chromosomes and even portions thereof.

This reproducibility of higher-order structure in mitotic chromosomes is also easily seen when specific DNA sequences are marked by in situ hybridization. When individual loci are highlighted by this method, they appear as pairs of spots on the sister chromatids (Fig. 13-15). The two spots are distributed symmetrically, indicating that the chromatin fiber is folded similarly in both chromatids.

Three broad classes of models try to explain how the chromatin fiber is organized in mitotic chromosomes. Hierarchical coiling models suggest that the 30-nm chromatin fiber coils on itself, reaching larger and larger diameters and higher degrees of compaction. Large chromatin fibers (~100 nm in diameter) can be seen in early prophase, as chromosome condensation begins (see Chapter 44). These models postulate that the final condensed mitotic chromosome forms by coiling up this fiber.

Loop domain models suggest that chromatin loops, containing an average of 15,000 to 100,000 base pairs, provide the structural basis for large-scale chromatin compaction in mitotic chromosomes. If metaphase chromosomes are swelled in hypotonic solutions, it is readily apparent that loops of chromatin radiate outward from the central chromatid axis (Fig. 13-16C). Similarly, if stripped of histones, isolated metaphase chromosomes consist of an enormous pool of DNA surrounding a residual structure that retains the general shape of chro-

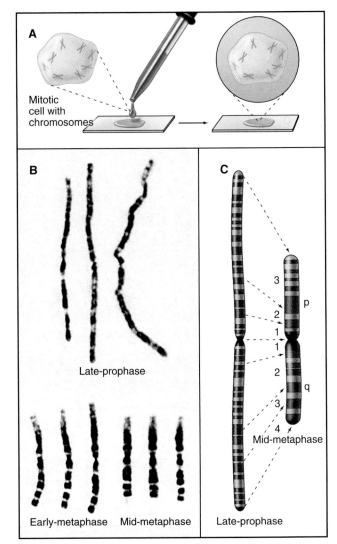

Figure 13-14 CHROMOSOME BANDING REVEALS THE COMPLEX AND REPRODUCIBLE MULTIDOMAIN SUBSTRUCTURE OF MITOTIC CHROMOSOME ARMS. **A,** Mitotic cells in a hyprotic medium are dropped on a slide to spread the chromosomes. In G-banding, chromosomes are given harsh treatments, such as exposure to concentrated sodium hydroxide, proteases, or high temperatures, and then are stained with Giemsa dye. The chromosome arms then exhibit a characteristic pattern of light and dark bands. **B,** Photographs of G-banded human chromosome 2 from cells in late prophase, early metaphase, and mid-metaphase. Several examples are shown for each stage, illustrating the reproducibility of the banding patterns. **C,** Diagram summarizing the metaphase and prophase patterns. Because G-banding patterns are reproducible, this technique provides a way to identify individual chromosomes unambiguously. This was a major factor in the development of the field of cytogenetics, which is the study of the correlation between the structure of the chromosomes and genetics. (B–C, Adapted from Yunis JJ, Sawyer JR, Ball DW: The characterization of high-resolution G-banded chromosomes of man. Chromosoma 67:293–307, 1978.)

mosome arms. In certain cases, it is possible to trace individual loops of DNA radiating outward from the central structure (Fig. 13-16B). Similar looped structures can be seen if interphase nuclei are depleted of histones.

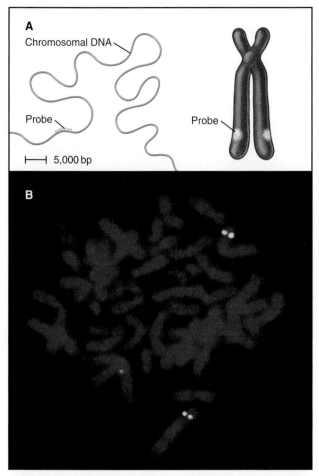

A

Chromosomal DNA

Probe

Probe

├──┤ 5,000 bp

B

Figure 13-15 FLUORESCENCE IN SITU HYBRIDIZATION PERFORMED ON MITOTIC CHROMOSOMES. **A,** Chromosomes are spread on a slide as in Figure 13-14. Following chemical fixation steps to preserve the chromosomal structure, the chromosomal proteins are removed by digestion with proteases and the genomic DNA strands are melted (separated) by heating. Next, a "probe DNA" *(yellow)* is added. This probe DNA is single-stranded so that it can base-pair (hybridize) to its complementary sequences in the chromosome. The probe DNA is chemically labeled with biotin. Next, the sites of hybridization on the chromosomes are detected with fluorescently labeled avidin, a protein from egg white that binds to biotin with extremely high affinity. The sites of avidin-binding appear *yellow,* whereas the remainder of the chromosomal DNA is counterstained with a *red* dye. **B,** The micrograph shows FISH analysis using a probe from near the von Hippel Lindau locus on chromosome 3. (B, Courtesy of Jeanne Lawrence, University of Massachusetts, Amherst.)

A third class of model combines aspects of the first two models. This proposes that most of the condensation of the chromatin occurs through hierarchical coiling or folding of the ~100-nm fiber. During the final stages of folding, key proteins that later make up the mitotic chromosome scaffold (see later) become concentrated along the axial regions of the condensing chromosome arms (Fig. 13-16A). These proteins cross-link chromatin into a network that stabilizes the overall structure. If cross-links form at intervals, the chromatin

between the cross-links forms loops that are seen if the chromosome is expanded or extracted. This model explains most available data, but the question of chromatin folding in chromosomes remains an area of active investigation and controversy.

Role of Nonhistone Proteins in Mitotic Chromosome Structure and Function

Mitotic chromosomes are composed of roughly equal weights of DNA, histones and **nonhistone proteins.** For many years, a controversy raged over whether mitotic chromosome structure was determined solely by levels of successive packing interactions of chromatin fibers (i.e., histones and DNA) or whether other specialized nonhistone proteins were involved. It is now clear that nonhistone proteins play an essential role in chromosome structure and function.

Early evidence suggesting that nonhistone proteins might contribute to mitotic chromosome structure came from experiments in which chromosomes were treated with nucleases to remove the DNA and extracted to remove most chromosomal proteins, including essentially all of the histones. The surviving remnant of the chromosome contained about 5% of the proteins and less than 0.1% of the DNA but still looked like a chromosome (Fig. 13-17). If the DNA was not digested, loops of DNA protruded from the protein mass (Fig. 13-16B). This protein remnant was called the **chromosome scaffold** because it looked like the structural backbone for the metaphase chromosome. This mechanical function is still disputed, but chromosome scaffold preparations contain a number of proteins with essential roles in the structure and maintenance of chromosomes.

The Nuclear Matrix

If isolated nuclei are subjected to the procedures that are used to isolate mitotic chromosome scaffolds (i.e., digestion with nucleases and extraction of the bulk of the histones), a residual structure is also obtained. This material has been termed the **nuclear matrix** or **nucleoskeleton.** The composition of nuclear matrix is distinct from the chromosome scaffold. A number of its most abundant components are proteins that package nuclear RNAs, which are absent from mitotic chromosomes. The function of the nuclear matrix remains controversial. It is possible that components of this remnant of the nucleus could be responsible for organizing chromosome territories and chromatin loops. On the other hand, many argue that the nuclear matrix is an artifact created by precipitation of nuclear proteins during the extraction procedure.

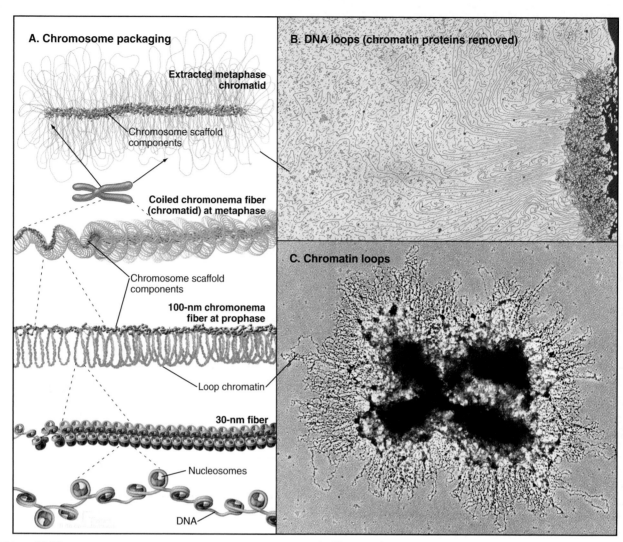

Figure 13-16 **CURRENT MODELS OF MITOTIC CHROMOSOME STRUCTURE. A,** Filament of nucleosomes, 30-nm fiber, chromonema fiber, coiled chromonema fiber. Nonhistone proteins complexes *(red dots)* bind and end up concentrated along the central axis of the chromatid arm. Cross-links between these complexes create the chromosome scaffold. When chromosomes are swollen or extracted, the scaffold remains compact, and loops of chromatin or DNA radiate out from it. **B,** DNA loops seen in a human mitotic chromosome from which the histones had been removed. **C,** Human chromosome showing loop domains. (B, From Paulson JR, Laemmli UK: The structure of histone-depleted chromosomes. Cell 12:817–828, 1977. C, Courtesy of William C. Earnshaw.)

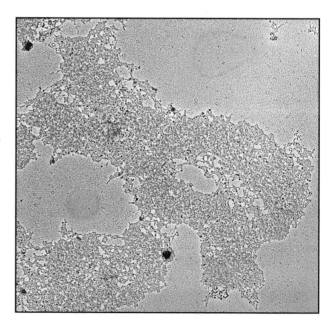

Figure 13-17 **ELECTRON MICROGRAPH OF THE ISOLATED HUMAN META-PHASE CHROMOSOME SCAFFOLD.** This preparation was centrifuged onto a thin carbon film and rotary-shadowed with Pt : Pd. This structure, which is about 95% protein, retains the overall shape of the mitotic chromosome. (Micrograph courtesy of William C. Earnshaw.)

DNA Sequences Associated with the Chromosome Scaffold and Nuclear Matrix

Loop domain models of mitotic chromosomes predict that the DNA might attach to the scaffold at specific sites. **Scaffold/matrix attachment regions (S/MARs)** are regions of DNA that associate preferentially with the nuclear matrix and chromosome scaffold in biochemical fractionation experiments (Fig. 13-18). In one example, when over 900,000 contiguous base pairs of the genome of the fruit fly *Drosophila melanogaster* were examined for the presence of S/MARs, 16 DNA regions, spaced 15,000 to 115,000 base pairs apart, showed a strong interaction with the nuclear matrix in vitro. The spacing to these sites roughly corresponds to the predicted size of loop domains in nuclei and chromosomes.

S/MARs contain runs of A or T, which give DNA a characteristically narrow minor groove, but they lack other conserved DNA sequences. Evidence for a functional role of S/MAR sequences in chromosome structure has come from experiments in which 20 copies of a protein domain that binds to runs of A and T (called an A-T hook) connected by flexible linkers were polymerized to make an artificial super–S/MAR-binding protein. This artificial protein inhibited mitotic chromosome condensation, suggesting that interactions between components bound to S/MARs may be important for higher-order organization of chromosomes.

Tests of the role of S/MARs in vivo have yielded equivocal results. S/MARs do not generally act as LCRs or insulators. S/MARs therefore remain enigmatic candidates for sequences that might possibly define structural domains within the chromosome.

Proteins of the Mitotic Chromosome and Chromosome Scaffold

One family of chromosome scaffold proteins called **SMC proteins** has several important roles in chromosome dynamics. The name derives from their roles in the *structural maintenance of chromosomes*. SMC proteins are components of multiprotein complexes that are essential for mitotic chromosome structure, the regulation of sister chromatid pairing, DNA repair and replication, and the regulation of gene expression. This section discusses two of these complexes: **condensin** and **cohesin.**

The name *condensin* is self-explanatory but is actually misleading. This complex of five polypeptides was originally thought to be essential for mitotic chromosome condensation. The role of the complex is now known to be more subtle, since chromosomes can condense in its absence. Condensin is composed of two SMC proteins (SMC2 and SMC4), plus three auxiliary

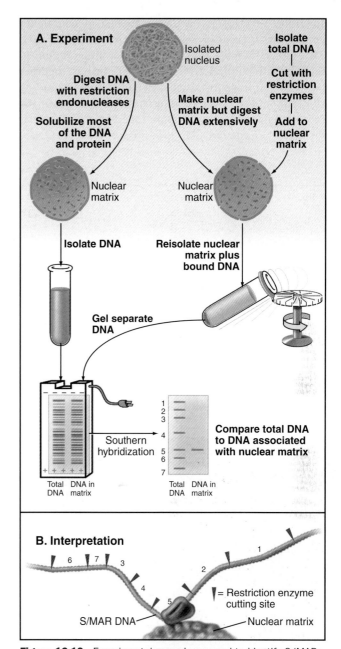

Figure 13-18 Experimental procedures used to identify S/MARs. These are regions associated with the nuclear matrix or chromosome scaffold in vitro. **A, left,** DNA of isolated nuclei is digested with restriction endonucleases. Most DNA and proteins are solubilized; the DNA that remains is separated by agarose gel electrophoresis and transferred to a membrane for analysis by Southern blotting. In this method, restriction fragments from a cloned region of genomic DNA (*numbers* in **A** and **B**) are labeled with radioactivity and hybridized to DNA on the membrane, similar to the method in Fig. 13-15. **Right,** DNA of isolated nuclei is digested extensively with restriction endonucleases. Most of the DNA and proteins are solubilized. Next, the same restriction fragments from the cloned region of genomic DNA used in the experiment on the left are mixed with the nuclear matrix under conditions where they can rebind to matrix proteins. Unbound DNA is washed away, and the bound sequences are detected by Southern blotting. **B,** From the restriction map of the chromosomal region used to prepare the probes, it is possible to identify the fragment(s) that bind preferentially to the nuclear matrix. Such fragments contain S/MARs. Both approaches give the same answer.

subunits. Vertebrates have two condensin complexes containing alternative sets of auxiliary subunits. Each SMC molecule folds back on itself at a hinge region to form an antiparallel coiled-coil. This brings together two globular domains, each with half of an ATP-binding site (Fig. 13-19C). ATP binding is thought to cause the two globular domains to come together. Condensin is formed when the two SMC proteins associate with each other via their hinges and the auxiliary subunits bind to the globular regions of the molecule.

Condensin binds to chromosomes only during mitosis when it is concentrated along the central axis of chromosome arms. The cell cycle kinase Cdk1:cyclin B (see Chapter 40) regulates condensin binding to chromosomes by phosphorylation of an auxiliary subunit. When condensin binds to naked DNA in a test tube, it is able

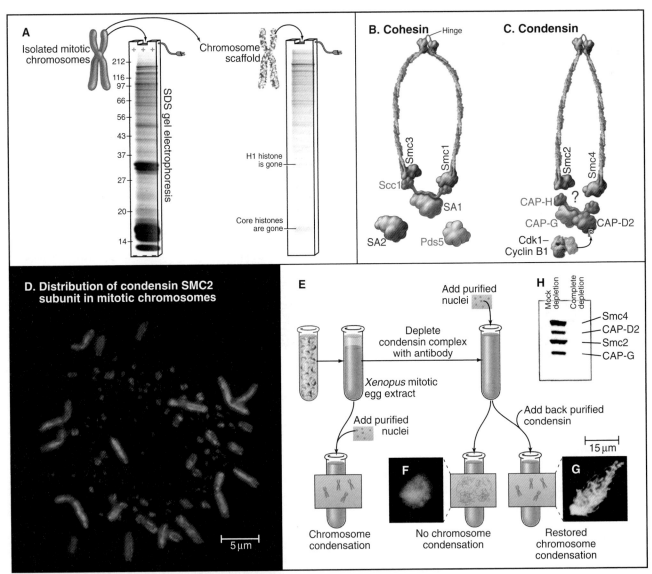

Figure 13-19 CONDENSIN AND COHESIN COMPLEXES HAVE ESSENTIAL ROLES IN CHROMOSOME STRUCTURE AND FUNCTION. **A,** Isolation of the mitotic chromosome scaffold. **Left,** SDS polyacrylamide gel of total chromosomal proteins (see Box 6-3). **Right,** Most proteins are solubilized by the protocol used to make chromosome scaffolds. Remaining proteins include components of the condensin complex and DNA topoisomerase IIα. **B–C,** Subunit composition and structural organization of the cohesin and condensin complexes. Condensin is regulated by phosphorylation of the CAP-D2 subunit by Cdk1:cyclin B kinase. **D,** Immunofluorescence micrograph showing the distribution of condensin subunit SMC2 on mitotic chromosomes of the chicken. The tiny chromosomes, called microchromosomes, are commonly seen in normal bird chromosomes. **E,** The experimental protocol showing that condensin is required for mitotic chromosome condensation in vitro. **F,** Chromatin lacking condensin does not form mitotic chromosomes in vitro, and this is restored by adding back condensin. **G–H,** SDS polyacrylamide gel reveals the members of the condensin complex and demonstrates that they can be depleted from egg extract using a specific antibody. (A [gel] and D [micrograph], Courtesy of William C. Earnshaw. F–H, From Hirano T, Kobayashi R, Hirano M: Condensins, chromosome condensation protein complexes containing XCAP-C, XCAP-E and a *Xenopus* homolog of the *Drosophila* Barren protein. Cell 89:511–521, 1997.)

to use the energy of ATP hydrolysis to supercoil the DNA, possibly by coiling DNA around itself. The role of this activity is unknown, because vertebrate chromosomes can condense to a normal extent in the absence of condensin. However, those chromosomes are fragile, lack a chromosome scaffold if extracted as described previously, and lose their orderly structure while trying to segregate in anaphase. It now appears that condensin regulates the timing of chromosome condensation and cooperates with other nonhistone proteins to stabilize chromosome structure throughout mitosis. Chromosomes lacking condensin can segregate normally at anaphase under specialized conditions.

Cohesin is the second major SMC-containing protein complex of mitotic chromosomes. Cohesin is a tetramer containing SMC1 and SMC3 plus two auxiliary subunits. One of these, Scc1, is cleaved by a protease called separase to initiate the separation of sister chromatids in mitotic anaphase (see Fig. 44-16). Cohesin, like condensin, is a ring-like molecule (Fig. 13-19). How cohesin holds the two sister chromatids together is not known, though given its ring-like structure, it might physically encircle two sister DNA molecules. Cohesin assembles on chromosomes during DNA replication and is recruited to regions of heterochromatin by HP1. Sister chromatid cohesion and mitotic segregation are defective in fission yeast with mutations in their HP1 ortholog.

DNA topoisomerase IIα, an enzyme that alters DNA topology by passing one double-helix strand through another, is also an abundant component of the mitotic chromosome scaffold fraction. In mitosis, topoisomerase IIα is concentrated at centromeres and in axial regions along the chromosome arms. Topoisomerase IIα is unlikely to have a structural role in chromosomes, as the protein is very dynamic in vivo, moving on and off of chromosomes in a time frame of seconds. Furthermore, mitotic chromosomes from cells lacking topoisomerase II look normal. However, topoisomerase II is required for replicated sister chromatids to separate from one another during mitotic anaphase. Presumably, the enzyme separates tangles and intertwinings of DNA created during DNA replication.

Chromosome scaffolds contain several hundred other proteins, including components of the kinetochore to be discussed next. Few other scaffold proteins have known functions.

Specialized Chromosomal Substructures: The Kinetochore

Embedded in the surface of the centromeric heterochromatin of most eukaryotes is a button-like structure called the **kinetochore,** which directs chromosomal movements in mitosis (Fig. 13-20). When a thin section of the centromere is examined by electron microscopy,

the kinetochore appears to have a number of layers. The **inner kinetochore** is continuous with the surface of the centromeric heterochromatin and is composed of a specialized form of chromatin. The **outer kinetochore** consists of an **outer plate** with a **fibrous corona** on its outer surface. It is constructed from protein complexes that link the chromatin to microtubules of the mitotic spindle. Kinetochores also include protein complexes that form signaling pathways to regulate the progression of the cell through mitosis without errors (see Fig. 44-11).

The multilayered kinetochore structure is visible only during mitosis. During interphase, the centromere persists as a condensed ball of heterochromatin that resembles other areas of condensed chromatin within the nucleus. The distinct kinetochore structure forms on the surface of the centromere during an early stage of mitosis called prophase (see Chapter 44), reaching its mature state following nuclear envelope breakdown when the chromosome comes into contact with microtubules at the onset of mitotic prometaphase.

Chapter 12 describes the three types of centromeres known in eukaryotes. Point centromeres found in budding yeasts assemble on defined DNA sequences and do not require epigenetic activation to function. They bind one microtubule. Regional centromeres, found in organisms ranging from fission yeast to humans, are based on preferred DNA sequences but require epigenetic activation in order to function. They bind 2 to 20 or more microtubules. In holocentromeres, as found in *Caenorhabditis elegans* and many insects, the underlying DNA sequences are unknown, and the microtubules (roughly 20 in *C. elegans*) bind all along the poleward-

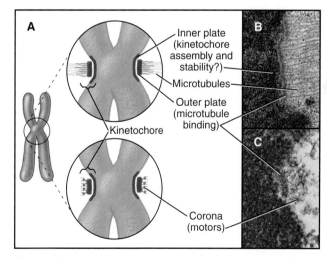

Figure 13-20 **KINETOCHORE STRUCTURE. A,** A diagram of the major layers of the kinetochore. **B,** Thin-section electron micrograph of a kinetochore with attached microtubules. **C,** Thin-section micrograph of an unattached kinetochore (B, Courtesy of J. B. Rattner, University of Calgary, Canada. C, Courtesy of Rebecca L. Bernat and William C. Earnshaw.)

facing surface of the mitotic chromosome. Given this diversity of centromeres, it is remarkable that the proteins responsible for centromere assembly and function are well conserved across evolution.

Centromere Proteins of the Budding Yeast

Binding of specialized proteins to CEN DNA sequences nucleates the formation of budding yeast kinetochores. Other protein complexes then bind, thereby establishing a structure that integrates the binding to microtubules with the signaling network that monitors this binding. Over 65 kinetochore-associated proteins are now known in budding yeast, giving the structure at least the size and complexity of a ribosome.

Two sorts of factors bind to centromere DNA. First are CBFs, DNA-binding complexes that recognize the specific CDE I and CDE III DNA sequences that specify the point centromere (see Fig. 12-7). This binding occurs on the surface of a specialized nucleosome, which is marked by a centromere-specific histone H3 variant related to CENP-A (Fig. 13-21). CDE I and CDE III are juxtaposed on this nucleosome and linked by a stretch of A : T-rich DNA called CDE II, which completes one turn around the nucleosome.

Several large complexes bind to this nucleosome/CBF platform (Fig. 13-21). Since the kinetochore is a large integrated structure, the exact complexes that are obtained when it is fractionated vary from study to study as different methods are employed. The 11-subunit Ctf19 complex links the inner and outer kinetochore. The four components of the NDC80 complex are highly conserved in organisms from budding yeast to humans and are required for chromosomes to make robust attachments to microtubules. The Dam1 complex (10 subunits) appears to make the final attachment to the microtubule. This complex has been poorly conserved during evolution, and its vertebrate counterpart has yet to be identified.

Another conserved group of proteins that bind to the kinetochore includes components of the mitotic checkpoint pathway—a signaling network that causes mitotic progression to pause until all chromosomes make suitable connections to both spindle poles of the mitotic spindle (see Fig. 44-11).

Mammalian Centromere Proteins

The first three specific centromere proteins identified in any species were discovered in humans using autoantibodies present in the sera of certain individuals with rheumatic disease (Figs. 13-22 and 13-23). These pro-

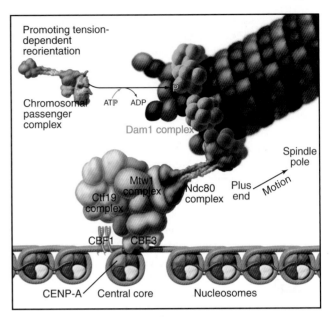

Figure 13-21 HYPOTHETICAL MODEL FOR THE ORGANIZATION OF THE BUDDING YEAST KINETOCHORE. The organization of the DNA in the budding yeast point kinetochore is discussed in Chapter 12.

teins, designated CENPs A–C, are conserved from humans to yeasts. CENPs A–C are components of the inner kinetochore, to which they remain bound throughout the cell cycle. As was mentioned previously, **CENP-A** is a histone H3 variant, so the regional centromere, like the point centromere, must be based on modified nucleosomes. How CENP-A selects the DNA that it assembles into kinetochore-specific nucleosomes is unknown.

CENP-B probably originated as the enzyme responsible for movement of an ancient transposon. CENP-B binds specifically to a 17–base pair sequence (the CENP-B box) in α-satellite DNA (Fig. 13-23A). CENP-B is required for the efficient establishment of the epigenetic state that favors kinetochore assembly on α-satellite DNA arrays, but how it acts is unknown.

CENP-C, the third protein recognized by the autoimmune sera, is an essential DNA-binding protein involved in assembly of the kinetochore plate. CENP-C requires prior binding of CENP-A to localize and function correctly. CENP-C appears to function as a bridge between the inner and outer kinetochore.

At present, at least 40 mammalian kinetochore proteins are known (Fig. 13-23B). As in the budding yeast, these are organized into protein complexes. One such complex of 10 proteins contains all four members of the NDC10 complex plus six other components. This NDC10-associated complex is found at both human and *C. elegans* kinetochores. Under some conditions, it is possible to find an association of CENP-C with this complex, raising the possibility that CENP-C might

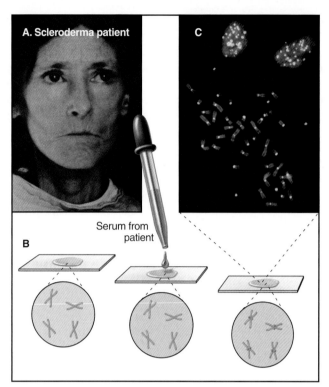

Figure 13-22 SOME PATIENTS WITH SCLERODERMA HAVE AUTOANTIBODIES THAT RECOGNIZE CENTROMERIC PROTEINS. Scleroderma ("hard skin") is a serious connective tissue disease associated with excessive deposition of collagen in the skin and walls of blood vessels. Note the "purse string" appearance of the skin surrounding the mouth of this patient **(A)**. When serum from a patient with anticentromere antibodies is added to chromosomes on a slide **(B)** and bound antibodies are detected with a fluorescent probe, the centromeric regions of the chromosomes "light up" **(C)**. Anticentromere antibodies are useful to identify patients who are at risk for serious autoimmune disease. Up to 20% of the population has a mild condition—Raynaud's phenomenon (hypersensitivity of the skin to cold)—that is occasionally a precursor to scleroderma. Sensitive assays for anticentromere antibodies revealed that patients with Raynaud's phenomenon who also have these autoantibodies have an increased risk of progression to scleroderma. (A, Reprinted from the American College of Rheumatology Clinical Slide Collection on the Rheumatic Diseases. Slide 21, Chapter 10. Atlanta, Georgia, ACR, 1997. C, Courtesy of William C. Earnshaw.)

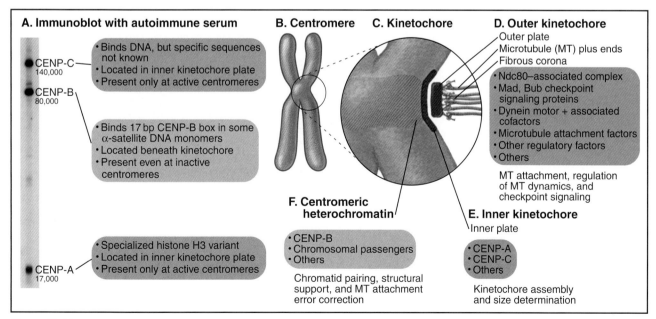

Figure 13-23 HUMAN CENTROMERE PROTEIN AUTOANTIGENS. **A,** Centrome proteins (CENPs) detected with anticentromere antibodies from a scleroderma patient on an immunoblot following SDS gel electrophoresis of chromosomal proteins. **B–F,** Localization of centromere protein complexes in the vertebrate kinetochore. (A, Immunoblot courtesy of William C. Earnshaw.)

anchor NDC10 to the specialized chromatin of the inner kinetochore.

Human NDC10-associated complex members associate with kinetochores during prophase, as cells are about to enter mitosis, and disappear from kinetochores at the end of mitosis. Functional analysis reveals that the NDC10-associated complex links the inner centromere to the microtubules of the mitotic spindle. Components of the complex are also required for the signaling components of the mitotic checkpoint to associate with kinetochores (see Fig. 44-11). The proteins that actually link kinetochores to the spindle microtubules remain unknown.

Role of RNAi at Centromeres

The fission yeast *Schizosaccharomyces pombe* has the simplest well-characterized regional centromere, and assembles a kinetochore that binds two to four microtubules. Fission yeast have orthologs of all the proteins and protein complexes described previously, together with a number of components that have yet to be described elsewhere. The fission yeast centromere provides the simplest example of centromeric heterochromatin. A major breakthrough came with the discoveries that the "silent" repeated DNA in the *S. pombe* centromere is transcribed and processed by the RNAi machinery and that this RNAi response is essential for assembly of centromeric heterochromatin. A wide range of *S. pombe* mutants affecting the RNAi machinery all compromise centromere function and mitotic chromosome segregation.

Whether RNAi is also essential for centromere function in metazoans has been more difficult to determine, as there are multiple redundancies in the genes encoding the RNAi machinery. This complicates genetic analysis. However, careful analysis reveals that centromeric satellite DNAs are indeed transcribed and that an essential component of the RNAi machinery is required for heterochromatin assembly in vertebrate cells. Cells that lack this component are defective at assembling heterochromatin and properly localizing the cohesin complex (see earlier discussion). The outcome is failure of chromosome segregation and cell death. Thus, the role of RNAi in assembly of centromeric heterochromatin is conserved from yeast to vertebrates.

Conclusions

The turn of the millennium was a very exciting time for the study of chromosome assembly and structure. Ironically, just as the sequence of euchromatic portion of the human genome was completed, an explosion in our understanding revealed that essential aspects of the control of gene activity and chromosome structure cannot be revealed by analysis of the DNA sequence alone, since these regulatory processes are "encoded" in transient epigenetic modifications of DNA and histones. Understanding the extraordinarily elaborate epigenetic code has only just begun, so watch this space for further exciting developments.

ACKNOWLEDGMENTS

Thanks go to Robin Allshire, Wendy Bickmore, Thomas Cremer and students, Irina Solovei, Bryan Turner, and Jerry Workman for their suggestions on revisions to this chapter.

SELECTED READINGS

Amor DJ, Kalitsis P, Sumer H, Choo KH: Building the centromere: From foundation proteins to 3D organization. Trends Cell Biol 14:359-368, 2004.

Belmont AS: Visualizing chromosome dynamics with GFP. Trends Cell Biol 11:250-257, 2001.

Belmont AS: Mitotic chromosome scaffold structure: New approaches to an old controversy. Proc Natl Acad Sci U S A 99:15855-15857, 2002.

Bird AP, Wolffe AP: Methylation-induced repression: Belts, braces, and chromatin. Cell 99:451-454, 1999.

Flaus A, Owen-Hughes T: Mechanisms for ATP-dependent chromatin remodelling: Farewell to the tuna-can octamer? Curr Opin Genet Dev 14:165-173, 2004.

Francis, NJ, Kingston RE: Mechanisms of transcriptional memory. Nat Rev Mol Cell Biol 2:409-421, 2001.

Gassmann R, Vagnarelli P, Hudson D, Earnshaw WC: Mitotic chromosome formation and the condensin paradox. Exp Cell Res 296:35-42, 2004.

Grewal SI, Moazed D: Heterochromatin and epigenetic control of gene expression. Science 301:798-802, 2003.

Henikoff A, Ahmad K: Assembly of variant histones into chromatin. Annu Rev Cell Dev Biol 21:133-153, 2005.

Hirano T: The ABCs of SMC proteins: Two-armed ATPases for chromosome condensation, cohesion, and repair. Genes Dev 16:399-414, 2002.

Khorasanizadeh S: The nucleosome: From genomic organization to genomic regulation. Cell 116:259-272, 2004.

Labrador M, Corces VG: Setting the boundaries of chromatin domains and nuclear organization. Cell 111:151-154, 2002.

Maiato H, Deluca J, Salmon ED, Earnshaw WC: The dynamic kinetochore-microtubule interface. J Cell Sci 117:5461-5477, 2004.

Naar AM, Lemon BD, Tjian R: Transcriptional coactivator complexes. Annu Rev Biochem 70:475-501, 2001.

Otte AP, Kwaks TH: Gene repression by polycomb group protein complexes: A distinct complex for every occasion? Curr Opin Genet Dev 13:448-454, 2003.

Strahl BD, Allis CD: The language of covalent histone modifications. Nature 403:41-45, 2000.

Swedlow JR, Hirano T: The making of the mitotic chromosome: Modern insights into classical questions. Mol Cell 11:557-569, 2003.

West AG, Gaszner M, Felsenfeld G: Insulators: Many functions, many mechanisms. Genes Dev 16:271-288, 2002.

Workman JL, Kingston RE: Alteration of nucleosome structure as a mechanism of transcriptional regulation. Annu Rev Biochem 67:545-579, 1998.

Nuclear Structure and Dynamics

The nucleus houses the chromosomes together with the machinery for DNA replication and RNA transcription and processing (Fig. 14-1). Immature RNAs must be kept apart from the translational apparatus because eukaryotic genes are transcribed into RNAs containing noncoding intervening sequences that must be removed by splicing to assemble mature RNA molecules with a continuous open reading frame. Sequestration of immature RNAs is one function of the nuclear envelope, two concentric membrane bilayers that separate the nucleus and cytoplasm. The nuclear envelope also regulates the movement of proteins, such as transcription factors, into and out of the nucleus.

This chapter describes what is known about the structure of the nucleus, the nuclear envelope, and the transport of macromolecules into and out of the nucleus.

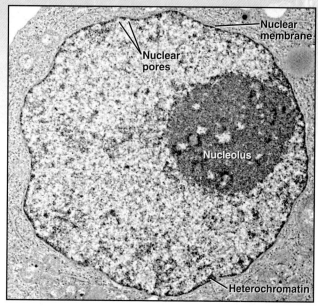

Figure 14-1 ELECTRON MICROGRAPH OF A THIN SECTION OF A NUCLEUS FROM A CANCER CELL WITH THE MAJOR FEATURES LABELED. (Courtesy of Scott Kaufmann, Mayo Clinic, Rochester, Minnesota.)

Much is known about the mechanisms of DNA replication (see Chapter 42), RNA transcription and processing (see Chapters 15 and 16), and nuclear trafficking of macromolecules. Currently, less is known about the structural organization of the nucleus and the role of its specialized subcompartments in these nuclear functions.

Overall Organization of the Nucleus

Studies in which entire individual chromosomes are labeled by in situ hybridization (chromosome painting; see Fig. 13-11) reveal that chromosomes tend to occupy discrete regions within the nucleus called **chromosome territories.** The boundaries of these territories are not absolute, as in some cases an active gene is located well outside its respective territory (see Chapter 13). The poorly defined region between adjacent territories is referred to as the **interchromosomal domain.** Most RNA transcription, processing, and transport are thought to occur either within or at the boundary of this domain. Although the nucleoplasm is very crowded with chromosomes and RNPs, many nuclear proteins can diffuse rapidly through the nucleus, possibly by moving in the interchromosomal domain.

Specialized Subdomains of the Nucleus

Cell nuclei contain numerous discrete subdomains or bodies with distinctive structural organizations and/or biochemical composition (Fig. 14-2 and Table 14-1). The most prominent of these is the nucleolus, discussed in the next section. Although these subdomains are often referred to as organelles, unlike cytoplasmic organelles, nuclear subdomains are not membrane bounded. In fact, many proteins that have been examined by the fluorescence recovery after photobleaching technique (see Fig. 6-3) exhibit a relatively rapid exchange between a respective body and a nucleoplasmic pool of the protein. Therefore, although these bodies are discrete at steady state, they represent highly dynamic associa-

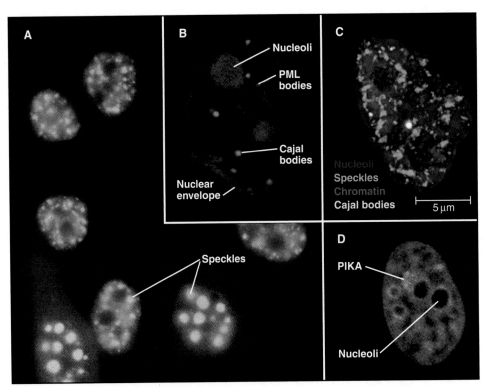

Figure 14-2   EXAMPLES OF MAJOR SUBNUCLEAR STRUCTURES. **A,** Components involved in RNA processing are scattered throughout the nucleus but concentrated in domains called speckles that are rich in interchromatin granules. Inhibition of RNA processing causes splicing components to accumulate in enormous concentrations of interchromatin granule clusters. Several cells were injected with a short oligonucleotide that disrupts the function of the U1 snRNP in RNA processing (see Chapter 16), and were then stained with an antibody recognizing the Sm splicing components (green). The injected cells were marked by introducing an inert fluorescent dextran marker into the cytoplasm (red). **B,** Nucleus with simultaneous staining of nucleoli (blue), PML nuclear bodies (red), Cajal bodies (green), and the nuclear envelope (purple). **C,** Nucleus with simultaneous staining of chromatin (blue), nucleoli (red), speckles (green), and Cajal bodies (white). **D,** Nucleus with simultaneous staining of DNA (blue) and the polymorphic interphase karyosomal association (PIKA)/ OPT domain (red). Nucleoli appear as unstained areas. A number of proteins involved in the sensing and repair of DNA damage concentrate in the PIKA. (A, Courtesy of David Spector, Cold Spring Harbor Lab, New York. B–C, Courtesy of Angus Lamond, University of Dundee, Scotland. D, Courtesy of William S. Saunders and William C. Earnshaw.)

Table 14-1

MAJOR NUCLEAR SUBDOMAINS

Structure	Comments
Cajal bodies	Formerly known as coiled bodies. About 0.2 to 1 µm in diameter, Cajal bodies have a coiled fibrous substructure. First identified by electron microscopy, up to 10 of these structures are seen per cell. They contain a characteristic protein called p80-coilin. They may be involved in snRNP and snoRNP assembly.
GEMs	GEMs are usually found paired with Cajal bodies, which they may overlap. They contain the survival of motor neurons (SMN) protein, which is encoded by the gene mutated in spinal muscular atrophy, a severe, inherited, human, muscular wasting disease. SMN and its cofactors appear to play an essential role in the assembly and maturation of snRNPs (see Chapter 16).
Nuclear bodies	Function unknown. 5 to 20 spots within the nucleus. Originally observed in electron micrographs of cells following hormonal treatments. However it is not clear that all nuclear bodies described in various cell types are structurally or functionally homologous. A marker antigen for some types of nuclear bodies (called PBC 95K—M_r 95 kD) is recognized by autoantibodies from patients with primary biliary cirrhosis. Some may correspond to PML bodies.
Nucleolus	The nucleolus (typically 1 to 5 structures of 0.5 to 5 µm diameter in mammalian cell nuclei) is the site of rRNA transcription and processing, as well as of preribosomal assembly. It is also the site of processing of several other noncoding RNAs, including the RNA component of the signal recognition particle (SRP—Chapter 20).
PIKA	The polymorphic interphase karyosomal association (PIKA) was later rediscovered and termed the OPT domain. The PIKA may be up to 5 µm in diameter during G_1 phase, but its morphology and number vary across the cell cycle. It appears to correspond to sites of sensing or repair of DNA damage as well as concentrations of certain transcription factors.
PML bodies	Also known as PODs and ND10, 10 to 30 of these structures are scattered throughout the nucleus. They are have links with human disease, and in some cases appear to be targeted during viral infections. Fusion of the marker protein PML to the α-retinoic acid receptor is often found in acute promyelocytic leukemia (hence the name PML), in which the PML bodies appear highly fragmented. The link with cancer appears significant, as treatments that are effective against PML appear to restore the normal morphology of PML bodies (see text).
Speckles	Speckles are concentrations of components involved in RNA processing. They often correspond to clusters of interchromatin granules seen by electron microscopy. They may serve as storage depots of splicing factors, or they may play a more active role in splicing factor modification and/or assembly.

tions of macromolecular complexes. These domains, like the nucleolus, reflect the functional compartmentalization of the nucleoplasm.

RNA transcription and processing occur at up to 10,000 discrete sites spread throughout the average mammalian nucleus. These sites likely correspond to structures, originally observed by electron microscopy on the surface of regions of condensed chromatin, called **perichromatin fibrils.** Perichromatin fibrils contain various splicing factors and RNA-packaging proteins.

When factors involved in RNA processing are detected by fluorescence microscopy, 20 to 50 bright **speckles** are seen against a diffuse background of nucleoplasmic staining (Fig. 14-2). The diffuse staining probably corresponds to splicing factors associated with perichromatin fibrils at the thousands of sites where RNA transcription and processing take place. Speckles are less prominent in cells that transcribe RNA at high levels, and they become strikingly prominent when RNA processing is inhibited (Fig. 14-2).

Most speckles correspond to clusters of **interchromatin granules,** particles 20 to 25 nm in diameter that are distributed throughout the interchromosomal domain. Proteomic analysis of isolated interchromatin granules reveals that they contain approximately 240 stably associated proteins, most involved with various aspects of RNA processing. Interchromatin granules may be sites for the assembly, modification, or storage of protein complexes involved in pre-mRNA processing. Consistent with this, a number of components involved in RNA processing were shown to be highly dynamic. When tagged with green fluorescent protein, these mRNA-processing proteins cycle between speckles and sites of transcription in less than 1 minute in vivo.

Metabolic labeling experiments indicate that speckles are not major sites of active transcription, and most messenger RNAs (mRNAs) are seldom or never seen associated with speckles. However, mRNAs for certain genes accumulate either within or immediately adjacent to speckles. These "speckles" could be highly active transcription sites that have recruited a significant population of splicing factors and are indistinguishable from interchromatin granule clusters by fluorescent microscopy.

When cells enter mitosis, speckles disperse as RNA-processing factors redistribute diffusely throughout the cytoplasm. During telophase, processing factors reaggregate in the cytoplasm into punctate structures termed *mitotic interchromatin granule clusters.* These factors are subsequently imported into the nucleus at the completion of mitosis.

Cajal bodies (formerly known as coiled bodies) are compact structures about 0.3 to 1.0 µm in diameter (Fig. 14-2) that resemble balls of tangled threads in the electron microscope. Nuclei contain 1 to 10 Cajal bodies, which accumulate many factors involved in mRNA processing, as well as a number of nucleolar components, but lack non-snRNP protein-splicing factors that are present in speckles. They also contain an 80-kD human autoantigen of unknown function, called p80-coilin. In contrast to speckles, Cajal bodies disperse when transcription and splicing are blocked, and they are particularly prominent in rapidly growing cells with high levels of gene expression. However, like speckles, some Cajal bodies disassemble during mitosis and reform during the G_1 phase after transcription is reinitiated. Cajal bodies are connected with the maturation of newly imported snRNP and snoRNP particles (see Chapter 16). They may also have other functions, including possibly regulating expression of snRNA gene clusters.

Mammalian nuclei also contain about 10 to 30 bodies, varying in size from 0.3 to 1 µm, known as **promyelocytic leukemia (PML) bodies** (other names are listed in Table 14-1) that are often juxtaposed with Cajal bodies (Fig. 14-2). PML bodies were initially defined by the presence of a protein called PML, and other components have since been identified. PML has a RING finger amino acid sequence motif and is therefore likely to be a ligase for ubiquitin or ubiquitin-like proteins (see Fig. 23-8). Its targets are unknown, but several components of PML bodies are conjugated to the ubiquitin-like protein SUMO-1.

The PML gene was identified by analysis of a chromosome translocation between chromosomes 15 and 17 found in patients with acute promyelocytic leukemia (APL). In many patients, this translocation produces a gene fusion between PML and the retinoic acid receptor alpha (RARα). The fusion protein is termed PML-RARα. Antibodies to PML protein stained subnuclear structures that were given the name *PML bodies*. In APL cells, PML bodies are "shattered" into many tiny punctate foci scattered throughout the nucleus. However, when APL cells are treated with drugs that are clinically effective in the treatment of patients with APL, such as retinoic acid and arsenic trioxide, the PML bodies reform, and the PML-RARα fusion protein is degraded. This reveals a tantalizing link between these structures and the cancerous phenotype. At present, the function of PML bodies remains uncertain.

The Nucleolus: The Most Prominent Nuclear Subdomain

The nucleolus, first described only five years after the nucleus, in 1835, is the most conspicuous and best-characterized nuclear subdomain (Fig. 14-3). Most mammalian cell nuclei have one to five nucleoli, which are specialized regions 0.5 to 5.0 µm in diameter surrounding transcriptionally active ribosomal RNA (rRNA) gene clusters. Within nucleoli occur the bulk of the steps for ribosome biogenesis, from the transcription and processing of rRNA to the initial assembly of ribosomal subunits. The ribosome is a complex macromolecular machine with four different structural RNA molecules and about 85 proteins that are assembled into two subunits (see Figs. 17-6 and 17-7). rRNA transcription by RNA polymerase I comprises nearly one half of total cellular RNA synthesis in some cell types. This high level of synthesis is necessary to produce about 5 million ribosomes in each cell cycle, more than 30 every second in budding yeast.

Over 690 proteins associate stably with human nucleoli. Many more may associate transiently, and this composition changes to reflect different metabolic states of the cell (Fig. 14-4). Many of these nucleolar proteins are involved with either ribosomal RNA synthesis and modification or with ribosome subunit assembly. Surprisingly, the functions of many (~80) other nucleolar proteins remain unknown and may reflect the involvement of nucleoli in other biological processes. Other stable RNAs, including the RNA component of the signal recognition particle (SRP; see Fig. 20-5), are also processed in the nucleolus, and the nucleolus might have other as yet undiscovered functions.

Ribosomal Biogenesis in Functionally Distinct Regions of the Nucleolus

The nucleolus contains three morphologically distinct regions in thin sections viewed by transmission electron microscopy (Fig. 14-3). **Fibrillar centers** contain concentrations of rRNA genes, together with significant amounts of RNA polymerase I and its associated transcription factors. Actively transcribed ribosomal genes are found near the border between the fibrillar centers and a **dense fibrillar component** that surrounds them. The **granular component** is the site for many steps in ribosome subunit assembly and is made up of densely packed clusters of preribosomal particles 15 to 20 nm in diameter.

Ribosomal RNA loci have a modular organization, with genes alternating with spacer regions in large tandemly arranged clusters (see Fig. 16-9). The repeat unit in this array (gene plus spacer) is approximately 40,000 base pairs in humans. Humans have approximately 300 to 400 copies of the ribosomal DNA (rDNA) repeat unit located in clusters on chromosomes 13, 14, 15, 21, and 22. Usually, only a fraction of these genes is actively transcribed. An additional rRNA, 5S, is encoded by distinct genes and transcribed by RNA polymerase III (see Fig. 15-10).

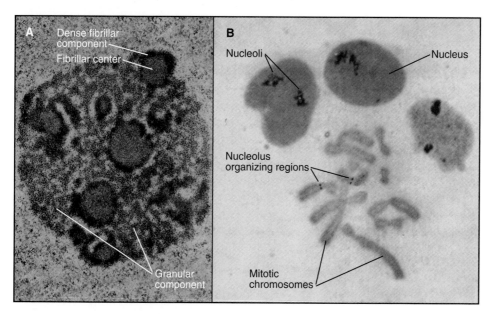

Figure 14-3 NUCLEOLUS AND NUCLEOLAR ORGANIZER REGION. **A,** Electron micrograph of a thin section of a typical nucleolus. The fibrillar centers, dense fibrillar component, and granular component are indicated. **B,** Use of silver staining to visualize the nucleolus in interphase nuclei and the nucleolar organizer regions on mitotic chromosomes of the rat kangaroo. (A, From Fawcett DW: The Cell. Philadelphia, WB Saunders, 1981. B, From Robert-Fortel I, Junera HR, Geraud G, et al: Three-dimensional organization of the ribosomal genes and Ag-NOR proteins during interphase and mitosis in PtK1 cells studied by confocal microscopy. Chromosoma 102:146–157, 1993.)

A simple yet efficient mechanism guarantees a balance between the RNA components of the two ribosomal subunits. The major rRNA components are encoded by a single precursor RNA molecule. In humans, this 13,000-base precursor is commonly described by its sedimentation coefficient in sucrose gradients as 45S. Following its transcription, the RNA precursor is processed in a series of cleavages to yield the 18S, 5.8S, and 28S rRNA molecules (see Fig. 16-9). In addition to the cleavages, rRNA processing also involves extensive base and sugar modifications, including approximately 100 2′-O-methyl ribose and approximately 90 pseudouridine residues per molecule. The earliest stages of rRNA processing probably occur in the dense fibrillar component of the nucleolus. Later stages take place in the granular component. Ribosomal protein synthesis occurs in the cytoplasm on free ribosomes, and the newly synthesized proteins are transported into the nucleus for assembly into ribosomes, predominantly in the granular component.

Disassembly of the Nucleolus during Mitosis

The nucleolus disassembles during each mitotic cycle, starting with the dispersal of the dense fibrillar and granular components during prophase. This disassembly is apparently driven by specific phosphorylation of nucleolar proteins. Ultimately, the fibrillar centers alone remain associated with the mitotic chromosomes, forming what are termed **nucleolus-organizing regions** (**NORs** [Fig. 14-3B]). NORs are often the sites of a prominent **secondary constriction** of the chromosome. (The primary constriction is the centromere.) The nucleolar proteins nucleolin and RNA polymerase

I remain bound at NORs as cells enter and exit mitosis.

Nucleolar reformation begins in telophase as processing factors and unprocessed pre-RNA remaining from the previous cell cycle associate with NORs (10 in human), which then cluster into one to five foci. Next, a wide variety of nucleolar components assemble into particles termed **prenucleolar bodies** that associate with the NORs in a process requiring transcription of the rRNA genes. Normally, nascent transcripts, rather than ribosomal genes, nucleate assembly of the nucleolus in each cell cycle. If antibodies to RNA polymerase I are microinjected into mitotic cells, rRNA

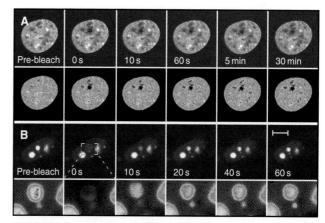

Figure 14-4 DYNAMIC ANALYSIS OF CHROMATIN AND A MAJOR NUCLEOLAR COMPONENT. **A,** Fluorescence recovery after photobleaching (FRAP) of H2B-GFP shows that chromatin is immobile within the cell nucleus. **B,** FRAP of fibrillarin-GFP shows that this major component of nucleoli is highly dynamic. Scale bar: 5 μm. (A–B, Courtesy of Tom Misteli. B, From Phair RD, Misteli T: High mobility of proteins in the mammalian cell nucleus. Nature 404:604–609, 2000.)

transcription is blocked, and nucleoli do not reform in the next G_1 phase.

Structure of the Nuclear Envelope

The nuclear envelope provides a selective permeability barrier between the nuclear compartment and the cytoplasm (Fig. 14-5). This barrier ensures that only fully processed mRNAs are delivered to ribosomes for translation into protein. In addition, various chromosomal events, including DNA replication and expression of certain genes, are regulated, at least in part, by changes in the ability of factors to move from the cytoplasm into the nucleus.

The nuclear envelope is composed of two concentric lipid bilayers termed the **inner** and **outer nuclear membranes.** The outer nuclear membrane is continuous with the rough endoplasmic reticulum and shares its functions. For example, it has ribosomes attached to its outer surface. A fibrous **nuclear lamina** of intermediate filaments supports the inner nuclear membrane in higher eukaryotes. These and other proteins of the inner nuclear membrane mediate interactions of the envelope with chromatin. The inner and outer nuclear membranes are separated by a **perinuclear space** of about 30 nm that is continuous with the lumen of the endoplasmic reticulum. **Nuclear pore complexes** bridging both nuclear membranes provide the sole route for communication between the nucleus and cytoplasm during interphase.

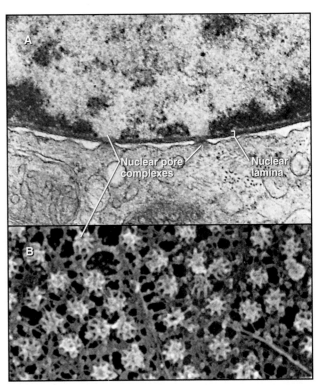

Figure 14-6 THE NUCLEAR LAMINA. **A,** Thin-section electron micrograph of a nuclear envelope with a prominent nuclear lamina and nuclear pores. **B,** Field emission scanning electron micrograph of the inner surface of an amphibian oocyte nuclear envelope. The nuclear pores are prominent, protruding above the underlying nuclear lamina. (A, Reference: Fawcett DW: The Cell. Philadelphia, WB Saunders, 1981, Fig. 156 [upper]. B, From Zhang C, Jenkins H, Goldberg MW, et al: Nuclear lamina and nuclear matrix organization in sperm pronuclei assembled in Xenopus egg extract. J Cell Sci 109:2275–2286, 1996.)

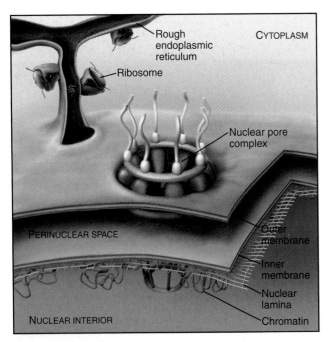

Figure 14-5 SUMMARY OVERVIEW OF THE ORGANIZATION OF THE NUCLEAR ENVELOPE.

Disassembly of the nuclear envelope is a critical aspect of mitosis in higher eukaryotes, as this releases the chromosomes so that they can be segregated to the daughter cells by the cytoplasmic mitotic spindle. Mitotic segregation of chromosomes to daughter cells takes place within the nucleus in some lower eukaryotes including yeasts.

Structure and Assembly of the Nuclear Lamina

The nuclear lamina is a protein meshwork, typically 20 to 40 nm thick, composed of type V intermediate filament proteins called **nuclear lamins** (Fig. 14-6). Mammalian lamins are generally divided into two families. **Lamin A** is encoded by a gene that gives rise to four polypeptides (including **lamin C**) by alternative splicing (see Fig. 16-6). Members of the **lamin B** family are the products of two distinct genes.

Lamin gene expression depends on the cell type and stage of development. All nuclei of higher eukaryotes, including early embryos, have a lamina that contains lamin B-family subunits, loss of which is lethal. Lamins A and C typically appear only later in development as cells begin to differentiate. This variation in lamina composition may affect chromosome organization, possibly contributing to different patterns of gene expression.

Like other intermediate filament proteins (see Fig. 35-2), nuclear lamins have a central, rod-like domain that is largely α-helical (Fig. 14-7). The basic building block of lamin assembly is an α-helical coiled-coil (see Fig. 3-10) of two identical parallel polypeptides. Two large globular C-terminal domains protrude from one end. Lamin dimers self-associate end to end to form polymers. In some cases, these polymers grow as thick as 10-nm intermediate filaments.

The C-terminal globular domain contains a nuclear localization sequence (see later section) that ensures the rapid import of newly synthesized lamin precursors into the nucleus through nuclear pores. Most lamin subunits acquire a hydrophobic posttranslational modification that targets them to the nuclear membrane. The modification involves the enzymatic addition of a hydrocarbon tail, a C15-isoprenoid group called **farnesyl** (see Figs. 7-9 and 20-13). The farnesyl group is added to a characteristic amino acid motif called the CaaX box (Ca_1a_2X, where C refers to cysteine located four amino

acids from the carboxyl terminus; a_1 refers to any aliphatic amino acid; a_2 refers to valine, isoleucine, or leucine; and X refers usually to methionine or serine) at the carboxyl terminus of the protein (Fig. 14-7). This motif was first recognized in the *Ras* proteins (see Fig. 25-7). Lamin subunits lacking a CaaX box form aggregates in the nuclear interior. Once at the nuclear membrane lamin A is processed by a specialized protease called FACE-1 (farnesylated protein-converting enzyme 1) that clips off the C-terminal 18 amino acids, removing the farnesyl group. The aaX residues are removed from B-type lamins, leaving a protein with the farnesyl group on its carboxyl terminal cysteine.

The assembled lamina appears to be tethered to the inner nuclear membrane by interactions with integral membrane proteins (see next section). The surface of the lamina facing the nuclear interior also interacts with the chromosomes. Thus, the lamina and its associated proteins not only may serve as a structural support for the nuclear envelope but also may influence chromosome distribution and function within the nucleus.

A diffuse network of lamins is spread throughout the nucleus of most cells, and local concentrations appear at particular times during the cell cycle. Intranuclear lamin A spots are most prominent in G_1, whereas those with lamin B are most prominent during S, when they colocalize with sites of DNA replication. Lamin B spots do not colocalize with lamin A spots. The role of these intranuclear concentrations of lamins is unknown, but they might be localized regions of nuclear matrix (see Fig. 13-18) with roles in RNA transcription and DNA replication.

Proteins of the Inner Nuclear Membrane

At least a dozen, and possibly over 80, integral membrane proteins are associated with the inner nuclear membrane. Most of those that have been characterized can both anchor the lamina to the membrane and interact with chromatin. However, the function of most is unknown, though sequence analysis suggests that many might be enzymes. For example, the hydrophobic region of the lamin B receptor (see later) resembles a yeast enzyme involved in cholesterol biosynthesis and has sterol C14 reductase activity when expressed in yeast.

Well-characterized lamin-binding proteins include the lamin B receptor, emerin, and the lamina-associated polypeptides (LAPs; Fig. 14-8). Two unrelated genes—LAP1 and LAP2—produce a number of polypeptides with distinct structural and functional properties as a result of extensive alternative splicing of the primary transcripts.

These four proteins also contribute to organizing chromatin at the nuclear periphery. For example, the lamin B receptor binds heterochromatin protein HP1

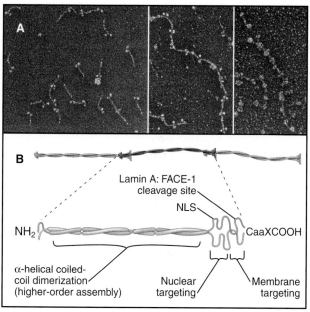

Figure 14-7 **LAMIN ORGANIZATION AND ASSEMBLY. A,** Several stages in the assembly of isolated lamin B dimers into filaments in vitro. The dimers at left have two globular heads at the C-terminal end of a rod that is 52 nm long. **B,** Diagram of the structural organization of the nuclear lamins. The sequence CaaXCOOH (see text) is a signal for the attachment of a farnesyl group. NLS, nuclear localization sequence. (A, From Heitlinger E, Peter M, Haner M, et al: Expression of chicken lamin B2 in *Escherichia coli*: Characterization of its structure, assembly, and molecular interactions. J Cell Biol 113:485–495, 1991.)

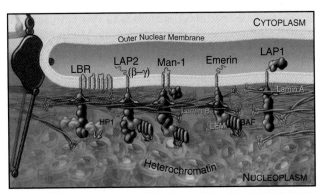

Figure 14-8 SEVERAL MAJOR INTEGRAL MEMBRANE PROTEINS OF THE INNER NUCLEAR MEMBRANE INTERACT WITH BOTH THE NUCLEAR LAMINA AND CHROMATIN. The lamin B receptor (LBR), lamina-associated protein 2 (LAP2), Man-1, and emerin all bind lamin B. LBR associates with chromatin via HP1. The other three associate with chromatin via BAF. Emerin and LAP1 also bind to lamin A. The α form of LAP2 is not membrane associated and is not shown here. (Modified from a slide by Roland Foisner.)

(see Fig. 13-9) and could thus link the envelope to condensed heterochromatin. The LEM domain, a degenerate 40-amino-acid motif common to LAP2, emerin, and MAN1, binds to an abundant small protein called barrier to autointegration factor (BAF) that also binds to DNA and has an important role in chromatin organization in both interphase nuclei and mitotic chromosomes. Despite their apparent roles in linking chromosomes to the nuclear envelope, live cell observations have shown that both HP1 and BAF are extremely mobile proteins.

Are these interactions between the chromosomes and the inner nuclear envelope functionally significant? This remains hotly debated, but a number of studies indicate that interactions with LAP2 and lamin A could be important in regulation of the cell cycle by the transcription factor E2F (see Fig. 41-8). Nuclear envelope proteins have been observed to interact with other transcriptional regulators, so (as is discussed later) alterations in gene expression might explain the link between mutations in nuclear envelope proteins and human disease.

Integral proteins of the inner nuclear membrane enter the nucleus by diffusion in the membrane. The lamin B receptor is highly mobile in the rough endoplasmic reticulum (ER), its site of synthesis, and rapidly diffuses to the nuclear envelope. Transit around the periphery of the nuclear pore complex requires energy. Once in the inner nuclear membrane, it becomes fixed in place, presumably by binding to the lamina or chromatin.

Nuclear Envelope Defects Lead to Human Diseases

In 1994, the gene that is mutated in human X-linked Emery-Dreifuss muscular dystrophy was found to encode a protein of the inner nuclear envelope named emerin. This link between the nuclear envelope and human disease was only the tip of an iceberg. Now genetic defects in nuclear envelope proteins are known to cause at least 14 disorders, including muscular dystrophies, lipodystrophies, and neuropathies (diseases of striated muscle, fatty tissue, and the nervous system). The most dramatic of these is Hutchinson-Gilford progeria (Fig. 14-9). Affected individuals are essentially normal at birth, but they appear to age rapidly and die in their early teens of symptoms (including atherosclerosis and heart failure) that are typically associated with extreme age.

Over 180 mutations scattered throughout the gene encoding both lamin A and C cause over 10 different diseases, collectively termed laminopathies (Fig. 14-9). At least two laminopathies are also linked to mutations in FACE-1, the membrane-associated protease that processes prelamin A. Some of the symptoms of laminopathies can be modeled in the mouse. Loss of lamin A causes disruption of the nuclear envelope and leads to a type of muscular dystrophy. Other mutations in mouse lamin A reproduce aspects of Hutchinson-Gilford progeria.

The most surprising aspect of the laminopathies is the fact that the defects are limited to a few tissues such as striated muscle, despite the fact that lamins A/C are ubiquitous in differentiated cells throughout the body. Lamin mutations appear to compromise the stability of the nuclear envelope, so it has been suggested that muscle nuclei might be particularly sensitive to these mutations, owing to mechanical stress during contraction. However, this mechanism cannot account for the link between lamin mutations and lipodystrophy—fat is not a force-generating tissue—neuropathy, or progeria.

An alternative suggestion is that these mutations cause disease by altering gene expression by compromising interactions between the inner nuclear membrane and chromatin. Cells from patients with Hutchinson-Gilford progeria show signs of aging in culture that are accompanied by dramatic alterations in heterochromatin (see Fig. 13-9), lending support to this model.

Nuclear Pore Complexes

In a typical growing cell, all traffic between the nucleus and cytoplasm passes through 3000 to 5000 channels, called **nuclear pore complexes,** that bridge both the inner and outer nuclear membranes (Fig. 14-10). Nuclear pore complexes have a central cylindrical core 90 nm long from which filaments project into the cytoplasm and nucleus. The central core consists of a massive multidomain **spoke ring** with eightfold symmetry surrounded by a **luminal ring** in the perinuclear space and sandwiched between **cytoplasmic** and **nuclear**

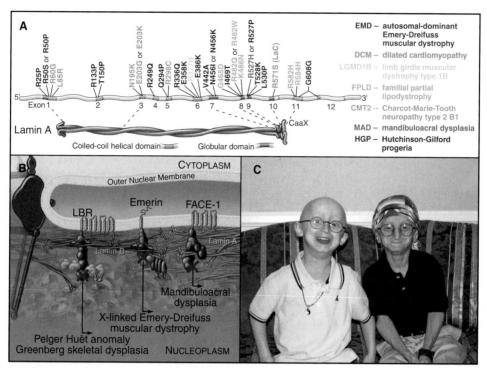

Figure 14-9 HUMAN DISEASES ASSOCIATED WITH NUCLEAR ENVELOPE ABNORMALITIES. **A,** Some of the mutations in the gene encoding lamin A that are associated with human disease. The G608G mutation makes no change in the protein sequence but creates a splice site leading to the loss of 50 amino acid residues from lamin A. This mutation causes Hutchinson-Gilford progeria. **B,** Mutations in three other nuclear envelope proteins also cause similar diseases. The structure of FACE-1 shown is hypothetical. **C,** Two young boys with the premature aging disorder Hutchinson-Gilford progeria. Sam Berns *(left)* with friend John Tacket, Progeria Research Foundation Youth Ambassador. (A, Modified from Mounkes L, Kozlov S, Burke B, Stewart CL: The laminopathies: Nuclear structure meets disease. Curr Opin Genet Dev 13:223–230, 2003. C, Courtesy of the Progeria Research Foundation, Peabody, Massachusetts, http://www.progeriaresearch.org.)

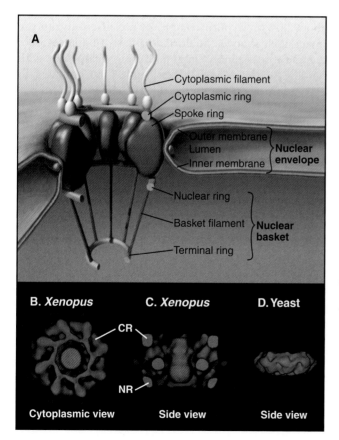

Figure 14-10 THREE-DIMENSIONAL MODEL OF THE NUCLEAR PORE COMPLEX. **A,** The pore has eightfold symmetry, with a central channel and eight peripheral channels. The cytoplasmic and nuclear filament networks contain components that function in docking of transport complexes to the pores. **B–D,** Three-dimensional reconstruction of the nuclear pore complexes from the frog *Xenopus laevis* and the budding yeast. The yeast pore complex is smaller than the amphibian complex. This structure is very difficult to observe by electron microscopy, partly because it is very fragile and partly because the structure contains both protein and lipid, which may limit access to stains. CR, cytoplasmic ring; NR, nuclear ring. (B–C, From Akey CW, Radermacher M: Architecture of the Xenopus nuclear pore complex revealed by three-dimensional cryo-electron microscopy. J Cell Biol 122:1–19, 1993. D, From Yang Q, Rout MP, Akey CW: Three dimensional architecture of the isolated yeast nuclear pore. Mol Cell 1:223–234, 1998.)

rings associated with the surfaces of the outer and inner nuclear membranes, respectively. The nuclear ring appears to be anchored to the nuclear lamina. The minimum diameter of the central channel through the spoke ring is 45 to 55 nm.

A "plug" occupies the central channel in many (although not all) pore complexes. Although originally thought to be an intrinsic component of pores, it is most likely cargo in transit through the pore.

Eight filaments project outward from each nuclear and cytoplasmic ring. The cytoplasmic filaments are often highly kinked in appearance. By comparison, the longer nuclear filaments are joined at their outer ends by a terminal ring, much like the wire that secures the cork on a champagne bottle. This structure is called the **nuclear basket.** Both sets of filaments are involved in docking of macromolecules to be transported through the pore.

Vertebrate nuclear pore complexes are large structures with a mass of approximately 90 million to 120 million daltons. Yeast nuclear pores are similar in overall structure but about half the mass. Given their large mass, it was originally believed that vertebrate nuclear pore complexes would contain multiple copies of 100 or more proteins. In fact, the core protein composition of yeast and mammalian pore complexes is remarkably similar. Both are composed of about 30 core proteins known as **nucleoporins** (Fig. 14-11). These are present in multiples of eight copies. With an average size of more than 100 kD, they can account for the observed mass of the pore. Proteomic analysis of rat and yeast nuclear pore complexes identified 94 and 174 polypeptides, respectively. The additional polypeptides are primarily transport factors and other auxiliary subunits that do not have a key structural role.

About one third of nucleoporins contain up to 40 or more repeats of the dipeptide FG (phenylalanine-glycine). Two common examples include XFXFG and GLFG, but other repeats also are found. These repeats occur in highly flexible and unstructured regions of the proteins and are thought to mediate interactions with nuclear transport receptors as they transit the pores (see later). Some FG nucleoporins are localized primarily to the cytoplasmic or nuclear surface of the pore, but most are distributed symmetrically. At least one nuclear-localized FG-nucleoporin has a flexible FG "arm" long enough to extend through the pore and into the cytoplasm.

Three experiments show that nucleoporins are required to transport proteins into the nucleus. First, antibodies to nucleoporins inhibit transport either when added to isolated nuclei or when injected into live cells. Second, lectins such as wheat germ agglutinin (which binds specifically to sugars attached to many nucleoporins) inhibit transport in similar experiments. Third, nuclear pore complexes assembled in *Xenopus* egg extracts (see Box 40-3) in the absence of the highly conserved nucleoporin **p62,** a component of the central region of the cytoplasmic and nuclear faces of the pore complex, appear structurally normal but are inactive in transport.

Nuclear pore complexes are assembled de novo during S phase, and in higher eukaryotes, they are disassembled to soluble subcomplexes during mitosis and reassembled in earliest G1 phase. Nothing is known about how new pore complexes are inserted into the intact nuclear envelope during S phase. In mitosis, pore complex reassembly begins during telophase with binding of the nine-member Nup107-160 complex to chromatin. If this complex is depleted from *Xenopus* egg extracts, nuclear membranes form around added nuclei but are devoid of pores. The stages in pore formation after binding of Nup107-160 to chromatin are under study.

Traffic between Nucleus and Cytoplasm

The nuclear pore complex is a highly efficient conduit that can allow the passage of up to 1000 macromolecules per second. Traffic heading out of the nucleus includes mRNPs, ribosomal subunits, and transfer RNAs (tRNAs), all of which must be transported to the cytoplasm to function in protein synthesis. Traffic headed into the nucleus includes transcription factors, chromatin components, and ribosomal proteins. Other molecules follow more complex routes. snRNAs are exported to the cytoplasm to acquire essential protein components; they are then reimported into the nucleus, where they undergo further maturation steps before function-

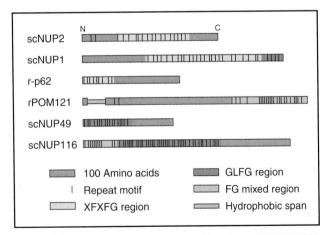

Figure 14-11 SEQUENCE ORGANIZATION OF SEVERAL NUCLEOPORINS, THE STRUCTURAL COMPONENTS OF THE NUCLEAR PORES. Nucleoporins contain combinations of repeated sequences as shown. Letters refer to the amino acids (see Fig. 3-2). They may be somehow involved in helping cargo to traffic through the pores.

ing in RNA processing. Individual pores can simultaneously transport components in both directions.

Nuclear pores have a constitutive channel through which solutes and small proteins of up to approximately 60 kD can diffuse passively. However, they can also actively transport much larger macromolecular complexes. Surprisingly, despite the presence of the constitutive channels, almost all physiological traffic through the pores, even of small molecules, is a facilitated process that involves specific carrier proteins. For example, the 28-kD NTF2 dimer (the Ran transporter; see later) traverses the pore about 120 times more rapidly than does the 27-kD green fluorescent protein.

The pore gate opens to a maximum of 30 to 40 nm, but larger particles can squeeze through, provided that they are deformable. This is well documented for export of a well-studied enormous RNA that associates with roughly 500 packaging proteins to make an RNP particle about 50 nm in diameter. The RNP is deformed into a rod-shaped structure as it squeezes through the pore (Fig. 14-12). Rigid particles cannot usually exceed the 30- to 40-nm limit.

Proteins that are imported into the nucleus bear a **nuclear localization sequence (NLS),** also called a nuclear localization *signal,* that is recognized by specific carrier proteins called transport receptors (Figs. 14-13 and 14-14). Known types of NLS vary in complexity. The best studied is a patch of basic amino acids

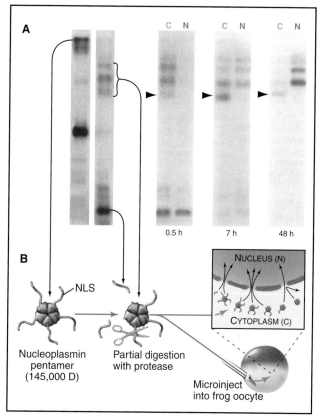

Figure 14-13 IDENTIFICATION OF A NUCLEAR LOCALIZATION SEQUENCE ON THE PROTEIN NUCLEOPLASMIN. This 29,000-kD protein exists in vivo as a pentameric complex with a molecular weight of 145,000. The monomer is small enough to diffuse passively through the nuclear pores, but the pentamer is too large to do so. **A,** Gentle cleavage of the pentamer with a protease removes a relatively small peptide from one end of the protein *(left two lanes).* When the cleaved pentamers were labeled with radioactivity and injected into the cytoplasm of a *Xenopus* oocyte, it was found that four species were produced that could still migrate into the nucleus and one species was produced that could not *(right three pairs of gel lanes).* **B,** The interpretation of this experiment is that each nucleoplasmin polypeptide contains a "tail" that can be removed by proteolysis and that this tail contains a nuclear localization sequence. Each pentamer can migrate into the nucleus as long as it retains at least one polypeptide with a tail. Tailless pentamers remain stuck in the cytoplasm. C, cytoplasm; N, nucleus. (A, From Dingwall C, Sharnick SV, Laskey RA: A polypeptide domain that specifies migration of nucleoplasmin in the nucleus. Cell 30:449–458, 1982.)

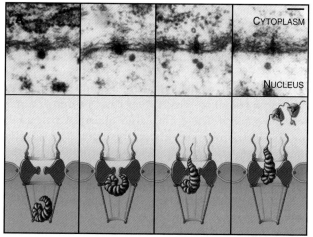

Figure 14-12 Electron micrographs *(upper panels)* and an artist's rendition *(lower panels)* show deformation of a large RNP particle as it passes through the nuclear pore complex (cytoplasm *[top];* nucleus *[bottom]).* This RNA encodes a secreted protein, with a molecular weight of about 1,000,000 D, from the salivary gland of the fly *Chironomus tentans.* Once in the cytoplasm, the 5' end of the RNA docks with ribosomes and begins synthesis of its protein even before the passage of the remainder of the RNP through the pore has been completed. (From Mehlin H, Daneholt B, Skoglund U: Translocation of a specific premessenger ribonucleoprotein particle through the nuclear pore studied with electron microscope tomography. Cell 69:605–613, 1992, Fig. 2. Copyright 1992.)

similar to the sequence PKKKRKV (single-letter amino acid code; see Fig. 3-2), first identified on the simian virus 40 (SV40) large T antigen. A point mutation, yielding PK*N*KRKV, inactivates this sequence as a signal for nuclear transport. A related type of bipartite NLS features two smaller patches of basic residues separated by a variable spacer (KRPAATKKAGQAKKKK [critical residues are underlined]). These two types of sequences are referred to as basic NLSs. Basic NLSs function autonomously and can direct the migration of a wide range of molecules into the nucleus in vivo. In one extreme

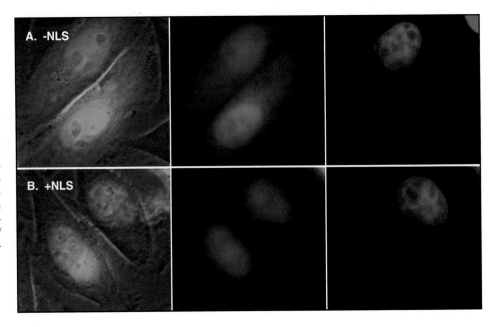

Figure 14-14 ICAD protein (the inhibitor of CAD nuclease; see Chapter 46) was fused to the green fluorescent protein (GFP) and expressed in cultured cells. **A,** A mutant form of the ICAD: GFP fusion protein lacking the ICAD nuclear localization sequence (NLS) accumulates randomly throughout the cell. **B,** The intact ICAD:GFP fusion protein with NLS accumulates quantitatively in the nucleus. (Courtesy of K. Samejima, University of Edinburgh, Scotland.)

example, when coated with nucleoplasmin, a protein with a bipartite basic NLS, colloidal gold particles up to 23 nm in diameter are transported through nuclear pores (Fig. 14-15). An alternative type of NLS is not basic but instead is rich in glycine. Proteins with this NLS are imported by a similar mechanism (see later) but are recognized by a different transport receptor.

Many proteins exported from the nucleus bear a **nuclear export sequence (NES)** that is recognized by carriers related to those used for nuclear import (Fig. 14-16). Like import signals, these signals vary in size and complexity. The human immunodeficiency virus I Rev

protein provides one example of a leucine-rich sequence (LQLPPLERLTL) that is recognized by the carrier CRM1. Certain RNA sequences or structures may also serve as NESs.

A third type of signal—a nuclear retention signal (NRS)—is present on a number of proteins that bind to immature RNAs. These proteins hold immature RNAs in the nucleus and must be removed before mature RNAs can be exported to the cytoplasm. This mechanism allows the nuclear envelope to segregate immature, unprocessed RNAs from the protein synthetic machinery in the cytoplasm.

The following is a brief thumbnail of protein import into the nucleus (Fig. 14-17). A protein with an NLS (known as **cargo**) binds to an **import receptor** either by itself or in combination with an **adapter** molecule, forming a complex, which then passes through pores into the nucleus. There, the cargo and adapter (if used) are displaced from the import receptor. The adapter then releases its cargo and is transported back to the cytoplasm as the cargo of an export receptor. Import receptors also shuttle back through pores, where they can meet more cargo or cargo/adapter complexes. Molecules exported from the nucleus use a variation of this cycle, being picked up by the transport machinery in the nucleus and discharged in the cytoplasm.

The key to this system is that it is *vectorial:* Nuclear components are transported into the nucleus while components that function in the cytoplasm are transported out. This means that each carrier picks up its cargo on one side of the nuclear envelope and deposits it on the other. This directionality is regulated by a simple yet elegant system involving Ran, a small guanine triphosphatase (GTPase [see Figs. 4-6 and 4-7 for background material on GTPases]), and associated factors.

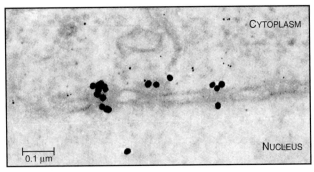

CYTOPLASM

NUCLEUS

0.1 μm

Figure 14-15 The nuclear localization sequence of nucleoplasmin can even cause large colloidal gold particles to be transported into the cell nucleus. A thin-section electron micrograph shows gold particles coated with nucleoplasmin crossing the nuclear envelope by passing through the nuclear pore complexes. Much smaller gold particles coated with bovine serum albumin (BSA) remain in the cytoplasm. Both sets of gold particles were microinjected into the cytoplasm of *Xenopus* oocytes, and the cells were processed 1 hour later for electron microscopy. Scale bar: 0.1 μm. (From Dworetzky SI, Lanford RE, Feldherr CM: The effects of variations in the number and sequence of targeting signals on nuclear uptake. J Cell Biol 107:1279–1287, 1988.)

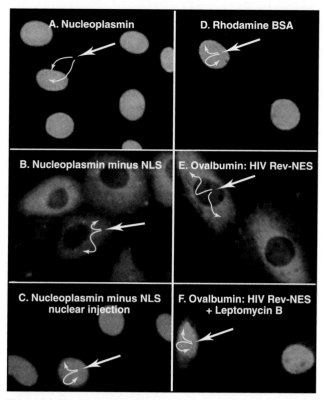

Figure 14-16 DEMONSTRATION OF THE EXISTENCE OF SPECIFIC NUCLEAR IMPORT AND EXPORT SIGNALS ON PROTEINS. **Left,** Nuclear import. **A,** Nucleoplasmin microinjected into the cytoplasm rapidly migrates into the nucleus. **B,** Nucleoplasmin lacking its NLS, when microinjected into the cytoplasm, stays in the cytoplasm. **C,** Nucleoplasmin lacking its NLS microinjected into the nucleus stays in the nucleus. **Right,** Nuclear export. **D,** Fluorescently labeled bovine serum albumin (BSA) microinjected into the nucleus stays in the nucleus. **E,** When ovalbumin, to which the NES of the HIV (the virus that causes AIDS) Rev protein has been conjugated, is microinjected into the nucleus, it rapidly migrates into the cytoplasm. **F,** In the presence of leptomycin B (a drug that inhibits the activity of the nuclear export receptor CRM1), ovalbumin to which the NES of the HIV Rev protein has been conjugated, if microinjected into the nucleus, stays in the nucleus. (**A–C,** From Dingwall C, Robbins J, Dilworth SM, et al: The nucleoplasmin nuclear location sequence is larger and more complex than that of SV-40 large T antigen. J Cell Biol 107:841–849, 1988, by copyright permission of the Rockefeller University Press. **D–F,** From Fukuda M, Asano S, Nakamura T, et al: CRM1 is responsible for intracellular transport mediated by the nuclear export signal. Nature 390:308–311, 1997, Fig. 1b [without lower right panel].)

Components of Nuclear Import and Export

The nuclear import and export system involves many components, but the general principles of its operation are simple. To understand how it works, this section first introduces several of the components (Table 14-2) and then describes one transport event in detail.

Adapters

Adapters bind to the NLS or NES sequences on some cargo molecules and also to particular regions on receptors. The best-known adapter is **importin α,** which is responsible for recognition of small basic NLS sequences and works together with the transport receptor importin β (see later) in nuclear transport. Importin α consists of a highly flexible N-terminal NLS-like importin β-binding domain followed by 10 repeats of a helical motif (the Armadillo repeat [Fig. 14-17D]) that give the structured portion of the molecule a slug-like shape. The importin β-binding motif can bind either the NLS-binding region on importin β or the NLS-binding domain on importin α itself (the "belly" of the slug). The latter provides an autoinhibitory mechanism that is thought to be important in regulating the release of cargo in the nucleus at the end of an import cycle. Binding to importin β uncovers the NLS binding site on importin α so that it can bind cargo more efficiently.

Other nuclear trafficking pathways use different adapters. For example, two adapters bridge between snRNA and the export receptor CRM1 during snRNA export from the nucleus.

Receptors

With the exception of mRNP export from the nucleus (which uses special transport factors), all nuclear trafficking receptors are related to **importin β,** the import receptor for proteins bearing a basic NLS. At least 20 members of the importin β family are known in vertebrates (14 in yeast). These proteins are also called **karyopherins.** Some of these function in nuclear import, whereas others function in export. Importin β consists entirely of 19 copies of a helical protein interaction motif called a HEAT repeat, giving the protein the shape of a snail-like superhelix with the potential to interact with a large number of protein ligands. All importin β family members have a binding site for the Ran GTPase that encompasses several HEAT repeats at the N-terminus (Fig. 14-17D). Importin β binds many NLSs directly but also interacts with other cargoes via the importin α adapter. Other importin β HEAT repeats bind to FG repeats of the nucleoporins.

Directionality/Recycling Factors

Ran GTPase and its bound nucleotides inform nuclear trafficking receptors about whether they are located in the nucleus or cytoplasm. Ran-GTP (Ran with bound GTP) *dissociates* import complexes but is required to *form* export complexes. The system imparts directionality because Ran-GTP is converted to Ran-GDP in the cytoplasm and Ran-GDP is converted to Ran-GTP in the nucleus.

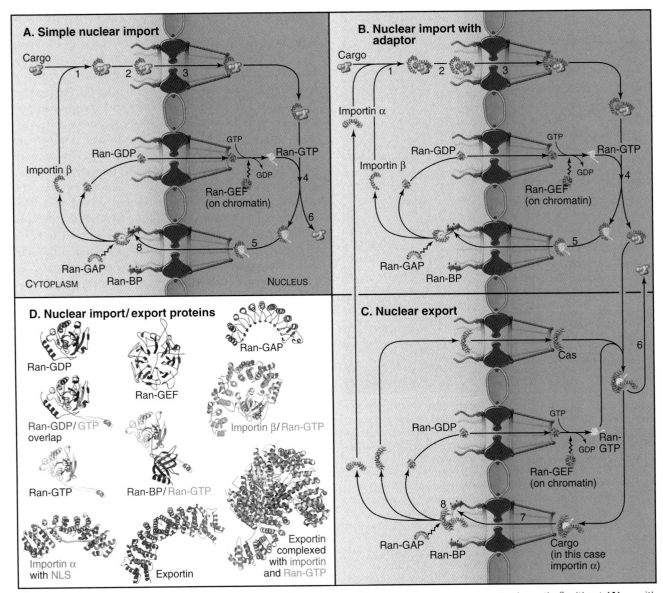

Figure 14-17 **NUCLEAR TRAFFICKING OF MACROMOLECULES.** Nuclear import of a cargo by the import receptor importin β without **(A)** or with **(B)** the use of an adapter protein. **C,** Export of a cargo by the importin β-related export receptor Cas. In this case, the cargo is the import adapter importin α. Directionality is given by Ran. Ran-GTP releases import cargoes in the nucleus and is required for formation of the export complex. Numbers refer to the steps described in the text. **D,** Crystal structures of several of the components involved in nuclear transport. (Ribbon models courtesy of F. Wittinghoffer, MPI Dortmund, Germany.)

Like other small GTPases, Ran has low intrinsic GTPase activity, but interactions with binding proteins (Ran-BP1 or Ran-BP2) and a GTPase-activating protein called **Ran-GAP1** stimulate GTP hydrolysis. Ran-BP1 is anchored in the cytoplasm. Ran-BP2 is a component of the fibers projecting from the nuclear pore into the cytoplasm. This huge (>350 kD) protein can bind up to four Ran molecules as well as Ran-GAP1 and may provide a structural scaffold for the conversion of Ran-GTP into Ran-GDP at the surface of the pore. Because Ran-BP1 and Ran-BP2 are both anchored in the cytoplasm, Ran-GTP is efficiently converted to Ran-GDP only in the cytoplasm, yielding a nuclear/cytoplasmic ratio of Ran-GTP of ~200:1.

Ran-GDP must reenter the nucleus to be recharged with GTP. Efficient Ran-GDP transport into the nucleus requires nuclear transport factor 2 (NTF2). Back in the nucleus, Ran must release its bound GDP to acquire GTP. GDP dissociation is slow but is stimulated by a guanine nucleotide exchange factor (GEF). This protein, called **regulator of chromosome condensation 1 (RCC1),** is tightly associated with chromatin throughout the cell cycle. This allows nuclear import to resume immediately after the nuclear envelope reforms at the end of mitosis. Since Ran is involved in essential every nuclear trafficking event, the flux of this small protein across the nuclear envelope is

Table 14-2

SEVERAL KEY PROTEINS INVOLVED IN NUCLEAR TRAFFICKING

Adapters

Importin α*	An import adapter, importin α interacts with importin β during nuclear transport and binds basic NLSs. Humans have at least six distinct importin α genes, expressed in a tissue-specific manner.
Snurportin 1	This adapter binds the trimethyl G cap structure on snRNPs during import. It also interacts with importin β during nuclear transport.
hnRNP A1	This protein has a major role in the export of mRNA from the nucleus. The molecule is extremely abundant (10^8 copies/cell) and active (10^5 copies/min shuttling between the nucleus and cytoplasm).

Importin β—Related Molecules Involved in Import*

Importin β	A founder member of the large family of nuclear trafficking receptors, importin β binds various adapters and interacts with nucleoporins during import. Ran-GTP regulates binding to adapters.
Transportin	Transportin imports mRNA-binding proteins into the nucleus.

Importin β—Related Molecules Involved in Export

CAS	CAS recycles importin α and snurportin 1 to the cytoplasm.
CRM1	CRM1 exports proteins with leucine-rich NESs and also U snRNAs. It is a target of the fungal toxin leptomycin B.
Exportin-t	This protein is involved in tRNA export.

Directionality Factors

Ran	A small Ras-family GTPase, Ran binds importin-related nuclear trafficking receptors, as well as a number of regulatory proteins.
Ran-GAP1	This protein stimulates GTP hydrolysis by Ran in cytoplasm (GAP = GTPase-activating protein).
RCC1	RCC1 is the nuclear GTP exchange factor (GEF) for Ran. It stimulates release of GDP from Ran.
Ran-BP1	Ran-BP1 is a cytoplasmic protein that binds Ran-GTP and acts with Ran-GAP1 to stimulate GTP hydrolysis by Ran.
Ran-BP2	A major component of the cytoplasmic filaments of the nuclear pore, Ran-BP2 has four Ran-binding domains. It also binds Ran-GAP1 and may locally convert cytoplasmic Ran-GTP to Ran-GDP so that it can return to the nucleus.
NTF2	NTF2 binds RanGDP and promotes its recycling back to the nucleus.

*The importin molecules (humans have 14 genes) were discovered independently and termed karyopherins.

enormous—several million molecules per minute in cultured cells.

Description of a Single Import Cycle in Detail

Consider the import into the nucleus of a typical protein (Fig. 14-17):

1. In the cytoplasm, the import complex forms as importin β binds to cargo with high affinity. Many cargoes bind directly to importin β. Other cargoes, including those containing the very widely studied basic NLS, consist of the target protein bound to an importin α adapter. Here both are referred to simply as *cargo.*

2. In a process known as docking, the import complex binds to the cytoplasmic filaments of the nuclear pore.

3. The complex is transferred through the pore in a process that involves interactions of importin β with FG repeats on nucleoporins. These interactions might be rather nonspecific, since it is pos-

sible to delete about half of the FG domains from yeast nucleoporins without killing the cell. The mechanism of transport through the pore is unknown, but most models propose that multiple weak interactions concentrate the import complex in the lumen of the pore and that movement through the pore itself occurs by simple Brownian motion (thermal motion of particles in solution). Nucleoside triphosphate hydrolysis is not required for the complex to cross the pore.

4. In the nucleus, the import complex encounters Ran-GTP. Ran-GTP binds to importin β, displacing the cargo from it.

5. Importin β/Ran-GTP then shuttles back through the pore to the cytoplasm.

6. In the nucleus, if the cargo was bound directly to importin β, it is now free to function. If it was actually a cargo/importin α complex, this now encounters a nuclear export receptor called **CAS.** Ran-GTP and CAS bind tightly to importin α, displacing the cargo.

7. CAS then carries importin α and Ran-GTP through the nuclear pores back to the cytoplasm. Importin

α functions as an adapter in one direction and cargo in the other.

The cargo is now in the nucleus, but the system is stalled. The import receptor, importin β, is back in the cytoplasm, but in a complex with Ran-GTP that is unable to bind further cargo. The import adapter, importin α, is also in the cytoplasm, but it is locked in a complex with the CAS export receptor and Ran-GTP. The solution to this problem is simple.

8. To keep the cycle going, the complex of Ran-BP1, Ran-BP2, and Ran-GAP1 associated with cytoplasmic filaments of the nuclear pore catalyze the hydrolysis of GTP bound to Ran. Ran-GDP dissociates from importin α, which is now ready for further cycles of nuclear import. In addition, after hydrolysis of GTP, the importin α/CAS/Ran-GDP complex dissociates, allowing CAS to return to the nucleus for further work as an export receptor and making importin α available in the cytoplasm to bind more cargo and function as an import adapter. The hydrolysis of GTP on Ran appears to be the only source of chemical energy required to drive the accumulation of proteins in the nucleus against a concentration gradient.

Although there are several names to remember, the nuclear trafficking system is actually quite straightforward, being regulated by the state of the guanine nucleotide bound by Ran. The key point is that the guanine nucleotide exchange factor that charges Ran-GDP with GTP is in the nucleus and the Ran-GAPs that promote hydrolysis of GTP bound to Ran are cytoplasmic. Cargo that is meant to be imported into the nucleus is released from its carriers in the presence of high levels of nuclear Ran-GTP. Conversely, cargo that is destined for export to the cytoplasm is picked up by its carriers only in the presence of high levels of nuclear Ran-GTP and is released when the Ran is converted to Ran-GDP in the cytoplasm. In this way, the directionality of transport is defined by the different concentrations of Ran-GDP and Ran-GTP in the cytoplasm and nucleus.

Regulation of Transport across the Nuclear Envelope

Cells regulate nuclear trafficking in several ways. The first of these is to change the number of pores. In rat liver, there are 15 to 20 pores per square micrometer of nuclear envelope (~4000 per nucleus). This number can be shifted up or down depending on the transcriptional activity in the nucleus.

Nuclear trafficking is most commonly regulated by phosphorylation near the NLS on the cargo. Phosphorylation adjacent to a basic NLS inhibits nuclear import. This provides a mechanism to regulate the ability of a particular cargo to enter the nucleus in response to cell

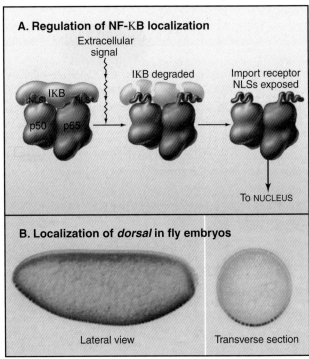

Figure 14-18   REGULATION OF NF-κB LOCALIZATION. **A,** The transcription factor NF-κB is kept in the cytoplasm as a result of interactions with its inhibitor IκB. IκB holds NF-κB in the cytoplasm in two ways. When it binds NF-κB, it covers up the NF-κB NLS. Second, IκB contains a nuclear export signal, so that any NF-κB associated with it that happens to enter the nucleus is rapidly exported to the cytoplasm. **B,** Localization of the *dorsal* transcription factor (a relative of NF-κB) in *Drosophila* embryos. These images represent a longitudinal *(left)* and cross-sectional *(right)* view of wild-type embryos. The *dorsal* protein is stained with specific antibody, which appears as dark spots where it has become concentrated in the cell nuclei in the ventral portion of the embryo. (B, From Roth S, Stein D, Nusslein-Volhard C: A gradient of nuclear localization of the dorsal protein determines dorsoventral pattern in the Drosophila embryo. Cell 59:1189–1202, 1989.)

cycle (see Fig. 43-6) or other cues that can be coupled to specific protein kinase activation.

Traffic across the nuclear envelope may be also regulated by masking or unmasking nuclear localization sequences. A "nuclear" protein with a masked NLS is trapped in the cytoplasm. A good example is the regulation of transcription factor NF-κB by IκB (Fig. 14-18). IκB binds to NF-κB and covers up its NLS. Because IκB also has a nuclear export signal, the NF-κB : IκB complex is entirely cytoplasmic. Following an appropriate signal (see Fig. 15-22C), IκB is degraded. This uncovers the NLS on NF-κB, allowing it to enter the nucleus.

Disorders Associated with Defective Nuclear Trafficking

In many instances, protein function appears to be regulated by adjusting its location in the cell, and nuclear transport is one mechanism controlling localization. Thus, a myriad of examples undoubtedly exist in which disruption of transport leads to disease. This area has yet to be explored systematically, but in one interesting example, human sex determination is disrupted by mutations of a NLS on the SRY transcription factor, a master regulator of sex determination. These NLS mutants apparently disrupt the accumulation of SRY in the nucleus at a critical stage during development, causing individuals with a 46XY karyotype (normal male) to develop as females.

Other Uses of the Importin/Ran Switch

The ability of Ran-GTP to release substrates bound to importin β provides a highly efficient switch for regulating protein availability. Cells use this system to regulate a number of supramolecular assembly processes, including assembly of the nuclear envelope, nuclear pore, and mitotic spindle, as well pairing of centrosomes.

In these processes, importin β (and occasionally importin α) acts as a negative regulator of assembly by binding to and sequestering key proteins. In the case of mitotic spindle assembly in large cells such as eggs that lack centrosomes, sequestration of these proteins blocks spindle assembly. In eggs, this block is overcome in the vicinity of chromosomes, which bind high concentrations of the guanine nucleotide exchange factor RCC1. Conversion of Ran-GDP to Ran-GTP near the chromosomes results in Ran-GTP binding to importin β and release of bound "cargo," which triggers formation of the mitotic spindle. Of course, spindle assembly is triggered only after nuclear envelope breakdown, when the chromosomes come in contact with the cytoplasm. In fact, the transport of components required for spindle assembly into the nucleus (and away from the microtubules) during interphase may be a second level of control.

Importin β and Ran appear to regulate nuclear pore assembly in a similar way by sequestering key pore components, including the Nup107-160 complex, until release by Ran-GTP. Importin β also sequesters an un-

known component required for vesicle fusion during nuclear reassembly following mitosis. The importin β switch appears to have other roles at centrosomes and kinetochores, but these are less well characterized.

ACKNOWLEDGMENTS

Thanks go to Roland Foisner, Angus Lamond, Erich Schirmer, and David Spector for their suggestions on revisions to this chapter.

SELECTED READINGS

Azuma Y, Dasso M: The role of Ran in nuclear function. Curr Opin Cell Biol 12:302-307, 2000.

Harel A, Forbes D: Importin beta: Conducting a much larger cellular symphony. Mol Cell 16:319-330, 2004.

Hetzer MW, Walther TC, Mattaj, IW: Pushing the envelope: Structure, function, and dynamics of the nuclear periphery. Annu Rev Cell Dev Biol 21:347-380, 2005.

Hood JK, Silver PA: In or out? Regulating nuclear transport. Curr Opin Cell Biol 11:241-247, 1999.

Hutchison CJ, Alvarez-Reyes M, Vaughan OA: Lamins in disease: Why do ubiquitously expressed nuclear envelope proteins give rise to tissue-specific disease phenotypes? J Cell Sci 114:9-19, 2001.

Lamond AI, Earnshaw WC: Structure and function in the nucleus. Science 280:547-553, 1998.

Lamond AI, Spector DL: Nuclear speckles: A model for nuclear organelles. Nat Rev Mol Cell Biol 4:605-612, 2003.

Lewis JD, Tollervey D: Like attracts like: Getting RNA processing together in the nucleus. Science 288:1385-1389, 2000.

Matera AG: Nuclear bodies: Multifaceted subdomains of the interchromatin space. Trends Cell Biol 9:302-309, 1999.

Mattaj IW, Englmeier L: Nucleocytoplasmic transport: The soluble phase. Annu Rev Biochem 67:265-306, 1998.

Mounkes L, Kozlov S, Burke B, Stewart CL: The laminopathies: Nuclear structure meets disease. Curr Opin Genet Dev 13:223-230, 2003.

Nigg EA: Nucleocytoplasmic transport: Signals, mechanisms and regulation. Nature 386:779-787, 1997.

Pemberton LF, Blobel G, Rosenblum JS: Transport routes through the nuclear pore complex. Curr Op Cell Biol 10:392-399, 1998.

Spector DL: The dynamics of chromosome organization and gene regulation. Annu Rev Biochem 72:573-608, 2003.

Stuurman N, Heins S, Aebi U: Nuclear lamins: Their structure, assembly, and interactions. J Struct Biol 122:42-66, 1998.

Suntharalingham M, Wente SR: Peering through the pore: Nuclear pore complex structure, assembly and function. Dev Cell 4:775-789, 2003.

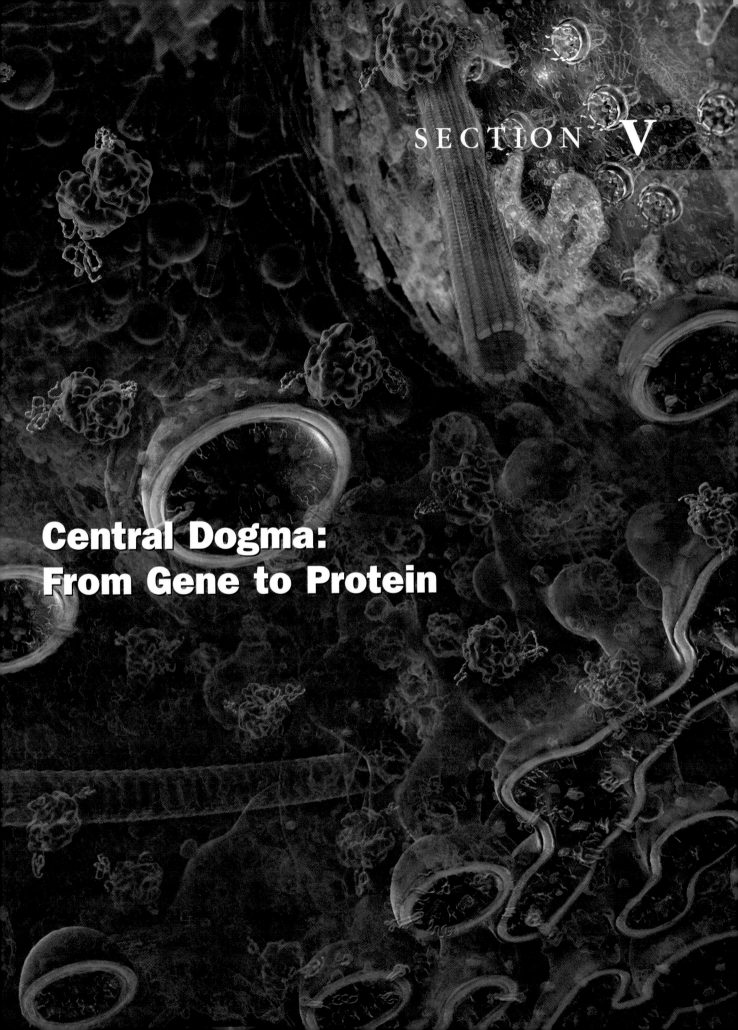

Central Dogma:
From Gene to Protein

SECTION V OVERVIEW

The hugely important prediction of a structure for DNA not only led Crick and Watson to propose a general strategy for the replication of DNA (discussed in Chapter 42) but also led Francis Crick to propose the central dogma of molecular biology: that DNA is transcribed into RNA and that this RNA is then translated into protein. Chapters 15 to 17 present the cell biology of this central dogma, with one crucial addition that could not have been foreseen by Crick. This new element is the complex battery of processing events that RNAs undergo before they function as messengers, transfer vehicles, processing machines, or protein synthesizing machines in the ribosome.

Chapter 15 discusses RNA transcription, the initial step in recovering the information encoded in the chromosomal DNA. Three cellular RNA polymerases have distinct specialized tasks: **Polymerase I** transcribes ribosomal RNAs; **polymerase II** transcribes all messenger RNAs (mRNAs) plus a number of small RNA molecules that are involved in RNA processing; and **polymerase III** transcribes transfer RNAs (tRNAs) and the smallest ribosomal RNAs. These three polymerases evolved from a common ancestor and retain many shared features. However, they have acquired significant differences in the ways they act on their target genes.

Eukaryotic genes contain both upstream (5′) and downstream (3′) regulatory regions that are not transcribed into RNA. Each gene has a **promoter** located just upstream from the site where transcription begins. **Enhancers** are DNA sequences that regulate transcription from a distance. Both promoter and enhancer sequences form binding sites for regulatory proteins that either stimulate or repress transcription. The chromatin organization of the DNA template and its location within the nucleus also influence the efficiency of transcription.

Fundamental differences in the ways in which eukaryotes and prokaryotes store their genomes have had a profound influence on the structure of genes and the fate of cellular RNAs. In prokaryotes, the DNA occupies a distinct region of cytoplasm that is not bounded by a membrane. This means that transcription of DNA sequences into mRNAs and translation of mRNAs into proteins can be coupled directly, with ribosomes attaching to nascent mRNAs even before they are fully copied from the DNA template. In contrast, eukaryotes house their genomes and the machinery for RNA transcription and processing in a nucleus bounded by a nuclear envelope. Eukaryotic protein-coding RNAs must be transported across the nuclear membrane prior to their translation by ribosomes in cytoplasm. This geographic segregation, in which mRNAs are created in one subcellular compartment and used in another, has allowed the evolution of structurally complex genes whose RNA products must be spliced before use.

The initial RNA products of transcription of most eukaryotic genes require extensive modifications by **RNA processing** before they are ready to function. Chapter 16 explains that most protein-coding genes of higher eukaryotes contain protein-coding regions called **exons** separated by noncoding **intron** regions. Consequently, the initial RNA copy of these genes must be processed to remove the introns before the finished mRNA is exported from the nucleus.

The nucleus is the site of many other essential RNA-processing events. These include the addition of 5′ cap structures to mRNAs, polyadenylation of the 3′ end of mRNAs, cleavage of some RNAs into functional pieces, modification of RNA bases, and a host of sometimes

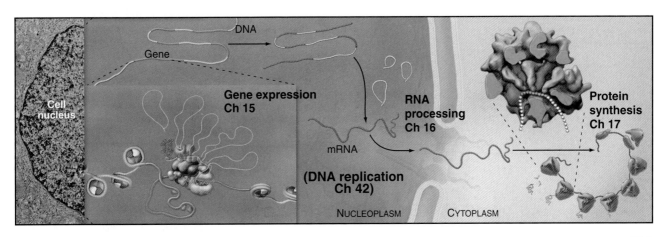

bizarre editing events. Both the RNA substrates for these events and many enzymes that carry out the reactions are packaged into ribonucleoprotein particles by specific proteins, but RNAs themselves carry out a number of enzymatic reactions, including catalysis of peptide bond formation by the ribosome.

Cells also contain enzymes that fragment double-stranded RNAs into small pieces, used by other proteins to direct the silencing of the genes that encoded them. This process of **RNAi** is critical for defense against RNA viruses and chromatin regulation. Cell biologists also use RNAi as a technique to study gene function in the laboratory.

Chapter 17 describes how ribosomes translate the sequence of nucleotide triplets in mRNAs into proteins. Transfer RNAs act as adapters, matching specific amino acids with triplet codons in the mRNA. The RNA component of ribosomes catalyzes the transfer of each successive amino acid from its tRNA onto the C-terminus of the growing polypeptide. Every step in the process is carefully regulated to ensure quality control of the finished polypeptide. Initiation factors select the proper AUG codon in the mRNA to begin the polypeptide with

a methionine residue (or formylmethione in the case of bacteria). Elongation factors check that the proper tRNA is matched with each codon before peptide bonds are formed. In spite of the fact that polypeptides grow at 20 residues per second, errors occur at a rate of less than one residue in a thousand. Termination factors bring protein synthesis to a close at the C-terminus of the polypeptide and recycle the ribosomal subunits for another round of translation.

Although some proteins fold spontaneously into their mature form following release from a ribosome, many proteins require a helping hand to reach their properly folded state. Chapter 17 covers four types of chaperones that help proteins fold by different mechanisms. Trigger factor, which is associated with ribosomes, provides a hydrophobic groove for protein folding. Hsp70 and Hsp90 chaperones bind hydrophobic residues in nascent polypeptides, prevent the unfolded protein from aggregating, and thereby promote folding. Cycles of binding and release are accompanied by hydrolysis of ATP. Chaperonins related to GroEL provide chambers to protect proteins during folding. ATP hydrolysis releases the protein from this chamber.

CHAPTER 15

Gene Expression

Each organism, whether it has 600 genes *(Mycoplasma)*, 6000 genes (budding yeast), or 25,000 genes (humans), depends on reliable mechanisms to turn these genes on and off. This is called regulation of gene expression. In simple organisms, such as bacteria and yeast, environmental signals, such as temperature or nutrient levels, control much of gene expression. In multicellular organisms, genetically programmed gene expression controls development from a fertilized egg. Within these organisms, cells send each other signals that control gene expression either through direct contact or via secreted molecules, such as growth factors and hormones.

Given the vast numbers of genes, even in simple organisms, regulation of gene expression is complicated. Control is exerted at multiple steps, including production of mRNA, translation, and protein turnover. This chapter focuses on the first of these regulatory steps: the transcription mechanisms that lead to the production of messenger RNA (mRNA) and other RNA transcripts. The past decade has seen the discovery of hundreds of key components in this process.

Proteins called **transcription factors** turn genes on or off by binding to particular DNA sequences adjacent to the sequences encoding the protein or RNA product of the gene. The paradigm of this level of regulation is the bacterial repressor that controls expression of genes required for lactose metabolism in *Escherichia coli*. In eukaryotes, transcription factors are numerous, representing approximately 6% of human genes. They are also quite diverse, binding to a wide range of DNA regulatory sites. Fortunately, they fall into a limited number of families with similar structures and binding mechanisms. Three types of eukaryotic DNA-dependent RNA polymerases respond to these regulatory proteins and copy DNA sequence into RNA. Regulation of transcription factors is achieved by variations in a limited number of mechanisms that control their synthesis, transport from the cytoplasm into the nucleus, and activity through posttranslational modifications or binding to small molecular ligands.

One key level of regulation is transcription initiation, the first step in production of RNA transcripts. This chapter examines the basic features of both prokaryotic and eukaryotic transcription units and the transcription machinery. Regulatory transcription factors that control the expression of several selected genes are discussed in the context of how external signals can reprogram patterns of gene expression. Finally, the chapter addresses the mechanisms by which mutation of transcription factor genes leads to human disease.

This chapter was written by Jeffrey L. Corden.

The Transcription Cycle

Synthesis of RNA by **RNA polymerases** is a cyclic process that can be broken down into three sets of events: initiation, elongation, and termination (Fig. 15-1). Each of these events consists of multiple individual steps. In the first step of the **initiation** process, RNA polymerase locates and binds to the chromosome near the beginning of the gene, forming a **preinitiation complex** at a sequence termed a **promoter.** This binding must be highly specific to distinguish promoter from nonpromoter DNA. Next, a conformational change in the polymerase-promoter complex results in formation of an **open complex** in which the DNA duplex is unpaired, allowing RNA polymerase access to nucleotide bases that are complementary to the start of the message. After formation of a phosphodiester bond between the first two complementary ribonucleotides, the polymerase translocates one base and repeats the process of phosphodiester bond formation, resulting in **elongation** of the nascent RNA. The elongation reaction cycle continues at an average rate of about 20 to 30 nucleotides per second until the complete gene has been transcribed. Elongation is not a uniform reaction, however, as RNA polymerase pauses at certain sequences. These pauses are important for regulation of transcription. The final step in the transcription cycle, **termination,** occurs when the polymerase reaches a signal on DNA that causes an extended pause in elongation. Given enough time and the appropriate sequence context, the nascent transcript dissociates from the elongating RNA polymerase, and the DNA template returns to a base-paired duplex conformation. Ultimately, RNA polymerase dissociates from the template and is free to begin a new search for a promoter.

Each of the steps in the transcription cycle can potentially serve as the target of regulatory molecules. The frequency of initiation varies among different promoters as dictated by the need for the gene product. The initiation reaction is most often regulated, presumably because this prevents synthesis of messages that encode unneeded products. Elongation and termination can also be regulated, as can splicing and further processing of mRNAs (see Chapter 16). In eukaryotes, the sum of these nuclear regulatory steps, together with cytoplasmic regulation of mRNA stability and translation efficiency, contributes to the wide variation seen in the abundance of different mRNAs and proteins in particular types of cells.

The Transcription Unit

Coding information in genomes is transcribed in increments corresponding to one or a few genes. Gene-coding and regulatory (*cis*-acting) DNA sequences that direct transcription initiation, elongation, and termination are collectively called a **transcription unit.** Prokaryotic transcription units, called **operons,** contain more than one gene, often encoding physiologically related proteins (Fig. 15-2A). Operons are flanked by sequences that direct the initiation and termination of transcription. Figure 15-2B shows a simple eukaryotic transcription unit encoding the human hemoglobin β-chain. Although only a small fraction of this region encodes the β-globin polypeptide, the adjacent regulatory sequences are crucial for proper expression of β-globin. Genetic defects resulting in decreased β-globin production are called β-thalassemias. Such mutations can occur either in the coding region, resulting in an unstable or truncated polypeptide, or in the adjacent control regions, leading to low levels of transcription or aberrant processing of the newly synthesized RNA (see Chapter 16). Thus, the transcription unit can be thought of as a linked series of modules, all of which must be functional for the gene to be transcribed at the correct level.

Biogenesis of RNA

A typical cell contains more RNA than genomic DNA. This RNA consists of molecules ranging typically from several hundred to several thousand nucleotides long. In prokaryotes, newly synthesized mRNA is immediately translated by ribosomes that initiate translation even before transcription has terminated. In eukaryotes, RNA is distributed between the nucleus, where RNA synthesis occurs, and the cytoplasm, where most RNA is used to synthesize proteins. Eukaryotic cells have four different types of RNA:

1. **Ribosomal RNA (rRNA** [see Fig. 16-9]), the most abundant type, making up about 75% of the total

2. Small, stable RNAs, such as **transfer RNA (tRNA** [see Fig. 17-3]), **small nuclear RNAs (snRNA** [see

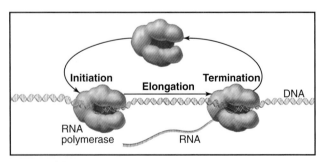

Figure 15-1   THE TRANSCRIPTION CYCLE. The transcription reaction consists of three basic steps in which the RNA polymerase initiates transcription at the promoter, elongates the nascent RNA copy of one of the DNA strands, and terminates transcription on completion of the message.

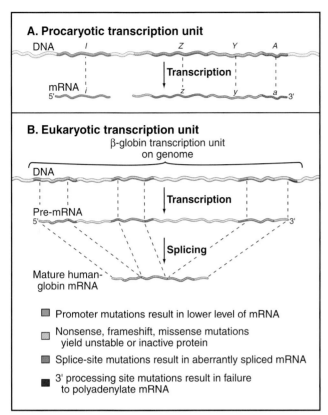

A. Procaryotic transcription unit

DNA   *I*   *Z*   *Y*   *A*

Transcription

mRNA
5'   *z*   *y*   *a* 3'

B. Eukaryotic transcription unit

β-globin transcription unit
on genome

DNA

Transcription

Pre-mRNA
5'   3'

Splicing

Mature human-
globin mRNA

◻ Promoter mutations result in lower level of mRNA

◻ Nonsense, frameshift, missense mutations
yield unstable or inactive protein

◼ Splice-site mutations result in aberrantly spliced mRNA

◼ 3' processing site mutations result in failure
to polyadenylate mRNA

Figure 15-2 PROKARYOTIC AND EUKARYOTIC TRANSCRIPTION UNITS. **A,** The two transcription units required for regulation of lactose metabolism in *E. coli*. The *I* gene encodes the lac repressor, while the *Z*, *Y*, and *A* genes encode β-galactosidase, lactose permease, and thiogalactoside transacetylase. All three genes are required for the cell to grow on media containing lactose and are coregulated as the *lac* operon. **B,** The nucleotide sequence of one of the two DNA strands is transcribed into a complementary pre-mRNA copy. The pre-mRNA is processed by removing introns and splicing together the protein-coding exons *(orange)*. The DNA sequences required for expression of a functional β-globin protein are indicated in different colors (see key). Mutations in any of these sequences can lead to decreased β-globin expression.

Chapter 16]) involved in splicing, and **5S rRNA,** which makes up about 15% of the total

3. **mRNA** and its precursor **heterogeneous nuclear RNA (hnRNA),** which account for only 10%

4. **Small noncoding (ncRNAs)** or **micro RNAs (miRNA),** which are involved in a variety of regulatory processes.

Transcription of eukaryotic DNA in the nucleus is linked to subsequent steps that process the nascent transcript in preparation for its eventual function (see Chapter 16 for a complete discussion of these steps). For mRNA precursors, this includes capping and methylation of the 5′ end of the nascent transcript. Most messages are also spliced to remove introns; the 3′ end of the message is then cleaved, and a stretch of adenosine

residues is added. The mRNA is then transported to the cytoplasm, where it serves as the template for protein synthesis.

Eukaryotic ribosomal RNA is synthesized from a set of tandemly repeated genes as a single molecule, which is cleaved and modified to give the final 28S, 5.8S, and 18S RNAs (Fig. 15-3). These are assembled, together with 5S RNA and about 80 proteins, into ribosomes in the nucleolus. Transfer RNA is synthesized in the nucleus and transported to the cytoplasm, where it is charged with amino acids prior to participating in protein synthesis (see Chapter 17). snRNAs are synthesized and processed in the nucleus. From there, they migrate to the cytoplasm, where they acquire essential proteins, and then return to the nucleus, where they function in the enzymatic reactions of RNA processing (splicing; see Chapter 16). The postsynthetic processing pathway that a particular transcript follows is dictated, in part, by the transcription machinery that is used to initiate and elongate the transcript and by certain features of the nascent RNA.

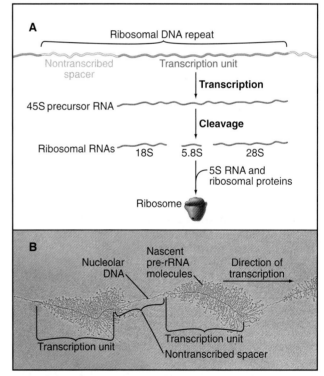

A

Ribosomal DNA repeat

Nontranscribed
spacer   Transcription unit

Transcription

45S precursor RNA

Cleavage

Ribosomal RNAs   18S   5.8S   28S

5S RNA and
ribosomal proteins

Ribosome

B

Nascent
Nucleolar   pre-rRNA   Direction of
DNA   molecules   transcription

Transcription unit
Transcription unit
Nontranscribed spacer

Figure 15-3 RIBOSOMAL RNA TRANSCRIPTION UNIT. Ribosomal RNA is transcribed from a set of transcription units arrayed as tandem copies of the same transcription unit. **A,** Map showing the arrangement of sequences in a typical ribosomal DNA repeat. **B,** Electron micrograph showing two active rRNA transcription units. Note that each transcription unit is transcribed by multiple RNA polymerases. As the polymerases traverse the gene, the attached nascent RNA is extended, giving a tree-like appearance. (B, Courtesy of Yvonne Osheim, University of Virginia, Charlottesville.)

RNA Polymerases

RNA polymerases synthesize a new strand of nucleic acid that is complementary to one of the chromosomal DNA strands. While the enzymatic reaction is similar to DNA replication (see Chapter 42), there are several important differences. First, RNA polymerases synthesize a strand of ribonucleotides. Second, unlike DNA polymerase, RNA polymerases can initiate transcription without a primer. Finally, unlike replication, the newly transcribed sequences do not remain base-paired with the template but are displaced after reaching a length of about 10 nucleotides. These properties are common to RNA polymerases in all cells; therefore, it is not surprising that all cellular RNA polymerases share common structural features.

Bacteria have a single RNA polymerase containing six polypeptides. Two copies of the α subunit and one each of the β, β', and ω subunits form a five-subunit **core enzyme** that synthesizes RNA. The sixth subunit, σ, binds to the core enzyme to form a **holoenzyme** that is able to recognize promoter sequences and initiate transcription.

Most eukaryotes have three different RNA polymerases (some species of plants contain four). The largest subunits of the three eukaryotic RNA polymerases are closely related to the bacterial β and β' subunits. RNA polymerases I, II, and III have up to 10 additional subunits, most of which are unique to each enzyme (Fig. 15-4A). The subunits of both prokaryotic and eukaryotic enzymes assemble into a structure that is roughly spherical, with a diameter of approximately 150 Å and a 25-Å-wide cleft, large enough to accommodate the DNA template (Fig. 15-4B). The site of nucleotide addition is located on the back wall of the cleft. The framework of this structure is provided by the two largest subunits, which make up the two lobes that clamp down on the template DNA.

The eukaryotic polymerases can be distinguished experimentally on the basis of their sensitivity to the fungal toxin α-**amanitin**, RNA polymerase II being the most sensitive and RNA polymerase I being the most resistant. RNA polymerase I localizes to the nucleolus, where it synthesizes rRNA. RNA polymerase II synthesizes mRNA and several snRNAs involved in RNA splicing in the nucleoplasm. RNA polymerase III synthesizes tRNA, 5S rRNA, and the 7S RNA of the signal recognition particle (see Fig. 20-5). The newly described RNA polymerase IV is present in plants, where it is involved in heterochromatin formation and gene silencing.

The multiple eukaryotic RNA polymerases apparently originated through duplication of primordial subunit genes, followed by evolution of specialized functions. For example, RNA polymerase I synthesizes one species, whereas RNA polymerase III synthesizes several hundred species of highly abundant transcripts. The pool of mRNAs is more complex, however. Human cells have approximately 20,000 different species of mRNA. The relative abundance of individual mRNAs can vary widely, often in response to external signals, from just a few copies to more than 10,000 copies per cell. Thus, RNA polymerase II must recognize thousands of different promoters and transcribe them with widely varying efficiencies. In contrast, RNA polymerases I and III are specialized for the high rates of transcription necessary to produce rRNAs (>100,000 copies per cell) and other abundant small, stable RNAs.

Specialization has been balanced, however, by the need to retain the structural elements required for RNA synthesis. In each eukaryotic RNA polymerase, the largest subunits are homologous to the bacterial β'- and β-subunits that make up the catalytic core of prokaryotic RNA polymerases (Fig. 15-4C). The structure of a bacterial RNA polymerase reveals that the most conserved residues are located on the inner surfaces of the enzymes, where they are likely to be involved in the synthesis of RNA (Fig. 15-4D).

Transcription does not necessarily require such large enzymes. Bacteriophages have evolved structurally distinct, DNA-dependent RNA polymerases that are one fifth the size of the eukaryotic enzymes yet are able to carry out complete transcription cycles. The complexity of the eukaryotic enzymes is likely attributable to the need for regulation, with additional subunits acting as sites for interaction with regulatory proteins. Domains that differ among the three types of eukaryotic RNA polymerase are likely to interact with cofactors that are unique to a particular class of polymerase. One example of a class-specific domain is found in the largest subunit of RNA polymerase II, which has an unusual repetitive **carboxyl-terminal domain (CTD)** made up of tandem repeats of the consensus heptapeptide TyrSerProThrSer-ProSer. This domain has been implicated in the formation of an RNA polymerase II complex that contains many of the cofactors needed for initiation. The CTD is highly phosphorylated in vivo, and the timing of CTD phosphorylation suggests that this modification may be involved in the transition between the initiation and elongation steps of transcription. The CTD also binds to pre-mRNA processing factors, suggesting that it plays a role in coupling transcription and the subsequent processing of the nascent mRNA.

RNA Polymerase Promoters

Initiation of transcription requires RNA polymerase loading onto the chromosome at the promoter of a gene or operon. The promoter can be loosely defined as the sum of DNA sequences necessary for transcription initiation. This definition is not sufficient, however, as most genes are regulated (positively or negatively) at the transcription initiation level. In eukaryotic cells, packag-

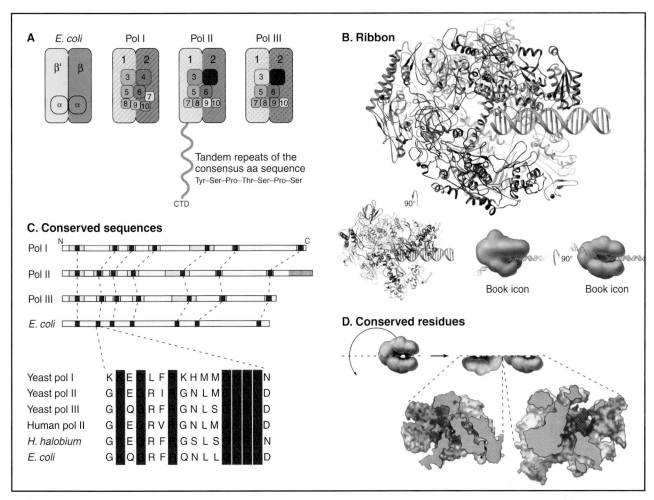

Figure 15-4 MULTIPLE RNA POLYMERASES. **A,** Eukaryotic cells have three different polymerases that share three common subunits (numbers 5, 6, and 8) and have a number of other related, but distinct, subunits (indicated by *related colors* and *distinct shading*). **B,** A ribbon diagram of the structure of RNA polymerase II showing the arrangement of different subunits (colored as in part A). Metal ions are indicated as *red balls.* A prominent cleft, large enough to accommodate a DNA template, is formed between the two largest subunits. The model DNA fragment is shown for size comparison only. **C,** Conserved amino acid sequences are dispersed throughout the largest subunits. *Red* indicates sequences that are conserved among both prokaryotes and eukaryotes. *Yellow* represents sequences that are conserved among the three different eukaryotic RNA polymerases. *H. halobium* is *Halobacterium halobium.* **D,** Conserved residues are located on the inner surface of the RNA polymerase cleft. (B, PDB file: 1I50. Reference: Cramer P, Bushnell DA, Kornberg RD: Structural basis of transcription: RNA polymerase II at 2.8 angstrom resolution. Science 292:1863–1876, 2001. D, From Zhang G, Campbell EA, Minakhin L, et al: Crystal structure of *Thermus aquaticus* core RNA polymerase at 3.3 Å resolution. Cell 98:811–824, 1999.)

ing into chromatin represses most promoters, and activator proteins are required for recruiting RNA polymerase to the site of initiation. In prokaryotes, both activators and repressors modulate the frequency of initiation at promoters. Strong promoters drive the expression of genes whose products are required in abundance, whereas weaker promoters are selected for expression of rare proteins or RNAs. In multicellular organisms, a promoter may direct expression at an intermediate level in some cells, at an activated level in others, and at a repressed level in yet others.

Promoters in bacteria are recognized by direct interactions between specific DNA sequences and the RNA polymerase σ factor. The most common σ factor in *E. coli* (σ 70) recognizes two conserved six-base sequences located 10 bases (minus 10) and 35 (minus 35) upstream of the transcription start site (Fig. 15-5A). Once initiation has occurred, σ is no longer required and can dissociate from the core enzyme. Bacterial cells have several distinct σ factors, each of which binds the core enzyme and direct RNA polymerase to a subset of promoters that contain different recognition sequences, thereby promoting transcription of genes with related functions.

Eukaryotic RNA polymerase I and II promoter sequences are also situated upstream of the transcription start site. In contrast, RNA polymerase III promoters contain key promoter elements within the transcribed sequences. RNA polymerase I recognizes a single type of promoter located upstream of each copy of the long

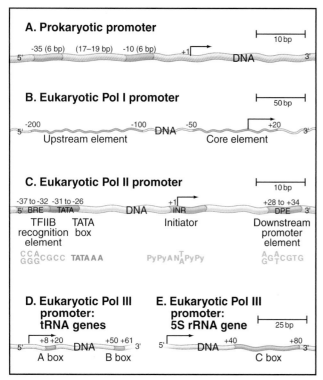

Figure 15-5 PROKARYOTIC AND EUKARYOTIC PROMOTERS. The prokaryotic **(A)** and three eukaryotic **(B–E)** RNA polymerases recognize different promoter sequences. Positions of promoter elements are indicated with respect to the start of transcription (+1). For the RNA polymerase II promoter elements, the consensus sequences are shown. Not all polymerase II promoters contain all of these elements.

tandem array of pre-rRNA coding sequences (Fig. 15-5B). The core element of this promoter overlaps the transcription start site, while an upstream control element located approximately 100 base pairs (bp) from the start site stimulates transcription. RNA polymerase I is not required in yeast cells that contain a pre-rRNA gene under control of an RNA polymerase II promoter. Therefore, if RNA polymerase I does recognize other promoters, these transcripts are not required for viability.

Comparison of the first eukaryotic protein-coding gene sequences revealed a conserved consensus sequence located approximately 30 bp upstream of the transcription start site of many RNA polymerase II–transcribed genes (Fig. 15-5C). This consensus sequence—TATAAAA—called a **TATA box,** shows some similarity to the bacterial −10 sequence. In addition to the TATA box, a less conserved promoter element, the **initiator,** is found in the vicinity of the transcription start site of many genes. RNA polymerase II–transcribed genes that do not contain TATA boxes often contain strong initiator elements. Together, these two elements account for the basal promoter activity of most protein-coding genes.

Both types of RNA polymerase III promoters have key elements within the transcribed sequences (Fig. 15-5D–E). tRNA genes contain two 11-bp elements, the

A box and B box, centered about 15 bp from the 5′ and 3′ ends of the coding sequence, respectively. The 5S-rRNA gene contains a single internal element, the C box, located in the center of the coding region. Given the differences in classes of eukaryotic promoters, it is not surprising that different polymerases use different proteins to recognize the promoter sequences.

Transcription Initiation

The loading of RNA polymerase onto the double-stranded genomic DNA at a promoter sequence is best understood in prokaryotes and is discussed first before the discussion of eukaryotes. Initiation takes place in a series of defined steps (Fig. 15-1). First, holoenzyme binds to the double-stranded promoter, forming what is called the **closed complex.** The specificity and strength of this interaction are dictated by sequence-specific contacts between the σ factor and the bases in the −10 and −35 elements of the promoter (Fig. 15-6). The second step in initiation is the formation of an **open complex** in which a 14-bp region around the transcription start site is unpaired producing a transcription bubble. This unpairing is accompanied by a conformational change in the polymerase that positions the single-strand DNA template in the active site and narrows the DNA-binding cleft, effectively closing the polymerase clamp. In the next step, the DNA template in the active site base-pairs with the first two ribonucleotides, and the first phosphodiester bond is catalyzed. This process is repeated until the nascent RNA reaches a length of eight to nine bases, at which point addition of bases to the growing RNA chain results in the unpairing of one base of the RNA-DNA hybrid, and the nascent RNA begins to exit through a channel on the surface of the polymerase. The resulting conformational change in polymerase leads to the release of σ factor and formation of a stable ternary (three-way) complex containing RNA polymerase, the DNA template, and the nascent RNA.

General Eukaryotic Transcription Factors

Purified eukaryotic RNA polymerase on its own cannot initiate transcription from promoters in vitro. Specific transcription can be obtained in vitro using extracts from nuclei, and fractionation of such extracts has led to the identification of additional factors necessary for specific transcription by purified RNA polymerase in vitro. Rather than a σ factor, eukaryotic RNA polymerases require multiple initiation factors. Most of these factors are unique to each RNA polymerase, and because they are required for transcription of most promoters (within each class), they are termed **general transcription factors (GTFs).** GTFs are remarkably conserved

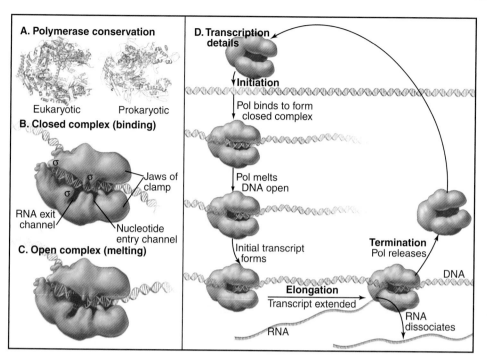

A. Polymerase conservation

Eukaryotic   Prokaryotic

B. Closed complex (binding)

σ
σ
σ

Jaws of
clamp

RNA exit
channel

Nucleotide
entry channel

C. Open complex (melting)

**D. Transcription
details**

Initiation

Pol binds to form
closed complex

Pol melts
DNA open

Initial transcript
forms

Elongation
Transcript extended

RNA

Termination
Pol releases

DNA

RNA
dissociates

Figure 15-6 RNA POLYMERASE INITIATION. **A,** While initiation of prokaryotic transcription is more completely understood, the conservation of RNA polymerase structure implies that the fundamental steps in initiation are conserved. **B,** In the closed complex, the double-stranded promoter DNA is recognized by σ factor domains on the surface of the holoenzyme. **C,** The open complex forms by unwinding DNA surrounding the transcription start site and positioning the single-stranded template in the active site of the polymerase. **D,** The initiation reaction in the context of the transcription cycle.

among different eukaryotes. Although most factors required for transcription by each class of polymerase are distinct, one of them, first identified as the **TATA box–binding protein,** participates in different protein complexes involved in each of the three polymerase systems. The next sections compare transcription by the three forms of eukaryotic RNA polymerase.

RNA Polymerase II Factors

The RNA polymerase II GTFs comprise more than 20 polypeptides with an aggregate molecular weight of more than 10^6 D (Table 15-1). Before RNA polymerase II can initiate transcription in vitro, an ordered assembly of factors at the promoter must occur. Assembly of the RNA polymerase II **preinitiation complex** begins with the binding of **TFIID,** a large factor (~700 kD) consisting of TATA box–binding protein (TBP) and a set of **TBP-associated factors** called **TAFIIs** (Fig. 15-7A). TBP alone is sufficient for basal transcription, while TAFs apparently serve as targets for further activation of transcription (see subsequent sections). TBP is the first polypeptide in the basal transcription machinery to recognize a specific DNA sequence during the initiation process. DNA binding is provided by a highly conserved C-terminal 180-amino-acid domain, which forms a saddle-shaped monomer with an axis of dyad symmetry (Fig. 15-7B). The underside of the TBP "saddle" binds to the minor groove of the TATA sequence, which is splayed open in the process. A pronounced DNA bend is produced at each end of the TATAAA element by the intercalation of phenylalanine side chains (Fig. 15-7C).

Table 15-1

SUMMARY OF EUKARYOTIC RNA POLYMERASE II GENERAL TRANSCRIPTION FACTORS

Factor	Number of Subunits	Subunit M (KD)	Functions
TFIIA	3	12, 19, 35	Stabilizes binding of TBP and TFIIB
TFIIB	1	25	Binds TBP, selects start site, and recruits polymerase II
TFIID	12	15-250	Interacts with regulatory factors
(TBP)	1	38	Subunit of TFIID; specifically recognizes the TATA box
TFIIE	2	34, 57	Recruits TFIIH
TFIIF	2	30, 74	Binds polymerase II and TFIIB
TFIIH	9	35-98	Unwinds promoter DNA; phosphorylates CTD (C-terminal domain of RNA polymerase II)
Polymerase II	12	10-220	Catalyzes RNA synthesis
TOTALS	42	~1000	

TBP, TATA box–binding protein.

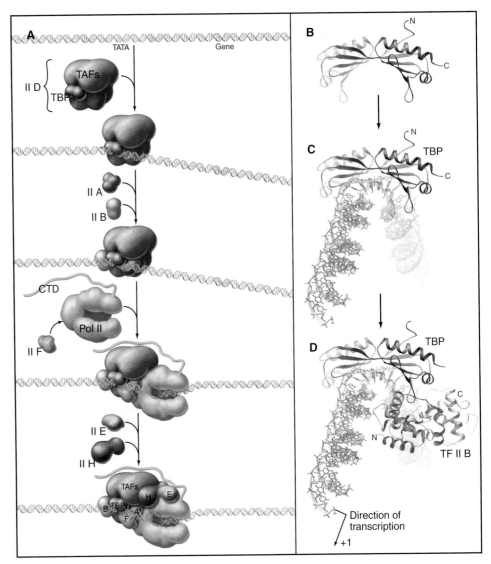

Figure 15-7 RNA POLYMERASE II PREINITIATION COMPLEX ON THE ADE-NOVIRUS-2 MAJOR LATE PROMOTER DNA. **A,** The sequential assembly of general transcription factors leads to a preinitiation complex with the promoter region in the closed complex. Helicase activities present in TFIIH use the energy of ATP to unwind the promoter, leading to formation of an open complex. **B,** Binding of TBP leads to **C,** a pronounced bend in the DNA. **D,** TFIIB interacts both upstream and downstream of the TATA box and directs RNA polymerase to the transcription start site. (B–D, PDB file: 1VOL. TBP + DNA coordinates courtesy of Stephen Burley, Rockefeller University, New York.)

The TFIID-TATA box complex serves as a binding site for additional positive and negative regulators. **TFIIA** binding stabilizes the TBP-DNA interaction and prevents the binding of repressors that arrest further initiation complex formation.

The next step in assembly of the initiation complex is binding of **TFIIB,** which binds to one side of TBP and makes contacts with DNA upstream and downstream of the TATA box (Fig. 15-7D). Mutations in the yeast gene that encodes TFIIB show altered mRNA start-site selection, indicating that TFIIB establishes the spacing between the TATA box and the transcription start site. TFIIB interacts directly with TBP and RNA polymerase II and is thus essential for the next steps in initiation complex assembly.

RNA polymerase II enters into the preinitiation complex (see Fig. 15-7A) in association with **TFIIF.** This factor is related to bacterial σ factor and acts to stabilize the interaction of RNA polymerase II with TFIIB and TBP. In addition, TFIIF binds to free polymerase and prevents interactions with nonpromoter DNA sites.

TFIIH and its stimulatory factor **TFIIE** are the final general factors to enter the preinitiation complex. Binding of these factors results in more stable protein DNA contacts in the vicinity of the transcription start site. TFIIH contains eight polypeptides, several of which also have functions outside of transcription initiation. TFIIH-associated **helicases** use the energy from ATP hydrolysis to unwind a short stretch of promoter DNA at the transcription start site. This unpairing of DNA allows RNA polymerase II to recognize the template strand, bind the complementary nucleotides, and synthesize the first few phosphodiester bonds. RNA polymerase II initiation requires hydrolysis of the β-γ phosphate bond in ATP, a reaction that is also catalyzed by TFIIH.

TFIIH also contains a protein kinase that phosphorylates the CTD. This is Cdk-activating kinase, itself a Cdk-cyclin complex that phosphorylates and activates other cyclin-dependent kinases (see Fig. 40-14). In the initiation complex, phosphorylation of the CTD is thought to release it from interactions with GTFs and allow the transition to the transcription elongation

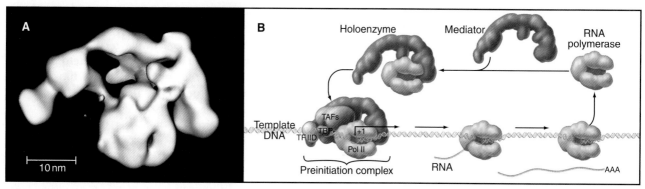

Figure 15-8 RNA POLYMERASE II HOLOENZYME. **A,** The three-dimensional structure of the yeast holoenzyme, reconstructed from electron micrographs of particles preserved in negative stain. **B,** The mediator complex assists RNA polymerase II in locating promoters through interactions with factors bound to promoter proximal and/or enhancer sequences. Interaction with TFIID, bound at the TATA box, is important in assembling a productive complex. TFIID is thought to remain bound to the TATA box and to facilitate subsequent rounds of initiation. (A, Courtesy of Joshua Davis and Francisco Asturias, Scripps Research Institute, La Jolla, California.)

phase. Other TFIIH subunits have been identified as components of the DNA repair machinery. Several genes encoding TFIIH subunits are mutated in the human DNA excision repair disease xeroderma pigmentosa, suggesting that TFIIH might serve to link transcription to DNA repair (see later section).

Mediator and the Holoenzyme

In vivo, many of the steps described previously involve the assembly of large macromolecular complexes containing RNA polymerase II, several of the GTFs, other factors that alter chromatin structure, and various additional transcription factors. One of these complexes, the **mediator,** contains over 20 polypeptides (many with unknown function) but lacks RNA polymerase II and the GTFs. Mediator reversibly interacts with RNA polymerase II and other factors to form a **"holoenzyme,"** which requires additional factors to be competent for initiation (Fig. 15-8). RNA polymerase II holoenzyme responds to transcription activators (described in a subsequent section) in vitro, suggesting that one role for the multitude of proteins in this complex is to offer multiple interaction sites for recruitment of holoenzyme to the promoter. Alternatively, a mediator lacking RNA polymerase II can be recruited to the promoter, where it subsequently attracts the polymerase. Thus, the mediator links DNA-bound activators to the basal transcription machinery. In this sense, the mediator acts as a **coactivator.** Other coactivators present in the holoenzyme act as chromatin remodeling factors (see subsequent section) that act to control access of the transcription machinery to the DNA template.

RNA Polymerase I Factors

Initiation at RNA polymerase I promoters can also proceed through an ordered assembly of transcription factors (Fig. 15-9). The upstream binding factor

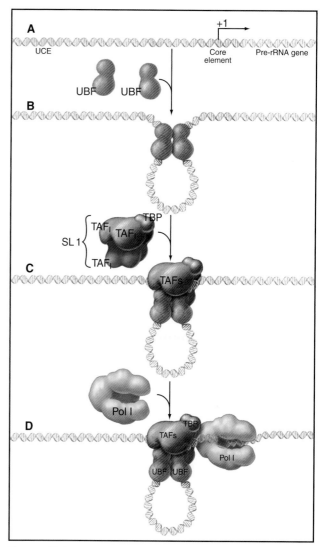

Figure 15-9 RNA POLYMERASE I PREINITIATION COMPLEX. **A,** Ribosomal RNA promoters assemble a preinitiation complex. (UCE, upstream control element.) **B,** This complex consists of an upstream binding factor (UBF) and a multisubunit factor called SL1 **(C)** that contains TBP. **D,** Together, these factors recruit RNA polymerase I.

binds to the upstream control element and to part of the core element. This initial complex is stabilized by the SL1 complex of TBP with three RNA polymerase I–specific TAFs.

RNA Polymerase III Factors

The assembly of RNA polymerase III initiation complexes differs at various promoters (Fig. 15-10). Initiation at tRNA genes begins with the binding of TFIIIC to the A and B boxes. TFIIIB then binds upstream of the A box at a sequence determined both by an interaction with TFIIIC and through the DNA-binding capacity of TBP. Once the TFIIIC-TFIIIB complex has been assembled, RNA polymerase III can initiate transcription. Multiple rounds of initiation can occur on the stable tDNA-TFIIIC-TFIIIB complex.

Transcription of 5S rRNA genes requires an additional factor called TFIIIA. This protein was the first transcription factor and the first zinc finger protein to be identified. TFIIIA recognizes the C box located near the center of the 5S rRNA coding region. TFIIIC then binds by making contacts on each side of TFIIIA, in much the same way that the A and B boxes are contacted on tRNA genes. Finally, TFIIIB binds through interactions with TFIIIC and DNA, and the resulting preinitiation complex is recognized by RNA polymerase III.

Other Initiation Pathways

In addition to the three classical initiation pathways, transcription can be initiated in other ways. First, some

RNA polymerase II promoters lack the TATA box element. In these cases, the initiator element provides the primary sequence target, and its recognition requires the function of one of several auxiliary factors that are thought to bind to the initiator. Despite the lack of a TATA box, these promoters still require TBP, presumably because it serves to stabilize the binding of required TAFs.

Another unusual set of promoters drives expression of the snRNA genes. These promoters contain binding sites for both RNA polymerase II and RNA polymerase III factors, and they can be transcribed by either polymerase. Like other eukaryotic promoters TBP is required for transcription. Unlike the other systems, the snRNA promoters recruit a novel TBP complex, which contains a unique set of TAFs.

Summary of the Eukaryotic Basal Transcription Machinery

Despite the evolutionary divergence of the multiple eukaryotic RNA polymerases and the specialization of each polymerase for a unique set of promoters, the fundamental mechanisms of transcription have been conserved. This conservation is reflected not only in similar sequences of the subunits of the polymerases themselves but also in the presence of TBP and TFIIB homologs among the GTFs used by each class of polymerase. Indeed, Archaea, which have only a single RNA polymerase, contain both TBP and TFIIB. This observation suggests that initiation mechanisms employing GTFs evolved before the duplication of the RNA polymerases.

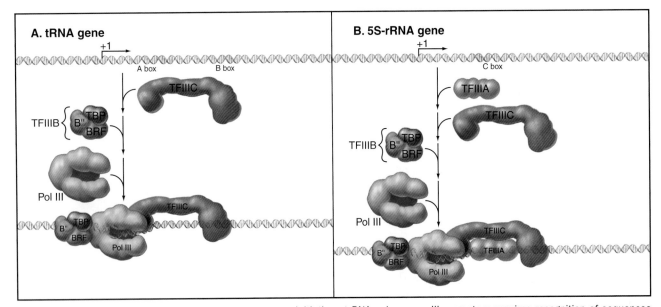

Figure 15-10   RNA POLYMERASE III PREINITIATION COMPLEXES. Initiation at RNA polymerase III promoters requires recognition of sequences within the transcribed sequences. These sequences differ for tRNA and 5S ribosomal genes. **A,** In the case of tRNA genes, only TFIIIC is required for specific binding. **B,** For 5S genes, the internal element is recognized by the specific DNA-binding factor TFIIIA. BRF, TFIIB-related factor.

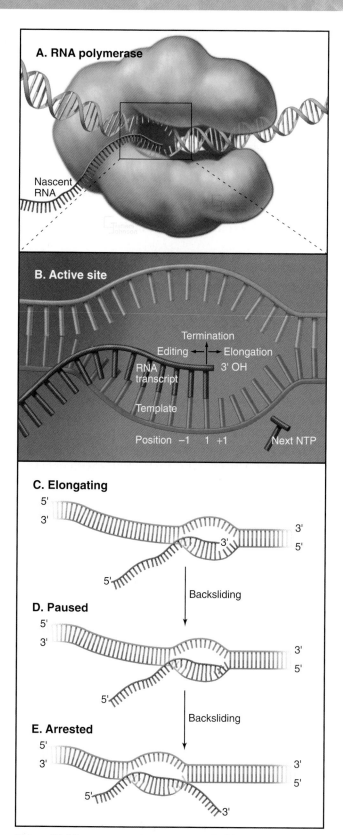

A. RNA polymerase

Nascent
RNA

B. Active site

Termination

Editing ←→ Elongation

RNA
transcript 3' OH

Template

Position −1 1 +1 Next NTP

C. Elongating

5'
3'
3'
5'
5'

Backsliding

D. Paused

5'
3'
3'
5'
5'

Backsliding

E. Arrested

5'
3'
3'
5'
5'
3'

Why are so many factors required to make a transcript? Part of the complexity might be necessary to generate multiple sites for interaction with regulatory factors that could either activate or repress the assembly or function of the preinitiation complex. A second role for the complex set of factors could be to target polymerases to specific sites in the nucleus. Finally, some factors could help load elongation, splicing, or termination factors onto the RNA polymerases.

Transcription Elongation and Termination

The final stage of initiation leads to elongation and movement of the polymerase away from the promoter. This process of **promoter clearance** is associated with structural changes in the polymerase, which prepare the enzyme for efficient RNA synthesis and render it susceptible to the action of factors that regulate the elongation process. Such regulatory factors, together with structural features of the nascent transcript, influence elongation and can trigger the termination of transcription and the dissociation of the ternary elongation complex containing the DNA template, nascent RNA, and RNA polymerase. This termination reaction typically occurs at the 3′ end of the gene or operon and serves both to recycle RNA polymerase for additional initiation reactions as well as to ensure that adjacent genes are not inadvertently transcribed.

The Catalytic Cycle

The DNA-dependent RNA polymerases catalyze synthesis of an RNA polymer from ribonucleoside 5′-triphosphates (ATP, guanosine triphosphate [GTP], cytidine triphosphate [CTP], and uridine triphosphate [UTP]) according to the following reaction:

$$(NMP)_n + NTP \rightarrow (NMP)_{n+1} + PPi$$

where $(NMP)_n$ is the RNA polymer; NTP is ATP, UTP, CTP, or GTP; and PPi is pyrophosphate. Polymerase extends the RNA chain in the 5′ to 3′ direction by adding ribonucleotide units to the chain's 3′ end. Selection of the incoming NTP is directed by the DNA template and takes place at the transcription bubble, an unpaired segment of the DNA template (Fig. 15-11). The 3′ hydroxyl

Figure 15-11 TRANSCRIPTION ELONGATION. A, Model of the transcription elongation complex consisting of RNA polymerase, template DNA, and nascent RNA transcript. RNA polymerases interact with the template upstream and downstream of the transcription bubble. **B,** The active site of RNA polymerase positions the growing end of the nascent transcript in the appropriate location for the addition of the next nucleoside triphosphate (NTP). After each single nucleotide addition, the polymerase may translocate forward and repeat the nucleotide addition **(C),** slide backward and pause for a variable time **(D),** or slide further backward, allowing removal of the transcript and termination of transcription **(E).**

group acts a nucleophile, attacking the α-phosphate of the incoming NTP in a reaction similar to that seen in DNA replication (see Fig. 42-1). This reaction proceeds in vivo at a rate of 30 to 100 nucleotides per second.

The Transcription Elongation Complex

Efficient synthesis of RNA requires balancing two competing demands. First, the elongation complex must be very stable, because premature dissociation from DNA produces defective partial transcripts and requires the polymerase to restart transcription from the promoter. The complex must also be loosely bound so that the polymerase can easily translocate along the DNA template. The structure of RNA polymerase has evolved to meet these needs. The cleft formed at the interface between the two largest subunits is open when the polymerase is in the initiation complex. Once the first few RNA phosphodiester bonds are formed, the polymerase undergoes a conformational change. Subunits at the outer edge of the cleft close like jaws to encircle the DNA template. In this structure, the front end of the transcription bubble is positioned at the back wall of the cleft, close to the catalytic center. This structure is highly efficient and can function continuously for the 17 hours that are required to transcribe the >2 million bp mammalian dystrophin gene.

Pausing, Arrest, and Termination

Following the addition of each nucleotide, RNA polymerase may add an additional nucleotide, pause, move in reverse, or terminate (Fig. 15-11B). The relative probabilities of these alternative reactions depend on interactions between the transcription complex and the template, the nascent RNA transcript, and regulatory transcription factors.

RNA polymerase does not elongate at a constant rate but rather synthesizes RNA in short spurts between pauses. A pause of short duration can be caused by low NTP concentrations or alternatively by the transient unpairing of the 3'-end of the nascent transcript and template. Longer pauses are provoked by the formation, in the nascent RNA, of short (~20 base) self-complementary sequences that can fold to form a stem-loop or hairpin, or the presence of a weak RNA-DNA hybrid. The presence of an unstable RNA-DNA hybrid can arise from the misincorporation of an NTP leading to an unpaired base in the hybrid. In this case, the RNA polymerase can backtrack or slide backward on the template (Fig. 15-11C). This backward movement of the transcription bubble is accompanied by a zippering movement of the RNA-DNA hybrid in which the nascent RNA in

the exit channel rehybridizes with upstream template sequences while the 3' end of the transcript unpairs from the hybrid and is extruded through the same channel that NTPs use to enter the active site. The backtracked transcription complex is said to be arrested. Transcription elongation factors bind in the NTP channel of arrested complexes and activate the RNA polymerase to cleave the backtracked RNA. The new 3' terminal residue is correctly positioned for incorporation of the next complementary NTP. This editing process increases the fidelity of transcription. Pausing also occurs following transcription of U-rich sequences, and this is often associated with transcription termination.

Termination

When elongating RNA polymerase reaches the end of a gene or operon, specific sequences in the RNA trigger the release of the transcript and dissociation of the RNA polymerase. Bacteria have two types of termination signals, called terminators. The first are called **intrinsic (or rho-independent) terminators,** because they function in the absence of any protein factors (Fig. 15-12A). Intrinsic terminators consist of two sequence elements: a stable GC-rich hairpin and a run of about eight consecutive U residues. As the first of these elements is synthesized, it forms a hairpin, causing polymerase to pause with unstable U : A bps (with only two H-bonds [see Fig. 3-14]) in the hybrid. The nascent transcript is released from this unstable transcription complex. The second type of prokaryotic termination requires a protein factor called rho (Fig. 15-12B). Rho is a hexameric protein that binds cytosine-rich sequences and uses ATP hydrolysis to translocate along the nascent transcript in the 5' to 3' direction, essentially chasing the RNA polymerase. When polymerase pauses, rho can catch up and use the energy derived from ATP hydrolysis to pull the RNA out of the transcription elongation complex.

Eukaryotic RNA polymerases have evolved distinct mechanisms for termination. RNA polymerase III requires no protein factors but terminates efficiently after transcribing four to six consecutive U residues, presumably owing to instability of the RNA-DNA hybrid in the enzyme active site. RNA polymerase I terminates in response to a protein factor that blocks further elongation by binding to a DNA sequence downstream of the termination site, leaving an inherently unstable U-rich RNA-DNA hybrid in the active site. The RNA polymerase II termination mechanism is more complex, requiring a large multiprotein complex that recognizes the poly(A) addition in the nascent transcript (see Fig. 16-3 for pre-mRNA processing). Deletion or mutation of the poly(A) signal results in a failure to terminate messages at the appropriate site, indicating that RNA polymerase II termination is coupled to 3'-end processing.

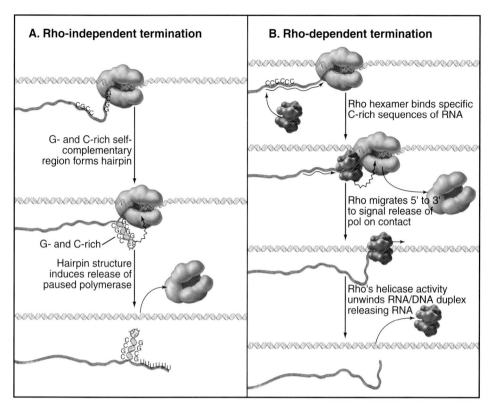

A. Rho-independent termination

G- and C-rich self-complementary region forms hairpin

G- and C-rich

Hairpin structure induces release of paused polymerase

B. Rho-dependent termination

CCCCCC

Rho hexamer binds specific C-rich sequences of RNA

Rho migrates 5' to 3' to signal release of pol on contact

Rho's helicase activity unwinds RNA/DNA duplex releasing RNA

Figure 15-12 PROKARYOTIC TRANSCRIPTION TERMINATION. **A,** Rho-independent termination is directed by sequences in the nascent transcript that operate in the absence of any additional factors. **B,** The bacterial termination factor rho translocates along the nascent RNA and on reaching the RNA polymerase causes the disassembly of the elongation complex.

Gene-Specific Transcription

Transcription initiation is the critical first step in determining which genes are expressed in which cells and at what level. Depending mainly on the sequence of the promoter, expression can be constitutive or influenced by regulatory proteins. This section discusses transcription regulatory proteins that either positively or negatively regulate specific genes. The discussion starts with a prokaryotic example and then expands to include a variety of eukaryotic regulators. Although the details differ in prokaryotes and eukaryotes, many of the basic principles are the same.

Regulation of Transcription Initiation in Prokaryotes

Prokaryotes typically regulate gene expression in response to signals that are produced in response to the internal metabolic state and to environmental cues such as the presence of nutrients in the growth medium (see Fig. 27-11). These signals inside the organism are transmitted to the appropriate genes through transcription regulatory proteins that bind to specific sequences near the genes they control to either activate or repress transcription. Both of these regulatory mechanisms come into play in regulation of the *E. coli* lactose (lac) operon (Fig. 15-2A). The genes expressed from this operon are

required for cells to metabolize lactose but are not expressed in the absence of lactose. Genetic studies in the 1960s showed that the gene upstream of the lac operon (*I* in Fig. 15-2A) encodes a repressor (lac repressor) that blocks expression of the lac operon in the absence of lactose (Fig. 15-13). The lac repressor binds to a site called an operator that overlaps the RNA polymerase binding site in the lac promoter. In the presence of lactose, the repressor undergoes a conformational change that eliminates DNA binding allowing the recruitment of RNA polymerase to the promoter. Full expression of the lac operon requires the catabolite activator protein (CAP), which is also an allosteric DNA-binding protein that binds just upstream of the lac promoter. If cellular glucose levels diminish, the cAMP concentration rises, and CAP binds cAMP. This induces a structural alteration in CAP, allowing it to dimerize and bind specific DNA sequences. CAP bound to its site stabilizes the otherwise weak interaction of RNA polymerase with the promoter. The resulting activation allows maximum expression of the lac operon in the presence of lactose and the absence of glucose.

In summary, control of lac gene expression by opposing repressor and activator function is an example of regulation at the first step in transcription initiation, binding of RNA polymerase to the promoter. Regulating access of RNA polymerase to promoters is a common form of transcription regulation in both prokaryotes and eukaryotes.

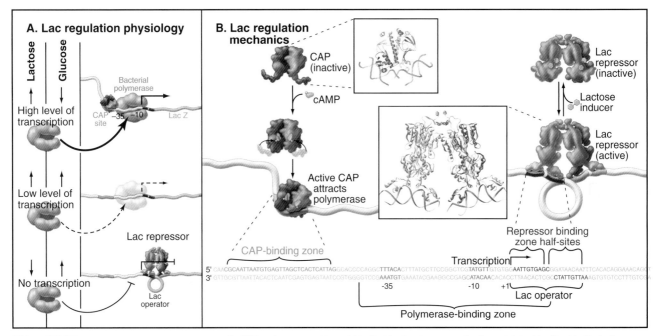

Figure 15-13 **REGULATION OF THE LAC OPERON. A,** RNA polymerase *(green)* binding to the lac promoter is regulated by the binding of repressor or activator (CAP). **B,** Binding sites for CAP and the repressor at the lac operon. The main repressor-binding site overlaps the promoter and blocks access of RNA polymerase. Additional lac repressor-binding sites are located upstream and downstream of the promoter. Lac repressor can form a tetramer and thus bind two operators, forming a loop in the lac operon DNA. Inducer binding dramatically alters the conformation of the lac repressor diminishing its affinity for the operator. CAP binds just upstream of the promoter where it can stabilize the bound RNA polymerase.

Eukaryotic Promoter Proximal and Enhancer Elements

In vivo techniques for analyzing eukaryotic promoter function led to the discovery of a number of regulatory elements in addition to the basal promoter elements. In these experiments, transgenes containing a promoter or its mutated derivative are introduced into eukaryotic cells by transfection or microinjection. Transcription directed by the cloned promoter is detected by various approaches that allow the transgene product to be identified from among the background of cellular transcripts. In one approach (Fig. 15-14A), the promoter drives expression of a bacterial **reporter** gene such as chloramphenicol acetyl-transferase (CAT), β-galactosidase, or luciferase. Eukaryotes lack these enzymes, so their expression can be assayed in extracts of transfected cells with little or no background activity. This approach applies only to RNA polymerase II, which produces translatable mRNAs. A more direct analysis, applicable to transcription by all three RNA polymerases, makes use of specific RNA or DNA probes to quantify RNAs transcribed from the transgene.

Such transgene experiments demonstrated that basal promoter elements are insufficient for full expression of these reporter genes. Deletion or mutation of regions upstream of the transcription start site revealed the existence of additional promoter elements. For RNA polymerase II, these elements fall into two classes; the

elements in the first class are located from 50 to 100 bp upstream of the start of transcription and have been termed *promoter proximal elements,* while those in the second class, enhancers, are located at distances up to 10 kilobase (kb) from the start of transcription. All of these elements are composed of multiple binding sites for transcription regulatory proteins.

Promoter proximal elements are short (~10 bp) sequences located within a few hundred bp upstream of the TATA box. One example of a promoter proximal element is the CCAAT box in the promoter of the herpes simplex virus thymidine kinase gene. This site was identified by a technique called linker-scanning, in which clustered mutations are introduced at regular intervals in the promoter (Fig. 15-14A). Mutations that result in a decrease in transcription define important sequences. In the case of the thymidine kinase promoter, the CCAAT and TATAAA sequences are required for full transcription. Thymidine kinase expression also requires the sequence GGCGCC, which serves as the binding site for SP1, a transcription factor involved in expression of a number of so-called housekeeping genes, whose products are involved in normal cellular functions. These promoter proximal elements are present in many different genes, where they are necessary for constitutive expression. Other promoter proximal elements are involved in regulated expression, for example, in response to cellular stress or exposure to heavy metals. Most promoters contain several different promoter proxi-

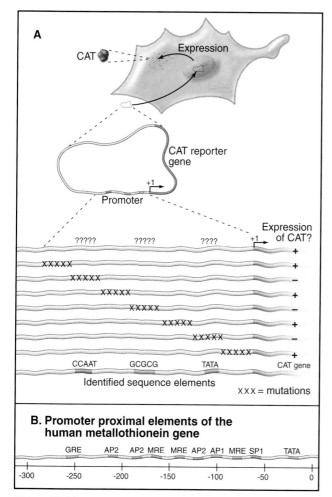

Figure 15-14 RNA POLYMERASE II PROMOTER REGULATORY ELEMENTS. **A,** In vivo assays are used to identify key regulatory sequences. In the example shown, a promoter is placed in front of a gene encoding chloramphenicol acetyltransferase (CAT), and the resulting plasmid is transfected into cultured cells. This bacterial enzyme is easily assayed in eukaryotic cells because there is no endogenous activity. Targeted clusters of mutations, strategically placed throughout the promoter region, are tested for their effect on expression of the reporter gene. Mutations that reduce expression define important regulatory elements. **B,** The region immediately upstream of the metallothionein gene contains binding sites for several transcription factors. The elements are named for the factor that binds there: GRE (glucocorticoid response element), MRE (metal response element), and AP1, AP2, and SP1 (which bind protein factors with the same names as the DNA elements).

mal elements. This allows for combinatorial regulation of transcription levels by varying the relative abundance or activity of the various factors. The location of numerous regulatory elements directly upstream of the human metallothionein gene, whose product protects cells from the toxic effects of metals (Fig. 15-14B) suggests that a variety of different mechanisms regulate this gene.

Enhancers are clusters of regulatory elements in the DNA similar to promoter proximal elements, but they are considerably more complicated and have several distinguishing features. First, an enhancer increases the

rate of initiation from a basal promoter even if it is located up to 10 kb away from the promoter. Second, enhancers work even if located internal to or downstream of the promoter. Finally, the enhancer element will work in either orientation relative to the promoter (Fig. 15-15A). Figure 15-15B shows an example of an enhancer sequence with a number of transcription factors (see the following section) bound, forming a complex called an enhanceosome. Enhancer elements are found in the vicinity of many but not all genes. In most cases, the enhancer works in a cell type–specific fashion. An example is a sequence in an intron of the immunoglobulin heavy chain gene that enhances transcription in lymphocytes but not in other cells. This regulation of enhancer function is likely to be accomplished by changes in the levels of various enhancer-binding factors in different tissues.

Both enhancers and promoter proximal elements can be grafted onto different basal promoters and maintain their function. Even though an enhancer may be more than 1000 bp away from the start site of transcription, it is thought that proteins bound to the enhancer create a loop in the intervening DNA and therefore make direct physical contact with proteins that are bound near the transcription start site.

Gene-Specific Eukaryotic Transcription Factors

Eukaryotic transcription factors bind specific DNA sequences located near the genes they regulate. This

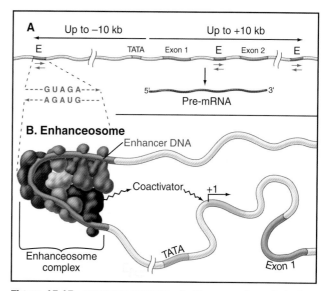

Figure 15-15 ENHANCER ELEMENTS. **A,** These condensed clusters of factor-binding sites can influence expression when located far from the promoter in either the upstream or downstream position. In addition, they work in either orientation with respect to transcription. **B,** Model enhancer showing the tight packing of several different DNA-binding proteins. These complexes fold into structures that have been called enhanceosomes.

binding leads to activation or repression of expression by mechanisms more varied than in prokaryotes. In the simplest cases, the transcription factor interacts directly with the basal machinery. In more complex cases, this interaction may involve a coactivator or corepressor. Transcription factors may also act on the chromatin template rather than the basal transcription machinery. The 1990s witnessed the identification and characterization of hundreds of eukaryotic gene-specific transcription factors. Current estimates indicate that approximately 6% of the coding capacity of the human genome is devoted to transcription factors that recognize specific DNA sequences. The following sections discuss the identification of transcription factors, the functional organization of these proteins, and regulation of the basal transcription machinery and the chromatin template by transcription factors.

Methods for Identifying, Isolating, and Localizing Transcription Factors

Identifying and characterizing transcription factors requires techniques to detect and characterize specific DNA-protein complexes. In one such technique, DNA footprinting, protein is mixed with DNA that is radioactively labeled at one end (Fig. 15-16A–B). The resulting DNA-protein complex is then lightly digested with deoxyribonuclease to give, on average, one random cut per DNA molecule. The population of cleaved DNA molecules thus produced is then stripped of protein and separated by gel electrophoresis. The area protected from cleavage by a specific DNA-binding protein appears as a blank area or "footprint" that results from the protein's blocking access to the nuclease, thus leaving a gap in the family of digestion products of differing lengths. A less precise but more versatile method of visualizing protein-DNA complexes is the DNA mobility shift assay (Fig. 15-16C). The principle of this technique is that fragments of DNA with a bound protein move more slowly during gel electrophoresis than the same DNA fragments without bound protein.

Both techniques allow detection of specific DNA-binding proteins in crude cellular extracts and thus can be used as assays for protein purification. Transcription factors can also be cloned directly by screening expression libraries with labeled DNA oligonucleotides corresponding to the sequence of the regulatory element and detecting proteins that bind to them. These approaches have been used to isolate hundreds of specific DNA-binding proteins that play specific roles in transcription regulation.

The DNA sites that bind known transcription factors in vivo can be determined by using a technique called chromatin immunoprecipitation (ChIP; Fig. 15-16D). By using this approach, a transcription factor can be localized to a specific promoter at a specific time. The combination of ChIP with microarray approaches allows the distribution of the factor across the genome to be determined.

DNA-Binding Domains

Binding of proteins to specific DNA sequences requires recognition of a pattern of bases along the monotonous double helix. The richest source of DNA sequence variation comes from the chemical groups exposed in the major groove. Most specific DNA-binding proteins probe the major groove of double helix with a small structural element (usually, an α-helix) with a shape that is complementary to the surface topography of a particular DNA sequence. The correct DNA sequence is recognized through multiple interactions between amino acid side chains in the recognition helix and the chemical groups on the edges of DNA bases in the major groove. Single amino acid changes in the recognition helix can change the DNA sequence that is recognized. Protein-DNA complexes are stabilized by additional contacts between amino acid side chains and deoxyribose rings and phosphate groups or by bending of the DNA.

DNA recognition domains of specific transcription factors typically interact with only 3 to 6 bp of DNA. Given the size and complexity of the typical mammalian genome, a sequence must be approximately 16 bp long to occur by chance only once. How then can genes be specifically recognized among the very large number of close but nonidentical sequences? Two strategies increase the length of the specific sequence to be recognized. The recognition protein can either use several recognition elements or it can dimerize with itself or other DNA-binding proteins. Binding of protein dimers can lead to recognition of sequences with twofold rotational symmetry.

DNA-binding proteins can be grouped into families based on the structure of the domains used for DNA sequence recognition (Fig. 15-17 and Table 15-2). These include the **helix-turn-helix (HTH)** proteins, **homeodomains, zinc finger** proteins, **steroid receptors, leucine zipper** proteins, and **helix-loop-helix** proteins. Although these families include most of the known transcription factors, there remain other, uncharacterized recognition domains. Within a given family, the recognition domain of each transcription factor has an amino acid sequence that targets the protein to a particular DNA sequence. Conversely, different families of transcription factors can recognize the same promoter element. The following sections discuss some of the more common eukaryotic DNA-binding domains.

Homeodomain

This 60-amino-acid motif was discovered in *Drosophila* proteins that regulate development and has been found

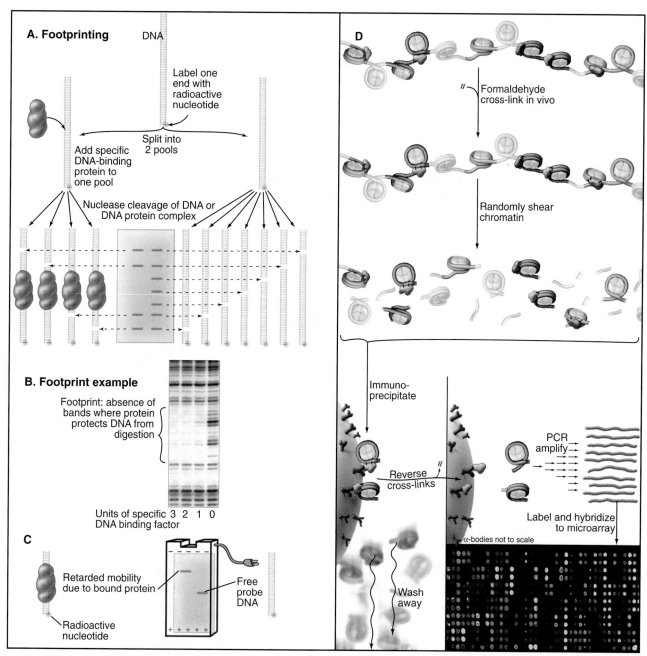

Figure 15-16 TECHNIQUES FOR STUDYING PROTEINS THAT BIND TO SPECIFIC DNA SEQUENCES. **A–B,** Footprinting assay. A fragment of DNA thought to contain a specific protein-binding site is radiolabeled at one end of one strand. The labeled probe is then split into two fractions, and the DNA-binding protein is added to one fraction. The two samples are then randomly cleaved with nuclease or chemical reagents in such a way as to cleave only one bond per DNA fragment. High-resolution electrophoresis is used to separate the cleaved fragments, and auto-radiography reveals a ladder of fragments that differ in length by a single base. **B,** Protein bound to DNA protects a limited region of DNA (its footprint) from cleavage, as revealed by the absence of bands in the radioactive ladder. **C,** Electrophoretic mobility shift assay. A short (20- to 50-bp), double-stranded DNA fragment is radiolabeled and bound to a protein sample. The complex is electrophoresed in a nonde-naturing gel. The large protein bound to the DNA retards its mobility in the gel compared with the free DNA. **D,** Chromatin immunoprecipita-tion. Proteins are covalently cross-linked to DNA with formaldehyde and then randomly sheared to yield chromatin fragments containing a few hundred bp of DNA. These chromatin fragments are then immunoprecipitated with antibodies to a DNA-binding protein and the enrich-ment of particular sequences is examined by quantitative PCR or by hybridization to a microarray. (D, Based on data from Stephen Hartman and Michael Snyder, Yale University, New Haven, Connecticut.)

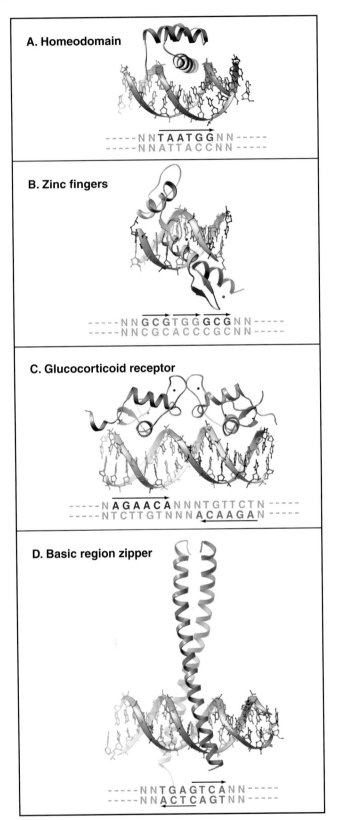

A. Homeodomain

```
-----NNTAATGGNN-----
-----NNATTACCNN-----
```

B. Zinc fingers

```
-----NNGCGTGGGCGNN-----
-----NNCGCACCCGCNN-----
```

C. Glucocorticoid receptor

```
-----NAGAACANNNTGTTCTN-----
-----NTCTTGTNNNACAAGAN-----
```

D. Basic region zipper

```
-----NNTGAGTCANN-----
-----NNACTCAGTNN-----
```

Table 15-2

MUTATION OF TRANSCRIPTION FACTOR GENES CAUSES HUMAN DISEASE

Transcription Factor	Factor Class	Activity	Disease
Pit-1	Gene-specific activator	DNA binding homeodomain	Combined pituitary hormone deficiency
POU4F3	Gene-specific activator	DNA binding homeodomain	Inherited progressive hearing loss
HNF4a	Gene-specific activator	DNA binding Nuclear receptor	Maturity-onset diabetes
AIRE	Gene-specific activator	DNA binding Zinc finger	Autoimmune disease
P53	Gene-specific activator	DNA binding	Cancer
ATRX	Chromatin remodeling	ATPase/ helicase	α-thalassaemia, mental retardation
CBP (CREB-binding protein)	Coactivator	Histone acetylase	Developmental abnormalities

in a wide range of eukaryotic transcription factors, including more than 150 in the human genome. Recognition is provided by a helix-turn-helix (HTH) motif composed of two helices, one of which sits in the major groove of the DNA-binding site contacting a recognition sequence of 6 bp (Fig. 15-17A). The HTH structure is not a stable domain on its own but exists as part of a larger DNA-binding domain, such as the homeodomain. Additional binding affinity is provided in the homeodomain by a flexible arm that interacts with the minor groove.

Zinc Finger Proteins

The zinc finger protein sequence motif (Fig. 15-17B), first identified in the RNA polymerase III basal factor

Figure 15-17   **MOLECULAR STRUCTURES OF TRANSCRIPTION FACTOR DNA-BINDING DOMAINS.** Recognition of specific DNA sequences requires interactions between amino acid side chains in the protein and chemical groups on the DNA bases. In each of the examples shown here, an α-helix interacts with specific bases through contacts in the major groove. **A,** The homeodomain α-helix recognizes a specific six-base sequence. **B,** A protein with three zinc fingers recognizes three consecutive three-base sequences. **C,** The glucocorticoid receptor forms a dimer that recognizes the same six-base sequence (a hormone response element) in opposite orientations spaced three bases apart. **D,** A leucine zipper factor dimerizes to recognize a pair of four-base sites with opposite orientation spaced one base apart.

TFIIIA, has since been found in a variety of different RNA polymerase II factors, including more than 600 human transcription factors. Each "finger" consists of a 30-residue sequence with conserved pairs of cysteines and histidines that bind a single zinc ion. The tip of the finger sticks into the DNA major groove, where it contacts three bases. Most zinc finger proteins contain multiple fingers, allowing longer sequences to be recognized to increase specificity. A related structure is present in the steroid hormone receptor family, although in this case, four cysteine residues coordinate the zinc ion and the finger is composed of two helices rather than one. Steroid hormone receptors also contain a dimerization domain, allowing recognition of sequences with dyad symmetry (Fig. 15-17C).

Leucine Zipper Proteins

Leucine zipper domains are made up of two motifs: a basic region that recognizes a specific DNA sequence and a series of repeated leucine residues (leucine zipper) that mediate dimerization. These motifs form a continuous α-helix that can dimerize through formation of a coiled-coil structure involving specific contacts between hydrophobic leucine zipper domains (Fig. 15-17D; also see Fig. 3-10). CAAT/enhancer-binding protein, the factor that recognizes the CCAAT sequence, was the first member of this family to be discovered. Dimers of leucine zipper proteins recognize short, inverted, repeat sequences. The zipper family comprises many members, some of which can cross-dimerize and recognize asymmetrical sequences. Another family of factors comprises the helix-loop-helix proteins, which have the same type of basic region but differ in that they have two helical dimerization domains separated by a loop region.

Factor Interactions

An important aspect of transcription factor function is the ability to associate with other factors. Such associations can expand the repertoire of DNA sequences that can be specifically recognized. In the case of the leucine zipper proteins, formation of a heterodimer leads to recognition of a site that is different from either of the sites recognized by the two homodimers (Fig. 15-18). Thus, a diverse set of binding sites can be recognized by using a relatively small set of interacting factors. Such interactions need not be limited to related proteins, and small interactions surfaces involving only a few specific contacts often suffice.

Transcription Factors as Modular Proteins

In addition to interaction with specific DNA sequences, transcription factors may also interact with regulatory molecules and/or the basal transcription machinery. Functional domains in transcription factors have been mapped by testing various domains in vivo (Fig. 15-19). Such chimeric factors will stimulate transcription as long as two functions are maintained: specific DNA binding and transcription activation. The surprising result of this type of analysis is that many transcription factors are modular proteins with discrete functional domains that can be exchanged without impairing activity. For example, exchanging the DNA-binding domains of the glucocorticoid and estrogen receptors creates a hybrid factor that recognizes estrogen-responsive promoters but activates transcription in response to glucocorticoid hormone.

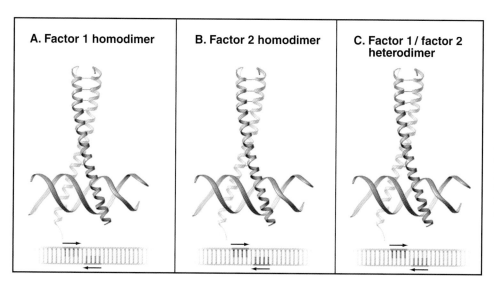

| **A. Factor 1 homodimer** | **B. Factor 2 homodimer** | **C. Factor 1 / factor 2 heterodimer** |

Figure 15-18 TRANSCRIPTION FACTOR DIMERS THAT RECOGNIZE NOVEL TARGETS. **A–B,** The homodimers of transcription factors 1 and 2 recognize different sites containing inverted four-base recognition elements. **C,** Heterodimers formed by factors 1 and 2 recognize a novel class of asymmetrical sites consisting of two different half-sites.

Transcriptional Activation

Binding of a transcription factor to DNA per se does not activate transcription (Fig. 15-19). A separate domain provides this function by interacting directly or indirectly with the basal transcription machinery to elevate the rate of transcription. The best-characterized activation domain is an acidic region derived from the herpesvirus VP16 protein. Acidic activation domains are generally disordered segments of polypeptide consisting of multiple acidic residues dispersed among a few key hydrophobic residues. Such domains activate transcription when experimentally grafted to a wide variety of different DNA-binding domains in a number of different cell types. Other types of activator domains have been characterized as being proline-rich or glutamine-rich.

The diverse activation domains use several mechanisms to promote transcription (Fig. 15-20). The most direct mechanism is recruitment of the basal transcription machinery. Recall that RNA polymerase II requires a number of additional factors for specific transcription. TFIID binds the TATA box and recruits the polymerase in a complex with the mediator. Interactions between activation domains and mediator or TFIID components in these complexes stabilize the preinitiation complex

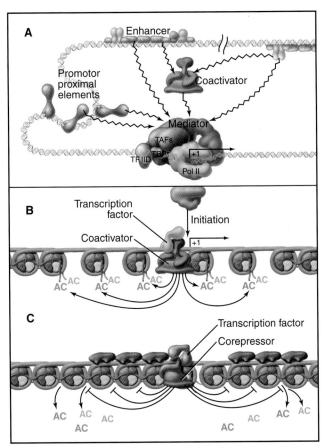

Figure 15-20 TRANSCRIPTION ACTIVATION MECHANISMS. **A,** Contact between transcription activators and mediator or TAF subunits, or both, leads to stable preinitiation complexes and elevated transcription. In some cases, a coactivator acts as an intermediary in this process. **B,** Histone acetylases in a coactivator loosen chromatin in the vicinity of the promoter, allowing assembly of preinitiation complexes. **C,** Recruitment of histone deacetylases in a corepressor represses transcription by compacting the chromatin in the vicinity of the promoter.

and produce higher rates of RNA polymerase II initiation. The chromatin immunoprecipitation technique (Fig. 15-16D) has been used to demonstrate recruitment of the transcription machinery to specific genes.

Transcriptional Repressors

As in prokaryotes, some eukaryotic transcription factors repress transcription. Unlike the lac repressor, however, the eukaryotic repressors generally do not act by blocking binding of RNA polymerase. Some eukaryotic repressors act by competing with activators for the same DNA sequence. Often, these repressors are related to the activator they block but simply lack the activation domain. Another type of eukaryotic repressor binds near the activator and interacts with the activator to mask its activation domain. Some repressors bind to specific sites on DNA and interact with coactivators in a manner that blocks their function. Finally, some repres-

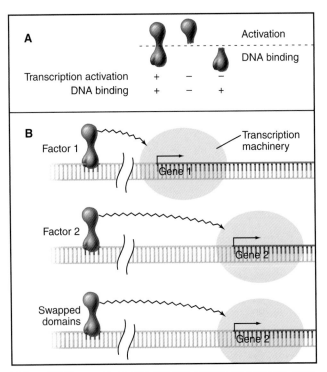

Figure 15-19 TRANSCRIPTION FACTORS CONSIST OF DISCRETE, FUNCTIONAL MODULES. **A,** Domain characterization. Although the entire factor is required for activation, the bottom domain is sufficient for DNA binding. **B,** Domain swapping. The activation domain of one factor (activating gene 1) can be fused to the DNA-binding domain of a heterologous factor (activating gene 2). The resulting chimeric factor will activate only genes containing the recognition site for the DNA-binding domain (gene 2).

sors bind corepressors that can alter chromatin structure in a way that the transcription machinery is denied access.

Chromatin and Transcription

DNA in eukaryotic cells associates with an equal mass of protein to form chromatin (see Chapter 13). Packaging DNA in arrays of nucleosomes compacts the DNA, and the most obvious influence of chromatin on transcription is the ability of nucleosomes to restrict access of transcription proteins to the DNA template. Thus, if histone synthesis is artificially shut off, there is an increase in the basal expression of many genes. Additional evidence of the repressive nature of chromatin is seen in the resistance to nuclease digestion of unexpressed genes and the localization of unexpressed genes in highly condensed heterochromatin.

Gene activation often involves disruption or displacement of nucleosomes located on specific genes. Before the discussion of specific mechanisms, it is useful to consider some aspects of nucleosome structure. The nucleosome consists of DNA wrapped in a left-handed helix around an octamer of histone subunits (see Fig. 13-1). The histone core makes numerous contacts with the DNA minor groove and phosphate backbone, leading to tight binding that is not sequence specific. This aspect of the nucleosome allows for a dynamic association with DNA because binding to one position along the DNA strand is as energetically favorable as another. The N-terminal histone "tails" are highly conserved and play multiple roles in chromatin structure and gene regulation. Histone tails are important sites of modifications that regulate chromatin structure and transcription. Both the nonspecific nature of interactions between histones and DNA and the ability to modify the histone tails are exploited to regulate the ability of nucleosomes to block access of the transcription machinery to the DNA template.

Nucleosome remodeling complexes use the energy of ATP hydrolysis to alter the location of nucleosomes on the DNA template. These multiprotein complexes destabilize interactions between histones and DNA and "remodel" the chromatin to allow increased access to the template. In addition to facilitating transcription initiation through coactivator function, some remodeling complexes are required for transcription elongation and termination.

SWI/SNF complexes (see Chapter 13) are recruited to a specific subset of genes through interactions with transcription activators. The resulting remodeling of nucleosomes in the vicinity of the promoter is required for stable preinitiation complex formation at SWI/SNF-regulated genes. Other remodeling complexes are thought to regulate distinct sets of genes in a similar manner. SWI/SNF can also repress transcription at some promoters, presumably by repositioning nucleosomes to restrict access to the promoter.

Gene activation by nucleosome disruption can also be counteracted by factors that stabilize chromatin. In one example, broad regions of chromatin are **silenced** by recruitment of histone deacetylases that maintain heterochromatin domains (see Fig. 13-9).

Histone Modification and Chromatin Accessibility

The pattern of modification of the histone N-terminal tails forms the basis of a "histone code" that is read by the gene expression machinery. Modification of the histone tails is carried out by enzymes that are specific both for a particular modifying group and for specific residues within the tail of particular histones. For example, the histone methyl transferase SET1 is specific for lysine 4 in the histone H3 tail. The modifying enzymes are generally part of large complexes (Table 15-3) that are recruited to chromatin through interactions with gene regulatory proteins and thus, like the mediator, are considered coactivators (or corepressors).

Proteins containing **bromodomains** or **chromodomains** interact with acetylated or methylated tails, respectively. Many of the protein complexes involved in gene regulation contain one or more of these domains. For example, the SAGA histone acetyltransferase complex contains a bromodomain that anchors the com-

Table 15-3

NUCLEOSOME-MODIFYING COMPLEXES

Name	Subunits	Catalytic Activity	Histone-interacting Domain	Target Histone(s)
SAGA	15	Histone acetylase	Bromodomain	H3, H2B
NuA4	6	Histone acetylase	Chromodomain	H4
P300	1	Histone acetylase	Bromodomain	H2A, H2B, H3, H4
NuRD	9	Histone deacetylase	Chromodomain	?
SIR2	3	Histone deacetylase	Neither	H4
MLL	7	Histone methylase	Neither	H3 (lysine 4)

plex to chromatin, facilitating further modification of regions that are already acetylated. A subunit of TFIID also contains a bromodomain that can facilitate the binding of TFIID to acetylated nucleosomes associated with active chromatin. Similarly, a number of histone methyltransferases contain chromodomains and are therefore targeted to their substrates by preexisting histone methylation.

Combinatorial Control

The complexity of eukaryotic regulatory systems allows for the integration of multiple regulatory signals at individual genes. Such combinatorial control is seen in a limited way in prokaryotes. For example, the *E. coli* lac genes are regulated by both lactose and glucose. Only when glucose is absent and lactose is present do the activator (CAP) and repressor (lac repressor) function to maximize lac expression. Regulation of transcription initiation in eukaryotes is based on similar principles with DNA-binding activators and repressors controlling individual genes. For each eukaryotic gene, however, there are often binding sites for many more factors. Integration of the individual binding events can take place in several ways. First, there is a degree of synergism to the binding of multiple factors. The enhanceosome is an example in which binding of proteins that bend the DNA can lead to more efficient binding of additional proteins. The key characteristic of the resulting complex is that the activation of transcription provided by the enhanceosome is greater that the stimulatory effect predicted from the sum of individual transcription factors. Synergy can also result from multiple interactions between activators bound to DNA at different upstream sites or different enhancers and targets in coactivators such as the mediator or nucleosome remodeling complexes. Many of the same mechanisms also can occur with repressors.

Combinatorial control also can result from the interplay between factors that alter chromatin structure. For example, modification of histone tails by a histone acetyltransferase tethered to a DNA-bound transcription factor can result in the loosening of chromatin at a particular site and creation of binding sites for additional factors. Subsequent binding of a nucleosome remodeling complex can render sequences accessible to the transcriptional machinery.

Modulation of Transcription Factor Activity

Regulation of transcription initiation is of fundamental importance in controlling gene expression. In many cases, the availability of factors that bind to specific sites in promoters is the switch that turns a gene on. Various strategies to control the binding of specific factors have

been discovered (Fig. 15-21). One of the most straightforward is de novo synthesis of the specific factor (Fig. 15-21A). This requires an additional level of transcription regulation and translation of the mRNA that encodes the specific factor. All of these steps take some time; therefore, this regulatory scheme is not used in situations in which rapid responses are required. Instead, it is used more commonly in regulating developmental pathways.

Several mechanisms are used for rapid regulation of the activity of existing transcription factors. One mechanism involves the formation of an active factor from two inactive subunits (Fig. 15-21D). This association can be regulated through synthesis or by modification of preexisting subunits, leading to their association. Binding of small-molecule ligands is another means of controlling transcription factor activity (Fig. 15-21B). In this case, the binding of the ligand induces a conformational change that leads to DNA binding and transcription activation. Interaction of transcription factors with inhibitory subunits is also used to regulate factor activity (Fig. 15-21E). The DNA binding or activation poten-

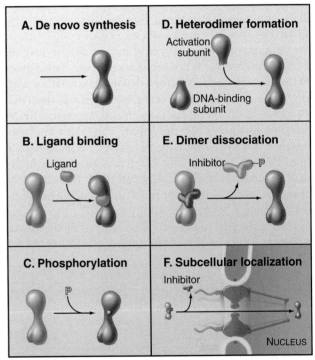

Figure 15-21 REGULATION OF TRANSCRIPTION FACTOR ACTIVITY. Many strategies have evolved to regulate transcription factors in response to specific signals. **A,** The availability of a factor may be controlled by expressing it, de novo, only when it is needed. **B,** Factors may be synthesized in an inactive state and depend on a small molecule (ligand) for activity. **C,** Transcription factors that are synthesized in an inactive state can be activated by postsynthetic modification, such as phosphorylation. **D,** Some factors require an appropriate partner for activity. **E,** Constitutively active factors can be held in check by associating with inhibitory subunits. **F,** Active factors can be sequestered in the cytoplasm by blocking their transport to the nucleus.

tial is held in check until the appropriate signal leads to dissociation of the inhibitory factor. Covalent modification—for example, by phosphorylation—is also used to convert inactive transcription factors to a functional form (Fig. 15-21C). Finally, the ability of transcription factors to bind DNA may be regulated by restricting their localization to the cytoplasm (Fig. 15-21F). These regulatory schemes are not mutually exclusive, and many regulatory pathways (see the examples that follow) employ several different levels of regulation.

Transcription Factors and Signal Transduction

One of the hallmarks of eukaryotic gene regulation is the ability of cells to respond to a wide range of external signals. Cells detect the presence of hormones, growth factors, cytokines, cell surface contacts, and many other signals. This information is then transmitted to the nucleus, where appropriate changes in expression of specific genes are executed. Transcription factors represent the final step in these signal transduction pathways; the following sections discuss several specific examples. Chapter 27 covers several other signaling pathways that regulate gene expression (see Fig. 27-4 for the three types of signaling pathways to the nucleus).

Steroid Hormone Receptors

Regulation of gene expression by steroid hormone receptors involves both ligand-binding and inhibitory subunits. This family of nuclear receptors includes transcription factors with a common sequence organization consisting of a specific DNA-binding domain, a ligand-binding domain that regulates DNA binding, and one or more transcription activation domains. The ligands that regulate these factors are small, lipid-soluble hormone molecules that diffuse through cell membranes and bind directly to the transcription factor (Fig. 15-22A).

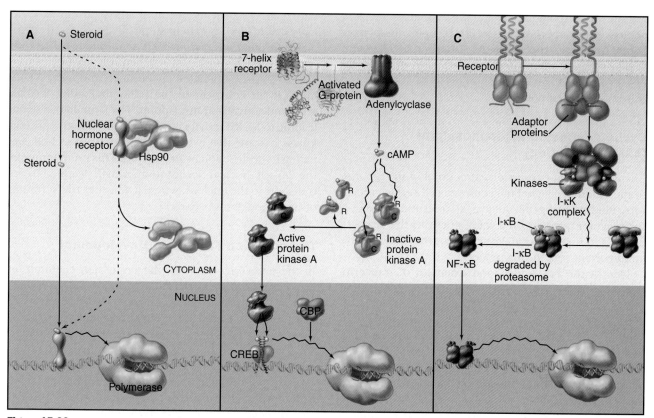

Figure 15-22 TRANSCRIPTION FACTORS AS TARGETS OF SIGNAL TRANSDUCTION PATHWAYS. External signals are transmitted by a variety of pathways that eventually impinge on transcription factors. **A,** Steroid hormones diffuse through the cell membrane and bind to the hormone receptor in the cytoplasm (estrogen) or, more commonly, the nucleus. Hormone binding induces a conformational change that renders the receptor competent to activate transcription. **B,** Ligands bound to the extracellular surface of seven-helix receptors initiate a pathway that leads to the activation of protein kinase A that moves to the nucleus, where it phosphorylates transcription factor CREB. (C, catalytic subunit of PKA. R, regulatory subunit of PKA that is dissociated from C by binding cAMP [R is shown smaller than actual size].) **C,** In a third strategy, constitutively active transcription factors are kept sequestered in the cytoplasm until a signaling pathway is activated. In this example, the transcription factor NF-κB is bound to an inhibitor called I-κB. Activation of the pathway leads to phosphorylation of I-κB, which targets the inhibitory subunit for destruction by the proteasome. The free NF-κB is transported to the nucleus, where it activates the transcription of target genes.

The steroid hormones, retinoids, thyroid hormone, and vitamin D bind to distinct members of the nuclear receptor family, enabling them to recognize sequences in the promoters of a range of target genes. The specific sites of action in promoter DNA, termed **hormone response elements,** are related to either AGAACA or AGGTCA (Fig. 15-17C). Specificity of the response is generated by the spacing and relative orientation of the binding sites. Steroid receptors usually bind to inverted repeats separated by three nucleotides, whereas some other related receptors prefer direct repeats of similar sites. The nuclear receptors can bind as homodimers, although recent evidence suggests that heterodimers actually prevail in vivo. In addition to heterodimerizing with other members of the nuclear receptor family, interactions with other types of transcription factors could serve to link the steroid response to other pathways that signal through cell surface receptors.

Inactive steroid hormone receptors are blocked from interacting with DNA by heat shock protein 90 (Hsp90; Fig. 15-22A). This protein is a molecular chaperone that keeps the receptor ligand-binding domain in a conformation ready to bind the ligand but unable to enter the nucleus. Hormone binding to the receptor dissociates Hsp90 and frees the receptor's DNA-binding domain. The free ligand–bound receptor moves from the cytoplasm to the nucleus, where it binds its DNA target and activates transcription.

Cyclic Adenosine Monophosphate (cAMP) Signaling

Changes in gene expression often develop in response to the binding of signal molecules to cell surface receptors. Binding of ligand induces a structural change in the receptor that sets off a chain of events that leads to changes in transcription. Protein phosphorylation plays an important role in this process.

One of the best-understood examples of transcriptional regulation through cell surface receptor signaling is the adenyl cyclase system. The binding of ligand to some seven-helix receptors results in an increase in synthesis of **cAMP,** which, in turn, activates **protein kinase A** (see Fig. 27-3). The promoters of cAMP-regulated genes contain a conserved DNA sequence element, called a **cAMP response element,** that mediates the transcriptional response to cAMP. A transcription factor, termed cAMP response element–binding **(CREB)** protein, binds this sequence specifically. CREB protein is a member of the leucine zipper family and binds the DNA as a dimer. The DNA-binding domain of CREB protein can be exchanged with other DNA-binding domains without loss of cAMP responsiveness. This indicates that cAMP does not work by altering the DNA binding of CREB protein; rather, it suggests that cAMP alters the transcription activation function. Recent experiments have identified a site in the activation domain of CREB protein that is phosphorylated by protein kinase A. Mutation of serine 133 to alanine results in a CREB protein that cannot be phosphorylated and cannot activate transcription of target genes. Phosphorylation of serine 133 leads to a conformational change in CREB protein that allows it to interact with a protein adaptor that recruits the transcription machinery leading to transcription of target genes. Thus, the signal generated by binding of a ligand to a cell surface receptor is transduced to a DNA-binding factor that activates transcription of genes containing the appropriate regulatory elements.

NF-κB Signaling

NF-κB proteins are a family of related transcription factors present in many cell types. These factors control a diverse set of cellular processes, including immune and inflammatory responses, development, cell growth, and apoptosis. The activity of NF-κB is normally tightly controlled as persistently active NF-κB is associated with cancer, arthritis, asthma, and heart disease. In most cells, NF-κB is held in an inactive form in the cytoplasm through interaction with an inhibitor called **I-κB** (see Figs. 14-18 and 15-22C). When B lymphocytes (see Fig. 28-9) are stimulated to produce antibody, NF-κB binds to an enhancer in the immunoglobulin κ-chain gene and activates transcription. The stimulatory signal leading to NF-κB activity is transmitted through a protein kinase cascade that eventually phosphorylates I-κB, signaling its destruction by proteolysis. This event unmasks the NF-κB nuclear localization signal, leading to its transport to the nucleus, where it activates transcription of immunoglobulin genes.

Transcription Factors in Development

In the preceding sections, the discussion centered on how external signals can lead to changes in gene expression in the nucleus, which, in turn, lead to changes in cell function. A critical step in this genetic program is the regulation of one transcription factor by another. Such cascades of transcription factor activity are fundamental to gene regulation in development.

Early cell divisions in multicellular organisms create different types of daughter cells that express distinct sets of genes. In this case, two types of information govern the expression of a gene. First, the environment of the cell sends signals that are transduced to the nucleus and change the pattern of gene expression. How the nucleus interprets the transduced signals depends on the set of transcription factors that preexist within it. Thus, in addition to external signals, the history of the cell dictates which genes will respond to which signals.

The exact program of transcription factor interaction during development is extremely complicated and is certainly beyond the scope of this chapter. The underlying principles of these pathways are worth considering, however. One important observation is that developmentally regulated transcription factors are often autoregulatory. For factors that activate their own expression, this form of regulation acts as a switch that leads to continued expression after the initial stimulus is gone. Another important property of developmentally regulated transcription factors is that they are, in turn, regulated by several different factors. This allows complicated combinatorial signals to dictate expression. For example, some transcription factors activate certain promoters while repressing others. The basis of this contradictory property is thought to be the ability of transcription factors to cooperate with each other when bound at the same promoter. This cooperation can be either positive or negative. This allows the expression of a target gene to be regulated both by external signals (e.g., proximity of an adjacent cell that expresses a signaling molecule) and by the preexistence of a given factor in the cell. In this way, only cells of a certain lineage that are located in a certain area of an embryonic segment are able to express the gene. As new transcription factors involved in development are discovered, the challenge will be to decipher the complicated combinatorial interactions among them.

Transcription Factors and Human Disease

Advances in genomics and human genetics have demonstrated that mutations within specific genes are responsible for the pathogenesis or clinical features of particular human diseases. Multicellular organisms devote a significant fraction of their genome to encoding the transcription apparatus and attendant regulatory factors. Therefore, it is not surprising that mutations in some of the thousands of genes involved in transcription result in clinical phenotypes. The following examples indicate that mutations in either gene-specific or general transcription factors can contribute to disease.

Androgen Receptor

A nuclear hormone receptor, androgen receptor, binds to testosterone and regulates expression of genes involved in the development of male secondary sexual characteristics. Like other transcription factors, the androgen receptor has DNA-binding and transcription activation domains. In addition, the androgen receptor has a ligand-binding domain that binds testosterone and regulates the DNA-binding properties of the factor. Because the androgen receptor gene is located on the X chromosome, recessive mutations of the gene have a phenotype in males (which have only one copy of the X).

Mutations that alter different parts of the androgen receptor cause different clinical phenotypes. The most severe mutations cause **androgen insensitivity syndrome,** a condition in which individuals with a 46,XY chromosome constitutionally develop secondary female sexual characteristics. In this syndrome, androgens are synthesized, but the receptor fails to respond. Single missense mutations in the ligand-binding domain can weaken or eliminate ligand binding. Alternatively, ligand binding may be normal, but the mutation may weaken or eliminate DNA binding. Some androgen insensitivity syndrome mutations are associated with male breast cancer.

Another type of mutation in the androgen receptor causes a neuromuscular disease called spinal and bulbar muscular atrophy (Kennedy's syndrome). This X-linked disease involves wasting of the proximal limb muscles as well as changes in facial muscles. The molecular basis of the disease is an expansion of a series of repeated CAG (glutamine) codons in the amino-terminal transcription activation domain. Normally, this region encodes 11 to 31 consecutive glutamine residues in different individuals. The number of repeats in patients with Kennedy's syndrome ranges from 40 to 52. The mechanism by which the expanded polyglutamine domain results in motor neuron damage has not been determined.

TFIIH and Human Disease

As was discussed in a previous section, the general RNA polymerase II transcription factor TFIIH is a multisubunit factor that contains both RNA polymerase II CTD kinase and DNA helicase activities. In addition to its role as a transcription factor, TFIIH plays a role in DNA repair and might serve to direct DNA repair to transcriptionally active regions in the genome.

Mutations in TFIIH subunits are associated with a set of rare human disorders (**xeroderma pigmentosum,** Cockayne's syndrome, and trichothiodystrophy), each linked to defects in nucleotide excision repair of DNA damaged by ultraviolet light or chemical mutagens (see Box 43-1). Mutations in these diseases map to the genes encoding two different TFIIH helicase activities. Presumably, the alterations in these activities cause changes in DNA unwinding, either in the transcription initiation reaction or in the process of nucleotide excision repair. Some mutations are more selective for the DNA repair function, whereas other TFIIH mutations cause little or no DNA repair phenotype but rather seem to affect the TFIIH transcription function. The latter mutations cause wide-ranging defects, as might be expected for a defect in a general transcription factor.

ACKNOWLEDGMENT

Thanks go to Richard Treisman for his suggestions on revisions to this chapter.

SELECTED READINGS

Asturias FJ: RNA polymerase II structure, and organization of the preinitiation complex. Curr Opin Struct Biol 14:121-129, 2004.

Bai L, Santangelo TJ, Wang MD: Single-molecule analysis of RNA polymerase transcription. Annu Rev Biophys Biomol Struct 35:343-360, 2006.

Bracken AP, Ciro M, Cocito A, Helin K: E2F target genes: Unraveling the biology. Trends Biochem Sci 29:409-417, 2004.

Cramer P, Bushnell DA, Kornberg RD: Structural basis of transcription: RNA polymerase II at 2.8 angstrom resolution. Science 292:1863-1876, 2001.

Davidson I: The genetics of TBP and TBP-related factors. Trends Biochem Sci 28:391-398, 2003.

Dilworth FJ, Chambon P: Nuclear receptors coordinate the activities of chromatin remodeling complexes and coactivators to facilitate initiation of transcription. Oncogene 20(24):3047-3054, 2001.

Garvie CW, Wolberger C: Recognition of specific DNA sequences. Mol Cell 8:937-946, 2001.

Gnatt AL, Cramer P, Fu J, et al: Structural basis of transcription: An RNA polymerase II elongation complex at 3.3 Å resolution. Science 292:1876-1882, 2001.

Holmberg CI, Tran SEF, Eriksson JE, Sistonen L: Multisite phosphorylation provides sophisticated regulation of transcription factors. Trends Biochem Sci 27:619-627, 2002.

Kornberg RD: Mediator and the mechanism of transcriptional activation. Trends Biochem Sci 30:235-239, 2005.

Le Hir H, Nott A, Moore MJ: How introns influence and enhance eukaryotic gene expression. Trends Biochem Sci 28:215-220, 2003.

Lemon B, Tjian R: Orchestrated response: A symphony of transcription factors for gene control. Genes Dev 14:2551-2569, 2000.

Levsky JM, Singer RH: Gene expression and the myth of the average cell. Trends Cell Biol 13:4-6, 2003.

Pombo A: Cellular genomics: Which genes are transcribed, when and where? Trends Biochem Sci 28:6-9, 2003.

Ptashne M, Gann A: Transcriptional activation by recruitment. Nature 386:569-577, 1997.

Reinberg D, Orphanides G, Ebright R, et al: The RNA polymerase II general transcription factors: Past, present, and future. Cold Spring Harb Symp Quant Biol 63:83-103, 1998.

Roeder RG: Role of general and gene-specific cofactors in the regulation of eukaryotic transcription. Cold Spring Harb Symp Quant Biol 63:201-218, 1998.

Shilatifard A, Conaway RC, Conaway JW: The RNA polymerase II elongation complex. Annu Rev Biochem 72:693-715, 2003.

Spector DL: The dynamics of chromosome organization and gene regulation. Annu Rev Biochem 72:573-608, 2003.

Steinmetz ACU, Renaud J-P, Moras D: Binding of ligands and activation of transcription by nuclear receptors. Annu Rev Biophys Biomol Struct 30:329-359, 2001.

Steitz TA: The structural basis of the transition from initiation to elongation phases of transcription, as well as translocation and strand separation, by T7 RNA polymerase. Curr Opin Struct Biol 14:4-9, 2004.

Eukaryotic RNA Processing

In all organisms, the genetic information is encoded in the sequence of the DNA. However, to be used, this information must be copied, or transcribed, into the related polymer, RNA. Eukaryotes synthesize many different types of RNA, but none of these RNAs is simply transcribed as a finished product. The mature, functional forms of all eukaryotic RNA species are generated by posttranscriptional processing, and these processing reactions are the major topic of this chapter.

The major RNAs can be assigned to three major classes: (1) The cytoplasmic messenger RNAs (mRNAs) and their nuclear precursors (pre-mRNAs) carry the information that is used to specify the sequence, and therefore the structure, of all proteins in the cell. (2) Other RNAs do not encode protein but function directly, playing major roles in several metabolic pathways, including protein synthesis. These include the ribosomal RNAs (rRNAs) and transfer RNAs (tRNAs), which are the key components of the protein synthesis machinery; the small nuclear RNAs (snRNAs), which form the core of the pre-mRNA splicing system; and the small nucleolar RNAs (snoRNAs), which are important factors in ribosome biogenesis. These RNAs are generally much longer-lived than are the mRNAs and therefore often are referred to as *stable* or *nonprotein coding* RNAs (ncRNAs). (3) The third and most recently identified class of RNA comprises several structurally related groups of very small (21 to 25 nucleotides) RNA species that play important roles in regulating gene expression. Base pairing between endogenous micro-RNAs (miRNAs) and target mRNAs in the cytoplasm represses their translation into protein. The packaging of DNA into a nontranscribed form termed *heterochromatin* (see Fig. 13-9) is promoted by a class of nuclear, small heterochromatic RNAs (shRNAs). Finally, the introduction of small double-stranded RNAs into many cell types and organisms results in cleavage of the target mRNA and consequent silencing of gene expression. This phenomenon is described as RNA interference (RNAi), and the RNAs are referred to as small interfering RNAs (siRNAs).

Synthesis of mRNAs

An overview of mRNA synthesis and degradation is shown in Figure 16-1.

This chapter was written by David Tollervey and includes some text and figures from a chapter in the first edition written by Barbara Sollner-Webb, with contributions from Christine Smith.

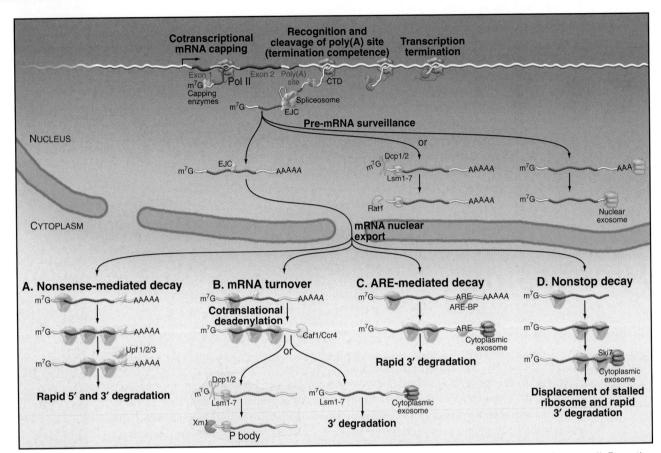

Figure 16-1   Synthesis and degradation of eukaryotic mRNAs. Nascent mRNA transcripts are transcribed by RNA polymerase II. Formation of the 5' cap structure and cleavage and polyadenylation of the 3' end of the mRNA both occur cotranscriptionally and involve factors that are recruited by the C-terminal domain (CTD) of the transcribing polymerase (see Fig. 15-4). The termination of transcription requires both the recognition of the site of polyadenylation and the activity of the 5'-exonuclease Rat1, which degrades the nascent RNA transcripts. Rat1 binds to the polymerase CTD via Rtt103. Pre-mRNA splicing can either be cotranscriptional or occur shortly after transcript release, and recruitment of splicing factors is not strongly dependent on the CTD. In human cells, the spliceosome deposits the exon-junction complex (EJC) around 24 nucleotides upstream of the site of splicing. Several steps in nuclear mRNA maturation also are subject to surveillance. In yeast, nuclear pre-mRNAs can be either 3' degraded by the nuclear exosome complex or decapped and 5' degraded by the exonuclease Rat1. Nuclear decapping requires the Lsm2–8 complex and is probably performed by the Dcp1/2 decapping complex. Once in the cytoplasm, the mRNA is translated into proteins and undergoes degradation. Several different mRNA degradation pathways have been identified. **A, Nonsense-mediated decay (NMD).** If the EJCs all lie within or very close to the ORF, they will be displaced by the translating ribosomes. However, if an EJC lies beyond the end of the ORF, it will remain on the translated mRNA. This is taken as evidence that translation has terminated prematurely and triggers the NMD pathway. Recognition of the EJC requires the Upf1/2/3 surveillance complex, which also interacts with the ribosomes as they terminate translation. In yeast, NMD triggers both rapid decapping and 5' degradation, without prior deadenylation, and 3' degradation by the exosome. **B, General mRNA turnover.** During translation, most mRNAs undergo progressive poly(A) tail shortening. Loss of the poly(A) tail leads to rapid degradation. As in the nucleus, cytoplasmic mRNAs can be degraded from either the 5' or the 3' end. 5' degradation occurs largely in a specialized cytoplasmic region termed the P body in yeast or cytoplasmic foci in human cells. Here, the mRNAs are decapped by the Dcp1/2 heterodimer and then degraded by the cytoplasmic 5'-exonuclease Xrn1. Both activities are strongly stimulated by the cytoplasmic Lsm1–7 complex. Alternatively, deadenylated mRNAs can be 3' degraded by the cytoplasmic exosome. **C, ARE-mediated decay.** In this pathway, specific A+U rich elements (AREs) are recognized by ARE-binding proteins (ARE-BP) in the nucleus. These are transported to the cytoplasm in association with the mRNA and recruit the cytoplasmic exosome to rapidly degrade the RNA. **D, Nonstop decay.** If the mRNA lacks a translation termination codon, the first translating ribosome will stall and be trapped at the 3' end of the RNA. The Ski7 protein, which is associated with the cytoplasmic exosome complex, is believed to release the stalled ribosome and target the RNA for 3' degradation by the exosome. Note that this legend provides detail beyond the text.

mRNA Capping and Polyadenylation

Two distinguishing features set mRNA apart from other RNAs: a 5' cap structure and a 3' poly(A) tail. Both of these elements help to protect the mRNA against degradation and act synergistically to promote translation in the cytoplasm.

The mRNA cap is an unusual structure. It consists of an inverted 7-methylguanosine residue, which is joined onto the body of the mRNA by a 5'-triphosphate-5' linkage (Fig. 16-2). Cap addition involves three enzymatic activities: A 5' RNA triphosphatase cleaves the 5' triphosphate on the nascent transcript to a diphosphate; RNA guanylyltransferase forms a covalent enzyme–GMP

A. Chemical structure of 5' capped mRNA

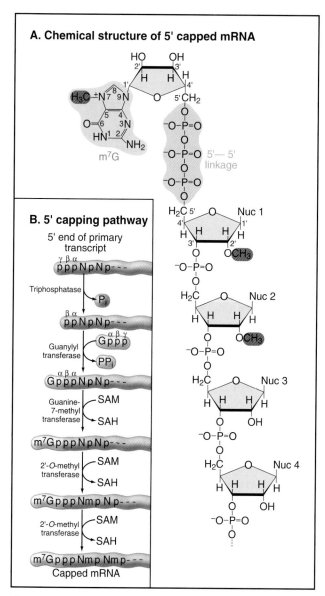

B. 5' capping pathway

Figure 16-2 mRNAs have a distinctive 5' cap structure. **A,** The 5' ends of mRNAs are blocked by an inverted guanosine residue that is attached to the body of the mRNA by a 5'–5' triphosphate linkage. The N7 position of the guanosine is methylated *(red)*. The first encoded nucleotide of the mRNA (Nuc 1) is also methylated on the 2'-hydroxyl of the ribose ring. The second nucleotide (Nuc 2) may also be methylated. **B,** Capping of mRNAs is a multistep process.

250 A residues are added to mRNAs in human cells, and around 70 to 90 are added in yeast. Cleavage and polyadenylation are performed by a large complex containing approximately 20 proteins that recognizes sequences in the mRNA, of which the best defined is a highly conserved AAUAAA motif located upstream of the site of polyadenylation (Fig. 16-3).

Links between mRNA Processing and Transcription

The processes of cap addition and 3' cleavage and polyadenylation are both linked to transcription of the mRNA by RNA polymerase II and occur cotranscriptionally on the nascent RNA (Fig. 16-1). The **C-terminal domain (CTD)** of the largest subunit of RNA polymerase II (RNA pol II) consists of many copies of a seven-amino-acid repeat (YSPTSPS), which undergo reversible modification by phosphorylation (see Fig. 15-4). A pronounced change in the CTD phosphorylation pattern coincides with the release of the polymerase from initiation mode into processive elongation mode. Immediately following transcription initiation, the repeats are largely phosphorylated on the serine residue at position 5. This modification is lost, while serine 2 phosphorylation increases, as the polymerase moves along the transcript. Capping of the 5' end of the mRNA occurs by the time the transcript is approximately 25 to 30 nucleotides long, and the capping enzyme interacts

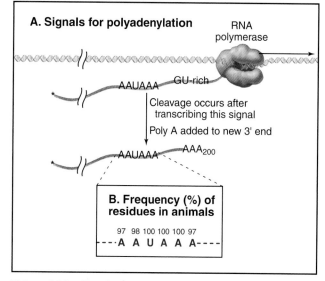

Figure 16-3 Signals for pre-mRNA polyadenylation. **A,** Poly(A) tails are added to pre-mRNAs following transcription. After pol II transcribes the protein-coding region of the mRNA, it encounters two sequence elements: AAUAAA and a GU-rich element. These act as signals for the assembly of a large 3' processing complex that cleaves the nascent pre-mRNA, releasing it from the transcription complex, and adds a tail of up to 200 adenosine residues. **B,** The poly A signal is highly conserved in vertebrates.

complex and then caps the RNA by transferring this to the diphosphate; and RNA (guanine-7) methyltransferase covalently alters the guanosine base by methylation, generating m^{7}G. In addition, the first encoded nucleotides are frequently modified by methylation of the 2' hydroxyl position on the ribose group, but the functional significance of these internal modifications is currently unclear.

During 3' processing, the nascent pre-mRNA is cleaved by an endonuclease, and a tail of adenosine residues is added by poly(A) polymerase. Around 200 to

with the serine 5 phosphorylated CTD. This and other interactions with the polymerase result in strong allosteric activation of capping activity. In contrast, the cleavage and polyadenylation factors involved in 3′ end processing are recruited by interaction with the CTD phosphorylated at serine 2.

The termination of transcription by RNA polymerase II is dependent on RNA processing. Termination requires recognition of the poly(A) site by the cleavage and polyadenylation factors. These are carried with the transcribing polymerase, and their offloading might make the polymerase competent for termination. Cleavage of the nascent transcript also allows the entry of a **5′ exonuclease**—an enzyme that can degrade RNA from the 5′ end in a 3′ direction. This enzyme, which is called Rat1 in yeast and Xrn2 in humans, then chases after the transcribing polymerase, degrading the newly transcribed RNA strand as it goes. When the exonuclease catches the polymerase, it stimulates termination of transcription. This is referred to as the *Torpedo model* for transcription termination.

Human β-globin mRNA precursors contain an additional cleavage site (termed the cotranscriptional cleavage site) downstream of the site of polyadenylation. The cotranscriptional cleavage site RNA sequence has intrinsic self-cleavage activity in the absence of proteins. Such an RNA is referred to as a **self-cleaving ribozyme.** This cleavage provides an entry site for the Xrn2 nuclease, allowing more efficient termination.

Regulated 3′ End Formation on Histone mRNAs

A different 3′ end processing system is seen for mRNAs encoding the major, replication-dependent histone proteins. These are highly expressed only during DNA replication, when they must package the newly synthesized DNA. A sequence in the **3′ untranslated region (3′ UTR)** of these mRNAs is recognized by base pairing to a small RNA: the U7 snRNA. In addition, a specific stem-loop structure is recognized by a protein that is referred to as the stem-loop binding protein. Endonuclease cleavage generates the mature 3′ end of the mRNA, which is not polyadenylated but is protected by the stem-loop binding protein. The efficiency of histone mRNA synthesis is increased during DNA replication at least in part by increased abundance of stem-loop binding protein. Minor histone variants that are synthesized throughout the cell cycle are polyadenylated like other mRNAs.

Pre-mRNA Splicing

Important experiments in the 1950s and 1960s established that genes were collinear with their protein products. It therefore came as a considerable surprise when,

in the late 1970s, it emerged that genes in animals and plants frequently had numerous strikingly large inserts whose sequence was not included in the mature mRNA or the protein product. It turns out that most human pre-mRNAs undergo **splicing** reactions, in which specific regions are cut out and the remaining RNA is covalently rejoined. The regions that will form the mRNA are termed **exons,** and the bits that are cut out (and are normally degraded) are called **introns.** In unicellular eukaryotes, introns are generally a few hundred nucleotides in length or shorter. In metazoans, however, they are often several kilobases in length, and pre-mRNAs can contain many introns. It is therefore remarkable that all of the sites can be precisely identified and spliced.

Signals for Splicing

The signals in the pre-mRNA that identify the introns and exons are recognized by a combination of proteins and a group of small RNAs called the **small nuclear RNAs** (snRNAs). The snRNAs function in complexes with proteins in small nuclear ribonucleoprotein (**snRNP**) particles. Splicing occurs in a large complex termed the spliceosome, within which the pre-mRNA assembles together with five **snRNAs (U1, U2, U4, U5, and U6)** and around 100 different proteins. Particularly important protein-splicing factors are members of a large group of **SR-proteins**—so named because they contain domains rich in serine-arginine dipeptides.

Three conserved sequences within introns play key roles in their accurate recognition by the splicing machinery (Fig. 16-4). These lie immediately adjacent to the **5′ splice site** and **the 3′ splice site** and surrounding an internal region that will form the **intron branch point** during the splicing reaction. The U1 and U6 snRNAs have sequences that are complementary to the 5′ splice site, while U2 is complementary to the branch point region.

While the spliceosome will finally bring together the sequences at each end of the intron, it is believed that the splicing machinery initially recognizes the *exons* in a reaction termed **exon definition.** This makes sense because mRNA exons are generally quite small—up to a few hundred nucleotides in length—whereas the introns can be many kilobases long.

No sequences in the exons are strictly required for splicing, but there are important stimulatory elements termed **exonic splicing enhancers (ESEs),** which generally bind members of the SR-protein family. The ESEs have two major functions: They stimulate the use of the flanking 5′ and 3′ splice sites, promoting exon definition, and they prevent the exon in which they are located from being included in an intron. This latter function is particularly important in ensuring that all introns are spliced out without the splicing machinery

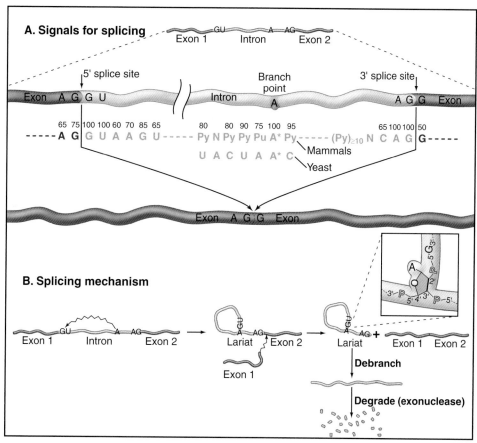

Figure 16-4 Signals and mechanism of pre-mRNA splicing. The precursors to most mRNAs in humans and other eukaryotes contain regions (introns) that will not form part of the mature mRNA and do not encode protein products. During pre-mRNA splicing, the introns are removed and the flanking regions (exons) are ligated. **A,** Introns contain three conserved sequence elements that are recognized during splicing. These lie at the 5′ and 3′ splice sites and surrounding the branch-point adenosine within the intron. Numbers indicate the degree of conservation at each position in mammalian pre-mRNAs. The branch point sequence is much more highly conserved between different pre-mRNAs in yeast. The region between the branch point and the 3′ splice site frequently contains a run of pyrimidine residues, which is referred to as the polypyrimidine tract. **B,** Pre-mRNA splicing involves two catalytic steps. An attack by the branch-point adenosine on the 5′ splice site releases the 5′ exon and intron as a circularized molecule (referred to as the intron lariat) joined to the 3′ exon. In the second step, the 3′ end of the 5′ exon attacks the 3′ splice site releasing the joined exons and the free intron lariat. The lariat is subsequently linearized (debranched) and degraded.

skipping from the 5′ end of one intron to the 3′ end of a downstream intron.

The Pre-mRNA Splicing Reaction

The splicing reaction proceeds in two steps (Fig. 16-4). In the first, the 5′–3′ phosphate linkage that joins the 5′ exon to the first nucleotide of the intron—at the 5′ splice site—is attacked and broken. This reaction leaves the 5′ end of the intron attached to the adenosine residue via an unusual 5′–2′ phosphate linkage. Since this adenosine remains attached to the flanking nucleotides by conventional 5′ and 3′ phosphodiester bonds, this creates a circular molecule with a tail that includes the 3′ exon. This structure is termed the intron **lariat,** and the adenosine to which the 5′ end of the intron is attached is termed the **branch point,** because it has a

branched structure. In the second step of splicing, the free 3′ hydroxyl on the 5′ exon is used to attack and break the linkage between the last nucleotide of the intron and the 3′ exon—at the 3′ splice site. This leaves the 5′ and 3′ exons joined by a conventional 5′–3′ linkage and releases the intron as a lariat. This is linearized by the **debranching enzyme** and is probably rapidly degraded from both ends by exonucleases.

The initial steps in splicing are the recognition of the 5′ splice site by the U1 snRNA and the binding of U2 snRNA to the branch-point region, assisted by SR-proteins (Fig. 16-5). Base pairing between U2 and the pre-mRNA leaves a single adenosine bulged out of a helix and available for interaction with the 5′ splice site. The U4 and U6 snRNAs then join the spliceosome as a base-paired duplex, within a large complex that also contains the U5 snRNA. The U4 and U6 base pairing is

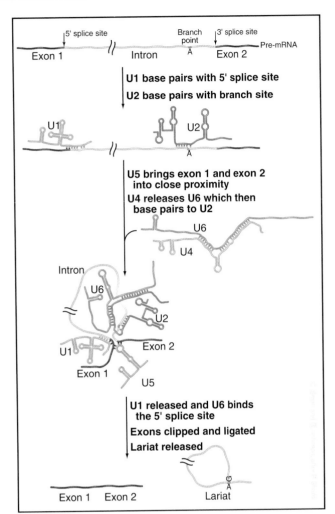

Figure 16-5 Small nuclear RNAs play key role in pre-mRNA splicing. Although shown as RNAs, the snRNAs function in large RNA-protein complexes termed snRNPs. Despite this fact, the major steps in both intron recognition and catalysis are believed to be performed by the snRNAs. The 5′ splice site and intron branch point are recognized by base pairing to the U1 and U2 snRNAs, respectively. The U5 snRNA enters the spliceosome in a complex with U4 and U6, which are tightly base-paired. U5 forms contacts with both the 5′ and 3′ exons. U4 releases U6, which base-pairs to U2 and then displaces U1 in binding to the 5′ splice site. Within this very complex RNA structure, the 2′ hydroxyl group on the branch point adenosine, which is bulged out of the duplex between U2 and the pre-mRNA, attacks the phosphate group at the junction between the 5′ exon and the intron. In a transesterification reaction, the phosphate backbone is broken at the 5′ splice site. The 5′ exon is released with a 3′ OH group, and the 5′ phosphate of the intron is transferred onto the 2′ position of the ribose on the branch point adenosine, creating the intron lariat structure. U5 retains the 5′ exon and aligns it for a second transesterification reaction, during which the 3′ hydroxyl on the 5′ exon attacks the 3′ splice site, joining the exons and releasing the intron lariat.

opened, and the liberated U6 sequences displace U1 at the 5′ splice site. They also bind to U2—bringing the 5′ splice site and branch point into close proximity. At this point, the first enzymatic step of splicing occurs. This reaction is believed to be directly catalyzed by the intri-

cate structure of the snRNA/pre-mRNA interactions rather than by the protein components of the spliceosome. The 5′ splice site is attacked and broken by the ribose 2′ hydroxyl group of the adenosine residue that is bulged out of the U2-intron duplex. The U5 snRNA and its associated proteins are responsible for holding onto the now free 5′ exon and correctly aligning it with the 3′ exon for the second catalytic step of splicing.

Both catalytic steps in splicing are technically termed **transesterification** reactions, because nucleotides are linked by phosphodiester bonds, and the new bond is made at the same time as the old bond is broken. For this reason, the splicing reactions do not, in principle, require any input of energy. However, the assembly and subsequent disassembly of the spliceosome require numerous ATPases. Most of these belong to a family of proteins that are generally termed **RNA helicases.** These are believed to use the energy of ATP hydrolysis to catalyze structural rearrangements within the assembling and disassembly spliceosome.

AT-AC Introns

The large majority of human mRNA splice sites have a GU dinucleotide at the 5′ splice site and AG at the 3′ splice site (Fig. 16-4). However, a minor group of introns contain different consensus splicing signals and are termed AT-AC (pronounced "attack") introns because of the identities of the nucleotides located at the 5′ and 3′ splice sites. The splicing of the AT-AC introns involves a distinct set of snRNAs—U11, U12, $U4_{ATAC}$, and $U6_{ATAC}$—which replace U1, U2, U4, and U6, respectively. Only U5 is common to both spliceosomes. However, the underlying splicing mechanism is believed to be the same for both classes of intron.

Alternative Splicing

A surprising finding from the human genomic sequencing project was the relatively low number of predicted protein-coding genes, currently estimated at around 30,000. This result has caused increased interest in the phenomenon of alternative splicing, which allows the production of more than one mRNA, and therefore more than one protein product, from a single gene. Several general forms of alternative splicing are commonly found. Exons can be excluded from the mRNAs, or introns can be included. Some genes have arrays of multiple alternative exons, only one of which is included in each mRNA. In addition, the use of alternative splice sites can generate longer or shorter forms of individual exons (Fig. 16-6).

Current estimates for the proportion of human genes that are subject to alternative splicing range from 30% to 75%. In some cases, this could potentially give rise to a very large number of different protein **isoforms.**

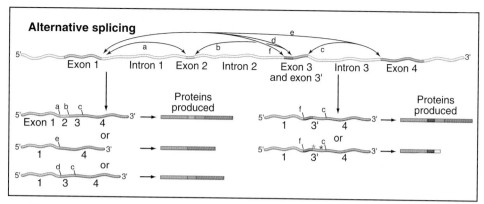

Figure 16-6 ALTERNATIVE SPLICING CAN GENERATE MULTIPLE DIFFERENT PROTEINS FROM A SINGLE GENE. Here are some of the possible mRNA and protein products of a gene whose pre-mRNA is subject to alternative splicing. **Left,** Examples show the other effects of skipping one or more internal exons, which produces a set of related proteins with different combinations of "modules." **Right,** Examples show the effects of alternative splice sites. In the case shown, the use of alternative 3' splice sites redefines the 5' end of the downstream exon. This can lead to the inclusion of additional amino acids in the protein product. Use of an alternative splice site can also cause the exon to be read in a different reading frame *(green asterisk),* changing the amino acid sequence. If the alternative reading frame contains a translation stop codon *(red asterisk),* a truncated protein will be produced, and the mRNA will generally be targeted for rapid degradation by the NMD pathway (Fig. 16-1).

In other cases, alternatively spliced proteins can have antagonistic functions, such as transcription activation versus transcription repression. For the vast majority of human genes, no information is available on the relative activities of different spliced isoforms. Compounding the difficulty in understanding is the fact that many genes show tissue-specific splicing. Thus, a gene could be transcribed in, say, both the liver and brain but generate products with substantially different functions in each tissue. In addition to generating protein diversity, alternative splicing can generate mRNAs with premature translation termination codons—"nonsense" codons. These are subject to rapid degradation by the nonsense-mediated decay (NMD) surveillance pathway (see later). Switching splicing into a pathway that generates an NMD target is therefore a means of downregulating gene expression.

It is likely that alterations in the activities of many different factors can lead to the preferential use of alternative splice sites. In at least some cases, changes in the abundance of a general splicing factor generates tissue-specific patterns of splicing. Modulation of the activities of exonic splicing enhancers is also important in regulating alternative splicing.

Localization of Pre-mRNA Splicing

The location of the splicing reaction within the nucleus was long a contentious topic. The snRNAs can be detected dispersed in the nucleoplasm but concentrate in small structures referred to as **nuclear speckles** or **interchromatin granules,** as well as in discrete larger structures known as **Cajal bodies** (see Fig. 14-2). It is now widely accepted that most splicing is performed by the dispersed snRNA population and can occur either cotranscriptionally or immediately following transcript release. Consistent with this, there is evidence that the recruitment of some splicing factors is promoted by association with the CTD of the transcribing polymerase. The speckles are likely to represent sites at which splicing factors are stockpiled ready for use. The Cajal bodies, in contrast, represent sites of maturation in which the snRNAs undergo site-specific nucleotide modification and perhaps assembly with specific proteins.

Editing of mRNAs

The term *RNA editing* in humans refers to covalent modifications that are made to individual nucleotides, which alter the base-pairing potential. Since the process of translation involves base pairing between mRNA and tRNAs, editing of the mRNA can have the effect of changing the amino acid that is incorporated and therefore the function of the protein. Like alternative splicing, this increases the diversity of protein products that can be synthesized from the genome.

Slightly confusingly, the term *editing* is also used for quite different mechanisms that insert and delete nucleotides from RNAs in some single-celled eukaryotes. The best-characterized example is in the mitochondria of trypanosomes, which are protozoans that cause major human diseases, including African trypanosomiasis, Chagas' disease, and leishmaniasis. Uracil residues are added and, less frequently, deleted from the mitochondrial mRNAs at many sites. These changes are specified by a large number of small guide RNAs. This form of editing is not known to occur in higher eukaryotes.

C-to-U Editing

Deamination of cytosine to uracil is performed by an editing complex, sometimes referred to as the editosome, which includes the deaminase Apobec-1 (Fig. 16-7). Only a small number of nuclear-encoded targets have been identified to date, and in these, editing generates translation termination codons, producing shorter forms of the encoded proteins. The best-characterized example of C-to-U RNA editing involves the mRNA encoding intestinal apolipoprotein B (ApoB), where CAA-to-UAA editing in the loop of a specific stem-loop structure generates a stop codon. The truncated protein, ApoB48, has an important role in lipoprotein metabolism. In other cases editing may generate mRNAs that are targets for NMD (see later), leading to down-regulation of protein expression.

A-to-I Editing

The enzyme **ADAR** (adenosine deaminase acting on RNA) can convert adenine residues to inosine by deamination of the base (Fig. 16-7). Inosine acts like guanosine and base-pairs with cytosine rather than uracil, potentially altering the protein encoded by the mRNA. Most of the transcripts that are edited by ADAR encode receptors of the central nervous system, and RNA editing is required to create the full receptor repertoire. The amino acid substitutions that result from editing of the mRNAs can greatly alter the properties of ion channels, and aberrant editing occurs in various disorders ranging from epilepsy to malignant brain gliomas. ADAR binds as a dimer to imperfect double-stranded RNA duplexes, which are formed between the target site and sequences in a flanking intron. Editing is generally not 100% efficient, so heterogeneous populations of proteins are generated.

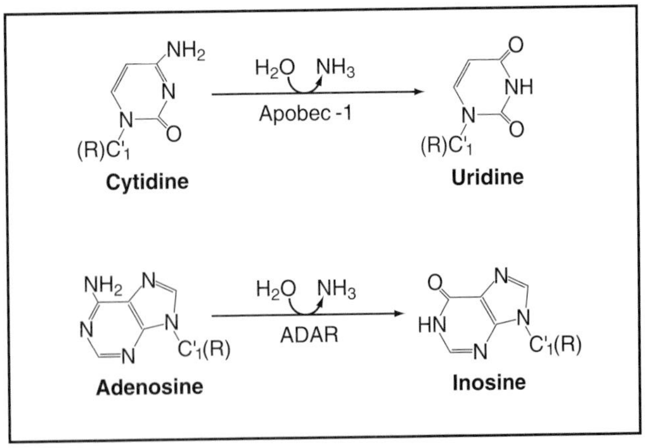

Cytoplasmic Polyadenylation

The early steps of embryogenesis in metazoans occur before transcription of the genome commences. All the mRNAs that are present in early embryos were therefore inherited from the mother. These "maternal messages" are frequently translationally inactive, at least in part because they lack a poly(A) tail. They can be activated for translation by polyadenylation in the cytoplasm. Cytoplasmic polyadenylation events are critical for many developmental decisions in oocytes and embryos. In addition, regulated cytoplasmic polyadenylation at synapses controls local translation in neuronal cells. This involves a family of cytoplasmic polymerases that are distinct, and their association with substrates and activity are both regulated by specific RNA-binding proteins.

mRNA Degradation and Surveillance

The Exosome Complex

The exosome is a protein complex composed of multiple different 3′ to 5′ exonucleases. Nuclear and cytoplasmic forms of the complex share 10 common components, some of which have proven or predicted exonuclease activity. The nuclear complex is associated with an additional 3′ to 5′ exonuclease (Rrp6 in yeast, PM-Scl100 in humans), whereas the cytoplasmic complex is associated with a GTPase (Ski7) that is homologous to translation factors. The nuclear exosome participates in RNA maturation, notably in the processing of the 5.8S rRNA, but its major functions are probably in the surveillance and degradation of nuclear RNAs. The cytoplasmic exosome functions in several different mRNA turnover pathways.

Degradation of mRNA

Most analyses of the regulation of gene expression have concentrated on changes in the levels of mRNA transcription. However, the rate at which mRNAs are degraded is also important, influencing both the total amount of protein synthesized and the timing of protein synthesis following a transcription event. mRNAs are frequently described as having half-lives, but this is generally quite misleading. Degradation is not stochastic, and it is probably better to think of mRNA lifetimes. There are enormous variations in the lifetimes of different human mRNAs—from a very few minutes to many days—which have a large impact on protein expression levels.

Different pathways of mRNA degradation can be classified as (1) the default pathway (i.e., when we do not

Figure 16-7 RNA EDITING CHANGES NUCLEOTIDE BASE PAIRING. The coding potential of an mRNA can be altered by deamination. In C-to-U editing, the amino group at position 4 of the cytosine base is replaced with a carbonyl group, creating uracil. In A-to-I editing, replacement of the amino group at position 2 of adenosine creates inosine, which base-pairs with C residues rather than with U.

yet know of any specific activator or repressor of degradation), (2) regulated degradation pathways that respond to developmental or other signals, and (3) surveillance pathways that identify and rapidly degrade aberrant mRNAs or pre-mRNAs. A theme emerging from studies of all mRNA decay pathways is that RNA-binding proteins, which associate with the newly transcribed precursor in the nucleus, can be retained when the mRNA is exported to the cytoplasm. These proteins maintain a record of the nuclear history of the RNA that can be "read" by the cytoplasmic degradation machinery, and this plays a key role in determining the cytoplasmic fate of the mRNA.

A key step in the timing of degradation of most mRNA is the slow, stepwise removal of the poly(A) tail by enzymes called **deadenylases.** The intact poly(A) tail is bound by multiple copies of the poly(A)-binding protein (PABP), at a stoichiometry of around one molecule per 10 to 20 A residues. Surprisingly, PABP antagonizes 5' cap removal, probably via interactions with the translation initiation factor eIF4G, which in turn stabilizes the cap-binding protein eIF4E. These interactions effectively circularize the mRNA and strongly stimulate translation initiation (see Fig. 17-9). When the tail becomes too short for the last PABP molecule to bind, these interactions are lost. The cap can then be removed by a **decapping complex,** which cleaves the triphosphate linkage to the body of the mRNA, releasing m^7GDP. Cap removal allows rapid 5' to 3' degradation of the mRNA by the 5' exonuclease Xrn1. In addition, loss of the PABP/poly(A) complex allows 3'-degradation of the mRNA by the cytoplasmic exosome.

ARE-Mediated Degradation

The degradation of many mRNA species in human cells is triggered by the presence of sequence motifs referred to as A+U-rich elements (AREs) (Fig. 16-1C). These are generally located in the 3' UTR of the mRNA, where bound proteins will not be displaced by the translating ribosomes. This pathway plays an important regulatory role in gene expression, as it targets for rapid turnover mRNAs that encode proteins such as cytokines, growth factors, oncogenes, and cell-cycle regulators, for which limited and transient expression is important. Computational analyses indicate that up to 8% of human mRNAs carry AREs, and there is evidence that alterations in the activity of this pathway are associated with both developmental decisions and cancer. ARE-binding proteins associate with the nuclear pre-mRNAs and are exported to the cytoplasm, where they can either activate or repress ARE-mediated decay. Some ARE-binding proteins that activate degradation function by directly recruiting the exosome complex to degrade the mRNA from the 3' end.

Surveillance of mRNAs

Nonsense-Mediated Decay

The surveillance of mRNA integrity is important because defective molecules can encode truncated proteins, which are frequently toxic to the cell. The presence of a premature translation termination signal (or nonsense codon) strongly destabilizes mRNA via the **nonsense-mediated decay (NMD)** pathway (Fig. 16-1A). In human cells, termination codons are identified as being located in a premature position by reference to the sites of pre-mRNA splicing. Normal termination codons are within, or very close to, the 3' exon, so no former splice sites lie far downstream. If any former splice site is located more than about 50 nucleotides downstream of the site of translation termination, the mRNA is targeted for degradation. The sites of former splicing events can be identified in the spliced mRNA product, because the spliceosome deposits a specific protein complex on the mRNA during the splicing reaction (Fig. 16-1). This is called the **exon-junction complex (EJC),** and it binds to the 5' exon sequence ~24 nucleotides upstream of the splice site. Several of the EJC components remain associated with the mRNA following its export to the cytoplasm. In normal mRNAs, the EJCs will all be displaced by the first translating ribosome, so if one (or more) remains on the mRNA, then translation has terminated too soon.

The identification of premature termination codons in yeast and *Drosophila* does not rely on cues provided by splice sites but probably involves recognition of other nuclear RNA-binding proteins that are retained on the cytoplasmic mRNAs. In all organisms tested, NMD also requires a **surveillance complex,** which bridges interactions between the terminating ribosome and the "place markers" on the mRNAs.

In yeast and probably in humans, recognition of an mRNA as prematurely terminated activates both 5' and 3' degradation. The mRNA can be decapped and 5'-degraded by Xrn1 without prior deadenylation or can be rapidly deadenylated and 3'-degraded by the exosome. In contrast, the degradation of mRNAs targeted by the NMD pathway in *Drosophila* is initiated by an endonuclease cleavage.

Nonstop Decay

Some mRNAs lack any translation termination codon, because they have been inappropriately polyadenylated, inaccurately spliced, or partially 3'-degraded. Translating ribosomes efficiently stall at the ends of such **nonstop mRNAs,** and this inhibits the repeated synthesis of truncated proteins (Fig. 16-1D). The cytoplasmic form of the exosome complex is associated with Ski7p, which is homologous to the GTPases that function in translation. The interaction of Ski7p with the stalled ribosome is believed to both release the ribosome and target the mRNA for rapid degradation.

Nuclear RNA Degradation

Analyses of RNA degradation have focused largely on cytoplasmic mRNA turnover, but most RNA synthesized in a eukaryotic cell is actually degraded within the nucleus. Pre-mRNAs are predominantly composed of intronic sequences, and almost all stable RNAs are synthesized as larger precursors that undergo nuclear maturation. In contrast to the role of poly(A) tails in stabilizing mRNAs in the cytoplasm, there is evidence that poly(A) tails can act as *destabilizing* features during RNA degradation in the nucleus. In yeast, complexes that include nuclear poly(A) polymerases activate the exosome complex during surveillance and degradation of many defective nuclear RNAs, including tRNAs and pre-rRNAs. In Bacteria such as *Escherichia coli,* poly(A) tails are added to RNAs to make them better substrates for degradation. This has led to the proposal that the original function of polyadenylation was in RNA degradation, and this role is maintained in the eukaryotic nucleus. Following the appearance of the nuclear envelope in early eukaryotes, poly(A) tails took on a distinctly different function in promoting mRNA stability and translation in the cytoplasm.

Synthesis of Stable RNAs

Transfer RNA Synthesis

All tRNAs are processed from precursors (pre-tRNAs) that are extended at their 5′ and 3′ ends (Fig. 16-8). Some pre-tRNAs are polycistronic, with two or more tRNAs excised from the same precursor. In yeast, at least, the genes that encode tRNAs cluster around the surface of the nucleolus, and pre-tRNA processing appears to occur largely within the nucleolus.

The 5′ end of the mature tRNA is generated by cleavage by the ribozyme endonuclease RNase P, which recognizes structural elements that are common to all tRNAs. The 3′ ends of all mature tRNAs have the sequence Cp-Cp-A$_{OH}$, to which the aminoacyl group is covalently attached. However, this CCA sequence is not encoded by the tRNA gene in eukaryotes, although it is encoded by tRNA genes in many Bacteria. Instead, the pre-tRNA is initially trimmed, and the CCA sequence is then added by a specific RNA polymerase that belongs to the same family as the poly(A) polymerases that add tails to mRNAs.

Many pre-tRNAs contain a single, short intron, which is removed by splicing. The enzymology of tRNA splicing is quite different from that of pre-mRNA splicing. The pre-tRNA is cleaved at the 5′ and 3′ splice sites by a tetrameric protein complex containing two endonu-

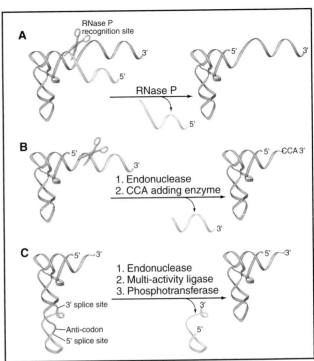

Figure 16-8 Mature tRNAs are generated by processing. **A,** Transcription by RNA polymerase III generates a pre-tRNA that is 5′ and 3′ extended and may also contain an intron. Cleavage by RNase P generates the mature 5′ end. **B,** The 3′ end is cleaved by an unidentified nuclease, and the sequence CCA is added by a specific RNA polymerase. This sequence forms a single stranded 3′ end on all tRNAs. **C,** If an intron is present, it is removed in a splicing reaction that is distinct from pre-mRNA and does not involve small RNA cofactors. The anticodon (*green*) is generally located 1 nucleotide away from the splice site.

cleases and two targeting factors. The cleavages leave products with 5′ hydroxyl residues and 2′-3′ cyclic phosphate. A separate tRNA ligase then recognizes these termini and rejoins the exons.

In addition, tRNAs are subject to a bewildering array of covalent nucleotide modifications. Almost 100 different modified nucleotides have been identified in tRNAs, ranging from simple methylation to the addition of very elaborate molecules. All are added without breaking the phosphate backbone of the RNA. The structures of all mature tRNAs are very similar, since each must fit exactly into the A, P, and E sites of the translating ribosome (see Fig. 17-7). It is likely that the modifications help the tRNAs fold into precisely the correct shape. They also aid accurate recognition of different tRNAs by the aminoacyl-tRNA synthases, which are responsible for charging each species of tRNA with the correct amino acid.

Ribosome Synthesis

The synthesis of ribosomes is a major activity of any actively growing cell. Three of the four rRNAs—the 18S,

5.8S, and 25S/28S rRNAs—are cotranscribed by RNA polymerase I as a polycistronic transcript. This pre-rRNA is the only RNA synthesized by RNA polymerase I (RNA pol I) and is transcribed from arrays of the ribosomal DNA (rDNA) repeated in tandem. In humans, approximately 300 to 400 rDNA repeats are present in five clusters (on chromosomes 13, 14, 15, 21, and 22). These sites often are referred to as *nucleolar organizer regions,* reflecting the fact that nucleoli assemble at these locations in newly formed interphase nuclei. The pre-rRNAs are very actively transcribed and can be visualized as "Christmas trees" in electron micrographs taken following spreading of the chromatin using low-salt conditions and detergent (Fig. 16-9A). The 5S rRNA is independently transcribed by RNA polymerase III. In the majority of eukaryotes, the 5S rRNA genes are present in separate repeat arrays.

The Nucleolus

Most steps in ribosome synthesis take place within a specialized nuclear substructure, the nucleolus (see Fig. 14-3). In micrographs, the nucleolus appears to be a very large and stable structure, but kinetic experiments indicate that it is in fact highly dynamic, with most nucleolar proteins rapidly exchanging with nucleoplasmic pools. There is little evidence that signals for the localization of proteins or mature snoRNAs to the nucleolus are distinct from the features that allow them to function there. A current view of the nucleolus is that its assembly is the consequence of many relatively weak and transient interactions between the nucleolar proteins. The result is a self-assembly process that greatly increases the local concentration of ribosome synthesis factors. This is envisaged to promote efficient preribosome assembly and maturation while allowing the rapid and dynamic changes in preribosome composition involved in this pathway. Similar mechanisms may generate other subnuclear structures such as Cajal bodies.

The key steps in ribosome synthesis are (1) transcription of the pre-rRNA, (2) covalent modification of the mature rRNA regions of the pre-rRNA, (3) processing of the pre-rRNA to the mature rRNAs, and (4) assembly of the rRNAs with the ribosomal proteins (Fig. 16-9D). During ribosome synthesis, the maturing preribosomes move from their site of transcription in the dense fibrillar component of the nucleolus, through the granular component of the nucleolus. They are then released into the nucleoplasm prior to transport through the nuclear pores to the cytoplasm. Here, the final maturation into functional 40S and 60S ribosomal subunits takes place.

Pre-rRNA Processing

The posttranscriptional steps in ribosome synthesis are very complex, involving approximately 200 proteins and approximately 100 snoRNA species, in addition to the four rRNAs and approximately 80 ribosomal proteins. Ribosome synthesis is best understood in budding yeast, but all available evidence indicates that it is highly conserved throughout eukaryotes. Many pre-rRNA processing enzymes have been identified, although others remain to be found (Fig. 16-9E). A combination of endonuclease cleavages and exonuclease digestion steps generates the mature rRNAs in a complex, multistep processing pathway. The remaining species, 5S rRNA, is independently transcribed and undergoes only 3′-trimming. Notably, all of the nucleases indicated in Figure 16-9E process other RNAs in addition to the pre-rRNAs. It seems very probable that when the enzymes responsible for the remaining processing activities are identified, they too will be found to process other substrates.

Modification of the Pre-rRNA

The rRNAs are subject to covalent nucleotide modification at many sites. Modification takes place on the pre-rRNA, either on the nascent transcript or shortly following transcript release. The majority of modifications are methylation of the 2′-hydroxyl group on the sugar ring (**2′-*O*-methylation**) and conversion of uracil to **pseudouridine** by base rotation. The sites of these modifications are selected by base pairing with two groups of **small nucleolar RNAs (snoRNAs).** The **box C/D snoRNAs** direct sites of 2′-*O*-methylation and carry the methyltransferase (called *fibrillarin* in humans and Nop1 in yeast) (Fig. 16-9B). The **box H/ACA snoRNAs** select sites of pseudouridine formation and carry the pseudouridine synthase (called dyskerin in humans and Cbf5 in yeast [Fig. 16-9C]).

A small number of snoRNAs do not direct RNA modification but are required for pre-rRNA processing. The best characterized is the U3 snoRNA, which binds cotranscriptionally to the 5′-external transcription factor (ETS) region of the pre-rRNA. Base pairing between U3 and the pre-rRNA is required for the early processing reactions on the pathway of 18S rRNA synthesis and directs the assembly of a large pre-rRNA processing complex called the small subunit processome. This complex can be visualized as a "terminal knob" in micrographs of spread pre-rRNA transcripts (Fig. 16-9A).

A subset of ribosome synthesis factors interacts with both the rDNA and RNA polymerase I. These interactions might promote both efficient pre-rRNA transcription and recognition of the nascent pre-rRNA. This is reminiscent of the association of mRNA processing factors with RNA polymerase II and suggests that maturation of different classes of RNA and their assembly with specific proteins might be functionally coupled to transcription.

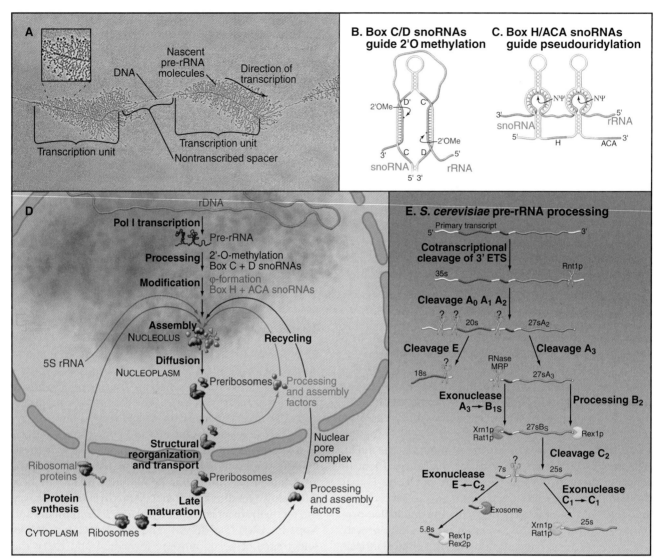

Figure 16-9 RIBOSOME SYNTHESIS. **A, "Christmas trees" of nascent pre-rRNA transcripts.** This electron micrograph shows rDNA genes in the process of transcription. Note the numerous molecules of RNA polymerase I along the rDNA, each associated with a pre-rRNA transcript. In the enlarged *inset,* the terminal balls can be seen on the transcripts. These large pre-rRNA-processing complexes (small subunit processomes) assemble around the binding site for the U3 snoRNA and are required for the early pre-rRNA processing steps. **B–C, Roles of the modification guide snoRNAs.** The pre-rRNAs undergo extensive covalent modification. Most modification involves methylation of the sugar 2′ hydroxyl group (2′-O-methylation) or pseudouridine (Ψ) formation, at sites that are selected by base pairing with a host of small nucleolar ribonucleoprotein (snoRNP) particles. Human cells contain well over 100 different species of snoRNPs, and each pre-rRNA molecule must transiently associate with every snoRNP. Sites of 2′-O-methylation are selected by base pairing with the box C/D class of snoRNAs, which carry the methyltransferase Nop1/fibrillarin. Sites of pseudouridine formation are selected by base pairing with the box H/ACA class of snoRNAs, which carry the pseudouridine synthase Cbf5/dsykerin. **D, Key steps in eukaryotic ribosome synthesis.** Following transcription of the pre-rRNAs, most steps in eukaryotic ribosome synthesis take place within the nucleolus. The preribosomes are then released from association with nucleolus structures and are believed to diffuse to the nuclear pore complex (NPC). Passage through the NPC is preceded by structural rearrangements and the release of processing and assembly factors. Further ribosome synthesis factors are released during late structural rearrangements in the cytoplasm that convert the preribosomal particles to the mature ribosomal subunits. During pre-rRNA transcription and processing, many of the approximately 80 ribosomal proteins assemble onto the mature rRNA regions of the pre-RNA. **E, The pre-rRNA processing pathway.** The pathway is presented for the budding yeast *Saccharomyces cerevisiae,* but extensive conservation is expected throughout eukaryotes. The mature rRNAs are generated by sequential endonuclease cleavage, with some of the mature rRNA termini generated by exonuclease digestion. Scissors with question marks indicate that the endonuclease responsible is unknown.

Small Nuclear RNA Maturation

The U1, U2, U4, and U5 snRNAs are encoded by individual genes transcribed by RNA polymerase II (Fig. 16-10C). Like mRNAs, the snRNA precursors undergo cotranscriptional capping with 7-methylguanosine, but they are not polyadenylated. In human cells, the newly synthesized precursors to these snRNAs are then exported to the cytoplasm. Once in the cytoplasm, the snRNAs form complexes with the **Sm-proteins.** This set of seven different, but closely related, proteins assembles into a heptameric ring structure. Sm-proteins are named after the human autoimmune serum that was initially used in their identification. On their own, the Sm-proteins show low substrate specificity in RNA binding. However, in human cells, the assembly of the snRNAs with the Sm-proteins is highly specific and is mediated by a large protein complex. This complex includes the **SMN** protein **(survival of motor neurons),** which is the target of mutations in the relatively common genetic disease spinal muscular atrophy. While in the cytoplasm the snRNAs are further processed; the 3′ end of the RNA is trimmed, and the cap structure undergoes additional methylation to generate 2,2,7-trimethylguano-

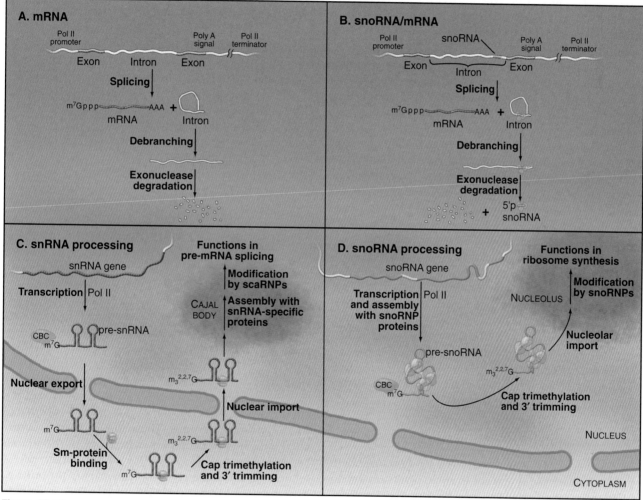

Figure 16-10 DIFFERENT PATTERNS OF STABLE RNA SYNTHESIS BY RNA POLYMERASE II. **A,** Primary transcripts encoding mRNAs generally contain one or more introns, which are removed and degraded to produce the mature mRNA. **B,** In human cells, the snoRNAs that are involved in rRNA modification are generally synthesized by excision from the introns of highly transcribed protein-coding genes. The snoRNP proteins bind to the snoRNA sequence within the pre-mRNA and protect it from degradation. **C,** The spliceosomal U1, U2, U4, and U5 snRNAs are transcribed by RNA polymerase II and, like mRNAs, are capped with 7-methylguanosine and are bound by the nuclear cap-binding complex (CBC). The pre-snRNA is exported to the cytoplasm, where it associates with the Sm-protein complex and is 3′ trimmed. The cap is then hypermethylated to 2,2,7-trimethylguanosine, and the RNA-protein complex is reimported into the nucleus. The newly imported snRNPs localize to the Cajal bodies, where the snRNA is covalently modified at sites selected by base pairing to the small Cajal RNAs (scaRNAs), a class of modification guide RNAs. Assembly with specific proteins then generates the mature snRNPs. **D,** Some snoRNAs, including U3, are individually transcribed by RNA polymerase II. Like the snRNAs, they are initially capped by with 7-methylguanosine and bind CBC. Following association with a set of snoRNA-specific proteins, they undergo cap-trimethylation and 3′ trimming. The snoRNPs then localize to the nucleolus, where they themselves undergo snoRNP-dependent modification and then participate in rRNA processing.

sine. This hypermethylated cap structure is also present on small nucleolar RNAs (see later) and might be important to allow resident nuclear RNAs to be distinguished from mRNA precursors.

Once the cap is trimethylated and bound by the Sm-proteins, the snRNAs can be reimported into the nucleus, where they initially localize to discrete subnuclear structures termed **Cajal bodies** (see Fig. 14-2). Within the Cajal bodies, specific nucleotides in the snRNAs are modified by 2′-O-methylation and pseudouridine formation. The sites of these modifications are selected by base pairing with a group of resident small **Cajal body RNAs (scaRNAs),** which carry the RNA-modifying enzymes. The scaRNAs closely resemble the snoRNAs except that single scaRNAs can frequently direct both 2′-O-methylation and pseudouridine formation.

Maturation of U6 snRNA is quite different from that of the other snRNAs. U6 is transcribed by RNA polymerase III and is not exported to the cytoplasm. Mature U6 retains the 5′ triphosphate and 3′ poly(U) tract that are characteristic of primary transcripts made by RNA pol III (see Chapter 15). However, the 5′ triphosphate is methylated on the γ-phosphate (i.e., the position furthest from the nucleotide), while the terminal U of the poly(U) tract carries a 2′ to 3′ cyclic phosphate. Both of these modifications may help to protect the RNA against degradation. U6 does not bind the Sm-proteins but instead associates with a related heptameric ring structure that is comprised of seven **Lsm-proteins** ("like sm"). Two distinct but related heptameric Lsm-complexes are present in the nucleus and cytoplasm. The nuclear Lsm2-8 complex binds to the U6 snRNA and also participates in the decapping of mRNA precursors that are destined for degradation in the nucleus (Fig. 16-1). In contrast, the Lsm1-7 complex participates in mRNA decapping and 5′ degradation in the cytoplasm. Nucleotides within the U6 snRNA are also modified at positions that are selected by guide RNAs, but this modification occurs in the nucleolus rather than the Cajal body.

Small Nucleolar RNA Maturation

The small nucleolar RNAs (snoRNAs) are all transcribed by RNA polymerase II (except in some plants in which pol III-transcribed snoRNAs can be found). However, the genes encoding snoRNAs can have a surprising variety of different organizations. In human cells, most snoRNAs are excised from the introns of genes that also encode proteins in their exons (Fig. 16-10B). The introns that encode snoRNAs are released by splicing and then linearized by debranching. The mature snoRNA is then generated by controlled exonuclease digestion. In contrast, most characterized snoRNAs in higher plants and several yeast snoRNAs are processed from polycistronic

precursors that encode multiple snoRNA species. Individual pre-snoRNAs are liberated by cleavage of the precursor by the double–strand-specific endonuclease RNase III (Rnt1 in yeast) and then trimmed at both the 5′ and 3′ ends. SnoRNAs can also be processed from single transcripts, and these have many features in common with snRNA transcripts. Like snRNAs, these individually transcribed snoRNAs carry trimethylguanosine cap structures (Fig. 16-10D). However, unlike snRNAs, which have a cytoplasmic phase, the maturation of snoRNAs and assembly of snoRNPs take place entirely within the nucleus, most steps probably occurring in the nucleolus.

Synthesis and Function of miRNAs

The terms **sRNAs** and **miRNAs** are used to describe recently identified groups of RNAs that are physically similar but have distinct functions and a variety of different names. All are around 22 nucleotides in length and associate with a protein complex called the **RNA-induced silencing complex (RISC).** Under different circumstances, sRNAs can lead to cleavage of target RNAs, repress translation of mRNAs, or inhibit transcription of target genes via formation of heterochromatin. It seems likely that miRNAs play major roles in regulating global patterns of gene expression in human cells.

Endogenous **micro-RNAs (miRNAs)** are encoded in the genomes of many eukaryotes, including humans (Fig. 16-11). These are frequently transcribed as polycistronic precursors called pri-miRNAs. Within the pre-miRNA, the precursors to the individual miRNAs (pre-miRNAs) form stem-loop structures. The stems are first cleaved by a nuclear double-strand-specific endonuclease called **Drosha,** releasing the individual pre-miRNAs. These are then exported to the cytoplasm, where cleavage by a second double-strand-specific endonuclease, **Dicer,** releases the miRNA in the form of a duplex with characteristic 2-nucleotide 3′ overhangs and 5′ phosphate groups. These duplexes are incorporated into the RISC complex, where one of the strands becomes the functional miRNA. If the target mRNA sequence is incompletely complementary to the miRNA, its translation is repressed (Fig. 16-11). This is likely to be the normal function of most endogenous miRNAs. It has recently been estimated that 30% or more of human mRNAs are targets of miRNA regulation. miRNAs show tissue-specific patterns of expression and dynamic changes in expression during differentiation. Individual miRNAs can modulate the expression of many different mRNAs.

If a target RNA sequence is found that is perfectly complementary to the miRNA, it is cleaved by a compo-

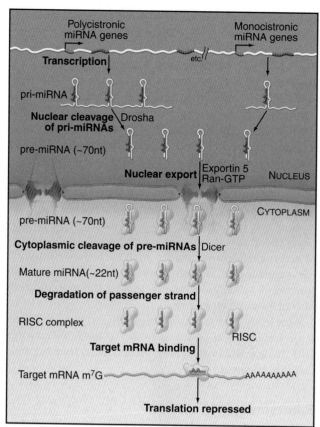

Figure 16-11   mRNA maturation. The polycistronic miRNA precursors (termed primary-miRNAs, or pri-miRNAs) are cleaved by the double-strand-specific endonuclease Drosha within the nucleus. The individual pre-miRNAs are then exported to the cytoplasm by the export factor Exportin 5 in complex with Ran-GTP (see Fig. 14-17). Once in the cytoplasm, the pre-miRNAs are cleaved by the double-strand-specific endonuclease Dicer. One strand of the resulting duplex is then incorporated into the RNA-induced silencing complex (RISC) and becomes the functional miRNA. Imperfect duplexes are formed between the miRNA and target mRNAs; this results in the inhibition of the mRNA translation.

nent of the RISC complex, Ago2 (**"Slicer"**). Target RNA cleavage occurs within the miRNA : mRNA duplex at a fixed distance (between nucleotides 10 and 11) from the 5′ end of the miRNA, which is specifically bound and used to precisely position the duplex relative to the catalytic site.

This pathway can be exploited in techniques for the specific inactivation of target mRNAs, termed **RNA interference (RNAi** [Fig. 16-12]). The technique uses exogenously provided RNAs that are generally fully complementary to the target, typically provided as 22-nucleotide RNAs termed **small interfering RNAs (siRNAs).** In many organisms (e.g., in *Drosophila* or the nematode *Caenorhabditis elegans*), RNAi can be performed by introducing long double-stranded RNAs. These are cleaved in vivo by Dicer into 22-base-pair fragments, which are then incorporated into the RISC

complex. In mammals, including human cells, long double-stranded RNAs cannot be used for RNAi, as they trigger an antiviral response and cell death. RNAi can, however, be performed in human cells by the introduction of precleaved 22-bp RNA fragments. Alternatively, small hairpin structures can be expressed that resemble endogenous pre-miRNAs and are processed into functional 22-nucleotide siRNAs in vivo. The small size, ease of use, and potent function of siRNAs have made RNAi the method of choice for many analyses of eukaryotic gene function.

In the nucleus, a closely related system is used to establish transcriptional silencing of RNA synthesis (Fig.

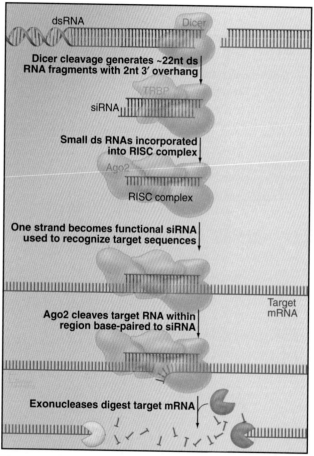

Figure 16-12   siRNA function in mRNA cleavage. In contrast to the endogenous miRNAs, exogenously added siRNAs are generally perfectly complementary to the target RNA, which is then cleaved by the Ago-2 component of the RISC complex. In many organisms (including the nematode worm *C. elegans* and insects such as *Drosophila*), long-double stranded RNAs can be used, which are processed to approximately 22-nucleotide duplexes. In human cells, siRNAs are generally introduced as preformed 22-nucleotide duplexes or as stem-loops with structures that resemble endogenous pre-miRNAs. In either case, the siRNAs associate with Dicer, the double-strand RNA-binding protein TRBP, and Argonaut 2 to form the RISC complex. One strand becomes the functional siRNA, while the "passenger" strand is lost from the complex.

16-13). Although important gaps remain in our understanding, it appears that transcription of a region of the chromosomal DNA on both strands, generating a double-stranded RNA, may be sufficient to induce its silencing. The double-stranded RNA is likely to be cleaved by Dicer and/or Drosha to generate 22-nucleotide fragments, in this case termed **small heterochromatic RNAs (shRNAs)**. These associate with a nuclear complex called **RITS (RNA-induced transcriptional silencing** [see Fig. 16-13]), which is related to the cytoplasmic RISC complex. These shRNAs identify the corresponding gene, possibly by binding to nascent RNA transcripts and, together with the RITS complex components, recruit a protein methyltransferase. This meth-

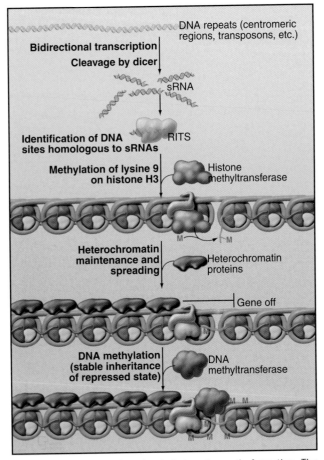

Figure 16-13   shRNA function in heterochromatin formation. The targets of miRNAs and siRNAs are cytoplasmic mRNAs. However, sRNAs can also function in the nucleus. Small double-stranded RNAs in the nucleus can associate with the RNA-induced transcriptional silencing (RITS) complex. The sRNA-RITS complex then identifies the genomic site of transcription, possibly by recognition of the nascent transcripts. This leads to the establishment of heterochromatin at this location, via the recruitment of protein methyltransferases that methylate lysine 9 on histone H3, a hallmark of repressive heterochromatin (see Fig. 13-9). In some organisms, this is followed by methylation of the DNA, which makes the repressed heterochromatic state more stable and heritable.

ylates histone H3 on lysine 9, a hallmark of repressive heterochromatin, which in turn recruits other heterochromatin proteins such as HP1 (see Fig. 13-9). The RITS complex includes an RNA-dependent RNA polymerase, and this may be able to generate new shRNAs, allowing the spreading of the heterochromatin into flanking sequences. The tendency of heterochromatin to spread into the flanking euchromatin has long been recognized and gives rise to the phenomenon of position effect variegation (see Fig. 13-9). In some eukaryotes, the methylated histone H3 can also recruit **DNA methyltransferases** that modify cytosine residues to 5′-methylcytosine. This reinforces heterochromatin formation and makes it heritable by daughter cells. It is likely that this system is important for the establishment of heterochromatin domains, such as those surrounding the centromeres in higher eukaryotes. It might also function as a defense system against the amplification of transposable elements.

The irony is that it now seems likely that the large-scale organization of the genome in many eukaryotes will involve RNAs that long eluded detection because they are so small.

Ribozymes

Some RNAs have catalytic activity in the absence of proteins. Such RNA enzymes are termed **ribozymes.** Only nine classes of ribozymes are known, so cells appear to have far fewer ribozymes than protein enzymes, but ribozymes play some key roles.

Group I and Group II Self-splicing Introns

Two classes of introns can catalyze their own excision from precursor RNAs. These ribozymes are referred to as **group I** and **group II self-splicing introns.** Both classes of RNA fold into complex structures that catalyze splicing via two-step transesterification pathways (Fig. 16-14).

The first group I intron was identified in 1981 as a 413-nucleotide fragment that was able excise itself from the pre-rRNA synthesized in the ciliate *Tetrahymena*. This was a major surprise, since at that time, all known enzymes were proteins. The demonstration that an RNA could function as an enzyme had a major impact on subsequent RNA research. Group I introns are found in the pre-rRNAs of other unicellular eukaryotes, in the mitochondria and chloroplasts of many lower eukaryotes, and in the mitochondria of higher plants.

Group II introns have been found in mitochondria of plants and fungi and in chloroplasts. The splicing mechanism of group II introns strikingly resembles nuclear pre-mRNA splicing (Fig. 16-14C–D). This led to the proposal that the nuclear pre-mRNA splicing

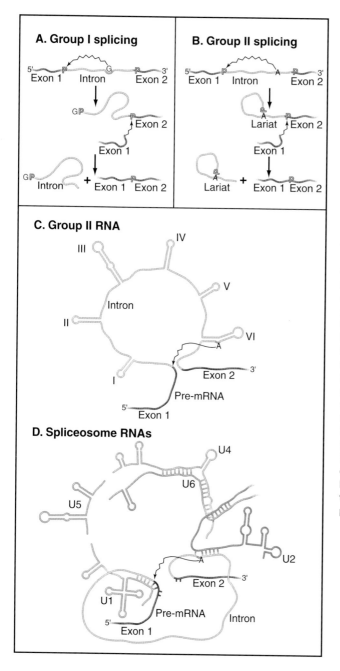

Figure 16-14 Comparison of self-splicing with pre-mRNA splicing. Groups I and II introns are catalytic RNAs or ribozymes that are able to excise themselves from precursor RNAs in the absence of proteins. **A,** The removal of group I introns is mechanistically distinct from nuclear pre-mRNA splicing and commences with the binding of an exogenous guanosine nucleotide (*red* G) within a pocket created by the intronic RNA structure. This G is used to attack and break the phosphate backbone at the 5′ splice site. Subsequently, the free 3′ end of exon 1 attacks the phosphodiester bond at the 3′ splice site, leading to exon ligation and the release of the linear intron. **B,** In contrast, the mechanism of splicing group II introns is very similar to pre-mRNA splicing. An adenine residue (A) near the 3′ end of the intron attacks the 5′ splice site, leading to the formation of a lariat intermediate. The subsequent attack of the free 3′ end of exon 1 on the phosphodiester bond at the 3′ splice site leads to exon ligation and the release of the intron lariat (compare to Fig. 16-4). **C–D,** Parallels can be drawn between structure and mechanism of group II self-splicing introns and pre-mRNA splicing. This suggested the model that group II introns gave rise to the nuclear pre-mRNA splicing system. The snRNAs may be derived from fragments of a group II intron, which developed the ability to function in *trans* (i.e., on other RNAs) rather than acting only in *cis* on its own sequence. Specifically, Domain VI of the group II introns functions like the U2-branch point duplex in activating the branch-point adenosine by bulging it out of a helix. Domain V acts like the U2-U6 duplex in bringing this adenosine to the 5′ splice site. Domain III resembles the U5 snRNA in base pairing to both the 5′ and 3′ exons at the splice sites.

system derived from ancestral group II introns. During early eukaryotic evolution, the catalytic center of the group II intron might have become fragmented and separated into the present spliceosomal snRNAs. This would have converted a system that could work only on its own transcript into a system that could process other RNAs, greatly increasing the potential range of spliced RNAs.

RNase P and RNase MRP

Shortly after the identification of the group I intron in *Tetrahymena*, the RNA component of RNase P was shown also to function as a ribozyme. RNase P is an RNA-protein complex that cleaves pre-tRNAs at the 5′ end of the mature tRNA sequence in all organisms. The bacterial enzyme has one RNA component and one protein, but the RNA can cleave pre-tRNAs in vitro in the absence of the protein. In eukaryotes, RNase P has become more complicated, with one RNA and nine protein components. The eukaryotic RNA has not been shown to be active in the absence of proteins, but it does show structural similarities to the bacterial RNA, and it is assumed to be the catalyst.

Eukaryotes also contain a second RNA-protein enzyme, called RNase MRP, which is closely related to

RNase P. The RNA components share common structural features, and the complexes share eight common proteins. RNase MRP cleaves the preribosomal RNA between the small and large subunit rRNAs (Fig. 16-9E). Notably, in many Bacteria, RNase P can cleave the pre-rRNA at a similar position because of the presence of a tRNA within the pre-rRNA transcript. This suggests that RNase MRP arose in an early eukaryote as a specialized form of RNase P, with a specific function in pre-rRNA processing. By analogy to RNase P, cleavage by RNase MRP is predicted to be RNA catalyzed. RNase MRP also functions in mRNA turnover, at least in yeast, initiating the cell-cycle-regulated degradation of a small number of mRNAs.

Large Subunit rRNA

The most important ribozyme is the rRNA component of the large ribosomal subunit, which does not participate in RNA processing but catalyzes peptide bond formation (see Fig. 17-10). During translation elongation, the peptidyl-transferase reaction (the reaction by which amino acid residues are attached to each other to form proteins) is catalyzed by the rRNA itself. The peptidyl-transfer reaction is energetically favorable, and it is currently believed that the catalytic activity derives primarily from the precise spatial positioning of the A-site and P-site tRNAs by the rRNA. The ribosomal proteins act as chaperones in ribosome assembly and as cofactors to increase the efficiency and accuracy of translation.

Conclusions

Eukaryotic cells have a bewildering array of RNA species that perform many different, key functions in gene expression. The mature forms of all of these RNAs are generated by RNA processing reactions, so the RNA processing machinery is of considerable importance. Probably for this reason, RNA-processing enzymes and cofactors are generally highly conserved during eukaryotic evolution. For many RNA species, transcription and maturation are closely coupled and can be thought of as an integrated system.

Finally, it is notable that many new species of RNA are being discovered as this book goes to press, so there is every reason to think that additional classes of RNA remain to be identified.

ACKNOWLEDGMENT

Thanks go to Jim Manley for his suggestions on revisions to this chapter.

SELECTED READINGS

Almeida R, Allshire RC: RNA silencing and genome regulation. Trends Cell Biol 15:251–258, 2005.

Fromont-Racine M, Senger B, Saveanu C, Fasiolo F: Ribosome assembly in eukaryotes. Gene 313:17–24, 2003.

Kiss T: Small nucleolar RNAs: An abundant group of noncoding RNAs with diverse cellular functions. Cell 109:145–148, 2002.

Parker R, Song H: The enzymes and control of eukaryotic mRNA turnover. Nat Struct Mol Biol 11:121–127, 2004.

Rodriguez MS, Dargemont C, Stutz F: Nuclear export of RNA. Biol Cell 96:639–655, 2004.

Sanford JR, Caceres JF: Pre-mRNA splicing: Life at the centre of the central dogma. J Cell Sci 117:6261–6263, 2004.

Wilusz CJ, Wilusz J: Bringing the role of mRNA decay in the control of gene expression into focus. Trends Genet 20:491–497, 2004.

Protein Synthesis and Folding

The nuclear genome contains information specifying many thousands of proteins. Whatever their final destination—nucleus, cytoplasm, membrane-bound organelles, or extracellular space—these proteins are synthesized in the cytoplasm. The few proteins encoded by genes in mitochondria and chloroplasts are synthesized in those organelles. The biochemical synthesis of proteins is called **translation,** as the process translates sequences of nucleotides in a **messenger RNA (mRNA)** into the sequence of amino acids in a polypeptide chain. Translation of mRNA requires the concerted actions of small **transfer RNAs (tRNAs)** linked to amino acids, **ribosomes** (complexes of RNA and protein), and many soluble proteins. GTP binding and hydrolysis regulate several proteins that orchestrate the interactions of these components. Ultimately, RNA bases in the ribosome catalyze the formation of peptide bonds. Some newly synthesized polypeptides fold spontaneously into their native structure in the cellular environment, but many require assistance from proteins called **chaperones.** It has been proposed that the bulk of the evolution of the translation apparatus occurred after the basic mechanisms were established, to provide greater precision. This perspective seems to explain the extraordinary complexity of the process.

Protein Synthetic Machinery

Messenger RNA

mRNAs have three parts: Nucleotides at the 5′ end provide binding sites for proteins that initiate polypeptide synthesis; nucleotides in the middle specify the sequence of amino acids in the polypeptide; and nucleotides at the 3′ end regulate the stability of the mRNA (see Figs. 15-1 and 16-1). Within the protein-coding region, successive triplets of three nucleotides, called **codons,** specify the sequence of amino acids. The **genetic code** relating nucleotide triplets to amino acids is, with a few minor exceptions, universal. One to six different triplet codons encode each amino acid (Fig. 17-1). An **initiation codon** (AUG) specifies methionine, which begins all polypeptide chains.

This chapter was revised using material from the first edition written by William E. Balch, Ann L. Hubbard, J. David Castle, and Pat Shipman.

		Second Position				
		U	**C**	**A**	**G**	
First Position (5′ end)	**U**	UUU ⎫ Phe UUC ⎭ UUA ⎫ Leu UUG ⎭	UCU ⎫ UCC ⎬ Ser UCA ⎪ UCG ⎭	UAU ⎫ Tyr UAC ⎭ ● UAA ⎫ Stop ● UAG ⎭	UGU ⎫ Cys UGC ⎭ ● UGA Stop UGG Trp	U C A G
	C	CUU ⎫ CUC ⎬ Leu CUA ⎪ CUG ⎭	CCU ⎫ CCC ⎬ Pro CCA ⎪ CCG ⎭	CAU ⎫ His CAC ⎭ CAA ⎫ Gln CAG ⎭	CGU ⎫ CGC ⎬ Arg CGA ⎪ CGG ⎭	U C A G
	A	AUU ⎫ AUC ⎬ Ile AUA ⎭ ● AUG Met	ACU ⎫ ACC ⎬ Thr ACA ⎪ ACG ⎭	AAU ⎫ Asn AAC ⎭ AAA ⎫ Lys AAG ⎭	AGU ⎫ Ser AGC ⎭ AGA ⎫ Arg AGG ⎭	U C A G
	G	GUU ⎫ GUC ⎬ Val GUA ⎪ GUG ⎭	GCU ⎫ GCC ⎬ Ala GCA ⎪ GCG ⎭	GAU ⎫ Asp GAC ⎭ GAA ⎫ Glu GAG ⎭	GGU ⎫ GGC ⎬ Gly GGA ⎪ GGG ⎭	U C A G

● = Chain-terminating codon
● = Initiation codon

Figure 17-1   THE GENETIC CODE. The location of the nucleotide in first, second, and third position defines the amino acid encrypted by the code.

(Right margin label: Third Position (3′ end))

In addition, any one of three **termination codons** (UAA, UGA, UAG) stops peptide synthesis.

Eukaryotic and bacterial mRNAs differ in three ways. First, eukaryotic mRNAs encode one protein, and bacterial mRNAs generally encode more than one protein. Second, most eukaryotic (and eukaryotic viral) mRNAs are capped by an inverted 7-methylguanosine residue joined onto the 5′ end of the mRNA by a 5′-triphosphate-5′ linkage (Fig. 17-2). This **5′ cap** is stable throughout the life of the mRNA and protects the 5′ end against attack by nucleases. Third, most eukaryotic mRNAs have a tail of 50 to 200 adenine residues added post-transcriptionally to the 3′ end (see Fig. 16-3). The

poly(A) tail may protect the mRNA from degradation in the cytoplasm and increase reinitiation of transcription. Bacterial mRNAs lack 5′ caps or 3′ poly(A) tails. Most eukaryotic mRNAs require processing to remove introns (see Fig. 16-4). Many single-stranded mRNAs have some secondary structure (see Fig. 3-19) stabilized by hydrogen bonding of complementary bases. This secondary structure must be disrupted during translation to allow reading of each codon.

Transfer RNA

tRNAs are adapters that deliver amino acids to the translation machinery by matching mRNA codons with their corresponding amino acids as they are incorporated into a growing polypeptide (Fig. 17-3). One to four different tRNAs are specific for each amino acid, generally reflecting their abundance in proteins. Specialized tRNAs carrying methionine (formylmethionine in Bacteria) initiate protein synthesis. Transfer RNAs consist of about 76 nucleotides that base-pair to form four stems and three intervening loops. These elements of secondary structure fold to form an L-shaped molecule stabilized by base pairing. A "decoding" triplet (the **anticodon**) is at one end of the L (the anticodon arm), and the amino acid acceptor site is at the other end of the L (the acceptor arm).

Enzymes called **aminoacyl-tRNA (aa-tRNA) synthetases** catalyze a two-step reaction that couples an amino acid covalently to its cognate tRNA but not to any other tRNA (Fig. 17-4). In the first step, adenosine tri-

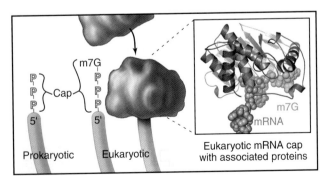

Figure 17-2   mRNA cap structures. Prokaryotic mRNAs end with a 5′ triphosphate. The 5′ cap of eukaryotic mRNAs consists of a 7-methylguanosine residue (m7G) linked to the mRNA by three phosphates. The protein eIF4E binds the cap and protects against degradation by nucleases. (PDB file: 1EJ1.)

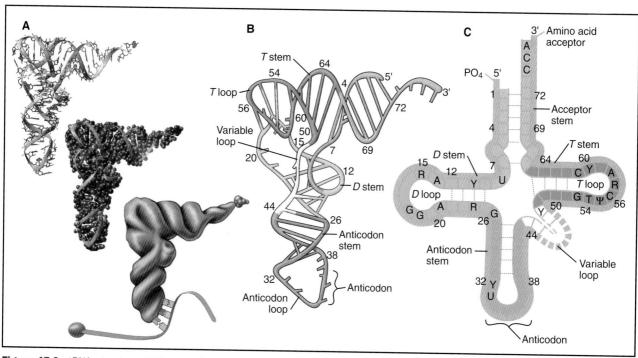

Figure 17-3 tRNA structure. tRNAs match an amino acid attached at the 3′ end with the mRNA triplet coding for that amino acid. **A,** Ribbon model, space-filling model, and textbook icon showing base pairing of the anticodon to an mRNA codon. **B,** Backbone model. **C,** Planar model showing stem loops of a generic tRNA. Single-letter code for the bases: adenine (A), any purine (R), any pyrimidine (Y), cytosine (C), guanine (G), pseudouridine (Ψ), thymine (T), and uracil (U). (PDB file: 6TNA.)

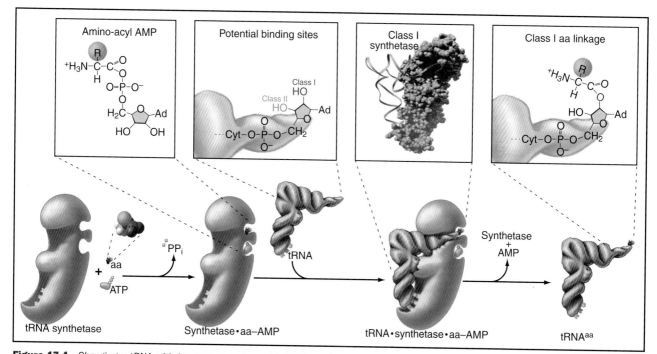

Figure 17-4 Charging a tRNA with its correct amino acid. tRNA synthetases (shown schematically and as a space-filling atomic model in *purple*) provide a docking platform for a specific amino acid and its cognate tRNA (shown in *orange* as a schematic model and as a ribbon model bound to a synthetase). The amino acid is first activated by reaction with ATP. The carboxyl group of the amino acid is coupled to the α-phosphate of AMP with the release of pyrophosphate. The synthetase then transfers the amino acid from the aminoacyl AMP (aa-AMP) to a high-energy ester bond *(red disk)* with either the 2′ (illustrated here) or 3′ hydroxyl of the adenine at the 3′ end of the tRNA. (PDB file: 1QTQ.)

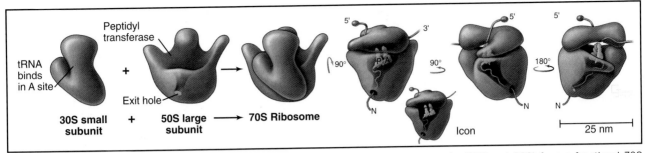

Figure 17-5 MODEL OF THE BACTERIAL RIBOSOME ILLUSTRATING OVERALL ORGANIZATION. Two subunits (30S and 50S) form a functional 70S ribosome. An mRNA threads between the subunits in association with the small subunit. tRNAs bind to two sites, designated the A site and P site, between the large and small subunits. Codons of the mRNA in the A and P sites on the small subunit specify which aa-tRNAs occupy these sites. The amino acids at the far end of the bound tRNAs are positioned for peptide bond formation by the peptidyl transferase site on the large subunit. The growing polypeptide chain (shown in *blue*) emerges from a tunnel in the large subunit.

phosphate (ATP) and the amino acid react to form a high-energy aminoacyl adenosine monophosphate (AMP) intermediate with release of pyrophosphate. The second step transfers the amino acid to the 3′ adenine of tRNA, forming an aa-tRNA. This reaction is appropriately called *charging,* since the high-energy bond between the amino acid and the tRNA activates the amino acid in preparation for forming a peptide bond with an amino group in the growing polypeptide chain. Each of the 20 aa-tRNA synthetases couples a particular amino acid to all of its corresponding tRNAs.

The fidelity of protein synthesis depends on near-perfect coupling of amino acids to the appropriate tRNAs. Synthetases make this selection by interacting with as many as three areas of their cognate tRNAs: anticodon, 3′ acceptor stem, and the surface between these sites (Fig. 17-4). To distinguish between appropriate and inappropriate amino acids, synthetases use proofreading steps, which remove incorrectly paired amino acids from tRNAs.

Ribosomes

Ribosomes are giant macromolecular machines that bring together an mRNA and aa-tRNAs to synthesize a polypeptide. Base pairing between mRNA codons and tRNA anticodons directs the synthesis of a polypeptide in the order specified by the mRNA codons. Ribosomes consist of a **small subunit** and a **large subunit** that bind together during translation of an mRNA (Fig. 17-5). Each subunit consists of one or more **ribosomal RNA (rRNA)** molecules and many distinct proteins (Fig. 17-6). The sizes of these subunits and rRNAs are traditionally given in units of S, the sedimentation coefficient measured in an ultracentrifuge.

Ribosomal RNAs constitute the structural core of each ribosomal subunit (Fig. 17-7). The 16S rRNA of the small subunit consists of 1500 bases, most of which are folded into base-paired helices. The large subunit contains two RNAs: 23S rRNA consisting of 2900 bases and

5S rRNA of 121 bases. The rRNAs fold into many based-paired helices, as predicted by phylogenetic analysis of sequences (Fig. 17-6). These helices and their intervening loops pack into a compact structure, as is seen in both surface views and cross sections. Although eukaryotic rRNAs differ in size and sequence from prokaryote rRNAs, their predicted secondary structures are similar, and they are expected to fold in similar ways. Many features of rRNAs have been conserved during evolution, including the surfaces where subunits and elements of RNA structure interact; sites that are required for binding tRNA, mRNA, and protein cofactors; and the residues involved with peptide bond formation.

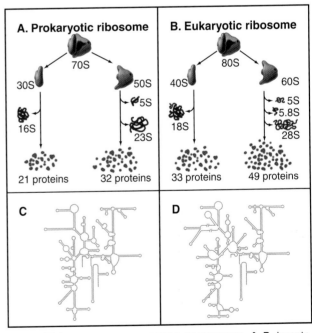

Figure 17-6 MOLECULAR COMPONENTS OF RIBOSOMES. A–B, Inventories of rRNAs *(middle)* and proteins *(bottom).* Prokaryotic and eukaryotic rRNAs and ribosomal proteins differ in size and number but are related by evolution and form similar structures. **C–D,** Secondary structures of prokaryotic 16S rRNA and 18S eukaryotic rRNA illustrate their similarities despite divergent sequences.

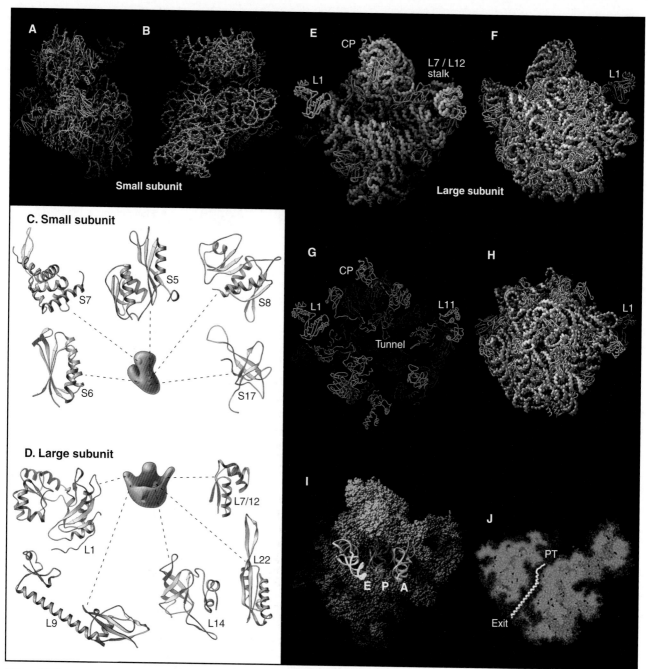

Figure 17-7   CRYSTAL STRUCTURES OF THE RIBOSOME SMALL AND LARGE SUBUNITS. RNA is shown in *gray,* and proteins are *gold,* except in panel G, which features various colors. **A–B,** Two views of the model of the small subunit of *Thermus thermophilus.* **C–D,** Representative structures of individual ribosomal proteins and their locations on the small and large subunits. (PDB file: 1FJF.) **E–J,** Structure of the large subunit of the ribosome of *Haloarcula marismortui.* **E,** Crown view from the perspective of the small subunit. **F,** View in panel C rotated 180 degrees around a vertical axis. **G,** Crown view of the proteins minus RNA. **H,** View in panel E rotated 180 degrees around a horizontal axis to show the exit from the nascent polypeptide tunnel, the dark patch in the middle. **I,** Crown view with models of tRNA in the A, P, and E sites. **J,** Cross section showing the tunnel for the nascent polypeptide extending from the peptidyl transferase (PT) site to the exit. (A–B, From Wimberly BT, Brodersen DE, Clemons WM, et al: Structure of the 30S ribosomal subunit. Nature 407:327–339, 2000. E–J, Courtesy of T. Steitz, Yale University, New Haven, Connecticut; adapted from the work of Ban N, Nissen P, Hansen J, et al: The complete atomic structure of the large ribosomal subunit at 2.4 Å resolution. Science 289:905–920, 2000; and Nissen P, Hansen J, Ban N, et al: The structural basis of ribosome activity in peptide bond synthesis. Science 289:920–930, 2000. A–C, PDB file: 1FJF. D–J, PDB file: 1FFK.)

Most ribosomal proteins associate with the surface of the rRNA core, although several extend peptide strands into the core (Fig. 17-7). Ribosomal proteins are generally small (10 to 30 kD) and basic, but each has a unique structure. With one exception, ribosomes have just one copy of each protein.

Decoding of the mRNA and synthesis of the polypeptide take place in the cavity between the subunits. The surfaces of this cavity are generally free of proteins, so rRNAs—not proteins—are largely responsible for mRNA binding, tRNA binding, and peptide bond formation. tRNAs move sequentially through three sites shared by the two subunits: the **A site** (aa-tRNA), the **P site** (for peptidyl-tRNA), and the **E site** (for exit). The growing polypeptide chain exits through a tunnel in the RNA core of the large subunit.

Soluble Protein Factors

Many soluble proteins cycle on and off ribosomes during protein synthesis, enhancing the rate or fidelity of the reactions. The following sections highlight the role(s) of these soluble factors.

Outline of Protein Synthesis

Organisms in all three domains of life use many homologous components and similar reactions for protein synthesis, but many of the details differ as is expected after 3 billion years of evolutionary divergence. In all three domains, protein synthesis takes place in four steps: initiation, elongation, termination, and subunit recycling (Fig. 17-8). Guanosine triphosphatase (GTPase) proteins regulate the progress and fidelity of many of the steps (see Fig. 4-6 for details on GTPase cycles). Initiation, elongation, and termination all depend on directed movement of molecular machinery along an mRNA and precise recognition between amino acids, tRNAs, adapter proteins, and the gene sequence encoded in the mRNA.

During **initiation,** a complex composed of a small ribosomal subunit and an initiator tRNA (carrying methionine) binds the initiation codon (AUG) of an mRNA. This ternary complex then associates with a large subunit to form a 70S ribosome in Bacteria and an 80S ribosome in eukaryotes. Eukaryotes use many more components than prokaryotes to regulate initiation.

During **elongation,** tRNAs bring amino acids to the ribosome in the order specified by the sequence of codons in the mRNA. The ribosome catalyzes formation of a peptide bond between the amino group of each new amino acid and the carboxyl group at the C-terminus of the growing polypeptide chain and then moves on to the next codon. The mechanism of elongation is conserved across the phylogenetic tree. More

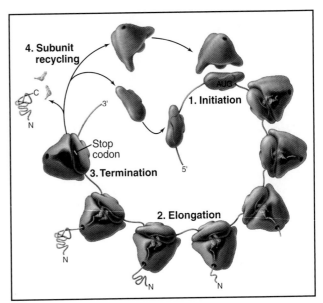

Figure 17-8 Overview of the translation cycle showing six ribosomes on a single mRNA. *1,* Initiation. Initiator tRNA^{Met}, mRNA, and accessory soluble factors assemble on the small subunit, which then joins with a large subunit. *2,* Elongation. The polypeptide chain is synthesized, in the order specified by the mRNA, in sequential steps by recruitment of new aa-tRNAs that match the mRNA-coding sequence, formation of peptide bonds, and dissociation of free tRNA. *3,* Termination. Release factors recognize the stop codon *(yellow)* and terminate translation. The ribosome releases the polypeptide for folding in the cytoplasm. *4,* Subunit recycling. The ribosomal subunits dissociate and are available for another round of translation.

than one ribosome is active on most mRNAs, as coding sequences are usually much longer than the 40 to 50 nucleotides associated with a single ribosome. Once a ribosome proceeds about 60 nucleotides beyond the initiation codon, another ribosome-tRNA complex can assemble on the mRNA and start translation. Messenger RNAs with multiple ribosomes are called **polysomes.** This multiple occupancy of mRNAs explains why ribosomes are more abundant than mRNAs and how one mRNA molecule guides the synthesis of several copies of its protein product simultaneously.

Termination occurs when the ribosome encounters a termination codon (UAA, UAG, or UGA) at the 3′ end of the coding sequence. At this point, a protein factor (not an aa-tRNA) binds to the mRNA, and the C-terminal amino acid of the polypeptide chain is hydrolyzed from its tRNA. After the polypeptide is released from the ribosome, the ribosomal subunits dissociate and are available for **recycling** to initiate translation of another mRNA.

Initiation Phase

The goal of initiation is to bring together the initiator tRNA carrying methionine (or *N*-formylmethionine, fMet, in Bacteria) and the AUG initiator codon of the mRNA on the ribosome (Fig. 17-9). In eukaryotes, more

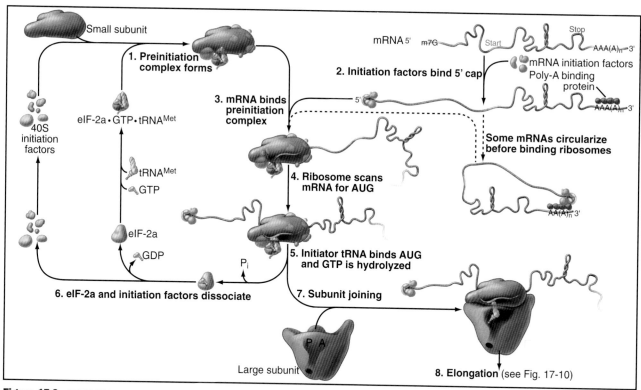

Figure 17-9 STEPS IN INITIATION IN EUKARYOTES. *1*, Initiation factors *(green)* assemble with mRNA, eIF-2a *(purple, activated with GTP),* and tRNA^Met on a small ribosomal subunit to form the preinitiation complex. *2*, Other initiation factors *(blue)* bind the 5′ cap of the mRNA. For some mRNAs, these 5′ cap-binding factors interact with poly(A)-binding proteins at the 3′ end of the mRNA. This circularization promotes initiation of some mRNAs and inhibits initiation of other mRNAs. *3*, The preinitiation complex binds an mRNA. *4*, The small subunit scans the mRNA for the AUG start codon *(green).* *5*, When the initiator tRNA binds the start codon, eIF-2a hydrolyzes its bound GTP. *6*, Phosphate, GDP, eIF-2a, and other initiation factors dissociate and recycle for further rounds of initiation. *7*, The small subunit binds a large subunit. *8*, Elongation begins.

than 10 soluble protein factors (eukaryotic **initiation factors,** or eIF) coordinate the interactions of the RNA molecules. Fewer protein factors (designated IF) participate in prokaryotes. In eukaryotes, several steps occur in succession:

Step 1. Initiator Met-tRNA and the GTPase eIF-2a (with bound guanosine triphosphate [GTP]) form a **preinitiation complex** on a small ribosomal subunit.

Step 2. Several protein initiation factors assemble on the 5′ cap of the mRNA. The RNA **helicase** eIF4A in this complex uses ATP hydrolysis to remove any secondary structure or bound proteins at the 5′ end of the mRNA. These cap recognition factors also interact with poly(A)-binding proteins on the other end of the mRNA, forming a circular complex that can either favor or inhibit initiation.

Step 3. The **cap recognition complex** targets the mRNA to a preinitiation complex. The order of these first three steps is still being investigated. mRNA may also bind to the small subunit before the initiation factors and Met-tRNA.

Step 4. The ribosome scans along the mRNA for the initiator AUG codon. This movement depends on ATP hydrolysis, but its role is not clear. Eukaryotic mRNAs tend to begin translation at the first AUG codon encountered, but the local sequence of the mRNA may also contribute to the specificity as in Bacteria.

Step 5. When Met-tRNA base-pairs with the initiator AUG codon, eIF-2a hydrolyzes its bound GTP.

Step 6. eIF-2a and the other initiation factors dissociate from the small subunit for recycling back to other preinitiation complexes and 5′ caps.

Step 7. A large ribosomal subunit binds the small subunit complexed with both the mRNA and Met-tRNA. Another GTPase called eIF5B hydrolyzes its bound GTP before elongation of the polypeptide begins.

Initiation is the most highly regulated step in protein synthesis, frequently involving phosphorylation of initiation factors. For example, phosphorylation increases the affinity of eIF-2a for its guanine nucleotide-exchange factor (eIF-2b). Strongly bound eIF-2b inhibits initiation by competing with initiator tRNA for binding eIF-2a. Cells that are subjected to various stresses utilize phosphorylation of eIF-2a to inhibit translation. In contrast, phosphorylation of eIF-4F favors translation by enhancing the interaction of this initiation factor with the 5′ cap of mRNAs. This modulation of affinity can even influence the selective translation of particular mRNAs, since the 5′ caps of mRNAs vary in affinity for eIF-4F.

Elongation Phase

Accurate protein synthesis depends on the fidelity of amino acid coupling to the correct tRNA and of codon-anticodon pairing between mRNA and tRNA. Both reactions occur in two steps by a mechanism that increases accuracy. Much of the energy invested in protein synthesis is used to achieve this accuracy, and elongation is the most expensive phase of translation in terms of energy expenditure.

Repetitive cycles of codon-directed incorporation of amino acids into the polypeptide chain begin once the two ribosomal subunits are joined with an initiator tRNA and mRNA properly in place (Fig. 17-10). Each cycle of elongation consists of four steps: (1) binding of an aa-tRNA to the A site on the ribosome; (2) proofreading to ensure that it is the correct aa-tRNA; (3) peptide bond formation; and (4) translocation, which advances the mRNA by one codon and moves the peptidyl-tRNA from the A site to the P site on the ribosome.

Elongation reactions occur in a cavity between the two ribosomal subunits. mRNA is threaded, codon by codon, between the subunits. aa-tRNAs enter on one side of the cavity and bind successively to three sites between the two ribosomal subunits. Having half of each site on each of the two subunits allows ribosomes to maintain contact with one end of the tRNA as it moves, step by step, from the A site to the P site to the E site prior to dissociation. Codon-anticodon recognition takes place at both the A and P sites on the small subunit, where the anticodons of the two tRNAs base-pair with mRNA. Peptide bonds form at the other end of the tRNAs, which position the amino acid and peptidyl chain on the A and P sites of the large subunit. **Elongation factors** (EF; eEF for eukaryotic elongation factors) and movements of the subunits relative to each other facilitate the movements of the tRNAs along the sequence of three sites. The growing polypeptide exits through a 10-nm-long tunnel in the large subunit.

Step 1. aa-tRNA binding. The GTPase eEF1A (EF-Tu in Bacteria; see Fig. 25-7) with bound GTP delivers aa-tRNAs to ribosomes with empty A sites. The nucleotide-exchange factor eEF-X (EF-Ts in Bacteria) prepares eEF1A to bind aa-tRNA by promoting the exchange of GDP for GTP. Cells contain enough

eEF1A-GTP to bind all of the aa-tRNA and protect the labile ester bond of the aa-tRNA.

Step 2. Proofreading. A proofreading mechanism in the A site checks each aa-tRNA to ensure that its anticodon matches the mRNA codon in the decoding site of the small subunit. Correct aa-tRNAs are retained; incorrect aa-tRNAs dissociate. A "kinetic proofreading mechanism" discriminates between correct and incorrect aa-tRNAs using two first-order reactions. First, eEF1A associated with the aa-tRNA hydrolyzes its bound GTP. Then GDP-eEF1A dissociates from the aminoacyl end of the aa-tRNA and the ribosome, allowing the aminoacyl end of the aa-tRNA to move into the peptidyl transfer site on the large subunit. Each reaction takes a few milliseconds. Correct base pairing between the aa-tRNA anticodon and the mRNA codon promotes GTP hydrolysis by eEF1A, so GDP-eEF1A can dissociate and allow the aa-tRNA to form a peptide bond. Those aa-rRNAs with weak, imperfect codon-anticodon pairs dissociate from the A site before eEF1A can hydrolyze GTP and dissociate from the aminoacyl end of the tRNA.

Step 3. Peptidyl transfer. The RNA of the large subunit forms the highly conserved active site that catalyzes the formation of peptide bonds (Fig. 17-10). This reaction eliminates water and transfers the carboxyl group esterified to the peptidyl-tRNA in the P site to the free amino group of the aa-tRNA in the A site. Catalysis of peptide bond formation depends on a combination of precise orientation of the substrates and stabilization of the transition state (just like protein enzymes). The chemistry is similar, but in reverse, to the hydrolysis of peptide bonds by proteolytic enzymes such as chymotrypsin. After formation of the new peptide bond, the tRNA in the A site has the polypeptide on one end and its anticodon arm still base-paired to its mRNA codon on the small subunit. The antibacterial agent **puromycin** can disrupt elongation by mimicking a tRNA^Phe or tRNA^Tyr (Fig. 17-11). Puromycin attacks the esterified carboxyl group of a peptidyl-tRNA in the P site, but lacking an appropriate acceptor site for further peptidyl transfer reactions, it terminates elongation, resulting in premature release of the polypeptide chain from the ribosome.

Step 4. Translocation. Three linked reactions, promoted by elongation factor eEF2 (and the homologous protein EF-G in Bacteria), complete each elongation cycle. eEF2 is a GTPase with domains similar to domains 1 and 2 of EF-Tu (see Fig. 25-7) plus three domains that mimic the size and shape of a tRNA. Domain 1 binds and hydrolyzes GTP. Domains 3 to 5 target GTP-eEF2 to an empty A site on the ribosome. Binding of GTP-eEF2 to an empty

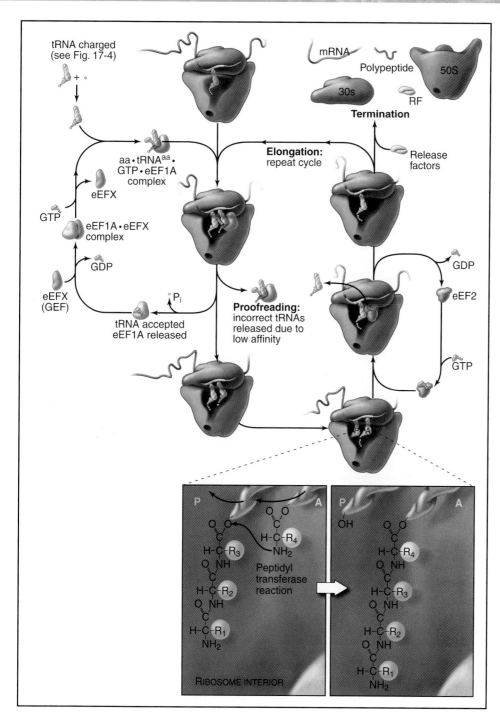

Figure 17-10 STEPS IN ELONGA-TION AND TERMINATION IN EUKARY-OTES. Starting in the *upper left*, elongation factor eEF1A (EF-Tu in Bacteria) forms a ternary complex with GTP and an amino acyl-tRNA^{aa} for delivery of the tRNA^{aa}, matching the mRNA codon in the A site to the ribosome. This ternary complex dissociates rapidly if the anticodon-codon match is incorrect. If the antico-don-codon match is correct, the ternary complex remains bound to the A site long enough for eEF1A to hydrolyze its bound GTP and dissociate from the tRNA still bound to the A site. The ribosome catalyzes formation of a new peptide bond *(inset)*. eEF2 (EF-G in Bacteria) binds the A site tran-siently after peptide bond forma-tion to facilitate movement of the tRNAs and mRNA through the ribosome. Release factors (RF, *green*) recognize the stop codon and terminate the polypeptide chain *(blue)*, allowing the mRNA and ribosomal subunits to disso-ciate. The guanine nucleotide-exchange factor eEFX promotes the exchange of GDP for GTP on eEF-1A.

A site promotes the movement of peptidyl-tRNA from the A site to the P site on the small subunit together with sliding of the mRNA three bases forward on the small subunit. At the same time, the deacylated tRNA in the P site is moved to the exit (E) site, where it dissociates from the ribo-some. Hydrolysis of the bound GTP releases eEF2 from the A site, initiating another round of elongation.

The growing peptide threads through a 10-nm-long tunnel in the large subunit lined with RNA (Figs. 17-5, 17-7, and 17-8). The tunnel accommodates an extended polypeptide about 40 residues long. The distal parts of the tunnel are wide enough to pass an α-helix. The N-ter-minus of longer peptides exits from the large subunit.

Cells balance speed and accuracy during translation to achieve an error rate of about 1 in 10^4 incorrect amino acids. As a result of this compromise, ribosomes

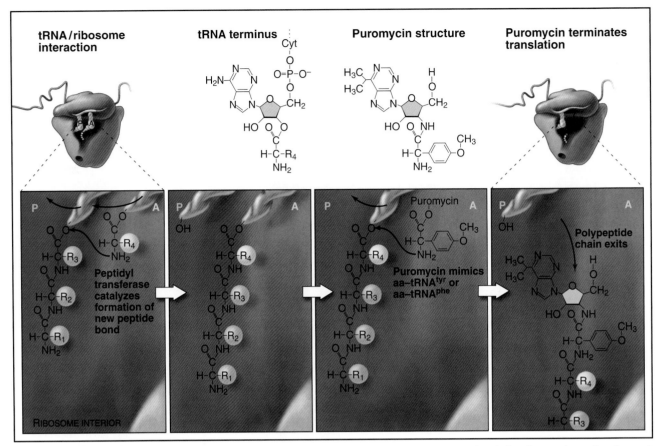

Figure 17-11   MECHANISM OF THE PUROMYCIN REACTION SHOWN IN FOUR STEPS. The antibiotic puromycin mimics the terminus of amino acyl-tRNA^{Tyr} or tRNA^{Phe}. It is incorporated on the C-terminus of the polypeptide and terminates translation prematurely, as it is not attached to a tRNA and lacks an activated carboxyl group.

add about 20 amino acids per second to a polypeptide at 37°C, so synthesis of a protein of average size (300 amino acids) takes only 15 seconds. Greater precision might be achieved by slowing translation, but slower cellular growth might be an evolutionary disadvantage.

Termination Phase

The assembly of a protein stops when a termination codon (UAA, UAG, or UGA) moves into the A site on the small subunit of the ribosome (Fig. 17-10). A release factor called eRF1 (RF1 or RF2 in Bacteria) recognizes stop codons, binds to the A site, and induces the ribosome active site to hydrolyze the peptidyl-tRNA ester in the P site. The completed polypeptide chain threads through the ribosome and is released. The large subunit dissociates from the mRNA and the small subunit, leaving both subunits ready to initiate another round of synthesis. Protein factors might contribute to these recycling reactions, but the details are still being investigated.

Spontaneous Protein Folding

Termination is the final step in translation but just the beginning for a new protein. A polypeptide begins to experience its new environment while still being synthesized. When it is about 40 residues long, its N-terminus emerges from the protected tunnel of the large ribosomal subunit into cytoplasm, where it must fold into a three-dimensional structure (see Fig. 3-5) and find its correct cellular destination.

The structure of folded proteins and the folding mechanism are both encoded in the amino acid sequence, making folding spontaneous under suitable conditions. For the soluble proteins, these conditions are aqueous solvent at physiological temperature, neutral pH, and moderate ionic strength. Folding of transmembrane proteins in a lipid bilayer is quite different (see Chapter 20). In test tube experiments, small soluble proteins can be denatured with high temperature, extremes of pH, or high concentrations of urea or guanidine. Denatured proteins exist as ensembles of unfolded polymers with little residual secondary structure.

When denatured polypeptides of modest length are transferred to physiological conditions, many fold spontaneously into their native three-dimensional structures on a microsecond to millisecond time scale. (Proteins that require isomerization of prolines, such as collagen, fold much more slowly; see Fig. 29-4.) Starting from many initial denatured states, the polypeptides converge toward a single low-energy native state (Fig. 17-12). The number of possible pathways to the native state is so numerous that if they were sampled individually, proteins would never fold. Thus, both theory and experiment indicate that folding involves a subset of the potential pathways, including an ensemble of loosely folded transition states with elements of secondary structure, certain turns, and hydrophobic contacts found in the core of the native protein.

Many proteins also fold spontaneously on their own during biosynthesis in vivo. Folding begins when the N-terminus of the nascent polypeptide emerges from the ribosome. The vectorial nature of this "cotranslational folding" has both advantages and liabilities. An advantage is that vectorial folding limits the routes to the folded state and might account for why many proteins fold more efficiently during biosynthesis than from the denatured state. On the other hand, vectorial folding precludes interactions between N-terminal sequences with C-terminal sequences until they have emerged from the ribosome. Such interactions are common in folded proteins.

Folding of larger proteins is more complicated, especially in the presence of other partially folded proteins with exposed hydrophobic segments that are buried in the core of native proteins. These exposed core elements are prone to aggregate irreversibly before completing folding. Many newly synthesized native proteins also need assistance to avoid irreversible denaturation, aggregation, or destruction by proteolysis during folding.

Misfolding of mutant proteins contributes to many human diseases. For example, the most common cause of cystic fibrosis is genetic deletion of a single amino acid in CFTR, resulting in failure of the protein to fold properly (see Fig. 11-4). Beyond lacking function, misfolded proteins also poison the assembly of native proteins in blistering skin diseases (see Fig. 35-6), hypertrophic cardiomyopathies (see Table 39-4), and other "dominant negative" conditions. Folding of proteins into nonnative states causes prion and amyloid diseases.

Chaperone-Assisted Protein Folding

Several families of molecular chaperones (Fig. 17-13) facilitate folding of newly synthesized and denatured proteins. These chaperones do not fold polypeptides by directing the formation of secondary or tertiary structure. Rather, by binding exposed hydrophobic segments of nonnative polypeptides or providing sequestered environments, chaperones inhibit aggregation. They release polypeptides in a folding-competent state for attempts at folding. If folding fails, the cycle of binding and release can be repeated. The following sections cover **trigger factor** (and other chaperones associated with ribosomes), **Hsp70, Hsp90,** and cylindrical **chaperonins.** In addition, specialized chaperones assist with the folding of particular proteins such as tubulin and actin. Mutations in several of these chaperones have been associated with human disease. See Fig. 20-10 for chaperones in the endoplasmic reticulum.

Trigger Factor

Hydrophobic segments of the nascent chain must be protected from aggregation until enough of the chain has emerged from the ribosome to participate in folding. Each growing polypeptide first encounters a chaperone bound next to the exit tunnel on the large ribosomal subunit. The chaperone associated with bacterial ribosomes is called trigger factor (Fig. 17-13). A structurally unrelated protein called nascent polypeptide-associated

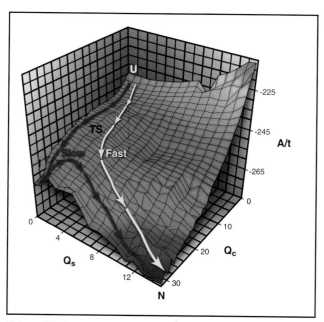

Figure 17-12 ENERGY CONSIDERATIONS IN PROTEIN FOLDING. As a protein matures from the unfolded state (U) through transition states (TS) to the native folded state (N), native-like contacts form, and the free energy of the system decreases. The two paths (folding trajectories) illustrate that fast protein folding (yellow line) is observed when more native-like contacts are made. When proteins become trapped in partially folded intermediate states, folding is slower (pink line) because energy barriers must be overcome. (Adapted from Radford SE, Dobson CM: Computer simulations to human disease: Emerging themes in protein folding. Cell 97:291–298, 1999.)

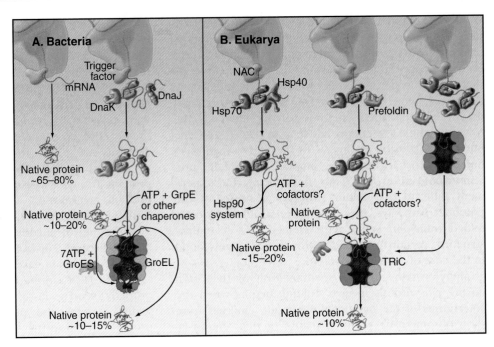

Figure 17-13 COMPARISON OF CHAPERONE-ASSISTED FOLDING PATHWAYS. **A,** Bacteria. **B,** Eukaryotes. The percentages refer to estimates of the fraction of proteins using each pathway. Most proteins fold without the assistance of chaperones. NAC, nascent polypeptide-associated complex. (Modified with permission from Hartl FU, Hayer-Hartl M: Molecular chaperones in the cytosol: From nascent chain to folded protein. Science 295:1852–1858, 2002. Copyright 2002 AAAS.)

complex has a similar function in Archaea and eukaryotes. Trigger factor has a hydrophobic groove that is suggested to cradle the growing polypeptide. The signal recognition particle binds on the other side of the exit tunnel, positioned so that its methionine-rich groove (see Fig. 20-5) also interacts with the growing polypeptide. Most bacterial polypeptides fold successfully after being released from trigger factor, while most eukaryotic polypeptides require assistance from additional chaperones.

Hsp70 Chaperones

The most widespread chaperones are members of the heat shock protein 70 (Hsp70) family (Fig. 17-14). Their name came from the observation that cells subjected to stresses, such as elevated temperature, increase the synthesis of these proteins to protect against denatured proteins. Hsp70s are present in Archaea, Bacteria (called DnaK), and most compartments of eukaryotes. The family includes Hsp70 in mitochondria and BiP in endoplasmic reticulum (see Fig. 20-4). Budding yeasts have genes for 14 Hsp70s; vertebrates have more.

Hsp70s bind and release peptides with 8 to 13 hydrophobic residues in a wide range of nascent or unfolded polypeptides. ATP binding and hydrolysis drive cycles of peptide binding and release, protecting hydrophobic peptides from aggregation during attempts at folding, delivery to mitochondria and chloroplasts, and import into these organelles (see Figs. 18-4 and 18-6).

Bacterial Hsp70 is a well-characterized model for other members of the family. A flexible hinge connects the N-terminal ATP-binding domain to the C-terminal peptide-binding domain. ATP binding favors release of the polypeptide, whereas ATP hydrolysis and phosphate release favors association with an unfolded polypeptide. DnaJ (Hsp40) delivers unfolded proteins to DnaK and promotes their binding by stimulating hydrolysis of ATP bound to DnaK. GrpE promotes exchange of ADP for ATP and release of the bound peptide. Animal Hsp70s have a mechanism of action similar to that of DnaJ except that they have intrinsic nucleotide-exchange activity and do not require a nucleotide-exchange protein such as GrpE.

Hsp90 Chaperones

Hsp90 cooperates with other chaperones to stabilize steroid-hormone receptors before they bind their ligands such as progesterone, glucocorticoids, estrogens, or androgens (Fig. 17-15). The chaperones use cycles of ATP hydrolysis to maintain receptors in an "open" state, ready to bind hydrophobic steroids. Steroid binding completes the folding of the receptors and displaces the Hsp90 complex. Then the receptors move to the nucleus to regulate gene expression (see Fig. 15-22). Hsp90 also interacts with other signaling proteins including protein kinases.

Chaperonins

The chaperonin family of barrel-shaped particles promotes efficient protein folding (Fig. 17-16). They allow nascent and denatured polypeptides to fold or refold

structure made of GroES. GroEL forms two rings of seven identical subunits. Mitochondrial (Hsp60/Hsp10), chloroplast (Cpn60/Cpn10), and eukaryotic chaperonins (TriC) are similar in design but more elaborate than GroEL/GroES, containing up to eight different gene products. This complexity represents evolutionary diversification for regulation of chaperonin function.

ATP binding and hydrolysis set the tempo for folding cycles. Unfolded polypeptides bind to hydrophobic patches on the inner wall of the GroEL cylinder. Cooperative binding of ATP to each of the subunits in one of the two rings of seven changes their conformation (compare the upper and lower rings in Fig. 17-16B), expanding the internal volume by twofold and favoring binding of a heptameric ring of 10-kD GroES subunits. This closes the top of the cylinder and creates a folding cavity for proteins up to about 70 kD. After ATP hydrolysis on the ring surrounding the folding protein and ATP binding to the opposite ring of seven GroEL subunits, the GroES cap releases, and the cage opens. Folded polypeptides escape into the bulk solution, whereas incompletely folded intermediates can rebind GroEL for another attempt at folding.

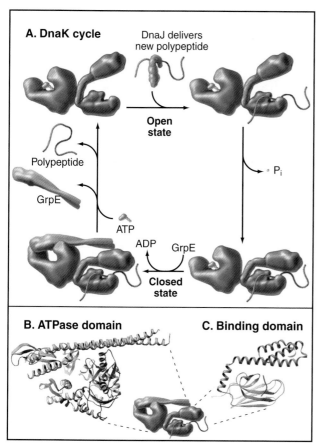

Figure 17-14 Hsp70 structure and function. **A,** The Hsp70 folding cycle with bacterial DnaK as the example. **B–C,** Atomic structures of DnaK *(blue)* and GrpE *(green)*. The ATPase domain and peptide-binding domain work together in a cyclical mechanism. DnaJ (Hsp40) delivers an unfolded peptide to the ATP-bound open state of DnaK and promotes ATP hydrolysis. The ADP-bound closed state of DnaK binds the peptide strongly. GrpE promotes dissociation of ADP. Rebinding of ATP dissociates GrpE and the peptide, which is free to attempt folding. Multiple Hsp70 cycles are usually required to complete protein folding. (PDB files: 1DKX and 1DKG. References: Zhu X, Zhao X, Burkholder WF, et al: Structural analysis of substrate binding by the molecular chaperone DnaK. Science 272:1606–1614, 1996; and Harrison CJ, Hayer-Hartl M, Hartl F, et al: Crystal structure of the nucleotide exchange factor GrpE bound to the ATPase domain of the molecular chaperone DnaK. Science 276:431–435, 1997.)

while sequestered in a cylindrical cavity protected from the complex environment of the cytoplasm. Although 85% of newly synthesized bacterial proteins fold spontaneously or with the assistance of Hsp70s, the remainder require the more isolated folding environment provided by chaperonins (Fig. 17-13). The mechanism of chaperonins is best understood for *Escherichia coli* **GroEL** and its co-chaperonin **GroES.** These assist with folding of nascent polypeptides, which in bacteria occurs largely after translation is complete.

The GroEL/GroES complex consists of a cylinder with a central cavity composed of GroEL and a cap

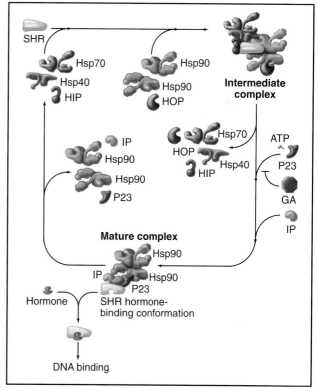

Figure 17-15 Stabilization of ligand-free steroid hormone receptors (SHRs) by Hsp70, Hsp90, and various accessory factors (HOP, HIP, P23, GA, and IP). Hormone binding releases the chaperones and allows the receptor-steroid complex to move to the nucleus. (Reference: Buchner J: Hsp90 & Co.: A holding for folding. Trends Biochem Sci 24:136–142, 1999.)

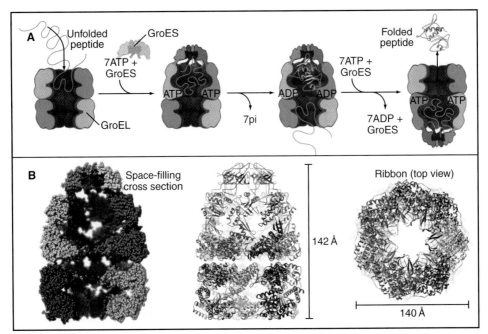

Figure 17-16   Chaperonin-mediated folding by GroEL and GroES. **A,** One folding cycle. **B,** Crystal structure of GroEL with a GroES cap bound to the upper, ATP-bound ring of seven subunits. Unfolded polypeptides bind the rim of an uncapped ring. Cooperative binding of ATP to each of the seven GroEL subunits in one ring changes their conformation, favors GroES binding, and doubles the volume of the central cavity, where the protein folds. Following ATP hydrolysis, binding of ATP and GroES to the lower ring structure dissociates the upper GroES and discharges the folded protein. (B, Based on the work of Xu Z, Horwich AL, Sigler PB: The crystal structure of the asymmetric GroEL-GroES-(ADP)7 chaperonin complex. Nature 388:741–750, 1997. PDB file: 1AON.)

ACKNOWLEDGMENT

Thanks go to Scott Strobel for his suggestions on revisions to this chapter.

SELECTED READINGS

Abbott CM, Proud CG: Translation factors: In sickness and in health. Trends Biochem Sci 29:25–31, 2004.

Andersen GR, Nissen P, Nyborg J: Elongation factors in protein biosynthesis. Trends Biochem Sci 28:434–441, 2003.

Chiti F, Dobson CM: Protein misfolding, functional amyloid, and human disease. Annu Rev of Biochem 75:333–366, 2006.

Daggett V, Fersht AR: Is there a unifying mechanism for protein folding? Trends Biochem Sci 28:18–25, 2003.

Dobson CM: Protein folding and misfolding. Nature 426:884–890, 2003.

Frydman J: Folding of newly translated proteins in vivo: The role of molecular chaperones. Annu Rev Biochem 70:603–647, 2004.

Ibba M, Curnow AW, Soll D: Aminoacyl-tRNA synthesis: Divergent routes to a common goal. Trends Biochem Sci 22:39–42, 1997.

Kapp LD, Lorsch JR: The molecular mechanics of eukaryotic translation. Annu Rev Biochem 73:657–704, 2004.

May BC, Govaerts C, Prusiner SB, Cohen FE: Prions: So many fibers, so little infectivity. Trends Biochem Sci 29:162–165, 2004.

Mazumder B, Seshadri V, Fox PL: Translational control by the 3′-UTR: The ends specify the means. Trends Biochem Sci 28:91–98, 2003.

Mitra K, Frank J: Ribosome dynamics: Insights from atomic structure modeling into cryoelectron microscopy maps. Annu Rev Biophys Biomolec Struct 35:299–317, 2006.

Moore PB, Steitz TA: The structural basis of large ribosomal subunit function. Annu Rev Biochem 72:813–850, 2003.

Myers JK, Oas TG: Mechanisms of fast protein folding. Annu Rev Biochem 71:783–815, 2002.

Nakamura Y, Ito K: Making sense of mimic in translation termination. Trends Biochem Sci 28:99–105, 2003.

Ogle JM, Carter AP, Ramakrishnan V: Insights into the decoding mechanism from recent ribosome structures. Trends Biochem Sci 28:259–266, 2003.

Pearl LH, Prodromou C: Structure and mechanism of the Hsp90 molecular chaperone machinery. Annu Rev Biochem 75:271–294, 2006.

Piper M, Holt C: RNA translation in axons. Annu Rev Cell Devel Biol 20:505–523, 2004.

Rodnina MV, Wintermeyer W: Peptide bond formation on the ribosome: Structure and mechanism. Curr Opin Struct Biol 13:334–340, 2003.

Saibil HR, Ranson NA: The chaperonin folding machine. Trends Biochem Sci 27:627–632, 2002.

Selkoe DJ: Folding proteins in fatal ways. Nature 426:891–899, 2003.

Sonenberg N, Dever TE: Eukaryotic translation initiation factors and regulators. Curr Opin Struct Biol 13:56–63, 2003.

Wilkie GS, Dickson KS, Gray NK: Regulation of mRNA translation by 5′- and 3′-UTR-binding factors. Trends Biochem Sci 28:182–188, 2003.

Young JC, Barral JM, Hartl FU: More than folding: Localized functions of cytosolic chaperones. Trends Biochem Sci 28:541–547, 2003.

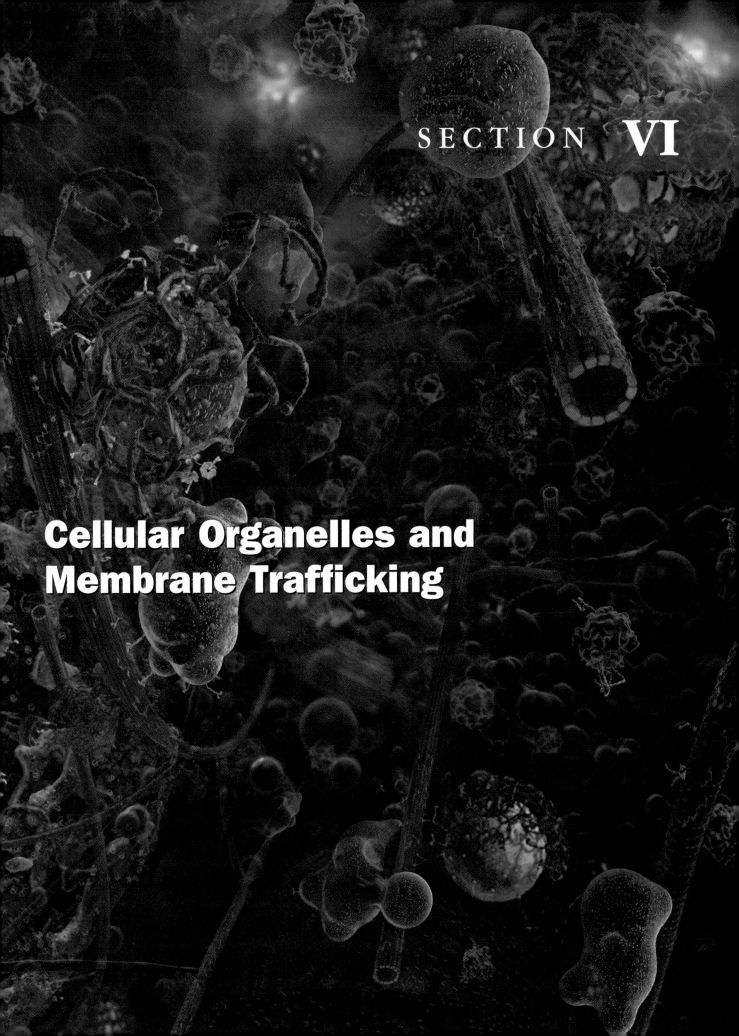

SECTION VI

Cellular Organelles and Membrane Trafficking

SECTION VI OVERVIEW

Eukaryotic cells evolved membrane-bounded compartments specialized to provide energy; to synthesize lipids, carbohydrates, proteins, and nucleic acids; and to degrade cellular constituents. These subcellular compartments, called **organelles,** have distinctive chemical compositions. Organelles vary in abundance and size in different cell types, even within multicellular organisms, in which each tissue and organ has specialized functions. An organelle often holds a monopoly on performing a given task; for example, **endoplasmic reticulum** (ER) synthesizes membrane proteins and certain membrane lipids, lysosomes contain enzymes to degrade many macromolecules, and mitochondria convert energy derived from the covalent bonds of nutrients into ATP to provide energy for diverse cellular functions.

A semipermeable membrane surrounds each organelle and establishes an internal microenvironment with concentrated enzymes, cofactors, and substrates to favor particular macromolecular interactions. Pumps (see Chapter 8), carriers (see Chapter 9), and channels (see Chapter 10) in each organelle membrane establish an internal chemical environment (pH, divalent cation concentration, redox potential) that is appropriate for particular biochemical functions. **Mitochondria** and **chloroplasts** utilize many enzymes embedded in their membranes to catalyze reactions that depend on the separation of reactants across the membrane or involve hydrophobic substrates and products soluble in the lipid bilayer (Chapter 19). Compartments also protect the rest of the cell from potentially dangerous activities, such as degradative enzymes in lysosomes and oxidative enzymes in **peroxisomes**.

This division of labor among organelles has many advantages but also presents cells with challenges in terms of coordination of cellular activities, organelle biosynthesis, and cell division. Organelles are not autonomous, so their activities must be integrated to benefit the whole cell. Therefore, mechanisms are required to transport material between compartments and across the membranes that surround them. Many functional pathways require macromolecules and lipids to move from one organelle to another in a vectorial manner.

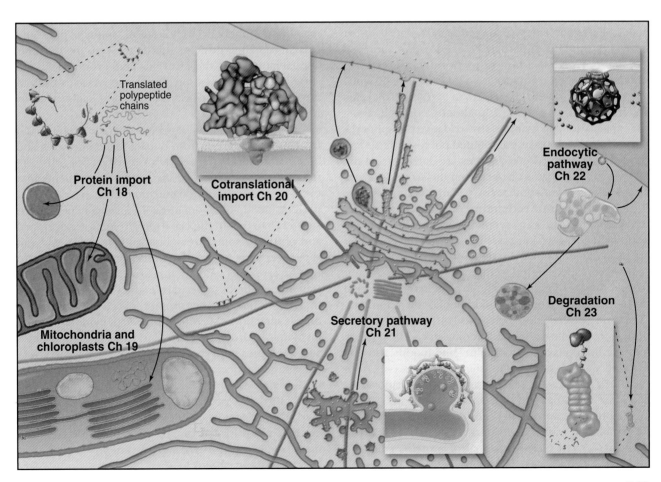

Translated polypeptide chains

Protein import
Ch 18

Cotranslational
import Ch 20

Endocytic
pathway
Ch 22

Mitochondria and
chloroplasts Ch 19

Secretory pathway
Ch 21

Degradation
Ch 23

This transport between organelles generally involves budding of vesicles from one membrane-bounded compartment followed by fusion with another, in a process collectively termed **vesicular trafficking.**

This section of the book focuses on two important processes as they pertain to the biogenesis and functions of the various organelles. The first is the targeting of proteins, either during or after translation to their home organelle. The second is the bidirectional movement of vesicular traffic between organelles and the plasma membrane. The exocytic or **secretory pathway** from the endoplasmic reticulum to the plasma membrane and lysosomes coordinates organelle biosynthesis and secretion. The **endocytic pathway** takes in molecules and microscopic particles from outside the cell along with plasma membrane components. Operating together, the two pathways coordinate the distribution pathways and turnover of membrane proteins and lipids.

Proteins that are synthesized in the cytoplasm either remain there or move to their final destinations in the nucleus (see Chapter 14), mitochondria, chloroplasts, and peroxisomes (Chapter 18). Hundreds of proteins destined for mitochondria and chloroplasts are synthesized in the cytoplasm and directed to these organelles by zip codes built into their polypeptide sequences. Most of these guide sequences are removed once the polypeptide has moved through channels into one of the membranes or compartments inside these organelles. Different sorts of targeting sequences target dozens of proteins to peroxisomes.

Chapter 19 explains how **mitochondria** and **chloroplasts** descended from bacteria that established symbiotic relationships with eukaryotes in two singular events about a billion years apart. Mitochondria brought along the capacity for ATP synthesis by oxidative phosphorylation, while chloroplasts contributed photosynthesis and oxygen production. **Peroxisomes** are derived from the ER by a process that is distinct from the secretory pathway. They carry out a number of oxidative reactions.

The **endoplasmic reticulum** (Chapter 20) generates the secretory pathway by synthesizing proteins for membranes and for secretion as well as many of the lipids that are used in membranes throughout the cell. Amino acid sequences called **signal sequences** direct ribosomes that synthesize integral membrane proteins and secreted proteins to receptors on the endoplasmic reticulum. Translation pushes these polypeptides through a protein pore into the lumen of the endoplasmic reticulum or into the lipid bilayer. After folding and modification by addition of oligosaccharides, these proteins exit from the ER in vesicles for transport to the Golgi apparatus and more distal parts of the secretory pathway.

Chapter 21 explains the mechanisms that are used for membrane trafficking. Under the direction of membrane-associated GTPases, a coat of proteins from the cytoplasm forms on a donor membrane and distorts the membrane into a vesicle that buds from the surface, carrying the proteins and lipids in the membrane and any material in the lumen. Sorting signals direct some proteins into these transport vesicles. Cells use three different types of coat proteins for budding from different organelles. After the vesicle moves by diffusion or by active transport along the cytoskeleton to a target membrane, different GTPases and peripheral proteins facilitate fusion of the vesicle with a target membrane. Such vesicle traffic moves membranes and content along the secretory pathway from the endoplasmic reticulum to the **Golgi apparatus,** lysosomes, and plasma membrane. Retrograde vesicle traffic mediated by other proteins retrieves membranes and proteins from the Golgi apparatus back to the ER. In spite of this heavy bidirectional traffic between organelles, the sorting mechanisms allow each organelle to maintain its identity.

Cells employ at lease five distinct mechanisms to internalize plasma membrane along with a wide range of extracellular materials (Chapter 22). Ingestion of small particles, including bacteria, takes place by **phagocytosis,** in which a veil of plasma membrane surrounds the particle and takes it into a vacuole inside the cell. Fusion of vesicles containing lysosomal enzymes initiates the degradation of the contents. A second endocytic pathway takes receptors and their ligands into cells in small vesicles coated with **clathrin.** Other forms of endocytosis take up extracellular fluid and patches of plasma membrane enriched in cholesterol, sphingolipids, and certain signaling proteins. Inside the cell, the contents and membranes of these various endocytic vesicles are sorted in **endosomes** for direction in vesicles back to the plasma membrane or onward to the Golgi apparatus or lysosomes.

Chapter 23 explains how cells degrade proteins and lipids, some taken in from outside by endocytosis and others from inside the cell. DNA is stable, but cells continuously replace most of their other constituents in a cycle of synthesis and degradation. Each type of RNA, protein, and lipid has a natural lifetime, generally much shorter than that of the cell itself. Proteins are degraded and replaced, some every hour, others every day and some every few weeks or months. Membrane lipids also turn over; some with lifetimes measured in minutes. Proteins and lipids taken in by endocytosis are degraded in **lysosomes.** In the process called **autophagy,** a double membrane surrounds a zone of cytoplasm, even including entire organelles. Fusion of late endosomes and lysosomes with these autophagic vacuoles delivers enzymes that degrade the contents. Cytoplasmic and nuclear proteins are degraded by a large protein complex called the **proteasome,** but only after they are marked for degradation by conjugation with the small protein, **ubiquitin.** A hierarchy of ubiquitin-conjugating enzymes controls the fate of proteins as they turn over during the cell cycle.

Posttranslational Targeting of Proteins

Protein synthesis is largely a monopoly of cytoplasmic ribosomes that provide all of the proteins for the nucleus, cytoplasm, peroxisomes, and secretory pathway. Even mitochondria and chloroplasts import most of their proteins from cytoplasm, despite the fact that they originated as bacterial endosymbionts and have retained the capacity to synthesize a few of their proteins. Most of the original bacterial genes moved to the nucleus of the eukaryotic host.

Given a common site of synthesis, accurate addressing is essential to direct proteins to their sites of action and to maintain the unique character of each cellular compartment. This is achieved by "zip codes" built into the structure of each protein (Fig. 18-1). Residues in the sequence of each protein—often, but not necessarily, contiguous amino acids—form a signal for targeting.

Targeting signals are both necessary and sufficient to guide proteins to their final destinations. Transplantation of a targeting signal, such as a presequence from a mitochondrial protein, to a cytoplasmic protein reroutes the hybrid protein into the organelle specified by the targeting sequence, mitochondria in this example. Some targeting signals are transient parts of the protein. For example, most mitochondrial proteins are synthesized with N-terminal extensions that guide them to mitochondria and then are removed. Alternatively, signals may be a permanent part of the mature protein, in some cases serving repeatedly to target a mobile protein between different destinations. Permanent nuclear targeting signals can be located at the N-terminus, the C-terminus, or even the middle of a protein. Some proteins have more than one targeting signal: a primary code that directs the protein to the target organelle or pathway, and a second signal that steers the protein to its specific site of residence within the organelle or pathway.

Targeting signals direct proteins to their destination by binding to organelle-specific receptors or using soluble "escort" factors as intermediaries. When necessary, proteins cross membranes via channels called **translocons** formed by integral membrane proteins (Fig. 18-2). Like ion channels (see Chapter 10), these protein-translocating channels are gated to prevent indiscriminate transport of cellular constituents when not occupied by a polypeptide. Polypeptides fit so tightly in these channels during

This chapter was revised using material from the first edition written by William E. Balch, Ann L. Hubbard, J. David Castle, and Pat Shipman.

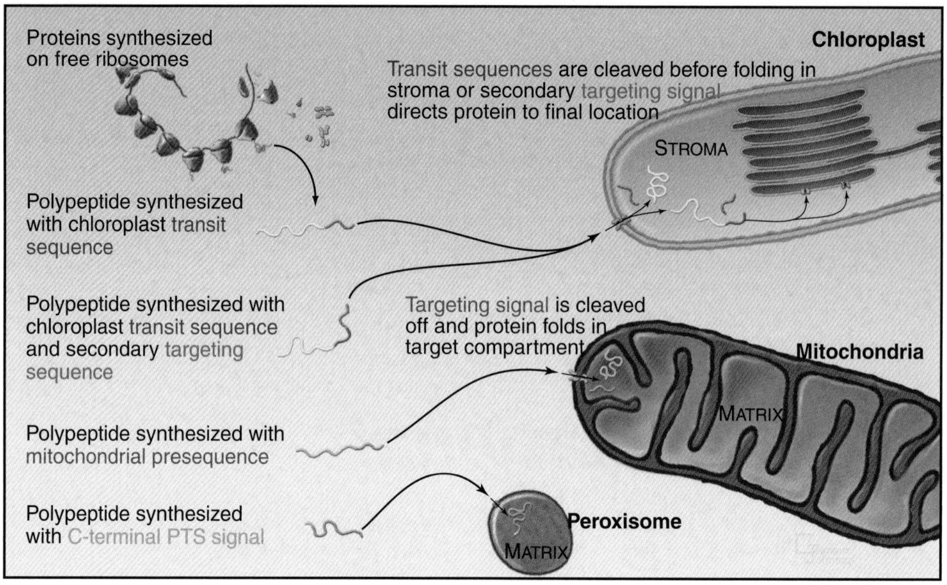

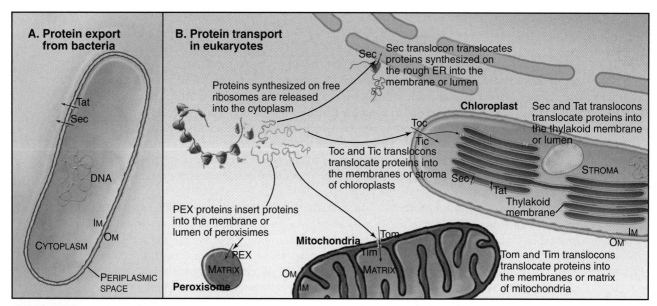

Figure 18-1 TARGETING SIGNALS THAT DIRECT POLYPEPTIDES SYNTHESIZED ON CYTOPLASMIC RIBOSOMES TO CHLOROPLASTS, MITOCHONDRIA, AND PEROXISOMES. Some but not all of these targeting signals are removed by signal peptidases after the polypeptide enters the organelle.

Proteins synthesized on free ribosomes

Polypeptide synthesized with chloroplast transit sequence

Polypeptide synthesized with chloroplast transit sequence and secondary targeting sequence

Polypeptide synthesized with mitochondrial presequence

Polypeptide synthesized with C-terminal PTS signal

Transit sequences are cleaved before folding in stroma or secondary targeting signal directs protein to final location

STROMA

Chloroplast

Targeting signal is cleaved off and protein folds in target compartment

Mitochondria

MATRIX

Peroxisome

MATRIX

translocation that ions do not leak through. Ions traverse ion channels in a microsecond, whereas polypeptides take tens of seconds to move through translocons. Protein synthesis, adenosine triphosphate (ATP) hydrolysis, or the membrane potential provides the energy to power protein translocation across membranes.

Three families of protein translocation channels are found in all three domains of life. Sec translocons direct proteins into the endoplasmic reticulum in eukaryotes and out of prokaryotes. The Tat family of pores translocate folded proteins into chloroplast thylakoids and out of prokaryotes. Membrane proteins related to Oxa1p help to insert proteins synthesized in the mitochondrial

matrix and prokaryotic cytoplasm into membranes. Mitochondria (Fig. 18-4), chloroplasts (Fig. 18-6), and prokaryotes (Fig. 18-10) have additional families of protein translocation channels.

Primary targeting can occur either cotranslationally, coincident with protein synthesis, or posttranslationally, after polypeptide synthesis. Chapter 20 covers protein targeting to endoplasmic reticulum where, with a few exceptions, targeting is cotranslational. This chapter covers **posttranslational targeting** mechanisms that move proteins across membrane bilayers into mitochondria, chloroplasts, and peroxisomes and out of Bacteria. Eukaryotes also secrete a few proteins directly

A. Protein export from bacteria

Tat
Sec

DNA

IM
OM

CYTOPLASM

PERIPLASMIC SPACE

B. Protein transport in eukaryotes

Proteins synthesized on free ribosomes are released into the cytoplasm

Sec

Sec translocon translocates proteins synthesized on the rough ER into the membrane or lumen

Chloroplast

Toc
Tic

Sec and Tat translocons translocate proteins into the thylakoid membrane or lumen

Toc and Tic translocons translocate proteins into the membranes or stroma of chloroplasts

STROMA

Sec
Tat

Thylakoid membrane

IM
OM

PEX proteins insert proteins into the membrane or lumen of peroxisimes

PEX

MATRIX

Peroxisome

Mitochondria

Tom

Tim

MATRIX

OM

IM

Tom and Tim translocons translocate proteins into the membranes or matrix of mitochondria

Figure 18-2 TRANSLOCONS USED BY POLYPEPTIDES TO CROSS MEMBRANES. **A,** Bacterium with Sec and Tat translocons in the inner membrane. **B,** Eukaryote translocons including Sec in the endoplasmic reticulum and thylakoid membrane of chloroplasts, Toc in the outer membrane of chloroplasts, Tic in the inner membrane of chloroplasts, Tat in the thylakoid membrane of chloroplasts, Tom in the outer membrane of mitochondria, Tim in the inner membrane of mitochondria, and PEX in peroxisomes.

across the plasma membrane. Chapter 14 covers post-translational movements of proteins into and out of the nucleus through a large aqueous channel in the nuclear pore.

Transport of Proteins into Mitochondria

Mitochondrial outer and inner membranes define two spaces: one between the **outer** and **inner membranes (intermembranous space)** and an interior space termed the **matrix** (Fig. 18-3). Each membrane and space has distinct functions and protein compositions, which are covered in Chapter 19. Targeting signals and specific translocation machinery guide more than 500 imported proteins selectively to these compartments.

Genetic and biochemical experiments on fungi defined the molecular machinery for proteins to enter mitochondria, including the **Tom complex** (translocase of the outer mitochondrial membrane), the **Sam complex** (sorting and assembly machinery of the outer membrane), and two **Tim complexes** (translocase of the inner mitochondrial membrane). See Figures 18-4 and 18-5. Although the distinction is not absolute, one Tim complex is specialized to transport proteins into the matrix, and the other is specialized for insertion of proteins into the inner membrane. Translocation requires energy and assistance from protein chaperones both outside and inside mitochondria.

Delivery of Protein to Mitochondria

After synthesis by cytoplasmic ribosomes, most proteins destined for mitochondria bind cytosolic chaperones of the **Hsp70** family (see Fig. 17-14). This interaction maintains proteins in unfolded configurations competent for import. Some imported proteins require additional factors, such as mitochondria-import stimulation factor, for targeting to the translocation machinery.

Targeting signals for proteins of the matrix are generally located at the N-termini of precursor polypeptides as contiguous sequences of 10 to 70 amino acids. These targeting motifs are called **presequences,** because they are usually removed by proteolytic cleavage in the mitochondrial matrix. Presequences are rich in basic, hydroxylated, and hydrophobic amino acids but share no sequences in common. The targeting sequences of many mitochondrial membrane proteins are in the middle of the polypeptide and are not cleaved after import. Cytochrome c, a component of the electron transport chain in the intermembranous space (see Fig. 19-5), also has an internal signal for import into mitochondria.

A succession of weak interactions with outer membrane receptors Tom20, Tom22, Tom5, and perhaps Tom70 guide presequences and other target signals to

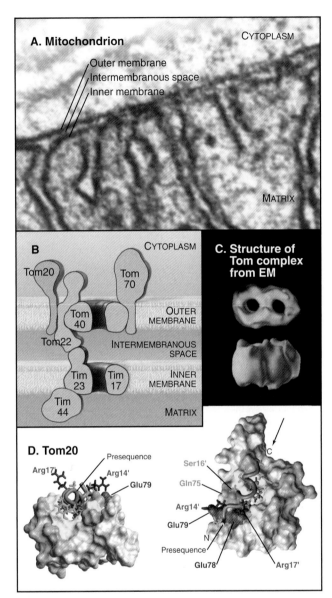

Figure 18-3 MITOCHONDRIAL IMPORT COMPONENTS. **A,** Electron micrograph of a thin section of a mitochondrion. **B,** The mitochondrial import apparatus, including Tom complex in the outer membrane and Tim complex in the inner membrane. **C,** Three-dimensional reconstruction from electron micrographs of Tom core complex, the translocase of the outer mitochondrial membrane. **D,** Structure determined by nuclear magnetic resonance spectroscopy of a presequence peptide bound to a hydrophobic patch on Tom20, a receptor from the mitochondrial outer membrane. Space-filling model of a cytoplasmic domain of Tom20. The presequence forms two turns of α-helix with two arginines exposed on the surface. N is the N-terminus and C is the C-terminus of the peptide. *Yellow* is a hydrophobic patch; *orange* is Gln-rich; *red* is Glu-rich. (A, Courtesy of Don W. Fawcett, Harvard Medical School, Boston, Massachusetts. C, Reproduced from Ahting U, Thun C, Hegerl R, et al: The Tom core complex: The general protein import pore of the outer membrane of mitochondria. J Cell Biol 147:959–968, 1999. Copyright 1999 The Rockefeller University Press. D, Courtesy of D. Kohda, Kyushu University. From Abe Y, Shodai T, Muto T, et al: Structural basis of presequence recognition by the mitochondrial protein import receptor Tom20. Cell 100:551–560, 2000. PDB file: 1OM2.)

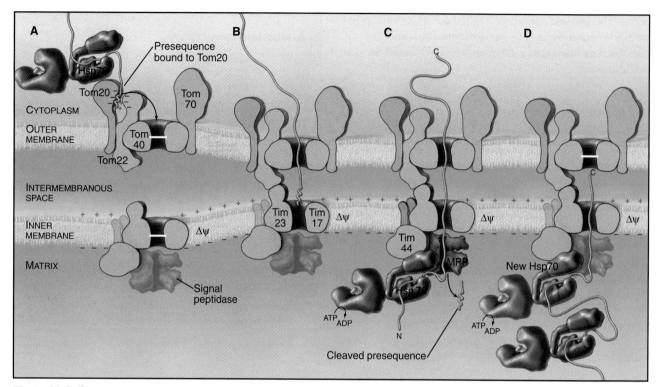

Figure 18-4 IMPORT OF MATRIX PROTEINS INTO MITOCHONDRIA. A *white bar* across a translocon indicates that it is closed. **A,** Hsp70 escorts polypeptides synthesized on cytoplasmic ribosomes to mitochondria where the presequence associates with Tom20/22. **B,** The basic presequence leads the polypeptide through the translocase of the outer membrane (Tom) across the intermembrane space to the translocase of the inner membrane (Tim). **C,** The potential across the inner membrane ($\Delta\Psi$) pulls the presequence through Tim into the matrix, where it is cleaved by the matrix protease MPP. The polypeptide binds matrix Hsp70. **D,** Cycles of Hsp70 binding to the peptide followed by ATP hydrolysis and dissociation of Hsp70 from Tim44 ratchet the translocating peptide into the matrix, where it folds.

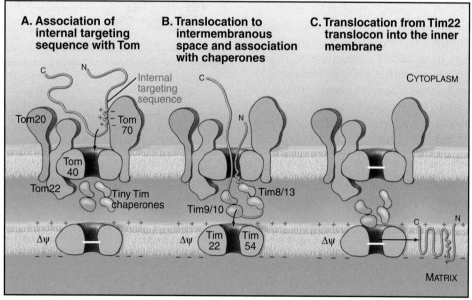

Figure 18-5 IMPORT OF THE ADP/ATP ANTIPORTER ACC AND INSERTION INTO THE INNER MEMBRANE BILAYER. A *white bar* across a translocon pore indicates that it is closed. **A,** An internal targeting sequence binds the ACC polypeptide to Tom70, which directs it into the Tom channel. **B,** In the intermembranous space, Tim9/10 and Tim8/13 capture the polypeptide and direct it to the Tim22/54 translocon that is used for import of matrix proteins. **C,** Tim22/54, in conjunction with the inner membrane potential ($\Delta\psi$), promotes insertion of the six transmembrane helices into the inner membrane bilayer.

the outer membrane translocon. The presequence initially contacts Tom20. Eight residues of the presequence fold into an amphipathic (hydrophobic on one side, hydrophilic on the other) α-helix that binds in a shallow hydrophobic groove on Tom20. Arginines on the surface of this helix interact with acidic residues on Tom22 (Fig. 18-4D). Other parts of the presequence are thought to interact with Tom40, the translocon itself. Although these associations are weak, collectively, they distinguish mitochondrial presequences from other proteins in the cytoplasm with high fidelity.

Translocation across the Outer Membrane

Outer membrane receptors transfer the presequence to the translocon channel, which is composed mainly of Tom40 along with three small subunits. Tom40 is an integral membrane protein that is predicted to span the bilayer exclusively as β-strands. Electron microscopy of purified Tom complex revealed two pores with diameters of approximately 2 nm, which agrees with the size of the pore calculated from ion conductance measurements of purified Tom40 inserted into lipid bilayers. Two molecules of Tom40 are postulated to form a channel and the complex may contain two or three of these channels. Proteins must be largely unfolded to fit through a pore of this size. Like Sec translocons of endoplasmic reticulum (see Fig 20-6) and bacteria (Fig. 18-9), Tom channels are likely to be gated, so they close when not occupied by a translocating polypeptide. After crossing the outer membrane, some proteins remain in the intermembranous space.

Assembly of Outer Membrane Proteins

Some simple outer membrane proteins transfer laterally into the bilayer while they are in transit through Tom, while more complicated outer membrane proteins, including Tom40 itself and porins (see Fig. 7-8), require assistance. Two protein complexes of the outer membrane called Sam I and Sam II mediate folding and insertion into the membrane.

Translocation across the Inner Membrane to the Matrix

Proteins use the Tim23 translocon to cross the inner membrane into the matrix. The channel across the inner membrane is formed by the integral membrane proteins Tim23 and Tim17 (Fig. 18-4). Interactions of the N-terminal presequences of matrix proteins with Tim50 and Tim23 guide the presequence into the translocation channel. Physical interactions of Tom and Tim complexes may facilitate the transfer of matrix proteins across both membranes. The MPP peptidase (matrix

processing protease) cleaves off the presequences once they enter the matrix.

Two energy sources—the electrical potential across the inner membrane and ATP hydrolysis by matrix chaperones—power polypeptide translocation across the inner membrane. The membrane potential (negative inside) pulls positively charged presequences across the membrane. Then the chaperone Hsp70 takes over and uses cycles of peptide binding and ATP hydrolysis to move the peptide into the matrix. One idea is that Hsp70 rectifies movements of the polypeptide in the pore, allowing movement forward into the matrix but not backward. Hsp70 binds when the polypeptide slides forward. After ATP hydrolysis, Hsp70 dissociates from the polypeptide and the exchange factor mGrp1 (see Fig. 17-14) rapidly recharges it with ATP, ready for another cycle of peptide binding, ATP hydrolysis, and release. This allows the polypeptide to slide forward into the matrix but not backward, so it eventually ends up as a folded protein in the matrix. Another model proposes that the energy from ATP hydrolysis is used to pull the polypeptide across the inner membrane.

Translocation into the Inner Membrane Bilayer

The integral proteins of the inner membrane lack cleaved targeting signals, depending instead on targeting information contained in the intact protein to reach their destination. One example is the most abundant protein of the inner membrane, the adenosine diphosphate (ADP)/ATP antiporter that spans the inner membrane six times (see Fig. 9-2). Its signal sequence is located in the middle of the polypeptide. A family of small "tiny Tim" chaperone proteins guide inner membrane proteins from Tom across the intermembranous space to the Tim22 translocon in the inner membrane (Fig. 18-4). This family of chaperones includes Tim8, Tim9, Tim10, Tim12, and Tim13. Complexes of Tim9/10 or Tim8/13 bind to hydrophobic segments of polypeptides during transit to the inner membrane.

The Tim22 translocon used by many inner membrane proteins is a 300-kD complex composed of Tim22, Tim54, Tim12, and Tim18, all different from the Tim23 complex used by most translocating matrix proteins. Tim22 forms the heart of the translocon, but little is known about its structure or mechanism. Insertion of transmembrane segments into the bilayer depends on membrane potential.

Export from the Matrix

Insertion of proteins synthesized in the matrix into the inner membrane depends on an inner membrane protein called Oxa1p, which forms a translocon similar to bacterial YidC and chloroplast Alb3 (see later sections).

Oxa1p interacts with mitochondrial ribosomes, so it might guide hydrophobic transmembrane segments directly into the bilayer. At least one other protein complex participates in export of proteins from the matrix.

Transport of Proteins into Chloroplasts

Eukaryotes acquired chloroplasts through symbiosis with a photosynthetic cyanobacterium (see Figs. 2-8 and 19-7). Over time, most of the bacterial genes moved to the nucleus, so most chloroplast proteins are synthesized on cytoplasmic ribosomes and imported into one of three chloroplast membranes or the compartments that they surround (Fig. 19-7). Chapter 19 covers chloroplast functions. The innermost thylakoid membranes contain the photosynthetic apparatus inherited from cyanobacteria. The outer membrane likely came from the eukaryotic host, whereas the inner envelope membrane has both bacterial and eukaryotic features. Some

organisms acquired their photosynthetic plastids by secondary or even tertiary rounds of endosymbiosis, when a eukaryote such as the precursor of *Euglena* took up a green alga (see Fig. 2-8). These secondary or tertiary plastids are bounded by one or more additional membranes and have more complicated mechanisms to import the proteins expressed from nuclear genes.

Although both chloroplasts and mitochondria arose from symbiotic Bacteria, chloroplasts evolved a distinct mechanism of protein import (Fig. 18-6). The principles are similar, but the two systems share no common proteins. The closest known relatives of any protein component of the chloroplast import machine are found in the ancestors of chloroplasts, photosynthetic cyanobacteria, in which they appear to have a role in secretion.

In plants, N-terminal signal sequences called **transit sequences** target chloroplast proteins to the import machinery in the outer envelope. When added experimentally to the N-terminus of a test protein, transit sequences suffice to guide the test protein into the stroma of chloroplasts. These N-terminal targeting sequences are reminiscent of sequences that target pro-

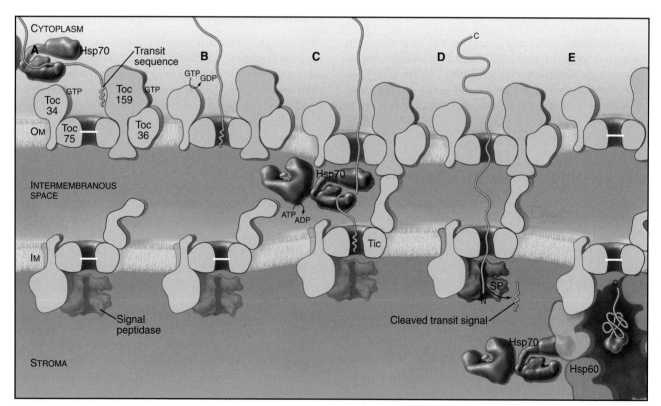

Figure 18-6 Chloroplast protein import pathway via Toc and Tic complexes. Proteins move from the cytoplasm to various chloroplast compartments in five stages. **A,** Energy-independent binding of the transit sequence to outer membrane lipids and proteins, especially Toc159. **B,** Insertion of the transit sequence through the outer membrane pore composed of Toc75 is dependent on GTP hydrolysis by Toc34 and perhaps Toc159. **C,** ATP-dependent formation of a translocation intermediate engaged with the Tic complex. **D,** ATP-dependent translocation across the inner membrane through a translocon, followed by removal of the N-terminal transit sequence by a stromal protease SP. **E,** Hsp60 and Hsp70 promote folding of stromal proteins, while other proteins are rerouted to other compartments, including thylakoids. (Modified from Chen X, Schnell D: Protein import into chloroplasts. Trends Cell Biol 9:222–227, 1999; and from May T, Soll J: Chloroplast precursor protein translocon. FEBS Lett 452:52–56, 2000.)

teins to endoplasmic reticulum and mitochondria, but the sequence determinants of the chloroplast transit sequences are much less well defined. They vary in length from 20 to 120 residues, and the amino acid sequences have little in common beyond a net positive charge and numerous serines and threonines.

All imported proteins use the same "general import pathway" to cross the outer and inner envelope membranes. The machinery consists of different protein complexes in each membrane called **Toc** (translocon at the outer envelope membrane of chloroplasts) and **Tic** (translocon at the inner envelope membrane of chloroplasts) (Fig. 18-6). These complexes were identified in biochemical experiments in which isolated chloroplasts imported precursor proteins synthesized in vitro. Chemical cross-linking of these imported proteins to translocon proteins identified the subunits that bind the transit sequence and contact imported polypeptides as they cross both membranes. Other subunits account for the requirements for ATP and guanosine triphosphate (GTP) hydrolysis. Both Toc and a "super complex" of Toc with Tic can be isolated for analysis of their composition. Mutations that compromise chloroplast import have also contributed to understanding the process.

The journey of a protein from its site of synthesis in cytoplasm into the stroma is understood in broad outline. Transit sequences target chloroplast preproteins to two outer membrane receptors Toc159 and Toc34. Both receptors are members of a family of related guanosine triphosphatases (GTPases) with overlapping functions. Bound GTP favors binding of transit sequences. Formation of a ternary complex of transit sequence with both Toc159 and Toc34 stimulates GTP hydrolysis and transfer of the transit sequence to the translocon. GTP hydrolysis may open the translocation pore or promote binding of Toc to Tic to form a continuous pore across both membranes for translocation into the stroma. The β-barrel protein Toc75 is the prime candidate for the channel across the outer membrane. A homologous protein Omp85 translocates proteins in the opposite direction across the outer membrane of gram-negative bacteria. The pore seems narrower than those in the α-helical Sec translocons, so polypeptides are thought to be unfolded during transit. However, some small, folded, protein domains might fit through the pore. The existence of small gene families encoding proteins related to Toc34 and Toc159 suggests that variations of the general import pathway might exist to accommodate the import of distinct classes of chloroplast preproteins.

The pore across the inner membrane consists of a complex of at least seven Tic proteins. The abundant protein Tic110 not only forms some or all of the pore but also binds Hsp70 chaperones on the stromal side of the membrane. The structure of the pore and the roles of the other subunits are under investigation. As in mitochondria, ATP hydrolysis by Hsp70 in both the intermembranous space and stroma promotes translocation of the imported protein.

As proteins emerge into the stroma, a signal peptidase cleaves off the transit peptide before the proteins fold or redistribute to their final locations. Some proteins fold with the help of Hsp70, an Hsp100 chaperone, and an Hsp60 chaperone similar to GroEL (see Fig. 17-16) and remain in the stroma. Other proteins move on to thylakoid membranes or the thylakoid lumen using at least four different pathways.

Some photosynthesis proteins insert directly into thylakoid membranes from the stroma. Others require help from proteins homologous to parts of the signal recognition particle (SRP) system used for export from bacteria (Fig. 18-10) and into the endoplasmic reticulum of eukaryotes (see Fig. 20-3). Although chloroplasts lack SRP RNA, GTPases similar to an SRP protein and the SRP receptor cooperate with a protein that is homologous to Oxa1p to mediate insertion into the thylakoid membrane.

Hydrophilic proteins destined for the thylakoid lumen retain a secondary N-terminal signal sequence after the transit sequence is cleaved in the stroma. Some move across the thylakoid membrane into the thylakoid lumen through a translocon homologous to bacterial SecYE, powered by ATP hydrolysis by a homolog of SecA (Fig. 18-9). Other proteins with tightly bound redox factors cross the thylakoid membrane while compactly folded using translocon factors similar to the bacterial Tat system (Fig. 18-2). Secondary signal sequences with two arginine residues direct these proteins to a Tat translocon and the proton gradient drives the polypeptide across the membrane. After translocation, a peptidase in the thylakoid lumen removes both types of secondary signal sequences.

Transport of Proteins into Peroxisomes

Peroxisomes are simple organelles with a single membrane limiting a lumen containing many **oxidative enzymes** (see Fig. 19-10). Nuclear genes encode all proteins found in the membrane and lumen of peroxisomes. Their mRNAs are translated on cytoplasmic ribosomes, and the proteins are incorporated posttranslationally into peroxisomes (Fig. 18-1).

Two types of targeting signals direct proteins to the peroxisome lumen (called matrix). The type-1 **peroxisomal targeting signal (PTS1)** is found at the extreme C-terminus of most peroxisomal enzymes (Fig. 18-7). PTS1 is just three amino acids long, and it conforms to the consensus sequence of serine-lysine-leucine-COOH, or a conservative variant. For example, alanine or

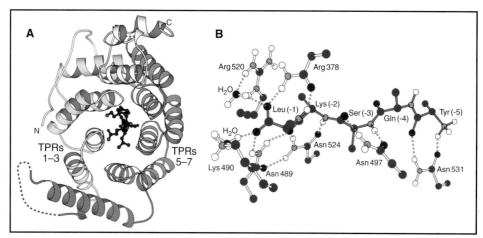

Figure 18-7 STRUCTURE OF A PEX5-PTS1 COMPLEX. **A,** PEX5 binds PTS1 via its C-terminal tetratricopeptide repeat (TPR) domain. The C-terminal, 40-kD TPR domain of PEX5, shown as a ribbon diagram, surrounds the PTS1 peptide, shown as a stick figure. Note TPRs 1 to 3 *(yellow ribbons)* and TPRs 5 to 7 *(blue ribbons)*. An α-helical span *(green ribbon)* links the two triplet TPRs at the bottom of this structure; the C-terminal extension *(white ribbons)* also connects the two triplet TPRs. **B,** Detailed view of PEX5-PTS1 interactions between the PTS1 backbone *(brown bonds)* and PEX5 side chains *(white bonds)*; the putative hydrogen bonds are shown as *dashed green lines.* This structure revealed the chemical basis of PEX5-PTS1 binding, as well as the sequence constraints of PTS1. (A, PDB file: 1FCH. Courtesy of S. J. Gould, Johns Hopkins Medical School, Baltimore, Maryland. Reprinted by permission from Macmillan Publishers Ltd. from Gatto GJ Jr, Geisbrecht BV, Gould SJ, Berg JM: Peroxisomal targeting signal-1 recognition by the TPR domains of human PEX5. Nature Struct Biol 7:1091–1095, 2000. Copyright 2000.)

cysteine can substitute at the −3 position, arginine or histidine can function at the penultimate position, and methionine can substitute for the C-terminal leucine. PTS1 is always located at the extreme C-terminus, and amidation of the C-terminal carboxylate inactivates the signal. The type-2 peroxisomal targeting signal **(PTS2)** also targets proteins to the peroxisome matrix but is found on few proteins (only four are known in humans, one in yeast). PTS2 sequences are located at or near the N-terminus and have a loose consensus sequence of RLXXXXXH/QL (where X is any amino acid).

Proteins called **peroxins** recognize newly synthesized peroxisomal proteins and deliver them to peroxisomes for insertion into the peroxisomal membrane or translocation across the membrane into the lumen (Fig. 18-8 and Appendix 18-1). Loss of function mutations in humans and yeast revealed the genes for more than 20

peroxins that are crucial for the biogenesis and proliferation of peroxisomes. Mutations of these *PEX* genes in humans cause a number of devastating human diseases known as the **peroxisomal biogenesis disorders** (see Chapter 19).

After synthesis in the cytoplasm, PTS1-containing enzymes bind the import receptor, PEX5. Binding of a PTS1 signal dissociates the PEX5 tetramer into a dimer that carries the protein to the peroxisomal membrane. A similar mode of action is proposed for PEX7, the import receptor for PTS2 proteins. In fact, in higher eukaryotes, PEX5 and PEX7 form a complex that may function as a single, oligomeric import receptor for all peroxisomal matrix proteins. Mutations in the PEX5 gene cause some cases of peroxisomal biogenesis disorders, and some of these mutations alter residues that are critical for binding PTS1.

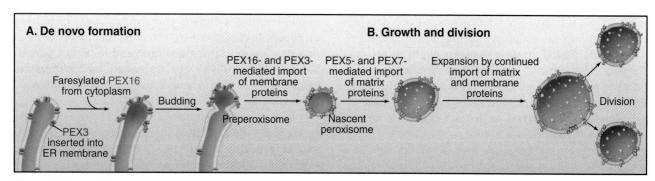

Figure 18-8 PEROXISOME BIOGENESIS. **A,** De novo formation by budding of a vesicle containing PEX3 and PEX16 from endoplasmic reticulum to form a preperoxisome. **B,** Growth and division of peroxisomes. PEX3 and PEX16 mediate the import of membrane proteins. The PEX5–PTS1 receptor, PEX7, and other peroxins mediate the import of proteins with PTS1 and PTS2 into peroxisomes.

Both PTS receptors and their cargo proteins interact with PEX14 and other peroxins on the peroxisomal membrane, but the mechanism that translocates proteins into the lumen is not well characterized. The translocon itself has not yet been identified, and it is not clear how large folded proteins can cross the membrane. Following translocation of a peroxisomal enzyme into the lumen, the receptors recycle back to the cytoplasm for further rounds of import.

Peroxisomal membranes form from lipids made in the endoplasmic reticulum and proteins imported from the cytoplasm. The mechanism that transports lipids from the endoplasmic reticulum (ER) to peroxisomes is not known. Peroxisomal membrane proteins lack motifs similar to PTS1 or PTS2 and instead utilize a different **membrane peroxisomal targeting sequence (mPTS)** for delivery to peroxisomes by different peroxins. The consensus sequence within the mPTS varies widely but consists of basic amino acids along with a transmembrane domain. Some peroxisomal membrane proteins possess more than one mPTS.

Cells depend on a different set of peroxins, including PEX3, PEX16, and PEX19, to insert proteins into the peroxisomal membrane (Fig. 18-8). Cells that are deficient in any of these three peroxins lack peroxisomal membranes and the peroxisomal membrane proteins are degraded or mislocalized to other cellular membranes, particularly mitochondria. PEX3 is an integral protein of the peroxisomal membrane. Some PEX16 is in the cytoplasm; some is attached to the cytoplasmic side of the membrane by a farnesyl tag. PEX19 plays a dual role: As a cytoplasmic chaperone, it binds and stabilizes peroxisomal membrane proteins in cytoplasm; and as an import receptor, it recruits proteins with mPTS sequences to the peroxisomal membrane.

Peroxisomes may arise by either of two pathways (Fig. 18-8). Peroxisomes can form de novo by budding from the ER. PEX3 is inserted into the ER, where it recruits PEX16 and other peroxins. This specialized domain of ER then pinches off for delivery to peroxisomes or to form a nascent peroxisome de novo. By originating from the ER in this manner, peroxisomes can arise in cells that lack them without a preexisting peroxisome as template. Preexisting peroxisomes can grow by importing proteins and lipids and then divide by a process of fission dependent on the GTPase dynamin (see Fig. 22-11).

Translocation of Eukaryotic Proteins across the Plasma Membrane by ABC Transporters

Most proteins that are secreted by eukaryotic cells travel to the cell surface through the classical secretory pathway, including the endoplasmic reticulum and Golgi apparatus (see Chapters 20 and 21). But budding yeast use an **ABC transporter** (see Fig. 8-9) to transport their a-type mating factor directly from the cytoplasm across the plasma membrane. The a-factor is synthesized in the cytoplasm as part of a precursor, excised from the precursor by proteolytic cleavage, and then prenylated on its C-terminus before transport across the plasma membrane. This mechanism has been invoked to explain the secretion of a few mammalian proteins that lack the "signal sequences" that direct proteins to the classic ER secretory pathway. These include some cytokines, fibroblast growth factor, and some blood-clotting factors. This is a well-characterized route for secretion of some bacterial proteins (Fig. 18-10).

Targeting to the Surfaces of the Plasma Membrane

Many proteins synthesized in the cytoplasm are targeted to the cytoplasmic side of organelle and plasma membranes (see Fig. 7-9). These include peripheral membrane proteins that bind to cytoplasmic domains of integral membrane proteins or bind directly to the lipid bilayer.

Other proteins are tethered to membrane bilayers by a covalently attached lipid added as a posttranslational modification following synthesis on cytoplasmic ribosomes. Lipid modifications on tethered proteins include long-chain, saturated fatty acids and isoprenoids. The saturated fatty acids are either myristate (14 carbons), which is added through amide linkage to amino-terminal glycine residues, or palmitate (16 carbons), which is usually added through a thioether linkage to cysteine residues found toward the C-terminus. The isoprenoids farnesyl (15 carbons) and geranylgeranyl (20 carbons) are added through thioether linkages to cysteine residues located at or near the C-terminus in specific structural motifs. Attachment of a lipid helps to stabilize membrane association, but does not guarantee permanent anchoring to the membrane. Some proteins, such as the catalytic subunit of cyclic AMP–dependent protein kinase, are fatty acylated but mostly soluble in cytoplasm.

Proteins attached to the external surface of plasma membranes by glycosylphosphatidylinositol anchors arrive by a different route. These proteins are synthesized on ribosomes associated with the endoplasmic reticulum and then translocated into the ER lumen anchored by a C-terminal transmembrane segment. Inside the ER the protein is cleaved from its membrane anchor and transferred enzymatically to glycosylphosphatidylinositol before transport to the cell surface (see Fig. 20-7C).

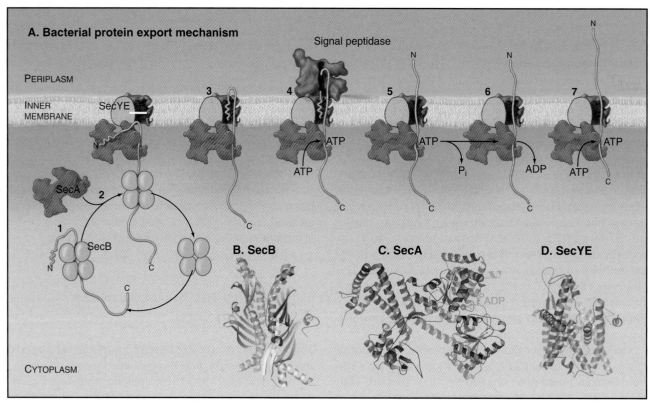

Figure 18-9 Secretion of proteins from bacteria through the SecYE translocon. **A,** Pathway of secretion. *1,* After synthesis by a cytoplasmic ribosome, the polypeptide associates with the SecB chaperone. *2,* SecA binds the presequence (*blue*) and docks on the SecYE translocon. *3,* The presequence inserts into the translocon. *4,* ATP-binding to SecA promotes insertion of the associated polypeptide into the translocon, followed by cleavage of the signal sequence. *5-7,* The membrane potential and cycles of ATP hydrolysis by SecA drive the polypeptide across the inner membrane. **B,** Ribbon diagram of *Haemophilus influenzae* SecB. **C,** Ribbon diagram of *Bacillus subtilis* SecA. **D,** Ribbon diagram of *Methanococcus jannaschii* SecY complex translocon. (A, Modified from Danese PN, Silhavy TJ: Targeting and assembly of periplasmic and outer-membrane proteins in *E. coli.* Annu Rev Genet 32:59–94, 1999. B, PDB file: IOZB. Reference: Zhou J, Xu Z: Structural determinants of SecB recognition by SecA in bacterial protein translocation. Nature Struct Biol 10:942–948, 2003. C, PDB file: 1TF2. Reference: Osborne AR, Clemons WM, Rapoport TA: A large conformational change of the translocation ATPase SecA. PNAS 101:10937–10942, 2004. D, PDB file: 1RHZ. Reference: van de Berg B, Clemons WM, Collinson I, et al: X-ray structure of a protein-conducting channel. Nature 427:36–44, 2004.)

Bacterial Protein Export

Bacteria employ at least 10 distinct strategies to transport proteins from the cytoplasm across the inner membrane and beyond. Seven of these pathways use a common pore across the inner membrane called the Sec translocon. These pathways are important because some contribute to human disease. In addition, they serve as important model systems, as eukaryotes use a homologous translocon to move proteins into the bilayer or lumen of the endoplasmic reticulum (see Fig. 20-6). This section begins with a discussion of six branches of the Sec secretory pathway and finishes with three distinct pathways.

Pathways Dependent on the SecYE Translocon

Organisms in all three domains of life use Sec translocons to move proteins synthesized in the cytoplasm across membranes. Translocons in the plasma membranes of Bacteria and Archaea consist of two transmembrane proteins called SecY and SecE in Bacteria (Fig. 18-9). The translocons of the endoplasmic reticulum of eukaryotes consist of homologous protein subunits called Sec61α and γ (see Fig. 20-6). The narrow pore for translocating the secreted polypeptide is located in the middle of a bundle of α-helices. Loss of function mutations of SecY or SecE compromise the secretion of most proteins by Bacteria or Archaea. Several accessory subunits assist in translocation, but they are not essential in Bacteria or present in eukaryotes.

Posttranslational Protein Translocation

Bacteria use **Sec-signal sequences** to direct many proteins to the SecYE translocon for transport across the plasma membrane or for insertion into the plasma membrane. Gram positive bacteria such as *Bacillus subtilis* lack an outer membrane, so the proteins leave the cell after crossing the plasma membrane. In gram-negative bacteria, translocated proteins enter the periplasm, insert into the outer membrane, or leave the cell.

Proteins targeted to the Sec translocon are synthesized in the cytoplasm with an N-terminal Sec-signal sequence. These targeting sequences consist of about 25 residues beginning with methionine, followed by a few basic residues, 10 to 15 hydrophobic residues, and a site for cleavage by a proteolytic enzyme called signal peptidase after translocation across the inner membrane. Chaperones such as **SecB** bind newly synthesized proteins to prevent folding and maintain a state that is competent for translocation (Fig. 18-9). Unlike most other chaperones (see Fig. 17-13), SecB does not require ATP hydrolysis for cycles of interaction with substrates. Hsp70 homologs (DnaK) have a secondary role in chaperoning precursors for translocation.

Translocation of many bacterial membrane and secreted proteins with cleavable signal sequences depend on the adenosine triphosphatase (ATPase) **SecA.** SecA binds proteins associated with SecB in the cytoplasm and targets the signal sequence to the Sec translocon. A system reconstituted from purified SecA, SecY, and SecE can translocate precursor proteins across lipid membranes in the presence of ATP. Remarkably, Archaea lack SecA, despite the fact that they depend on translocon components that are homologous to SecYE. Eukaryotes use SecA only for translocation into chloroplast thylakoids (Fig. 18-2).

The actual translocation step requires ATP hydrolysis by SecA. ATP binds SecA between two domains similar to DNA helicases, and other domains create a potential binding site for an extended peptide substrate. SecA can assume several different conformations. It is postulated that SecA ratchets the polypeptide through SecY and across the membrane during a cycle of conformational changes that couple ATP binding and hydrolysis with binding substrate peptides. The details are still being investigated, but the passage through SecY is so narrow that SecA cannot itself insert into the translocation pore. SecY also "proofreads" the signal sequence associated with SecA, releasing those with defects prior to translocation.

Signal peptidases located on the outer surface of the plasma membrane cleave signal peptides from translocated proteins soon after they cross the plasma membrane. Some bacterial signal peptidases are similar to eukaryotic homologs. Other bacterial signal peptidases are specialized to cleave lipoproteins just before an invariant cysteine. This cysteine is then conjugated to diacylglycerol, which anchors the lipoprotein to the outer surface of the plasma membrane or to the outer membrane of gram-negative bacteria. Signal peptidases also degrade cleaved signal peptides.

Translocation Dependent on the Signal Recognition Particle

In eukaryotes, the **signal recognition particle** (SRP) is the adapter between signal sequences and the translocon of endoplasmic reticulum (see Fig. 20-3), but in bacteria, only a minority of integral membrane proteins and secreted proteins depend on SRP for targeting to the Sec translocon. Eukaryotic and archaeal SRPs consist of a 7S RNA and several proteins, whereas *Escherichia coli* SRP consists of a smaller 4.5S RNA and a single protein called Ffh (for "fifty-four homologue," after its eukaryotic counterpart) (see Fig. 20-5). SRP binds Sec-signal sequences and signal-anchor sequences as they emerge from the ribosome. This interaction stops translation until SRP docks on the cytoplasmic surface of the inner membrane with its receptor FtsY and the Sec translocon. Resumption of translation drives the polypeptide through the translocon. See Chapter 20 for more details on SRP and eukaryotic cotranslational translocation.

Proteins inserted into the inner membrane depend on another protein, YidC, to move laterally out of the translocon into the lipid bilayer. A subset of proteins uses YidC to insert into the inner membrane independent of the Sec translocon. Homologs of YidC called Oxa1p and Alb3 direct proteins into the inner membrane of mitochondria and thylakoid membranes of chloroplasts.

Insertion of Proteins in the Outer Membrane of Gram-Negative Bacteria

Outer membrane proteins are synthesized in the cytoplasm and directed to the Sec translocon by signal sequences. The signal sequence is cleaved from the unfolded protein after crossing the inner membrane into the periplasm. No specific targeting signals are known for outer membrane proteins, so their localization likely depends on their tertiary structure. Individual protein subunits fold and then associate to form dimers and trimers (see Fig. 7-8C) before, or possibly after, insertion into the outer membrane. Several periplasmic assembly factors participate in protein folding, including enzymes that catalyze the isomerization of proline peptide bonds and oxidation/reduction of cysteine thiol groups.

Outer Membrane Autotransporter Pathway

Some proteins, including secreted proteolytic enzymes and toxins as well as membrane-anchored adhesins and invasins, hitch a ride to the cell surface on their own

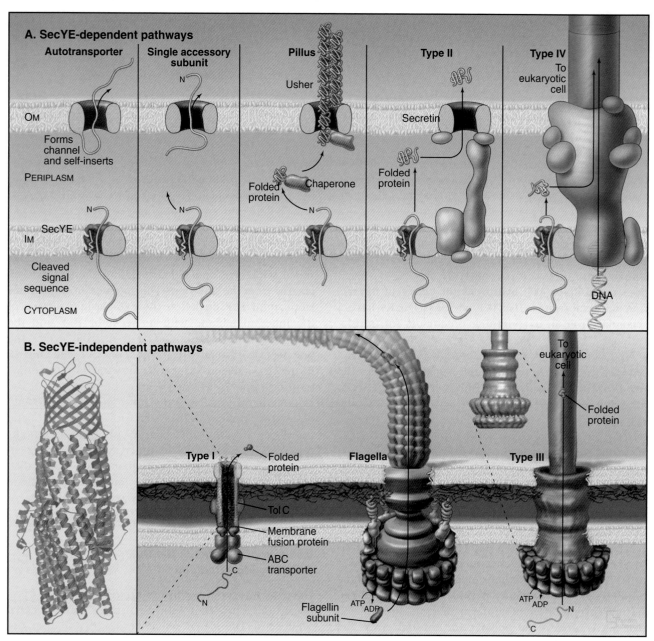

Figure 18-10 SECRETION ACROSS THE OUTER MEMBRANE OF GRAM-NEGATIVE BACTERIA. **A,** Pathways dependent on SecYE. The cleaved signal sequence is shown in *blue*. The β-domain of autotransporters forms a pore for the translocation of part of its own chain, which may remain attached, as shown, or be cleaved for escape from the cell. Single accessory proteins form a pore for secretion of separate proteins. Usher forms a pore for the translocation and assembly of pili. Type II secretion uses a secretin pore for translocation. Type IV secretion employs a large translocon similar to that used by *Agrobacterium* for secretion of DNA. **B,** Pathways independent of SecYE. Type I secretion uses an ABC transporter to cross the inner membrane and additional subunits to cross the periplasm and outer membrane. **Left panel,** Ribbon model of TolC, one type of translocon that spans the periplasm and outer membrane. **Right panel,** Each TolC subunit contributes four β-strands to a porin-like structure that spans the outer membrane. α-Helical continuations of these β-strands form a tube having an internal diameter of 3.5 nm for transport of proteins across the periplasm. Bacterial flagella transport flagellin subunits across both membranes and then through the central channel of the flagellar filament for incorporation at the growing tip. Type III secretion uses components similar to the basal body of flagella. *Gray* illustration *(far right)* shows a three-dimensional reconstruction of the type III secretion apparatus from *Salmonella typhimurium.* IM, inner membrane; OM, outer membrane. (A–B, Drawings based on Thanassi DG, Hultgren SJ: Multiple pathways allow protein secretion across the bacterial outer membrane. Curr Opin Cell Biol 12:420–430, 2000. B, TolC ribbon diagram based on PDB file: 1EK9. Reference: Koronakis V, Sharff A, Koronakis E, et al: Crystal structure of the bacterial membrane protein TolC central to multidrug efflux and protein export. Nature 405:914–919, 2000. Reconstruction of the type III secretion complex from *S. typhimurium* based on Marlovits TC, Kubori T, Sukhan A, et al: Structural insights into the assembly of the type II secretion needle complex. Science 306:1040–1042, 2004.)

outer membrane transporters (Fig. 18-10A). These proteins are fused to a C-terminal β-domain that is thought to be similar to a porin (see Fig. 7-8). The protein uses the Sec pathway to cross the inner membrane and inserts into the outer membrane. The N-terminal functional domain then translocates across the outer membrane through its β-domain pore. An outer membrane protease releases toxins and proteases, whereas adhesins that follow this route remain on the surface attached to the β-domain.

Outer Membrane Single Accessory Pathway

Some hemolysins and hemagglutinins move to the periplasm through the Sec pathway and then use a single accessory protein to translocate across the outer membrane. The accessory protein is thought to form an outer membrane pore like the β-domain of autotransporters, but there is no sequence homology except with chloroplast outer membrane porins that transport peptides.

Chaperone/Usher Pathway

Gram-negative bacteria use a novel mechanism, downstream of the Sec pathway, to transport and assemble pili on their outer surface. These appendages are involved with bacterial pathogenesis, including urinary tract infections. A periplasmic chaperone binds the pillus peptide and promotes folding. The pilus subunit is folded similar to an immunoglobulin (Ig) domain (see Fig. 3-13), but lacking the seventh β-strand. This exposes core hydrophobic residues. The chaperone consists of two immunoglobulin-like domains, one of which donates a strand to complete the immunoglobulin domain of the pilus subunit. The chaperone delivers a pilus subunit to an outer membrane translocon called usher (Fig. 18-10A). There, it transfers its bound subunit to the end of a growing chain of pilus subunits, all bound together, head to tail, by strands that complete the seven-strand β-sheet of the adjacent subunit. On the outer surface, the pilus subunits rearrange into a helical pilus. The assembly reaction is thought to provide the energy for translocation. The chaperone prevents premature assembly of the pilus.

Type II Secretion

Bacteria use an alternate route downstream of the Sec pathway to secrete other toxins and enzymes with cleaved signal sequences (Fig. 18-10A). At least a dozen protein subunits participate in this complicated pathway. The pore in the outer membrane is composed of a secretin, a protein with relatives that also participate in type III secretion, phage biogenesis, and formation of one type of pilus. The secretin pore is a ring of 12 to 14 subunits around a large but gated channel that is 5 to 10 nm in diameter.

Type IV Secretion

Bacteria secrete a few proteins using an apparatus similar to that used for DNA transfer between two bacteria during conjugation and for DNA injection into plant cells by *Agrobacterium*. DNA is transferred directly from the cytoplasm of one bacterium to the cytoplasm of another bacterium or plant cell. Proteins that are secreted by this pathway include pertussis toxin by *Borditella pertussis* and another toxin by *Helicobacter pylori*. This pathway starts with synthesis in the cytoplasm and translocation across the plasma membrane by the Sec translocon. If present, the signal sequence is cleaved before translocation across the outer membrane by the type IV secretion system (Fig. 18-10A).

Pathways Independent of the SEC Translocon

Type I ABC Transporters

Bacteria use ABC transporters (see Fig. 8-9) to secrete a small number of toxins (e.g., *E. coli* hemolysin), proteases, and lipases. C-terminal signal sequences of 30 to 60 residues target these proteins to the ABC transporter, the only component required for secretion by gram-positive bacteria. Gram-negative bacteria require not only a transporter in the inner membrane but also two proteins that form a continuous channel across the periplasm and outer membrane (Fig. 18-10B). ATP hydrolysis by the ABC transporter provides energy for translocation. Protein conduits across the periplasm and outer membrane engage ABC transporters presenting substrates for export and then disengage when translocation is complete. Genes for secreted proteins are generally in the same operon as the export machinery.

Flagellar and Type III Secretion Systems

The basal bodies of bacterial flagella transport flagellin subunits through a central pore that crosses both membranes (Fig. 18-10B) and extends the length of the flagellar shaft to the tip, where subunits add to the distal end (see Fig. 5-9). This flagellar pathway transports a few other proteins, including a phospholipase that contributes to the virulence of *Yersinia*, the cause of the black plague.

Pathogenic gram-negative bacteria, such as *Yersinia*, use the syringe-like type III apparatus, similar to a bacterial flagellum, to transport toxins from the cytoplasm into the medium or directly into target cells. In the target cell, these toxins disrupt cellular physiology, including formation of pores in target cell membranes. The type III secretion complex consists of about 20 different protein subunits. A complex base consisting of several protein rings spans the periplasm and both membranes. A polymer of a single protein forms a hollow needle up to 40 nm long for injection of toxins directly into target animal or plant cells.

Several signals direct proteins to this pathway. One signal is a protein sequence that binds a chaperone dedicated to targeting toxins to the type III pathway. Remarkably, the mRNA itself might direct some proteins to this pathway. A cytoplasmic ATPase provides energy for transport.

Double Arginine Pathway

Many but not all Bacteria and Archaea use proteins homologous to chloroplast Tat proteins to translocate proteins across the plasma membrane. In both prokaryotes and chloroplasts, some of these cargo proteins participate in redox reactions and have bound cofactors such as flavins or FeS clusters. These cofactors are incorporated as the proteins fold in the cytoplasm or chloroplast stroma. So in contrast to the Sec translocon, the Tat translocon accommodates (or might even require) folded proteins. The N-terminal signal sequences for this pathway have a pair of arginines (RR) in a conserved sequence (Ser/Thr-Arg-Arg-X-Phe-Leu-Lys, where X is any amino acid) adjacent to a stretch of at least 13 uncharged residues. Translocation of these proteins in *E. coli* requires three Tat proteins. One forms the transmembrane pore, and the others appear to participate in targeting.

ACKNOWLEDGMENT

Thanks go to Mecky Pohlschroder for suggestions on revisions to this chapter.

SELECTED READINGS

Chen X, Schnell DJ: Protein import into chloroplasts. Trends Cell Biol 9:222-227, 1999.

Danese PN, Silhavy TJ: Targeting and assembly of periplasmic and outer-membrane proteins in *E. coli*. Annu Rev Genet 32:59-94, 1999.

Gutensohn M, Fan E, Frielingsdorf S, et al: Toc, Tic, Tat et al.: Structure and function of protein transport machines in chloroplasts. J Plant Physiol 163:333-347, 2006.

Keegstra K, Cline K: Protein import and routing systems of chloroplasts. Plant Cell 11:557-570, 1999.

Keegstra K, Froehlich JE: Protein import into chloroplasts. Curr Opin Cell Biol 2:471-476, 1999.

Koehler CM: New developments in mitochondrial assembly. Annu Rev Cell Devel Biol 20:309-335, 2004.

Koehler CM: The small TIM proteins and the twin Cx3C motif. Trends Biochem Sci 29:1-4, 2004.

Lazarow PB: Peroxisome biogenesis: Advances and conundrums. Curr Opin Cell Biol 15:489-497, 2003.

Nassoury N, Morse, D: Protein targeting to the chloroplast of photosynthetic eukaryotes: Getting there is half the fun. Biochim Biophys Acta 1743:5-19, 2005.

Pfanner N: Protein sorting: Recognizing mitochondrial presequences. Curr Biol 10:R412-415, 2000.

Pohlschroeder M, Dilks K, Hand NJ, Rose RW: Translocation of proteins across archaeal cytoplasmic membranes. FEMS Microbiol Rev 28:3-24, 2003.

Thanassi DG, Hultgren SJ: Multiple pathways allow protein secretion across the bacterial outer membrane. Curr Opin Cell Biol 12:420-430, 2000.

APPENDIX 18-1

*Peroxin Features and Known Roles**

Peroxin	Features	Functions	Relation to Disease
PEX1	AAA ATPase	Matrix protein import	Mutated in CG1
PEX2	Zinc-binding PMP	Matrix protein import	Mutated in CG10
PEX3	Orphan PMP	Membrane biogenesis	Mutated in CG12
PEX4	UBC	Matrix protein import	?
PEX5	PTS1 receptor	Matrix protein import	Mutated in CG2
PEX6	AAA ATPase	Matrix protein import	Mutated in CG4
PEX7	PTS2 receptor	Matrix protein import	Mutated in CG11
PEX8	PMP	Matrix protein import	?
PEX9	PMP	Matrix protein import	?
PEX10	Zinc-binding PMP	Matrix protein import	Mutated in CG7
PEX11	PMP	Peroxisome division	?
PEX12	Zinc-binding PMP	Matrix protein import	Mutated in CG3
PEX13	SH3 PMP	Matrix protein import	Mutated in CG13
PEX14	Docking PEX5/7	Matrix protein import	?
PEX15	Orphan PMP	Matrix protein import	?
PEX16	Orphan PMP	Membrane biogenesis	Mutated in CG9
PEX17	Orphan PMP	Matrix protein import	?
PEX18	PEX7 binding	Matrix protein import	?
PEX19	PMP receptor	Membrane biogenesis	Mutated in CG14
PEX20	Thiolase binding	Matrix protein import	?
PEX21	PEX7 binding	Matrix protein import	?
PEX22	PEX4 binding	Matrix protein import	?
PEX23	PMP	Matrix protein import	?

*PEX5 and PEX7 are import receptors for newly synthesized peroxisomal enzymes. Most other peroxins are also required for matrix enzyme import. Peroxins PEX3, PEX11, PEX16, and PEX19 are implicated in peroxisome membrane biogenesis rather than matrix protein import. AAA, AAA family of ATPases; CG, complementation group of patients with peroxisomal biogenesis disorders; PMP, peroxisomal membrane protein; SH3, Src-homology-3 domain; UBC, ubiquitin-conjugating enzyme. "Orphans" are novel proteins.

CHAPTER 19

Mitochondria, Chloroplasts, Peroxisomes

This chapter considers three organelles formed by posttranslational import of proteins synthesized in the cytoplasm. Mitochondria and chloroplasts both arose from endosymbiotic bacteria, two singular events that occurred about one billion years apart. Both mitochondria and chloroplasts retain remnants of those prokaryotic genomes but depend largely on genes that were transferred to the nucleus of the host eukaryote. Both organelles brought biochemical mechanisms that allow their eukaryotic hosts to acquire and utilize energy more efficiently. In **oxidative phosphorylation** by mitochondria and **photosynthesis** by chloroplasts, energy from the breakdown of nutrients or from absorption of photons is used to energize electrons. As these electrons tunnel through transmembrane proteins, energy is partitioned off to create proton gradients. These proton gradients drive the rotary ATP synthase (see Fig. 8-5) to make adenosine triphosphate (ATP), which is used as energy currency to power the cell. Peroxisomes contain no genes and depend entirely on nuclear genes to encode their proteins. Their evolutionary origins are obscure. Peroxisomes contain enzymes that catalyze oxidation reactions that are essential for normal human physiology. Patients who lack peroxisomes have severe neural defects.

Mitochondria

Evolution and Structure of Mitochondria

Mitochondria (Fig. 19-1) arose about 2 billion years ago when a Bacterium fused with an archaeal cell or established a symbiotic relationship with a primitive eukaryotic cell (see Fig. 2-5 and associated text). The details are not preserved in the fossil record, but the bacterial origins of mitochondria are apparent in their many common features (Fig. 19-2). The closest extant relatives of the Bacterium that gave rise to mitochondria are *Rickettsia*, aerobic α-proteobacteria with a genome of 1.1 megabase pairs. These intracellular pathogens cause typhus and Rocky Mountain spotted fever. However, some evidence argues that the actual progenitor bacterium had the genes required for both aerobic and anaerobic metabolism.

As primitive eukaryotes diverged from each other, most of the bacterial genes were lost or moved to the nuclei of the host eukaryotes. The pace of the gene transfer to the nucleus varied considerably depending on the species, but all known mitochondria retain some bacterial genes. A very few eukaryotes, such as *Entamoeba*, that branched

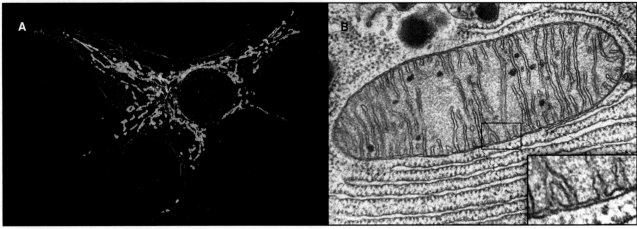

Figure 19-1 CELLULAR DISTRIBUTION AND STRUCTURE OF MITOCHONDRIA. **A,** Fluorescence light micrograph of a Cos-7 tissue culture cell with mitochondria labeled with *green* fluorescent antibody to the β-subunit of the F1-ATPase and microtubules labeled *red* with an antibody. **B,** Electron micrograph of a thin section of a mitochondrion. (A, Courtesy of Michael Yaffee, University of California, San Diego. B, Courtesy of Don Fawcett, Harvard Medical School, Boston, Massachusetts.)

well after their ancestors acquired mitochondria lost the organelle, leaving behind a few mitochondrial genes in the nucleus.

Chromosomes of contemporary mitochondria vary in size from 366,924 base pairs (bp) in the plant *Arabidopsis* to only 5966 bp in *Plasmodium*. These small, usually circular genomes encode RNAs and proteins that are essential for mitochondrial function, including some subunits of proteins responsible for adenosine triphosphate (ATP) synthesis. The highly pared-down human mitochondrial genome with 16,569 bp encodes only 13 mitochondrial membrane proteins, two ribosomal RNAs, and just enough tRNAs (22) to translate these genes. The number of proteins encoded by other mitochondrial genomes ranges from just 3 in *Plasmodium* to 97 in a protozoan. Nuclear genes encode the other 600 to 1000 mitochondria proteins, including those required to synthesize proteins in the matrix. All mitochondrial proteins that are encoded by nuclear genes are synthesized in the cytoplasm and subsequently imported into mitochondria (see Figs. 18-2 and 18-3).

Mitochondria consist of two membrane-bounded compartments, one inside the other (Fig. 19-2). The **outer membrane** surrounds the **intermembranous space**. The **inner membrane** surrounds the **matrix.** Each membrane and compartment has a distinct protein composition and functions. **Porins** in the outer membrane provide channels for passage of molecules of less than 5000 D, including most metabolites required for ATP synthesis. The highly impermeable inner membrane is specialized for converting energy provided by breakdown of nutrients in the matrix into ATP. Four complexes (I to IV) of integral membrane proteins use the transport of energetic electrons to create a gradient of protons across the inner membrane. The F1F0 ATP

synthase (see Fig. 8-5) utilizes the proton gradient to synthesize ATP. The area of inner membrane available for these reactions is increased by folds called **cristae** that vary in number and shape depending on the species, tissue, and metabolic state. Cristae may be tubular or flattened sacs. Contacts between the inner and outer membranes are sites of protein import (see Fig. 18-4).

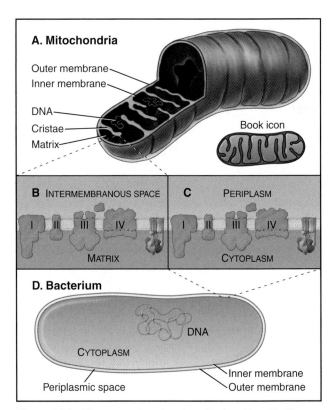

Figure 19-2 The compartments of a mitochondrion **(A–B)** compared with a Bacterium **(C–D).** Respiratory chain complexes I to IV are labeled with roman numerals.

Proteins in the intermembranous space participate in ATP synthesis but, when released into the cytoplasm, trigger programmed cell death (see Fig. 46-15).

Biogenesis of Mitochondria

Mitochondria grow by importing most of their proteins from the cytoplasm and by internal synthesis of some proteins and replication of the genome (Fig. 19-3). Targeting and sorting signals built into the mitochondrial proteins that are synthesized in the cytoplasm direct them to their destinations (see Fig. 18-4).

Similar to cells, mitochondria divide, but unlike most cells, they also fuse with other mitochondria. These fusion and division reactions were first observed nearly one hundred years ago. Now it is appreciated that a balance between ongoing fusion and division determines the number of mitochondria within a cell. Both fusion and division depend on proteins with guanosine triphosphatase (GTPase) domains related to dynamin (see Fig. 22-11). In fact, eukaryotes might have acquired their dynamin genes from the bacterium that became mitochondria.

One dynamin-related GTPase is required for division of mitochondria. This GTPase self-assembles into spirals that appear to pinch mitochondria in two. During apoptosis (see Chapter 46), this GTPase also participates in the fragmentation of mitochondria.

Fusion involves two GTPases, one anchored in the outer membrane and the other in the inner membrane, both linked by an adapter protein in the intermembrane space. Fusion of the outer membranes requires a proton gradient across the inner membrane, while fusion of the inner membranes depends on the electrical potential across the inner membrane. Loss of function mutations in fusion proteins lead to cells with numerous small mitochondria, some lacking a mtDNA molecule. Human

mutations in the genes for fusion proteins result in defects in the myelin sheath that insulates axons (one form of Charcot-Marie-Tooth disease) and the atrophy of the optic nerve. Mitochondrial fusion proteins are also required for apoptosis.

Synthesis of ATP by Oxidative Phosphorylation

Mitochondria use energy extracted from the chemical bonds of nutrients to generate a proton gradient across the inner membrane. This proton gradient drives the F1F0 ATP synthase to synthesize ATP from ADP and inorganic phosphate. Enzymes in the inner membrane and matrix cooperate with pumps, carriers, and electron transport proteins in the inner membrane to move electrons, protons, and other energetic intermediates across the impermeable inner membrane. This is a classic chemiosmotic process (see Fig. 11-1).

Mitochondria receive energy-yielding chemical intermediates from two ancient metabolic pathways, **glycolysis** and **fatty acid oxidation** (Fig. 19-4), that evolved in the common ancestor of living things. Both pathways feed into the equally ancient **citric acid cycle** of energy-yielding reactions in the mitochondrial matrix:

- The glycolytic pathway in cytoplasm converts the six-carbon sugar glucose into pyruvate, a three-carbon substrate for pyruvate dehydrogenase, a large, soluble, enzyme complex in the mitochondrial matrix. The products of pyruvate dehydrogenase (carbon dioxide, the reduced form of nicotinamide adenine dinucleotide [**NADH**], and acetyl coenzyme A [-CoA]) are released into the matrix. NADH is a high-energy electron carrier. **Acetyl-CoA** is a two-carbon metabolic intermediate that supplies the citric acid cycle with energy-rich bonds.

- Breakdown of lipids yields fatty acids linked to acetyl-CoA by a thioester bond. These intermediates are transported across the inner membrane of mitochondria, using carnitine in a shuttle system. In the matrix, acyl-carnitine is reconverted to acyl-CoA. Enzymes in the matrix degrade fatty acids two carbons at a time in a series of oxidative reactions that yield NADH, the reduced form of flavin adenine dinucleotide (**FADH$_2$**, another energy-rich electron carrier associated with an integral membrane enzyme complex), and acetyl-CoA for the citric acid cycle.

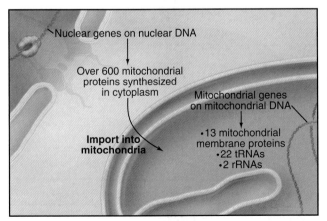

Figure 19-3 **BIOGENESIS OF MITOCHONDRIA.** The drawing shows the relative contributions of nuclear and mitochondrial genes to the protein composition.

Breakdown of acetyl-CoA during one turn of the citric acid cycle produces three molecules of NADH,

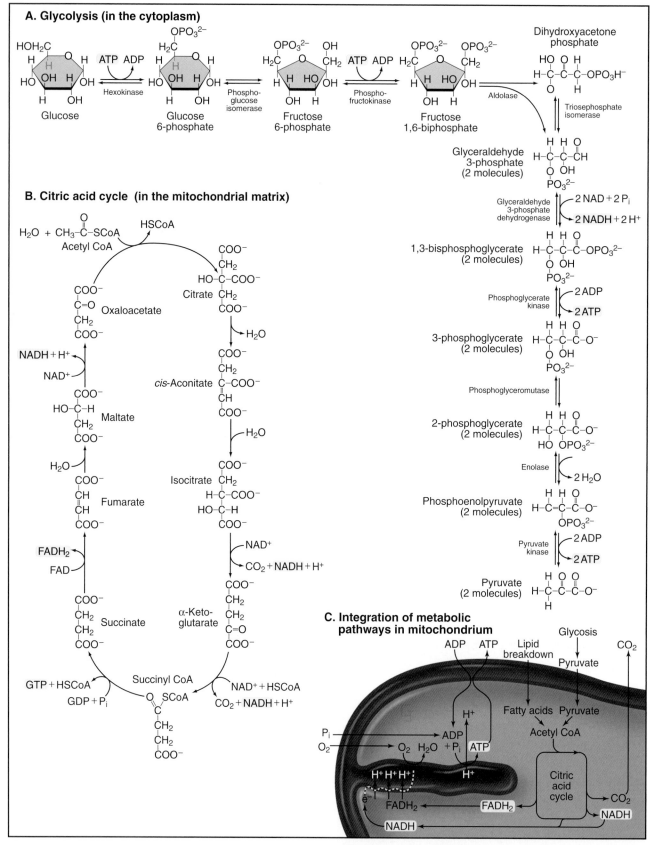

Figure 19-4 METABOLIC PATHWAYS SUPPLYING ENERGY FOR OXIDATIVE PHOSPHORYLATION. **A,** Glycolysis. **B,** Citric acid cycle. Production of acetyl-CoA by the glycolytic pathway in cytoplasm and fatty acid oxidation in the mitochondrial matrix drive the citric acid cycle in the mitochondrial matrix. This energy-yielding cycle is also called the Krebs cycle after the biochemist H. Krebs. NADH and FADH$_2$ produced by these pathways supply high-energy electrons to the electron transport chain. **C,** Overview of metabolic pathways. Note energy-rich metabolites *(yellow)*.

one molecule of $FADH_2$, and two molecules of carbon dioxide. Energetic electrons donated by NADH and $FADH_2$ drive an **electron transport pathway** in the inner mitochondrial membrane that powers a chemiosmotic cycle to produce ATP (Fig. 19-5). Electrons use two routes to pass through three protein complexes in the inner mitochondrial membrane. Starting with NADH, electrons pass through complex I to complex III to complex IV. Electrons from $FADH_2$ pass through complex II to complex III to complex IV. Along both routes, energy is partitioned off to transfer multiple protons (at least 10 electrons per NADH oxidized) across

the inner mitochondrial membrane from the matrix to the inner membrane space. The resulting electrochemical gradient of protons drives ATP synthesis (see Fig. 8-5).

This process is called **oxidative phosphorylation,** since molecular oxygen is the sink for energy-bearing electrons at the end of the pathway and since the reactions add phosphate to ADP. Eukaryotes that live in environments with little or no oxygen use other acceptors for these electrons and produce nitrite, nitric oxide, or other reduced products rather than water. Oxidative phosphorylation is understood in remarkable detail,

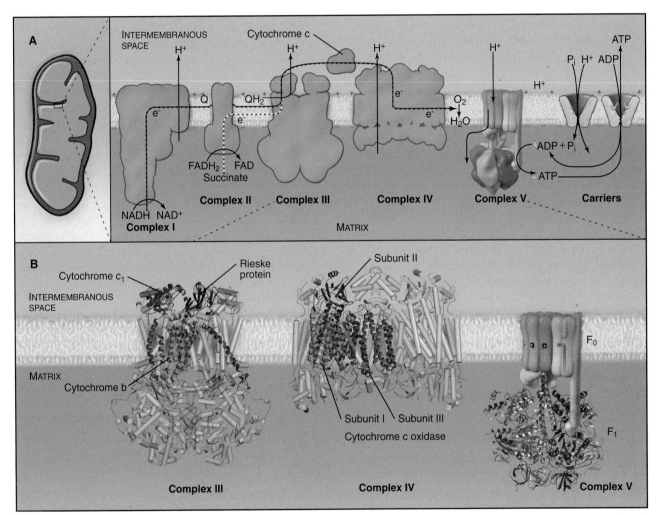

Figure 19-5 CHEMIOSMOTIC CYCLE OF THE RESPIRATORY ELECTRON TRANSPORT CHAIN AND ATP SYNTHASE. **A, left panel,** A mitochondrion for orientation. **Right panel,** The electron transport system of the inner mitochondrial membrane. Note the pathway of electrons through the four complexes (*red* and *yellow arrows*) and the sites of proton translocation between the matrix to the intermembranous space (*black arrows*). The stoichiometry is not specified, but at the last step, four electrons are required to reduce oxygen to water. ATP synthase uses the electrochemical proton gradient produced by the electron transport reactions to drive ATP synthesis. **B,** The available atomic structures of the electron transport chain are shown. In the cytochrome bc_1 complex III, the 3 of 11 mitochondrial subunits used by bacteria are shown as ribbon models. The supporting subunits found in mitochondria are shown as cylinders. The four subunits of complex IV encoded by the mitochondrial genome are shown as ribbon models. They form the functional core of the complex, which is supported by additional subunits shown as cylinders. See Figure 8-4 for further details of ATP synthase (complex V). (B, Images of complex III and complex IV courtesy of M. Saraste, European Molecular Biology Laboratory, Heidelberg, Germany. Reference: Zhang Z, Huang L, Schulmeister VM, et al: Electron transfer by domain movement in cytochrome bc_1. Nature 392:677–684, 1998. PDB file: 1BCC. Reference: Yoshikawa S, Shinzawa-Itoh K, Nakashima R, et al: Redox-coupled crystal structural changes in bovine heart cytochrome c oxidase. Science 280:1723–1729, 1998. PDB file: 2OCC.)

thanks to atomic structures of ATP synthase and three of the four electron transfer complexes. Nuclear genes encode most of the protein subunits of these complexes, but mitochondrial genes are responsible for a few key subunits.

Bacteria and mitochondria share homologous proteins for the key steps in oxidative phosphorylation (Fig. 19-2), but the machinery in mitochondria is usually more complex. Thus, bacteria are useful model systems with which to study the common mechanisms. Plasma membranes of bacteria and inner membranes of mitochondria have equivalent components, and the bacterial cytoplasm corresponds to the mitochondrial matrix (Fig. 19-2).

Energy enters this pathway in the form of electrons that are produced when NADH is oxidized to NAD^+, releasing one H^+ and two electrons (Fig. 19-5). If the proton and electrons were to combine immediately with oxygen, their energy would be lost as heat. Instead, these high-energy electrons are separated from the protons and then passed along the electron transport pathway before finally recombining to reduce molecular oxygen to form water. Along the pathway, electrons associate transiently with a series of oxidation/reduction acceptors, generally metal ions associated with organic cofactors, such as hemes in cytochromes and iron-sulfur centers (2Fe2S) and copper centers in complex IV. Electrons move along the transport pathway at rates of up to $1000 \ s^{-1}$. To travel at this rate through a transmembrane protein complex spanning a 35-nm lipid bilayer, at least three redox cofactors are required in each complex, because the efficiency of quantum mechanical tunneling of electrons between redox cofactors falls off rapidly with distance. Two cofactors, even with optimal orientation, would be too slow.

Step by step, electrons give up energy as they move along the transport pathway. In three complexes along the pathway, this energy is used to pump protons from the matrix to the inner membrane space. This establishes an electrochemical proton gradient across the inner mitochondrial membrane that is used by **ATP synthase** to drive ATP production. Direction is provided to the movements of electrons by progressive increases in the electron affinity of the acceptors. The final acceptor, oxygen (at the end of the pathway), has the highest affinity.

The first component of the electron transport pathway is called **complex I** (or NADH:ubiquinone oxidoreductase). Vertebrate mitochondrial complex I with 46 different protein subunits is more complex than bacterial complex I with 14 subunits. NADH donates two electrons to flavin mononucleotide associated with protein subunits located on the matrix side of the inner membrane. A crystal structure of the cytoplasmic domain of the bacterial complex shows the path for the electrons from flavin mononucleotide through seven iron sulfur clusters to quinone in the lipid bilayer. For each molecule of NADH oxidized, the transmembrane domains of complex I transfer four protons from the matrix into the inner membrane space.

The second component of the electron transport pathway is **complex II** or succinate:ubiquinone reductase, a transmembrane enzyme that makes up part of the citric acid cycle. Complex II couples oxidation of succinate (a four-carbon intermediate in the citric acid cycle) to fumarate with reduction of flavin adenine dinucleotide (FAD) to $FADH_2$. Complex II does not pump protons but transfers electrons from $FADH_2$ to ubiquinone. Reduced ubiquinone carries these electrons to complex III.

The third component of the electron transport pathway is **complex III**, also called **cytochrome bc_1.** This well-characterized, transmembrane protein complex consists of 11 different subunits. The homologous bacterial complex has only three of these subunits, the ones that participate in energy transduction in mitochondria. Eight other subunits surround this core. Complex III couples the oxidation and reduction of ubiquinone to the transfer of protons from the matrix across the inner mitochondrial membrane. Energy is supplied by electrons that move through the cytochrome b subunit to a subunit with a 2Fe2S redox center. This subunit then rotates into position to transfer the electron to cytochrome c_1, another subunit of the complex. Cytochrome c_1 then transfers the electron to the water-soluble protein cytochrome c in the intermembranous space (or periplasm of bacteria).

Cytochrome oxidase, complex IV, takes electrons from four cytochrome c molecules to reduce molecular oxygen to two waters as well as to pump four protons out of the matrix. Mitochondrial genes encode the three subunits that form the core of this enzyme, carry out electron transfer, and translocate protons. Nuclear genes encode the surrounding 10 subunits.

The electrochemical proton gradient produced by the electron transport chain provides energy to synthesize ATP. Chapter 8 explained how the rotary ATP synthase (complex V) can either use ATP hydrolysis to pump protons or use the transit of protons down an electrochemical gradient to synthesize ATP (see Figs. 8-5 and 8-6). The proton gradient across the inner mitochondrial membrane drives rotation of the γ-subunit. The rotating γ-subunit physically changes the conformations of the α- and β-subunits, bringing together ADP and inorganic phosphate to make ATP. An antiporter in the inner membrane exchanges cytoplasmic ADP for ATP synthesized in the matrix (see Fig. 9-2A).

Mitochondria and Disease

As expected from the central role of mitochondria in energy metabolism, mitochondrial dysfunction contributes to a remarkable diversity of human diseases (Fig. 19-6) including seizures, strokes, optic atrophy, neuropathy, myopathy, cardiomyopathy, hearing loss, and Type 2 diabetes mellitus. These disorders arise from mutations in genes for mitochondrial proteins encoded by both mitochondrial DNA (mtDNA) and nuclear DNA. More than half of the known disease-causing mutations are in genes for mitochondrial transfer RNAs.

The existence of about 1000 copies of mtDNA per vertebrate cell influences the impact of deleterious mutations. A mutation in one copy would be of no consequence, but segregation of mtDNAs may lead to cells in which mutant mtDNAs predominate, yielding defective proteins. For example, a recurring point mutation in a subunit of complex I causes some patients to develop sudden onset of blindness in middle age owing to the death of neurons in the optic nerve. Patients with the same mutation in a larger fraction of mtDNA molecules suffer from muscle weakness and mental retardation as children. Mutations in the genes for subunits of ATP synthase cause muscle weakness and degeneration of the retina. Slow accumulation of mutations in mtDNA may contribute to some symptoms of aging.

Mutations in nuclear genes for mitochondrial proteins cause similar diseases (Fig. 19-6A). A mutation in one subunit of the protein import machinery (see Fig. 18-5), Tim8, causes a type of deafness.

Chloroplasts

Structure and Evolution of Photosynthesis Systems

Photosynthetic Bacteria and chloroplasts of algae and plants (Fig. 19-7) use **chlorophyll** to capture the remarkable amount of energy carried by single photons to boost electrons to an excited state. These high-energy electrons drive a chemiosmotic cycle to make NADPH and ATP, energy currency that is used by all cells. Photosynthetic organisms use ATP and the reducing power of NADPH to synthesize three-carbon sugar phosphates from carbon dioxide. Glycolytic reactions (Fig. 19-4) running backward use this three-carbon sugar phosphate to make six-carbon sugars and more complex carbohydrates for use as metabolic energy sources and structural components. Some Archaea, such as *Halobacteria halobium*, and some recently discovered Bacteria use a completely different light-driven pump lacking chlorophyll to generate a proton gradient to synthesize ATP. Retinol associated with bacteriorhodopsin absorbs light to drive proton transport (see Fig. 8-3).

Photosynthesis originated approximately 3.5 billion years ago in a Bacterium, most likely a gram-negative purple bacterium (see Fig. 2-4). These bacteria evolved

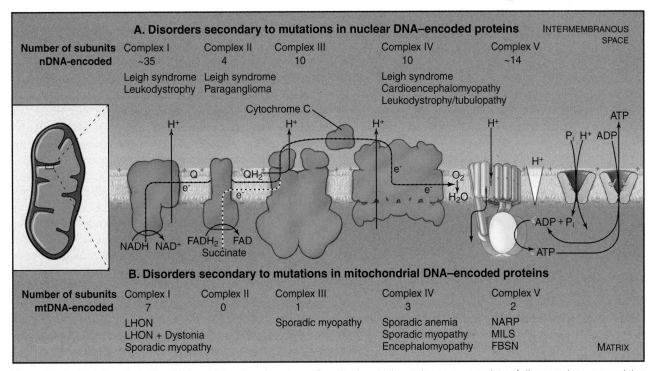

Figure 19-6 Mutations in both mitochondrial and nuclear genes for mitochondrial proteins cause a variety of diseases by compromising the function of particular mitochondrial subsystems. FBSN, familial bilateral striatal necrosis; LHON, Leber hereditary optic neuropathy; MILS, maternally inherited Leigh syndrome; NARP, neurogenic muscle weakness, ataxia, retinitis pigmentosa. (Adapted from Schon EA: Mitochondrial genetics and disease. Trends Biochem Sci 25:555–560, 2000.)

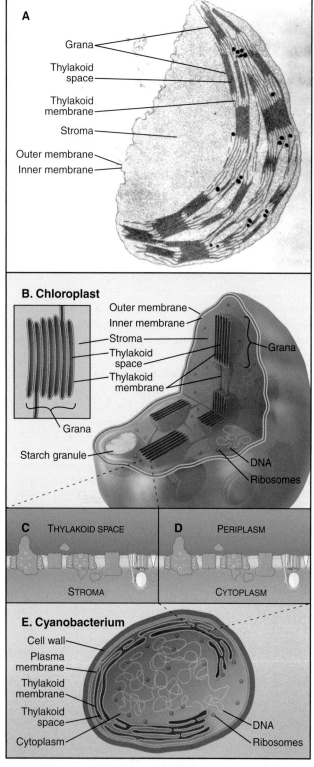

Figure 19-7 MORPHOLOGY OF CHLOROPLASTS AND CYANOBACTERIA. **A,** Electron micrograph of a thin section of a spinach chloroplast. **B,** Chloroplast. **C–D,** Comparison of the machinery in the photosynthetic membranes of chloroplasts and cyanobacteria. **E,** Drawing of a cyanobacterium illustrating the internal folds of the plasma membrane to form photosynthetic thylakoids. (A, Courtesy of K. Miller, Brown University, Providence, Rhode Island.)

components to assemble a transmembrane complex of proteins, pigments, and oxidation/reduction cofactors called a **reaction center** (Fig. 19-8). Reaction centers absorb light and initiate an electron transport pathway that pumps protons out of the cell. Such photosystems turn sunlight into electrical and chemical energy with 40% efficiency, better than any human-made photovoltaic cell. Given their alarming complexity and physical perfection, it is remarkable that photosystems emerged only a few hundred million years after the origin of life itself.

Broadly speaking, photosynthetic reaction centers of contemporary organisms can be divided into two different groups (Fig. 19-8). The reaction centers of purple bacteria and green filamentous bacteria utilize the pigment pheophytin and a quinone as the electron acceptor, similar to **photosystem II** of cyanobacteria and chloroplasts. The reaction centers of green sulfur bacteria and heliobacteria have iron-sulfur centers as electron acceptors, similar to **photosystem I** of cyanobacteria and chloroplasts.

Cyanobacteria are unique among Bacteria in that they have both types of photosystems as well as a manganese enzyme that splits water, releasing from two water molecules four electrons, four protons, and oxygen (Fig. 19-7E). Coupling this enzyme to photosynthesis was a pivotal event in the history of the earth, as this reaction is the source of most of the oxygen in the earth's atmosphere.

Chloroplasts of eukaryotic cells arose from a symbiotic cyanobacterium (see Fig. 2-8). Much evidence indicates that this event occurred just once, giving all chloroplasts a common origin. However, to account for chloroplasts in organisms that diverged prior to the acquisition of chloroplasts, one must also postulate lateral transfer of chloroplasts from, for example, a green alga to *Euglena*. Less likely, but not ruled out conclusively, cyanobacteria may have colonized eukaryotic cells on up to three different occasions, giving rise to organelles that evolved into chloroplasts.

Chloroplasts have retained up to 250 original bacterial genes on circular genomes, whereas many bacterial genes were lost or moved to the nucleus of host eukaryotes. Chloroplast genomes encode subunits of many proteins responsible for photosynthesis and chloroplast division, ribosomal RNAs and proteins, and a complete set of tRNAs. Chloroplast proteins encoded by nuclear genes are transported posttranslationally into chloroplasts (Fig. 18-6) after their synthesis in cytoplasm.

The organization of cyanobacterial membranes explains the architecture of chloroplasts (Fig. 19-7C–E). In cyanobacteria, light-absorbing pigments, as well as protein complexes involved with electron transport and ATP synthesis, are concentrated in invaginations of the

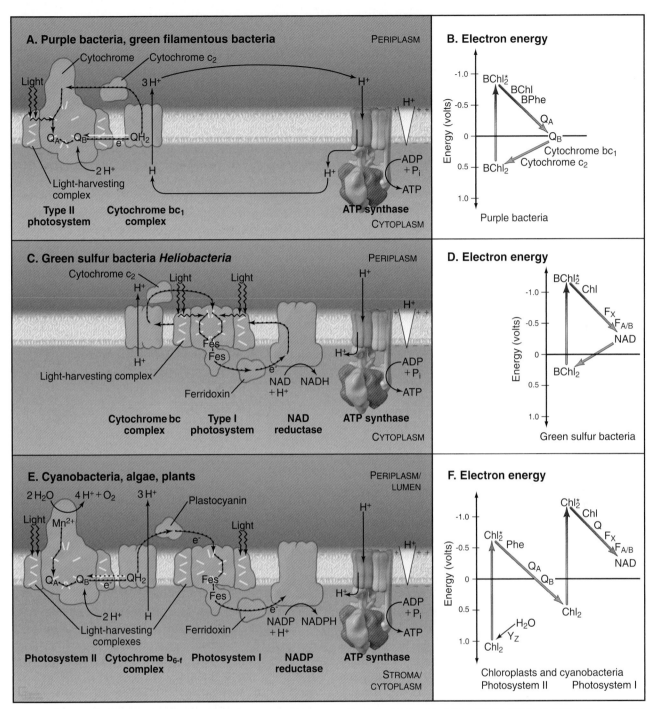

Figure 19-8 COMPARISON OF PHOTOSYNTHETIC COMPONENTS, ELECTRON TRANSPORT PATHWAYS, AND CHEMIOSMOTIC CYCLES TO MAKE ATP. **A–B,** Type II photosystem only. **C–D,** Type I photosystem only. **E–F,** Both photosystem II and photosystem I. **Right diagrams,** The energy levels of electrons in the three types of photosynthetic organisms, showing excitation of an electron by an absorbed photon *(vertical arrows),* electron transfer pathways through each reaction center *(arrows sloping right),* and electron transfer steps outside the reaction centers *(arrows sloping left).* (A, C, and E, Reference: Kramer DM, Schoepp B, Liebl U, Nitschke W: Cyclic electron transfer in *Heliobacillus mobilis.* Biochemistry 36:4203–4211, 1997. B, D, and F, Reference: Allen JP, Williams JC: Photosynthetic reaction centers. FEBS Lett 438:5–9, 1998.)

plasma membrane. The F1 domain of ATP synthase faces the cytoplasm, and the lumen of this membrane system is periplasmic. This internal membrane system remains in chloroplasts but is separated from the inner membrane (the former plasma membrane). These **thylakoid** **membranes** contain photosynthetic hardware and enclose the thylakoid membrane space. Like the bacterial plasma membrane, the chloroplast "**inner membrane**" is a permeability barrier, containing carriers for metabolites. The inner membrane surrounds the

stroma, the cytoplasm of the original symbiotic bacterium, a protein-rich compartment devoted to synthesis of three-carbon sugar phosphates, chloroplast proteins, and all plant fatty acids. The stroma also houses the genomes and stores starch. The **outer membrane,** like the comparable bacterial and mitochondrial membranes, has large pore channels that allow free passage of metabolites.

Light and Dark Reactions

Photosynthetic mechanisms capture energy from photons to drive two types of reactions:

- **Light reactions** depend on continuous absorption of photons. These reactions occur in or on the surface of thylakoid membranes. They include generation of high-energy electrons, electron transport to make NADPH, creation of a proton gradient across the thylakoid membrane for the chemiosmotic synthesis of ATP, and generation of oxygen.

- **Dark reactions** convert carbon dioxide into three-carbon sugar phosphates. These reactions continue for some time in the dark. However, they depend on ATP and NADPH produced by light reactions, so they eventually stop when ATP and NADPH are exhausted in the dark. These reactions account for most of the carbon dioxide converted to carbohydrates on earth. (Alternatively specialized prokaryotes drive carbon fixation by oxidation of hydrogen sulfide and other inorganic compounds.)

All photosynthetic systems use similar mechanisms to capture energy from photons (Fig. 19-8). Pigments associated with transmembrane proteins in photosynthetic reaction centers absorb photons and use the energy to boost electrons to a high-energy, **excited state.** Subsequent electron transfer reactions partition this energy in several steps to generate a proton gradient across the membrane. Generation of this proton electrochemical gradient and chemiosmotic production of ATP are similar to oxidative phosphorylation (Fig. 19-5).

Specific photosynthetic systems differ in the complexity of the hardware, the source of electrons, and the products (Fig. 19-8). Most photosynthetic bacteria use either a type I photosystem or a type II photosystem to create a proton gradient to synthesize ATP. Cyanobacteria and green plants use both types of reaction centers in series to raise electrons to an energy sufficient to make NADPH in addition to ATP. These advanced systems also use water as the electron donor and produce molecular oxygen as a by-product.

Energy Capture and Transduction by Type II Photosystems and Photosystem II

The reaction center from the purple bacterium *Rhodopseudomonas viridis* (Fig. 19-9A) is a model for the more complex photosystem II of cyanobacteria and chloroplasts. This bacterial reaction center consists of just four subunits. A cytochrome subunit on the periplasmic side of the membrane donates electrons. Two core subunits form a rigid transmembrane framework to bind 10 cofactors in orientations that favor transfer of high-energy electrons from two "special" **bacteriochlorophylls** through **chlorophyll b** and **bacteriopheophytin b.**

Photosynthesis begins with absorption of a photon by the special pair bacteriochlorophylls. Photons in the visible part of the spectrum are quite energetic, 40 to 80 kcal mol^{-1}, enough to make several ATPs. The purple bacterium reaction center absorbs relatively low-energy, 870-nm red light. The energy elevates an electron in the special pair bacteriochlorophylls to an excited state (Fig. 19-8B). In an organic solvent, the excited state would decay rapidly (10^9 s^{-1}), and the energy would dissipate as heat or emission of a less energetic photon by fluorescence or phosphorescence. However, reaction centers are optimized to transfer excited-state electrons rapidly and efficiently from the special pair bacteriochlorophylls to bacteriopheophytin (3×10^{-12} s) and then to tightly bound quinone A (200×10^{-12} s). Transfer is by **quantum mechanical tunneling** right through the protein molecule. Because the tunneling rate falls off quickly with distance, four redox centers must be spaced close together to allow an energetic electron to transfer across the lipid bilayer faster than spontaneous decay of the excited state.

On the cytoplasmic side of the membrane, two electrons transfer from quinone A to loosely bound quinone B (100×10^{-9} s), where they combine with two protons to make a high-energy **reduced quinone,** QH$_2$ (Fig. 19-8A). In purple bacteria, these cytoplasmic protons are taken up through water-filled channels in the reaction center, contributing to the proton gradient.

QH$_2$ has a low affinity for the reaction center and diffuses in the hydrophobic core of the bilayer to the next component in the pathway, the chloroplast equivalent of the mitochondrial cytochrome bc$_1$ complex III (Fig. 19-8A). As in mitochondria, passage of energetic electrons through this complex releases protons from QH$_2$ on the periplasmic side of the membrane, adding to the electrochemical gradient. The electron circuit is completed by transfer of low-energy electrons from complex bc$_1$ to a soluble periplasmic protein, cytochrome c$_2$. Electrons then move to the cytochrome subunit of the reaction center, which supplies special

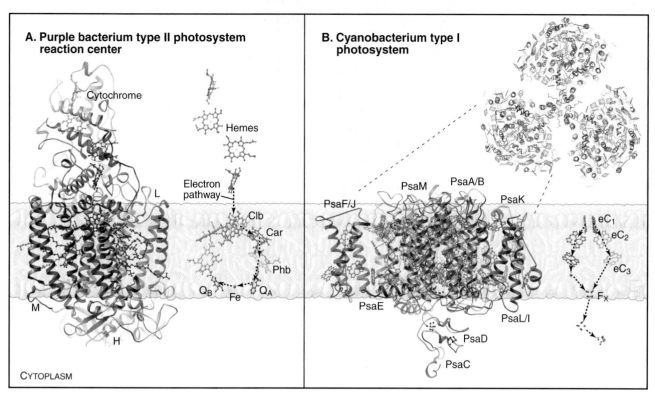

Figure 19-9 STRUCTURES OF PHOTOSYSTEM HARDWARE. **A,** Ribbon diagram of type II photosystem from the purple bacterium *Rhodopseudomonas viridis,* with ball and stick models of bacteriochlorophyll and other cofactors to the right in their natural orientations. Similar core subunits L and M each consists of five transmembrane helices. This pair of subunits binds four molecules of chlorophyll b (Clb), two molecules of bacteriopheophytin b (Phb), one nonheme iron (Fe), two quinones (Q_A, Q_B), and one carotenoid (Car) in a rigid framework. A cytochrome with four heme groups binds to the periplasmic side of the core subunits. Subunit H associates with the core subunits via one transmembrane helix and with their cytoplasmic surfaces. The atomic structure of this photosynthetic reaction center was the Nobel Prize work of J. Diesenhoffer, R. Huber, and H. Michel. **B,** Ribbon diagram of photosystem I of *Synechococcus elongatus,* with ball and stick models of chlorophyll and other cofactors to the *right* in their natural orientations. This trimeric complex consists of three identical units, each composed of 11 polypeptide chains. Within each of these units, this 4-Å resolution structure includes 43 α-helices, 89 chlorophylls, a quinone, and three iron-sulfur centers, but other details (e.g., amino acid side chains) are not resolved. The photosynthetic reaction center consists of the C-terminal halves of the two central subunits *(PsaA/PsaB, red-brown)* associated with six chlorophylls, one or two quinones, and a shared iron-sulfur cluster. Plastocyanin or cytochrome c_6 on the lumen side donates electrons to reduce the P700 special pair chlorophylls (eC_1) of the reaction center. Light energizes an electron, which passes successively through two other chlorophylls, a quinone, and the shared iron-sulfur cluster *(red)*, F_x. The electron then transfers to the iron-sulfur clusters of the accessory subunit PsaC on the stromal side of the membrane. The surrounding eight subunits *(red, gray)*, associated with about 80 chlorophylls, compose the core antenna system, forming a nearly continuous ring of α-helices around the reaction center. Absorption of light by additional light-harvesting complexes and these antenna subunits puts chloroplast electrons into an excited state. This energy passes from one pigment to the next until it eventually reaches the reaction center. (A, Copyright of Diesenhoffer & Michel, Nobel Foundation, 1988. Reference: Diesenhoffer J, Michel H: The photosynthetic reaction center from the purple bacterium *Rhodopseudomonas viridis*. Science 245:1463–1473, 1989. PDB file: 1PRC. A 3.5 Å crystal structure [PDB file: 1IZL] of the PSII complex from the cyanobacterium *Thermosynechococcus elongatus* including 19 subunits is now available. Reference: Ferreira KN, Iverson TM, Maghlaoui K, et al: Architecture of the photosynthetic oxygen-evolving center. Science 303:1831–1838, 2004. B, PDB file: 2PPS. Reference: Schubert W-D, Klukas O, Krauss N, et al: Photosystem I of *Synechococcus elongatus* at 4 Å resolution: Comprehensive structure analysis. J Mol Biol 272:741–769, 1997.)

pair chlorophylls with electrons for the photosynthetic reaction cycle.

The net result of this cycle is the conversion of the energy of two photons into transport of three protons to the periplasm. A diagram of the energy levels of the various intermediates in the cycle (Fig. 19-8B) shows how energy is partitioned after an electron is excited by a photon and then moves, step by step, through protein-associated redox centers back to the ground state.

The proton electrochemical gradient established by photosynthetic electron transfer reactions is used to drive an ATP synthase (see Fig. 8-5) similar to those of nonphotosynthetic prokaryotes and mitochondria.

Light Harvesting

Reaction center chlorophylls absorb light themselves, but both chloroplasts and bacteria increase the efficiency of light collection with proteins that absorb light and transfer the energy to a reaction center. Most of these **light-harvesting complexes** are small, transmembrane proteins that cluster around a reaction center, although some bacteria and algae also have soluble light-harvesting proteins. Transmembrane, light-harvesting proteins consist of a few α-helices associated with multiple chlorophyll and carotenoid pigments (Figs. 19-8A and C and 19-9B). The use of different pigments broadens the range of wavelengths absorbed. Multiple pigments increase the efficiency of photon capture. Leaves are green because chlorophylls and carotenoids absorb purple and blue wavelengths (<530 nm) as well as red wavelengths (>620 nm), reflecting only yellow-green wavelengths in between.

Light that is absorbed by light-harvesting proteins boosts pigment electrons to an excited state. This energy (but not the electrons) moves without dissipation by **fluorescence resonance energy transfer** from one closely spaced pigment molecule to another and eventually to the special pair chlorophylls of a reaction center. This rapid (10^{-12} s), efficient process transfers energy captured over a wide area to a reaction center to initiate a cycle of electron transfer and energy transduction.

Energy Capture and Transduction by Photosystem I

The reaction centers of green sulfur bacteria and heliobacteria are similar to photosystem I of cyanobacteria and chloroplasts. Generation of a proton gradient by photosystem I has many parallels with photosystem II. Direct absorption of light or resonance energy transfer from surrounding light-harvesting complexes excites special pair chlorophylls in photosystem I (Fig. 19-8C–D). Excited-state electrons move rapidly within the reaction center from these chlorophylls through two accessory chlorophylls and to an iron-sulfur center. The pathway includes a quinone in cyanobacteria and chloroplasts. Electrons then move to the iron-sulfur center of a subunit on the cytoplasmic side of the membrane. The subsequent events in green sulfur bacteria and heliobacteria are still under investigation but are thought to include electron transfer by the soluble protein ferridoxin to an NAD reductase, followed by transfer by a lipid intermediate to cytochrome bc complex, and then back to the reaction center via a cytochrome c.

Oxygen-Producing Synthesis of NADPH and ATP by Dual Photosystems

Chloroplasts and cyanobacteria combine photosystem II and photosystem I in the same membrane to form a system capable of accepting low-energy electrons from the oxidation of water and producing both a proton gradient to drive ATP synthesis and reducing equivalents in the form of NADPH (Fig. 19-8E–F). Both photosystems are more elaborate in dual systems than in single systems. Although plant photosystem II, with more than 25 protein subunits, is much more complicated than is the homologous reaction center of purple bacteria, the arrangement of transmembrane helices and chlorophyll cofactors in the core of the plant reaction center is similar to the simple reaction center of purple bacteria.

Photosynthesis involves a tortuous electron transfer pathway powered at two way stations by absorption of photons. This process begins when the special pair chlorophylls of photosystem II are excited by direct absorption of light or by resonance energy transfer from surrounding light-harvesting complexes (Fig. 19-8E–F). Electrons come from splitting two waters into molecular oxygen and four protons. Excited-state electrons tunnel through the redox cofactors and combine with protons from the stroma (or cytoplasm in bacteria) to reduce quinone QB to QH_2, a high-energy electron donor. QH_2 diffuses to complex b_{6-f}, the chloroplast equivalent of the mitochondrial bc_1 complex. Passage of electrons through complex b_{6-f} releases protons from QH_2 into the thylakoid lumen (or bacterial periplasm), contributing to the proton gradient across the membrane.

Complex b_{6-f} donates electrons from QH_2 to photosystem I. Direct absorption of 680-nm light or resonance energy transfer from surrounding light-harvesting complexes boosts special pair chlorophyll electrons to a very high-energy, excited state (Fig. 19-8F). Excited-state electrons pass through chlorophyll and iron-sulfur centers of photosystem I to the iron-sulfur center of the redox protein, ferridoxin, on the cytoplasmic/stromal surface of the membrane. The enzyme NADP reductase combines electrons from ferridoxin with a proton to form NADPH, the final product of this tortuous electron transfer pathway powered at two way stations by absorption of photons. Uptake of stromal protons during NADPH formation contributes to the transmembrane proton gradient for the synthesis of ATP. Antiporters in the inner membrane exchange ATP for ADP, as in mitochondria.

Synthesis of Carbohydrates

ATP and NADPH produced by light reactions drive the unfavorable conversion of carbon dioxide into sugars. This is the first step in the earth's annual production of about 10^{10} tons of carbohydrates by photosynthetic organisms. This process is very expensive, consuming three ATPs and two NADPHs for each carbon dioxide added to the five-carbon sugar ribulose 1,5-bisphosphate. The responsible enzyme, **ribulose phosphate carboxylase** (called RUBISCO), is the most abundant protein in the stroma and might be the most abundant protein on the earth. The products of combining the five-carbon sugar with carbon dioxide are two molecules of the three-carbon sugar 3-phosphoglycerate.

An antiporter in the inner chloroplast membrane exchanges 3-phosphoglycerate for inorganic phosphate, so 3-phosphoglycerate can join the glycolytic pathway in the cytoplasm (Fig. 19-4). Driven by this abundant supply of 3-phosphoglycerate, the glycolytic pathway runs backward to make six-carbon sugars, which are used to make disaccharides such as sucrose to nourish nonphotosynthetic parts of the plant, the glucose polymer **starch** to store carbohydrate, and **cellulose** for the extracellular matrix (see Figs. 3-25A and 32-12).

Peroxisomes

Peroxisomes are organelles bounded a single membrane (Fig. 19-10), named for their content of enzymes that produce and degrade hydrogen peroxide, H_2O_2. Oxidases produce H_2O_2 and peroxidases such as catalase break it down. Peroxisomes also contain diverse enzymes for the metabolism of lipids and other metabolites, including the β-oxidation of fatty acids and oxidation of bile acids and cholesterol. Peroxisomes lack nucleic acids, and there is no evidence that they arose from a bacterial ancestor. All peroxisomal proteins are encoded by nuclear genes, translated on cytoplasmic ribosomes, and then subsequently incorporated into peroxisomes (see Fig. 18-8).

Peroxisomes form in two different ways: de novo synthesis by budding from the endoplasmic reticulum and growth and division of preexisting peroxisomes (see Fig. 18-8). Cells that lack preexisting peroxisomes can form peroxisomes without a template by differentiation and budding of ER membranes. PEX3 and PEX16 target to the ER, where they recruit other peroxins to form a specialized domain that pinches off to form a nascent peroxisome. In addition to arising by outgrowth from the ER, new peroxisomes can form by fission of preexisting peroxisomes.

Defects in peroxisomal biogenesis cause a spectrum of lethal human diseases known as the **peroxisomal biogenesis disorders** (see Appendix 18-1). These diseases include Zellweger syndrome, neonatal adrenoleukodystrophy, infantile Refsum's disease, and rhizomelic chondrodysplasia punctata. They are moderately rare, occurring in approximately 1 in 50,000 live births. Most patients with peroxisomal biogenesis disorders display no defect in peroxisome membrane synthesis or import of peroxisomal membrane proteins, but they do have mild-to-severe defects in matrix protein import. However, in rare cases, patients lack peroxisome membranes altogether. Studies of both yeast *pex* mutants and cells from patients with peroxisomal biogenesis disor-

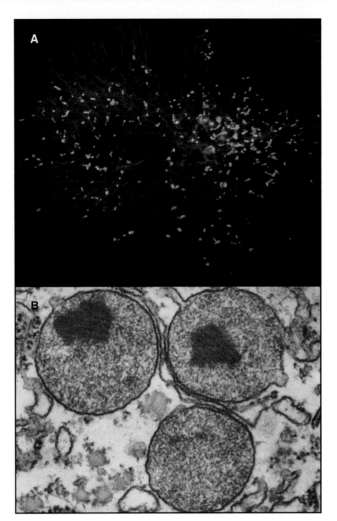

Figure 19-10 PEROXISOMES. **A,** Fluorescence micrographs of a CV1 cell expressing *green* fluorescent protein fused to PTS1, which labels peroxisomes *green*. Microtubules are stained *red* with labeled antibodies, and nuclear DNA is stained *blue* with propidium iodide. **B,** Electron micrograph of a thin section of a tissue culture cell showing three peroxisomes. Peroxisomes have a single bilayer membrane and a dense matrix, including a crystal (in some species) of the enzyme urate oxidase. (A, Courtesy of S. Subramani, University of California, San Diego. Reference: Wiemer EAC, Wenzel T, Deernick TJ, et al: Visualization of the peroxisomal compartment in living mammalian cells. J Cell Biol 136:71–80, 1997. B, Courtesy of Don W. Fawcett, Harvard Medical School, Boston, Massachusetts.)

ders have provided clues regarding peroxisome biogenesis (see Fig. 18-7).

ACKNOWLEDGMENT

Thanks go to Gary Brudvig for his suggestions on revisions to this chapter.

SELECTED READINGS

Blankenship RE, Hartman H: The origin and evolution of oxygenic photosynthesis. Trends Biochem Sci 23:94–97, 1998.

Cecchini G: Function and structure of complex II of the respiratory chain. Annu Rev Biochem 72:77-109, 2003.

Deisenhofer J, Michel H: The photosynthetic reaction center from the purple bacterium *Rhodopseudomonas viridis.* Science 245:1463-1473, 1989.

Frey TG, Mannella CA: The internal structure of mitochondria. Trends Biochem Sci 25:319-324, 2000.

Gray MW, Burger G, Lang BF: Mitochondrial evolution. Science 283:1476-1481, 1999.

Hosler JP, Ferguson-Miller S, Mills DA: Energy transduction: Proton transfer through the respiratory complexes. Annu Rev Biochem 75:165-187, 2006.

Iwata S, Barber J: Structure of photosystem II and molecular architecture of the oxygen-evolving centre. Curr Opin Struct Biol 14:447-453, 2004.

Lazarow PB: Peroxisome biogenesis: Advances and conundrums. Curr Opin Cell Biol 15:489-497, 2003.

Lowell BB, Shulman, GI: Mitochondrial dysfunction and type 2 diabetes. Science 307:384-387, 2004.

Meeusen SL, Nunnari J: How mitochondria fuse. Curr Opin Cell Biol 17:389-394, 2005.

Moser CC, Keske JM, Warncke K, et al: Nature of biological electron transfer. Nature 355:796-802, 1992.

Osteryoung KW, Nunnari J: The division of endosymbiotic organelles. Science 302:1698-1704, 2003.

Rhee K-H: Photosystem II: The solid structural era. Annu Rev Biophys Biomol Struct 30:307-328, 2001.

Rhee K-H, Morris EP, Barber J, Kuhlbrandt W: Three-dimensional structure of the plant photosystem II reaction centre at 8 Å resolution. Nature 396:283-286, 1998.

Rutherford AW, Boussac A: Water photolysis in biology. Science 303:1782-1784, 2004.

Scheffler IE: Mitochondria. New York, Wiley & Sons, 1999.

Schubert W-D, Klukas O, Krauss N, et al: Photosystem I of *Synechococcus elongatus* at 4 Å resolution: Comprehensive structure analysis. J Mol Biol 272:741-769, 1997.

Schultz BE, Chan SI: Structures and proton-pumping strategies of mitochondrial respiratory enzymes. Annu Rev Biophys Biomol Struct 30:23-65, 2001.

Smith JL, Zhang H, Yan J, et al: Cytochrome bc complexes: A common core of structure and function surrounded by diversity in the outlying provinces. Curr Opin Struct Biol 14:432-439, 2004.

Tielens AGM, Rotte C, van Hellemond JJ, Martin W: Mitochondria as we don't know them. Trends Biochem Sci 27:564-572, 2002.

Wallace DC: Mitochondrial diseases in man and mouse. Science 283:1482-1488, 1999.

Wanders RJ, Waterham HR: Biochemistry of mammalian peroxisomes revisited. Annu Rev Biochem 75:295-332, 2006.

Wittenhagen LM, Kelley SO: Impact of disease-related mitochondrial mutations on tRNA structure and function. Trends Biochem Sci 28:605-611, 2003.

CHAPTER

Endoplasmic Reticulum

One of the key distinguishing features of eukaryotic cells is the presence of the **endoplasmic reticulum (ER),** the largest of numerous membrane-delineated intracellular compartments. The ER is thought to have evolved from the prokaryotic plasma membrane by expansion, internalization, and subdivision (Fig. 20-1A–D; see also Fig. 2-6). It provides both an expanded membrane surface (up to 30 times that of the plasma membrane) for carrying out vital cellular functions, including protein and lipid biosynthesis, and an internal compartment (or lumen) that collects proteins synthesized in the cytoplasm for modification and delivery into the secretory pathway. About one third of all cellular proteins are imported into the lumen of the ER or integrated into its membranes. Consisting of an extensive array of tubules or flat saccules called cisternae (*cisterna* means "reservoir"), the ER forms a continuous three-dimensional network (a reticulum) stretching from the nuclear envelope to the cell surface (Fig. 20-1E). Microtubules and their associated motors generate this extended network in

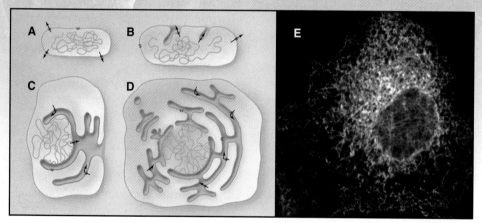

Figure 20-1 MODEL FOR ORIGIN OF ENDOPLASMIC RETICULUM/NUCLEAR ENVELOPE AND FLUORESCENT IMAGE OF ENDOPLASMIC RETICULUM DISTRIBUTION WITHIN A CELL. **A–D,** The ER may have originated by invagination of regions of the plasma membrane containing protein translocation channels (*red* complexes), which transfer newly synthesized proteins across the membrane. The invaginated membranes then proliferated into a reticular network. Wrapping of this network around DNA led to the formation of the nuclear envelope and nucleus. **E,** Fluorescent micrograph of a cell expressing an ER marker tagged with *green* fluorescent protein (appears *white* in this image). (Courtesy of Dr. Erik Snapp, Albert Einstein College of Medicine, Bronx, New York.)

This chapter was revised using material from the first edition written by William E. Balch, Ann L. Hubbard, J. David Castle, and Pat Shipman

animal cells by pulling ER membranes out toward the periphery of the cell. This allows the ER to coordinate diverse processes over large regions of the cytoplasm. The ER's size and shape are maintained over time despite a continuous flow of proteins and lipids into and out of this compartment. The flow results from the large rate of synthesis of lipids and proteins (between 2 million and 13 million new proteins per minute) occurring at the ER membrane, as well as from the continuous export of these molecules into the secretory pathway and their selective retrieval back to the ER from the Golgi apparatus.

This chapter describes the following: (1) the overall functions and organization of the ER; (2) insertion of proteins into and across the ER membrane; (3) the mechanisms of folding, assembly, and degradation of proteins in the ER; and (4) the synthesis and metabolism of lipids by the ER.

Endoplasmic Reticulum Functions and Organization

The membrane surface of the ER performs several functions for cells. Foremost is the production of the proteins and lipids that will make up the membranes of the other organelles, including the Golgi apparatus, nucleus, endosomes, lysosomes, and plasma membrane, as well as nearly all proteins that will be secreted from the cell. The membranes of mitochondria and peroxisomes also depend on the ER to supply much of their lipid. Another key function of the ER membrane is to form the nuclear envelope, which encloses the nucleus (see Fig. 14-5). The surface of the ER forming the outer nuclear envelope (which faces the cytoplasm) is indistinguishable from the rest of the ER except for the presence of nuclear pores that span both inner and outer nuclear envelope to allow passage of molecules between the nucleus and cytoplasm. By contrast, the ER surface forming the inner nuclear envelope, which faces the nucleus, contains specialized proteins that interact with the nuclear lamina and chromatin. ER membranes also detoxify endogenous steroids, carcinogenic compounds, and lipid-soluble drugs (xenobiotics) from the environment. This occurs by an electron transfer process carried out by ER membrane proteins such as the cytochrome P450 family of enzymes.

The lumen of the ER also performs numerous essential functions. Specialized for receiving proteins transported from the cytoplasm across ER membranes, the ER lumen is enriched in a dense meshwork of chaperones and other modifying enzymes (estimated to be 200 mg/mL in concentration) that catalyze the folding and assembly of newly synthesized proteins. These transported proteins, including both soluble and transmembrane forms, are exported from the ER for secretion or for delivery to the lumen or membrane of the Golgi apparatus, lysosome, or endosome. Proteins that are incorrectly folded or misfolded can be exported back into the cytoplasm, where they are degraded. Misfolded proteins, when accumulated in the ER at high levels, can trigger an unfolded protein response, which activates specific genes in the nucleus whose products help to modify or destroy the misfolded proteins and compensate for the decreased capacity of ER folding. The ER lumen is one of the major Ca^{2+} storage sites in cells, owing to ER membranes being rich in calcium pumps (see Fig. 8-7) and many Ca^{2+}-binding proteins in the lumen. Such Ca^{2+} stores can be released by calcium channels in response to cellular signals such as IP_3 (see Fig. 26-13). Carefully regulated release and uptake of Ca^{2+} by the ER control muscle contraction (see Fig. 39-15) and many other cellular processes. The lumen of the ER is also an oxidizing environment that favors disulfide bond formation, which helps to stabilize proteins after they are exported from the ER to the outside of the cell.

The diverse functions carried out by the membrane and in the lumen of the ER (Table 20-1) occur in distinctive ER regions (Fig. 20-2A). The **rough ER** is studded with ribosomes on its cytoplasmic surface, defining areas that are specialized for protein synthesis, folding, and degradation (Fig. 20-2B). The **smooth ER,** composed of tubular elements lacking ribosomes, is dedicated to enzyme pathways involved in drug metabolism (hepatocytes), steroid synthesis (endocrine cells), or calcium uptake and release (see Fig. 26-12). The **cytochrome P-450** family of heme-containing membrane proteins is found in the smooth ER. Other regions of the ER that lack ribosomes, called **ER export domains** consist of tubulovesicular membranes that bud during export of secretory cargo to the Golgi apparatus (see Chapter 21). Regions of the ER surrounding the nucleus compose the nuclear envelope.

The abundance of a particular ER region varies in specialized cells. Cells dedicated to the production, storage, and regulated secretion of proteins (such as exocrine cells and activated B cells) are rich in rough ER. By contrast, smooth ER is abundant in endocrine cells that synthesize steroid hormones and in muscle cells owing to their requirement to store and release Ca^{2+} to control contraction. In mitosis, the ER maintains its morphology as an interconnected network, whereas the nuclear envelope either disassembles (in cells undergoing open mitosis) or remains intact (in cells undergoing closed mitosis). In cells whose nuclear envelope disassembles, integral membrane proteins of the nuclear envelope diffuse into surrounding ER membranes on nuclear pore disassembly.

Table 20-1

SUBDOMAINS OF THE ENDOPLASMIC RETICULUM

ER Domain	Function	Associated Proteins
Rough ER	Protein translocation Protein folding and oligomerization Carbohydrate addition ER degradation	Sec61 complex, TRAP, TRAM, BiP PDI, Calnexin, Calreticulin, BiP Oligosaccharide transferase EDEM, Derlin1
Smooth ER	Detoxification Lipid metabolism Heme metabolism Calcium release	Cytochrome P450 enzymes HMG-CoA reductase Cytochrome b(5) IP3 receptors
Nuclear envelope	Nuclear pores Chromatin anchoring	POM121, GP210 (see Fig. 14-8) Lamin B receptor
ER export sites	Export of proteins and lipids into secretory pathway	Sar1p, Sec12p, Sec16p
ER contact zones	Transport of lipids	LTPs

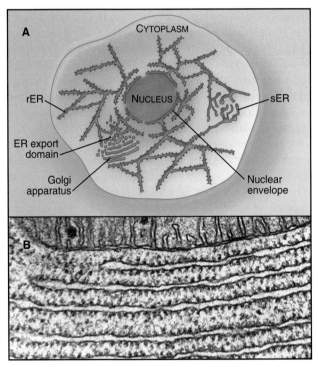

Figure 20-2 ENDOPLASMIC RETICULUM SUBDOMAIN ORGANIZATION WITHIN THE CELL. **A,** ER membranes containing ribosomes, called rough ER (rER), extend from the nuclear envelope to the cell periphery. ER membranes lacking ribosomes, called smooth ER (sER), include membranes specialized for drug metabolism and steroid synthesis, as well as tubulovesicular elements composing ER exit sites. The nuclear envelope consists of ER membrane that has wrapped around DNA and other nuclear elements to compartmentalize them. Its double membrane is studded with nuclear pores, which provide a passageway for nuclear components to move between the nucleus and cytosol. (See Fig. 14-17 for more details.) **B,** Electron micrograph of a thin section of rough ER and neighboring mitochondrion from the pancreas. (Micrograph by Keith R. Porter; courtesy of Don W. Fawcett, Harvard Medical School, Boston, Massachusetts.)

Overview of Protein Translocation into the Endoplasmic Reticulum

All proteins are synthesized in the cytoplasm and must be specifically targeted to the ER, where they are either fully translocated across the ER membrane and released into the ER lumen (soluble proteins) or only partly translocated across the ER membrane and embedded in the lipid bilayer of the ER membrane (transmembrane proteins). This transport to the ER can happen either as the protein is being made (**cotranslational translocation**) or after synthesis is complete (**post-translational translocation**). The orientation of a protein in the lipid bilayer or its localization to the lumen is established during protein translocation and maintained as the protein is transferred by membrane-bound carriers through the secretory pathway (see Fig. 21-2). Thus, domains of transmembrane proteins to be exposed on the cell surface must be inserted into the ER membrane, facing the lumen. Similarly, secreted soluble proteins must be fully translocated into the lumen of the ER.

Because the lumen of the ER is topologically equivalent to the extracellular space, transport of proteins into the ER is analogous to transport into or across a prokaryotic plasma membrane. The two processes face similar challenges in that substrates to be transported must be (1) recognized, (2) targeted from the cytoplasm to the membrane, and (3) translocated across the membrane through a protein channel without causing leakage of molecules across the membrane surface. Each of these obstacles is overcome by core protein translocation machinery that is conserved across eukaryotic cells.

Signal Sequence Recognition

Soluble and membrane proteins destined for ER translocation contain a hydrophobic sequence either at their N-terminus or in transmembrane segments that serve as recognition signals for direction to the ER membrane. N-terminal leader sequences (termed **signal sequences**) are typically 15 to 35 amino acids long and contain a hydrophobic core of at least 6 residues, while transmembrane signal segments have a hydrophobic stretch of 16 to 25 residues. Aside from hydrophobicity, these signal sequences have no other features in common (Table 20-2). Nevertheless, when attached to proteins that are not normally targeted to the ER, these signal sequences direct the protein to the ER and not to other organelles such as to mitochondria or peroxisomes, which use unique targeting signals (see Fig. 18-1).

A protein containing a signal sequence or transmembrane signal segment is guided to the ER membrane by either a cotranslational pathway or a posttranslational pathway. In the cotranslational pathway, substrates are translocated across the ER concurrent with their synthesis by membrane-bound ribosomes. In the posttranslational pathway, the substrate is first fully synthesized in the cytoplasm and then translocated in a ribosome-independent fashion. These pathways operate in several qualitatively different ways.

Cotranslational Translocation

In the cotranslational pathway, the **signal recognition particle (SRP)** recognizes and binds the first hydrophobic domain of either the signal sequence or the transmembrane signal segment as it emerges from the ribosome slowing translation of the polypeptide (Fig. 20-3A). Then the complex consisting of ribosome, nascent chain, and SRP associates with the ER membrane by binding the **SRP receptor (SR),** a heterodimer consisting of one subunit that binds SRP and another that spans the ER membrane. Both the SRP and the SR have guanosine triphosphatase (GTPase) domains (Fig. 20-3B) similar to Ras (see Fig. 4-6). GTP binding and hydrolysis by SRP and SR provide directionality and order to the sequence of reactions that bring the nascent chain to the translocation channel. Once the ribosome-nascent chain–SRP complex is bound to SR at the ER membrane, SRP releases the signal sequence, allowing the ribosome–nascent chain complex to be transferred to the protein-conducting channel across the ER membrane. SRP and SR then dissociate after hydrolyzing their bound guanosine triphosphate (GTP), releasing SRP into the cytoplasm and allowing SR to diffuse away in the membrane. The targeting cycle delivers the ribosome–nascent chain complex to the protein-conducting channel (called the **translocon**) and recycles the targeting machinery (i.e., SRP and SR).

The nascent chain emerging from the ribosome must then engage and open the translocon for transport across the ER membrane. The central component of the translocon is the evolutionarily conserved heterotrimeric Sec61 protein complex **(Sec61 complex).** The Sec61 complex provides a high-affinity docking site for the ribosome–nascent chain complex. Binding of the signal sequence to the Sec61 complex is facilitated by additional factors, including the protein TRAM (translocating chain-associating membrane protein) and the protein complex TRAP (translocon-associated protein). Once bound, the ribosome–nascent chain complex inserts the nascent chain into the Sec61 channel. The channel then opens toward the lumen, providing the nascent chain a continuous path from the peptidyl transferase center in the ribosome, through the translocation channel and into the ER lumen. Elongation of the polypeptide chain by the ribosome "pushes" the nascent chain through the channel and across the membrane. In this way, the energy used for protein synthesis is harnessed to drive translocation of the polypeptide across the membrane. Inside the ER lumen binding and release of chaperones help to "pall" the polypeptide across the membrane.

Table 20-2			
SIGNAL SEQUENCES WITHIN PROTEINS			
Protein	**Signal Sequence**	**Length**	**Charge**
BiP	MKLSLVAAMLLLLSAARA	18	+1
Apo-A1	MKAAVLTLAVLFLTGSQA	18	+1
TGF-β2	MHYCVLSAFLILHLVTVAL	19	0
Interferon γ	MKYTSYILAFQLCIVLG	17	+1
Glucagon	MKSIYFVAGLFVMLVQG	19	+1
Choriogonadotropin	MEMFQGLLLLLLLSMGGTWA	20	−1
EGF-receptor	MRPSGTAGAALLALLAALCPRA	24	+1
Growth hormone	MATGSRTSLLLAFGLLCLPWLQEGSA	26	+1

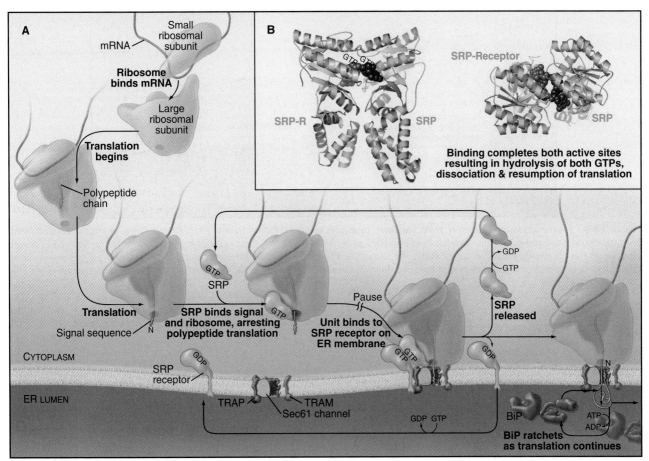

A

mRNA

Small ribosomal subunit

Ribosome binds mRNA

Large ribosomal subunit

Translation begins

Polypeptide chain

Translation

Signal sequence

N

SRP binds signal and ribosome, arresting polypeptide translation

GTP

SRP

GTP

Pause

Unit binds to SRP receptor on ER membrane

GTP

GTP

GDP

GDP

SRP released

GTP

N

CYTOPLASM

SRP receptor

GDP

ER LUMEN

TRAP

Sec61 channel

TRAM

GDP GTP

BiP

ATP

ADP

BiP ratchets as translation continues

B

GTP GTP

SRP-R

SRP

SRP-Receptor

SRP

Binding completes both active sites resulting in hydrolysis of both GTPs, dissociation & resumption of translation

Figure 20-3   COTRANSLATIONAL PATHWAY FROM RIBOSOME TO ENDOPLASMIC RETICULUM LUMEN. **A,** Signal recognition particle (SRP) and SRP-receptor use a cycle of recruitment and hydrolysis of GTP to control delivery of the ribosome-mRNA complex to the ER translocon. SRP binds a signal sequence emerging from a ribosome and arrests polypeptide translation. SRP also directs the ribosome to the SRP-receptor on the ER membrane, where the ribosome docks on the translocon and continues translation. (GDP, guanosine diphosphate.) **B,** Ribbon diagram of SRP and SRP-receptor-binding complex showing the close association between each protein's GTPase domain, which permits the GTPases to undergo reciprocal activation.

Posttranslational Translocation

Posttranslational translocation (prevalent in fungi such as yeast) differs because neither cotranslational targeting machinery (SRP and SR) nor ribosomes participate. Instead, other components fulfill the functions provided by SRP, SR, and ribosomes (with the Sec61 complex serving as channel, as it does in cotranslational translocation). Signal-containing polypeptides destined for posttranslational insertion into the ER are held in a largely unfolded state by cytoplasmic chaperones until they can be delivered to the tetrameric Sec62/63 protein complex at the ER membrane (Fig. 20-4). A similar strategy is used to import proteins into the mitochondria (see Fig. 18-4). During posttranslational translocation, the signal sequence engages and opens the Sec61 channel in a fashion similar to cotranslational translocation. Since protein synthesis is already complete, another energy source must be exploited to move the substrate through the channel into the ER. **BiP,** a luminal ER

chaperone belonging to the Hsp70 family, binds the substrate in the ER lumen, thereby preventing it from sliding back into the cytoplasm. Repeated rounds of substrate binding and release, catalyzed by ATP hydrolysis, allow BiP to act as a molecular ratchet to drive substrate transport into the lumen. The transmembrane protein Sec63 regulates the ATPase activity of BiP and helps to recruit BiP to the translocation channel. Thus, the peptide is "pulled" across the membrane from the luminal side instead of being "pushed" from the cytoplasmic side, as during cotranslational translocation. Hsp70 family members perform a similar function during import of proteins into mitochondria and chloroplasts (see Fig. 18-4).

Universality of Protein Translocation

In both cotranslational and posttranslational translocation, the Sec61 complex translocation channel is closed

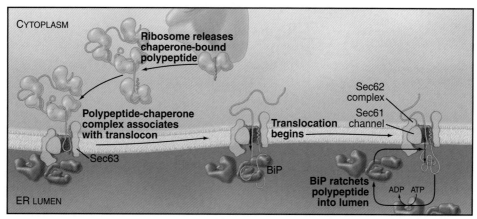

Figure 20-4   POSTTRANSLATIONAL PATHWAY FROM RIBOSOME TO ENDOPLASMIC RETICULUM LUMEN. As the polypeptide emerges *(purple thread)* from the ribosome in the cytosol, it is bound by chaperones *(green)* that prevent it from aggregating and guide it to the Sec62/63 protein complex at the ER membrane. After signal sequence engagement with the Sec63 protein-conducting channel, the polypeptide is pulled across the membrane from the lumenal side by repeated binding to and release from BiP (i.e., ratcheting). The signal sequence is the *blue* portion of the polypeptide.

until opened by interacting with binding partners, including the translocated polypeptide. This ensures that only specific types of proteins pass through the ER membrane and that the permeability barrier of these membranes is maintained at all times. In cotranslational translocation, interactions with a ribosome and a signal sequence open the channel, and protein synthesis provides the energy for translocation. In posttranslational translocation, the Sec62/63 complex operates on both sides of the membrane. On the cytoplasmic side, it contributes to the interactions of the signal sequence that open the translocon. On the lumenal side, it recruits BiP to provide the driving force for translocation. This theme applies to protein translocation across the plasma membrane by prokaryotes. There, a homolog of the Sec61 complex (the SecYE complex) interacts with the cytoplasmic SecA adenosine triphosphatase (ATPase), a partner that drives translocation across the plasma membrane (see Fig. 18-9).

Molecular Machinery for Protein Translocation into the Endoplasmic Reticulum

Signal Recognition Particle and Signal Recognition Particle–Receptor

Human SRP is a ribonucleoprotein composed of six proteins (named by their apparent molecular weights and a 300-nucleotide RNA (Fig. 20-5). The SRP54 protein subunit and a portion of the RNA compose the minimal hardware for targeting to the translocon and are found in both prokaryotic and eukaryotic cells. SRP54 binds signal sequences in a deep, hydrophobic groove lined

by the flexible side chains of several methionines. Like bristles of a brush, the methionines accommodate the various shapes of the hydrophobic side chains of the residues of different signal sequences. Phosphates of the SRP RNA near one end of this groove may interact with basic residues that are often (but not always) adjacent to the hydrophobic core of signal sequences and transmembrane signal segments.

SRP binding to a signal sequence slows translation, a phenomenon that is termed *elongation arrest* (Fig. 20-3A). The mechanism appears to involve occlusion of the elongation factor binding site on the ribosome by the SRP9 and SRP14 subunits of SRP, which structurally resembles a portion of eEF2. Slowing translation provides time to target the ribosome to the translocation channel before excessive polypeptide synthesis precludes cotranslational transport.

Interaction of SRP with SR directs the SRP–ribosome–nascent chain complex to the translocation channel (Fig. 20-3A). This interaction is regulated by GTP binding and hydrolysis by SRP and SR, whose GTPase cycles are a notable exception to the GTPase switch paradigm of Ras-like GTPases that involve GTP exchange factors (GEFs) and GTPase-activating proteins (GAPs; see Fig. 25-8). No external GEFs or GAPs are known for SRP and SR GTPases. Instead, these proteins readily exchange GDP for GTP and are in the GTP-bound state as they enter the targeting cycle. On formation of a complex, SRP and SR reciprocally activate each other's GTPase activity, thereby obviating the need for an external GAP to drive the conversion of GTP to GDP on these proteins. Upon GTP hydrolysis, the conformations of SR and SRP change in a way that reduces their affinity. They dissociate from each other as well as from the ribosome–nascent chain and translocation channel. This

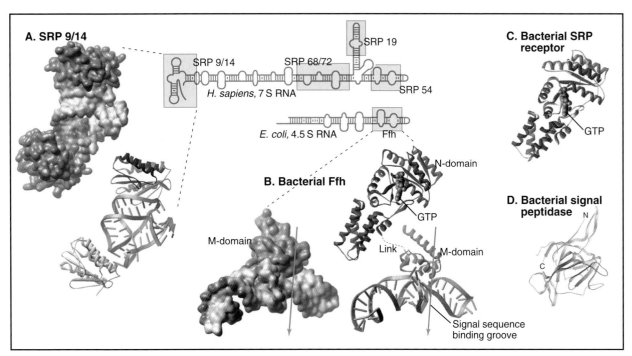

Figure 20-5 ATOMIC STRUCTURES OF COTRANSLOCATION HARDWARE. **A–B,** Comparison of bacterial and human signal recognition particles, showing the base pairing of human 7S SRP RNA and bacterial 4.5S SRP RNA and indicating protein-binding sites *(blue boxes)*. Atomic structures of elements of the RNA and associated proteins are shown as space-filling and ribbon diagrams. Ffh GTP-binding and N-domains (PDB files: 3NG1, 2NG1), Ffh M-domain bound to RNA (PDB file: 1DUL), RNA (PDB file: 1E9S), SRP9/14 bound to RNA (PDB file: 1E80). **C,** Bacterial SRP-receptor subunit FtsY. (PDB file: 1FTS.) **D,** Bacterial signal peptidase. (PDB file: 1B12.)

frees SRP and SR for further rounds of ribosome–nascent chain targeting. Release of SRP and SR occurs only after the ribosome has become properly engaged with the translocation channel in the ER membrane, thereby ensuring that the channel is closed until the ribosome has bound.

Sec61 Complex: The Protein-Conducting Channel

The protein-conducting channel consists of three or four copies of the Sec61 complex, appearing as a donut-like structure (Fig. 20-6A). Each Sec61 complex is a heterotrimer of three transmembrane polypeptides: an α subunit with 10 transmembrane segments, and smaller β and γ-subunits, each with single transmembrane sequences. The homologous bacterial proteins are called SecY, SecE, and SecG. They form the SecY complex (Fig. 20-6C), the channel for translocating proteins across the plasma membrane of bacteria.

Reconstructions of Sec61 complex from electron micrographs revealed a large central hole that might have been the pore for translocation of proteins across the ER bilayer. However, reconstructions at higher resolutions showed that the hole is not an aqueous channel, but a low-density region filled with lipid. This suggested that the pore was formed somewhere else, possibly within the Sec61 complex itself.

Crystal structures of the archaeal SecY complex revealed a small, hourglass-shaped pore within a single SecY complex (Fig. 20-6D). This pore is flanked on its luminal and cytoplasmic sides by funnels. The narrow constriction between the two funnels is only about 5 to 8 Å in diameter and lined by several hydrophobic side chains that together form the pore ring. Because of their small size and flexibility, the side chains forming the pore ring could fit snugly around a translocating peptide, preventing passage of ions or other small molecules. Another segment of SecY protein (termed the *plug domain*) occludes the pore in its inactive state and is proposed to shift away from the pore in its active state. The arrangement of the polypeptide allows the pore to open sideways, providing a lateral gate from the aqueous interior of the channel into the hydrophobic environment of the lipid bilayer that transmembrane domains of proteins use to access the lipid bilayer.

The structures strongly suggest that a single Sec61 complex functions as the pore for proteins to translocate across the ER. Several identical Sec61p complexes compose the translocon, but owing to its large size, only one ribosome can bind a translocon. Thus, only one Sec61p complex could be active for translocation. Why then is the translocon an oligomer of several Sec61 complexes? One possibility is that this creates binding sites for components associated with the translocon, such as

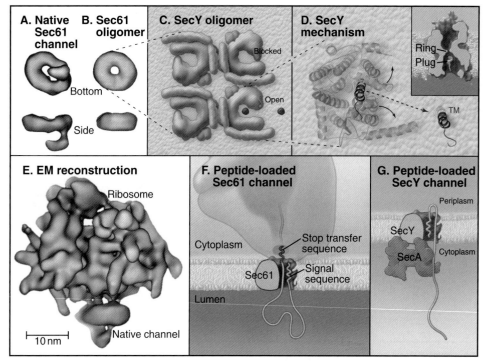

Figure 20-6   Structure of the Sec61 protein-conducting translocon. **A–B,** Three-dimensional reconstructions from electron micrographs: native translocon (channel) isolated from the ER and purified recombinant Sec61 oligomer. **C,** Tetrameric assembly of SecY complexes, as seen from electron micrographs. **D,** Ribbon diagram of SecY oligomer, showing potential path for lateral movement of the transmembrane segment of the translocated protein out of the channel. **Inset,** Side view of the channel with the front half of the model cut away. The pore ring represents the narrowest constriction between the two funnels of the channel. A segment of the SecY protein ("plug") occludes the pore until the polypeptide causes it to open. **E,** A ribosome bound to the Sec61 channel. **F–G,** Orientation of the signal sequence within the Sec61 channel or SecY channel. The signal sequence is the *blue* portion of the *purple* polypeptide that threads through each channel.

the ER signal peptidase, the oligosaccharide transferase, TRAP, or TRAM. Oligomerization might also stabilize ribosome binding to the ER by increasing the number of binding sites that are made between Sec61 complex and the ribosome.

Signal Sequence

Binding of a signal sequence to the Sec61p complex opens or "gates" the translocon in preparation for protein translocation. Current evidence suggests that the signal sequence forms a loop in the channel with its N-terminus exposed to the cytoplasm (Fig. 20-6F). This occurs by signal sequence binding to transmembrane helices 2 and 7 on Sec61p.

The ability to recognize signal sequences allows Sec61 to discriminate substrates for translocation from other proteins. Traditionally, this has been thought to be a constitutive process that is predetermined by the sequences on the substrate. However, various cell types differ in the efficiency with which they recognize particular signal sequences. This can be explained if additional factors at the translocation site might influence signal sequence recognition. For example, proteins at or

near the site of translocation (i.e., Sec62, Sec63, p180, p34, TRAM, or TRAP complex) might stimulate or inhibit the translocation of selected substrates by recognizing diversity within the signal sequence. Selective changes in expression or modifications of these accessory components in different cell types could then affect the outcome of translocation for different substrates.

Protein Insertion into the Endoplasmic Reticulum Bilayer or Lumen

Translocation of Soluble Proteins into the Lumen of the Endoplasmic Reticulum

Soluble proteins destined for secretion or retention in the lumen of the ER are translocated fully across the Sec61 protein-conducting channel into the lumen of the ER (Fig. 20-7A). Once the polypeptide has grown to about 150 residues during this process, a **signal peptidase** in the ER lumen removes the signal sequence from

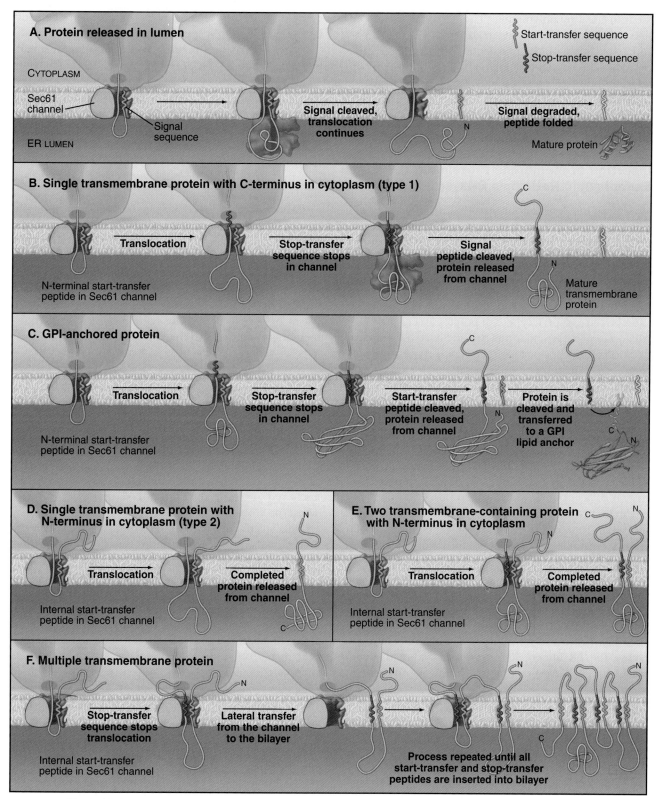

A. Protein released in lumen

Start-transfer sequence
Stop-transfer sequence

CYTOPLASM

Sec61 channel

Signal sequence

ER LUMEN

Signal cleaved, translocation continues

N

Signal degraded, peptide folded

Mature protein

B. Single transmembrane protein with C-terminus in cytoplasm (type 1)

Translocation

Stop-transfer sequence stops in channel

Signal peptide cleaved, protein released from channel

C

N-terminal start-transfer peptide in Sec61 channel

N

Mature transmembrane protein

C. GPI-anchored protein

Translocation

Stop-transfer sequence stops in channel

Start-transfer peptide cleaved, protein released from channel

Protein is cleaved and transferred to a GPI lipid anchor

C

N

N-terminal start-transfer peptide in Sec61 channel

C N

D. Single transmembrane protein with N-terminus in cytoplasm (type 2)

N

Translocation

Completed protein released from channel

Internal start-transfer peptide in Sec61 channel

C

E. Two transmembrane-containing protein with N-terminus in cytoplasm

C   N

N

Translocation

Completed protein released from channel

Internal start-transfer peptide in Sec61 channel

F. Multiple transmembrane protein

N

Stop-transfer sequence stops translocation

N

Lateral transfer from the channel to the bilayer

N

N

N

Internal start-transfer peptide in Sec61 channel

C

Process repeated until all start-transfer and stop-transfer peptides are inserted into bilayer

Figure 20-7 Targeting of Sec61-dependent proteins to the lumen and membrane of the endoplasmic reticulum.

the translocating polypeptide. The signal peptidase consists of five subunits ranging in size from 12 kD to 25 kD and associates with the translocon. After signal peptide cleavage, the new N-terminus of the growing polypeptide continues to pass through the translocon until it is released into the ER lumen. The remaining cleaved signal peptide either is degraded or has other functions elsewhere in the cell.

Insertion of Membrane Proteins in the Endoplasmic Reticulum Bilayer

Most proteins destined for insertion into the bilayer of the ER membrane use the Sec61 protein-conducting channel. During translocation of transmembrane proteins, some parts of the polypeptide chain are translocated across the lipid bilayer, whereas others are not. Depending on how the transmembrane protein is translocated and oriented across the bilayer, the protein is categorized as type 1, type 2, or polytopic (Fig. 20-7B–F). All copies of a particular polypeptide have the same orientation after translocation (i.e., type 1, type 2, or polytopic), and this orientation is usually maintained as the protein is carried to different membrane destinations in the cell through membrane budding and fusion events (see Chapters 21 and 22).

In **type 1 transmembrane proteins,** the N-terminal signal sequence initiates translocation, similar to soluble proteins (Fig. 20-7B). In the crystal structure of the archaeal SecY complex, the signal sequence binds to two adjacent helices that are proposed to open laterally to let hydrophobic segments of transmembrane proteins exit from the pore into the bilayer (see Fig. 20-6D). A stop-transfer signal (usually the future transmembrane domain) stops the transfer process before the type 1 polypeptide chain is completely translocated. The signal sequence (also called a start-transfer signal) is then cleaved off by the ER signal peptidase, and the polypeptide slides out of the translocon through the lateral exit site. The protein is now oriented with its N-terminus facing the ER lumen, its C-terminus facing the cytoplasm, and its transmembrane segment spanning the ER membrane.

Some type 1 proteins, called **GPI-anchored proteins,** exchange their carboxyl terminal transmembrane segment for an oligosaccharide anchored to the lipid phosphatidylinositol (Fig. 20-7C; also see Fig. 7-9). An enzyme in the ER lumen cleaves off the transmembrane segment and transfers the new C-terminus to a preassembled **glycosylphosphatidylinositol (GPI)** membrane anchor. Many cell surface proteins are attached to the plasma membrane in this manner. This allows them to be readily released from the cell when specific phospholipases in the plasma membrane are activated. For example, during sperm capacitation, many GPI-anchored proteins are cleaved and released from the sperm plasma membrane. This reorganization of the sperm's cell surface is essential for a sperm to fertilize an egg.

Type 2 transmembrane proteins use a transmembrane domain as an internal signal sequence (Fig. 20-7D). Once such an internal signal sequence emerges from a ribosome, it is recognized by SRP and brought to the ER membrane, where it serves as a start-transfer signal to initiate protein translocation. When the protein is fully synthesized, the start-transfer signal, which is not cleaved off, slides out of the translocation channel into the surrounding lipid bilayer, where it serves as a transmembrane anchor.

Polytopic proteins that span the membrane multiple times (such as ion channels and carriers) utilize multiple stop-transfer signals, none of which are cleaved by signal peptides (Fig. 20-7E–F). SRP is probably required to target the first signal sequence to the ER membrane. Thereafter, the dynamics of the channel must accommodate sequences that specify translocation of loops in the cytoplasm or lumen alternating with the transfer of transmembrane segments to the lipid bilayer.

Association of Tail-Anchored Proteins with the Endoplasmic Reticulum Membrane

Although most integral membrane proteins that integrate into the ER bilayer do so by being targeted to and translocated through the Sec61 translocation channel, a group of integral membrane proteins known as C-tail-anchored proteins **(tail-anchored proteins)** do not. These proteins are held in the phospholipid bilayer by a single stretch of hydrophobic amino acids close to the C-terminus and have their entire functional N-terminus facing the cytoplasm (Fig. 20-8).

Tail-anchored proteins lack an N-terminal signal sequence and their membrane-interacting region is so close to the C-terminus that it emerges from the ribosome only on termination of translation. Because of this, tail-anchored proteins do not bind to SRP, which recognizes only signal peptides or signal anchors as long as they are part of a nascent polypeptide chain (i.e., still attached to the ribosome). Tail-anchored proteins also do not posttranslationally target to the Sec61 channel. Instead, they use a still unclear mechanism for membrane insertion that involves ATP, cytosolic factors, and membrane components, and that requires that the C-terminal anchor of the protein be hydrophobic. The C-terminus of a tail-anchored protein that crosses the bilayer doubles as a transmembrane anchor after insertion into the appropriate bilayer with only two to three hydrophilic residues translocated across the membrane. By contrast, most other transmembrane and soluble proteins translocate a much larger hydrophilic region across the membrane during their biogenesis.

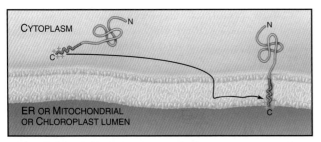

Figure 20-8 TARGETING OF TAIL-ANCHORED PROTEINS TO THE ENDOPLAS-MIC RETICULUM OR MITOCHONDRIAL MEMBRANE. Tail-anchored proteins have a short, hydrophobic transmembrane domain flanked on one or both sides by positively charged residues. The charged residues at the C-terminus and hydrophobic domain directly cross the bilayer with the aid of cytosolic factors and ATP. After insertion, the majority of the protein faces the cytoplasm with only the C-terminal charged residues in the lumen.

Tail-anchored proteins have diverse roles in membrane biogenesis and traffic, as well as in cell metabolism (Table 20-3). They include SNARE proteins, such as syntaxins and synaptobrevins, which are responsible for membrane fusion events within cells (see Chapter 21); Sec61γ and β of the translocation channel; cytochrome b$_5$, which participates in lipid metabolism; and Bcl and Bax, which are found on the mitochondrial outer membrane and regulate apoptosis.

Association of Lipid-Anchored Proteins with the Cytoplasmic Surface of the Endoplasmic Reticulum

Many classes of lipid-anchored proteins, including N- and H-Ras GTPases, are targeted from the cytoplasm to the cytoplasmic leaflet of the ER bilayer by posttranslational modification of a C-terminal cysteine-alanine-alanine-x (CAAX) motif. The first step in this process is prenylation, in which a soluble prenyltransferase attaches a farnesyl or geranylgeranyl lipid to the protein via a stable thioether linkage to the cysteine residue in CAAX. A prenyl-CAAX protease localized in the ER bilayer then cleaves the AAX residues, leaving the prenylcysteine as the new C terminus. The modified cysteine is then recognized by a prenylcysteine carboxyl methyltransferase (pcCMT) also in the ER bilayer that methylesterifies the α carboxyl group. (In the case of N- and H-Ras, a further modification occurs whereby one or two other cysteine residues upstream of the CAAX motif are modified by palmitic acid via a labile thioester linkage.) These hydrophobic C-terminal modifications anchor the otherwise hydrophilic molecule to the cytoplasmic surface of the ER membrane. To reach the plasma membrane, the lipid-anchored proteins follow the secretory pathway out of the ER.

Protein Folding and Oligomerization in the Endoplasmic Reticulum

Once proteins that translocate across the ER bilayer through the Sec61 translocation channel emerge into the ER lumen, they encounter a wealth of proteins that interact with the nascent polypeptide. The proteins remove the signal sequence, add oligosaccharides, and direct folding by catalyzing disulfide bond formation and oligomerization. One such factor, **BiP,** binds unfolded polypeptides by interacting with hydrophobic regions that are normally sequestered in the interior of a protein. This prevents newly synthesized proteins from aggregating and promotes their folding, and it helps to bias the movement of the polypeptide into the lumen but not back out. Another factor involved in protein folding and assembly is **oligosaccharyl transferase,** which adds core sugars to the growing chain when an asparagine in an appropriate sequence passes by. An additional factor is **protein disulfide isomerase (PDI),** which catalyses disulfide exchange between sulfhydryl (SH) groups on cysteines allowing the formation of disulfide (S-S) bonds. The oxidizing equivalents to form disulfide bonds flow from flavin adenine dinucleotide (FAD) through two pairs of cysteines of an ER membrane protein called Ero1p, which oxidizes a pair of cysteines in the active site of PDI. PDI then mediates correct formation of disulfide bonds by forming reversible mixed disulfides with polypeptide substrates until the correct disulfides are formed. Retention of these folding factors in the ER depends on the sequence lysine–aspartic acid–glutamic acid–leucine (KDEL), present at the C-termini of these proteins. If this sequence is deleted, the mutated protein is transported

Table 20-3	
EXAMPLES OF TAIL-ANCHORED PROTEINS	
Protein	**Function**
ER-Inserted	
Target SNAREs (syntaxin)	Target membrane for vesicle insertion
Vesicle SNAREs (synaptobrevin)	Target membrane for vesicle insertion
Giantin	Golgi tethering protein
Sec61γ, Sec61β	ER protein translocation
Cytochrome b(5)	Heme metabolism
Heme oxygenase I and II	Heme metabolism
UBC 6	ER degradation
Mitochondrial-Inserted	
Bcl-2	Apoptosis
Bax	Apoptosis
Tom5, Tom6	Mitochondrial protein translocation

to the Golgi apparatus and secreted from the cell. Addition of KDEL to a normally secreted protein results in its accumulation in the ER.

Folding and assembly factors interact with proteins throughout their lifetimes in the ER. The following sections describe machinery that controls protein folding and assembly in the ER, mechanisms for sensing correctly folded or misfolded proteins, and pathways for disposing of misfolded proteins that accumulate in the ER.

N-linked Glycosylation

The majority of proteins synthesized in association with the ER are glycoproteins with covalently attached carbohydrates. One class of protein glycosylation takes place cotranslationally in the ER by the addition of a preformed oligosaccharide complex to asparagine residues (Fig. 20-9). These asparagine or N-linked oligosaccharides form flexible hydrated branches that can extend 3 nm or more out from the polypeptide. They frequently make up a sizable portion of the mass of a glycoprotein and cover a large fraction of its surface. Because the oligosaccharides are polar, glycosylation makes the protein more hydrophilic and is less likely to aggregate. By avoiding aggregation, the protein has a higher probability of folding into its correct conformation. Hence, oligosaccharides on proteins play a key role in enabling a newly synthesized protein to fold properly. Once correctly folded, the protein can leave the ER and move through the secretory pathway, where the sugars can be modified further. The great diversity of oligosaccharides found on secreted proteins is also crucial for their functions outside the cell.

A single, preformed oligosaccharide precursor, composed of 14 sugars (three glucoses, nine mannoses, and two N-acetyl glucosamines) ($Glc_3Man_9GlcNAc_2$), serves as the core for N-linked oligosaccharides. This precursor is synthesized in a stepwise fashion while attached to the ER membrane by **dolichol phosphate** (a long-chained, unsaturated isoprenoid alcohol with pyrophosphate at one end; Fig. 20-9). Assembly of the oligosaccharide precursor involves 14 separate transfer reactions: seven on the cytoplasmic face of the ER and seven in the lumen. The mechanism that flips the glycolipid across the bilayer is unknown. The enzyme oligosaccharyltransferase recognizes dolichol and transfers the complete oligosaccharide to asparagine side chains on the nascent polypeptide contained in the sequences Asn-X-Ser/Thr, where X is any amino acid other than proline. The sequence must have emerged a distance of 12 to 14 residues out of the translocon into the ER lumen before it can be recognized.

Calnexin/Calreticulin Cycle

Once the core oligosaccharide has been added to the protein, the glycoprotein begins a cycle of modifications that help it to achieve its fully folded state. This **calnexin cycle** (Fig. 20-10) starts when glucosidases I and II remove the first two glucose residues of a core glycan. The resulting monoglucosylated transmembrane or soluble proteins bind to **calnexin,** a type I transmembrane protein in the ER lumen (Fig. 20-10). Monoglucosylated soluble proteins also bind to **calreticulin,** a soluble protein in the ER lumen similar to calnexin. Both proteins are related to sugar-binding lectin proteins from legumes. Both are monomeric, calcium-

Figure 20-9 DOLICHOL PATHWAY. A core oligosaccharide consisting of mannose and N-acetylglucosamine is synthesized in the cytoplasm, attached through high-energy pyrophosphate bonds to dolichol in the ER membrane. Following transfer across the ER bilayer, the addition of sugars imported into the ER completes the core structure. The oligosaccharide-transferase complex transfers the completed oligosaccharide to the consensus Asn-X-Ser/Thr motif of a nascent chain as it enters the lumen of the ER.

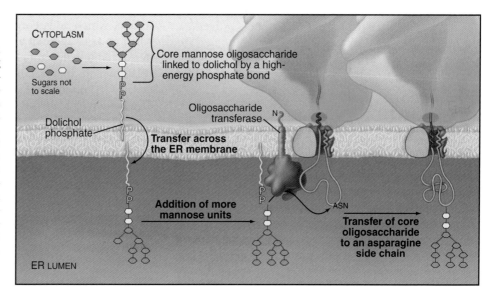

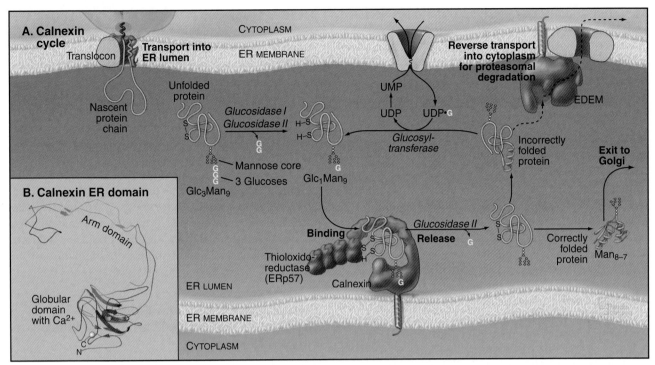

Figure 20-10 CALNEXIN CYCLE OF PROTEIN FOLDING IN THE LUMEN OF THE ENDOPLASMIC RETICULUM AND PROTEIN DEGRADATION FROM THE ENDOPLASMIC RETICULUM. **A,** Glucosidases I and II rapidly remove two of three glucoses from newly synthesized, unfolded glycoprotein. The calnexin-thioloxidoreductase complex binds the monoglucosylated protein. Glucosidase II removes the remaining glucose, releasing the protein. If the released protein is folded, it can exit the ER. If unfolded, it is recognized by glucosyltransferase and reglucosylated so that it reenters the folding cycle until folding is complete, or it enters the degradation pathway by interacting with EDEM and a retrograde translocation channel, which deliver the unfolded polypeptide to the proteasome for degradation. Thioloxidoreductases catalyze rearrangements of disulfide bonds during folding. (Glc, glucose; Man, mannose; UDP, uridine diphosphate; UMP, uridine monophosphate.) **B,** Three-dimensional structure of calnexin showing a globular, lectin-binding domain and an extended arm composed of four repeat modules that folds around a sugar residue after it binds to the globular domain.

binding proteins. Binding to calnexin or calreticulin sequesters the glycoprotein and prevents its aggregation. It also exposes the glycoprotein to ERp57, a thiol-disulfide oxidoreductase. A close homolog of protein disulfide isomerase, ERp57 forms a complex with calnexin and calreticulin and specifically interacts with glycoproteins. ERp57 catalyzes intramolecular disulfide bond interchange during the folding process.

Release of bound glycoprotein chains from calnexin/ERp57 occurs once glucosidase II removes the remaining glucose residue on the core glycan. The glycoprotein is now free to leave the ER unless recognized by a soluble enzyme, UDP-Glc:glycoprotein glucosyltransferase (GT). GT reglucosylates only incompletely folded glycoproteins, so it serves as a folding sensor in the cycle. When reglucosylated by GT, the glycoprotein rebinds to calnexin or calreticulin. The glycoprotein stays in the cycle until it is properly folded and oligomerized, in which case it enters the secretory pathway. If the protein cannot fold or oligomerize properly, it is removed from the cycle by being translocated out of the ER into the cytoplasm, where it is degraded. When association with the cycle is inhibited, for example, by blocking the action of the glucosidases, the folding efficiency decreases. In this case, the glycoprotein may associate with BiP, which cooperates with the calnexin cycle in helping the protein to fold correctly.

Protein Degradation in the Endoplasmic Reticulum and the Unfolded Protein Response

Many polypeptides transferred to the ER are subunits of homo-oligomeric or hetero-oligomeric protein complexes. Oligomer assembly generally occurs prior to ER export and involves chaperones such as BiP that protect hydrophobic surfaces found at subunit interfaces. Because each polypeptide is synthesized on its own ribosome and because the synthesis of the chains composing a complex may be unbalanced, additional chaperones promote subunit interactions and prevent premature export or degradation. For example, chaperones play a critical role in antigen presentation by ensuring that only peptide-loaded major histocompatibility complex type I proteins exit the ER. These chaperones also protect cell surface receptors and other secreted proteins from binding potential ligands that are also imported into the ER and that could activate them prematurely.

Protein Degradation in Endoplasmic Reticulum

The ER has a highly regulated mechanism to prevent the export of dysfunctional proteins into the secretory pathway. Improperly folded polypeptides, excess subunits of oligomeric assemblies, or incorrectly assembled oligomers are degraded rather than being exported from the ER (Fig. 20-10). The degradation process, termed **ER-associated degradation (ERAD),** prevents accumulation of unsalvageable, misfolded proteins in the ER. ERAD occurs in four sequential steps: a misfolded glycoprotein is first recognized, retrotranslocated across the ER membrane to the cytoplasm, ubiquitinated (see Fig. 23-8), and then degraded by a proteasome in the cytoplasm.

For a protein to be targeted for ERAD, it must be misfolded or unassembled. The cell distinguishes a misfolded or unassembled protein subunit from a bona fide folding intermediate by linking degradation of glycoproteins to the trimming of mannoses (Fig. 20-10). The longer an unfolded glycoprotein remains in the ER, the more likely it will be exposed to mannosidases, which trim terminal mannose residues from the core oligosaccharide. When such trimming occurs, the glycoprotein becomes a substrate for ERAD and is recognized by a membrane-bound ER protein called **EDEM** (for "ER degradation-enhancing α-mannosidase-like protein"), which helps to direct the glycoprotein to the retrotranslocation channel. (Elimination of the EDEM homolog in yeast retards ERAD of glycoproteins but not of nonglycosylated proteins, which use a different pathway for degradation.) Because the concentration of mannosidases in the ER is low, newly synthesized proteins and nascent chains have time to fold correctly and thereby avoid having their terminal mannoses trimmed. Once mannose trimming on these molecules has occurred, EDEM begins to compete for these substrates with the calnexin/calreticulin cycle. The channel that exports ERAD substrates back into the cytoplasm for degradation (termed the **retrotranslocon**) remains to be identified.

Endoplasmic Reticulum Stress Responses and Endoplasmic Reticulum Folding Diseases

The folding pathway in the ER is tightly linked to the physiological state of the cell. Conditions that flood the ER with excess protein or result in accumulation of misfolded proteins trigger the **unfolded protein response** (**UPR**; Fig. 20-11). Essentially, any condition that exceeds the protein-folding capacity of the ER triggers the unfolded protein response: misfolding of mutant proteins, inhibition of ER glycosylation (by the drug

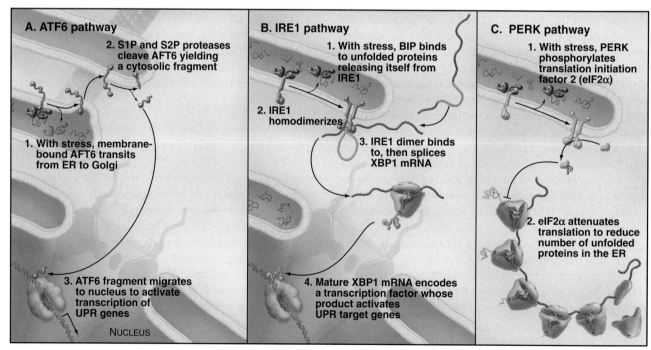

Figure 20-11   UNFOLDED PROTEIN RESPONSE PATHWAYS TO STRESS IN THE LUMEN OF THE ENDOPLASMIC RETICULUM. **A,** ATF6 pathway. **B,** IRE1 pathway. **C,** PERK pathway.

tunicamycin), inhibition of disulfide formation (by reducing agents), or even overproduction of normal proteins. To compensate for these events, this stress-induced signaling pathway upregulates genes that are required to synthesize the entire ER, including folding machinery. In yeast, the unfolded protein response activates more than 300 genes involved with all aspects of ER function, including lipid synthesis, protein translocation, protein folding, glycosylation, and degradation, as well as export to and retrieval from the Golgi apparatus. Developmental programs might work through the same genetic controls to determine the abundance of ER in differentiated cells, producing, for example, extensive ER in secretory cells such as plasma, liver, and pancreatic acinar cells.

The Unfolded Protein Response

The response to ER stress (i.e., UPR) is regulated by three key ER transmembrane proteins: **IRE1** (inositol requiring 1), **PERK/PEK** (PKR-like endoplasmic reticulum kinase/pancreatic eIF2a kinase), and **ATF6** (activating transcription factor 6). These proteins serve as stress sensors to regulate the production of **bZIP (basic leucine zipper) domain–containing transcription factors** (see Fig. 15-17) that upregulate genes involved in ER function. This allows cells to adjust the capacity of the ER to promote ER folding depending on the demand. Whereas only IRE1 is present in yeast, all three transmembrane proteins are present and function in metazoan cells.

Accumulation of unfolded proteins in the ER lumen of metazoan cells results in activation of ATF6, IRE1, and PERK, each by a different mechanism (Fig. 20-11). Under normal conditions, free BiP is thought to inhibit the UPR pathway. BiP binds to the lumenal domains of IRE1 and PERK, preventing their dimerization. BiP also associates with ATF6, retaining it in the ER. When unfolded proteins accumulate during ER stress, BiP binds to them rather than to IRE1, ATF6, and PERK.

When released from BiP, ATF6 is transported to the Golgi, where it is cleaved by S1P and S2P proteases to produce a cytoplasmic fragment. The fragment moves to the nucleus, where it activates the transcription of responsive genes, including XBP1.

Freed of BiP, IRE1 dimerizes. This activates IRE1's cytoplasmic endoribonuclease activity allowing it to remove a small intron from the XBP1 mRNA. This alters the translational reading frame of XBP1 to make a protein that is a potent transcriptional activator.

When dissociated from BiP, PERK phosphorylates the **eukaryotic translation initiation factor 2 (eIF2).** This reduces the frequency of AUG codon recognition and thereby slows the rate of translation initiation on many mRNAs. The mRNAs that are preferentially translated under these conditions are all involved in cell survival and ER functions.

Aspects of the UPR pathway involving IRE1 and PERK are also important for promoting differentiation in higher eukaryotic cells. For example, IRE1 is activated during B-lymphocyte differentiation into a plasma cell (see Fig. 28-9), in which the ER expands 5-fold to accommodate immunoglobulin synthesis. Activation of the innate immune response (i.e., the inflammatory response), for example by lipopolysaccharide (LPS) treatment, also activates IRE1. Furthermore, PERK activity is required for B-cell differentiation and/or survival. These findings have led to the view that the UPR allows cells to respond to ER stress, to provide a way to sense nutrients and to promote differentiation.

Endoplasmic Reticulum Folding Diseases

Given the central role of the ER in the synthesis of proteins for the entire exocytic and endocytic pathways, it is not surprising that many inherited diseases are a direct consequence of proteins failing to pass ER quality control. Many metabolic disorders, including some lysosomal storage diseases (see Appendix 23-1), are a direct consequence of key enzymes failing to be exported from the ER. The most common form of **cystic fibrosis** is due to the inability of cells to export a mutant form of the cystic fibrosis transmembrane regulator (CFTR) to the cell surface, where it would normally function as a chloride channel for the respiratory system and pancreas (see Fig. 11-4). Similarly, the inability of the liver to secrete mutated forms of α1-antitrypsin predisposes to the lung disease emphysema. Normally, α1-antitrypsin protects tissues by inhibiting extracellular proteases such as elastase, which is produced by neutrophils. Mutations prevent α1-antitrypsin folding in the ER, resulting in its degradation. The resulting deficiency in α1-antitrypsin circulating in the blood allows elastase to destroy lung tissue, leading to emphysema. In severe cases, mutant forms of the protein not only fail to be exported from the ER but also elude degradation pathways, accumulating as insoluble aggregates that induce stress responses and liver failure.

In some conditions, the ER uses the unfolded protein response to compensate, in part, for mutations in cargo proteins. In congenital **hypothyroidism,** mutant thyroglobulin (the precursor of thyroid hormone) is not exported efficiently from the ER. Excess protein accumulates as insoluble aggregates in the ER. Feedback pathways trigger massive proliferation of ER in an attempt to produce normal levels of circulating hormone. Similarly, in mild forms of **osteogenesis imperfecta** (see Chapter 32), osteoblasts assemble and secrete defective procollagen chains for bone synthesis, even though the resulting bone tissue is weak. The alternative, complete loss of procollagen by retention and degradation of the mutant procollagen in the ER would be lethal. Faulty ER quality control may also contribute to diseases of the central and peripheral nervous systems, including Alzheimer's disease.

Lipid Biosynthesis, Metabolism, and Transport within the Endoplasmic Reticulum

The ER membrane synthesizes all the major classes of lipids or their precursors that are formed within cells. These include phosphoglycerides, cholesterol, and ceramide. ER enzymes participating in phosphoglyceride synthesis have their active sites facing the cytoplasm, the site of synthesis of most lipid precursors. Synthesis begins with the conjugation of two activated fatty acids to glycerol-3 phosphate to form phosphatidic acid, which can be dephosphorylated to produce diacylglycerol (DAG; see Fig. 26-4). Neither phosphatidic acid nor DAG is a bulk component of membranes; however, both are used in the synthesis of the four major phospholipids: **phosphatidylcholine** (PC), **phosphatidylethanolamine** (PE), **phosphatidylserine** (PS), and **phosphatidylinositol** (PI) (see Fig. 7-2). The most abundant phospholipids, PC and PE, are produced with the activated head groups, cytidine diphosphate (CDP)–choline, and CDP-ethanolamine. PI synthesis is by a distinct route using inositol and CDP-DAG produced from phosphatidic acid (see Fig. 26-7). PS synthesis (in mammalian cells) is an energy-independent exchange of polar head groups of PE. Head group exchange of phospholipids occurs primarily in the ER but may also occur in other organelles.

Like other types of biosynthesis carried out in the ER, phospholipid synthesis creates a topologic problem: Synthesis occurs in the cytoplasmic leaflet, restricting membrane growth to that leaflet. Phospholipids move to the luminal leaflet by individual molecules flip-flopping across the bilayer (Fig. 20-12). Flip-flopping of phospholipids across the ER bilayer is much faster than that in vesicles of pure phospholipids, owing to protein translocators called flippases. ER flippases function independently of metabolic energy and catalyze the transverse movement of most phospholipid classes in both directions promoting a symmetric lipid distribution across the ER bilayer (Fig. 20-12A). Catalysis of flip-flopping in the ER is probably not the role of one specific protein, as peptides that mimic the α-helices of transmembrane proteins can stimulate flip-flopping of phospholipids in liposomes. Cholesterol inhibits helix-induced flip-flopping. Cholesterol is a minor component of the ER but abundant in the plasma membrane. Because of this, the mechanism of transbilayer lipid movement in the plasma membrane, in contrast to that for ER membrane, involves tightly controlled translocation

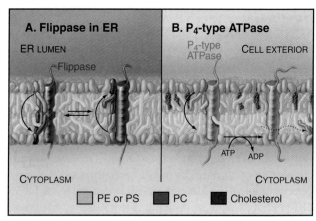

Figure 20-12   TRANSVERSE MOVEMENT OF PHOSPHOLIPIDS ACROSS THE MEMBRANE BILAYER. **A,** Flippases in the ER catalyze the exchange of lipids between leaflets promoting lipid symmetry across the ER bilayer. **B,** P4-type ATPases at the plasma membrane use ATP hydrolysis to transfer PS and PE from the exoplasmic to the cytoplasmic leaflet of the plasma membrane.

mechanisms, including energy-dependent inward and outward flippases (Fig. 20-12B).

Energy-dependent inward flippases, such as aminophospholipid translocase (i.e., a **P4-type ATPase**), use ATP hydrolysis to mediate a fast ($t_{1/2}$ min) exchange of PS and PE from the exoplasmic to cytoplasmic leaflet of the plasma membrane. This process keeps PS in the *exoplasmic* leaflet of the plasma membrane low. Exoplasmic PS can trigger blood coagulation or signal engulfment of apoptotic cells by macrophages. By keeping PE levels high in the *cytosolic* leaflet, it further facilitates endocytic budding events at the plasma membrane due to PE's cone-like shape, which causes expansion of the cytoplasmic leaflet relative to the exoplasmic leaflet.

Energy-dependent outward flippases at the plasma membrane include the family of **ABC transporters** (e.g., ABCA1, MDR1, MDR3) that facilitate the outward translocation of PC, glycosphingolipids, and cholesterol. This is important in liver cells, which mediate lipid extrusion into the bile by outward translocation of lipid at the apical plasma membrane and its subsequent desorption from the cell surface into the bile duct.

Cholesterol Synthesis and Metabolism

Cholesterol is maintained in animal cells by a combination of de novo synthesis (Fig. 20-13) in the ER and receptor-mediated endocytosis of lipoprotein particles containing esterified cholesterol (see Chapter 22). Coordinated regulation of these two processes precisely maintains the physiological level of cholesterol in cellular membranes. Peroxisomes also may participate in aspects of cholesterol synthesis and metabolism.

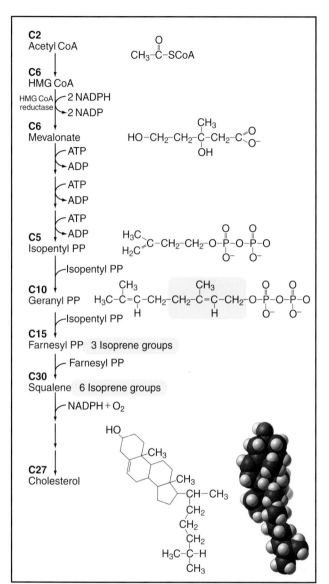

Figure 20-13 Key steps in the biosynthesis of cholesterol from acetyl CoA. Synthesis of mevalonate from 3-hydroxy-3-methylglutaryl CoA is closely regulated by controlling the concentration of the enzyme, HMG-CoA reductase, as shown in Figure 20-14. Five-carbon isoprene groups are the building blocks (yellow) for making a 10-carbon geranyl-pyrophosphate (PP), a 15-carbon farnesyl-pyrophosphate, and 30-carbon squalene intermediates. Several reactions add a hydroxyl group and join squalene into four rings to make cholesterol. ADP, adenosine diphosphate; NADP, nicotinamide adenine dinucleotide phosphate.

key step. Enzymes in the ER bilayer catalyze the subsequent condensation of farnesyl-PP to make squalene, and cyclization to cholesterol, progressively less-polar molecules. Although the final steps leading to cholesterol take place in the ER, cholesterol is not a resident ER lipid and is rapidly exported to post-ER membranes, including the plasma membrane, where it constitutes up to 50% of the bilayer. Chapter 21 discusses the distribution of cholesterol in different organelles and current ideas regarding its transport.

Feedback loops sense the cholesterol content of the ER membrane and regulate both the synthesis and degradation of enzymes that synthesize cholesterol (Fig. 20-14). High cholesterol levels inhibit the synthesis and stimulate the destruction of key synthetic enzymes. A novel transcription factor precursor, steroid regulator element-binding proteins **(SREBP)**, controls the expression of these genes. When cholesterol is abundant, SREBP cleavage-activating protein **(SCAP)**, a partner protein with cholesterol-sensing transmembrane segments, retains SREBP in the ER owing to interactions with the protein Insig. When the membrane cholesterol level is low, SCAP and Insig proteins do not interact. The SREBP-SCAP complex is then free to move to the Golgi apparatus, where two successive proteolytic cleavages release the N-terminal domain of SREBP, a basic helix-loop-helix leucine zipper transcription factor, into the cytoplasm. (The Golgi proteases that are responsible for cleaving SREBP are SP1 and SP2, the same ones used to process ATF6 during UPR.) In the nucleus, the transcription factor binds steroid regulatory elements, enhancers for a wide range of genes encoding enzymes that synthesize cholesterol and other lipids, as well as low-density lipoprotein receptors that take up cholesterol from the medium (see Fig. 23-9). Cholesterol also regulates degradation of HMG-CoA reductase, which has cholesterol-sensing transmembrane domains similar to SCAP. Abundant cholesterol targets HMG-CoA reductase for degradation by the proteolytic pathway that disposes of unfolded proteins through the proteasome (Fig. 20-10 and Chapter 23). The enzyme **acyl-CoA-cholesterol transferase (ACAT)** helps to lower cholesterol levels in the ER bilayer by catalyzing the formation of cholesterol esters, a storage form of cholesterol.

Ceramide Synthesis

Ceramide, the backbone of all sphingolipids (see Fig. 7-3), also begins its synthesis on the cytoplasmic face of ER membranes. It is made through sequential condensation of the amino acid serine with two fatty acids. Ceramide is transported to the Golgi apparatus by a nonvesicular pathway (see later), where enzymes on the lumenal leaflet either add oligosaccharide chains to it to form glycosphingolipids or add a choline head group to form sphingomyelin (see Chapter 21).

Enzymes in the cytoplasm and ER use 22 sequential steps to synthesize cholesterol from acetate (Fig. 20-13). Cytoplasmic enzymes catalyze the initial steps, using water-soluble molecules to produce **farnesyl-pyrophosphate** (farnesyl-PP) from acetyl coenzyme A (acetyl CoA). An important exception is the step going from 3-hydroxy-3methylglutaryl CoA (HMG-CoA) to mevalonate. A carefully regulated, integral membrane protein of the ER (Fig. 20-13), **HMG-CoA reductase,** catalyzes this

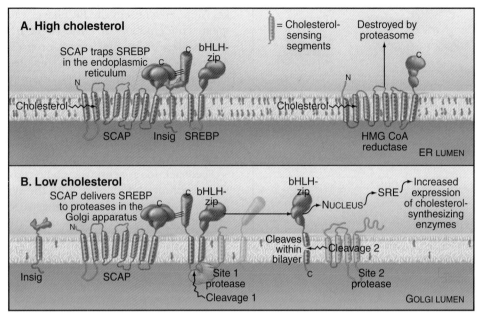

Figure 20-14   CONTROL OF CHOLESTEROL BIOSYNTHESIS BY PROTEOLYSIS. **A,** High-cholesterol conditions. Cholesterol-sensing transmembrane segments *(pink)* of SCAP (SREBP cleavage-activation proteins) retain intact SREBP in the ER through an interaction with Insig. Similar cholesterol-sensing transmembrane segments of HMG-CoA reductase stimulate its destruction by proteolysis. **B,** Low-cholesterol conditions. Insig dissociates from SCAP and SREBP, allowing these molecules to move to the Golgi apparatus where the membrane-anchored site 1 serine protease cleaves the loop of SREBP in the lumen. Subsequently, an unusual transmembrane zinc-protease cleaves SREBP at a second site within the bilayer, releasing the basic helix-loop-helix-zip (bHLH-zip) transcription factor. This factor enters the nucleus, where it activates genes for cholesterol biosynthetic enzymes by steroid-response elements (SREs).

Lipid Movement between Organelles

While lipids can rapidly diffuse along one side of the bilayer as well as flip-flop across the bilayer, the hydrophobic nature of lipids makes free diffusion between adjacent bilayers thermodynamically unfavorable. Thus, lipids use two other mechanisms to move between organelles (Fig. 20-15). The major pathway is movement through the use of vesicle carriers (see Chapter 21). In addition, small, soluble phospholipid exchange proteins promote movements between membranes by a nonvesicular mechanism. These proteins—called **lipid-transfer proteins (LTPs)**—have a common overall structure and are specific for particular phospholipids. One example of an LTP is **ceramide transport protein (CERT),** which mediates ceramide transport to the Golgi apparatus by extracting newly synthesized ceramide from the ER and carrying it to the Golgi apparatus. To accomplish this, CERT has a domain that recognizes ceramide and mediates its intermembrane transfer. CERT also has a motif for targeting to the ER and a PH domain (see Fig. 25-11) for binding polyphosphoinositides in the Golgi apparatus.

LTPs catalyze lipid exchange but not net transfer. When the protein delivers a lipid to a target membrane, the protein exchanges that lipid for another one and returns with the second lipid (Fig. 20-15). The lipid-binding pocket of LTPs is largely lined with hydrophobic residues that stabilize the internal lipid. In the open

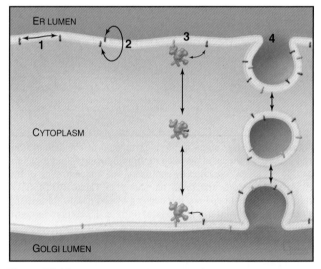

Figure 20-15   MECHANISMS OF LIPID MOVEMENT WITHIN, ACROSS, AND BETWEEN MEMBRANE BILAYERS. Membrane lipids can (1) laterally diffuse within the bilayer, (2) translocate between two leaflets of the bilayer, (3) move through the cytosol from one bilayer to another by attaching to a cytosolic lipid-transfer protein, or (4) be transported from one membrane compartment to another by incorporating into membrane-bound transport carriers.

conformation, a hinged cover projects outward away from the protein, allowing the LTP to embed itself partially into the cytosolic leaflet of the bilayer. Interactions with other membrane components (either lipids or proteins) dictate what compartments the LTP targets to.

Zones of close apposition between the ER and other organelles—such as mitochondria, chloroplasts, lipid droplets, TGN, endosomes, and lysosomes—are enriched in certain types of LTPs, suggesting that lipid trafficking occurs across these sites. Some proteins with lipid transfer domains might function as lipid sensors rather than as lipid carriers.

ACKNOWLEDGMENTS

Thanks go to Ramanujan Hegde, Carolyn Ott, and Peter Kim for their suggestions on revisions to this chapter.

SELECTED READINGS

Borgese N, Colombo S, Pedrazzini, E: The tale of tail-anchored proteins: Coming from the cytosol and looking for a membrane. J Cell Biol 161:1013-1019, 2003.

Choy E, Chiu VK, Silletti J, et al: Endomembrane trafficking of Ras: The CAAX motif targets proteins to the ER and Golgi. Cell 98:69-80, 1999.

Clemons WM, Menetret J-F, Akey CW, Rapoport TA: Structural insight into the protein translocation channel. Curr Opin Struct Biol 14:390-396, 2004.

Egea PF, Stroud RM, Walter P: Targeting proteins to membranes: Structure of the signal recognition particle. Curr Opin Struct Biol 15:213-220, 2005.

Helenius A, Aebi M: Roles of N-linked glycans in the endoplasmic reticulum. Annu Rev Biochem 73:1019-1049, 2004.

Holthuis JCM, Levine TP: Lipid traffic: Floppy drives and a superhighway. Nat Rev Mol Cell Biol 6:209-220, 2005.

Meusser B, Hirsch C, Jarosch E, Sommer T: ERAD, the long road to destruction. Nat Cell Biol 7:766-772, 2005.

Osborne AR, Rapoport TA, van den Berg B: Protein translocation by the Sec61/SecY channel. Annu Rev Cell Dev Biol 21:529-550, 2005.

Rawson RB: The SREBP pathway: Insights from insigs and insects. Mol Cell Biol 4:631-640, 2003.

Schröder M, Kaufman RJ: The mammalian unfolded protein response. Annu Rev Biochem 24:739-789, 2005.

Sitia R, Braakman I: Quality control in the endoplasmic reticulum protein factory. Nature 426:891-894, 2003.

Sprong H, van der Sluijs P, van Meer G: How proteins move lipids and lipids move proteins. Nat Rev 2:804-813, 2001.

Secretory Membrane System and Golgi Apparatus

Eukaryotic cells transport newly synthesized proteins destined for the extracellular space, the plasma membrane, or the endocytic/lysosomal system through a series of functionally distinct, membrane-bound compartments, including the **endoplasmic reticulum (ER), Golgi apparatus,** and vesicular transport intermediates. This is the secretory membrane system (Fig. 21-1), which allows eukaryotic cells to perform three major functions: (1) distribute proteins and lipids synthesized in the ER to the cell surface and other cellular sites, (2) modify and/or store protein and lipid molecules after their export from the ER, and (3) generate and maintain the unique identity and function of the ER, Golgi apparatus, and plasma membrane. This chapter describes how the secretory membrane system is organized and operates to fulfill these functions. It also provides a detailed description of the Golgi apparatus whose conserved features are central for the operation of the secretory membrane system.

Overview of the Secretory Membrane System

The secretory membrane system uses membrane-enclosed transport carriers to move thousands of diverse macromolecules—including proteins, proteoglycans, and glyco-proteins—efficiently and precisely among different membrane-bound compartments (i.e., the ER, Golgi apparatus, and plasma membrane). Within the large cytoplasmic volume of the eukaryotic cell (up to 10^3 times that of the volume of a prokaryotic cell), this is essential for coordinating cellular needs in response to the constantly changing environment and organismal physiology.

Newly synthesized transmembrane and lumenal proteins transported through the secretory system are called **cargo.** These include lumenal proteins destined to be stored within a compartment or secreted to the cell exterior, as well as transmembrane proteins that are retained in a particular compartment (e.g., Golgi processing enzymes), delivered to the plasma membrane, or recycled among compartments (e.g., transport machinery). Transfer of cargo molecules through the secretory system begins with their cotranslational insertion into or across the ER bilayer (see Fig. 20-7). The cargo molecules are next folded and assembled into forms that can be sorted and concen-

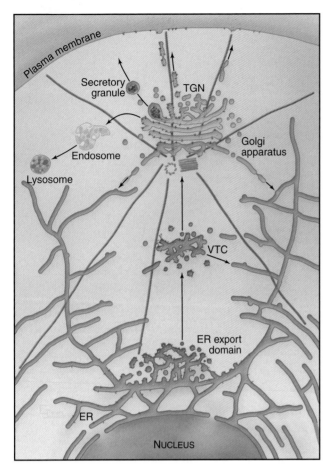

Figure 21-1 OVERVIEW OF THE SECRETORY MEMBRANE SYSTEM. The three principal organelles of the secretory pathway—the ER, Golgi apparatus, and plasma membrane—communicate with one another and the cell exterior by way of transport carriers. The carriers (either small vesicles or larger vesicle-tubule elements) move along cytoskeletal elements (*red lines*) to transfer newly synthesized proteins, called cargo, from the ER to the Golgi, and from the Golgi to the plasma membrane (or to the endosome/lysosomal system). Carriers form from the ER at specialized regions, called ER export domains, producing pre-Golgi structures called vesicular tubular carriers (VTCs) that move to the Golgi. Retrograde transport carriers bud off from the VTC or Golgi apparatus to retrieve proteins and lipids back to the ER for repeated use and to balance the anterograde flow of membrane to the plasma membrane. The lumenal spaces enclosed by the carriers and organelles of the secretory membrane system are all topologically equivalent to the outside of the cell.

trated within membrane-bound transport intermediates (called **vesicular tubular carriers [VTCs]**) destined for the Golgi apparatus. Once packaged into and transported by such a carrier, cargo enters the Golgi apparatus, which serves as the central processing and sorting station in the secretory membrane system. Within the Golgi apparatus, numerous enzymes modify the cargo molecules by trimming or elongating the cargo's glycan side chains or cleaving its polypeptides. Processed cargo is then sorted into membrane-bound carriers that bud out from the Golgi apparatus and move to the plasma membrane, to the endosome/lysosomal system, or back

to the ER. In specialized cell types, the Golgi apparatus can sort certain classes of cargo into secretory granules (for storage and later release to the cell exterior in response to specific stimuli) or give rise to transport carriers that target to different polarized plasma membrane domains.

Membrane-enclosed **carriers** mediate transport within the secretory membrane system (Fig. 21-2). Carriers are shaped as tubules, vesicles, or larger structures. The carriers are too large to diffuse freely in the crowded cytoplasm but are transported over long distances along microtubules or actin filaments by molecular motor proteins. Each carrier selects certain types of cargo before budding from a donor compartment and fuses only with an appropriate target membrane. Molecular markers on the cytoplasmic surface of the carrier, as well as on the acceptor membrane, steer the carrier through the cytoplasm and ensure that it fuses only with the correct target compartment. The carriers continuously shuttle among ER, Golgi apparatus, and plasma membranes, enabling cargo to be distributed to its appropriate target organelle.

Sorting of cargo into transport carriers is facilitated by the presence of specialized lipids in the donor organelle membrane (such as sphingomyelin, glycosphingolipids, and phosphoinositides in the Golgi apparatus) and by the recruitment of protein-based sorting and transport machinery (e.g., coat proteins and tethering/fusion factors). Together, the specialized lipids and protein-sorting machinery generate membrane microdomains that concentrate or exclude cargo. The domains then pinch off the membrane bilayer as membrane-enclosed carriers and travel to target membranes.

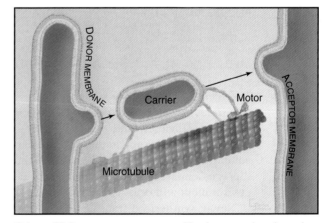

Figure 21-2 CARRIER TRANSPORT. Membrane-enclosed carriers (shaped as vesicles, tubules, or vesicle-tubule elements) bud off from a donor compartment after packaging both lumenal and transmembrane cargo proteins. Carriers are moved through the cytoplasm along cytoskeletal elements (e.g., microtubules in mammalian cells) by motor proteins until they fuse with a target compartment. During this process, the relative topology of the lipids and transmembrane proteins is maintained.

During transport of a carrier, the relative orientation (called topology) of lipid and protein in the membrane bilayer, established during synthesis in the ER, is maintained (Fig. 21-2). Hence, one side of the membrane always faces the cytoplasm. The other side initially faces the lumen of the ER. This side remains inside each membrane compartment along the secretory pathway but is exposed on the cell surface if the carrier fuses with the plasma membrane. Selection of proteins and lipids by a carrier, budding of the carrier, and subsequent fusion of the carrier with an acceptor compartment all also occur without leakage of contents from the carrier or the donor and target compartments.

The flow of cargo and lipid forward through the secretory system toward the plasma membrane (**antero-grade traffic**) is balanced by selective **retrograde traffic** of cargo and lipids back toward the ER (Fig. 21-1). Retrograde traffic allows proteins and lipids involved in membrane transport and fusion to be retrieved for repeated use. Retrograde traffic also returns proteins that have been inadvertently carried forward through the secretory system so they can be redirected to their proper destination. Both anterograde and retrograde flows of membrane within the secretory system are necessary for the ER, Golgi apparatus, and plasma membrane to generate and maintain their distinct functional and morphologic identities.

Advantages of the Secretory Membrane System

The secretory membrane system, found in all eukaryotic cells, offers numerous advantages over the simpler secretory process in prokaryotic cells, which involves insertion of newly synthesized proteins directly into or across the plasma membrane. First, synthesizing, folding, and processing membrane and secretory proteins within a series of distinct compartments provides a protective environment for cells to modify proteins before they are exposed on the cell surface. Newly synthesized proteins within the ER, for example, can fold into complex shapes and assemble into multisubunit complexes. Within the Golgi apparatus, the cargo molecules can be further modified by glycan processing and proteolytic cleavage. The resulting repertoire of protein structures that are expressed at the cell surface is significantly larger and capable of performing more diverse functions than that found in prokaryotes.

A second advantage is the capacity of the secretory membrane system to regulate protein secretion and expression at the cell surface. Eukaryotic cells can store proteins in membrane compartments before releasing them at the cell surface in response to internal or external signals. By exploiting these capabilities, eukaryotic cells have evolved elaborate ways to control the types of proteins located on or secreted from the cell surface.

A third advantage relates to the differentiation of the plasma membrane. Prokaryotic cells synthesize their proteins at the plasma membrane, so they must keep this surface enriched in loosely packed glycerophospholipids that are pliable enough that newly synthesized proteins can enter into and fold in a hydrophobic environment. Consequently, prokaryotic cells secrete a rigid cell wall as a protective barrier to the outside. In eukaryotes, concentrating protein synthesis in the ER frees the plasma membrane to become enriched in lipids such as cholesterol and sphingolipids that can arrange into highly ordered, flexible arrays. The ordered, flexible arrays of cholesterol and sphingolipids in the plasma membrane provide mechanical stability and an impermeable barrier to water-soluble molecules. As a consequence, eukaryotic cells do not require a cell wall to survive (although some eukaryotes, such as plant and fungal cells, make cell walls) and can employ their plasma membrane in a wide range of functions, such as membrane protrusion for engulfing large extracellular objects (see Chapter 22) and for crawling (see Chapter 38).

Building and Maintaining the Secretory Membrane System

Effective operation of the secretory membrane system depends on several features. The system must generate and maintain the specialized character of each secretory compartment (including the different lipid and protein environments of the ER, Golgi apparatus, and plasma membrane) in the face of continual exchange of protein and lipid components. Cargo must be concentrated selectively in or excluded from each transport carrier. Each carrier must be directed along a specific route and fuse only with an appropriate target membrane.

Two mechanisms, described in more detail in the following sections, play important roles in accomplishing these tasks. First, a lipid-based sorting mechanism uses the inherent capacity of lipids to self-organize into different domains to create a gradient of phospholipid composition across the secretory pathway. On the basis of the length of their transmembrane segments, transmembrane proteins partition into particular membranes that differ in the thickness of the lipid bilayer. Second, protein-based sorting machinery generates transport carriers capable of concentrating specific cargo proteins and targeting to appropriate acceptor membranes, where they fuse and deliver their cargo.

Protein Sorting by the Lipid Gradient across the Secretory Membrane System

A conserved feature of the secretory membrane system is the differential distribution of various classes of lipids

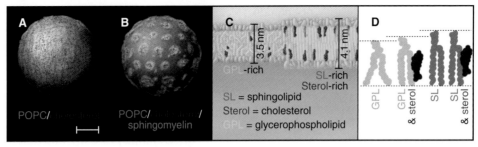

Figure 21-3 PROPERTIES OF LIPIDS WITHIN MEMBRANES. **A–B,** Cartoon depiction of an artificial bilayer containing a POPC/cholesterol mixture of 2:1 **(A)** and a POPC/cholesterol/sphingomyelin mixture of 2:1:1 (POPC, 1-palmitoyl-2-oleoyl-*sn*-glycero-3-phosphocholine) **(B).** The *blue spherical spots* in part **B** are cholesterol- and sphingomyelin-enriched domains that have segregated from POPC because of the affinity between sphingomyelin and cholesterol. **C,** A bilayer enriched in cholesterol and sphingomyelin has a greater thickness than a bilayer composed mainly of glycerophospholipids, owing to the long saturated hydrocarbon chains of glycosphingolipids that attract proteins with longer transmembrane domains. **D,** Glycerophospholipid-containing membranes with high concentrations of cholesterol have a greater thickness than those with low concentrations, owing to a tighter alignment of the hydrocarbon chains. Scale bar is 5 μm.

along the pathway. These classes of lipids include **glycerophospholipids** (phosphoglycerides), **sphingolipids** (e.g., sphingomyelin and glycosphingolipids), and **cholesterol** (see Figs. 7-4 and 20-13). These lipids play a major role in the sorting of proteins within the secretory membrane system because of their immiscibility (i.e., the property of not mixing) in membranes with different lipid compositions. By not mixing with some lipids while mixing with others, these lipid classes form lateral lipid assemblies, termed *microdomains,* that can concentrate or exclude specific membrane proteins.

Studies using artificial membranes have demonstrated how lipid immiscibility allows a continuous lipid bilayer to self-organize into distinct **lipid domains** with unique lipid compositions and biophysical properties. A prime example is an artificial bilayer containing glycerophospholipids and cholesterol to which sphingolipid is added; after sphingolipid is added, the cholesterol and glycerophospholipids partition into distinct domains (Fig. 21-3A–B). Because of van der Waals attraction between the sphingolipid's long, saturated hydrocarbon chain and cholesterol's rigid, flat-cylindrical steroid backbone, the cholesterol and sphingolipids associate in the plane of the membrane, whereas glycerophospholipids, which have unsaturated, kinked hydrocarbon chains with much less affinity for cholesterol, are largely excluded from the cholesterol/sphingolipid domains. The domains enriched in cholesterol/sphingolipid are thicker than the surrounding membrane composed of shorter, unsaturated, kinked glycerophospholipids (Fig. 21-3C). Tension on the bilayer (i.e., from binding of proteins that bend or curve the membrane) enhances the tendency of lipids that have different physical properties to separate into distinct phases.

In addition to prompting separation of sphingolipids from glycerophospholipids, cholesterol can affect a bilayer composed of glycerophospholipids alone (Fig. 21-3D). In this case, the cholesterol fills the space between the floppy hydrocarbon chains of glycerophospholipids in the bilayer. This forces the glycerophospholipids into a tighter alignment and increases the distance between their head groups. As a result, the bilayer becomes thicker, resembling the thickness of bilayers enriched in sphingomyelin alone or sphingomyelin plus cholesterol.

Sphingolipids (e.g., glycosphingolipids and sphingomyelin) are synthesized in the Golgi apparatus, while the ER produces cholesterol and glycerophospholipids. Synthesis of these lipids at two different sites, combined with the self-organizing capacity of sphingolipids, cholesterol, and glycerophospholipids, gives rise to a pattern of lipid circulation within the secretory system that plays important roles in membrane sorting (Fig. 21-4A). Newly synthesized cholesterol is continually removed from the ER and redistributed to the Golgi apparatus, where high affinity interactions with sphingolipids prevent it from returning to the ER. The association of cholesterol with sphingolipids in the Golgi apparatus, in turn, triggers the lateral differentiation of domains enriched in these lipids. Through the additional activity of protein-based sorting and trafficking machinery, these domains bud off the Golgi apparatus and move to the plasma membrane, redistributing sphingolipids and cholesterol to the cell surface.

The forward flow of cholesterol, sphingolipids, and glycerophospholipids toward the plasma membrane is balanced by selective retrograde flow. Glycerophospholipids transferred from the ER to the Golgi apparatus are recycled back to the ER. Similarly, sphingolipids delivered to the plasma membrane from the Golgi apparatus are returned to the Golgi apparatus. Cholesterol, in contrast, is not returned through these retrograde pathways to either the ER or the Golgi apparatus but enters and circulates within the endocytic pathway leading to lysosomes. This pattern of lipid circulation creates a gradient of cholesterol, sphingolipids, and glycerophospholipids across the secretory membrane system. Within this gradient, the ER has a low concen-

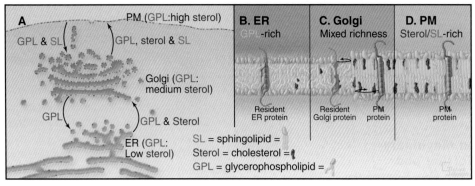

Figure 21-4   A LIPID GRADIENT ARISES ACROSS THE SECRETORY PATHWAY AS A RESULT OF THE SELF-ORGANIZING PROPERTIES OF GLYCEROPHOSPHOLIPIDS, SPHINGOLIPIDS, AND CHOLESTEROL AND THEIR DIFFERENTIAL SITES OF SYNTHESIS. The gradient helps to sort and transport proteins to different sites within the secretory system. **A,** Lipid circulation and sorting within the secretory membrane system. Glycerophospholipids (GPL) and cholesterol (sterol) are synthesized in the ER, whereas sphingolipids (SL), including sphingomyelin and glycosphingolipids, are synthesized in the Golgi apparatus. Cholesterol that moves to the Golgi from the ER associates with SL and is carried to the plasma membrane. This gives rise to different concentrations of these lipids in these organelles at steady state and results in lipid environments in the ER and plasma membrane that are compatible with their functions (e.g., protein translocation for the ER and low permeability for the plasma membrane). **B–D,** Sorting of transmembrane proteins based on the length of their transmembrane domains. The distinct lipid compositions of the ER, Golgi apparatus, and plasma membrane result in bilayers that differ in thickness (with the ER bilayer depleted of SL/sterols and thin, the plasma membrane bilayer enriched in SL/sterols and thick, and the Golgi bilayer intermediate in SL/sterol content and having mixed thickness). To avoid hydrophobic mismatch, transmembrane proteins move to the organelle whose bilayer thickness best matches that of the protein's transmembrane domain length.

tration of cholesterol (e.g., sterols) and sphingolipids, the Golgi apparatus has an intermediate concentration, and the plasma membrane has a high concentration (Fig. 21-4A).

The lipid gradient serves two important functions. First, it generates different lipid environments in the ER, Golgi apparatus, and plasma membrane compatible with their distinct functions. The low concentration of sterols and sphingolipids in the ER membrane means that it is composed primarily of glycerophospholipids (i.e., phosphatidylcholine, PC; phosphatidylserine, PS; and phosphatidylethanolamine, PE). The loosely packed acyl chains of PC, PS, and PE are readily deformable, permitting newly synthesized membrane proteins to insert into and fold in the ER bilayer. This feature explains why the ER is used as the sole site of cotranslational protein synthesis in the cell. By contrast, the high concentration of sterols and sphingolipids makes the plasma membrane bilayer thicker and less permeable to small molecules. This allows the plasma membrane to form a flexible but impermeable barrier between the cytoplasm and cell exterior. The intermediate concentration of sterols and sphingolipids in the Golgi apparatus allows it to serve as a membrane-sorting station.

A second function of the lipid gradient is to promote sorting of transmembrane proteins within the secretory system. Each integral membrane protein seeks a lipid bilayer with a thickness that matches the lengths of its transmembrane segments (Fig. 21-4B–D). Because most transmembrane segments are stiff hydrophobic α-helices, it is energetically unfavorable to expose hydro-

phobic residues of a transmembrane polypeptide to the aqueous environment of the cytoplasm or vesicle lumen or to bury hydrophilic amino acids with the lipid acyl chains in the interior of the membrane. To avoid such hydrophobic mismatches, integral membrane proteins of the secretory system have evolved with transmembrane segments that are matched to the thickness of their target membranes. Hence, resident membrane proteins in the ER and Golgi apparatus typically have shorter transmembrane segments (around 15 amino acids) than do resident plasma membrane proteins (approximately 20 to 25 amino acids). Retention and/or transport of these proteins occurs because the lipid bilayers of carriers budding out from either the ER (toward the Golgi apparatus) or the Golgi apparatus (toward the plasma membrane) are thicker than the bilayers of the donor organelles. Only transmembrane proteins with transmembrane segments long enough to span this thickness enter such carriers.

If the transmembrane segment of a plasma membrane protein is shortened experimentally by using recombinant DNA techniques, the new protein is retained in the thinner bilayers of the ER and/or Golgi apparatus rather than moving on to the thicker plasma membrane. Similarly, when the transmembrane segment of a Golgi protein is extended, the protein is no longer retained in the Golgi apparatus but is transported to the plasma membrane.

This lipid-based protein sorting mechanism takes advantage of the lipid gradient established by the self-organizing properties of glycerophospholipids, cholesterol, and sphingolipids to sort and transport proteins within the secretory system. It is not, however, the only mechanism used by cells to organize and transport proteins along the secretory pathway. In addition, a complex protein-based machinery is relied on to bring far greater specificity and efficiency to these processes.

Protein-Based Machinery for Protein Sorting and Transport within the Secretory Membrane System

Sorting and transporting proteins within the secretory membrane system depend on several types of proteins (Fig. 21-5): Specialized "coats" help to generate both small and large transport carriers and sort proteins into them; motor proteins move carriers along the cytoskeleton; "tethering factors" attach carriers to the cytoskeleton and to their destination organelles prior to fusion; and fusion proteins mediate fusion of the carrier with an acceptor membrane. These components also associate with specific organelles, providing organelles with an identity that is both unique and dynamic. Many of the components are peripheral membrane proteins that

lack transmembrane domains, so they must be recruited to the cytoplasmic surface of appropriate membranes by binding to either specific lipids, such as phosphoinositides, or to activated GTPases. Cells regulate the distributions of these organelle-specific lipids and GTPases. When infectious agents or stressful conditions disrupt these targeting molecules, secretory membrane trafficking can be disorganized and/or inhibited. The following sections describe the six major protein-based mechanisms that are used for sorting, transport, and fusion in the secretory membrane system.

Arf GTPases

The Arf family of **GTPases** includes **Sar1, Arf1-6** and several distantly related Arf-like GTPases. These small GTPases mediate the association of a wide variety of protein effectors with specific membranes, which, in turn, leads to the differentiation of membrane domains that give rise to transport carriers and create compartmental identity.

Like other GTPases (see Figs. 4-6 and 4-7), Arfs are molecular switches that alternate between a GTP-bound active form that interacts with effector targets and a GDP-bound inactive form that does not (Fig. 21-6). Active Arf GTPases associate with membranes, whereas inactive GTPases are cytoplasmic. Specific **GTP exchange factors** (GEFs) recruit Arf proteins to particular membrane surfaces and then catalyze the exchange of GDP for GTP. When associated with particular membranes active Arfs bind their effectors until a **GTPase-activating protein** (GAP) induces hydrolysis of GTP, reversing membrane association and effector binding. The distribution of GEFs on particular membranes determines the location of specific active Arfs. Similarly, the location of GAPs determines where each type of Arf is inactivated.

Activation of Arfs by exchange of GDP for GTP not only creates a binding site for target proteins (i.e., effectors) but also promotes interaction with the lipid bilayer. A myristoyl group covalently bound to the N-terminus of most Arfs allows them to interact transiently and nonspecifically with membranes. When a specific Arf-GEF on a membrane catalyzes the exchange of GDP for GTP, an amphipathic (hydrophobic on one side, hydrophilic on the other) N-terminal, α-helix is released from a hydrophobic pocket on the GTPase so that the hydrophobic side of the helix can interact with the bilayer (Fig. 21-6D). The membrane-associated GEFs that are responsible for activating Arfs all contain an evolutionarily conserved domain (referred to as the Sec7 domain). Association of this domain with Arf1-GDP is stabilized in the presence of the toxic fungal metabolite **brefeldin A** (BFA [Fig. 21-6D]). This prevents Arf1 conversion to its active, GTP-bound state and thereby blocks Arf1 activity, similar to that of a GDP-locked Arf1 mutant.

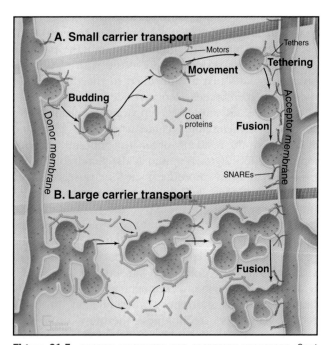

Figure 21-5 PROTEIN MACHINERY FOR SECRETORY TRANSPORT. Coat proteins that cluster into polymerized arrays help to sort soluble cargo and transmembrane proteins into a coated bud that pinches off a donor membrane as a coated vesicle (**A**) or larger vesicular tubular carriers (**B**). The carriers move by motor proteins along either microtubules or actin. Tethering factors, including long coiled-coil proteins or multimeric tethering complexes, tether the carriers to an acceptor membrane. SNARE proteins on the carrier and acceptor membrane then form a complex that drives membrane fusion, leading to delivery of the carrier's content to the acceptor membrane.

Figure labels: A. Small carrier transport · Motors · Tethers · Tethering · Movement · Budding · Coat proteins · Fusion · Donor membrane · Acceptor membrane · SNAREs · B. Large carrier transport · Fusion

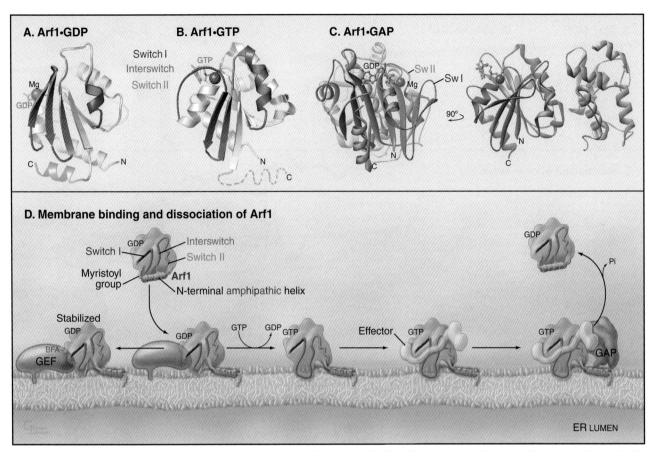

Figure 21-6 Arf-GTPase cycle. **A–C,** Ribbon diagrams of Arf1-GDP **(A),** Arf1-GTP **(B),** and free Arf1 and Arf1 bound to its GAP **(C).** **D,** Membrane binding and dissociation of Arf1. In the cytoplasm, Arf1 exists in its GDP-bound form with its N-terminal amphipathic helix tucked into a hydrophobic pocket. An N-terminal myristoyl group allows Arf1 to reversibly bind to membranes for activation by a GEF. The exchange of GDP for GTP induces a conformational change in switch 1 and 2, as well as in the interswitch loop, which displaces the N-terminal helix out of its pocket. This causes Arf1-GTP to bind tightly to membranes, since both the hydrophobic residues of the N-terminal helix and the myristoyl anchor associate with the bilayer. Arf1-GTP then recruits effectors. Association of a GAP with the Arf1-GTP-effector complex stimulates GTP hydrolysis. Arf1-GDP returns to the cytoplasm, and GAP and effector proteins dissociate from the membrane. Note that GDP-bound Arf1 has its N-terminal amphipathic helix *(striped blue and pink)* retracted into a hydrophobic pocket and its interswitch region *(purple)* retracted. The N-terminal myristoyl group *(green)* is still free to associate with membrane, but the binding is weak, resulting in reversible binding. On exchange of GDP for GTP, the switch 1 and 2 domains move, and the interswitch toggles out of the hydrophobic pocket, allowing tighter membrane binding. The drug BFA interferes with exchange of GDP for GTP on Arf1 by stabilizing the association between Arf1-GDP and its GEF. As a result, Arf1 cannot recruit effectors to the membrane, leading to disruption of membrane traffic between the ER and Golgi apparatus.

Arf GTPases of the secretory pathway, in particular Sar1 and Arf1, recruit to membranes many types of effector proteins. These include the coat protein complexes of **COPII, COPI,** and **clathrin/adapters** plus other effectors such as phospholipid modifiers (e.g., phospholipase D, a lipid metabolizing enzyme), phosphoinositides, and cytoskeletal components. The coat protein complexes assemble into large polymeric structures (called **protein coats**) at the cytoplasmic surface of ER, pre-Golgi, and Golgi membranes, from which they sort cargo and promote the budding of transport carriers. The other Arf effectors play roles in differentiating the membrane environment of these carriers and enabling them to move to different locations within the cell. The four other mammalian Arf proteins (Arfs 2 to 6) regulate vesicle formation at other locales in the exocytic and endocytic pathways.

Sar1 assembles the COPII coat complex that is involved in differentiating ER export domains, which are the sites from which transport carriers bud out from the ER. Arf1, by contrast, assembles the COPI coat complex that is involved in the creation of retrograde transport carriers that bud from pre-Golgi and Golgi structures. Arf1 also recruits the clathrin/adapter coat complexes that are involved in budding of transport carriers from the Golgi en route to the endosome/lysosomal system. Disruption of the GTPase cycles of either Sar1 or Arf1 has dramatic consequences for secretory transport and the organization of the secretory pathway (Fig. 21-14). When the GTPase cycles of Sar1 or Arf1 are disrupted, the Golgi apparatus disassembles, and Golgi enzymes return to the ER or to ER exit sites with all secretory transport out of the ER inhibited.

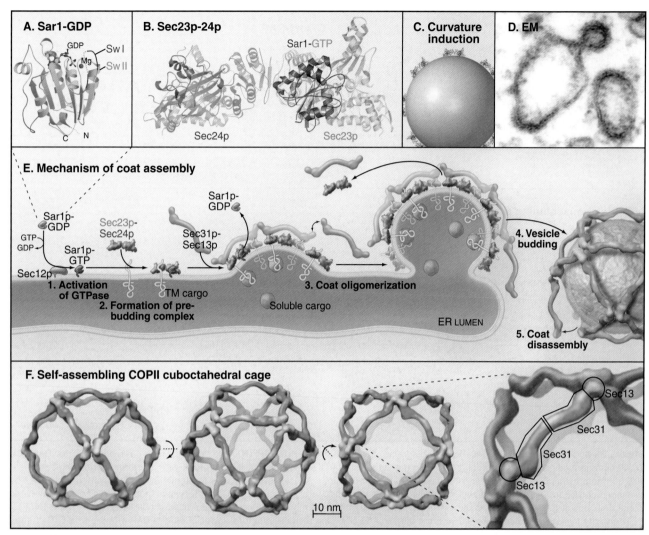

Figure 21-7 COPII COAT ASSEMBLY ON ENDOPLASMIC RETICULUM MEMBRANE. **A–B,** Ribbon diagrams of Sar1-GDP (PDB file: 1F6B) and the Sec23p-24p complex with Sec24p bound to Sar1-GTP. **C,** The bow-tie structure of Sec23p-Sec24p provides an extensive membrane-interaction surface that is concave, positively charged, and suitable for curving the bilayer when the subcomplex is bound to a membrane surface. **D,** Electron micrograph of a thin section illustrates the formation of a typical COPII vesicle when ER membranes are incubated in a test tube with cytosol and ATP. **E,** Sec12p activates Sar1 by promoting exchange of GDP for GTP, bringing Sar1 to the membrane. Sar1p-GTP then recruits the Sec23p·Sec24p subcomplex. Binding of Sec13p·Sec31p to Sec23p·Sec24p clusters these complexes into a coat. Transmembrane cargo is recruited into the coat by binding to Sec24p. Coat complexes dissociate from the lattice after Sar1-GTP converts to Sar1-GDP and releases into the cytosol. As long as coat oligomerization occurs faster than Sar1-dependent coat complex release, the lattice grows into a coated bud that can pinch off the membrane as a coated vesicle. Coat disassembly on the coated vesicle results from continued Sar1-dependent coat complex release in the absence of further coat complex addition due to Sec12 not being packaged into the coated vesicle membrane. **F,** Three-dimensional reconstruction of COPII cage at 30-Å resolution using cryoelectron microscopy and single-particle analysis. (C, Adapted from Bickford LC, Mossessova E, Goldberg J: A structural view of the COPII vesicle coat. Curr Opin Struct Biol 14:147–153, 2004, with permission from Elsevier. D, Courtesy of W. Balch, Scripps Research Institute, La Jolla, California. F, Adapted by permission from Macmillan Publishers Ltd. from Stagg SM, Gurkan C, Fowler DM, et al: Structure of the Sec13/31 COPII cage. Nature 439:234–238, 2006. Copyright 2006.)

The COPII Coat

The COPII coat complex (Fig. 21-7) is essential for sorting and trafficking secretory cargo out of the ER. It consists of Sar1p GTPase, the Sec23p•Sec24p subcomplex, and the Sec13p•Sec31p subcomplex. These components self-assemble into a polymeric, two-dimensional scaffold (called a coat) that then collects specific types of cargo. The intrinsic curvature of the coat promotes the formation of membrane buds that are capable of pinching off the membrane as coated vesicles.

COPII coats assemble by a sequential process (Fig. 21-7E). A GEF called Sec12p recruits Sar1p-GDP from the cytoplasm to the ER membrane and activates it by exchanging GDP for GTP. Activated Sar1p-GTP then recruits the two COPII subcomplexes: Sec23p•Sec24p, which is embedded within the ER membrane, and Sec13p•Sec31p, which is soluble in the cytoplasm. The Sec13p•Sec31p subcomplexes bound to Sec23p•Sec24p polymerize into a mesh-like scaffold that coats the membrane. The coat starts as a small aggregate but grows larger as more Sec23p•Sec24p subcomplexes (which are in direct contact with Sar1p in the membrane) diffuse in from surrounding membrane and become cross-linked by Sec13p•Sec31p subcomplexes recruited from the cytoplasm. As the lattice grows in size, it bends the patch of membrane into a coated bud that recruits specific types of proteins. The coated bud pinches off as a coated carrier (containing concentrated proteins) or remains as a "metastable" coated structure that participates in the differentiation of membrane domains at ER exit sites.

Two proteins regulate COPII coat disassembly: a GAP, Sec23p, enhances hydrolysis of GTP bound to Sar1p, and Sec13p stimulates the GAP activity of Sec23p. Inactivation by GTP hydrolysis releases Sar1p from the COPII lattice, followed by dissociation of the other COPII coat components and disassembly of the coat.

Localization of the GEF for Sar1p (i.e., Sec12p) in the ER membrane and the GAP for Sar1p (i.e., Sec23p) in the coat provides a mechanism for the continuous, self-regulated assembly and disassembly of the COPII coat. Coat subcomplexes associated with Sar1p-GTP add to the lattice rim, while units without Sar1p are released from the lattice interior. As long as subcomplex addition is faster than unit release, the coat lattice grows and deforms the membrane into a coated carrier. The carrier vesicle leaves behind the Sec12p GEF for Sar1p when it detaches from the membrane, so coat dissociation then dominates, leading automatically to carrier uncoating.

The Sec24p component of COPII coats recognizes several types of sorting signals in the cytoplasmic domains of transmembrane cargo proteins (Fig. 21-8). These include diacidic motifs that fit the consensus asp-glu-x-asp-glu (DExDE) and short hydrophobic motifs such as phe-phe (FF), phe-tyr (FY), leu-leu (LL), or ile-leu (IL). Some transmembrane cargo proteins lack these sorting signals, raising the question of how these cargo proteins (as well as luminal cargo proteins) are sorted into COPII-coated buds at ER export sites. One possibility is that transmembrane proteins containing these sorting signals escort cargo proteins lacking COPII-sorting signals to COPII-containing ER exit domains. Other transmembrane proteins may be exported from the ER by virtue of having longer transmembrane segments that partition into the potentially thicker bilayers of ER export domains.

The COPI Coat

The COPI coat complex (Fig. 21-9) is found on the cyto-plasmic face of pre-Golgi (also called vesicular tubular

VSV-G	TM–18aa–**YTDIE**MNRLGK
CFTR (NBD1)	TM–212aa–**YKDAD**LYLLD –287aaTM
GLUT4	TM–36aa–**YLGPDEND**
LDLR (prox. Yxxφ)	TM–17aa–**YQKTTEDE**VHICH–20aa
CI-M6PR	TM–26aa–**YSKVSKEEE**TDENE–127aa
E-cadherin	TM–95aa–**YDSLLVFDYE**GSGS –42aa
EGFR	TM–58aa–**YKGLWIPE**GEKVKIP–467aa
ASGPR H1	MTKE**YQDLQHLDNE**ES–24aaTM
NGFR	TM–65aa–**YSSLPPAKREE**VEKLLNG–74aa
TfR	19aa–**YTRFSLARQVDG**DNSHV–26aaTM

Figure 21-8 EXAMPLES OF TRANSMEMBRANE PROTEINS WITH TYROSINE-LINKED DIACIDIC ENDOPLASMIC RETICULUM EXIT CODES (ACIDIC-X-ACIDIC) THAT DIRECT THEIR INCORPORATION INTO COPII-COATED BUDS. ASGPRH1, asialoglycoprotein receptor; CFTR, cystic fibrosis transmembrane regulator; C1-M6PR, mannose 6-phosphate receptor; EGFR, epidermal growth factor receptor; GLUT4, a glucose carrier; LDLR, low-density lipoprotein receptor; NGFR, nerve growth factor receptor; TfR, transferrin receptor; VSV-G, vesicular stomatitis virus glycoprotein.

carrier [**VTC**]) and Golgi compartments and helps to mediate protein sorting and retrograde transport from these structures back to the ER. This is crucial for these structures to functionally and morphologically differentiate from the ER. Like the COPII coat complex, the COPI coat complex assembles into a lattice (i.e., COPI coat) on a patch of membrane, recruits specific proteins, deforms the membrane patch into a coated bud, and then pinches off as a coated carrier or remains as a "metastable" coated structure.

The formation of the COPI coat (Fig. 21-9B) begins with a small, soluble GTPase, Arf1, binding to the membrane and recruiting a preformed **coatomer complex** (Fig. 21-9A) from the cytoplasm. The coatomer complex consists of at least seven subunits, ranging in mass from 25 to more than 100 kD. Coatomer bound to Arf1 then attracts from the cytoplasm Arf-GAP1, the GTPase-activating protein for Arf1. This complex of a GTPase, a GAP and coatomer is the basic building unit of the COPI coat on membrane. Interactions between coatomer subunits and the cytoplasmic tail of transmembrane cargo proteins concentrates the cargo proteins as the coat polymerizes.

COPI units (consisting of Arf1, coatomer, and GAP) polymerize into a coat by addition of other COPI units diffusing in the plane of the membrane. The COPI coat bends the membrane as it forms a basket-like lattice. Arf-GAP1 is inactive during diffusion of individual units, but curved membranes favor its interaction with Arf1-GTP and hydrolysis of the GTP. (Sar1 and its GAP respond similarly to membrane curvature.) Thus, assembly of the COPI coat on membranes automatically inactivates Arf1, which is released from membranes, destabilizing the

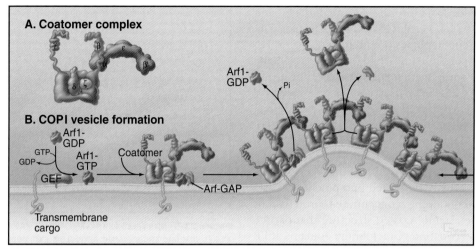

Figure 21-9 COPI COAT ASSEMBLY ON MEMBRANES. **A,** Depiction of COPI subunits within the coatomer complex. **B,** Activation of Arf1 to the GTP-bound form by the Sec7 domain of Arf1-specific GEFs results in the coupled recruitment of cargo, vesicle tethering factors, and fusion factors through binding of the cytoplasmic coatomer complex. Low-affinity interactions among Arf1, coatomer, and GAP cause them to polymerize into a coat that bends the patch of membrane to which they are associated. The increased curvature activates the GAP that stimulates Arf1 to hydrolyze GTP triggering its release from the membrane. After Arf1 is released, coatomer and GAP are destabilized and dissociate from the coat. The continuous cycle of coatomer binding, polymerization, and dissociation mediated by Arf1 GTPase activity leads to the formation of a coated bud that can pinch off the membrane as a coated vesicle or remain as a meta-stable coated bud that imparts curvature and tension to the membrane.

lattice of coatomer and Arf-GAP1. This leads to coat disassembly.

A consequence of these dynamic events is that COPI units move into the lattice from the rims and are released from the interior after Arf1 hydrolyzes its GTP, paralleling events occurring in the COPII coat. This results in a continuous flux of coat units through the lattice whether or not a coated vesicle detaches from the membrane. This dynamic behavior of coat units allows for several outcomes (Fig. 21-10A–C). The lattice can grow, disassemble (after budding off the membrane as a coated vesicle), or persist as a coated bud. In the latter case,

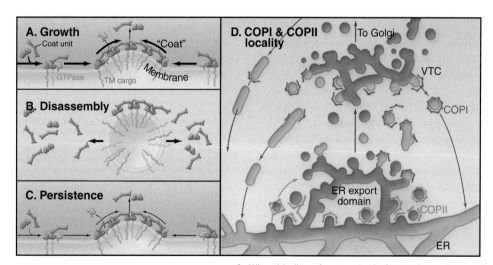

Figure 21-10 POTENTIAL FATES OF COAT COMPLEXES ON MEMBRANES. **A,** When binding of coat units is faster than release, the coat grows and forms a coated vesicle. **B,** After a coated vesicle forms, coat binding becomes slower than release (owing to GEF not being incorporated into the coated bud), and the coat disassembles. **C,** When coat units bind at the same rate as they release, then the coat is metastable (it neither shrinks nor grows but imparts curvature to the membrane). By increasing curvature in the membrane, metastable coats increase membrane tension, which can cause lipid partitioning. **D,** Cartoon diagram of the distribution of COPII and COPI coats on ER export domains and VTCs. COPII coats are restricted to ER membranes, where they recruit cargo into the ER export domain. COPI coats are present on the vesicular/tubular elements of the ER export domain, VTC and Golgi apparatus, where they orchestrate retrieval of proteins back to the ER.

the rate of addition of coat units to the bud is equal to the rate of unit loss. These behaviors of the coat lattice play key roles in orchestrating the protein sorting and morphologic events that occur at ER export domains to allow for VTC formation (Fig. 21-10D).

Incorporation of recycling proteins into COPI coated buds requires a specific sorting motif. Generally, this is a dilysine motif in a sequence of Lys-Lys-x-x-COOH (KKxx), where x is any amino acid. Two arginine residues substitute for the lysines in some proteins. Dilysine motifs are generally found at the cytoplasmic C-terminus of transmembrane proteins. They function in retrieval and possibly in retention of proteins within post-ER compartments by interacting with specific subunits of the COPI complex.

Rab GTPases

The Rab family of GTPases are the molecular switches that control the protein-protein interactions between transport carriers and docking complexes on target membranes (Fig. 21-11). These complexes recruit motor proteins that transport carriers on actin filaments or microtubules and then tether carrier vesicles to an organelle prior to fusion. Mammals express about 70 different Rab proteins to provide specificity at numerous transport steps in the secretory membrane systems of various cell types.

Rab proteins are posttranslationally modified by two geranylgeranyl lipids on conserved cysteine residues at their C-termini. This modification is essential for function and facilitates Rab association with the membrane bilayer. The cysteines are included in a variable segment of 30 amino acids that targets each Rab to its correct subcellular location.

Rab proteins cycle between the cytoplasm, where they are found in the GDP-bound form, and membranes, where they contain bound GTP (Fig. 21-11). In the cytoplasm, Rabs are complexed with a carrier protein called a **guanine nucleotide dissociation inhibitor** (GDI), which prevents exchange of GDP to GTP. GDI also sequesters the hydrophobic geranylgeranyl groups. Proteins called GDI displacement factors facilitate Rab recruitment to membranes by displacing GDI.

Rab-specific GEFs activate and recruit Rabs to form carrier vesicles. Rab-GTP then recruits the targeting and docking components to be used subsequently to recognize the target membrane and initiate bilayer fusion. Following fusion, a Rab-specific GAP stimulates GTP hydrolysis, recycling Rab-GDP back to the cytoplasm through binding to GDI. Using this GTPase cycle, Rab proteins regulate the timing of the assembly and disassembly of diverse multiprotein complexes involved in the trafficking of transport containers.

Tethering Factors

Tethering factors are rod-shaped proteins that extend about 15 nm from membranes into the cytoplasm (Fig. 21-11). They tether membrane carriers to target organelles prior to fusion and play structural roles as components of a Golgi matrix or scaffold for the assembly of other factors important for fusion and/or cargo sorting. Heterogeneous in sequence and structure, tethering factors can be divided into two general classes:

- Coiled-coiled tethering factors interact exclusively with active Rabs and function as Rab effectors. For example, the tethering factor p115/Uso1p functions in ER-Golgi transport. It is a homodimer with a long tail consisting of a coiled-coil of parallel α-helices and two globular heads at the C-terminus, reminiscent of myosin II (see Fig. 36-1). An internal hinge-like region in the tail collapses once the tether brings the membrane-enclosed carrier close to an acceptor membrane.

- Multisubunit tethering factors, such as TRAPI/II, the exocyst, and COG, bind to inactive Rabs and participate in their activation (functioning as GEFs). The TRAPP I (transport protein particle)

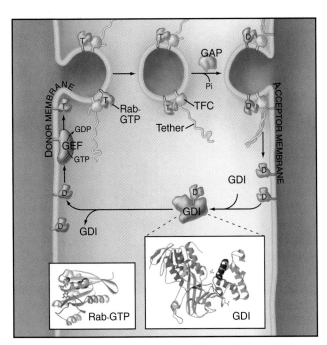

Figure 21-11 Rab GTPase cycle. Rab GTPases in their GDP-bound form are complexed with GDI in the cytoplasm. Following delivery to the membrane involving interactions with a GTPase dissociation factor, they are activated by a membrane-associated, Rab-specific GEF. In the GTP-bound form, they recruit effectors, such as tethering factor complexes (TFCs), which aid in targeting and docking the vesicle. Rab-GTP is returned to the GDP-bound form by a GAP, wherein it binds again to GDI. *Insets* show ribbon diagrams of Rab-GTP and GDI (PDB files: 3RAB and 1D5T). Pi, inorganic phosphate.

complex contains seven subunits, whereas the COG (conserved oligomeric Golgi) complex contains eight subunits. Recent structural studies suggest that the mechanism for TRAPP association with membranes involves a membrane-interacting surface that is flat, wide, and decorated with positively charged residues. Cells that are defective in COG function exhibit pleiotropic defects in virtually all N-linked, O-linked and lipid-linked conjugates, suggesting that the COG complex regulates glycosylation reactions in the Golgi in addition to interacting with Rabs.

SNAP Receptor Components

The SNAP receptor (SNARE) family of proteins participates in the fusion of carriers with their appropriate acceptor compartment (Fig. 21-12). Most SNAREs are transmembrane proteins with their functional N-terminal domains in the cytoplasm and their C-termini anchored to the bilayer. Each contains a heptad repeat (i.e., "SNARE motif") of 60 to 70 amino acids that can form a coiled-coil. Multiple SNAREs assemble a SNARE complex consisting of a bundle of α-helices. Members of the SNARE protein family were originally grouped according to whether they were v-SNAREs or t-SNAREs, referring to whether they conferred function to the vesicle (**v-SNARE**) or target (**t-SNARE**) compartment. For example, synaptobrevin is a v-SNARE found on synaptic vesicles involved in neurotransmission (see Fig. 11-9), whereas syntaxin 1 is a t-SNARE found on presynaptic densities to which synaptic vesicles fuse to trigger neurotransmitter release.

The formation of a SNARE complex occurs by the pairing of cognate v- and t-SNAREs. This generates a four-helix bundle with one α-helix contributed by one

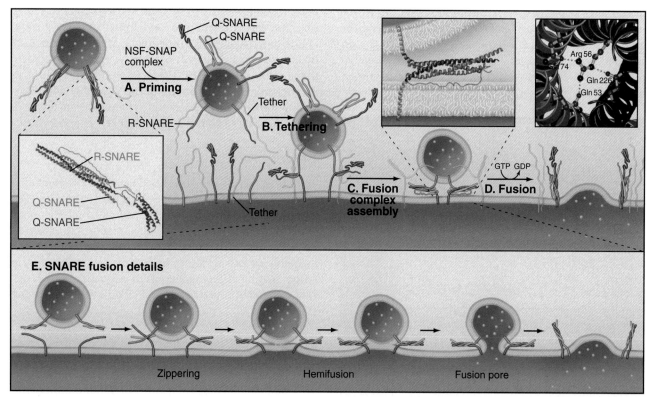

Figure 21-12 GENERIC SNAP RECEPTOR TARGETING AND DOCKING MACHINERY. **A,** Tethering factors and SNAP receptor (SNARE) proteins form *cis*-SNARE complexes during carrier formation. The *lower left inset* shows a ribbon diagram of a SNARE complex of a synaptic vesicle involved in neurotransmitter release involving R-SNARE (synaptobrevin, *blue*) and Q-SNARE (syntaxin, *red*) and SNAP25 (*green*) SNARE. (PDB file:1SFC.) **B–C,** Interaction of a vesicle with its target membrane through tethers results in the formation of *trans*-SNARE pairs involving extensive coiled-coiled regions of the interacting SNARE proteins. The *middle inset* shows the *trans*-SNARE pair. The *upper right panel* is a ribbon diagram looking down the coiled-coil, illustrating the critical Arg (arginine) residue of R-SNAREs that stabilizes interaction with glutamines (Glns) of Q-SNAREs forming the four-helix bundle in a SNARE complex. **D,** Following *trans*-SNARE pairing, hydrolysis of GTP bound to Rab (not shown) leads to vesicle fusion. This results in the incorporation of the *trans*-SNARE pair into the bilayer of the target membrane, where it and tethering complexes are disassembled for reuse. **E,** Overview of SNARE-mediated fusion. (*Top right inset,* Adapted from Ossig R, Schimtt HD, de Groot B, et al: Exocytosis requires asymmetry in the central layer of the SNARE complex. EMBO J 22:6000–6010, 2000, by permission of Oxford University Press.)

SNARE and the other three α-helices contributed by an oligomerized t-SNARE. The four-helix bundle of SNAREs depends on interactions of an arginine from one helix with glutamines from three other helices. This requirement has led to an alternative classification of these proteins as either R-SNAREs or Q-SNAREs, based on the presence of these critical arginine (R) or glutamine (Q) residues.

The v-SNAREs and t-SNAREs in separate membranes can pair to form a *trans*-SNARE complex, or v-SNAREs and t-SNAREs in the same membrane can pair to form a *cis*-SNARE complex. Assembly of a *trans*-SNARE complex, also called the "SNAREpin," is thought to supply the free energy needed to bring two membranes close enough to fuse. This is similar to the operation of viral fusion proteins.

Fusion of a carrier with a target membrane transforms a *trans*-SNARE complex into a *cis*-SNARE complex on the cytoplasmic face of the fused membrane. Following completion of fusion, the *cis*-SNARE complex is disassembled by a ubiquitous AAA ATPase (see Box 36-1) called **NSF** (for *N*-ethyl maleimide [NEM]–sensitive factor). The sulfhydryl alkylating reagent NEM inactivates NSF and prevents all carrier transport in the cell. SNAP proteins recruit NSF to the membrane. NSF uses the energy from ATP hydrolysis to dissociate the *cis*-SNARE complex and recycles the SNAREs for another round of membrane fusion.

Most SNARE proteins are anchored to membranes by a transmembrane segment that inserts into ER membranes after translation (i.e., they are tail-anchored proteins; see Chapter 20). Thus, SNARES must traverse the secretory pathway to reach specific organelles, but little is known about the mechanism they use. The length of their transmembrane domains and their capacity to interact with protein coats are likely to be important. For example, SNAREs involved in ER to Golgi transport are packaged into COPII coats at ER export sites for delivery to the Golgi apparatus, where they mediate homotypic fusion (i.e., fusion of two like transport containers that have identical *cis*-SNARE pairs) among incoming carriers as well as heterotypic fusion (i.e., fusion of two distinct membrane structures that have different *cis*-SNARE pairs) of these carriers with the Golgi membrane. The SNAREs are then packaged into COPI coats for retrieval to the ER. This allows them to function repeatedly in ER-to-Golgi apparatus transport.

Particular v-SNARE and t-SNARE complexes help to ensure the specificity of fusion at different steps along the secretory membrane pathway. SNAREs do not work alone in membrane fusion. Tethering factors assembled with the aid of Rab GTPases link specific apposing membranes prior to SNARE complex formation. Thus, SNAREs, tethers, and Rabs work together to ensure that membranes fuse at the correct time and place within the secretory system.

Secretory Transport from the Endoplasmic Reticulum to the Golgi Apparatus

Transport of newly synthesized proteins out of the ER takes place in specialized areas called **ER export domains.** These structures are approximately 1 to 2 μm in diameter and appear in fluorescent images as dispersed, punctate structures that are scattered over the surface of the ER (Fig. 21-13A). An individual ER export domain is organized into two zones (Fig. 21-13B–C). One is a region of smooth ER membrane studded with COPII-coated buds and uncoated tubules. The other is a central cluster of vesicles and tubules with the capacity to detach and traffic to the Golgi apparatus. The ER membrane is continuous between these two zones until the vesicle-tubule cluster and its associated cargo detach from the ER and move to the Golgi apparatus as a transport intermediate, called vesicular tubular carrier (VTC) (Fig. 21-10D). Cargo proteins are actively sorted into ER export domains through binding of signal motifs within their cytoplasmic tails to the COPII coat, and/or by lateral partitioning into the specialized lipid environment of this region. Partitioning is thought to occur once the transmembrane segments of the cargo proteins match the thickness of the ER exit site lipid bilayer.

The morphologic and biochemical differentiation of the ER export domain into a motile VTC is a multistep process orchestrated by the sequential action of the Sar1, Rab1, and Arf1 GTPases and their effectors (Fig. 21-14). Sar1 GTPase initiates ER export domain formation through COPII-mediated sorting of specific integral membrane proteins (including the p24 family proteins and SNAREs) and the formation of coated buds. The presence of coated buds and specialized cargo in this region, together with the membrane tension produced by the coated buds, leads to changes in bilayer lipid composition. This, in turn, promotes partitioning of other transmembrane proteins into the ER export domain, including proteins with longer-than-average transmembrane domains that lack COPII recognition motifs in their cytoplasmic domains. Additional cytoplasmic proteins are then also recruited to the ER exit site, including Rab1 and p115, which interact with tethering factors (such as GM130 and giantin), SNARE proteins, and GBF1 (the GEF for Arf1). Together, these molecules stimulate the membrane budding and fusion events that differentiate the ER export domain and VTC. The SNARE proteins, for example, allow the COPII-coated vesicles and membrane tubules that bud out

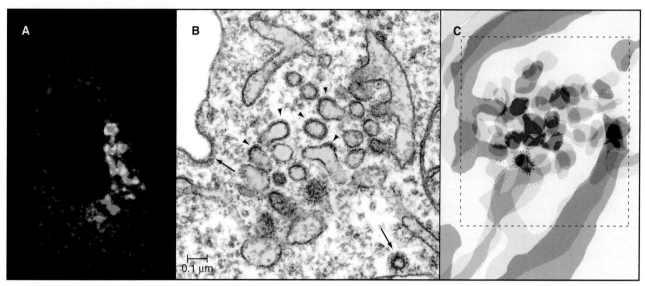

Figure 21-13 MORPHOLOGY AND OVERALL DISTRIBUTION OF ENDOPLASMIC RETICULUM EXPORT DOMAIN AND VESICLE-TUBULE CARRIER. **A,** Light micrograph showing the distribution of ER export domains and Golgi apparatus within a fibroblast cell. The cell was transfected with cDNAs encoding an ER export domain marker, Sec31-YFP *(red),* and Golgi marker, galactosyltransferase-CFP *(green),* which were labeled with different color variants of *green* fluorescent protein. Note that the ER exit sites are distributed throughout the cytoplasm as punctate structures, whereas the Golgi apparatus is localized in a juxtanuclear site. **B,** Electron micrograph of a thin cross section of a typical ER export domain containing a central vesicle tubule carrier that can detach and traffic to the Golgi apparatus. ER is *green,* ER-associated-coated buds are *blue,* the VTC is *red, arrowheads* mark COPI coats, and *arrows* mark clathrin-coated vesicles from the plasma membrane. **C,** Reconstruction from four consecutive serial-thin sections illustrating the three dimensional organization of ER export domain demarcated by the box. (A, Adapted from Altan-Bonnet N, Sougrat R, Liu W, et al: Golgi inheritance in mammalian cells is mediated through endoplasmic reticulum export activities. Mol Biol Cell 17:990–1005, 2006. B–C, From Bannykh SI, Nishimura N, Balch WE: Getting into the Golgi. Trends Cell Biol 8:21–25, 1998.)

from the smooth ER to fuse with themselves to form a tubule cluster; GM130 and giantin tether these membranes to the cytoskeleton; and Arf1 effectors differentiate the membrane further by initiating retrieval of specific proteins back to the ER. Disruption of the GTPase cycle of Sar1 through expression of a GDP-locked form prevents ER export domain formation, whereas disruption of the GTPase cycle of Arf1—through expression of a GDP-locked form of Arf1 or by BFA treatment—blocks VTC formation (Fig. 21-14). By blocking membrane delivery into the secretory pathway, both treatments also cause the disappearance of the Golgi apparatus, which depends on continuous membrane input to maintain its structure.

Detachment of the VTC from the ER export domain and its maturation and delivery to the Golgi apparatus are the next steps in protein trafficking from ER to Golgi apparatus. Mammalian cells use motors to detach VTCs from ER export domains and to carry them along microtubules toward the Golgi apparatus located near the microtubule-organizing center (Fig. 21-1). During this process, the VTC matures by a process that is orchestrated by Arf1 and its effectors. Activated Arf1 recruits dozens of cytoplasmic proteins to VTCs (and to Golgi membranes). Among these, the COPI coat binds to and clusters specific proteins, enabling them to be retrieved back to the ER. Lipid-modifying enzymes such as

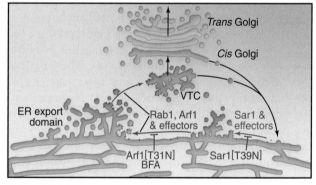

Figure 21-14 TRANSPORT FROM THE ENDOPLASMIC RETICULUM TO THE GOLGI APPARATUS. ER to Golgi transport is orchestrated by the combined activities of many molecules. Sar1 and its effectors initiate COPII-coated bud formation and clustering of cargo at regions called ER export domains. This induces p115 and Rab1 to bind to these regions, which in turn recruits GBF1, the GEF for Arf1. Subsequent recruitment of Arf1 and its effectors further differentiates the ER export domain into a VTC. The VTC detaches from the ER and targets the Golgi apparatus, where it fuses with the cis face of the Golgi. The cargo in the VTC is then released into the Golgi and moves to the *trans* Golgi (where it will exit from the TGN). Expression of a constitutively inactive Sar1 mutant, Sar1[T39N], blocks COPII recruitment, and no ER exit sites form. Expression of an inactive Arf1 mutant, Arf1[T31N], or BFA treatment blocks recruitment of Arf1 effectors, which prevents ER exit sites from differentiating into VTCs. This causes the shrinkage and disappearance of the Golgi apparatus because new membrane from the ER cannot be delivered to the Golgi.

phosphatidylinositol kinases and phosphatases create a lipid environment that is distinct from that in the ER membrane, permitting tethering factors and matrix proteins to bind to the motile VTC membrane. Ankryrin and spectrin proteins (see Fig. 7-10) form a scaffold for other cytoskeletal proteins, including actin, tubulin, dynactin, and dynein. Among these, the dynactin complex (see Fig. 37-2) mediates dynein-dependent clustering of VTCs by movement on microtubules toward centrioles at the center of the cell.

After VTCs have clustered by movement inward along microtubules, they undergo fusion with the Golgi apparatus. This occurs at the *cis* **or entry face** of the Golgi apparatus, also called the *cis*-Golgi network (CGN) because of its elaborate tubular appearance. The membrane fusion releases cargo proteins and lipids of the VTC into the Golgi system for processing by enzymes that modify the cargo's oligosaccharide side chains.

Exactly how biosynthetic cargo is then transferred through the Golgi apparatus system has not been clarified experimentally, but three mechanisms are likely to contribute. The first mechanism uses vesicular transport to transfer cargo between the distinct cisternal elements that make up the Golgi apparatus. Vesicles derived from one cisternum transfer cargo to a neighboring cisternum. In a second mechanism, cargo is conveyed across the Golgi system by directed maturation of cisternal elements. A third mechanism involves diffusion and/or lateral partitioning of cargo within the membrane or lumenal spaces between interconnected cisternal Golgi elements. The contributions of each

mechanism are still unclear and may vary depending on the cargo being transported through the Golgi system.

Sorting from the *Trans*-Golgi Network

After transport through the Golgi system, cargo leaves the *trans* or exit face of the Golgi apparatus (Fig. 21-15). The exit region is called the *trans*-**Golgi network (TGN)** because of its tubular network organization. This organization is characteristic of other sorting compartments, such as that of the VTC, the *cis* Golgi, and sorting endosomes (see Chapter 22). Depending on the cell type, the cargo that arrives in the TGN can be distributed, via distinct transport carriers, to several different intracellular locations, including the plasma membrane or cell exterior, the endosome/lysosomal system, or specialized secretory organelles or granules. The intracellular route taken by each protein depends on sorting properties that are encoded in the polypeptide chain.

Constitutive Transport of Cargo to the Plasma Membrane or Cell Exterior

A steady stream of both proteins and lipids from the TGN to the cell surface occurs constitutively through tubular transport carriers that bud out from the TGN (Fig. 21-16). No known coat proteins function in the formation of these structures. Instead, cargo proteins conveyed to the plasma membrane by these structures

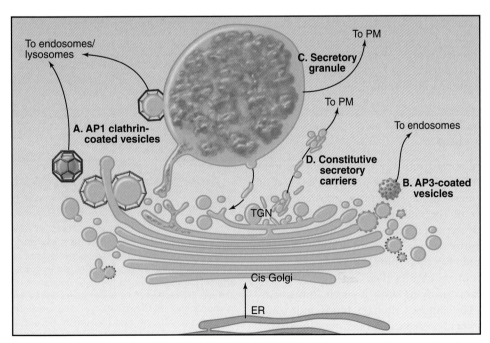

Figure 21-15 DIVERGENCE OF BIOSYNTHETIC/EXOCYTIC CARGOES AT THE *TRANS*-GOLGI NETWORK. A–D, Cargo destined for secretion or distinct intracellular locations is sorted and packaged into distinct transport carriers. The tubular/vesicular geometry of the TGN plays an important role in protein sorting. PM, plasma membrane.

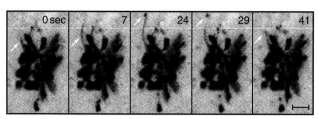

Figure 21-16 FLUORESCENCE MICROGRAPHS OF A TISSUE CULTURE CELL EXPRESSING A FLUORESCENTLY TAGGED TRANSMEMBRANE PROTEIN, VSVG-GFP, EN ROUTE TO THE PLASMA MEMBRANE. The images were collected over time and show long tubules enriched in the labeled protein *(arrows)* emanating from the Golgi apparatus. The tubules later detach from the Golgi and traffic to the plasma membrane. Scale bar is 5 μm. (Reproduced from Hirschberg K, Miller CM, Ellenberg J, et al: Kinetic analysis of secretory protein traffic and characterization of Golgi to plasma membrane transport intermediates in living cells. J Cell Biol 143:1485–1503, 1998. Copyright 1998 The Rockefeller University Press.)

have transmembrane segments that partition into lipid domains containing sphingolipids and cholesterol. Activation of specific lipid-modifying enzymes such as phosphatidylinositol 4-kinase in the sphingolipid/cholesterol-enriched sorting domain of the TGN then results in the domains forming tubules that pinch off the TGN. Because the tubules have a higher volume-to-surface ratio than small vesicles, bulk soluble markers are also carried to the plasma membrane by these structures. Tubule extension is facilitated by motors moving on microtubules and/or by actin filaments, while tubule severing is mediated by dynamin-2, a GTPase localized in TGN. In mammalian cells, motor proteins such as kinesins move the constitutive membrane carriers outward from the Golgi apparatus along microtubules. Fusion of the carriers with the plasma membrane releases cargo within the lumen of the carrier vesicle into the extracellular space. After fusion, membrane lipids and proteins redistribute laterally by diffusion in the plane of the plasma membrane.

Sorting to the Endosome/Lysosomal System

Proteins that are sorted into the endosome/lysosomal system (Fig. 21-17) include a large and diverse class of hydrolytic enzymes contained within lysosomes, the digestive centers of the cell (see Chapter 23). Newly synthesized hydrolytic enzymes are prevented from entering constitutive tubular carriers destined for the plasma membrane by their binding to **mannose-6-phosphate receptors (MPRs** [Fig. 21-17A]). MPRs are integral membrane proteins with a single transmembrane domain. The luminal domain binds individual prohydrolase molecules that have been modified with mannose-6-phosphate (M6P), whereas the cytoplasmic domain encodes sorting motifs that interact with the clathrin/adapter sorting machinery (see Chapter 22)

that directs packaging into carriers as they leave the TGN destined for endosomes. After MPRs discharge their cargo, other carriers transfer the unoccupied MPRs back from the endosome to the TGN (Fig. 21-17).

AP1 complexes direct clathrin coat assembly at the TGN (Fig. 21-17B). They interact directly with either tyrosine-based or dileucine sorting motifs on the MPR receptor tail. Recruitment and assembly of the AP1-containing clathrin coat on the TGN occur through direct interaction with the same small guanosine tri-

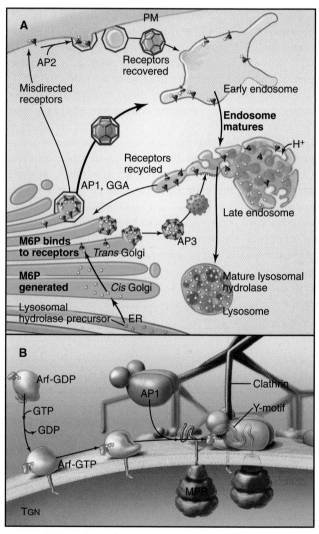

Figure 21-17 SORTING PATHWAYS USED BY MANNOSE 6-PHOSPHATE RECEPTORS AND COAT ASSEMBLY AT THE *TRANS*-GOLGI NETWORK. **A,** MPRs carry newly synthesized lysosomal hydrolases containing mannose-6-phosphate (M6P) from the TGN, via endosomes, to lysosomes, after which they return to the TGN. Receptors missorted to the cell surface are recovered by endocytosis and returned to the pathway in endosomes. **B,** Coordination of coat assembly and cargo recruitment at the TGN. An exchange factor activates the small GTPase Arf to bind GTP, which triggers recruitment of AP1 coat constituents to the TGN membrane. The MPR is concentrated in the emerging coated vesicle through interactions between a tyrosine-based sorting motif in its cytoplasmic domain and the μ-subunit of AP1.

phosphate (GTPase) Arf1 that also triggers COPI assembly (Fig. 21-6). The assembly of the clathrin-AP1 coat drives receptor clustering and budding off the TGN membrane of clathrin-coated transport vesicles. Several lysosomal membrane proteins are also sorted into these clathrin-coated vesicles by virtue of tyrosine-based sorting motifs on the cytoplasmic domains of the membrane protein. After budding off the TGN in clathrin-AP1-coated vesicles, both lysosomal hydrolases and lysosomal membrane proteins are delivered to lysosomes by way of endosomal intermediates.

Secretory Granule Formation and Transport

An additional sorting pathway from the TGN occurs in specialized endocrine, exocrine, or neuronal cells that concentrate and package selected proteins in storage granules for eventual mobilization and discharge from the cell in response to hormonal or neural stimulation. This is the so-called **regulated secretory pathway** (Fig. 21-18), which is used for discharging most of the body's polypeptide hormones, enzymes used in the digestive tract, and many other products that are needed intermittently rather than continuously.

Our mechanistic understanding of secretory granule formation and sorting processes is hindered by the apparent lack of a universal sorting signal on proteins that are destined for inclusion into regulated secretory granules. Instead, secretory granule formation appears to involve physical sorting, selective retention, and condensation (Fig. 21-19). Condensation of luminal content during secretory granule biogenesis involves charge neutralization, protein aggregation and active extrusion of ions.

In some cells that produce and store peptide hormones, aggregation involves only selected products of proteolytic processing of hormone precursors. For example, production of **insulin** requires proteolytic enzymes in immature granules that cleave proinsulin at two sites, generating insulin and C-peptide. Insulin condenses with zinc ion in the granule core, whereas C-peptide is excluded and so accumulates around this core. As a consequence, more C-peptide is shed into unstimulated secretory pathways that originate from the immature granule. Very tight regulation of insulin secretion is important for controlling the glucose

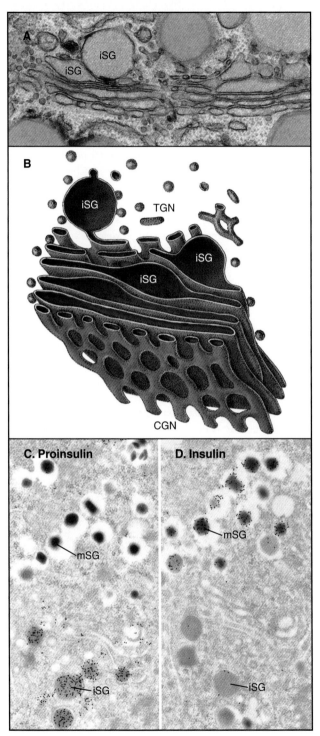

Figure 21-18 FORMATION OF SECRETORY GRANULES. Transmission electron micrograph of a thin section (**A**) and a diagram (**B**) show immature secretory granules (iSG) as they emerge from the TGN. Much of the TGN surface is consumed by forming immature secretory granules. **C–D,** Cryoelectron micrographs of frozen sections reacted with gold-labeled antibodies to proinsulin (**C**) or insulin (**D**). Proinsulin is concentrated in immature secretory granules. After processing, insulin is concentrated in mature, dense-core secretory granules (mSG). (A, Courtesy of J. Clermont, McGill University but by permission of Wiley-Liss, Inc. B, Redrawn from Clermont Y, Rambourg A, Hermo L: *Trans*-Golgi network (TGN) of different cell types: Three-dimensional structural characteristics and variability. Anat Rec 242:289–301, 1995. Copyright © 1995. Reprinted with permission of Wiley-Liss, Inc., a subsidiary of John Wiley & Sons, Inc. C–D, Courtesy of L. Orci, University of Geneva, Switzerland.)

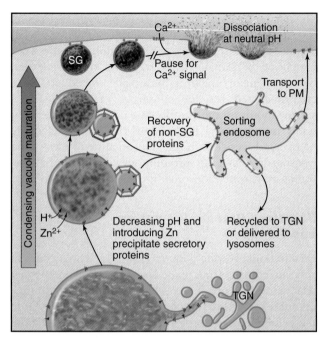

Figure 21-19   MATURATION OF NASCENT SECRETORY GRANULES/CONDENSING VACUOLES. The vacuolar H^+-ATPase in the secretory granule (SG) membrane lowers the internal pH. This drives condensation and concentration of the contents. Dense-core, mature secretory granules are stored in the cytoplasm until a Ca^{2+}-mediated signaling event triggers fusion and release of their contents. Proteins inadvertently included in large, immature secretory granules emerging from the TGN are captured by clathrin-coated vesicles and recycled to endosomes and the TGN. PM, plasma membrane.

concentration in the blood plasma. This regulation is compromised in certain forms of **diabetes.**

Trafficking to the Plasma Membrane in Polarized Cells

In contrast to nonpolarized cells, polarized cells have functionally (and thus compositionally) distinct apical and basolateral domains separated by tight junctions that cement neighboring cells together and prevent diffusion between the domains (Fig. 21-20). Most of our knowledge of membrane sorting in polarized cells has come from studying epithelial cells. As expected, the trafficking complexity increases as destination options increase, and three distinct mechanisms for the polarized sorting of plasma membrane proteins have been revealed (Fig. 21-21). One mechanism involves selective packaging of apically or basolaterally destined proteins into distinct carrier vesicles at the TGN for delivery to the appropriate surface. A second mechanism involves the random delivery of newly synthesized proteins to both surfaces, followed by selective retention or depletion so that, at steady state, they become differentially abundant because they are more stable at one surface than at the other. A third mechanism

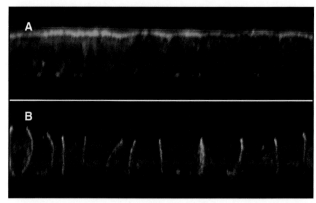

Figure 21-20   FLUORESCENCE MICROGRAPHS SHOW THE RESTRICTION OF PROTEINS TO THE APICAL OR BASOLATERAL COMPARTMENTS OF COLUMNAR EPITHELIAL CELLS. Tight junctions (marked with *red* fluorescence in both **A** and **B**) seal the boundary between these domains. **A,** E-cadherin (*green*) is restricted to the apical plasma membrane. **B,** Syntaxin-3 (*green*) is restricted to the basolateral surface. Cell nuclei are stained *red*. (Courtesy of T. Weimbs and S. H. Low, Cleveland Clinic Foundation, Ohio.)

involves delivery of newly synthesized proteins to the basolateral surface, followed by selective internalization, sorting in the endosomal compartment, and delivery to the apical surface in a process termed transcytosis. Most epithelial cells use different combinations of these three mechanisms to generate and maintain cell polarity.

Direct targeting uses basolateral targeting signals in the cytoplasmic domains of proteins to sort these molecules during secretory transport or during endocytosis

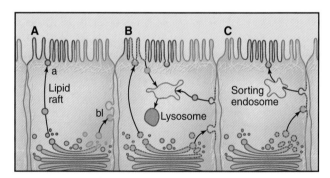

Figure 21-21   Three pathways for the distribution of integral membrane proteins destined for either the apical (*a* [*red*]) or basolateral (*bl* [*blue*]) membranes of polarized epithelial cells. **A,** Direct sorting from the TGN to either the apical or basolateral surface. Apical transport involves inclusion into lipid rafts, whereas proteins destined for direct transport to the basolateral surface carry a cytoplasmic sorting motif for inclusion into specific transport vesicles. **B,** Indirect pathway. Newly synthesized proteins are randomly targeted to both surfaces followed by selective retention and/or selective degradation from one surface or the other, resulting in a polarized distribution. **C,** Indirect pathway. Newly synthesized proteins are transported to the basolateral surface, followed by retention of basolateral proteins and selective transcytosis of apical proteins to the apical surface.

by recycling the proteins from endosomes back to the appropriate membrane domain. Examples include receptors for low-density lipoprotein, transferrin, MPRs, and polymeric immunoglobulin receptor. Alternatively, direct targeting occurs by lateral partitioning of proteins into sphingomyelin- and cholesterol-rich subdomains (called **lipid rafts**) (see Fig. 7-7) formed in the TGN or at the plasma membrane. GPI-anchored proteins or other integral membrane proteins that directly associate with these lipid rafts based on physical properties of their transmembrane domains are selectively targeted to the apical surface. The unique physical properties of these lipid subdomains render them resistant to detergent solubilization.

The second sorting mechanism—random delivery followed by selective rearrangements—is particularly relevant to establishing polarity during cellular differentiation. In this case, uniformly distributed proteins that preexist on a nonpolarized cell will redistribute themselves in a polarized fashion in response to cell-cell contacts that initiate polarization. Often, this occurs by the selective retention of a specific protein at the appropriate surface through intracellular (cytoskeletal) or extracellular (cell-cell or cell-matrix) interactions, or both. Proteins that are not actively retained on the other cell surface are internalized and degraded in lysosomes. Examples of proteins that are polarized in this way include Na^+K^+-ATPase and the cell adhesion molecule uvomorulin, an immunoglobulin-like cell adhesion molecule.

Regulated Fusion with the Plasma Membrane

All transport carriers leaving the TGN contain components of the vesicle targeting and fusion machinery (i.e., v-SNAREs, members of the synaptobrevin/VAMP family, Rab proteins) required to direct their fusion with the appropriate target organelle containing cognate t-SNAREs (members of the syntaxin, SNAP, and Sec1p families). Secretory granules carry additional regulatory factors that are superimposed on this constitutive machinery for docking and fusion. This ensures that fusion takes place only on demand. Regulated fusion has been studied extensively in the context of synaptic vesicle release, in endocrine cells, and in mast cells. In all cases, regulated secretion can be divided into three steps: docking, priming, and fusion (Fig. 21-22). Docking is the slowest step and is believed to involve interactions of v-SNARE and t-SNAREs regulated by Rab GTPases. In vitro reconstitution studies have suggested a role for a phosphatidylinositol transfer protein, a phosphatidylinositol 5-kinase, and phosphatidylinositol 4,5-bisphosphate (PIP$_2$, the product of PI-5 kinase), in priming steps required for regulated secretion in neuroendocrine cells. A cytoplasmic protein, CAPS (calcium activator protein for secretion), is recruited to the secretory vesicle via interactions with PIP$_2$ and is required for calcium-triggered fusion of dense core secretory granules. In most cases, fusion is triggered by an influx of Ca^{2+}, a process called *calcium-secretion coupling.* Synaptotagmins, part of a family of transmembrane vesicle proteins that also bind calcium and interact with the fusion machinery, are believed to act as clamps, inhibiting fusion until calcium triggers their release.

Diverse signals lead to the calcium influx that triggers fusion. These include ligand activation of G-protein-coupled receptors on neuroendocrine cells, activation of immunoglobulin E receptors and kinase cascades in mast cells (see Fig. 28-5), and membrane depolarization in neurons (see Figs. 11-8 and 11-9).

The Golgi Apparatus: Function, Structure, and Dynamics

The Golgi apparatus (Fig. 21-23) performs three primary functions within the secretory membrane system. First,

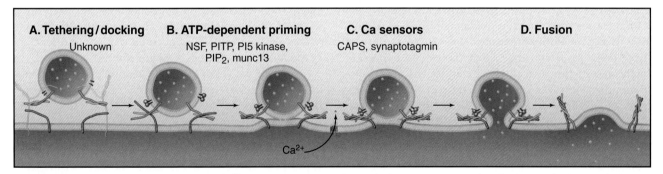

A. Tethering/docking
Unknown

B. ATP-dependent priming
NSF, PITP, PI5 kinase, PIP$_2$, munc13

C. Ca sensors
CAPS, synaptotagmin

D. Fusion

Ca^{2+}

Figure 21-22 Four terminal steps (**A–D**) in Ca^{2+}-triggered membrane fusion during regulated secretion. Docking/tethering and fusion are mechanistically similar to other vesicle fusion events (Fig. 21-15). Additional steps prepare proteins on both the secretory vesicles and plasma membrane to respond rapidly to Ca^{2+} influx, which triggers fusion. CAPS, calcium activator protein for secretion; munc 13, mammalian homolog for *Caenorhabditis elegans* UNC13 (unknown function, critical for Ca^{2+}-triggered fusion of primary vesicles); NSF, NEM-sensitive factor; PTP, phosphatidylinositol transfer protein.

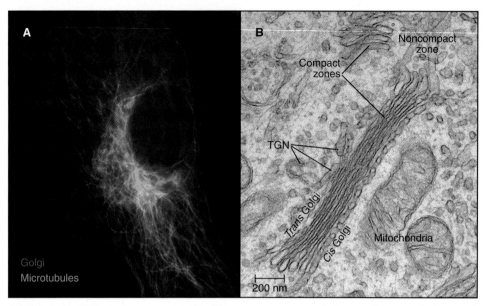

Figure 21-23   LOCALIZATION AND MORPHOLOGY OF THE GOLGI APPARATUS IN ANIMAL CELLS. **A,** Immunofluorescent micrograph of a rat fibroblast stained with antibodies to galactosyltransferase (a Golgi enzyme) *(red)* and antibodies to tubulin *(green)*. The Golgi typically extends as a ribbon-like structure around the microtubule organizing center, which is localized to one side of the nucleus. **B,** Electron micrograph of a rat epithelial cell showing a single Golgi stack of cisternae cut transversely. The *cis* and *trans* faces of the Golgi are at opposite ends of the stack, with the TGN extending off from the *trans* face. The compact zones are the stacked regions of the Golgi, whereas the noncompact zones are tubular-vesicular regions of the Golgi that interconnect stacks and participate in membrane trafficking through the Golgi apparatus. (Courtesy of J. Lippincott-Schwartz and Rachid Sougrat, National Institutes of Health, Bethesda, Maryland. Reprinted from Zaal K, Smith CL, Polishchuk RS, et al: Golgi membranes are absorbed into and reemerge from the ER during mitosis. Cell 99:589–601, 1999. Copyright 1999, with permission from Elsevier.)

it acts as a carbohydrate factory in which glycoproteins, polysaccharides (in plants) and proteoglycans received from the ER are further processed. Such processing permits these molecules to participate in numerous specialized biological functions at the cell surface. Second, the Golgi apparatus functions as a protein-sorting station for the delivery of proteins to many different destinations within the cell. This includes transport to the plasma membrane, secretion to the cell exterior, sorting to the endosome/lysosomal system, or retrieval back to the ER. Third, the Golgi apparatus serves as the site where sphingomyelin and glycosphingolipids are synthesized within the cell. These lipids are capable of packing tightly in the membrane, which causes the bilayer to thicken and be less permeable to water-soluble molecules (Fig. 21-3). Affinity of these lipids for each other when cholesterol is present furthermore results in the formation of discrete membrane microdomains called lipid rafts that can concentrate or exclude specific membrane proteins. Such domains can serve as platforms for the association of diverse signaling molecules and can initiate the formation of transport carriers that bud out from the Golgi apparatus.

Golgi Morphology and Dynamics

The Golgi apparatus in many animal cells appears as a ribbon-like structure adjacent to the nucleus and close to centrosomes, which are the microtubule organizing centers of the cell (Fig. 21-23A). In electron microscope images, the Golgi apparatus exhibits a distinctive morphology consisting of a series of stacked, flattened, membrane-enclosed cisternae that resemble a stack of pancakes (Fig. 21-23B). Cross-linking of cisternae by Golgi-associated tethering factors results in their tight, parallel alignment within the stack. Tubules and vesicles at the rims of the stacks interconnect the stacks into a single ribbon-like structure by a process dependent on microtubules. If microtubules are experimentally depolymerized, the ribbon-like Golgi structure reorganizes into single stacks (i.e., fragments) found at ER exit sites (Fig. 21-24). This distribution resembles the distribution of Golgi stacks in plant cells. There, hundreds of single stacks are localized adjacent to ER exit sites rather than being joined together as a single ribbon.

The stacks of Golgi cisternae in animal and plant cells all exhibit a *cis* to *trans* polarity that reflects the passage of cargo through this organelle. As was mentioned before, proteins from the ER enter at the stack's *cis* face (entry face). After passing through the cisternae in the middle of the stack, cargo then leaves the Golgi at the *trans* face, which is at the opposite end of the stack. Membrane sorting and transport activities of the Golgi are thought to be especially high at the *cis* and *trans* faces and within the tubular-vesicular elements (noncompact zone) that interconnect the stacks (Fig. 21-23B).

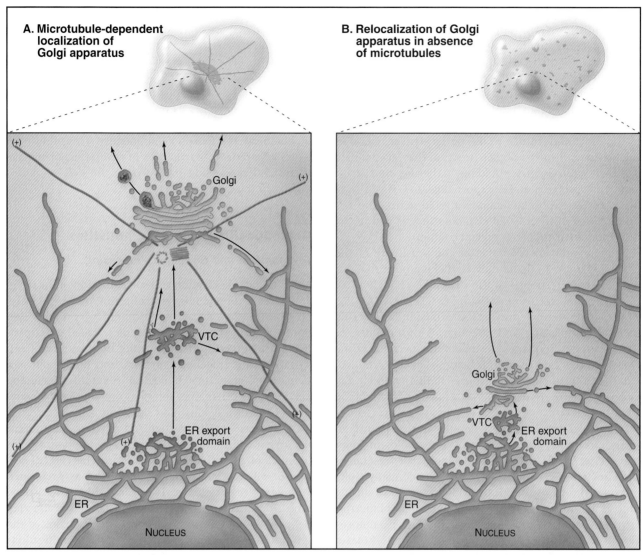

Figure 21-24 **EFFECT OF MICROTUBULE DISRUPTION ON THE DISTRIBUTION OF THE GOLGI APPARATUS. A,** Microtubules radiating out from the centriole *(red barrels)* with their plus ends at the cell periphery help localize the Golgi apparatus in many animal cells by serving as tracks for the inward movement of membrane-bound carriers (VTC) derived from the ER. The carriers deliver secretory cargo, as well as Golgi enzymes, to the Golgi apparatus. Retrograde transport of Golgi enzymes back to the ER is not dependent on microtubules (since the ER is widely distributed throughout the cytoplasm). Because of this, when microtubules are disassembled **(B),** the Golgi apparatus reforms at sites adjacent to ER export domains, owing to the accumulation of cycling Golgi enzymes at these sites.

The size, the appearance, and even the existence of the Golgi apparatus depend on the amount and speed of cargo movement through the secretory pathway. The yeast *Saccharomyces cerevisiae,* for example, has a poorly developed Golgi apparatus because secretory transport is normally too fast for elaborate Golgi structures to accumulate. However, conditions that slow cargo transport out of the Golgi apparatus in these cells lead to the Golgi apparatus enlarging and rearranging into compact stacks similar to those seen in most animal and plant cells.

The Golgi apparatus is a continuously renewed organelle rather than a permanent cellular structure because both its proteins and lipids move continuously along various pathways. No class of Golgi protein is stably associated within this organelle. Integral membrane proteins associated with the Golgi apparatus, including processing enzymes and SNAREs, continuously exit and reenter the Golgi apparatus by membrane-trafficking pathways leading to and from the ER. Peripheral membrane proteins associated with the Golgi apparatus (including Arf1, coatomer, Rab proteins, matrix proteins, tethering factors, and GEFs) exchange constantly between Golgi membranes and cytoplasmic pools. Newly synthesized secretory cargo coming from the ER enters the Golgi apparatus on the *cis* face of the stack, traverses across the stack, and then leaves from the *trans* face.

The transient and dynamic association of molecules with the Golgi apparatus makes this organelle sensitive to malfunctions of many cellular systems. As mentioned before, experimental depolymerization of microtubules causes the pericentriolar Golgi apparatus of a mammalian cell to become relocated adjacent to ER export domains (Fig. 21-24B). This occurs because Golgi enzymes that are undergoing continuous recycling back to the ER cannot return to the pericentriolar region in the absence of microtubules. Instead, they accumulate together with Golgi scaffolding, tethering, and structural coat proteins at ER export domains. Given hundreds of ER export domains scattered across the ER, hundreds of distinct Golgi elements appear within the cell upon microtubule depolymerization.

A more dramatic example of the sensitivity of the Golgi apparatus to membrane trafficking perturbations is the Golgi's response to the drug BFA (brefeldin A). BFA prevents Arf1 from exchanging GTP for GDP (Fig. 21-6D) and thereby prevents the membrane recruitment of cytoplasmic Arf1 effectors. Within minutes of BFA treatment, resident transmembrane proteins of the Golgi are recycled to the ER where they are retained, and the Golgi apparatus vanishes. On BFA washout, the Golgi apparatus reforms by outgrowth of membrane from the ER.

The Golgi apparatus disassembles during mitosis in many eukaryotic cells and then reassembles in interphase (Fig. 21-25). This process superficially resembles the effects of BFA and BFA washout, since many Golgi enzymes return to the ER or to ER export sites during mitosis and reemerge from the ER at the end of mitosis. Furthermore, Arf1 is inactivated during mitosis. However, mitotic cells also inactivate mitotic kinases (see Chapter 40) that phosphorylate tethering factors

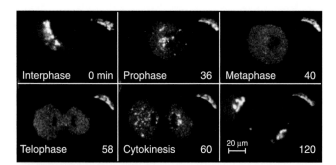

Figure 21-25 TIME-LAPSE IMAGING OF A CELL EXPRESSING A FLUORESCENTLY TAGGED GOLGI ENZYME, GALACTOSYLTRANSFERASE-GFP, THAT IS PROGRESSING THROUGH MITOSIS. As the cell in the *left* of the image passes through prophase and metaphase, its Golgi membranes fragment and then disperse. During cytokinesis, the Golgi membranes reappear as fragments. These fragments then coalesce into a juxtanuclear Golgi ribbon at the end of mitosis. (From Zaal K, Smith CL, Polishchuk RS, et al: Golgi membranes are absorbed into and reemerge from the ER during mitosis. Cell 99:589–601, 1999.)

and other matrix proteins of the Golgi apparatus. This has led to a competing explanation for Golgi disassembly during mitosis in which the Golgi undergoes a direct breakdown into small vesicles and fragments without being absorbed into the ER.

Although the Golgi apparatus is highly dynamic and continually exchanges its protein and lipid components with other cellular compartments, it maintains a unique biochemical and morphologic identity. This allows the Golgi apparatus to participate in several major biosynthetic and processing pathways in the cell, as is discussed in the next section.

Golgi-Specific Processing Activities

Glycoprotein and Glycolipid Processing

Much of the organization and specialization of the Golgi apparatus is directed toward achieving the correct **glycosylation** (i.e., sugar modification) of proteins and lipids. The sugar-modified molecules, called **glycoproteins and glycolipids,** constitute the majority of cell surface and extracellular proteins and lipids, and participate in numerous biological functions, including cell-cell and cell-matrix interactions, intracellular and intercellular trafficking, and signaling.

The most widely recognized glycosylation event occurring within the Golgi involves the modification of *N*-linked oligosaccharides on glycoproteins (Fig. 21-26). These *N*-linked sugar chains are added as preformed complexes (consisting of 14 sugar residues) to asparagine side chains of the protein in the ER. Following delivery to the Golgi, the *N*-linked sugar chains of the glycoprotein undergo extensive further modifications in an ordered sequence. The first modification is the removal of mannose residues. This is followed by the sequential addition of *N*-acetylglucosamine, the further removal of mannoses, the addition of fucose and more *N*-acetylglucosamine, and the final addition of galactose and sialic acid residues. Cell biologists have used the *N*-linked glycan-processing steps that take place in the mammalian Golgi apparatus as experimental signposts for the passage of glycoproteins through the secretory pathway.

Many oligosaccharides are further chemically modified after growing by simple addition of monosaccharide units. Enzymes add substituents such as phosphate, sulfate, acetate or methyl groups or isomerize specific carbons. These modifications as well as differential processing of *N*-linked oligosaccharide structures (producing high-mannose type, complex type, and hybrid structures) contribute to the diversity of sugar residues exposed at the cell surface and can impart specific functions to the sugar chains.

More than 200 Golgi enzymes participate in the biosynthesis of glycoproteins and glycolipids. Enzymes

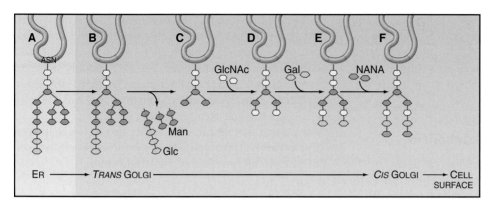

Figure 21-26 PROCESSING OF *N*-LINKED CORE OLIGOSACCHARIDES IN THE GOLGI APPARATUS. **A–F,** Sequential steps trim the mannose (Man)/glucose (Glc) core and then add *N*-acetylglucosamine (GlcNAc), galactose (Gal), and sialic acid (NANA) to form a variety of complex oligosaccharides, one of which is shown here. ASN, asparagines.

called **glycosyltransferases** add specific sugar residues to glycans, while enzymes called **glycosidases** remove specific sugar residues. All of these enzymes are type II transmembrane proteins with a short cytoplasmic amino terminal domain followed by a transmembrane segment and catalytic domain within the Golgi lumen. Additional constituents involved in Golgi oligosaccharide processing include **transporters,** donor sugar-nucleotides, and pyrophosphatases.

Transporters first transfer sugar-nucleotide donors made in the cytoplasm into the lumen of the Golgi apparatus (see Chapter 9). They function as antiporters (see Fig. 9-4), exchanging nucleotide sugars (such as UDP-*N*-acetylglucosamine, UDP-galactose, and CMP-*N*-acetylneuraminic acid) for nucleoside monophosphates formed during glycosyl transfer. Glycosyltransferases then use the high-energy sugar-nucleotides as substrates to add new sugars to an oligosaccharide chain. Most glycosyltransferases are specific for sugar-nucleotide donors and particular oligosaccharide acceptors, but the oligosaccharides are synthesized without a template, so they vary more than polypeptides and polynucleotides, which are synthesized on templates. Finally, glycosidases trim sugars from the branched core oligosaccharides prior to addition of other sugars. They include mannosidase I and II, which clip outer-branch mannose residues on *N*-linked oligosaccharides prior to the addition of *N*-acetylglucosamine.

The Golgi enzymes also add oligosaccharides to the hydroxyl groups of serine and threonine residues of selected proteins, such as **proteoglycans,** heavily glycosylated proteins in secretory granules, and the extracellular matrix (see Figs. 29-13 and 29-14). This process, called **O-linked glycosylation,** begins with the addition of one of three short oligosaccharides to selected serine and threonine residues of a proteoglycan core protein. Glycosyltransferases in the Golgi then add many copies of the same disaccharide unit to the growing polysaccharide. Other enzymes then add sulfates to a few of the sugar residues before the molecule exits the Golgi system.

Enzymes in the Golgi apparatus also mark specific proteins for transport to lysosomes by phosphorylation of the 6-hydroxyl of mannose. This modification, as was mentioned before, is the sorting signal that enables lysosomal enzymes to interact with MPRs in the *trans* Golgi for targeting to lysosomes. The *N*-linked oligosaccharides on these enzymes are initially processed within the ER by trimming of glucose and mannose residues. However, on transport to the Golgi, they become the unique substrates for two enzymes that act sequentially to generate terminal mannose 6-phosphates, which are the lysosomal targeting signal. Human patients with the fatal disease mucolipidosis II (called I-cell disease) fail to phosphorylate the mannose residues required for targeting to lysosomes (see Chapter 23). As a result, the lysosomal enzymes are secreted from the cell, and lysosomes fail to degrade waste materials. Lysosomes become engorged with undigested substrates, leading to fatal cell and tissue abnormalities.

Enzymes in the Golgi stacks further load noncovalently associated cholesterol and phospholipids onto high-density and **low-density lipoproteins** for secretion by liver cells into the blood. Golgi enzymes are also involved in the synthesis of complex polysaccharides in plant cells, which are an important constituent of the plant cell wall.

Proteolytic Processing of Protein Precursors

A number of proteins, particularly peptide hormones, are cleaved into active fragments in the Golgi apparatus and its secretory vesicles. Such proteins are synthesized as large precursors with one or more small hormones embedded in long polypeptides. One example is a yeast mating pheromone. Another is pro-opiomelanocortin, the precursor to no less than six small peptide hormones. Proteolytic enzymes called **prohormone convertases** cleave the precursor proteins into active hormones in the TGN and post-TGN transport intermediates. The mixture of products depends on the prohormone convertases expressed in particular cells. Proteolysis in the Golgi also affects the final folding state and activity of many other proteins. Inherited defects in these processing pathways lead to a number of diseases, including hormone insufficiency and a hereditary amyloid disease.

Lipid Biosynthesis and Metabolism

Another Golgi-specific processing activity is the synthesis of sphingolipids. Sphingolipids, including **sphingomyelin** (SM) and the **glycosphingolipids** glucosylceramide and galactosylceramide, play central roles in membrane sorting within the Golgi apparatus as well as sorting within post-Golgi compartments. As was described earlier, these lipids have affinity for cholesterol, act as donors of intermolecular hydrogen bonds, and have saturated lipid chains, resulting in the denser packing of these lipids compared to glycerophospholipids. When densely packed, the sphingolipids and cholesterol form long cylinders that cause an increase in the thickness of the bilayer relative to a bilayer containing glycerophospholipids alone (e.g., ER [Fig. 21-3]). An enrichment of sphingolipids and cholesterol along the secretory pathway from Golgi to plasma membrane results in an increased thickness of the membranes along this route relative to the ER. This plays a vital role within the secretory system because of a protein's tendency to match the length of its transmembrane domain with that of the lipid bilayer.

The backbone of all sphingolipids, ceramide (see Chapter 20), is synthesized in the ER and then transported to the Golgi complex, where it is modified to form glucosylceramide and sphingomyelin. Glucosylceramide synthesis is catalyzed on the cytoplasmic surface of Golgi membranes by the enzyme UDP-glucose: ceramide glucosyltransferase. Glucosylceramide can then be transported to the plasma membrane or translocated to the luminal leaflet of Golgi membranes, where galactosylation of the head group results in the formation of lactosylceramide. Sequential glycosylation of lactosylceramide by glycosyltransferases of the Golgi lumen generates complex glycolipids and gangliosides for the plasma membrane.

Sphingomyelin synthesis is catalyzed by sphingomyelin-synthase, an enzyme on the luminal leaflet of Golgi membranes. The enzyme transfers phosphorylcholine from phosphatidylcholine to ceramide, releasing the signaling lipid diacylglycerol (DAG) in the process. This mechanism therefore couples consumption of the signaling lipid ceramide (see Fig. 26-11) with the production of the signaling lipid DAG (see Fig. 26-8). If DAG accumulates in the Golgi apparatus, phosphorylcholine can be transferred from sphingomyelin back to DAG, forming phosphatidylcholine and ceramide. Alternatively, DAG can be digested by lipases.

Glycosphingolipid microdomains, or rafts, are thought to form spontaneously by lateral lipid-lipid associations in the luminal leaflet of Golgi membranes. GPI-anchored proteins (see Fig. 7-7), doubly acylated proteins, and many transmembrane proteins physically partition into these microdomains and are thereby enriched in lipid structures that sort preferentially to the plasma membrane. The ability of the Golgi apparatus to drive glycosphingolipid synthesis therefore contributes to its function as a sorting station.

ACKNOWLEDGMENTS

Thanks go to Juan Bonifacino, William Balch, Catherine Jackson, Sean Munro, Kathryn Howell, and Suliana Manley for their suggestions on revisions to this chapter.

SELECTED READINGS

Altan-Bonnet N, Sougrat R, Lippincott-Schwartz J: Molecular basis for Golgi maintenance and biogenesis. Curr Opin Cell Biol 16(4):364–372, 2004.

Antonny B: Membrane deformation by protein coats. Curr Opin Cell Biol 18:1–9, 2006.

Bankaitis VA, Morris AJ: Lipids and the exocytic machinery of eukaryotic cells. Curr Opin Cell Biol 15:389–395, 2003.

Barlowe C: Signals for COPII-dependent export from the ER: What's the ticket out? Trends Cell Biol 13:295–300, 2003.

Baumgart T, Hess ST, Webb WW: Imaging coexisting fluid domains in biomembrane models coupling curvature and line tension. Nature 425:821–824, 2003.

Behnia R, Munro S: Organelle identity and the signposts for membrane traffic. Nature 438:597–604, 2005.

Bi X, Corpina RA, Goldberg J: Structure of the Sec23/24-Sar1 pre-budding complex of the COPII vesicle coat. Nature 419:271–277, 2002.

Bonifacino JS, Glick BS: The mechanisms of vesicle budding and fusion. Cell 116:153–166, 2004.

Bonifacino JS, Lippincott-Schwartz J: Coat proteins: Shaping membrane transport. Nat Rev Mol Cell Biol 4:409–414, 2003.

Bretscher MS, Munro S: Cholesterol and the Golgi apparatus. Science 261:1280–1281, 1993.

Godi A, DiCampli A, Konstantakopoulos A, et al: FAPPs control Golgi-to-cell-surface membrane traffic by binding to Arf and PtdIns(4)P. Nat Cell Biol 6:393–404, 2004.

Gurkan C, Stagg SM, Lapointe P, Balch WE: The COPII cage: Unifying principles of vesicle coat assembly. Nature Rev Mol Cell BIol 7:727–738, 2006.

Holthius JCM, Pomorski T, Raggers RJ, et al: The organizing potential of sphingolipids in intracellular membrane transport. Physiol Rev 81:1689–1723, 2001.

Keller P, Simons K: Post-Golgi biosynthetic trafficking. J Cell Science 110:3001–3009, 1997.

Kepes F, Rambourg A, Satiat-Jeunemaitre B: Morphodynamics of the secretory pathway. Int Rev Cytol 242:55–120, 2005.

Killian JA: Hydrophobic mismatch between proteins and lipids in membranes. Biochim Biophys Acta 1376:401–416, 1998.

Lee MCS, Miller EA, Goldberg J, et al: Bi-directional protein transport between the ER and Golgi. Annu Rev Cell Dev Biol 20:87–123, 2004.

Lippincott-Schwartz J, Roberts TH, Hirschberg K: Secretory protein trafficking and organelle dynamics in living cells. Annu Rev Cell Dev Biol 16:557–589, 2000.

Miller EA, Beilharz TH, Malkus PN, et al: Multiple cargo binding sites on the COPII subunit Sec24p ensure capture of diverse membrane proteins into transport vesicles. Cell 114:497-509, 2003.

Nishimura N, Balch WE: A di-acidic signal required for selective export from the endoplasmic reticulum. Science 277:556-558, 1997.

Palmer KJ, Stephens DJ: Biogenesis of ER-to-Golgi transport carriers: Complex roles of COPII in ER export. Trends Cell Biol 14:57-61, 2004.

Renault L, Gulbert B, Cherfils J: Structural snapshots of the mechanism and inhibition of a guanine nucleotide exchange factor. Nature 426:525-530, 2003.

Van Meer G, Sprong H: Membrane lipids and vesicular traffic. Curr Opin Cell Biol 16:373-378, 2004.

Varki A: Factors controlling the glycosylation potential of the Golgi apparatus. Trends Cell Biol 8:34-40, 1998.

Whyte JRC, Munro S: Vesicle tethering complexes in membrane traffic. J Cell Science 1152627-2637, 2002.

CHAPTER 22

Endocytosis and the Endosomal Membrane System

Regulated entry of small and large molecules into eukaryotic cells occurs at the plasma membrane, the interface between the intracellular and extracellular environments. Small molecules such as amino acids, sugars, and ions traverse the plasma membrane through the action of integral membrane protein pumps (see Chapter 8), carriers (see Chapter 9), or channels (see Chapter 10), but macromolecules can enter cells only by being captured and enclosed within membrane-bound carriers that invaginate and pinch off the plasma membrane in a process known as **endocytosis.** Cells use endocytosis to feed themselves, to defend themselves, and to maintain homeostasis. Some toxins, viruses, pathogenic bacteria, and protozoa "hijack" this process to enter cells.

Endocytosis was discovered more than a century ago in white blood cells (macrophages and neutrophils), the body's "professional phagocytes" (see Fig. 28-8). Endocytosis by these cells is very active, as they internalize the equivalent of their entire plasma membrane surface every hour. It was discovered that when macrophages internalize small particles of blue litmus paper, the color changes, revealing that endocytic vacuoles are acidic. Investigators still use molecules tagged with fluorescent dyes, green fluorescent protein, or electron-dense markers to follow endocytosis in living or fixed cells by light or electron microscopy. Subcellular fractionation, sometimes aided by loading cells with tracers that alter the density of the endocytic compartments or with ferromagnetic tags, has enabled the isolation and biochemical characterization of distinct classes of endocytic structures. In vitro reconstitution systems have also helped to decipher the mechanisms governing membrane trafficking along the endocytic pathway.

Cells utilize many different mechanisms for endocytosis (Fig. 22-1). These differ in mode of uptake and in the type and intracellular fate of internalized cargo. The mechanisms include **phagocytosis, macropinocytosis, clathrin-mediated endocytosis, caveolae-dependent uptake,** and **nonclathrin/noncaveolae endocytosis.** The protrusions or invaginations of the plasma membrane that are formed during these diverse endocytic processes all require coordinated interactions between a variety of protein and lipid molecules that dynamically link the plasma membrane and cortical actin cytoskeleton.

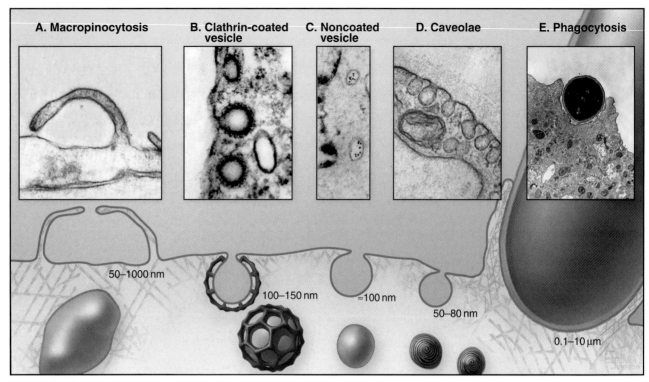

Figure 22-1   A–E, Electron micrographs and diagrams illustrating five structurally and mechanistically distinct pathways for entry into the cell. The endocytic vesicles that are generated differ in size and structure, as shown. (A and D, Courtesy of D. Fawcett, Harvard Medical School, Boston, Massachusetts. B, Courtesy of C-M Chang and S. Schmid, Scripps Research Institute, La Jolla, California. C, Courtesy of S. Hansen and B. van Deurs, University of Copenhagen, Denmark. E, Courtesy of Blair Bowers, National Institutes of Health, Bethesda, Maryland.)

In phagocytosis and clathrin-mediated endocytosis, cell surface receptors selectively bind macromolecules (ligands) to be internalized. Ligands can be proteins, glycoproteins, or carbohydrates. In phagocytosis, the ligands are usually membrane constituents of other cells, bacteria, or viruses. After ligand-receptor complexes are concentrated into patches in the membrane, the membrane is then either pinched off to form small vesicles (in clathrin-mediated endocytosis) or zippered up around the particle to form a large vacuole inside the cell (in phagocytosis).

All other forms of endocytosis are less selective. In these cases, cells take up bulk fluid through small, pino-cytic vesicles or through macropinocytosis, in which the cell extends its membrane and sweeps up extracellular fluid indiscriminately. Alternatively, ligands and molecules associated with lipid rafts are taken up at the plasma membrane through caveolae-mediated or non-clathrin/noncaveolar endocytosis.

Endocytic carriers produced by the various endocytic mechanisms are transported into the cytoplasm away from the plasma membrane, where they fuse with each other and with other membrane compartments comprising the **endosomal membrane system.** Among the different compartments of the endocytic

membrane system are **early/recycling endosomes, multivesicular bodies, late endosomes,** and **lysosomes.** Each has a distinct role in the sorting, processing, and degradation of internalized cargo, and they communicate with each other and/or the plasma membrane by mechanistically diverse and highly regulated pathways. The endosomal system controls important physiological processes, including nutrient absorption, hormone-mediated signal transduction, immune surveillance, and antigen presentation.

This chapter describes the molecular mechanisms of the major types of endocytosis and the functions of the endosomal system.

Phagocytosis

Phagocytosis is the ingestion of large particles such as bacteria, foreign bodies, and remnants of dead cells (Fig. 22-2). Cells use the actin cytoskeleton to push a protrusion of the plasma membrane to surround these particles.

Some cells, including macrophages, dendritic cells, and neutrophils, are specialized for phagocytosis. The presence of bacteria or protozoa in tissues attracts pro-

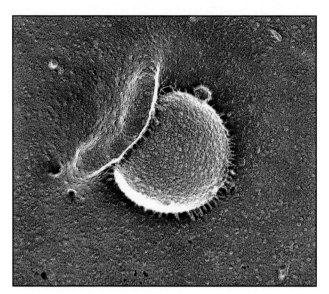

Figure 22-2 ELECTRON MICROGRAPH OF AN AMOEBA INGESTING A LATEX BEAD BY PHAGOCYTOSIS. Note the numerous sites of attachment between the amoeba cell surface and the bead. (Courtesy of John Heuser, Washington University, St. Louis, Missouri.)

the particle to be ingested. Growth of these actin filaments supports the plasma membrane as it zippers tightly around the particle to form a cup-like protrusion, called the **phagocytic cup.** The signaling pathways that give rise to these events are dependent on polyphosphatidylinositides and phosphatidylinositol (PI) kinases (Box 22-1 and Fig. 22-4). In the phagocytic cup, PI(3) kinase generates **PI(3,4,5)P$_3$ (PIP$_3$).** Effectors of this lipid include a group of PH-domain containing GEFs for the small GTPases Rac1, Arf6, and Cdc42. Once these GTPases are activated, they stimulate the cytoskeletal rearrangements of actin, leading to phagocytic cup growth. The requirement of PI(3) kinase is restricted to the stage at which the phagocytic cup seals to form a phagosome. Following this, PIP$_3$ levels in the newly formed phagosome decline rapidly owing to the activity of PI phosphatases. The phosphatase activity leads to

fessional phagocytes from the blood (see Fig. 30-13), where they ingest the microorganisms and initiate inflammatory and immune responses. Other cell types use phagocytosis to remove dead neighboring cells, while amoeba use phagocytosis for feeding.

Phagocytosis proceeds through four steps: attachment, engulfment, fusion with lysosomes, and degradation (Fig. 22-3). These steps are highly regulated by cell surface receptors, phospholipids, and signaling cascades mediated by Rho-family GTPases.

Attachment

Attachment depends on the ability of the phagocytic cell to recognize the particle to be ingested. Such specific interactions trigger ingestion of the particle. Vertebrates use proteins, collectively called "opsonins," to mark bacteria and other foreign particles for phagocytosis. Opsonins include antibodies, which bind to foreign antigens on bacteria, and complement proteins, which tag infected or dying cells. Phagocytes such as macrophages use plasma membrane receptors to bind particles coated with opsonins. For example, **immunoglobulin Fc receptors** bind to the constant regions of immunoglobulin G molecules (see H3 and H4 domains in Fig. 3-13B) coating pathogenic bacteria and viruses.

Engulfment

Binding of receptors such as the Fc receptor to a foreign particle generates localized signals on the cytoplasmic side of the plasma membrane. These signals trigger the assembly of the actin filaments immediately adjacent to

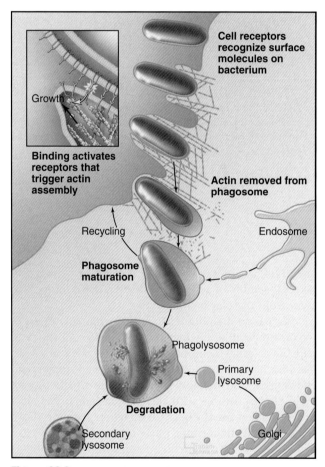

Figure 22-3 THE MOLECULAR MECHANISM FOR PHAGOCYTOSIS OF A BACTERIUM BY A MACROPHAGE. Macrophage surface receptors are activated by contact with a bacterium; this triggers actin rearrangements that lead to protrusion of the plasma membrane to engulf the bacterium. The actin filaments encasing the newly formed phagosome depolymerize, and membrane traffic to and from the phagosome leads to its maturation. Hydrolytic enzymes are delivered to the mature phagosome through fusion with primary and secondary lysosomes, and the bacterium is degraded.

Polyphosphatidylinositides in Endocytosis

Phosphatidylinositol (PI) is a glycerolphospholipid with a cyclohexanol head group (Fig. 22-4D) that can be phosphorylated on carbons 3, 4, and 5 either singly or in combination to produce **polyphosphoinositides** (see Fig. 26-7). Polyphosphoinositides are minor lipids in the cytoplasmic leaflet of the plasma membrane (~1% of total lipids) and endocytic membranes, but lipid kinases and phosphatases can change polyphosphoinositide levels rapidly at local sites in membranes (Fig. 22-4E). This local synthesis of particular polyphosphoinositides regulates membrane remodeling during exocytosis, endocytosis, and vesicular trafficking by recruiting and/or activating proteins that sense the curvature of the lipid bilayer, form scaffolds on the membrane (e.g., clathrin and dynamin), or regulate actin assembly.

The most important polyphosphoinositide for endocytosis is phosphatidylinositol(4,5)bis-phosphate (**PI(4,5)P$_2$**) with phosphates on carbons 4 and 5 of the head group. Two lipid kinases synthesize PI(4,5)P$_2$ by adding phosphate first to the hydroxyl on carbon 4 and then on carbon 5 (Fig. 22-4E; also see Fig. 26-7). The second enzyme, **phosphatidylinositol-4-P-5 kinase,** is activated by another glycerolphospholipid, phosphatidic acid (PA; see Fig. 7-2). Since PI(4,5)P$_2$ activates the phospholipase D (see Fig. 26-7) that makes PA, the two enzymes make a positive feedback loop that enriches PI(4,5)P$_2$ locally in the membrane. Interactions of PI(4,5)P$_2$ with proteins from the cytoplasm retard its mobility in the plane of the membrane, raising its local concentration until it is depleted by removal of the head group or by dephosphorylation (see Fig. 26-7).

PI(4,5)P$_2$ participates in clathrin-mediated endocytosis, phagocytosis, and macropinocytosis (Fig. 22-4A–C). The formation of the clathrin lattice and its tethering to the plasma membrane relies on several proteins that interact with PI(4,5)P$_2$, including AP180/CALM, epsin, and AP2 (Fig. 22-9). The GTPase dynamin, which is essential for the scission of clathrin-coated vesicles, also binds to PI(4,5)P$_2$ (Fig. 22-10). Dephosphorylation of PI(4,5)P$_2$ into PI(4)P is mediated by synaptojanin, which plays an important role in clathrin uncoating.

In phagosome biogenesis, high-affinity binding between ligands and plasma membrane receptors attracts P(3)kinase, which produces PIP$_3$. Activation of Rac, Arf6, and Cdc42 by PIP$_3$ leads to cortical actin assembly and protrusion of the plasma membrane around the phagocytosed particle. The plasma membrane then zippers up around a phagocytosed particle. After plasma membrane closure, PI(4,5)P$_2$ in the phagosome membrane promotes the assembly of actin filaments that drive the vesicle away from the plasma membrane.

Whereas PI(4,5)P$_2$ helps to regulate endocytosis, PI(3)P is important for early endosome dynamics. It is found on the limiting and intralumenal membranes of endosomes, where it recruits effector molecules. These include EEA1, which is responsible for endosome-endosome fusion through its interaction with Rab5, and Hrs, which recognizes ubiquitinated endocytic cargo and facilitates the formation of intralumenal endosomal vesicles through the assembly of ESCRT-I, -II, and -III. PI(3)kinase Class II or III is responsible for generating PI(3)P on membranes (Fig. 22-4E).

---

more PI(4,5)P$_2$ in the phagosome membrane, which promotes assembly of actin filaments that drive the vesicle away from the plasma membrane.

The plasma membrane alone was originally thought to contribute all of the membrane to make a phagocytic cup, but internal membranes are now known to contribute. Internal membranes from recycling endosomes, late endosomes, and possibly ER contribute to the phagocytic cup by fusing with the plasma membrane in a process called **focal exocytosis.** When secretory lysosomes fuse at the forming phagocytic cup, they release cytokines that contribute to inflammation. This couples phagocytosis to the immune response. Focal exocytosis relies on the same steps that are involved in other membrane fusion events, including transport of internal membranes along cytoskeletal tracks and their fusion by compartment-specific SNAREs under the control of Rab GTPases (see Fig. 21-12).

Closure of the phagocytic cup occurs when the membrane zippers up around the particle fuse together.

Phagosome closure coincides with local depletion of PIP$_3$ by PI phosphatases and phospholipase Cγ.

Fusion with Lysosomes

After closure, the actin filaments surrounding the phagosome disassemble, and motors direct the phagosome along microtubules deep into the cell during a process termed **directed maturation.** A series of fusion and fission reactions remove plasma membrane components and replace them with endosome-specific components including proteins (e.g., SNAREs) required for selective fusion with acidic lysosomes containing active hydrolytic enzymes. Fusion with lysosomes creates a hybrid vacuole called a **phagolysosome** (Fig. 22-3).

Alternative Fates of Ingested Particles

Many ingested particles are degraded in phagolysosomes to their constituent amino acids, monosaccharides and

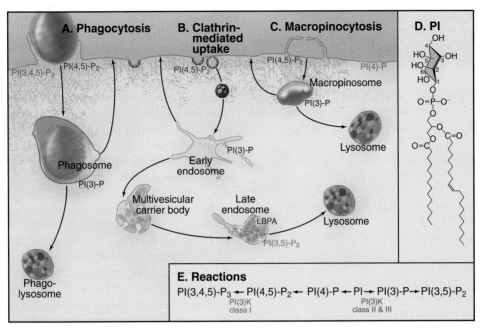

Figure 22-4   DISTRIBUTION OF PHOSPHOINOSITIDES AMONG ENDOCYTIC COMPARTMENTS. **A–C,** Polyphosphoinositol territories within the endocytic system. Localized $PI(4,5)P_2$ at the plasma membrane plays a role in phagocytosis **(A),** clathrin-mediated endocytosis **(B),** and macropinocytosis **(C).** $PI(3,4,5)P_3$ at the plasma membrane plays an additional role in phagocytosis. $PI(3)P$ is enriched in endosomes, whereas $PI(3,5)P_2$ and LBPA are enriched in late endosomes. Various proteins, including clathrin adapters, bind specifically to the polyphosphoinositides depicted here, providing a mechanism for their targeting. **D,** Phosphatidylinositol can be phosphorylated on the 3, 4, or 5 position of its inositol ring, with all seven combinations possible. The polyphosphatidylinositides that are so generated embed in the cytoplasmic leaflets of membranes. **E,** Biochemical pathways that generate different polyphosphatidylinositides. Three classes of PI(3)-kinases participate: Class I PI(3)-kinase uses $PI(4,5)P_2$ as substrate yielding $PI(3,4,5)P_3$ (involved in phagocytosis); Class II and III PI(3)-kinases use PI yielding $PI(3)P$ (involved in endosome maturation). PI(3)-kinase inhibitors such as wortmannin and 3-methyladenine have helped to characterize the function of these PI(3)-kinases. The inhibitors compete for ATP binding in the active site of the kinase domain.

disaccharides, nucleotides, and lipids by lysosomal hydrolases. These small products of digestion are transported across the phagolysosomal membrane into the cytoplasm, where they can be reused to synthesize new macromolecules. Any undegraded material remains within the lysosome, which is called a **residual body.**

Antigen-presenting phagocytic cells, such as dendritic cells, cleave proteins of ingested microorganisms into small peptides for loading onto membrane receptors called major histocompatibility complex (MHC) class II molecules. This transfer occurs in phagolysosomes called the **antigen-presenting compartment** in these cells. MHC Class II molecules loaded with peptides recycle back to the surface of phagocytic cells, where they activate CD4+ T-lymphocytes (see Fig. 27-8).

Ingested microorganisms are killed by a combination of factors in phagolysosomes. The reduced form of nicotinamide-adenine dinucleotide phosphate oxidase in the phagosomal membrane produces a lethal barrage of toxic oxidants. Proteases and acid hydrolases in the lumen of the phagolysosome digest the ingested organism. Small peptides called **defensins** bind and disrupt microbial membranes.

Some pathogens have counterstrategies to avoid destruction by phagocytes. These include mechanisms to inhibit fusion of phagosomes with lysosomes, to resist the low pH environment of the lysosome, and to escape to the cytoplasm by lysing the phagolysosome membrane (Table 22-1). For example, in tuberculosis, macrophages in the lung phagocytose the bacterium *Mycobacterium tuberculosis,* but the bacterium evades destruction by secreting a phosphatase that dephosphorylates phosphatidylinositol (3P) and thus halts phagosome maturation.

Macropinocytosis

Many cells ingest extracellular fluid in large endocytic structures called **macropinosomes.** Growth factors or other signals stimulate actin-driven protrusions of the plasma membrane in the form of ruffles (Fig. 22-5). These protrusions close around extracellular fluid, forming a macropinosome, which is then carried along microtubules toward the center of the cell. This allows cells to internalize fluid continuously from their surroundings without concentrating particular molecules, which is useful for bulk nutrient uptake.

Table 22-1

SURVIVAL STRATEGIES FOR INTRACELLULAR PATHOGENS

"Escape"

Secretion of toxins that disrupt phagosomal membrane (*Shigella flexneri, Listeria monocytogenes, Rickettsia rickettsii*)

"Dodge"

Entrance through alternative, pathogen-specific pathway (*Salmonella typhimurium, Legionella pneumophila, Chlamydia trachomatis*)

Inhibition of phagosome-lysosome fusion (*S. typhimurium, Mycobacterium tuberculosis*)

Inhibition of phagolysosome acidification (*Mycobacterium* species)

"Stand and Fight"

Low pH-dependent replication (*Coxiella burnetii, S. typhimurium*)

Enhancement of DNA repair to survive oxidative stress (*S. typhimurium*)

Protective pathogen-specific virulence factors (*C. burnetii, S. typhimurium*)

Prevention of the processing and presentation of bacterial antigens (*S. typhimurium*)

Macropinosomes persist inside cells for only about 5 to 20 minutes, during which their membrane components either recycle back to the plasma membrane, potentially bypassing other organelles within the cell, or are delivered to lysosomes (Fig. 22-4). Although the membrane composition of macropinosomes resembles the plasma membrane ruffles from which they were derived, the ruffles themselves are believed to have a different composition from the rest of the plasma membrane by being enriched in both specific polyphosphoinositides and lipid raft markers. Internalization of these membranes during macropinocytosis, therefore, is likely to generate inhomogeneities in the plasma membrane that might influence cellular motility and responses to external stimuli.

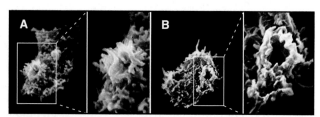

Figure 22-5 A–B, Scanning electron micrographs of *Acanthamoeba castellanii* showing membrane ruffling and macropinocytosis, the major pathway for nutrient uptake in this organism. (Courtesy of Steve Doberstein, Johns Hopkins Medical School, Baltimore, Maryland.)

Formation of macropinosomes depends on many of the same proteins that are used for phagocytosis. Phosphatidylinositol kinases and GTPases recruit and activate proteins that assemble the actin filaments supporting membrane ruffles. For example, the GTPase Arf6 activates phosphatidyl-4-phosphate-kinase, leading to production of $PI(4,5)P_2$ at plasma membrane sites of macropinocytosis (Fig. 22-4C). $PI(4,5)P_2$ then activates WASp-related proteins and the assembly of actin filaments. Overexpressing a constitutively active form of Arf6 increases ruffling and accumulation of macropinosomes that are enriched in $PI(4,5)P_2$.

Macropinocytosis serves diverse cellular functions. In some cases, macropinocytosis is induced by activation of plasma membrane receptors. Removal of these same receptors from the cell surface by macropinocytosis downregulates their signaling activity. Constitutive macropinocytosis allows cells to take up molecules from the medium. Examples include uptake of nutrients by amoeba, thyroglobulin by thyroid cells, and bulk extracellular fluid by dendritic cells for immune surveillance. Migrating cells use macropinocytosis for motility to coordinate insertion and uptake of plasma membrane with their direction of motion. Some pathogenic bacteria (e.g., *Salmonella typhimurium*) trigger macropinocytosis by injecting toxins into cells. They then use this triggered macropinocytosis to gain entry into the cell. Once in a macropinosome, the bacteria can replicate and avoid being destroyed by other cells engaged in phagocytosis.

Endocytosis Mediated by Caveolae

Caveolae are small (~50 nm), flask-shaped invaginations of the plasma membrane enriched in cholesterol, diverse signaling molecules, and membrane transporters (Fig. 22-6). They are especially abundant in endothelial cells (making up more than 10% of the plasma membrane), where they mediate transcellular shuttling of serum proteins and nutrients from the bloodstream into tissues. Caveolae in other cell types are generally static, but tyrosine phosphorylation can trigger internalization of these caveolae. Simian virus 40 (SV40), for example, use caveolae to enter cells by activating a signaling cascade that cross-links surface receptors in caveolae.

Caveolae are unique microdomains of the plasma membrane that are enriched in cholesterol and stabilized by the major protein **caveolin** (Fig. 22-7). Caveolin inserts as a loop into the inner leaflet of the plasma membrane, where it binds tightly to cholesterol in a 1 : 1 ratio. Caveolin also self-associates to form a striated coat on the cytoplasmic surface of the membrane invagination. The caveolin coat is believed to stabilize the membrane and to define the size and shape of caveolae.

Caveolin is immobilized in caveolae and does not diffuse laterally in the plasma membrane. This contrasts with the transient recruitment and regulated assembly of coat proteins involved in the formation of clathrin-coated pits (Fig. 22-11) and COP-coated buds (see Figs. 21-7 and 21-9). Cholesterol is also important, because depletion of cholesterol causes caveolae to flatten and caveolin to become mobile.

Association of transmembrane cargo proteins with caveolae on the cell surface involves interaction with caveolin and/or with components of the cholesterol-enriched membrane. Internalization of caveolae requires rearrangements of the actin cytoskeleton as well as the action of the GTPase **dynamin** (Fig. 22-8). The vesicles

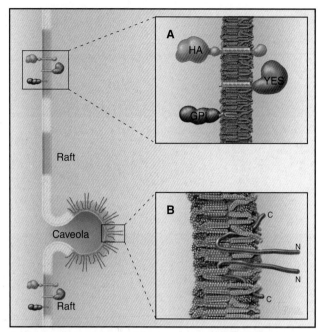

Figure 22-7 MICRODOMAINS OF THE PLASMA MEMBRANE ENRICHED IN CHOLESTEROL AND GLYCOSPHINGOLIPIDS AND HELD TOGETHER BY INTERACTIONS BETWEEN LIPID HEAD GROUPS AND LONG, SATURATED ACYL-CHAINS. **A,** "Lipid rafts" can exist independently of caveolin. Proteins that are enriched in these lipid rafts include those that are anchored to the outer leaflet by GPI tails or to the inner leaflet by acylation and some integral membrane proteins, depending on the composition of their transmembrane domains. **B,** Caveolae. Caveolin (*blue schematic*) binds cholesterol (*red*) and aids in forming and/or stabilizing these microdomains. HA, influenza virus hemagglutinin; YES, a Src-family tyrosine kinase.

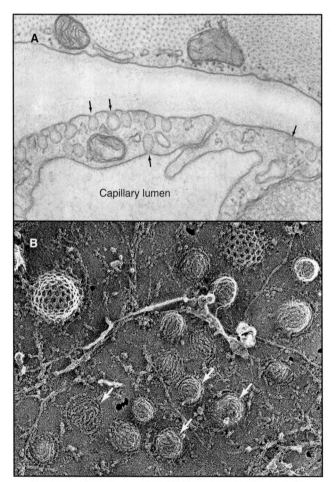

Figure 22-6 **A,** Electron micrograph of a thin section of a muscle capillary showing caveolae ("little caves"), which are abundant in endothelial cells that mediate transcytosis. *Arrows* show "cave" openings. **B,** Electron micrograph of the inside surface of a fibroblast prepared by quick-freezing, deep-etching, and rotary shadowing. The whorl-like coat on the caveolae formed by self-assembly of caveolin (*white arrows*). Caveolae are typically smaller than clathrin-coated pits shown in the *upper left and right*. (A, Courtesy of D. Fawcett, Harvard Medical School, Boston, Massachusetts. B, Courtesy of John Heuser, Washington University, St. Louis, Missouri.)

that form during this process are small (~60 nm in diameter) and interact transiently with endosomes or fuse with each other (forming a **caveosome**) while retaining their caveolae coat. In endothelial cells, where caveolae constitute a major portion of the cell surface, this permits extensive uptake of nutrients from the bloodstream. Endothelial cells in mice lacking caveolin I are unable to bind or take up serum albumin from the blood. Nonetheless, these mice are remarkably normal (except for excess cellular proliferation in some tissues and abnormal vasodilation of some blood vessels), since other pathways compensate for transport across endothelial cells.

Clathrin-Mediated Endocytosis

Clathrin-dependent endocytosis occurs at specialized patches on the plasma membrane, called **coated pits,** formed by a protein lattice of **clathrin** and adapter molecules on their cytoplasmic surface (Fig. 22-8). Eukaryotic cells use **clathrin-mediated endocytosis** to obtain essential nutrients, such as iron and cholesterol, and to remove activated receptors from the

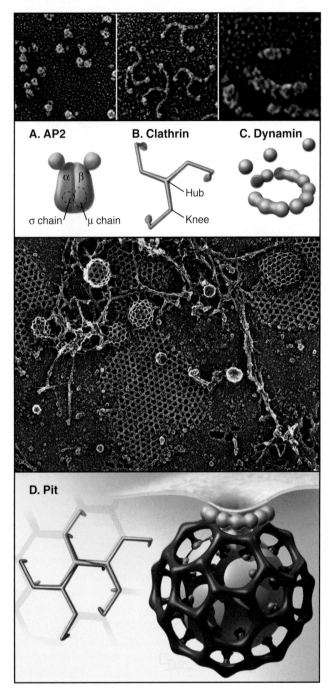

Figure 22-8 Electron micrographs and drawings of the major components of the endocytic clathrin-coated vesicle: AP2 complexes **(A)**, clathrin triskelions **(B)**, and dynamin **(C)**, visualized by platinum shadowing. **D,** Field of coated pits assembled on the cytoplasmic face of the plasma membrane viewed by quick-freeze, deep-etch microscopy. The diagrams are structural models of the major proteins and a model for their coassembly into a coated pit. AP2 complexes interact with docking sites on the membrane and mediate clathrin assembly into a polygonal lattice. Dynamin is targeted to the necks of deeply invaginated coated pits and can self-assemble into ring-like structures that are believed to regulate coated vesicle formation. (Micrographs courtesy of John Heuser, Washington University, St. Louis, Missouri.)

cell surface. Clathrin-coated vesicles also retrieve synaptic vesicle membrane at synapses following neurotransmitter release. In addition to its role in endocytosis at the plasma membrane, clathrin also participates in cargo sorting and membrane budding at other sites in cells, including endosomes and the *trans*-Golgi network (TGN).

Clathrin-dependent endocytosis concentrates many ligand-receptor complexes in small patches called **coated pits** on the cell surface. These patches invaginate and pinch off to form **clathrin-coated vesicles** carrying their cargo into the cell. Coated pits typically occupy 1% to 2% of the plasma membrane surface area and complete the budding process in approximately 1 minute. Therefore, depending on how effectively a receptor-ligand complex concentrates in coated pits (typically 10- to 20-fold), 20% to 40% of cell surface receptors can be internalized per minute. For other receptors that are not concentrated in coated pits, internalization is much slower, reflecting the rate of bulk membrane uptake into the clathrin-dependent pathway.

Structure of the Clathrin Coat

Clathrin forms a three-legged structure termed a triskelion (Fig. 22-8) consisting of three 190-kD heavy chains, each associated with one of two light chains of approximately 30 kD (LCα or LCβ). This hexameric complex can self-assemble empty cages under special conditions. The assembled empty cage is like a soccer ball, with clathrin forming the ribs or seams between adjacent faces. Each rib of the cage incorporates portions of four different triskelions, which are, in turn, arranged in pentagons and hexagons (Fig. 22-9A). (See Fig. 5-4 for an explanation of how pentagons and hexagons form closed shells.) The clathrin heavy chain contains an N-terminal β-propeller domain that binds several different cargo adapters and membrane attachment proteins (Fig. 22-10). Together with clathrin, these molecules help to drive curvature of the underlying membrane and promote vesicle formation.

While clathrin cages can assemble from clathrin alone in vitro, under physiological conditions, they require **assembly proteins (APs),** which are the other main clathrin coat constituent. Two classes of structurally and functionally distinct APs exist: the monomeric assembly protein AP180/CALM and **heterotetrameric adapter protein complexes (AP1-4).** AP2 is the only heterotetrameric AP that is involved in clathrin-coated vesicle formation at the plasma membrane, with the other heterotetrameric APs involved in vesicle formation at other distinct subcellular locations. The four subunits of the AP2 complex have distinct functions: the large α-adaptin subunit recruits accessory/regulatory proteins from the cytoplasm; the large β2 subunit

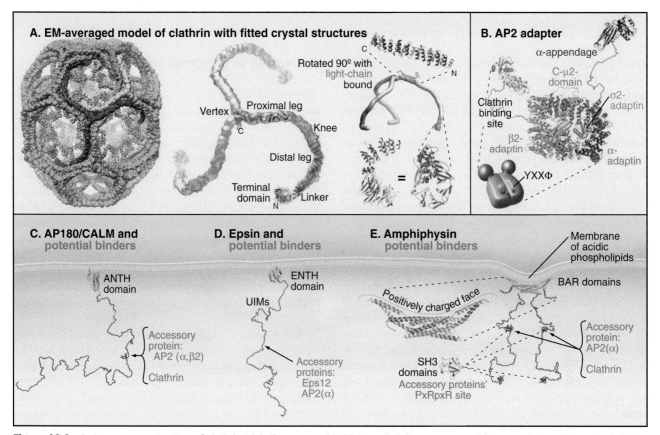

Figure 22-9 **A,** Image reconstruction of clathrin triskelions assembled into a clathrin cage seen at 2-nm resolution. The extended legs of clathrin triskelions are formed from multiple repeating units consisting of five helix hairpins that give them rigidity. These repeats continue into the linker region, which expands into the N-terminal domain, consisting of a seven-bladed β-propeller similar to a trimeric G protein β-subunit. **B,** Model of the AP2 complex from high-resolution structures of its individual subunits. The large subunits are helical solenoids of approximately 30 repeats of six- to eight-turn helices connected by short loops, whereas σ2 and μ2 are each five-stranded β-sheets flanked by α-helices. **C,** Model of AP180/CALM from its high-resolution structure. The α-helical solenoid domain at the N-terminus (called ANTH domain) binds $PI(4,5)P_2$ and has a similar structure to the epsin ENTH domain. The long C-terminal tail has no predicted secondary structure but contains binding motifs for Eps15, clathrin, and Dx[FW]. **D,** Model of epsin from a high-resolution structure. The ENTH domain binds $PI(4,5)P_2$, attaching epsin to the membrane. The long flexible arm contains a **ubiquitin-interacting motif (UIM)** and can bind AP2 and clathrin. When ubiquitin is bound to this motif, it serves as a signal for directing the membrane through the endocytic pathway, ending in incorporation into internal vesicles of multivesicular bodies that ultimately are degraded by hydrolytic enzymes stored in lysosomes. **E,** High-resolution structural model of amphiphysin. The molecule contains an N-terminal BAR domain and a C-terminal SH3 (Src homology region-3) domain. The BAR domains are banana-shaped dimers in which each subunit is composed of three long helices that wrap around each other to form a long, curved three-helical bundle. The concave surface of the dimer is positively charged, allowing it to bind to the phospholipid bilayer with no lipid specificity. Its concave shape results in preferential binding to curved membranes. The SH3 domain at the end of the extended region recruits SH3-binding proteins, while the extended region itself binds clathrin and AP2α. (A, Courtesy of Corinne Smith, Medical Research Council Laboratory of Molecular Biology, Cambridge, England. B–C, Courtesy of Frances Brodsky, University of California, San Francisco; Tomas Kirchhausen, Harvard Medical School, Boston, Massachusetts; and David Owen, Medical Research Council Laboratory of Molecular Biology, Cambridge, England.)

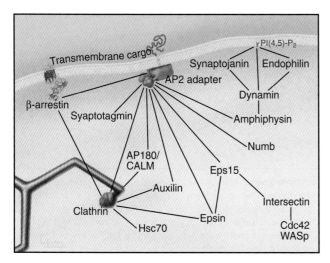

Figure 22-10 SCHEMATIC REPRESENTATION OF PROTEIN-PROTEIN INTERACTIONS AMONG THE PROTEINS INVOLVED IN CLATHRIN-COATED VESICLE FORMATION. Major components of the clathrin-coat include clathrin and AP2. Transmembrane cargo and $PI(4,5)P_2$ molecules are shown embedded in the plasma membrane bilayer. Single protein components of the endocytic machinery are indicated by name. Interactions between the components are indicated by a *solid line.*

binds to D/ExxxLL internalization signals (e.g., **dileu-cine-based sorting motifs**) of transmembrane receptors; the medium-sized μ2 subunit binds clathrin, β-arrestins, and the YxxΦ (where Φ is any bulky hydrophobic group) internalization signals (e.g., **tyrosine-based sorting motifs**) of transmembrane receptors; and a small σ chain stabilizes the AP complex. Multiple factors recruit AP2 to the plasma membrane. They include PI(4,5)P₂, AP180/CALM, tyrosine, and dileucine-based endocytic sorting motifs in the cytoplasmic tails of receptors, synaptotagmin, and other proteins.

APs belong to a general class of endocytic proteins called **adapters** that include epsin, amphiphysin, Hrs/Vps27p, and β-arrestin. These proteins help to coordinate clathrin coat formation by linking it with the selection and binding of cargo and with the recruitment of other proteins involved in creating and disassembling the clathrin coat. The adapter proteins all consist of one or more folded domains connected by long, flexible linkers (Fig. 22-9C–E). This "string and knots" design allows for multiple weak-binding sites on the long flexible polypeptide, which can sweep through a large volume of cytoplasm hunting for binding partners and recapturing dissociated ligands. Fast on/off rates for binding of ligands to the string-like region, furthermore, allow multiple ligands to be held in the same locale by continual and rapid exchange between free and bound states. Cooperative networks of weak interactions between multivalent binding partners (Fig. 22-10) create a positive amplification cascade that, once initiated, drives clathrin-coat formation. The network dissociates in a self-propagating fashion once these interactions are disrupted, leading to clathrin uncoating. In this manner, adapter proteins coordinate the assembly/disassembly cycle of clathrin lattices on membranes.

Formation of Clathrin-Coated Vesicles

The formation of clathrin-coated vesicles consists of several steps (Fig. 22-11). Clathrin first binds to AP2 complexes on the cytoplasmic surface of the plasma membrane and assembles into polyhedral lattices. In this process, the α-adaptin subunit of AP2 binds clathrin, whereas the β2 subunit mediates clathrin assembly. Once polyhedral lattices have begun to form, the μ2 subunit of AP2 interacts with sorting motifs on cargo molecules, resulting in the concentration of cargo molecules in the clathrin-coated region of the plasma membrane. These steps are facilitated by the ability of clathrin and AP2 to act as a binding scaffold for several other components that assist or regulate coated vesicle invagination (including Eps15, amphiphysin, and intersectin [Fig. 22-10]).

Once the coated pit becomes deeply invaginated, the neck narrows to form a constricted pit, which pinches off the plasma membrane as a clathrin-coated vesicle. The large (100-kD) GTPase **dynamin** coordinates the invagination, fission and internalization of clathrin-coated vesicles. In addition to a GTPase domain, dynamin has a PI(4,5)P₂ binding domain, a pleckstrin-homology domain (see Fig. 25-11), a GTPase effector domain, and a proline-rich domain. PI(4,5)P₂ recruits dynamin to coated pits, where it binds GTP and assembles into a helical "collar" around the necks of deeply invaginated coated pits. The proline-rich domain of dynamin binds a number of proteins with SH3 domains (see Fig. 25-11), including endophilin, cortactin, and amphiphysin. These proteins, together with dynamin, help to orchestrate coated pit invagination and budding. For example, the BAR domains of endophilin and amphiphysin (Fig. 22-9E) induce membrane curvature during

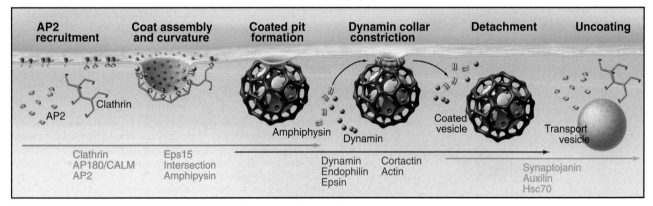

Figure 22-11 CYCLE OF RECEPTOR-MEDIATED ENDOCYTOSIS DRIVEN BY THE CLATHRIN-COATED VESICLE. AP2 complexes are targeted to docking sites on the plasma membrane and initiate clathrin assembly into a polygonal lattice. Receptors carrying cargo molecules are concentrated in coated pits through interactions between tyrosine-based sorting motifs on their cytoplasmic domains and the clustered μ subunits of AP2. The GTPase dynamin is targeted to coated pits through interactions with amphiphysin, which also binds AP2 and clathrin and, by mechanisms as yet unknown, regulates membrane invagination and fission to release coated vesicles carrying cargo into the cell. Synaptojanin and other uncoating factors disassemble the coat constituents and release the transport vesicles for fusion with endosomes.

coated pit constriction and coated vesicle release by dimerizing into crescent-shaped structures, which bind to highly curved, negatively charged membranes (Fig. 22-8). Epsin's lipid-binding domain (ENTH) and extended tail serve to retain clathrin and AP2 on membranes (Fig. 22-9D). Finally, actin-binding proteins such as cortactin promote assembly of actin filaments to drive internalization, whereas intersectin regulates actin assembly by recruiting the GTPase Cdc42 and N-WASP (Fig. 22-10).

Disassembly of Clathrin Coats

Soon after a clathrin-coated vesicle pinches off the plasma membrane, the clathrin coat begins to disassemble (Fig. 22-11). This uncoating reaction recycles coat components and frees the vesicle to fuse with other vesicles to form endosomes. An important protein that is involved in this uncoating reaction is synaptojanin, a lipid phosphatase. On being recruited to clathrin-coated membranes via endophilin, synaptojanin dephosphorylates $PI(4,5)P_2$, which weakens the attachment of coat proteins such as dynamin, Aps, and clathrin. Other proteins that are involved in clathrin uncoating include Hsc70, a member of the heat shock protein family of chaperones, and auxilin. Once the clathrin coat is removed from the vesicle, it undergoes rapid fusion with other similar vesicles or with early endosomes.

Nonclathrin/Noncaveolar Endocytosis

Endocytic pathways that do not depend on clathrin or caveoli were discovered when cells continued to take up certain proteins and lipids after clathrin function was disrupted by overexpression of domains from Eps15. Eps15 normally links several clathrin assembly proteins to AP-2, so individual Eps15 domains interfere with coat assembly. Surprisingly, these cells take up interleukin 2 (IL-2) receptors, an analog of sphingomyelin and GPI-anchored proteins. Uptake is less efficient without clathrin-mediated endocytosis, but it is sufficient to replace lipid raft markers in the plasma membrane every 2 to 3 hours.

The mechanism of this nonclathrin/noncaveolar endocytosis pathway is not well characterized. Rather than using coat complexes to recruit cargo and to bud from the membrane, this pathway is believed to exploit heterogeneity in the lipid and protein composition of the plasma membrane to form lipid microdomains with cargo that bud into the cell (Fig. 22-7A).

The nonclathrin/noncaveolar pathway takes up proteins found in lipid rafts, detergent-resistant regions of the plasma membrane enriched in cholesterol, glycosphingolipids, glycosylphosphatidylinositol (GPI) anchored proteins, and some membrane proteins (Fig 22–8; also see Fig. 7-9). Thus, the pathway might circulate membrane lipids and markers for lipid rafts between the cell surface and internal membranes. As sphingolipids are important for anterograde transport through the secretory membrane system (see Fig. 21-4), the non-clathrin/noncaveolar pathway might help to resupply the secretory pathway with sphingolipids. Another function might be to help differentiate the plasma membrane of epithelial cells into polarized apical (enriched with rafts) and basolateral (deficient in rafts) domains. By contrast, most proteins that are taken up by clathrin-mediated endocytosis, such as transferrin receptors and LDL receptors, are excluded from lipid rafts and do not enter the nonclathrin/noncaveolar endocytic pathway. Conditions that lead to depletion of cholesterol inhibit nonclathrin/noncaveolar endocytosis but not clathrin-mediated endocytosis.

Several bacterial toxins follow the nonclathrin/non-caveolar pathway, including Cholera and Shiga toxins. These toxins are also internalized by clathrin-coated pits, but only by passing through the nonclathrin/non-caveolar pathway do they exert their toxic effects on the cell. In the case of Shiga toxin, after being taken up within the nonclathrin/noncaveolar pathway, the toxin's A subunit is delivered to the Golgi apparatus and then to the ER, where it is translocated across the membrane bilayer into the cytoplasm. In the cytoplasm, the A subunit binds to the ribosome, disrupting protein translocation.

The Endosomal Compartment and the Endocytic Pathway

Endocytic transport intermediates, formed by clathrin-dependent or clathrin-independent mechanisms, fuse with and deliver their cargo to the endosomal compartment. Like the TGN in the biosynthetic pathway, endosomes are the major sorting compartments along the endocytic pathway toward lysosomes. Consistent with their sorting function, endosomes are structurally pleiomorphic and consist of a collection of vesicles, vacuoles, tubules, and multivesicular bodies.

In clathrin-mediated endocytosis, four classes of endosomes are distinguished based on the kinetics with which they accumulate endocytic tracers, their morphology, localization within the cell, and the presence of specific marker proteins (Fig. 22-12). Newly internalized proteins are first delivered to so-called **early endosomes,** which lie near the plasma membrane and appear as an anastomosing network of tubules and vacuoles. Receptors returning to the cell surface accumulate in so-called **recycling endosomes,** which are tubular portions of early endosomes located in the perinuclear Golgi region of the cell. Vacuolar structures or endosome carrier vesicles detach from the early endosomes and gradually acquire internal membrane vesicles. These so-called **multivesicular bodies** mature into **late endosomes** (Fig. 22-13). Late endosomes ultimately fuse with **lysosomes** (discussed in Chapter 23), whose acid hydrolases degrade internalized cargo.

The relationship among these four endosomal compartments is complex. Rather than each representing a distinct, stable organelle, the endosomal compartments exist as particular stages of a continuum in the sorting of endocytic cargo. Each compartment utilizes specific sorting mechanisms to separate cargo, receptors, and lipids for trafficking into different routes. These sorting mechanisms are linked to membrane differentiation events that allow particular compartments to fuse together, move apart, extend tubules, form invaginated intraluminal vesicles, or remain as vacuolar structures. The endosomal compartments are constantly being remodeled according to variations in the quan-

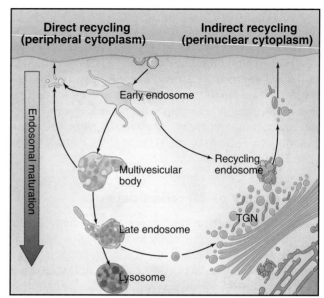

Figure 22-13 MEMBRANE TRAFFIC ALONG THE ENDOCYTIC PATHWAY. Cargo and membrane taken up by clathrin-mediated endocytosis are delivered to tubulovesicular early endosomes, which are mildly acidic. Most of the membrane, together with receptors, is recycled either by a rapid, direct route or by a slower, indirect route through perinuclear recycling endosomes. Ligands released from their receptors in the low pH environment accumulate in the vacuolar portions of early endosomes. During maturation, which involves the accumulation of internal membranes, continued recycling of receptors to the plasma membrane and TGN, delivery of newly synthesized lysosomal hydrolases from the TGN, and acquisition of targeting and fusion machinery, the late endosome prepares for fusion with lysosomes.

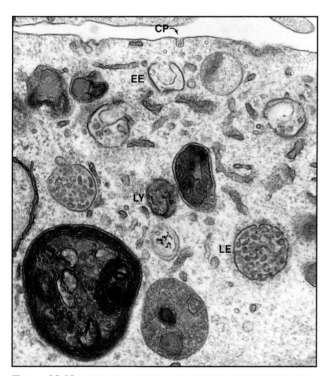

Figure 22-12 ELECTRON MICROGRAPH SHOWING INTERNALIZED GOLD-CONJUGATED PROTEIN BEING TRANSPORTED THROUGH THE STRUCTURALLY DIVERSE ORGANELLES OF THE ENDOSOMAL COMPARTMENT. The artificial gradient of colors reflects the maturation of early endosomes (EE) to late endosomes (LE) and lysosomes (LY). Gold particles *(tiny black dots)* are first delivered to early or sorting endosomes *(yellow)* that have both tubular and vacuolar regions and few intralumenal membranes. Tubular portions are recycled to the plasma membrane, whereas vacuolar portions undergo maturation. Late endosomes *(light brown)* are vacuolar and contain increasing amounts of intralumenal membrane. Lysosomes *(dark brown)* are very dense organelles, packed with internal vesicles and membrane whorls. CP, coated pit. (Courtesy of Mark Marsh, University College, London.)

tity and type of receptors and cargoes that traffic through them.

The Early Endosomal Compartment

Early endosomes are the first to receive the membrane proteins and lipids that enter the endosomal system through clathrin-mediated endocytosis. With bulk plasma membrane internalized at rates as high as 2% per minute and nutrient receptors internalized at rates exceeding 20% per minute, the amount of protein and lipid entering the early endosomal compartment is enormous. Remarkably, the majority of this internalized material (approximately 90% of internalized protein and lipid and 60% to 70% of all internalized fluid) is rapidly recycled to the cell surface from early endosomes.

The ability of early endosomes to sort proteins and lipids depends on the following features. First, early endosomal membranes readily fuse together, move apart, and extend/detach long membrane tubules that fuse with the plasma membrane.

Second, the geometry of the early endosome can affect protein and lipid sorting. Soluble ligands accumu-

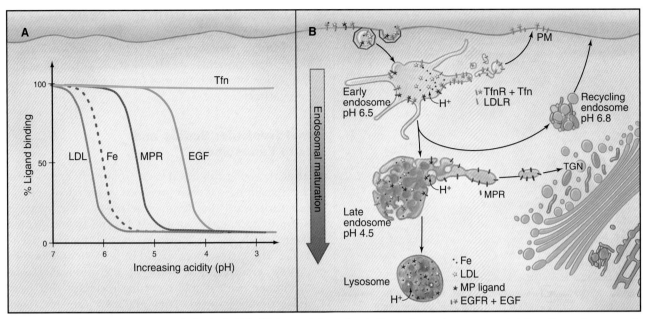

Figure 22-14 Progressive decrease in luminal pH facilitates protein sorting in the endosomal compartment. Interactions of many cargo molecules with their receptors are pH dependent **(B)**; dissociation places ligands in the luminal space, whereas receptors remain associated with membrane. Geometric considerations, as well as sorting motifs on the receptors, facilitate sorting of membrane from internal contents. Unoccupied receptors whose ligands, such as LDL, have dissociated under the relatively mild acidic conditions that are encountered in early endosomes are efficiently recycled back to the cell surface. Iron carried by transferrin (Tfn) dissociates at a pH of approximately 6, but apoTfn (transferrin without bound iron) remains bound to and recycles with its receptor. Mannose-6-phosphate receptors (MPRs) carry their ligands to late endosomes before dissociation at lower pH and recycling back to the TGN. EGF remains bound, and both ligand and receptor (EGFR) are delivered to and degraded in lysosomes. (PM, plasma membrane.) These differences in extents of ligand binding at different pH lead to a pH "signature" of each ligand-receptor system in ligand binding assays **(A),** reflecting the itinerary of the ligand within the endosomal system.

late in the volume-rich vacuolar portions of the early endosome, whereas receptors accumulate in the membrane-rich tubular portions. Tubules may recycle their content directly back to the plasma membrane or later through the recycling endosome, or they may carry their content back to the TGN, depending on when they detach from the endosomal membrane. Vacuolar portions of the early endosome undergo directed maturation first into a multivesicular body and then into a late endosome before eventually fusing with lysosomes where their contents are degraded.

A third feature of early endosomes that facilitates protein sorting is the presence of V-type proton pumps (see Fig. 8-5) in the membrane. This **vacuolar ATPase** lowers the luminal pH progressively along the endocytic pathway from approximately pH 6.5 in early endosomes to approximately pH 5.0 in late endosomes (Fig. 22-14). The interaction of many ligands with their sorting receptors is sensitive to pH. When receptor-ligand complexes reach their threshold pH for dissociation, the ligands are released into the lumen of the endosome and are carried in the vacuolar portion of the endosome toward lysosomes, while the receptors remain membrane-bound and are returned in tubules to the plasma membrane (Fig. 22-14). The pH gradient thus facilitates membrane

sorting within the endosomal system by providing spatial and temporal control over dissociation of ligand-receptor complexes and cargo degradation.

A fourth feature that influences early endosome sorting is the oligomerization or aggregation of transmembrane proteins (e.g., receptors). For example, monomeric Fc receptors recycle from endosomes to the plasma membrane, but Fc receptors cross-linked by binding antigen-antibody complexes on the cell surface are targeted from endosomes to lysosomes for degradation. Processing of internalized EGF receptors (see Fig. 27-6) is another example. The binding of EGF causes receptors to dimerize, followed by addition of a single ubiquitin (see Fig. 23-7). After internalization, EGF does not dissociate until the pH is less than 5.0, so the EGF–EGF receptor complex is targeted for degradation in lysosomes. This process, termed *downregulation* (see Fig. 23-2), is one of the negative feedback loops that allow cells to adapt to continuous stimulation (see Fig. 27-6).

In addition to these features, early endosomes exhibit a "mosaic" of specialized membrane domains that serves to orchestrate membrane fusion, tubulation, and invagination within this compartment (Fig. 22-15). The differentiated domains of lipids, protein-lipid, and

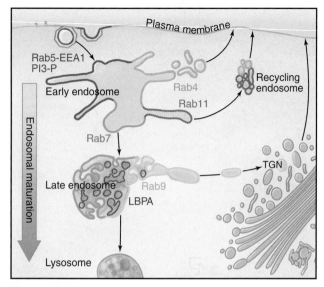

Figure 22-15 DOMAIN ORGANIZATION IN THE ENDOCYTIC PATHWAY. Subregions of endosomal membranes contain specific Rabs and Rab effectors (depicted in different colors). These subregions maintain their organization by the localized production of PIs, which recruit Rab-binding proteins such as EEA1. The domains allow the endosomal system to perform distinct functions. LBPA, lysobisphosphatidic acid.

protein-protein complexes on the early endosome are dynamically maintained. Localized production of PI(3)P by PI(3)-kinase on early endosomal membranes contributes to the formation of these domains. PI(3)P recruits the **early endosome antigen 1 (EEA1)** and then **Rab5** and its effectors, which together serve to organize the early endosome membrane.

EEA1 is a tethering factor in the early endosomal membrane. Homodimers of EEA1 have Rab5-binding sites at both ends of a long coiled-coil and a **FYVE-domain** to bind PI(3)P at the one end. This allows EEA1 to tether two Rab5-positive membranes, such as two early endosomes or an endocytic vesicle and early endosome. Rab5 recruits SNARE machinery (e.g., syntaxin 13 and NSF; see Fig. 21-12) to membranes forming dynamic oligomeric complexes that promote homotypic and heterotypic fusions of early endosomes. Inhibiting PI(3)-kinase with the drug wortmannin prevents the formation of such fusion assemblies, since PI(3)P is required to recruit EEA1. The absence of PI(3)P precludes fusion among early endosomes.

The binding of Rab5 effectors to early endosomes and the presence of Rab5 exchange factors in the effector complexes establishes a positive-feedback loop that amplifies the recruitment and the activation of Rab5 GTPases in specific regions of early endosomes. This feedback allows the generation and maintenance of domains that contain Rab5-EEA1-PI(3)P in early endosomes. Other Rabs are thought to operate in a similar

fashion in the endosomal system, with Rab4 and Rab11 in early/recycling endosomes and Rab7 and Rab9 in late endosomes (Fig. 22-15). Like Rab5, these other Rab proteins are thought to organize membrane domains with distinct functions within a single compartment.

Multivesicular Bodies and Late Endosomes

After recycling tubules detach from early endosomes, the remaining vacuolar portions move along microtubules toward the perinuclear region. The vacuoles begin to accumulate small vesicles and tubules within their lumen by invagination of the limiting membrane. These structures, called **multivesicular bodies (MVB),** gradually lose most of the residual plasma membrane markers and recycling receptors that were inadvertently trapped. They gradually gain lysosomal hydrolases as vesicles are delivered from the TGN along the biosynthetic pathway. Late in this maturation process, multivesicular bodies have a highly complex, intralumenal membrane system, and receptors are segregated into limiting or internal membranes. At this stage, they are called **late endosomes.** Late endosomes sort specific proteins and lipids to the TGN and back to the plasma membrane before fusing directly with lysosomes.

MVB formation begins on the vacuolar portions of early endosomal membranes by invagination of receptors destined for late endosomes or lysosomes (Fig. 22-16; see Fig. 23-2). Many downregulated receptors are ubiquitinated, and this modification is responsible for sorting of these receptors into newly forming MVBs through the action of **HRS (hepatocyte-growth-factor-regulated tyrosine kinase substrate)** and **ESCRT-I, -II, and -III (endosomal sorting complexes required for transport-I, -II, and -III).** When ubiquitinated receptors arrive in early endosomes, they bind HRS, which is retained at the membrane through its association with PI(3)P. Through interactions with clathrin, HRS sorts ubiquitinated receptors into clathrin-coated domains that form on new MVBs. These domains do not form clathrin-coated vesicles but instead sort ubiquitinated membrane proteins for transfer to ESCRT-1. Sequential transfer to ESCRT-II and -III on the cytoplasmic surface of the MVB drives both receptor incorporation into the membrane invaginations and invagination of the membrane itself. Wortmannin (the phosphatidylinositol 3-kinase inhibitor) inhibits the formation of intralumenal vesicles in MVBs.

Interestingly, ESCRT-1 is also involved in retrovirus budding at the plasma membrane (e.g., **Ebola and human immunodeficiency virus (HIV)),** a process that is topologically equivalent to membrane invagina-

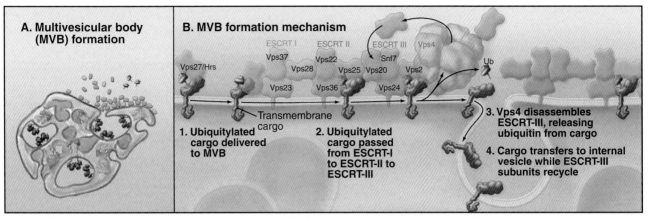

Figure 22-16   **A,** Protein sorting into multivesicular bodies. Ubiquitin on internalized membrane cargo proteins results in their being retained in Hrs- and clathrin-containing domains of the endosome membrane. Through the action of ESCRT-I, -II, and -III, the membrane proteins are sorted to intraluminal vesicles and targeted via MVBs for lysosomal degradation. **B,** Protein complexes involved in multivesicular body sorting and formation. A group of at least seven proteins are involved in MVE sorting and formation. The lipid PI(3)P mediates the localization of Hrs/Vps27 and its associated proteins, Eps15, STAM, and clathrin to endosomal membranes. The complex of Hrs, Eps15, and STAM binds to a ubiquitinated receptor and retains it in the endosomal membrane. The ubiquitinated receptor is then delivered to ESCRT-1 by an interaction between Hrs and the Vps23 subunit of ESCRT-1. The receptor is then relayed to ESCRT-II and then to ESCRT-III. Invagination of an intralumenal vesicle containing the receptor is mediated through polymerization of ESCRT-III complexes, which are small, highly charged coiled-coil proteins. A homomultimeric ATPase, Vps4, disassembles the multimeric ESCRT subunits, allowing them to be reutilized.

tion occurring in MVBs. This occurs because HIV Gag protein highjacks the ESCRT-1 complex by mimicking the binding activity of HRS.

In most cells, proteins destined for degradation are sorted into the intralumenal vesicles of the MVB. The MVB then matures into a late endosome, by fusion with preexisting lysosomes. However, under certain conditions, MVBs can fuse with the plasma membrane, releasing the intralumenal vesicles, termed **exosomes,** outside the cell. Exosomes have regulatory functions in the immune system. For example, antigen-presenting cells such as B-lymphocytes and dendritic cells secrete exosomes during exocytic fusion of MHC class II compartments with the plasma membrane. The released exosomes can stimulate proliferation of T-lymphocytes. Exosomes might also represent a novel method of intercellular communication. For example, **HIV particles** found in exosomes could represent a type of "Trojan horse" capable of transmitting the **HIV virus** on being taken up by other cells.

Late endosomes are structurally distinct from MVBs in being pleiomorphic, with cisternal, tubular, and multivesicular regions. Their protein/lipid composition is also distinct from MVBs in containing large amounts of lysosomal glycoproteins (in particular, **lysosome-associated membrane proteins Lamp1 and Lamp2**), which are very abundant in both late endosomes and lysosomes. In addition, late endosomes contain large amounts of **lysobisphosphatidic acid** (Fig. 22-15) that prefers to be in a hexagonal phase. This lipid structure

can promote positive or negative bilayer curvatures that are important for invagination and intralumenal vesicle formation. Interestingly, whereas Lamps are restricted to the limiting membranes of multivesicular, late endosomal elements, lysobisphosphatidic acid is enriched in their internal membranes.

In contrast to MVBs, which function primarily as an intermediate in late endosomes/lysosome delivery, late endosomes function as an important sorting station to the TGN and back to the plasma membrane (Fig. 22-15). The elaborate structure of late endosomes serves as a final station for determining which membrane constituents in the endocytic pathway will be degraded and which will be recycled. Among the proteins that are recycled from late endosomes to the TGN and back to the plasma membrane are acid hydrolase receptors (e.g., mannose 6-phosphate receptors) and transmembrane enzymes involved in the proteolytic processing of precursor proteins (e.g., the dibasic endopeptidase furin and carboxypeptidase D). Transport from late endosomes to TGN is thought to involve budding of membrane-enclosed carriers from late endosomes followed by fusion with the TGN. Genetic and biochemical analyses of this process has revealed an important role of **retromer,** a complex composed of five proteins that include members of the **sorting nexin** family of proteins. Mutations in any of the retromer proteins prevent acid hydrolase receptors from being retrieved to the TGN and result in secretion of acid hydrolases at the plasma membrane.

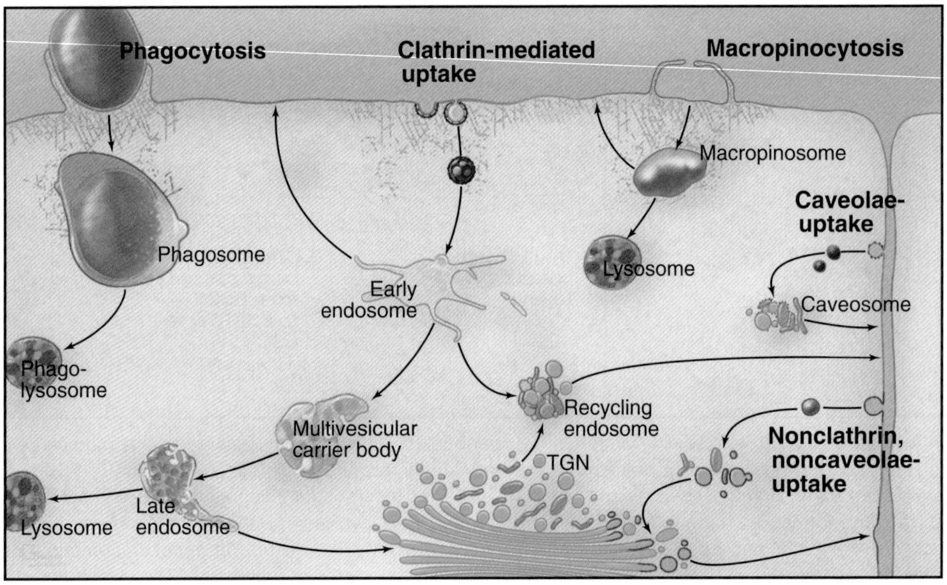

Figure 22-17 THE PATHWAYS FOLLOWED BY MOLECULES TAKEN UP BY DIFFERENT ENDOCYTIC MECHANISMS. *Arrows* depict the various routes followed by membrane-bound and soluble cargo molecules after uptake by each endocytic mechanism.

Other Endocytic Compartments and Pathways

Endocytic cargo and membrane taken up by phagocytosis, macropinocytosis, caveolae, and nonclathrin/noncaveolar pathways can follow distinct itineraries from that taken up by clathrin-mediated endocytosis (Fig. 22-17). For example, cargo molecules that are taken up into phagosomes during phagocytosis or into macropinosomes during macropinocytosis do not pass through multivesicular bodies or late endosomes. Instead, they remain within the phagosome or macropinosome as these structures mature into and/or fuse with lysosomes. Caveosomes that are formed during caveolae-mediated uptake do not mature into or fuse with lysosomes but serve as a conduit for movement of molecules to other regions of the plasma membrane. Nonclathrin, noncaveolar endocytotic structures also do not mature into multivesicular bodies or lysosomes. They traffic back to the TGN to resupply the Golgi with glycosphingolipids.

Viruses and Protein Toxins as "Opportunistic Endocytic Ligands"

The threat of infectious diseases throughout the world has made research on the survival tactics of intracellular pathogens and cellular defenses against them particularly crucial. Many enveloped viruses (i.e., those with a membrane bilayer) enter cells by catching a ride on membrane proteins capable of endocytosis. Once inside an endosome, specific viral membrane proteins undergo pH-dependent conformational changes that promote their insertion into and fusion with the organelle membrane. This places the viral nucleocapsid in the cytoplasm, where it has access to the cell's synthetic machinery, which it uses to replicate itself (Fig. 22-18).

Both bacteria and plants secrete protein toxins that kill animal cells efficiently by inhibiting cytoplasmic functions, such as protein translation. Some of these toxins bind to cell surface "receptors" (either integral proteins or glycolipids) via their B-chains; the toxins are endocytosed, and then the enzymatically active "A subunit" escapes into the cytoplasm (Fig. 22-18). Despite their structural similarities, various toxins enter the cytoplasm from different intracellular compartments, because their requirements for translocation differ. When pH is the trigger, toxins can be translocated directly across the endosomal membrane. Other toxins travel back to the endoplasmic reticulum and use the cell's translocation machinery in reverse to enter the cytoplasm.

Both clinicians and basic researchers benefit by studying these self-selected "hitchhikers." From them, much can be learned about which properties, sequences, and motifs to look for in endogenous, fusogenic proteins. Learning about something as esoteric as the action of a plant toxin can also have medical benefits, as in the treatment of cancer through coupling of the catalytic (A) subunits of toxins to antibodies and targeting of the toxic subunit to malignant cells. These chimeric proteins are called **immunotoxins.** Viruses have evolved efficient mechanisms for delivering their genome into host cells, so viruses are currently the leading candidates for therapeutic delivery of genes.

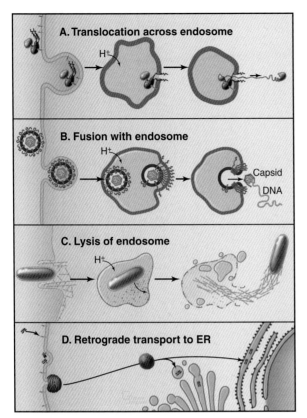

Figure 22-18 VIRUSES AND TOXINS HAVE SEVERAL MEANS TO GAIN ENTRY INTO THE CELL. Many viruses and toxins bind to cell surface receptors that are efficiently internalized. **A,** Once in endosomes, pH-dependent conformational changes can trigger the translocation of toxin subunits across the endosomal membrane into the cytoplasm. **B,** pH-dependent conformational changes can activate fusogenic viral coat proteins to mediate fusion of the viral envelope with the endosomal membrane releasing the nucleocapsid into the cytoplasm. **C,** Some bacteria secrete toxins after entering the endosome/phagosome; these intercalate into the membrane, creating large pores that disrupt endosomal compartments. Once in the cytoplasm, the bacterium can usurp the cell's actin *(yellow filaments)* assembly machinery for propulsion. (See Fig. 37-12.) **D,** Some toxins enter through alternative endocytic pathways (e.g., through caveolae) and are transported in a retrograde manner back to the endoplasmic reticulum (ER), where they can utilize the cell's translocation machinery—in reverse—to enter the cytoplasm.

ACKNOWLEDGMENTS

Thanks go to Harald Stenmark, Ben Nichols, Sandra Schmid, and Julie Donaldson for their suggestions on revisions to this chapter.

SELECTED READINGS

Connor SD, Schmid SL: Regulated portals of entry into the cell. Nature 422:37–44, 2003.

Finlay BB, Cossart P: Exploitation of mammalian host functions by bacterial pathogens. Science 276:718–725, 1997.

Gruenberg J, Stenmark H: The biogenesis of multivesicular endosomes. Nat Rev Mol Cell Biol 5:317–323, 2004.

Ikonen E: Roles of lipid rafts in membrane transport. Curr Opin Cell Biol 13:470–477, 2001.

Katzmann DJ, Odorizzi G, Emr SD: Receptor downregulation and multivesicular-body sorting. Nat Rev Mol Cell Biol 3:893–904, 2002.

Kirchhausen T: Clathrin. Annu Rev Biochem 69:699–727, 2000.

Lemmo SK, Traub LM: Sorting in the endosomal system in yeast and animal cells. Curr Opin Cell Biol 12:457–466, 2000.

Lindmo K, Stenmark H: Regulation of membrane traffic by phosphoinositide 3-kinases. J Cell Sci 119:605–614, 2005.

May RC, Machesky LM: Phagocytosis and the actin cytoskeleton. J Cell Sci 114:1061–1077, 2001.

McMahon HT, Gallop JL: Membrane curvature and mechanisms of dynamic cell membrane remodeling. Nature 438:590–596, 2005.

Meresse S, Steele-Mortimer O, Moreno E, et al: Controlling the maturation of pathogen-containing vacuoles: A matter of life and death. Nat Cell Biol 1:E183–E188, 1999.

Miaczynska M, Zerial M: Mosaic organization of the endocytic pathway. Exp Cell Res 272:8–14, 2002.

Mukherjee S, Maxfield FR: Role of membrane organization and membrane domains in endocytic lipid trafficking. Traffic 1:203–211, 2000.

Nichols BJ, Lippincott-Schwartz J: Endocytosis without clathrin coats. Trends Cell Biol 11:406–412. 2001.

Owen DJ, Collins BM, Evans PR: Adaptors for clathrin coats: Structure and function. Ann Rev Cell Dev Biol 20:153–191, 2004.

Pelkmans L, Helenius A: Endocytosis via caveolae. Traffic 3:311–320, 2002.

Piper RC, Luzio JP: Late endosomes: Sorting and partitioning in multivesicular bodies. Traffic 2:612–621, 2001.

Raiborg C, Rusten TR, Stenmark H: Protein sorting into multivesicular endosomes. Curr Opin Cell Biol 15:446–455, 2003.

Simonsen A, Wurmser AE, Emr SD, Stenmark H: The role of phosphoinositides in membrane transport. Curr Opin Cell Biol 13:485–492, 2001.

Degradation of Cellular Components

An individual cell can live for weeks, months, years, or even the entire lifetime of the organism, but the cell's constituent proteins, lipids, and RNA turn over continuously. This process of molecular degradation and replacement serves three functions. Constitutive turnover is a "housekeeping" function that ensures regular replacement of older molecules with newly synthesized ones or that removes misfolded, mislocalized, or otherwise damaged molecules so that they do not hinder the function of native molecules. Regulated or induced turnover results in rapid degradation of specific target molecules and functions in signal transduction, regulation of the cell cycle, and remodeling of cells and tissues during development. Finally, macroautophagy, a more global mechanism for degradation of cellular proteins or lipids, can be triggered under conditions of starvation, when the cell perceives a shortage of specific raw materials, such as amino acids. This chapter focuses primarily on the mechanisms that govern protein degradation and turnover, as these are the best studied; lipid turnover is also discussed. Chapter 16 covers RNA turnover.

Characteristics of Constitutive Protein Turnover

The turnover of cellular constituents at steady state arises from a careful balance of the rates of synthesis and degradation. Turnover can be massive. For example, approximately 40% of total cellular protein in rat liver is degraded every day. The rates of transcription and translation determine the rate of synthesis of each protein. Once synthesized, each type of protein turns over at a characteristic rate. Degradation is random, so older molecules are not selected over younger ones. The time course of degradation of the population of any specific protein follows a single exponential—strong evidence that chance, rather than aging, determines which copies of the protein are degraded (see Fig. 4-1 for first-order reactions). The rate is usually expressed as a half-life, the time for half of the molecules to be degraded.

The intrinsic rate of degradation of a given protein is determined by many factors, including its size, overall charge, thermal instability, flexibility, hydrophobicity, folding, and assembly with other protein subunits (if it is multimeric). Long-lived proteins have

This chapter was revised using material from the first edition written by Sandra L. Schmid, Ann L. Hubbard, J. David Castle, and Pat Shipman.

half-lives measured in days, while short-lived proteins have half-lives of hours or minutes. Small, basic proteins tend to have longer half-lives than do large, acidic proteins, and key enzymes of metabolic pathways often have very short half-lives. A protein may have specific sequences or structural motifs that are recognized by the proteolytic machinery. Phosphorylation marks some proteins for destruction. The rate at which a protein is degraded can be altered either by increasing the activity of its degradative pathway or by exposure or creation of "degradation motifs" on the protein to initiate destruction.

Proteolysis: A Compartmentalized Process

Unregulated proteolysis within a cell would be lethal. Therefore, cells compartmentalize intracellular proteolytic activity in two distinct ways so that access is denied to all but appropriate substrates. **Lysosomes** are membrane-bound compartments that sequester various hydrolases, including **proteases,** and provide a low pH environment in which these enzymes are optimally active. **Proteasomes** are proteolytic machines assembled from multiple protein subunits with the proteolytically active sites corraled inside on the walls of a small cylindrical chamber. The narrow internal diameter of the cylinder and regulatory complexes that guard the openings allow access only to selected polypeptide chains, which must be unfolded to enter.

Intracellular proteolysis depends on specific recognition of protein substrates and their translocation into a proteolytic compartment. Generally speaking, long-lived cytosolic proteins and integral membrane proteins circulating within the secretory and endosomal systems are degraded by lysosomes, whereas short-lived cytoplasmic proteins and ER membrane proteins are degraded by the proteasome. The small protein **ubiquitin** targets most (though not all) molecules for degradation by proteasomes and can also target proteins for degradation by lysosomes. Ubiquitin or a polyubiquitin chain is added posttranslationally to lysine residues on protein substrates and is recognized by the cellular machinery that targets them for proteolysis. These processes are tightly regulated. Energy in the form of adenosine triphosphate (ATP) is required for degradation of proteins, even though hydrolysis of a peptide bond actually releases energy.

Degradation in Lysosomes

Lysosomes, the major digestive organelles, contain at least 60 distinct hydrolytic enzymes, including proteases, lipases, phospholipases, glycosidases, and nucleases. Lysosomal hydrolases are tagged in the Golgi apparatus with mannose-6-phosphate groups on their

N-linked oligosaccharides. **Mannose-6-phosphate receptors** in the *trans*-Golgi network bind lysosomal hydrolases for diversion to **endosomes** and lysosomes (see Chapter 22). Most lysosomal hydrolases are synthesized as inactive precursors and are activated by proteolysis on arrival in lysosomes. The low pH of lysosomes, maintained by the vacuolar adenosine triphosphatase (ATPase) proton pump (see Fig. 8-5C), is essential for efficient degradation. Most lysosomal enzymes have maximal hydrolytic activity at pH 4 to 5 rather than at the cytoplasmic pH of 6.5 to 7.0. Moreover, the low pH helps to denature many proteins, increasing their susceptibility to degradation. It is important to note that the hydrolases themselves are more resistant than are most macromolecules to the harsh environment. Lysosomal enzymes degrade proteins, lipids, and nucleic acids to fragments that are small enough to be transported either actively or passively across the lysosomal membrane to the cytoplasm, where they are reused to synthesize new macromolecules.

Lysosomes degrade substrates that originate both outside and inside the cell. Extracellular substrates taken into the cell by endocytosis are delivered to lysosomes via the endocytic pathway (see Chapter 22). Lysosomes also degrade cellular constituents, accounting for 50% to 70% of cellular protein turnover. Substrates are delivered to lysosomes by endocytosis and by direct translocation from the cytoplasm. Degradation of intracellular substrates is generally termed **autophagy,** which occurs by three distinct mechanisms called **crinophagy, macroautophagy,** and **microautophagy,** which are described later.

The essential role of lysosomes as the primary site for constitutive degradation is revealed by the more than 30 distinct human lysosomal storage diseases (Appendix 23-1). Patients with these diseases lack the function of one or more lysosomal hydrolases. Consequently, undigested material accumulates in lysosomes and causes them to swell (Fig. 23-1), ultimately killing the cell.

Delivery to Lysosomes via the Endocytic Pathway

Lysosomal degradation of plasma membrane proteins internalized by endocytosis plays an important role in remodeling the plasma membrane in response to cell stimuli. For example, the half-life of the receptor for the epidermal growth factor (EGF) is normally approximately 10 hours. However, when circulating EGF binds, the activated receptor is more efficiently internalized and degraded in lysosomes with a half-time of less than 1 hour. This downregulates the biological response (see Fig. 27-6).

The degradation of lipids and membrane proteins in lysosomes poses a topologic problem, since fusion of lysosomes with other membrane compartments would

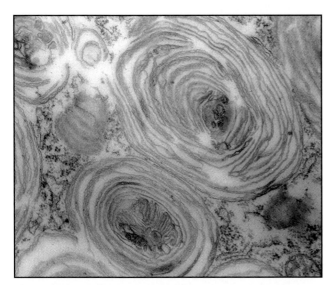

Figure 23-1 ELECTRON MICROGRAPH OF ABNORMAL LYSOSOMES IN THE NEURONS OF A PATIENT WITH GM$_1$ GANGLIOSIDOSIS. Similar lysosomes, called membranous cytoplasmic bodies, accumulate in the neurons of patients with GM$_2$ gangliosidosis (Tay-Sachs disease). (Courtesy of Kinuko Suzuki, University of North Carolina, Chapel Hill.)

simply merge the two membranes. This problem is solved by segregating the components to be degraded into regions of membrane that bud into endosomes, forming the intraluminal vesicles or tubules of **multivesicular** bodies (see Fig. 22-16). Fusion of a multivesicular body with a lysosome delivers the intraluminal vesicles to the lumen of the lysosome for digestion (Fig. 23-2). Resident lysosomal membrane proteins remain in the limiting membrane.

The formation of multivesicular bodies starts with a sorting process in endosomes (see Chapter 22). Proteins that are destined for degradation are tagged with single ubiquitin molecules, a process that is distinct from the polyubiquitination reaction required for targeting to proteasomes (see later). These monoubiquitinated proteins are gathered together in endosomes by ubiquitin-binding proteins that are localized there by interaction with phosphatidylinositol-3-phosphate (PI3-P), formed by PI3-kinase (see Fig. 26-7). A sequence of three multiprotein ESCRT complexes (endosomal complex required for transport [Fig. 22-16]) then further

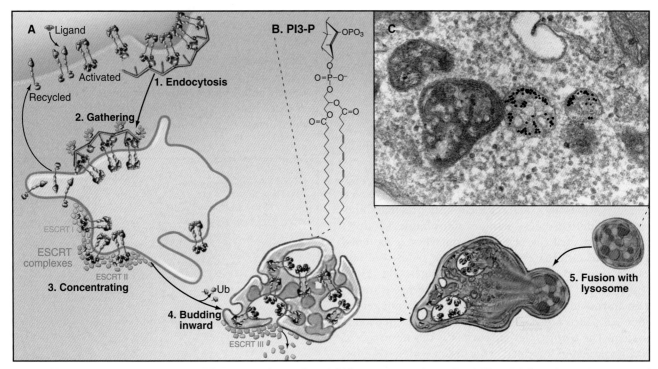

Figure 23-2 To limit the time course of EGF stimulation, activated EGF receptors are internalized **(A)** and delivered to endosomes and sequestered **(B)** with other membrane proteins to be destroyed within internal membrane vesicles that accumulate in late endosomes. Proteins destined for internalization and destruction are marked with single ubiquitin molecules, which are recycled prior to budding into the multivesicular body interior. Invagination of the late endosomal membrane is driven by the three ESCRT complexes and may involve production of the lipid species PI3-P by the enzyme PI3-kinase, which is activated by EGF receptors. After fusion with lysosomes, lysosomal proteases and lipases ensure that both the extracellular and cytoplasmic domains of the EGF receptor are degraded, a process termed receptor downregulation. Cytosolic proteins are also incorporated into the internal vesicles of multivesicular late endosomes and are degraded in a constitutive process termed microautophagy. **C,** EM of gold-labeled EGF receptor in multivesicular endosomes fusing with a lysosome. (C, Courtesy of Colin Hopkins, MRC Laboratory, University College, London, England.)

concentrates the monoubiquitinated proteins on regions of membrane that bud into the vesicle interior by an unknown mechanism. Components of the ESCRT complexes initially bind monoubiquitin but later recruit enzymes that remove and recycle the ubiquitin. Interestingly, budding of a number of viruses, including HIV-1, the virus that causes AIDS, resembles the process of multivesicular body formation. In fact, HIV hijacks two of the ESCRT complexes for this purpose.

Autophagy

Microautophagy and macroautophagy both describe the consumption of cytoplasmic constituents within lysosomes. Microautophagy occurs as a by-product of the formation of multivesicular bodies (Fig. 23-2; also see Fig. 22-16). Small volumes of cytoplasm are captured in the intraluminal vesicles and tubules that invaginate within endosomal or lysosomal membranes. The cytoplasmic components are degraded as the vesicles are consumed. However, studies in yeast suggest the existence of alternative pathways for the selective packaging and delivery of cytosolic proteins to lysosomes. When starved for glucose, *Saccharomyces cerevisiae* expresses several cytosolic enzymes and membrane transporters that are required to process more complex sugars. When glucose becomes available, the yeast switches metabolic pathways and degrades the enzymes it no longer needs. Transporters in the plasma membrane are internalized and delivered to the vacuole (the yeast lysosome equivalent) through the formation of multivesicular bodies and microautophagy. Unneeded cytoplasmic enzymes are selectively packaged into small vesicles that deliver their contents to the vacuole by fusion. Genetic studies of yeast are unraveling the mechanisms of these rapidly induced and selective degradation pathways.

Macroautophagy involves the engulfment of large regions of cytoplasm—that might include glycogen granules, ribosomes, and organelles, such as mitochondria and peroxisomes—into an **autophagic vacuole.** Autophagic vacuoles begin to form when a flattened membrane cisterna encircles a region of cytosol and closes into a vesicle with two membranes (Fig. 23-3). The origin of the smooth membrane cisternae is uncertain and could be either the smooth endoplasmic reticulum (ER), the *trans*-Golgi apparatus, or the endosomal system. The *trans*-Golgi apparatus has the advantage of having targeting information for fusion with lysosomes. Fusion of a nascent autophagic vacuole with late endosomes and lysosomes forms an **autolysosome** with acid hydrolases in the lumen to degrade the contents (Figs. 23-3 and 23-4). The end stage of an autolysosome is typically a **residual body** with a dense core of undegraded material. The process of formation and degradation of autophagic vacuoles in the liver requires less than 15 minutes.

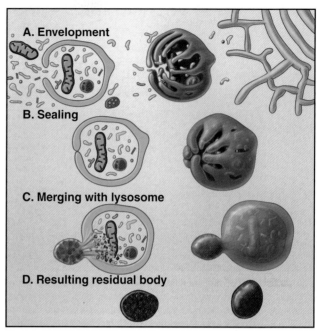

Figure 23-3 THE FOUR STAGES OF AUTOPHAGY. **A,** A membrane cisterna from an as-yet-undefined source envelops a large region of cytoplasm, including any organelles within this area. **B,** Membrane fusion results in formation of a nascent autophagosome. **C,** The nascent autophagosome fuses directly with a primary or secondary lysosome, which delivers hydrolytic enzymes that degrade the autophagosome contents. **D,** Undigested material remains in residual bodies.

Because large volumes of cytoplasm and entire organelles are destroyed, macroautophagy must be regulated precisely and directly. The intracellular signal that triggers macroautophagy is thought to be tied to the intracellular levels of particular amino acids, which are, in

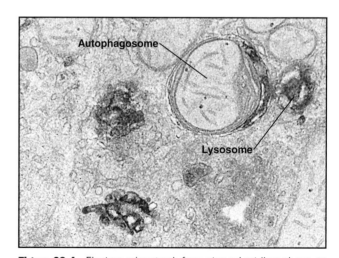

Figure 23-4 Electron micrograph from starved rat liver shows an autophagosome containing a mitochondrion that is fusing directly with a secondary lysosome. (Courtesy of William Dunn, University of Florida, Gainesville. Reproduced from Dunn WA Jr: Studies on the mechanisms of autophagy: Maturation of the autophagic vacuole. J Cell Biol 110:1935–1945, 1990, by copyright permission of The Rockefeller University Press.)

turn, related to the extracellular concentrations of these amino acids. Amino acids are potent inhibitors of autophagy. Circulating peptide hormones also regulate autophagy by binding receptors and activating signaling cascades that involve protein phosphorylation. For example, starvation increases the circulating levels of the hormone glucagon, which stimulates autophagy in liver cells. Feeding produces the opposite reaction by increasing the levels of insulin, which reduce autophagy. Diurnal feeding rhythms cause the numbers of autophagic vacuoles to vary along with the fluctuation of essential amino acids in the blood.

The mechanisms underlying autophagy are currently poorly understood. It is unclear how autophagosomal structures acquire membrane and how they target substrates. Genetic screens in budding yeast identified more than 15 gene products required for autophagosome formation and development. Two ubiquitin-like systems (Atg7 and Atg12) regulate the process by recruiting cytoplasmic autophagic components to target membranes. These reactions depend on enzymes that attach chains of the protein ubiquitin to proteins targeted for proteolysis (see later). This process and critical regulators of the pathway are conserved in higher eukaryotes.

Budding yeast use autophagy as a cell survival pathway during starvation, but autophagy can kill some cells. For example, autophagy can lead to death when a cell receives a lethal insult under conditions in which apoptotic pathways (see Chapter 46) are not functional. Whether autophagy is a physiological cell death pathway in addition to apoptosis remains controversial. Autophagy has also been implicated in the developmental programs of a number of higher organisms and in the destruction of intracellular protein aggregates.

Crinophagy

Fusion of lysosomes directly with secretory vesicles, a process known as crinophagy, results in the degradation of secretory proteins with a limited "shelf-life." This process is important in the anterior pituitary gland, which contains multiple types of regulated secretory cells that stockpile intracellular granules containing polypeptide hormones, such as prolactin. When suckling ends, and in response to an unknown signal, lysosomes fuse with granules to degrade the prolactin. Crinophagy might also function to remove aged granules that contain damaged proteins.

Selective Protein Uptake into Lysosomes

With prolonged starvation, autophagy diminishes, and a selective lysosomal degradative mechanism is initiated. This response perhaps reflects two competing needs: (1) the need to maintain critical levels of key cel-

lular proteins that might otherwise be destroyed through the nonselective process of autophagy and (2) the need to supply amino acids for the synthesis of essential proteins. The 20% to 30% of cytosolic proteins that are selected for degradation by this mechanism are normally long-lived and contain structural signals—in particular, the linear sequence KFPRQ—that are recognized by the molecular chaperone Hsc70, which escorts them to lysosomes. A lysosomal membrane glycoprotein might function as a receptor for these molecules, and a chaperone within lysosomes seems to be required for translocation across the lysosomal membrane. Although many questions remain to be answered, this process is important because it shows that soluble macromolecules can be transported selectively from the cytoplasm into lysosomes.

Degradation by Proteasomes

The proteasome is the second major cellular compartment for proteolysis. Proteasomes are multisubunit structures about half the size of a ribosome that are located in both the cytoplasm and nucleoplasm (Fig. 23-5). They are abundant, often accounting for up to 1% of total cellular protein. Proteasomes contain an array of proteolytic active sites arrayed on the interior wall of a cylindrical chamber. They degrade abnormal and misfolded proteins as well as selected normal proteins down to the level of small peptides (Fig. 23-6). Proteasomes degrade key substrates in response to signaling cascades or at key transitions of the cell cycle. One class of proteasomes processes intracellular antigens for presentation by the immune system.

The proteasome has two major structural components: the core and the cap. The core, referred to as the 20S proteasome (named according to its sedimentation coefficient; see Chapter 6) is structurally conserved from bacteria to mammals, although the subunit composition varies. In mammals, the cylindrical 20S core is assembled from two copies each of 14 different 25- to 35-kD subunits arranged into four seven-membered rings: α-type subunits form the top and bottom rings flanking the two rings of β-type subunits. Four constrictions divide the interior into three cavities: a central chamber surrounded by the β-subunits and two antechambers at either end of the cylinder (Fig. 23-5B). The proteolytic active sites on the β-subunits face the central chamber. An N-terminal threonine residue on the β-subunits is exposed by autocatalytic proteolysis and serves as the key active site residue for proteolysis. The antibiotic **lactacystin** reacts covalently and selectively with these threonine residues to inactivate the proteasome.

Eukaryotic proteasomes have multiple types of hydrolytic activities that can be ascribed to distinct β-type subunits (Fig. 23-6). In yeast and probably in

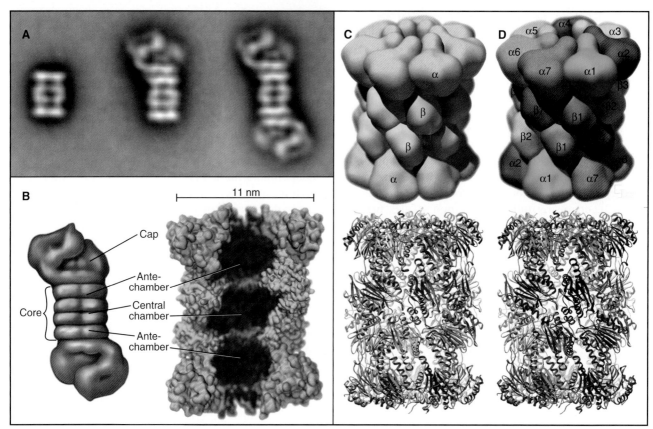

Figure 23-5 STRUCTURE OF THE PROTEASOME. **A,** Electron micrographs of negatively stained 20S proteasomes from bovine red blood cells alone *(left),* or singly *(middle),* or doubly *(right)* capped with PA700, the 19S regulator, to generate the 26S particle. These images were enhanced by computer processing. **B,** Model of the 26S proteasome compared with a space-filling model of the high-resolution crystal structure of the 20S particle on the right. The 20S proteasome, a cylinder 15 nm long and 11 nm in diameter, has a mass of about 700 kD. **C–D,** Ribbon diagrams and subunit compositions for the 20S proteasomes from *Thermoplasma acidophilum* **(C)** and from *S. cerevisiae* **(D).** Note the conservation of structure from Archaea to yeast to mammals. (A, Electron micrographs courtesy of Edward P. Gogol, University of Missouri, Kansas City. C, PDB file: 1PMA. Reference: Lowe J, Stock D, Jap B, et al: Crystal structure of the 20S proteasome from the archaeon T. acidophilum at 3.4 Å resolution. Science 268:533–539, 1995. D, PDB file: 1RYP. Reference: Groll M, Ditzel L, Lowe J, et al: Structure of 20S proteasome from yeast at 2.4 Å resolution. Nature 386:463–471, 1997.)

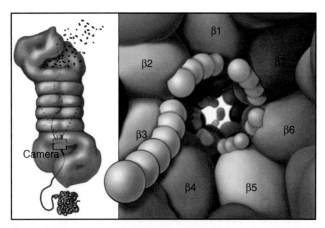

Figure 23-6 DRAWING OF A POLYPEPTIDE MOVING THROUGH THE CENTRAL CHANNEL OF THE 20S PARTICLE. Note that the distribution of protease sites varies with subunit composition, governing the size of the product peptides. Camera in *left panel* indicates the direction of view in the *right panel.*

mammalian proteasomes, the **caspase**-like activity of the β1-subunit cleaves after acidic residues, the trypsin-like activity of the β2-subunit cleaves after basic residues, and the chymotrypsin-like activity of the β5-subunit cleaves after hydrophobic residues (see Fig. 46-10 for a description of caspases). These three activities combine to give the proteasome broad specificity, allowing it to cleave diverse substrates into short peptides. Other β-type subunits in eukaryotic proteasomes are apparently not posttranslationally processed to mature, catalytically active enzymes. It was initially thought that the restricted length (seven to nine residues) of the final products of proteolysis reflected an "intrinsic molecular ruler," the length of which corresponded to the distance between active sites. However, mutagenesis to selectively inactivate individual β-subunits has no effect on product length, as would be predicted. Instead, the length of the peptides that are produced might be related to the kinetics of translocation of the unfolded substrate polypeptide through the proteasome.

The noncatalytic α-subunits are presumably involved in translocation of the substrate into the proteolytic chamber. The narrow dimensions of the chamber and constriction points limit access to unfolded polypeptide chains. The 20S proteasome degrades unfolded proteins into small peptides without hydrolyzing ATP. In cells, proteasome function requires ATP hydrolysis, presumably to unfold protein substrates.

The proteasomes of eukaryotes and Archaea are "capped" on one or both ends of the 20S barrel with regulatory complexes to form the 26S proteasome. The type of regulatory complex varies depending on the function of the proteasome. One such complex, called the 19S regulator or PA700, has a mass of approximately 700 kD (see Fig. 23-5A). Six of its subunits are members of the AAA ATPase family (see Box 36-1) and are believed to play a role in the dissociation of target protein oligomers, protein unfolding, and translocation into the central channels. Other subunits are involved in recognition of ubiquitinated proteins and in recycling ubiquitin from proteins destined for degradation (see the next section for more about ubiquitin).

A second regulator complex, the 11S cap or PA28 regulator, is associated with a subpopulation of 20S proteasome cores only in cells of higher vertebrates. This 20S/11S proteasome is induced by the cytokine **γ-interferon** as part of the immune response. This specialized **"immunoproteasome"** participates in ubiquitin-independent cleavage of intracellular antigens, such as those derived from an infecting virus, into peptides of uniform length for presentation on the cell surface of antigen-presenting cells (see Fig. 27-8). The 11S cap does not recognize ubiquitinated protein substrates and may be an adapter for the interaction of molecular chaperones with the immunoproteasome. Specialized catalytic β-subunits in the 20S core of the immunoproteasome generate somewhat longer peptides that are better suited for antigen presentation. The immunoproteasome is physically and functionally coupled to an **ABC transporter** (see Fig. 8-9) called the **TAP** (transporter associated with antigen presentation) that translocates peptides generated by the proteasome into the ER. Another integral membrane protein of the ER directly loads translocated peptides onto **class I major histocompatibility antigen I (MHC) molecules** for transport to the cell surface. On the cell surface, the MHC-peptide complex stimulates T-cells (see Fig. 27-8). To avoid detection by the immune system, some viruses commandeer this pathway and force the translocation of MHC molecules backward through TAP, out of the ER, and into the waiting jaws of the proteasome.

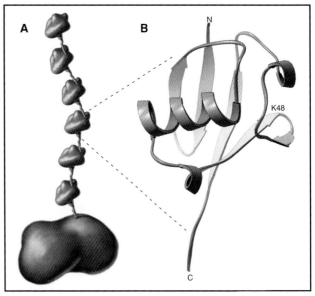

Figure 23-7 A polyubiquitin chain **(A)** is generated on a protein to target it for degradation in the proteasome by sequential conjugation of ubiquitin **(B),** shown in a ribbon diagram. With the C-terminal glycine and lycine (K48) indicated.

Ubiquitination Targets Proteins to Proteasomes

The key to regulating degradation by proteasomes is controlling access of molecules into the central proteolytic chamber. The best-characterized targeting mechanism involves the reversible, covalent linkage of a small protein, ubiquitin, onto the target protein. Ubiquitin is a very abundant and highly conserved protein of 76 residues. The C-terminal four amino acids extend from the compact globular structure, and its C-terminus is linked to target proteins (Fig. 23-7).

Ubiquitination directs the selective degradation of many different proteins: abnormally folded proteins; regulatory proteins, including some that control cell cycle progression; components of signal transduction systems; and regulators of transcription. Reversible ubiquitination is also involved in other cellular functions, such as the assembly of ribosomes, proteasomes, and other multimeric complexes, DNA repair, and chromosomal structure. Proteins with bound ubiquitin are directed to their various fates by interaction with proteins that contain ubiquitin-binding domains. Low-affinity interactions of ubiquitin-binding domains with ubiquitinated proteins allow the system a great degree of dynamic flexibility. Humans also have more than 80 deubiquitinating enzymes that remove ubiquitin from target proteins, thereby increasing the flexibility of ubiquitin-based signaling pathways. Disruption of the ubiquitination machinery is lethal in yeast.

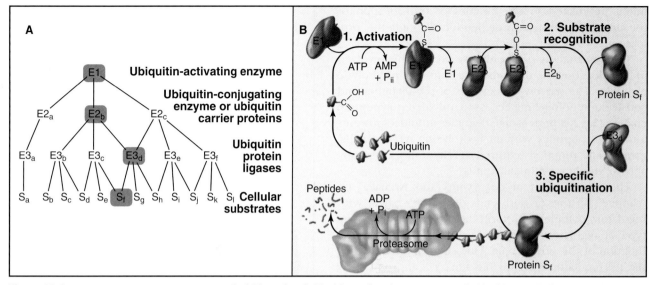

Figure 23-8   UBIQUITIN CONJUGATION MECHANISM. **A,** A hierarchy of ubiquitin-conjugating enzymes and ubiquitin protein ligases work together to recognize and ubiquitinate specific cellular substrates in a highly regulated manner. **B,** The three stages of ubiquitination for one representative set of enzymes. The common enzyme in each pathway is the ubiquitin-activating enzyme (E1). One of more than 40 (in human) E2 enzymes serves as an intermediate to transfer activated ubiquitin and works with one of more than 500 (in human) E3 enzymes to recognize the appropriate target protein (S_f) and to transfer the first ubiquitin molecule. Subsequent polyubiquitination targets the protein for degradation in the proteasome. ADP, adenosine diphosphate; AMP, adenosine monophosphate; P_{ii}, pyrophosphate.

Ubiquitination of protein substrates proceeds through a tightly regulated multistep pathway, which has been elucidated through biochemical purification of mammalian components and in vitro reconstitution of partial reactions. The overall scheme can be subdivided into three stages (Fig. 23-8):

- Activation of ubiquitin: The **ubiquitin-activating enzyme** E1 catalyzes the formation of a covalent thioester bond between the side chain of one of its own cysteine residues and the carboxyl group of the C-terminal glycine of ubiquitin. Humans have only a few E1 enzymes.

- Transfer of ubiquitin to an E2 enzyme: Activated ubiquitin is then transferred to a cysteine residue of an E2 or **ubiquitin-conjugating** (or carrier) **enzyme.** Humans have more than 40 E2 enzymes.

- Ubiquitination of target proteins: E3 **ubiquitin ligases** catalyze the transfer of ubiquitin from an E2-conjugate to the protein substrate, either directly or in two steps through an E3-ubiquitin intermediate. The ubiquitin C-terminus is usually attached to the target protein by an amide bond to the ε-amino group of a lysine residue or to the N-terminal amino group.

Humans have more than 500 E3 enzymes that confer specificity to the ubiquitination reaction. Many E3 enzymes contain a protein structural motif of 40 to 60 amino acids called a RING finger. This is a specialized type of Zn^{2+} finger (see Fig. 15-17) that mediates protein-protein interactions.

Additional ubiquitin molecules are then conjugated by an as yet unknown mechanism onto lysine 48 of the preceding ubiquitin to create a **polyubiquitin chain** (Figs. 23-7 and 23-8). In general, chains of four or more ubiquitins are sufficient for targeting to the proteasome. Subunits of the proteasome cap complete the cycle by deubiquitinating the substrates as they are fed into the proteolytic central chamber. The released ubiquitin is reutilized.

If polyubiquitin chains are assembled by linking ubiquitins between the C-terminal and lysine 63, rather than lysine 48, the modified protein is not targeted for destruction. Instead, this form of ubiquitination modulates other aspects of protein behavior. For example, such lysine 63–linked ubiquitin chains regulate the dynamic behavior of the chromosomal passenger protein Survivin at centromeres during mitosis (see Fig. 44-10) and are essential for normal chromosome segregation. Lysine 63–linked ubiquitin chains have also been implicated in signaling pathways, DNA repair, and vesicle trafficking.

In addition to ubiquitin, at least eight other highly conserved small proteins can be conjugated to ε-amino groups of lysine on target proteins. They are generally not involved in protein degradation and instead serve a variety of functions. The best known of these is called SUMO (small ubiquitin-like modifier). SUMO can be conjugated to the same residues on target proteins as ubiquitin, but it typically stabilizes the target protein rather than promoting degradation as ubiquitin does. The ubiquitin-like proteins are ligated to their targets by E1, E2, and E3 enzymes, which are distinct from those involved in conjugation of ubiquitin.

Motifs That Specify Ubiquitination

Tight regulation of ubiquitination pathways ensures that only the appropriate target proteins are recognized, ubiquitinated, and consequently degraded. The primary responsibility for substrate selectivity lies with the E3 family of enzymes. These ubiquitin ligases can bind directly to protein substrates or indirectly through adapter molecules. Although the 40 or more E2 enzymes can interact directly with substrate, in general, they recognize the E3-substrate complex. One E2 enzyme can cooperate with several different E3 enzymes in the ubiquitination reaction (Fig. 23-8). E2s accept substrates from a single E1 in yeast.

Particular E3 enzymes recognize different determinants on protein substrates, but only a few of the rules or motifs governing E3-substrate recognition signals have been identified (Table 23-1). The first and simplest signal to be identified is described by the **"N-end rule."** Through studies of chimeric and fusion proteins in yeast, researchers found that specific destabilizing amino acids at the N-terminus of a protein are recognized for ubiquitination by a specific E3 and subsequent destruction. Both the destabilizing N-terminal amino acid and a mobile lysine on the substrate are needed for ubiquitination and rapid degradation. The extent to which this simple rule governs proteolysis in vivo remains uncertain, although an increasing number of potential substrates that encode destabilizing amino acids at their N-terminus are being identified. One physiological substrate of the N-end rule is the C-terminal fragment of the Scc1 chromosome cohesin molecule that is produced by specific proteolysis at the outset of

anaphase (see Fig. 44-16). Interference with N-end rule degradation of this protein is lethal to the cell, presumably because chromosome segregation is disrupted during mitosis. The first known N-end rule substrate in metazoans was an IAP inhibitor of apoptosis in *Drosophila* (see Chapter 46). Cleavage of this protein by a caspase (see Fig. 46-10) exposes an N-terminal destabilizing residue. Subsequent destruction of the protein is essential for its function as an apoptosis inhibitor.

Amphipathic or hydrophobic stretches of amino acids also function as general recognition determinants for ubiquitination. Because hydrophobic surfaces are often buried in a folded protein or at the interface between subunits, exposure of this ubiquitination determinant is thought to assist in targeting misfolded proteins or excess subunits of oligomeric proteins for degradation. This pathway is especially prevalent in controlling the degradation of proteins that fail to fold in the ER (see later).

Regulated proteolysis is key in controlling cell cycle progression and transcription activation. In these cases, targeting signals for degradation can be generated by specific phosphorylation events. For example, phosphorylation of a conserved sequence near the N-terminus of several transcription factors or their regulatory subunits generates a determinant recognized by the SCF complex (a family of modular E3 enzymes named for their three core components: *skp1*, *cdc53/cullin*, and an *F*-box-containing protein; see Fig. 40-17). This phosphorylation is often performed by cyclin-dependent kinases (Cdks [see Fig. 40-14]) and is thereby tightly linked to the cell cycle. Phosphorylation of cell cycle proteins containing internal sequences that are rich in proline, glutamic acid, serine, and threonine (called PEST sequences) can also target these proteins via SCF family E3 enzymes for rapid degradation.

A second multisubunit class of E3 enzymes, designated the APC/C (anaphase-promoting complex/

Table 23-1

UBIQUITIN/PROTEASOME TARGETING SYSTEMS

Recognition Determinant	Cellular Substrates	Ubiquitin Ligases (E3)
The N-end rule ...N-terminal aa F,L,W,Y,R,K,H	Mislocalized proteins(?) Cleaved cohesion subunit Scc1	E3α (Ubr1p)
Amphipathic or hydrophobic peptides	α-2 transcription factor Misfolded proteins?	Unknown
Phosphorylated signals DS*GXXS* PES*T regions	Transcription factors (e.g. IκB, β-catenin) Cell cycle regulators (e.g. cyclins)	SCF complexes
Destruction Box R(A/T)(A)L(G)X(I/V)(G/T)(N)	Mitotic cyclins Cell cycle regulators	APC (anaphase-promoting complex)
KEN Box ...KEN...	Cell cycle regulators	APC

*Phosphorylation sites on serine residues.

cyclosome), recognizes a partially conserved, nine-residue "destruction box" sequence near the N-terminus of several cell cycle regulatory proteins that targets these proteins for degradation (see Chapter 40). The short amino acid sequence lysine, glutamic acid, asparagine (KEN), the "KEN-box," can also serve as a destruction signal for the APC/C. Deletion of the destruction box or the KEN box stabilizes the protein, whereas their transfer to a normally stable protein often results in cell cycle–dependent ubiquitination and rapid degradation. Destruction or KEN boxes are not themselves regulated, but APC/C activity and specificity are regulated by Cdk phosphorylation (see Chapter 40).

Because proteolysis is key for cell cycle progression, interference with the proteasome has been adopted as a strategy for treatment of cancer. One proteasome inhibitor, Bortezomib, is now used in the clinic to treat advanced multiple myeloma, a leukemia of B-lymphocytes.

Role of Proteasomes in Elimination of Misfolded Proteins from the Endoplasmic Reticulum

Integral membrane proteins and secretory proteins fold and assemble in the lipid bilayer or lumen of the endoplasmic reticulum (ER) (see Fig. 20-7). Proteins that fail to fold or assemble are retrieved from the ER and degraded by the proteasome in a pathway known as **ERAD** (ER-associated protein degradation). The ERAD pathway also regulates levels of a number of ER resident proteins. Interestingly, the E3 ligases responsible for ubiquitinating ERAD target proteins are localized in the cytoplasm, so a poorly understood mechanism must expose target proteins to the cytoplasm for ubiquitin tagging. After ubiquitination in the cytoplasm, association with ubiquitin-binding proteins appears to ensure the extraction of these proteins from the ER by AAA-ATPases, and their subsequent targeting to proteasomes.

The ERAD pathway is of considerable medical interest. Defects in ubiquitination of particular proteins are associated with the pathology of Parkinson's disease. Furthermore, the most common form of cystic fibrosis results from ERAD-mediated degradation of a slow-folding (but catalytically competent) variant of the CFTR ABC transporter (see Fig. 11-4).

Other Regulated Intracellular Proteolysis

Another form of regulated intracellular proteolysis is activation of inactive proenzymes or transcription factors (see Fig. 15-22 for NFκB) by proteolytic cleavage. An important example of activation by proteolytic cleavage is provided by **caspases.** Extracellular or intracellular signals trigger the cleavage of procaspases, turning on their proteolytic activity and initiating a cascade that leads to apoptosis (see Fig. 46-10). In all cases, intracellular proteolysis is tightly regulated through a combination of triggered activation of the protease, specific substrate recognition, and compartmentalization.

Lipid Turnover and Degradation

Distinct pathways exist for the turnover of the three classes of cellular lipids: phosphoglycerides, glycolipids, and cholesterol. Glycolipids, which are restricted to the extracellular leaflet of a lipid bilayer, are degraded primarily in lysosomes, as evidenced by their abnormal accumulation in lysosomal storage diseases (Appendix 23-1). Sphingomyelin and gangliosides are delivered to lysosomes via vesicular transport and degraded to the level of ceramide, sugars, and fatty acids by a series of lysosomal hydrolases. Recent evidence suggests that the specialized lipid composition of lysosomal membranes, including the phospholipid species **lysobisphosphatidic acid** (see Fig. 22-15), which is enriched in intraluminal vesicles of multivesicular bodies and lysosomes, may play a role in activating sphingomyelinases and restricting their hydrolytic activity to the intraluminal side of the membranes. Cell surface sphingomyelinases also exist, and their activation triggers production of ceramide, which can function in signal transduction pathways as a second messenger (see Fig. 26-11).

The turnover of phosphoglycerides is much more varied in mechanism and location. Some phosphoglycerides, particularly those found in the outer leaflet of the plasma membrane (and in topologically equivalent surfaces), are degraded in lysosomes to their fatty acids, head group, and glycerol constituents. More frequently, phosphoglyceride degradation is only partial, and the degradative products (e.g., fatty acids, lysophospholipids, and diacylglycerol) are salvaged and reutilized in "short-circuit pathways." In this way, "old" phospholipids are "remodeled," forming new ones with altered properties. These phospholipid-remodeling reactions are catalyzed by a variety of **phospholipases** that cleave distinct bonds in the phospholipid to generate distinct products (see Fig. 26-4). Localized lipid remodeling can generate specialized lipid subdomains that are required for vesicle fusion or fission or for the selective recruitment of proteins to the membrane. In addition, molecules released from partial degradation of phosphoglycerides, fatty acids, diacylglycerol, and some head groups function as second messengers in signaling cascades (see Fig. 26-4).

Cholesterol Homeostasis

Cholesterol metabolism in mammals involves multiple organs. Approximately 90% of the free cholesterol in animal cells is in the plasma membrane. Cholesterol is the precursor for steroid hormones, which are synthesized in specialized cells but utilized throughout the body for a myriad of essential functions. Cholesterol is also the precursor for bile acids, which are synthesized by the liver and transported to the gut, where they aid in the digestion of dietary fat. Unlike the case with virtually all other intracellular molecules, individual cells cannot degrade cholesterol. Instead, cellular levels of cholesterol are regulated by a complex balance of endogenous synthesis, uptake of extracellular cholesterol, and efflux of intracellular cholesterol to vascular fluids (Fig. 23-9). When present in excess, cholesterol accumulates as plaques in the walls of major arteries, contributing to atherosclerosis.

Cholesterol is insoluble and is transported through the body as cholesterol esters packaged with other lipids and proteins. The intestine assembles dietary cholesterol into particles called chylomicrons, which are transported through the blood and eventually taken up by the liver, the major site of cholesterol synthesis in mammals. The liver packages dietary and de novo–synthesized cholesterol into **low-density lipoproteins** (LDLs), which are secreted into the blood for transport to other tissues. Other cells take up LDL particles via receptor-mediated endocytosis and deliver them along the endocytic pathway to lysosomes (Fig. 23-9). Within the lysosome, cholesterol esters are hydrolyzed, and the bulk of free LDL-derived cholesterol is transported by a yet-to-be identified cytoplasmic carrier protein back to the plasma membrane. Importantly, a small portion of cholesterol is also transported to the ER, where the cholesterol level controls the activity of transcription factors that regulate genes involved with cholesterol metabolism.

Two key enzymes in the endoplasmic reticulum have sterol-sensing domains that allow them to respond to the cholesterol content of the membrane and control intracellular free cholesterol levels (Fig. 23-10). Accumulation of LDL-derived cholesterol in the ER activates acyl CoA : cholesterol acyltransferase (ACAT), the enzyme that converts free cholesterol to cholesterol esters for storage. Substantial increases in the levels of free cholesterol (or an oxygenated metabolite of it) trigger the destruction of the enzyme that catalyzes the first step in cholesterol biosynthesis, HMG-CoA reductase (Fig. 23-9). Cholesterol triggers the degradation of HMG-CoA

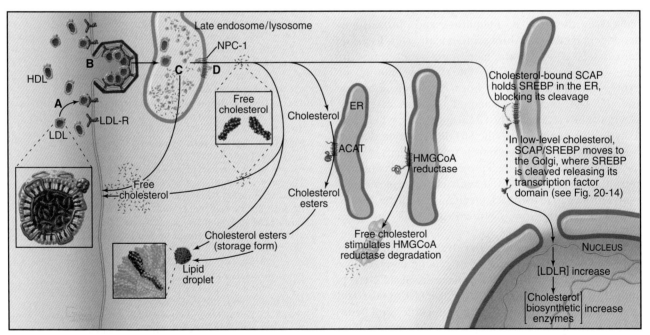

Figure 23-9   THE INTRACELLULAR PROCESSING AND REGULATION OF CHOLESTEROL BIOSYNTHESIS. **A,** Dietary cholesterol is delivered to cells in LDL particles. **B,** LDL particles are taken up by clathrin-mediated endocytosis. **C,** Free cholesterol is released in late endosomes/lysosomes and transported to the cell surface or internal membranes, depending, in part, on the activity of NPC-1 **(D),** an integral membrane protein. Excess cholesterol can be acylated by ACAT activity and stored in cytoplasmic lipid droplets as cholesterol esters. ACAT activity is increased by high intracellular cholesterol levels. At the same time, high cholesterol in the membrane decreases new cholesterol synthesis by triggering the proteasome-dependent degradation of the enzyme HMG-CoA reductase. Finally, high cellular cholesterol decreases the uptake of LDL particles and dietary cholesterol by blocking the proteolytic processing of the transcription factor, SREBP, required for LDL-receptor expression (see Fig. 20-14). Genetic defects that perturb steps **A** to **D** required for maintaining the delicate balance of cholesterol homeostasis cause several human diseases. Familial hypercholesterolemia is caused either by a lack of LDL receptor (LDL-R) **(A)** or by LDL-R that is defective in endocytic activity **(B).** Wolman disease is a lysosomal storage disease that is caused by defective lysosomal cholesterol esterase activity; Niemann-Pick disease type C, another lysosomal storage disease, results in defective trafficking of cholesterol out of late endosomes and lysosomes caused by mutations in NPC-1 **(D).**

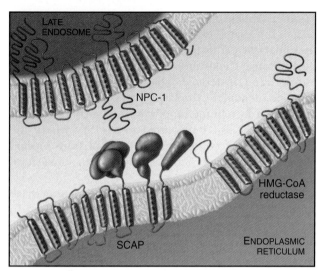

Figure 23-10 Proteins involved in cholesterol trafficking and homeostasis share a common sequence motif, the sterol-sensing domain. This is a region of the protein (red) that spans the membrane five times. Cholesterol binding to this domain in NPC-1 is required for normal cholesterol trafficking, whereas binding to the analogous domain inhibits the function of HMG-CoA reductase (which is ubiquitinated and destroyed) and of SCAP (which is retained in the ER as a complex with SREBP), thereby downregulating sterol production and uptake.

reductase through a ubiquitin- and proteasome-dependent pathway. A third protein with a sterol-sensing domain—SCAP—traps the membrane-bound transcription activator, SREBP, in the ER, thereby limiting the expression of the genes for both HMG-CoA reductase and the LDL receptor. When ER cholesterol is low, SCAP/SREBP escapes to the Golgi apparatus, where proteolytic cleavage liberates the SREBP activation domain (see Fig. 20-14). This then travels to the nucleus to drive the expression of LDL receptor, HMG-CoA reductase, and other proteins involved with cholesterol metabolism. This negative feedback mechanism reduces cholesterol input both from de novo synthesis and from extracellular sources (Fig. 23-9).

Cholesterol homeostasis is critical to human health, as is evidenced by the number of genetic diseases that result from defects in cholesterol metabolism. Defects in the LDL receptor reduce or eliminate LDL uptake, and LDL builds up in the blood, leading to cholesterol deposition in the walls of arteries and arteriosclerosis. Rare defects in the enzyme that hydrolyzes cholesterol esters in lysosomes lead to Wolman disease, which causes death within the first year of life. The devastating neurodegenerative disease called Niemann-Pick type C disease results from mutations in a multitransmembrane domain protein (designated NPC-1) that is required for transport of LDL-derived cholesterol from late endosomes to both the plasma membrane and ER. Cholesterol accumulates in lysosomes of diseased patients, and cholesterol homeostasis is impaired. Interestingly, NPC-

1 has a "sterol-sensing domain" found in enzymes that are regulated by the cholesterol composition of membranes (Fig. 23-10; also see Fig. 20-14).

ACKNOWLEDGMENTS

Thanks go to Margaret Robinson, Karin Römisch, and Sandra Schmidt for their suggestions on revisions to this chapter.

SELECTED READINGS

Abele R, Tampe R: Modulation of the antigen transport machinery TAP by friends and enemies. FEBS Lett 580:1156–1163, 2006.

Babst M: A protein's final ESCRT. Traffic 6:2–9, 2005.

Bonifacino JS, Weissman AM: Ubiquitin and the control of protein fate in the secretory and endocytic pathways. Annu Rev Cell Dev Biol 14:9–58, 1998.

Brown MS, Goldstein JL: A proteolytic pathway that controls the cholesterol content of membranes, cells, and blood. Proc Natl Acad Sci U S A 96:11041–11048, 1999.

Ciechanover A: Proteolysis: From the lysosome to ubiquitin and the proteasome. Nat Rev Mol Cell Biol 6:79–86, 2005.

Cuervo AM: Autophagy: In sickness and in health. Trends Cell Biol 14:70–77, 2004.

D'Azzo A, Bongiovanni A, Nastasi T: E3 ubiquitin ligases as regulators of membrane protein trafficking and degradation. Traffic 6:429–441, 2005.

Deshaies RJ: SCF and Cullin/Ring H2-based ubiquitin ligases. Annu Rev Cell Dev Biol 15:435–468, 1999.

Earnshaw WC, Martins LM, Kaufmann SH: Mammalian caspases: Structure, activation, substrates, and functions during apoptosis. Annu Rev Biochem 68:383–442, 1999.

Fineschi B, Miller J: Endosomal proteases and antigen processing. Trends Biochem Sci 22:377–382, 1997.

Hicke L, Dunn R: Regulation of membrane protein transport by ubiquitin and ubiquitin-binding proteins. Annu Rev Cell Dev Biol 19:141–172, 2003.

Klionsky DJ: The molecular machinery of autophagy: Unanswered questions. J Cell Sci 118:7–18, 2005.

McGrath ME: Lysosomal cysteine proteases. Annu Rev Biophys Biomol Struct 28:181–204, 1999.

Meusser B, Hirsch C, Jarosch E, Sommer T: ERAD: The long road to destruction. Nat Cell Biol 7:766–772, 2005.

Mizushima N, Yoshimori T, Ohsumi Y: Role of the Apg12 conjugation system in mammalian autophagy. Int J Biochem Cell Biol 35:553–561, 2003.

Pickart CM: Mechanisms underlying ubiquitination. Annu Rev Biochem 70:503–534, 2001.

Pines J: Mitosis: A matter of getting rid of the right protein at the right time. Trends Cell Biol 16:55–63, 2006.

Römisch K: Endoplasmic reticulum-associated degradation. Annu Rev Cell Dev Biol 21:435–456, 2005.

Schwartz DC, Hochstrasser M: A superfamily of protein tags: Ubiquitin, SUMO and related modifiers. Trends Biochem Sci 28:321–328, 2003.

Simons K, Ikonen E: How cells handle cholesterol. Science 290:1721–1726, 2000.

Sun L, Chen ZJ: The novel functions of ubiquitination in signaling. Curr Opin Cell Biol 16:119–126, 2004.

Varshavsky A: The ubiquitin system. Trends Biochem Sci 22:383–387, 1997.

Wolf DH, Hilt W: The proteasome: A proteolytic nanomachine of cell regulation and waste disposal. Biochim Biophys Acta 1695:19–31, 2004.

APPENDIX 23-1

Lysosomal Storage Diseases

Disease(s)	Enzyme Defect	Accumulated Material
Sphingolipidosis G_{M1} gangliosidosis	β-galactosidase	G_{M1} ganglioside glycoproteins
Tay-Sachs G_{M2} gangliosidosis	Hexosaminidase A	G_{M2} gangliosides
Sandhoff G_{M2} gangliosidosis	Hexosaminidase A and B	G_{M2} gangliosides
Krabbe . . . galactoceramide lipidosis	Galactosyl ceramide β-galactosidase	Galactocerebrosides
Niemann-Pick A and B . . . sphingomyelin lipidosis	Sphingomyelinase	Sphingomyelin Cholesterol
Gaucher Glucosylceramide lipidosis	β-glucocerebrosidase	Glucosylceramide
Fabry	α-galactosidase A	Trihexosylceramide
Glycoprotein storage diseases	α-fucosidase α-mannosidase α-aspartylglucosamine	Glycopeptides Glycolipids Oligosaccharides
Mucopolysaccharidosis Several types	α-iduronidase Iduronosulfate sulfatase N-acetyl-α-glucosaminidase Heparin sulfatase β-glucuronidase	Heparin sulfate
Sialidosis	Neuraminidase	Sialyoligosaccharides
Mucolipidosis II I cell disease	UDP-N-acetlyglucosmine (GlcNAc): glycoprotein GlcNAc-1- phosphotransferase	Glycoproteins Glycolipids

Signaling Mechanisms

SECTION VII OVERVIEW

Cells depend on signaling systems to adapt to changing environmental conditions. Free-living organisms, such as yeast and bacteria, respond to changes in temperature, osmotic stress, and nutrients by synthesizing the proteins that are required to optimize their survival. Motile cells respond to chemicals by migrating toward attractants and away from repellants. In vertebrate animals, the hormone adrenaline stimulates cellular energy metabolism, and growth factors stimulate cells to duplicate their genomes and divide. Developmentally regulated genetic programs equip each cell with the molecular hardware that is required to adapt to remarkably diverse stimuli.

The first three chapters in this section introduce the main molecular components of signaling pathways: receptors, protein messengers, and second messengers. With this background, the reader can appreciate nine well-characterized signal transduction pathways presented in Chapter 27 without being distracted by descriptions of the molecular components.

Cells use molecular **receptors** (Chapter 24) to detect physical stimuli. Physical interaction of the stimulus provides the energy to modify the structure of the receptor and initiate a signaling pathway. With the exception of RNA "riboswitches," all receptors are proteins. A few stimuli, including light, steroid hormones, and gases, penetrate the plasma membrane and react with receptors inside the cell. Most stimuli from outside the cell, including proteins, peptides, and charged biogenic amines, cannot penetrate the plasma membrane. These extracellular ligands bind transmembrane receptors on the cell surface that transfer the signal across the lipid bilayer.

Most stimuli act through one of about 20 families of receptor proteins, each coupled to distinct signal transduction mechanisms (Fig. 24-1). Multiple isoforms within each family provide thousands of different receptors,

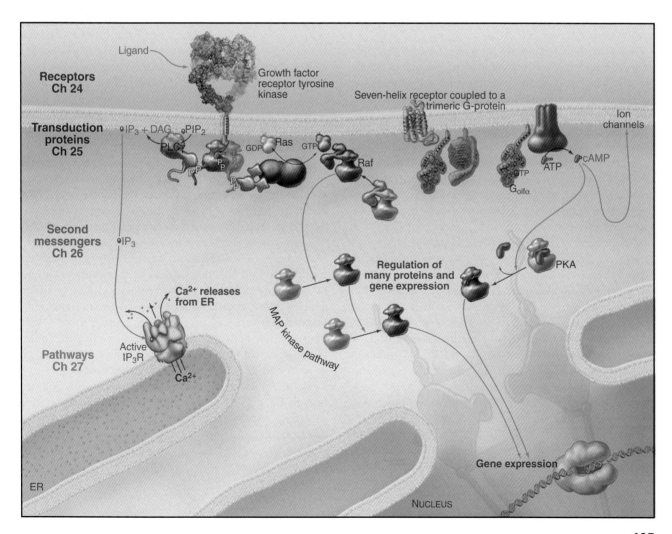

each with specificity for particular stimuli. For example, of 18,000 genes in the nematode genome, nearly 800 encode a large family of receptors with seven transmembrane helices. Presumably, all members of each receptor family arose from a common ancestor and acquired new specificities by multiple rounds of gene duplication and divergent evolution.

Active receptors generate a chemical signal inside the cell by interacting with one or more cytoplasmic proteins (Chapter 25). This **transduction** step converts one type of signal (stimulus) into another signal (messenger) and commonly amplifies the signal. Some receptors have a cytoplasmic domain with **protein kinase** activity or associate with a separate protein kinase. These enzymes transfer phosphate from ATP to specific amino acids on target proteins. The cytoplasmic domains of active seven-helix receptors catalyze the exchange of GDP for GTP on signal-transducing proteins, called G-proteins. GTP binding activates these **GTPases,** allowing them to bind and regulate target proteins. Adapter proteins also link active receptors to downstream effector proteins, including kinases and GTPases. Cytoplasmic signaling proteins often act in cascades, passing a signal from one to another. Amplification along these pathways allows small stimuli to generate biochemical responses inside the cell.

Many signaling pathways regulate the concentration of small molecules, called **second messengers** (Chapter 26). The most widely used second messengers are **Ca^{2+}, cyclic nucleotides,** and **lipids.** They modify the behavior of the cell by binding to and activating a wide range of effector proteins, regulating membrane physiology, metabolism, motility, and gene expression.

Signaling pathways regulate virtually all cellular processes (Chapter 27). Effector systems include transcription factors that control gene expression, proteins that regulate secretion, metabolic enzymes, structural elements of the cytoskeleton and associated motor, cell surface receptors, regulators of the cell cycle, and membrane ion channels. Multiple signaling pathways converge on each of these effector systems. Integration of these diverse signals determines cell behavior, whether it secretes or moves, grows, divides, or differentiates.

Understanding signaling pathways is challenging. First, cells employ hundreds of distinct signaling pathways, involving hundreds to thousands of different proteins. Second, few signal transduction mechanisms utilize simple linear pathways from a stimulus to a change in behavior. Rather, most pathways branch and converge multiple times, making it possible for information from several inputs to influence each effector system. This provides for integration of regulatory mechanisms but makes it difficult to predict how information flows through a system. Third, most pathways have positive or negative feedback loops that can either augment or inhibit responses. These **feedback loops** make many signals transient events. Fourth, the response of some pathways depends on both the strength and the temporal pattern of the stimulus. Ultimately, signaling pathways will be understood as integrated systems, like complex electrical circuits.

Two main approaches have revealed much about signaling mechanisms: biochemistry/pharmacology and genetic analysis. The biochemical approach generally starts with identification of a naturally occurring or synthetic chemical, such as a hormone, that modifies the activity of an organism, organ, or cell. These compounds are called **agonists.** Characterization of the biological effects of agonists is often aided by the discovery of chemicals that antagonize their action. In many cases, such **antagonists** prove to be useful as drugs, even before their mechanisms of action are understood. Aspirin is just one example. To define the mechanism, it is necessary to find and characterize the receptor that binds the chemical and then to trace the biochemical steps from receptor to effectors. Once a model mechanism has been defined for a particular class of receptors, the primary structure of a new receptor usually reveals (by homology with known receptors) the type of transduction mechanism and suggests the sorts of molecules that lie between the receptor and the effector systems in the cell.

The genetic approach involves characterization of mutants that affect the flow of information through a signaling pathway. By collecting enough mutants and testing for a hierarchy of effects, investigators can usually define the flow of information through a pathway. By cloning and sequencing the mutated genes, one can identify the proteins that are involved. Because one need make no assumptions about the nature of the biochemical hardware or how the components are connected, completely novel molecules emerge from genetic screens just as easily as familiar ones. One particularly fruitful genetic approach has been to analyze genes that predispose individuals to cancer or that cause naturally occurring heritable diseases in humans, mice, or other species. Many proteins that are responsible for regulating cell growth and proliferation cause cancer when constitutively activated by mutations. Inactivating mutations in other signaling proteins cause disorders of growth and development or endocrine diseases.

To understand the dynamics of a signaling system, one really needs to know all of the converging and diverging pathways and how the rates of the various reactions depend on the intensity and pattern of the stimuli. This has been achieved for one signaling system, bacterial chemotaxis.

CHAPTER 24

Plasma Membrane Receptors

Cells use about 20 different families of receptor proteins (Fig. 24-1) to detect and respond to the myriad of incoming chemical and physical stimuli (Appendix 24-1). Most receptors are plasma membrane proteins that interact with chemical **ligands** or are stimulated by physical events such as light absorption. A few chemical stimuli, including steroid hormones and the gas nitric oxide, cross the plasma membrane and bind receptors inside the cell.

Gene duplication and divergent evolution within each family have produced genes for multiple **receptor isoforms** that interact with different ligands. In multicellular organisms, selective expression of certain receptors and their associated cytoplasmic transduction machinery allows differentiated cells to respond specifically to particular ligands but not others (see Fig. 27-1). Fortunately, the mechanisms of the best-characterized receptors usually apply to the rest of their family. Thus, learning about a few examples provides a working knowledge of many related receptors.

Members of each family of receptors share one or more structurally homologous domains. In some families, the members share both ligand-binding and signal-transducing strategies (seven-helix receptors and cytokine receptors). Members of other families share either a similar ligand-binding structure (tumor necrosis factor [TNF] receptor family) or a common signal-transducing method (receptor tyrosine kinases) but differ in other respects. In families that share a common scaffold to bind similar ligands, amino acid substitutions on this scaffold allow each family member to recognize their specific ligands.

One cannot predict the type of receptor, signal transduction mechanism, or nature of the response from the chemical nature of a stimulus (Appendix 24-1). Although proteins and peptides are the only known ligands for receptor kinases and kinase-linked receptors, proteins and peptides also stimulate some seven-helix receptors and guanylyl cyclase receptors. A particularly wide range of stimuli activate seven-helix receptors, including photons, amino acids, nucleotides, biogenic amines, lipids, peptides, proteins, and hundreds of different organic molecules. Some ligands bind distinct receptors on different cells. For example, acetylcholine activates muscle contraction by opening a ligand-gated ion channel (see Fig. 10-12). It also binds seven-helix receptors on other cells, activating signaling pathways mediated by guanosine triphosphate (GTP)–binding proteins. Some ligands with similar names bind to different types of receptors. For example, several interleukins (IL-2 through IL-6) bind to cytokine

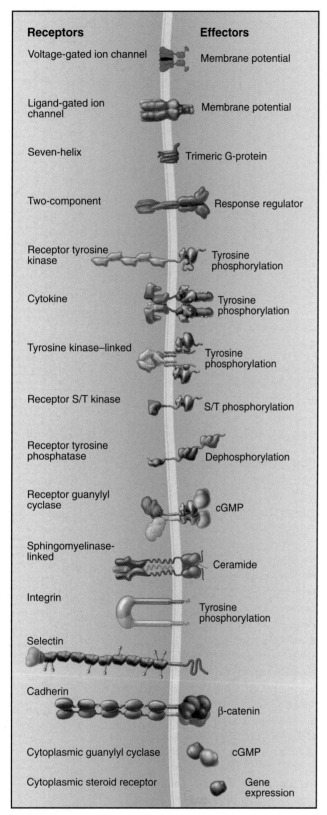

Figure 24-1   SIXTEEN CLASSES OF RECEPTORS WITH SIGNAL TRANSDUCTION MECHANISMS. S/T, serine/threonine.

receptors, but IL-1 activates a sphingomyelinase-linked receptor, and IL-8 binds a seven-helix, G-protein-coupled receptor.

Receptors use two different strategies to transfer energy from ligand binding across the plasma membrane to activate cytoplasmic signals. Ligand binding on the cell surface may change the conformation of the receptor, altering the structure of parts of the receptor in the cytoplasm. Seven-helix receptors use this strategy. Ligand binding also induces a conformational change in preformed dimers of cytokine receptors. Alternatively, ligand binding may cluster inactive receptor subunits diffusing in the plane of the membrane. Dimerization of some receptor tyrosine kinases by ligands brings the cytoplasmic kinase domains of the partners close enough together to activate each other.

Most signal-transducing pathways include one or more enzymes that amplify signals. In some receptor families, an enzyme is part of the receptor protein itself (receptor tyrosine kinases), but in others, the receptor interacts with a separate cytoplasmic enzyme (trimeric G-proteins, cytoplasmic protein kinases).

If extracellular stimulation is sustained, most signaling systems turn down their response. The literature variously calls this **adaptation,** attenuation, desensitization, tachyphylaxis, or tolerance. For example, rhodopsin and odorant receptors turn off within a second of continuous stimulation. This allows one to distinguish rapidly changing visual information and concentrations of odors.

This chapter covers nine families of well-characterized receptors that transfer signals across the plasma membrane. Other chapters describe additional receptor families: Chapter 10, ligand-gated and voltage-gated ion channels; Chapter 15, nuclear receptors for steroids and other ligands; Chapter 25, receptors with protein-phosphatase activity; Chapter 26, cytoplasmic nitric oxide receptors with guanylyl cyclase activity; Chapter 27, two-component receptors and tyrosine kinase–linked receptors; and Chapter 30, cell adhesion receptors, including integrins, cadherins, and selectins.

Seven-Helix Receptors

Members of the largest family of plasma membrane receptors are built from a serpentine arrangement of seven transmembrane α-helices. These diverse receptors use **trimeric GTP-binding proteins** (see Fig. 25-9) to relay signals to effector proteins inside cells. Seven-helix receptors are found in slime molds, so the genes for these proteins originated in early eukaryotes more than 1 billion years ago. Four percent of the genes of the nematode *Caenorhabditis elegans* (790) encode seven-helix receptors, the largest family of proteins in the organism. In mammals, olfactory cells alone use 500 to 1000 different seven-helix receptors to discriminate odorant molecules (see Fig. 27-1). Other cells are estimated to express another 375 seven-helix receptors to respond to light, amino acids, peptide and protein hormones, catecholamines, and lipids. The chemical ligand remains to be determined for about 40% of these 375 receptors, which are termed *orphan receptors.* A majority of medically useful drugs bind seven-helix receptors.

Seven hydrophobic sequences traverse the plasma membrane as α-helices (Fig. 24-2). The topology is the same as that of bacteriorhodopsin (see Fig. 7-8), but this might be an example of convergent evolution. Comparative analysis of amino acid sequences suggests that all seven-helix receptors have the same arrangement of helices. For example, the minimum length of sequences connecting the helices is compatible only with the helices being arranged sequentially from I to VII in a serpentine fashion as they cross the lipid bilayer. The N-terminus is outside the cell and varies from 7 to 6000 residues. Some of the larger N-terminal domains participate in ligand binding. The C-terminal segment of the polypeptide is in the cytoplasm and varies in length from 12 to more than 350 residues.

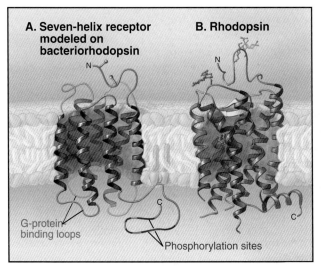

Figure 24-2 STRUCTURE OF SEVEN-HELIX RECEPTORS. **A,** Model of the generic seven-helix receptor, used throughout this text. The structure is based on the structure of bacteriorhodopsin and the amino acid sequence of a typical vertebrate seven-helix receptor. Seven hydrophobic segments cross the membrane as α-helices. Oligosaccharides are *blue.* The C-terminal cytoplasmic tail is anchored to the lipid bilayer by two fatty acids covalently bound to a pair of adjacent cysteines. **B,** Atomic structure of bovine rhodopsin, the receptor for photons in the retina. Covalently bound retinal pigment is *green.* Oligosaccharides on extracellular loops are *blue.* (PDB file: 1F88. Reference: Palczewski K, Kumasaka T, Hori T, et al: Crystal structure of rhodopsin: A G protein–coupled receptor. Science 289:739–745, 2000.)

Seven-helix receptors are shown throughout this book as individual proteins, but multiple lines of evidence show that many seven-helix receptors function as dimers or larger oligomers, allowing for cross talk between the subunits.

Most seven-helix receptors are activated by binding a soluble chemical ligand, but some interesting variations exist. Biochemical and mutagenesis experiments indicate that most small ligands bind in a central pocket among the extracellular ends of the helices. Residues lining this pocket are highly variable between receptors, providing specificity for each receptor to bind a particular ligand. The light-absorbing pigment **11-*cis* retinal,** of the photoreceptor protein **rhodopsin,** is the best-characterized "ligand." 11-*cis* retinal is unusual in that it is bound covalently to the receptor (Fig. 24-2B) and is activated by absorbing a photon (see Fig. 27-2). In other respects, it is a good model for other ligands (Fig. 24-3). **Neurotransmitters,** such as norepinephrine, and drugs also bind between the helices about one third of the way across the membrane. Peptide hormones bind deep in the helical pocket but probably also interact with residues that are more exposed on the cell surface. Receptors for some large ligands (pituitary glycoprotein hormones, such as luteinizing hormone, follicle-stimulating hormone, and thyroid-stimulating hormone) and some small ligands (glutamate, γ-amino butyric acid, calcium) bind with high affinity to extracellular N-terminal domains of their seven-helix receptor. The N-terminal domain with bound ligand then stimulates the transmembrane domain of the receptor. The blood-clotting enzyme thrombin activates its receptor on platelets by proteolysis of the receptor rather than by direct binding (see Fig. 30-14). The N-terminal peptide cleaved from the receptor dissociates and activates other receptors; what is left of the newly truncated N-terminus folds back and activates its own receptor.

Seven-helix receptors exist in an equilibrium between two conformations: a **resting state** and an **activated state** with the ability to catalyze the exchange of nucleotide bound to trimeric G-proteins (Fig. 24-3). Without bound ligand, the resting state is strongly favored. Ligand binding to the receptor (or the isomerization of retinal after absorbing light) initiates signal transduction by shifting the equilibrium to the active state. Activation involves movement of at least two transmembrane helices, but the structural details of this conformational change are not yet well defined. In any event, activation must rearrange the cytoplasmic ends of the helices and the loops connecting them to create a binding site for a target G-protein.

Active receptors transfer the signal to the cytoplasm by activating trimeric G-proteins. Cytoplasmic loops of active receptors catalyze the dissociation of guanosine diphosphate bound (EDP) to an inactive Gα

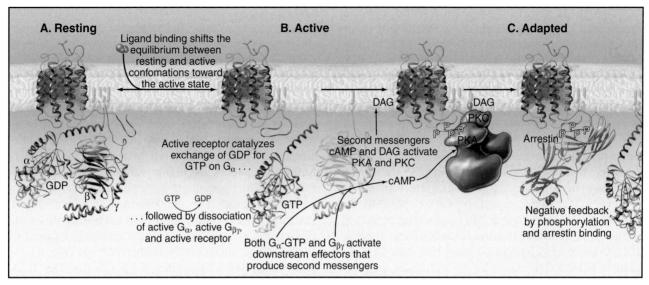

Figure 24-3 ACTIVATION AND ADAPTATION OF A SEVEN-HELIX RECEPTOR. **A,** Ligand binding shifts the equilibrium from the resting conformation toward the active conformation. **B,** The active receptor promotes dissociation of guanosine diphosphate from the α-subunit of multiple tri-meric G-proteins, allowing GTP to bind. Typically, this dissociates G_α from $G_{\beta\gamma}$, each of which activates downstream effectors that produce, for example, the second messengers cAMP and diacylgycerol (DAG). cAMP and DAG activate PKA and PKC, which phosphorylate active receptors on their C-terminus. **C,** This attracts arrestin, putting the receptor into the inactive adapted state. PKA, protein kinase A; PKC, protein kinase C. (PDB file for arrestin: 1CF1.)

subunit. GTP then binds and activates Gα (see Fig. 25-9). A single active seven-helix receptor can amplify the signal by activating up to 100 G-proteins. After dissociating from the receptor and each other, both Gα-GTP and Gβγ stimulate downstream effector proteins, further amplifying the signal (see Fig. 27-3 for an example of amplification).

Most seven-helix receptors adapt to sustained stimulation. In the short term, phosphorylation of the C-terminal tail of the receptor provides **negative feedback** that inactivates receptors with ligands still bound (Fig. 24-3C). Along one pathway, **second messengers**—produced in response to receptor activation—stimulate protein kinases, including cyclic adenosine monophosphate (cAMP)–activated protein kinase A and protein kinase C (see Fig. 25-4). These kinases phosphorylate the C-terminal tails of active receptors, inhibiting inter-actions with G-proteins. This mechanism allows for cross talk between receptors, as activation of one class of receptors can inactivate other receptors. A second pathway uses Gβγ subunits released in response to receptor stimulation to activate protein kinases specific for the receptors themselves, called **G-protein-coupled receptor kinases.** These kinases phosphorylate serines or threonines on the C-terminal tails of active (but not inactive) receptors.

Phosphorylation of receptor tails creates a binding site for **arrestin,** a protein with multiple functions. First, arrestin blocks interactions of the receptor with G-proteins, terminating signaling through the main pathway downstream of most seven-helix receptors. In some cases, arrestin initiates a new signal through the MAP kinase pathway (see Figs. 27-6 and 27-7 for two other pathways). Arrestin also promotes the removal of seven-helix receptors from the plasma membrane by endocytosis in clathrin-coated vesicles, a longer-term mechanism that turns down the response of a cell to continuous stimulation. Some internalized receptors recycle to the plasma membrane, but others modified by ubiquitin are directed to lysosomes for destruction. Chapter 27 covers three dramatic examples of seven-helix receptor adaptation.

Mutations of more than 30 seven-helix receptors have been linked to human diseases (Table 24-1). More than 600 mutations are known to inactivate seven-helix receptors in humans by every conceivable means from failure to synthesize the full length protein to reduced affinity for ligands to failure to activate G-proteins. These inherited loss of function mutations are recessive. For example, loss of function mutations in rhodopsin cause retinitis pigmentosa, a degeneration of photore-ceptor cells. Another example is severe obesity associ-ated with loss of function mutations of a seven-helix receptor that participates in the neural circuits control-ling eating. More than a hundred different mutations produce receptors that are constitutively active without ligand. Particular mutations of rhodopsin cause night blindness, and mutations in a calcium receptor cause dysfunction of the parathyroid gland. The physiology of these activating mutations is complicated, because cells use feedback mechanisms to compensate for the con-tinually active receptors.

Table 24-1

SEVEN-HELIX RECEPTORS AND DISEASE

Defective Receptor	Disease Phenotype
Activating Mutations	
Parathyroid Ca^{2+} sensor	Hypoparathyroidism
Rhodopsin	Night blindness
Thyroid hormone receptor	Hyperthyroidism, thyroid cancer
Loss of Function Mutations	
Cone cell opsin	Color blindness; no response to certain wavelengths
Parathyroid Ca^{2+} sensor	Hyperparathyroidism, failure to respond to high levels of serum Ca^{2+}
Rhodopsin	Retinitis pigmentosa, retinal degeneration
Thyroid hormone receptor	Hypothyroidism
Vasopressin receptor	Nephrogenic diabetes insipidus; failure of kidneys to resorb water

Receptor Tyrosine Kinases

Many polypeptide growth factors activate cells by binding plasma membrane receptors with cytoplasmic protein tyrosine kinase activity (Fig. 24-4). Ligand binding to extracellular domains allows the cytoplasmic kinase domains of pairs receptors to activate each other and to phosphorylate each other and downstream proteins that control cellular proliferation and differentiation. Mammals have 20 families of receptor tyrosine kinases with distinct structural features.

The growth factors that activate receptor tyrosine kinases regulate development and differentiation. For example, **epidermal growth factor** (EGF) stimulates proliferation and differentiation of epithelial cells. **Platelet-derived growth factor** stimulates growth of smooth muscle cells, glial cells, and fibroblasts (see Fig. 32-11). Some growth factors were discovered by biochemical purification of proteins that stimulate cellular growth or differentiation. EGF was discovered with a bioassay, as it causes the eyelids of newborn mice to open prematurely. A homolog of the EGF receptor, HER2/ErbB2, was discovered as the normal version of a cancer-causing viral oncogene. Other ligands and receptors were discovered as genes in flies or worms required for development. The *Drosophila sevenless* gene encodes a receptor tyrosine kinase that is related to insulin receptor. Mutations in the *sevenless* gene result in failure to develop photoreceptor cell number 7 in the fly's eye.

Receptor tyrosine kinases consist of an extracellular ligand-binding domain connected to a cytoplasmic tyrosine kinase domain by a single transmembrane helix (Fig. 24-4). The ligand binding is mediated by immunoglobulin domains, fibronectin III domains (see Fig. 3-13), cadherin domains (see Fig. 30-5), and less

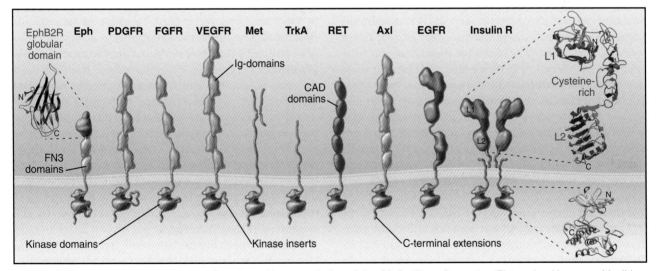

Figure 24-4 RECEPTOR TYROSINE KINASES. Domain architecture of nine of the 20 families of receptor (R) tyrosine kinases, with ribbon models of several domains. The globular domain of the EphB2 receptor is a β sandwich with a ligand-binding site that includes the exposed loop on the front of this model (PDB file: 1IGY). The extracellular part of the insulin-like growth factor consists of two similar β-helical domains connected by cysteine-rich domains (PDB file: 1IGR). The cytoplasmic kinase domain from the insulin receptor is similar to most known kinases (PDB file: 1IRK). Kinase inserts and C-terminal extensions contain tyrosine phosphorylation sites. **Receptor names:** EphR, receptor for ephrin, membrane-bound ligands in the nervous system, the largest class of receptor tyrosine kinases; PDGFR, platelet-derived growth factor receptor; FGFR, fibroblast growth factor receptor; VEGFR, vascular endothelial growth factor; Met, receptor for hepatocyte growth factor; TrkA, receptor for nerve growth factor; RET, a cadherin adhesion receptor; Axl, receptor for the growth factor Gas6; EGFR, epidermal growth factor receptor. **Domain names:** Ig, immunoglobulin; F3, fibronectin-III; CAD, cadherin. (References: Hubbard SR, Till JH: Protein tyrosine kinase structure and function. Annu Rev Biochem 69:373–398, 2000; Garrett TP, McKern NM, Lou M, et al: Crystal structure of the first three domains of the type-1 insulin-like growth factor receptor. Nature 394:395–399, 1998; and Hubbard SR, Wei L, Ellis L, Hendrickson WA: Crystal structure of the tyrosine kinase domain of the human insulin receptor. Nature 372:746–754, 1994.)

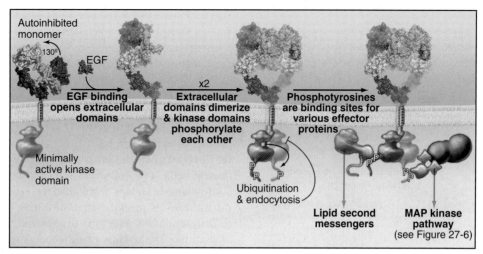

Figure 24-5 SUBUNIT DIMERIZATION MECHANISM FOR ACTIVATING THE EGF RECEPTOR TYROSINE KINASE. In the absence of EGF, intramolecular interactions preclude dimerization. EGF binding changes the conformation of the extracellular domains allowing dimerization of two receptors, bringing together two cytoplasmic kinase domains. Transphosphorylation activates both kinases and creates phosphotyrosine binding sites for SH2 and PTB domains of downstream signal transduction proteins. (PDB files: 2AHX and 2A91. Reference: Burgess AW, Cho HS, Eigenbrot C, et al: An open-and-shut case? Recent insights into the activation of EGF/ErbB receptors. Mol Cell 12:541–552, 2003.)

familiar domains such as β-helical and cysteine-rich domains. This domain architecture illustrates that genes for receptor tyrosine kinases were assembled from sequences for familiar domains followed by divergence to allow for interactions with diverse ligands.

Ligand binding activates all well-characterized receptor tyrosine kinases by bringing together a pair of kinase domains on the cytoplasmic face of the membrane. Dimeric ligands such as platelet-derived growth factor recruit a pair of receptors from the pool of subunits diffusing in the plane of the membrane and connect them physically. This **induced dimerization** juxtaposes two kinase domains in the cytoplasm. An EGF monomer binds a receptor and induces a conformational change that favors the formation of a receptor dimer but is not a physical part of the connection between the subunits (Fig. 24-5). Insulin binding induces a conformational change in a preformed receptor dimer held together by a disulfide bond. The conformational change brings together the kinase domains (see Fig. 27-7).

The juxtaposition of kinase domains allows the partners to activate each other by direct interaction and by phosphorylating each other on tyrosine residues. In most cases, phosphorylation of tyrosines on the **activation loop** of the catalytic domain refolds the loop into an active conformation (see Fig. 25-3D), although this is not required for the EGF receptor. In all cases, the paired kinases phosphorylate tyrosines on inserts and C-terminal extensions of the kinase domain, creating phosphotyrosine-binding sites for downstream effector and adapter proteins with **SH2** and **PTB** domains (Fig. 24-5; also see Figs. 27-6 and 27-7). Each SH2 and PTB domain

binds preferentially to a certain phosphotyrosine site by virtue of a pocket that recognizes both phosphotyrosine adjacent residues (see Fig. 25-11). For example, each of five phosphotyrosines of the platelet-derived growth factor receptor favors binding of a different effector or adapter protein.

Receptor tyrosine kinases activate effector proteins in two different ways. First, binding of an effector protein to a receptor phosphotyrosine favors its phosphorylation by the receptor kinase. In the case of **phospholipase Cγ**, tyrosine phosphorylation both activates its catalytic activity and dissociates the enzyme from its phosphotyrosine-binding site, allowing it to move to its site of action on the membrane. Second, binding to the receptor may promote activity by bringing an effector protein near its substrate. This applies to both **phosphoinositide-3-kinase,** which acts on lipid substrates in the membrane bilayer (see Fig. 27-7), and the nucleotide exchange protein that activates the **Ras** guanosine triphosphatase (GTPase), which is anchored to the membrane bilayer (see Fig. 27-6).

Multiple mechanisms turn off receptor tyrosine kinases. In the short term, lipid second messengers produced by phospholipase Cγ activate protein kinase C, which inhibits the kinase by phosphorylation. Active kinases are also targets for the addition of a single ubiquitin to one or more lysine side chains. These single ubiquitins are the signal for the receptor to be removed from the cell surface by endocytosis in clathrin-coated vesicles (see Fig. 23-2).

Mutations in receptor tyrosine kinases cause human disease. Many cancers have activating mutations or overexpression of EGF receptors. Activating mutations in a fibroblast growth factor receptor lead to a variety of congenital abnormalities of the skeleton, including a form of dwarfism and premature fusion of the sutures between the bones of the skull. Some of these mutations activate by promoting receptor dimerization through disulfide bonds or association of transmembrane helices. Others change ligand specificity.

Cytokine Receptors

Cytokines are a diverse family of polypeptide hormones and growth factors that regulate many cellular processes. Although they differ in detail, all cytokines are four-helix bundles. Pituitary **growth hormone** controls body growth and development of mammals, so loss of function receptor mutations cause one type of dwarfism. **Erythropoietin** regulates the proliferation and differentiation of red blood cell precursors (see Fig. 28-7). **Interleukins** modulate cells of the immune system, so loss of function receptor mutations result in deficient immune cells.

Cytokine receptors are homodimers or heterodimers, all with two extracellular fibronectin III domains that bind the ligand (Fig. 24-6). A single polypeptide segment, likely an α-helix, crosses the membrane. Cytoplasmic domains lack enzyme activity but bind one of several protein tyrosine kinases called **JAKs** ("just another

kinase"). It has not been settled whether inactive, ligand-free receptors diffuse separately in the plane of the membrane or form dimers with widely separated transmembrane domains, as observed in crystals of erythropoietin receptor without ligand (Fig. 24-6C). This separation of cytoplasmic domains could explain the lack of activity of ligand-free dimers.

Ligand binding activates cytokine receptors by bringing together two JAK kinases bound to the cytoplasmic domains—either by changing the conformation of preformed dimers or by inducing the dimerization of separate receptors (Fig. 24-7). A conformational change of a preformed dimer would explain how erythropoietin can activate cells with low concentrations of receptors on the cell surface. Close proximity allows JAKs to activate each other by transphosphorylation. The signal is then propagated to the nucleus when JAKs phosphorylate selected members of a family of transcription factors called **STATs,** which migrate to the nucleus to regulate gene expression (see Fig. 27-9).

Receptor Serine/Threonine Kinases

A third class of growth factor receptors uses cytoplasmic serine/threonine kinase domains to transduce signals (Figs. 24-8 and 24-9). Dimeric protein ligands bring together two different types of receptor subunits to turn on kinase activity. Humans have genes for seven

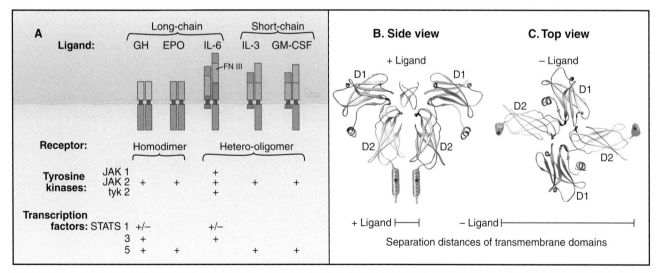

Figure 24-6 CYTOKINE RECEPTORS. **A,** Domain architecture and coupled signaling components of selected cytokine receptors. (EPO, erythropoietin; GH, growth hormone; GM-CSF, granulocyte-monocyte colony-stimulating factor; IL, interleukin.) **B–C,** Atomic structures of erythropoietin receptors. **B,** Side view of a receptor with a synthetic ligand called EMP1 *(green).* **C,** Top view of a receptor without ligand. D1 and D2 are the fibronectin III domains. The *pink helices* are models of the transmembrane segments. *Pink bars* indicate the separation of transmembrane segments. Association of erythropoietin and growth hormone with their receptors is remarkable, as a single, small, asymmetrical protein ligand binds between two identical receptor subunits using different sites on each receptor subunit. (A, Adapted from Wells JA, de Vos AM: Hematopoietic receptor complexes. Annu Rev Biochem 65:609–634, 1996. B–C, Reference: Livnah O, Stura EA, Johnson DL, et al: Crystallographic evidence for preformed dimers of erythropoietin receptor before ligand activation. Science 283:987–990, 1999. PDB files: 1EBP and 1ERN.)

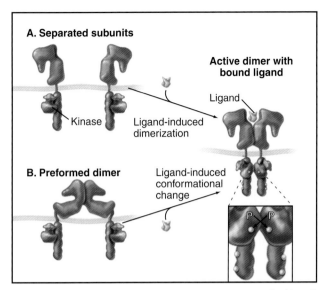

Figure 24-7 CYTOKINE RECEPTOR ACTIVATION MODELS. **A,** Ligand-induced dimerization of separate subunits. **B,** Ligand-induced conformational change in a preformed dimer. In either case, proximity of the cytoplasmic domains allows associated JAK tyrosine kinases to activate each other by transphosphorylation. See Fig. 27-9 for details. (Reference: Remy I, Wilson IA, Michnick SW, et al: Erythropoietin receptor activation by a ligand-induced conformational change. Science 283:990–993, 1999.)

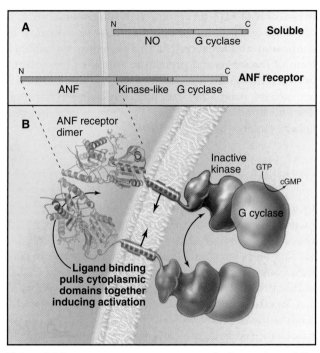

Figure 24-9 GUANYLYLCYCLASE RECEPTORS. **A,** Comparison of the domain architecture of the transmembrane atrial natriuretic factor (ANF) receptor and the cytoplasmic nitric oxide receptor. **B,** Ribbon model of the extracellular domains of a dimer ANF receptor showing how binding of ANF brings together the cytoplasmic domains, which activates the guanylylcyclase activity by an unknown mechanism. (PDB file: 1JDN. Reference: He X-L, Chow DC, Martick MM, Garcia KC: Allosteric activation of a spring-loaded natriuretic peptide receptor dimer by hormone. Science 293:1657–1662, 2001.)

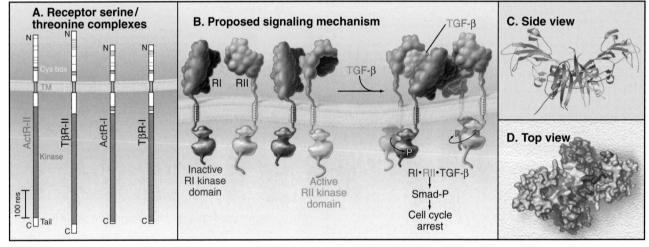

Figure 24-8 RECEPTOR SERINE/THREONINE KINASES. **A,** Drawing of domain architecture of activin and transforming growth factor-β (TGF-β) receptors. (TM, transmembrane domain.) **B,** Mechanism of activation of receptor serine/threonine kinases. Ligand binds two type II receptors (RII) and two type I receptors (RI). Within this hexameric complex, the type II receptor phosphorylates and activates the type I receptors, which in turn phosphorylate cytoplasmic transcription factors called Smads. Phosphorylated Smads move to the nucleus to activate particular genes. See Fig. 27-10 for details. **C–D,** Ribbon and space-filling models of BMP7 bound to type I and type II receptors. This model is based on crystal structures of dimeric BMP7 bound to two extracellular domains of the type II activin receptor and of BMP2 bound to two extracellular domains of BMP type I receptor. (References: Greenwald J, Groppe J, Gray P, et al: The BMP7/ActRII extracellular domain complex provides new insights into the cooperative nature of receptor assembly. Mol Cell 11:605–617, 2003; and Shi Y, Massague J: Mechanisms of TGFβ signaling from cell membranes to the nucleus. Cell 113:685–700, 2003. PDB files: 1LX5 and 1S4Y.)

type I receptors and five type II receptors. Active receptors phosphorylate transcription factors called **Smads,** stimulating their movement from cytoplasm into the nucleus, where they regulate genes controlling cellular proliferation and differentiation (see Fig. 27-10).

Humans have 40 proteins that bind receptor serine/threonine kinases, including **transforming growth factor-β (TGF-β), activin, inhibins,** and **bone morphogenetic proteins.** These dimeric growth factors are particularly important during embryonic development. Activin was discovered as a releasing factor for pituitary follicle-stimulating hormone but also has a strong influence on the differentiation of early embryonic cells into primitive germ layers. Bone morphogenetic proteins influence the differentiation of osteoblasts, which lay down bone matrix, among many other cells. TGF-β has two distinct effects. First, it inhibits proliferation of most adult cells. Mice with null mutations of one of their three TGF-β genes die with inflammation in multiple organs caused by excessive proliferation of lymphocytes. Second, TGF-β stimulates production of extracellular matrix, including collagen, proteoglycans, and adhesive glycoproteins (see Chapter 29). These proteins are essential for the development of organs. Overproduction of extracellular matrix is a common feature of many chronic inflammatory diseases, so inappropriate expression of TGF-β might provide a link between inflammation and the pathological fibrosis that scars diseased organs. On the other hand, loss of TGF-β receptors during progression of some tumors makes them unresponsive to growth inhibition by TGF-β and contributes, in part, to their ability to replicate autonomously.

Serine/threonine kinase receptors are composed of two types of subunits called type I receptors and type II receptors, which are present in small numbers on the cell surface. Single transmembrane sequences link the small ligand-binding domains to cytoplasmic serine/threonine kinase domains. Signal transduction requires the kinase activities of both subunits.

Four receptor subunits bind independently to a dimeric ligand, beginning with high-affinity binding of two type II receptors followed by lower-affinity interactions with two type I receptors (Fig. 24-8B). Within this complex, the constitutively active type II receptor kinases phosphorylate the cytoplasmic domain of the type I receptors on serine and threonine residues. This activates the type I receptor kinase, which phosphorylates cytoplasmic transcription factors called Smads. Phosphorylated Smads move to the nucleus, where they cooperate with other transcription factors to regulate gene expression (see Fig. 27-10).

In addition to these transducing receptors, cells have a greater abundance of another plasma membrane TGF-β-binding protein (type III receptors) that lacks signal transduction activity. A single transmembrane sequence links the large extracellular proteoglycan domain to a small cytoplasmic domain. This receptor may concentrate TGF-β on the cell surface. Even in the absence of TGF-β, type II receptors phosphorylate type III receptors, creating a binding site for β-arrestin and promoting endocytosis of both type II and type III receptors.

Guanylyl Cyclase Receptors

Animals have a family of cell surface receptors (Fig. 24-9) with intracellular domains that catalyze the formation of 3′-5′-cGMP from GTP. Vertebrates have at least seven guanylyl cyclase receptor isoforms; nematode worms have more than 25. The gases **nitric oxide** and carbon monoxide activate related cytoplasmic guanylyl cyclases that participate in additional signal transduction pathways (see Fig. 26-1). Regardless of its enzymatic origin, cGMP regulates the same targets: **cGMP-gated ion channels** (see Fig. 10-10), **cGMP-stimulated protein kinases** (see Fig. 25-4), and **cyclic nucleotide phosphodiesterases** (see Fig. 26-1).

All known ligands for guanylyl cyclase receptors are peptides, although the ligands for some receptors are not known. Most insights regarding function have come from knowledge about the ligands, the tissue distribution of receptors, and receptor gene disruptions, as highly specific inhibitors of the cell surface guanylyl cyclases are not available.

Guanylyl cyclase receptors are homodimers with novel, ligand-binding extracellular domains and two cytoplasmic domains—an enzymatically inactive kinase domain and a guanylyl cyclase domain (Fig. 24-9). The cyclase domain is closely related to adenylyl cyclases (see Fig. 26-2). In the absence of ligand, the extracellular domains hold the cytoplasmic domains apart. Ligand binding closes the cleft between the extracellular domains, pulling together the transmembrane and cytoplasmic domains in a way that stimulates guanylyl cyclase activity.

Guanylyl cyclase receptor A (GC-A) binds **atrial natriuretic factor,** a polypeptide hormone that is secreted mainly by the heart to control blood pressure. It stimulates excretion of salt and water by the kidney and dilates blood vessels. Mice with null mutations for GC-A have high blood pressure and enlarged hearts and fail to respond when overloaded with fluid and salt administered intravenously. Intestinal guanylyl cyclase receptor C (GC-C) binds bacterial **enterotoxin,** the mediator of fluid secretion in bacterial dysentery. The bacterial toxin mimics endogenous peptides of unknown function, which are secreted by various tissues but principally by the intestine. Mice with null mutations for GC-C are completely resistant to enterotoxin but have no apparent physiological defects. Guanylyl cyclase receptors E and F (GC-E, GC-F) are restricted to the eye; a null mutation for GC-E results in loss of cone visual receptor cells. Guanylyl cyclase receptor D is restricted to olfactory neuroepithelium. Sea urchin spermatozoa use a guanylyl cyclase receptor to respond to peptides secreted by eggs.

Tumor Necrosis Factor Receptor Family

TNF and its receptor are the prototypes for a diverse group of cell-signaling partners (Fig. 24-10). Lymphocytes produce three isoforms of TNF (also called lymphotoxin and cachectin), a trimeric lymphokine with many functions, including roles in shock and inflammation, protection from bacterial infections, killing tumor cells, and wasting in chronic disease. Mice with a genetic deletion of the lymphotoxin-α gene have no lymph nodes, so TNF participates in the development of the immune system. Other ligands for the TNF class of receptors are also trimers of subunits composed of β-strands, such as **nerve growth factor** and **Fas-ligand.** These ligands and receptors regulate many processes, including cell proliferation and death (see Fig. 46-17).

Human cells express two types of TNF receptors that bind the same ligands but generate different responses. The two receptors have similar ligand-binding domains coupled by single transmembrane segments to different cytoplasmic domains. The extracellular part of these receptors consists of four similar repeats of about 40 amino acids, each with six conserved cysteines (Fig. 24-10B). The cysteines form three disulfide bridges, arranged like the rungs of a ladder, to stabilize these small domains. In the absence of ligand, individual receptor subunits are presumed to diffuse independently in the plane of the membrane.

The structure of TNF bound to the extracellular domains of its receptor showed how the receptor works. Three finger-like receptors grasp one trimeric TNF molecule by binding along the interfaces between TNF subunits. The tapered shape of TNF brings together the transmembrane segments and cytoplasmic domains of three receptors. Something about this arrangement of TNF receptors activates a plasma membrane phospholipase that hydrolyzes sphingomyelin, producing the second messenger **ceramide** (see Fig. 26-11). Adapter proteins associated with active TNF receptors recruit protein kinases that alter gene expression by activating the transcription factor NF-κB (see Fig. 15-22). Other receptors with linear arrays of cysteine-rich subdomains, similar to the TNF receptor, also bind to multimeric ligands, so receptor activation by clustering their cytoplasmic domains might be a general theme. For example, Fas ligand triggers cell death by clustering Fas and activating a cascade of intracellular proteolysis (see Fig. 46-17).

TNF participates in the inflammation associated with autoimmune diseases such as rheumatoid arthritis. Intercepting TNF before it reaches its receptor is remarkably successful in blunting inflammation in these diseases. This is accomplished by injections of monoclonal antibodies to TNF or with constructs containing the extracellular domains of the TNF receptor.

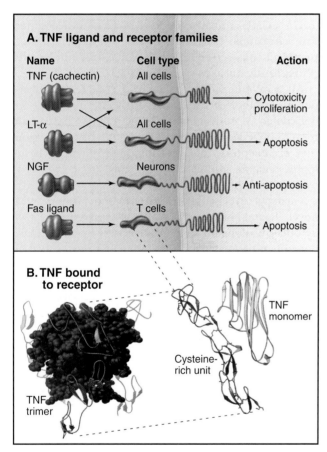

A. TNF ligand and receptor families

Name	Cell type	Action
TNF (cachectin)	All cells	Cytotoxicity proliferation
LT-α	All cells	Apoptosis
NGF	Neurons	Anti-apoptosis
Fas ligand	T cells	Apoptosis

B. TNF bound to receptor

TNF monomer

Cysteine-rich unit

TNF trimer

Figure 24-10   TUMOR NECROSIS FACTOR RECEPTOR FAMILY. **A,** Domain architecture of a sample of members from the TNF receptor family. (LT-α, lymphotoxin-α; NGF, nerve growth factor.) Fas and Fas ligand are presented in Chapter 46. **B,** Atomic model of TNF bound to its receptor. TNF is a trimer of three identical β sandwich subunits arranged in a pear-like structure. The four extracellular cysteine-rich domains of the receptor grasp TNF-like prongs. (A, Adapted with permission from Beutler B, vanHuffel C: Unraveling function in the TNF ligand and receptor family. Science 264:667–668, 1994. Copyright 1994 AAAS. B, Reference: Banner DW, D'Arcy A, Janes W, et al: Crystal structure of the soluble human 55 kD TNF receptor-human TNF beta complex: Implications for TNF receptor activation. Cell 73:431–445, 1993. PDB file: 1TNR.)

Toll-Like Receptors

Metazoan organisms use a small family of receptors named Toll-like receptors (TLRs) to sense and respond

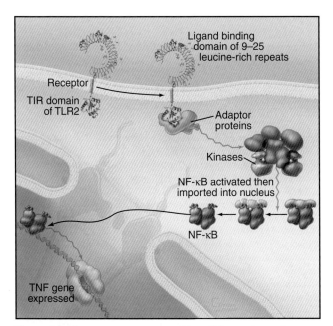

Figure 24-11 TOLL-LIKE RECEPTORS. Most TLRs are homodimers or heterodimers, but this figure shows a ribbon diagram of a single receptor molecule assembled from crystal structures of different receptors. Ribbon diagram of the extracellular domain of TLR3, an endosomal TLR consisting of 23 leucine-rich repeats that binds double-stranded RNAs released from viruses. A transmembrane helix connects to the cytoplasmic TIR domain from TLR2, a receptor for bacterial lipoproteins. Ligand binding to receptor dimers initiates a signal that is transmitted through adapter proteins to kinases, which activate cytoplasmic transcription factors including NF-κB. NF-κB moves to the nucleus and stimulates expression of TNF and other inflammatory mediators. (PDB file for the extracellular domain of TLR3: 1ZIW. PDB file for the cytoplasmic domain of TLR2: 1FYW.)

to infection by a wide variety of microorganisms including viruses, bacteria, fungi, and protozoa. The Toll gene was discovered in *Drosophila* encoding a receptor that was first linked to dorsal-ventral polarity in early development and was later found to be required for resistance to fungal infections. Mammals have about a dozen TLRs (Fig. 24-11) that bind certain macromolecules associated with microorganisms: double-stranded RNA from viruses, flagellin from bacteria, lipopolysaccharide from the outer membrane of gram-negative bacteria, and zymosan from the cell walls of fungi. Dimeric TLRs on the plasma membrane of white blood cells (including lymphocytes) and antigen-processing cells called dendritic cells sense these foreign macromolecules and stimulate the cell to respond by secreting inflammatory mediators such as TNF and interleukin-1 and -6. TLR3 is located in endosomes, where it can bind double-stranded RNA released from viruses. The signaling pathway from TLRs to TNF involves cytoplasmic adapter proteins and kinases that activate transcription factors

including NF-κB (see Fig. 15-22C). TNF and interleukins then alert distant cells to respond to the infection.

Notch Receptors

Components of the Delta/Notch signaling pathway have been identified by analysis of mutations affecting early development in flies and nematodes. Ligands are transmembrane proteins called **Delta** in flies and vertebrates and LAG-2 in worms. These ligands and **Notch receptors** regulate cellular fates during early embryonic development. Typically, cells expressing Delta interact with Notch receptors on adjacent cells to force the neighboring cells to chose a different fate than their own. The actual outcome depends on the context; in each tissue, Delta/Notch signals are integrated with the actions of other signaling pathways. As a general point, Delta/Notch signals tend to reinforce differences between cells in a particular tissue. For example, Delta on the earliest neurons directs adjacent cells to other fates. Defects in Delta or Notch result in excess neurons.

Genetic analysis established that Delta/Notch signaling is vital for animal development, but less is known about the mechanisms than those of the other receptors presented in this chapter. Some Delta is active as a cell surface protein that interacts locally with adjacent cells, but a matrix metalloproteinase (see Fig. 29-20) cleaves some Delta from the membrane, allowing it to act at a distance from its cell of origin. The receptors, called Notch (flies, vertebrates) or Lin-12 (worms), consist of several extracellular EGF-like domains and leucine-rich repeats, a single transmembrane span, and an intracellular region of ankyrin repeats that lacks any known enzyme activity. Notch is synthesized as a single polypeptide chain and is cleaved once before transport to the plasma membrane. The two polypeptides remain covalently associated, presumably by a disulfide bond. Cells carrying Delta activate Notch receptors on adjacent cells. This leads to proteolytic cleavage that frees the intracellular domains from the membrane. These cytoplasmic domains move into the nucleus and join a complex of proteins, including CSL, that activate transcription of certain genes.

Hedgehog Receptors

Genetic studies of *Drosophila* revealed a novel class of protein ligands, called **Hedgehog,** and two membrane proteins, called **Patched** and **Smoothened,** that are required for signal transduction during development. The Hedgehog receptor Patched consists of 12 transmembrane segments related to proton-driven bacterial antiporters, but the transported substrate, if any, is not known. Smoothened is an unusual seven-helix receptor, because it is constitutively active. Substoichiometric quantities of Patched inhibit the activity of Smoothened, perhaps by transporting out of the cell a ligand that binds and inhibits Smoothened. In flies, the Hedgehog pathway cooperates with the **Wnt** system (see Fig. 30-8) to establish boundaries between segments of the embryo and maintain a pool of stem cells.

Every aspect of this novel signaling pathway established new principles. A signal sequence guides Hedgehog protein into the secretory pathway, but before it reaches the cell surface, the protein cleaves itself in two pieces. The latter half of the protein carries out the cleavage reaction. This autocatalytic reaction also adds a molecule of **covalently bound cholesterol** to the new C-terminus of the first half of the protein, the domain with signaling activity. This was the first example of cholesterol being used for a posttranslational modification of a protein. Cholesterol and an N-terminal palmitic acid anchor the signaling domain to membranes and lipoprotein particles, which are secreted and act on cells up to 30 cell diameters distant from the source.

The Hedgehog signal transduction pathway is complicated, in part because activation is achieved by *inactivating inhibitors*. In the absence of Hedgehog, active Patched inhibits Smoothened. Hedgehog binding turns off Patched and relieves the inhibition of Smoothened (the first inactivation of an inhibitor in this pathway). Active Smoothened assembles a complex of several proteins that inhibits the proteolytic inactivation of a transcription factor called Ci (the second inactivation of an inhibitor in this pathway). Active Ci controls the expression of several genes required for cell fate specification and differentiation including Patched itself.

Vertebrate orthologs of the proteins that form the insect Hedgehog pathway have similar functions, regulating cellular differentiation in many tissues, including formation of the neural tube. Mutations in one of three mammalian Hedgehog genes (sonic hedgehog) cause widespread developmental defects that range from mild to grotesque, including a single eye in the middle of the face. Mutations in the gene for Patched cause basal cell carcinoma of the skin, the most common cancer in fair-skinned people. Human Smoothened is a proto-oncogene; activating mutations prevent its inhibition by Patched and cause skin tumors. The Ci ortholog Gli1 is an oncogene that was originally discovered in brain tumors.

ACKNOWLEDGMENTS

Thanks go to Senyon Choe, Dan Leahy, and Ruslan Medzhitov for their suggestions on revisions to this chapter.

SELECTED READINGS

Beutler B: Inferences, questions and possibilities in Toll-like receptor signalling. Nature 430:257-263, 2004.

Bray D: Signaling complexes: Biophysical constraints on intracellular communication. Annu Rev Biophys Biomol Struct 27:59-75, 1998.

Burgess AW, Cho H-S, Eigenbrot C, et al: An open-and-shut case? Recent insights into the activation of EGF/ErbB receptors. Mol Cell 12:541-552, 2003.

Carpenter G: Nuclear localization and possible functions of receptor tyrosine kinases Curr Opin Cell Biol 15:143-148, 2003.

Haglund K, Di Fiore PP, Dikic I: Distinct monoubiquitin signals in receptor endocytosis. Trends Biochem Sci 28:598-604, 2003.

Hubbard SR, Till JH: Protein tyrosine kinase structure and function. Annu Rev Biochem 69:373-398, 2000.

Kadesch T: Notch signaling: The demise of elegant simplicity. Curr Opin Genet Dev 14:506-512, 2004.

Krzysztof P: G protein-coupled receptor rhodopsin. Annu Rev Biochem 75:743-767, 2006.

Lefkowitz RJ, Whalen EJ: Beta-arrestins: Traffic cops of cell signaling. Curr Opin Cell Biol 16:162-168, 2004.

Lum L, Beachy PA: The Hedgehog response network: Sensors, switches and routers. Science 304:1755-1759, 2004.

Marchese A, Chen C, Kim Y-M, Benovic JL: The ins and outs of G protein-coupled receptor trafficking. Trends Biochem Sci 28:369-376, 2003.

Park PS, Filipek S, Wells JW, Palczewski K: Oligomerization of G protein-coupled receptors: Past, present, and future. Biochemistry 43:15643-15656, 2004.

Penn RB, Pronin AN, Benovic JL: Regulation of G protein-coupled receptor kinases. Trends Cardiovasc Med 10:81-89, 2000.

Sakmar TP: Structure of rhodopsin and the superfamily of seven-helical receptors: The same and not the same. Curr Opin Cell Biol 14:189-195, 2002.

Schoneberg T, Schulz A, Biebermann H, et al: Mutant G-protein-coupled receptors as a cause of human diseases. Pharmacol Ther 104:173-206, 2004.

Sebald W, Mueller TD: The interaction of BMP-7 and ActRII implicates a new mode of receptor assembly. Trends Biochem Sci 28:518-521, 2003.

Shi Y, Massague J: Mechanisms of TGFβ signaling from cell membranes to the nucleus. Cell 113:685-700, 2003.

Takeda K, Kaisho T, Akira S: Toll-like receptors. Annu Rev Immunol 21:335-376, 2003.

Wells JA, de Vos AM: Hematopoietic receptor complexes. Annu Rev Biochem 65:609-634, 1996.

Zhang G: Tumor necrosis factor family ligand-receptor binding. Curr Opin Struct Biol 14:154-160, 2004.

Zhang X, Gureasko J, Shen K, et al: An allosteric mechanism for activation of the kinase domain of epidermal growth factor receptor. Cell 125:1137-1149, 2006.

APPENDIX 24-1

Receptors and Ligands

Classes of Receptors Activators	Nature of Activation	Examples of Biological Function
Voltage-Gated Ion Channels→Membrane Depolarization or Repolarization		
Voltage-gated potassium channel	Electrical	Membrane repolarization
Voltage gated sodium channel	Electrical	Action potential
Ligand-Gated Ion Channels→Changes in Membrane Permeability		
Acetylcholine (nicotinic)	Biogenic amine	Action potential
Adenosine triphosphate	Nucleotide	Change in membrane potential
Glutamate (N-methyl-D-aspartate)	Amino acid	Change in membrane potential
Glutamate (non–N-methyl-D-aspartate)	Amino acid	Change in membrane potential
Glycine	Amino acid	Change in membrane potential
Serotonin	Biogenic amine	Change in membrane potential
Seven-Helix Receptors→Trimeric G Proteins→Diverse Responses		
Acetylcholine (muscarinic)	Biogenic amine	Slows heart; stimulates intestinal secretion
Adrencorticotropic hormone	Peptide	Stimulates adrenal cortisol production
Adenosine	Nucleoside	Dilates blood vessels
Angiotensin II	Peptide	Stimulates aldosterone secretion; contracts smooth muscle
Bradykinin	Protein	Stimulates intestinal secretion
Calcitonin	Protein	Inhibits calcium resorption from bone
Cholecystokinin	Peptide	Stimulates intestinal secretion
Complement (C5a, C3a)	Protein	Leukocyte chemoattractant
Dopamine	Biogenic amine	Neurotransmitter; inhibits prolactin secretion
Eicosanoids (prostaglandins)	Lipid	Promote or inhibit platelet aggregation, many other actions
Endothelins	Protein	Vasoconstriction
Epinephrine	Biogenic amine	Glycogenolysis; increases cardiac contractility
F-met-leu-phe	Peptide	Leukocyte chemotaxis
Follicle-stimulating hormone	Protein	Growth of ovarian follicle
γ-aminobutyric acid	Amino acid	Inhibitory neurotransmitter; stimulates intestinal secretion
Glucagon	Peptide	Glycogenolysis; stimulates intestinal secretion
Glutamate	Amino acid	Modulates synaptic transmission
Growth hormone–releasing factor	Peptide	Stimulates secretion of growth hormone
Histamine	Amino acid	Allergic responses; vasodilation; stimulates secretion
Interleukin, IL-8	Protein	Chemotaxis of leukocytes
Leutinizing hormone	Protein	Steroid production by ovarian granulosa cells
Light absorption by rhodopsin	Photon	Vision
Lysophosphatidic acid	Lipid	Fibroblast proliferation, neurite retraction
Melanocyte-stimulating hormone	Protein	Melanin synthesis
Neurokinins (substance P)	Peptide	Stimulates gastrointestinal and pancreatic secretion; neurotransmitter
Norepinephrine	Biogenic amine	Smooth muscle relaxation
Odorants	Organics	Olfaction

Classes of Receptors Activators	Nature of Activation	Examples of Biological Function
Opioids	Alkaloids	Alters mood
Oxytocin	Peptide	Contraction of uterus
Parathyroid hormone	Protein	Bone calcium resorption
Peptide-releasing factors	Protein	Secretion of pituitary hormones
Platelet-activating factor	Lipid	Platelet activation
Serotonin	Biogenic amine	Stimulates intestinal secretion
Somatostatin	Peptide	Inhibits secretion of growth hormone, insulin, and glucagon
Thrombin	Protein	Activates platelets
Thyroid-stimulating hormone	Protein	Thyroid hormone secretion
Vasoactive intestinal peptide	Peptide	Stimulates intestinal secretion
Melanocyte-stimulating hormone	Biogenic amine	Stimulates gastrointestinal and pancreatic secretion; neurotransm
Vasopressin	Peptide	Regulates the permeability of the renal tubule to water
Wingless (Wnt)	Protein	Modulates gene expression
Two-Component Systems: Receptor/Histidine Kinase→Response Regulator→Diverse Responses		
Aspartate	Amino acid	Controls flagellar motor and chemotaxis
Osmotic pressure	Physical	Regulates gene expression
Receptor Tyrosine Kinase→Ras, MAP Kinase, PLC, PI3 Kinase		
Epidermal growth factor	Protein	Epithelial cell proliferation and differentiation
Fibroblast growth factor-α	Protein	Mesoderm differentiation; fibroblast mitogen
Fibroblast growth factor-β	Protein	Fibroblast mitogen
Hepatocyte growth factor (scatter factor)	Protein	Epithelial cell mitogenesis, motility
Insulin	Protein	Glucose uptake; cell growth
Insulin-like growth factor I	Protein	General body growth
Macrophage colony-stimulating factor	Protein	Growth and differentiation of monocytes
Neurotrophins (nerve growth)	Protein	Neural growth; neuron survival
Platelet-derived growth factor	Protein	Smooth muscle, fibroblast, glial growth and differentiation
Steel ligand	Protein	Development of melanocytes, germ cells
Transforming growth factor-α	Protein	Differentiation of connective tissue
Vascular endothelial cell growth factor	Protein	Endothelial cell growth
Cytokine Receptors→JAK Kinase→STAT Transcription Factors→Gene Expression		
Ciliary neurotrophic factor	Protein	Survival/differentiation of neurons and glial cells
Erythropoietin	Protein	Growth and differentiation of red cell precursors
Granulocyte (colony-stimulating factor)	Protein	Growth and differentiation of granulocyte precursors
Granulocyte-monocyte (colony-stimulating factor)	Protein	Growth and differentiation of leukocyte precursors
Growth hormone	Protein	Cell growth and differentiation of somatic cells
Interleukin, IL-2	Protein	Growth factor for lymphocytes
Interleukin, IL-3	Protein	Growth factor for hematopoietic stem cells
Interleukin, IL-4	Protein	Regulates gene expression
Interleukin, IL-5	Protein	Regulates gene expression
Interleukin, IL-6	Protein	Regulates gene expression
Interferon α/β	Protein	Regulates gene expression
Interferon γ	Protein	Macrophage and lymphocyte gene expression
Prolactin	Protein	Stimulates milk synthesis
Tyrosine Kinase–Linked Receptors→Cytoplasmic Tyrosine Kinase→Gene Expression		
MHC-peptide complex→T-cell receptor	Protein	Growth and differentiation of T lymphocytes
Antigens→B-cell receptor	Various	Growth and differentiation of B lymphocytes

Classes of Receptors Activators	Nature of Activation	Examples of Biological Function
Receptor Serine/Threonine Kinase→Smad Transcription Factors→Control of Gene Expression		
Activin	Peptide	Mesoderm development
Bone morphogenetic protein	Protein	Mesoderm development
Inhibins	Protein	Inhibition of gonadal stromal mitogenesis
Transforming growth factor-β	Protein	Growth arrest, mesoderm development
Membrane Guanylyl Cyclase Receptors→cGMP→Regulation of Kinases and Channels		
Atrial natriuretic peptide	Peptide	Vasodilation; sodium excretion; intestinal secretion
Heat-stable endotoxin, guanylin		Unknown
Sea urchin egg peptides	Peptide	Fertilization
Sphingomyelinase-Linked Receptors→Ceramide-Activated Kinases→Gene Expression		
Interleukin, IL-1	Protein	Inflammation, wound healing
Tumor necrosis factor	Protein	Inflammation, tumor cell death
Integrins→Nonreceptor Tyrosine Kinases→Diverse Responses		
Fibronectin, other matrix proteins	Protein	Cell motility, gene expression
Selectins		
Mucins	Glycoproteins	Cell adhesion
Cadherins		
Like cadherins on another cell	Protein	Contact inhibition
Notch		
Delta	Cell surface protein	Cell fate determination
Cytoplasmic Guanylyl Cyclase Receptors→cGMP→Kinases, cGMP-Gated Channels		
Nitric oxide	Gas	Smooth muscle relaxation
Cytoplasmic Steroid Receptors→Active Transcription Factor→Gene Expression		
Retinoic acid	Organic	Cell growth and differentiation
Steroid hormones	Steroids	Cell growth and differentiation
Thyroid hormone	Amino acid	Cell growth and differentiation

CHAPTER 25

Protein Hardware for Signaling

This chapter introduces proteins that transduce signals in the cytoplasm: protein kinases, protein phosphatases, guanosine triphosphatases (GTPases), and adapter proteins. Remarkably, kinases and GTPases use the same strategy to operate molecular switches that carry information through signaling pathways: the simple addition and removal of inorganic phosphate. Protein kinases add phosphate groups to specific protein targets, and phosphatases remove them. GTPases bind guanosine triphosphate (GTP) and hydrolyze it to guanosine diphosphate (GDP) and inorganic phosphate, which dissociates. In both cases, the presence or absence of a single phosphate group switches a protein between active and inactive conformations.

Because addition of phosphate is reversible, both types of switches can be used as molecular timers that cycle on and off at tempos determined by the intrinsic properties of the switch and its environment. GTPases are active with bound GTP and switch off when they hydrolyze GTP to GDP. Similarly, phosphorylation activates many proteins but can inhibit others. In all of these examples, a single protein acts as a simple binary switch.

These molecular switches are often linked in series to form a **signaling cascade** that can both transmit and refine signals. Enzymes along signaling pathways (including kinases) often act as amplifiers. Turning on the binary switch of one enzyme molecule can produce many product molecules, each of which, in turn, may continue to propagate and amplify the original signal by activating downstream molecules. Other pathways involve negative feedback loops. Few signaling pathways are linear; instead, most branch and intersect, allowing cells to integrate information from multiple receptors and to control multiple effector systems simultaneously. Chapter 27 illustrates the functions of molecular switches in several signaling pathways.

Protein Phosphorylation

Phosphorylation is the most common posttranslational modification of proteins and regulates the activity of one or more proteins along most signaling pathways. Among other things, phosphorylation controls metabolic enzymes, cell motility, membrane channels, assembly of the nucleus, and cell cycle progression. Sometimes, phosphorylation turns a process on; sometimes, it turns one off. In either case, both the addition of a phosphate by a **protein kinase** and its removal by a **protein phosphatase** are required to achieve regulation.

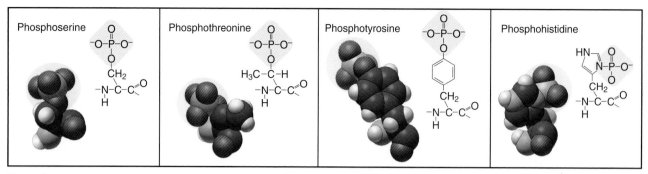

Figure 25-1 STRUCTURES OF PHOSPHOAMINO ACIDS. In addition to the N1 nitrogen illustrated, histidine is often phosphorylated on N3 at the upper left.

For historical and practical reasons, it has been easier to study protein kinases than protein phosphatases, so most research and accounts of regulation by phosphorylation emphasize kinases (witness the 361,167 PubMed hits for "protein kinase" compared with 127,267 for "protein phosphatase" in August 2006). Furthermore, many researchers assumed incorrectly that phosphatases are always active, leading to a lack of interest in their roles in signaling reactions. Readers should not forget that both directions are important on this two-way street.

In eukaryotes, more than 99% of protein phosphorylation occurs on **serine** and **threonine** residues, but phosphorylation of **tyrosine** residues regulates many processes in animals (Fig. 25-1). Bacteria and Archaea use **histidine** and **aspartate** phosphorylation for signaling (see Fig. 27-11), but these modifications are little known in eukaryotes. Phosphohistidine and phosphoaspartate are more difficult to assay than are other phosphorylated residues, so pathways using these phosphoamino acids might have escaped detection.

Effects of Phosphorylation on Protein Structure and Function

Despite its small size, phosphate is well suited to cause changes in the activity of proteins. The addition of a phosphate group with two negative charges to a single amino acid can change the conformation of a protein or alter interactions with other molecules, including the interaction of substrates with enzymes. A phosphate group can alter the activity of a protein in several ways:

- *Direct interference.* A phosphate group can directly block the binding site for a ligand. For example, phosphorylation inhibits the metabolic enzyme isocitrate dehydrogenase by blocking substrate binding to the active site (Fig. 25-2). Both direct steric hindrance and electrostatic repulsion between the negatively charged phosphate and

negatively charged substrates prevent substrate binding. Phosphorylation also can directly block protein assembly reactions, such as the polymerization of intermediate filaments (see Fig. 35-4) and binding of ADF/cofilin proteins to actin monomers and filaments (see Fig. 44-6).

- *Conformational change.* A phosphate group can participate in hydrogen bonds and electrostatic interactions distinct from those of the hydroxyl group that it replaces on an amino acid side chain. In many cases, these interactions of phosphorylated residues change the conformation of the protein. For example, phosphorylation activates the insulin receptor tyrosine kinases by inducing a dramatic change in a polypeptide loop on its surface (Fig. 25-3E). In the inactive conformation, this loop blocks the substrate-binding site and slows down the phosphorylation reaction. Phosphorylation of a single serine activates the metabolic enzyme glycogen phosphorylase by stabilizing a compact, active conformation.

- *Creation of binding sites.* Reversible phosphorylation controls interactions between partner proteins that require a phosphorylated residue to complete a binding site (Fig. 25-10A). Phosphorylated tyrosines are required for SH2 (Src homology) domains and phosphotyrosine-binding (PTB) do-

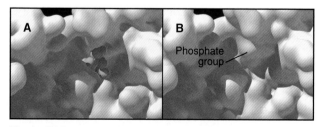

Figure 25-2 PHOSPHORYLATION BLOCKS SUBSTRATE BINDING TO ISOCITRATE DEHYDROGENASE. **A,** Surface representation with isocitrate (*blue*) bound to the active site. **B,** Phosphorylation of serine 113 (*yellow*) blocks isocitrate binding. (PDB files: 3ICD and 4ICD.)

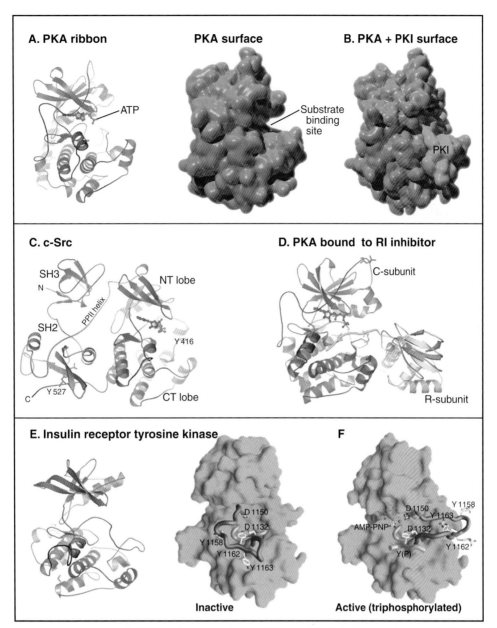

Figure 25-3 PROTEIN KINASE STRUCTURES. **A,** Ribbon diagram and space-filling model of cAMP-dependent protein kinase with a nonhydrolyzable ATP analog *(red)* bound to the active site. The adenine base of the ATP fits into a hydrophobic cleft formed by β-sheets lining the interface of the two lobes. The phosphates bind to conserved residues in loops connecting the β-strands. (PDB file: 1CPK.) **B,** Space-filling model of PKA with bound inhibitory peptide PKI. The location of this inhibitory peptide revealed the binding site for protein substrates. (PDB file: 1FMO.) **C,** Ribbon diagram of c-Src. When tyrosine-527 is phosphorylated, the SH2 domain binds intramolecularly to the C-terminus, locking the kinase in an inactive conformation. The N-terminal SH3 domain binds intramolecularly to a proline-rich sequence (PPII helix) connecting the SH2 and kinase domains. NT and CT are the N- and C-terminal lobes of the kinase domain. **D,** Ribbon diagram of PKA bound to the RIα regulatory subunit. The pseudo substrate peptide *(yellow)* sits in the active site. Binding of cAMP to two sites on the RIα subunit causes a conformational change that dissociates RIα from the catalytic subunit. (PDB file: 1U7E.) **E,** Insulin receptor tyrosine kinase. Ribbon diagram and space-filling model with the catalytic loop in *orange* and the activation loop in *green.* (PDB file: 1IRK.) **F,** Space-filling model of insulin receptor tyrosine kinase triphosphorylated on the activation loop. This rearranges the activation loop, allowing substrates *(pink with a white tyrosine side chain)* access to the active site. AMP-PNP is a nonhydrolyzable analog of ATP with nitrogen bridging the β- and γ-phosphates. (PDB file: 1IR3.) (E–F, Space-filling models courtesy of Steven Hubbard, New York University, New York.)

mains to recognize their protein ligands. A phosphoserine is required on protein ligands for binding 14-3-3 domains, some WW domains, and some FHA domains.

Protein Kinases

Protein kinases catalyze the transfer of the γ-phosphate from adenosine triphosphate (or, rarely, guanosine triphosphate) to amino acid side chains of proteins. Protein kinases are important, as is evident from the remarkable number of genes: 116 in budding yeast (second only to transcription factor genes), 409 in nematode worms (second only to seven-helix receptor genes), and 518 in humans. Most protein kinases in eukaryotes are either **serine/threonine kinases** or **tyrosine kinases** (Appendix 25-1). The difference is that most serine/threonine kinases phosphorylate either serine and threonine but not tyrosine, while most tyrosine kinases phosphorylate tyrosine but not serine or threonine.

Most serine/threonine and tyrosine kinases had a common evolutionary origin and share similar structures and catalytic mechanisms, despite differences in substrate specificity. Tyrosine kinases emerged in animals after their divergence from fungi. Nevertheless, fungi have phosphotyrosine owing to two families of serine/threonine kinases that also phosphorylate tyrosine and three protein tyrosine phosphatases to reverse these reactions. A family of 40 "atypical" protein kinases had a separate origin from the major family. **Lipid kinases** have a catalytic domain related to typical protein kinases. They phosphorylate inositol phospholipids (see Fig. 26-7) or a few proteins.

The catalytic domain of eukaryotic protein kinases consists of about 260 residues in two lobes surrounding the ATP-binding pocket (Fig. 25-3). Despite extensive sequence divergence, all of these kinases have a similar polypeptide fold with conserved residues at critical positions required for catalysis.

Each kinase has a restricted range of protein substrates, so activation of a particular protein kinase changes the phosphorylation and activity of a discrete set of target proteins. Substrate specificity is achieved by selective binding of substrates to a groove on the surface of the kinase (Fig. 25-3B). This groove recognizes amino acids that flank the phosphorylatable residue and position the acceptor amino acid side chain in the active site. Typically, all substrates that bind a particular kinase have similar residues surrounding the target serine, threonine, or tyrosine (a **consensus target sequence**). For example, the consensus sequence for protein kinase A (PKA) is Arg-Arg-Gly-**Ser/Thr**-Ile. The arginines and isoleucine flanking the target serine or threonine residue specify binding to PKA. Interactions outside the catalytic site may also contribute to specific binding.

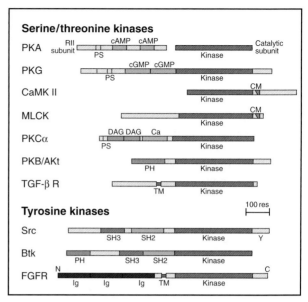

Figure 25-4 PROTEIN KINASE DOMAIN ARCHITECTURE. See Appendix 25-1 for definitions of the kinase names. Btk, Bruton tyrosine kinase; Ca, calcium-binding site; cAMP and cGMP, cyclic nucleotide–binding sites; CM, overlapping pseudosubstrate/calmodulin-binding site; DAG, diacylglycerol-binding site; FGFR, fibroblast growth factor receptor; Ig, immunoglobulin domains; PH, pleckstrin homology domain; PS, pseudosubstrate sequences; SH2 and SH3, Src-homology domains; TM, transmembrane domain.

In addition to the catalytic domain, most protein kinases have other domains for regulation or localization (Fig. 25-4). Adapter domains, such as SH2, SH3, and pleckstrin homology domains (Fig. 25-11), target kinases to specific sites in the cell. Such localization can either bring together a kinase and its substrates or limit their interaction. Transmembrane segments anchor receptor kinases to membranes. Receptor tyrosine kinases usually have additional residues inserted in the kinase domain and at the C-terminus. Phosphorylation of tyrosines in these inserts creates binding sites for effector proteins with SH2 domains (see Figs. 27-6, 27-7, and 27-8).

Prokaryotes generally lack serine/threonine/tyrosine kinases but use a large family of **histidine kinases** for signal transduction (see Fig. 27-11). These prokaryotic kinases differ in structure, mechanism and evolutionary origin from eukaryotic kinases. A few bacteria have acquired eukaryotic kinases by lateral transfer of genes.

Regulation of Protein Kinases

Each kinase has its own regulatory mechanism, but most involve one or more of three strategies: (1) phosphorylation, (2) interactions with intrinsic peptides or extrinsic subunits that may themselves be targets for second messengers or regulatory proteins, and (3) targeting to specific cellular locations, such as the nucleus, plasma membrane, or cytoskeleton, enhancing interaction with specific substrates.

Phosphorylation

Phosphorylation can either activate or inhibit protein kinases. In some cases, another kinase molecule of the same type carries out the phosphorylation, but often another type of kinase is responsible. When linked in series, different types of kinases form signaling cascades that can amplify and sharpen the response to a stimulus (see Fig. 27-5):

- *Activation by phosphorylation.* This is the most common way to regulate kinases. For example, phosphorylation of three tyrosines on an **activation loop** activates the insulin receptor kinase. Phosphorylation refolds the activation loop, allowing substrates access to the active site and bringing together the residues required for catalysis (Fig. 25-3D). Activation loop phosphorylation also turns on other receptor tyrosine kinases, Src-family tyrosine kinases (Fig. 25-3C; see also Box 27-1), mitogen-activated protein (MAP) kinases (see Fig. 27-5), cyclin-dependent kinases (see Fig. 40-14), and calcium-calmodulin–dependent kinases (Fig. 25-4).

- *Inhibition by phosphorylation.* Phosphorylation of myosin light-chain kinase by protein kinase A reduces its affinity for its protein substrate, and phosphorylation of platelet-derived growth factor receptor tyrosine kinase by protein kinase C inhibits its activity. Phosphorylation of a C-terminal tyrosine inhibits Src-family tyrosine kinases by creating an intramolecular binding site for an SH2 domain at the N-terminus (Fig. 25-3C). This interaction traps the kinase in an inactive conformation. Phosphorylation of certain residues also inhibits cyclin-dependent cell cycle kinases (see Fig. 40-14).

Regulation of Substrate Binding

Peptides that are intrinsic to the kinase or part of a separate protein can inhibit kinases by competing with protein substrates for binding to the enzyme (Figs. 25-3B and D and 25-4):

- *Extrinsic regulation by inhibitory subunits.* Separate **regulatory (R) subunits** inhibit PKA by blocking the protein substrate site with a **pseudosubstrate** (Figs. 25-3D and 25-4). Pseudosubstrates have consensus target sequences lacking the phosphorylated residue. For example, RI pseudosubstrate has the sequence Arg-Arg-Gly-**Ala**-Ile, which binds in the substrate groove but is not phosphory-

lated, as it has alanine or glycine, rather than serine, at the phosphorylation site. The RII pseudosubstrate has a serine, which is phosphorylated but then does not dissociate from the catalytic subunit as phosphorylated substrates do. Cyclic adenosine monophosphate (**cAMP**) regulates the affinity of these regulatory subunits for the catalytic subunit. In resting cells, the regulatory subunit is free of cAMP and binds the catalytic subunit with high affinity. With a rise in cAMP concentration (see Fig. 26-3), cAMP binds the regulatory subunit, dissociates it from the catalytic subunit, and allows substrates access to the active site.

- *Autoinhibition.* Many kinases have an intrinsic **pseudosubstrate** sequence (see Fig. 25-4) that binds intramolecularly to the active site, autoinhibiting the enzyme (Fig. 25-3B). **Ca²⁺-calmodulin** activates myosin light-chain kinase and calmodulin-activated kinase (CaMK) by binding immediately adjacent to the pseudosubstrate and displacing the inhibitory peptide from the kinase. Cyclic guanosine monophosphate (cGMP) binding to protein kinase G (PKG) displaces the autoinhibitory peptide from the catalytic domain, activating the enzyme.

- *Extrinsic regulation by activating subunits.* Regulatory subunits can also activate protein kinases. Regulatory subunits called **cyclins** bind and contribute to activating cyclin-dependent cell cycle kinases, **Cdks** (see Fig. 40-14).

- *Dual or triple regulation.* Multiple factors regulate most kinases. Both interaction of calcium-calmodulin with an intrinsic pseudosubstrate and activation loop phosphorylation activate CaMK. Both inhibitory and activating phosphorylation, as well as cyclins and inhibitory subunits, regulate **cyclin-dependent kinases.**

Targeting

Several mechanisms target kinases to specific cellular locations, bringing them close to particular substrates. This targeting helps to explain how kinases with broad specificity can have specific effects in particular target cells:

- The intracellular location of PKA is determined by both its RI and RII subunits and a family of **A kinase–anchoring proteins (AKAPs).** When the cAMP concentration is low, regulatory subunits bind and inhibit PKA. RII subunits also bind to AKAPs, which can target the inhibited PKA catalytic subunit to different cellular locations, including centrosomes, actin filaments, microtubules, endoplasmic reticulum, peroxisomes, mitochondria, or plasma membrane. An increase in cytoplasmic cAMP releases active PKA in close proximity to particular substrates. Once freed from RI or RII subunits by cAMP, the active PKA catalytic subunit can migrate into the nucleus, where it encounters a different array of substrates and regulates gene transcription (see Fig. 26-3F). The inhibitory protein PKI (Fig. 25-3B) is capable of capturing PKA in the nucleus, thereby targeting it for transport back to the cytoplasm. Some AKAPs bind other protein kinases, such as protein kinase C and phosphatases (PP2B). Similar to AKAPs, the inner centromere protein, INCENP, binds and targets aurora-B kinase to various structures during cell division: centromeres early in mitosis and the central spindle and cleavage furrow late in mitosis (see Chapter 44).

- **Pleckstrin homology (PH)** domains (Fig. 25-10A) and lipid tags target some kinases to lipid bilayers. A PH domain directs **PKB/Akt** to membrane polyphosphoinositides. This interaction with lipids opens up sites on the catalytic domain for phosphorylation and activation by PDK1, another kinase with a pleckstrin homology domain. An N-terminal myristic acid anchors Src tyrosine kinase to the plasma membrane.

- Phosphorylation induces the MAP kinase ERK2 to form homodimers, triggering movement of the dimer into the nucleus, where it regulates gene expression.

- A scaffolding protein called STE5, first identified in yeast, brings together three protein kinases that form part of the cascade of kinases that activate MAP kinases (see Fig. 27-5).

Kinases and Disease

Unregulated kinases—for example, the receptor tyrosine kinase RET in endocrine cancers and cyclin-dependent kinase Cdk4 in melanoma—can predispose individuals to cancer. Most patients with chronic myelogenous leukemia have a gene rearrangement that produces a fusion between the protein bcr and c-abl, a nonreceptor tyrosine kinase. The constitutively active fusion protein promotes the transformation of white blood cell precursors into cancer cells. The most effective treatment is with a small molecule called imatinib mesylate (Gleevec), which inhibits bcr-abl kinase activity and kills myelogenous leukemia cells. Inactivation of the serine/threonine kinase LKB1 causes Peutz-Jeghers syndrome with predisposition to various cancers.

Protein Phosphatases

Eukaryotes have several families of protein phosphatases that remove phosphate from amino acid side chains (Table 25-1 and Fig. 25-5). Like protein kinases, most protein phosphatases are active toward either phosphoserine/threonine or phosphotyrosine, although several dual-specificity phosphatases can dephosphorylate all three residues. The 90 active protein tyrosine phosphatases far outnumber the 20 serine/threonine phosphatase genes in the human genome. Each tyrosine phosphatase is thought to act on a limited number of substrates. The small number of serine/threonine phosphatases achieve specificity by associating with an array of accessory subunits, which regulate enzyme activity and target catalytic subunits to particular substrates. Domains flanking the catalytic domains also regulate enzyme activity (Fig. 25-6).

PPP Family of Serine/Threonine Phosphates

Members of the PPP family of **serine/threonine phosphatases** are found in Bacteria, Archaea, and all tissues of eukaryotes. PP1 and PP2A are two of the most evolutionarily conserved enzymes. All three PPP subfamilies share the same catalytic fold with a two-metal ion cluster (Fe^{2+} and Zn^{2+} in vivo) in the active site (Fig. 25-5A). Diverse regulatory subunits restrict the substrates for **PP1** and **PP2A** by targeting catalytic subunits to specific sites in the cell, as illustrated by the following examples:

- PP1: More than 50 associated proteins target a 38-kD catalytic subunit of PP1 to specific substrates. For example, M subunits target PP1 to myosin-II, where dephosphorylation of regulatory light chains relaxes smooth muscle (see Fig. 39-21). The complex of PP1 with an M subunit creates an active site that is specific for myosin-II light chains relative to other substrates. G subunits regulate glucose metabolism by targeting PP1 to glycogen particles, where it dephosphorylates two enzymes that control glycogen metabolism. Dephosphorylation inactivates glycogen phosphorylase, turning off glycogen breakdown, and activates glycogen synthase. The hormone adrenaline stimulates cells to mobilize energy stores by breaking down glycogen (see Fig. 27-3). Adrenaline activates PKA, which phosphorylates the G subunit. The phosphorylated G subunit allows PP1 to dissociate from the glycogen particle, allowing phosphorylase to break down glycogen into glucose-6-phosphate.

- PP2A: This phosphatase usually associates with a 65-kD scaffold subunit and one of several diverse B subunits. PP2A dephosphorylates many substrates, including kinases in the MAP kinase cascade (see Fig. 27-5). The inhibitors okadaic acid (a polyketide from dinoflagellates) and microcystin (a cyclic peptide from cyanobacteria) block access of substrates to the active site of PP2A.

Table 25-1

PROTEIN PHOSPHATASES

Catalytic Subunit	Regulatory Elements	Inhibitors	Regulated Functions
Serine-Threonine Phosphatases			
PPP Family			
PP1C subfamily = catalytic subunit + regulatory subunit	>50 regulatory subunits that target and regulate catalytic subunit	Okadaic acid Microcystin	Glycogen metabolism, muscle contraction, cell cycle, mRNA splicing
PP2A subfamily = catalytic subunit + 65-kD A subunit + B subunit	B subunits target and regulate core enzyme	Okadaic acid Microcystin	MAP kinase pathway, metabolism, cell cycle
PP2B (calcineurin) = catalytic A subunit + one of two B subunits	Calcium-calmodulin activates by binding autoinhibitory peptide	Cyclosporin-cyclophilin FK506-FKBP	T-lymphocyte activation, brain NMDA receptor signaling
PPM Family			
PP2C	Integral N- or C-terminal peptides	Unsaturated fatty acids	Antagonism of stress-activated kinases
Protein Tyrosine Phosphatases			
PTP Family			
Cytosolic PTPs (PTP1B, SHP1, SHP2)	SH2 and other domains target to substrates	Vanadate	Various signaling pathways
Transmembrane PTPs (CD45, RPTPμ, RPTPα)	Homodimerization may inhibit activity	Vanadate	Lymphocyte activation
Dual-specificity Family (MAP kinase phosphatases, etc.)			MAP kinase pathway
Cdc25 Family	Polo kinase, Chk1 kinase, phosphatases	Sulfirein, coscinosulfate	Cell cycle
Low-molecular-weight (Acid phosphatases)	Located in lysosomes	—	Unknown

mRNA, messenger RNA; NMDA, *N*-methyl-D-aspartate.

PP2B, also known as **calcineurin,** is the only cytoplasmic phosphatase regulated by Ca^{2+}. PP2B consists of two subunits: an A subunit with the phosphatase active site and a B subunit that is similar to calmodulin (see Fig. 3-12C) but does not participate in the response to Ca^{2+}. At low concentrations of Ca^{2+}, a C-terminal autoinhibitory segment of the A subunit blocks its own active site. An increase in cytoplasmic Ca^{2+} activates PP2B by first binding to calmodulin. Calcium-calmodulin then binds the autoinhibitory segment and displaces it from the active site. The transcription factor **NF-AT** (nuclear factor–activated T cells) is the best known

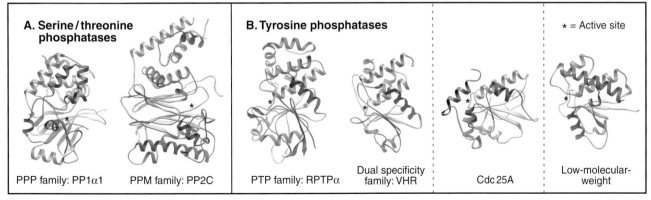

Figure 25-5 PROTEIN PHOSPHATASE STRUCTURES (*RED ASTERISKS* MARK THE ACTIVE SITES). **A,** Serine/threonine phosphatases: PP1α1 (PDB file: 1FJM) and PP2C (PDB file: 1A6O). **B,** Four families of protein tyrosine phosphatases: receptor tyrosine phosphatase RPTPα (PDB file: 1YFO), dual-specificity phosphatase VHR (PDB file: 1VHR), Cdc25A (PDB file: 1C25), and low-molecular-weight phosphatase (PDB file: 1PNT).

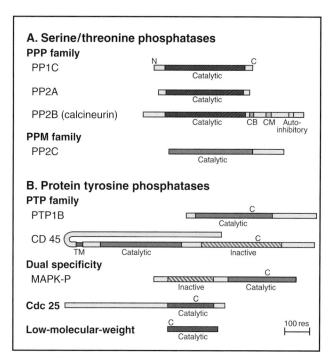

Figure 25-6 PROTEIN PHOSPHATASE DOMAIN ARCHITECTURE. SCALE LINEAR MODELS. **A,** Serine/threonine phosphatases. **B,** Protein tyrosine phosphatases. The five different catalytic domain folds are coded with different colors. CB, calcium binding; CM, calmodulin-binding; TM, transmembrane segment.

substrate (see Fig. 27-8). Activation of T-cell receptors on T lymphocytes releases Ca^{2+} in the cytoplasm and turns on PP2B. Dephosphorylation permits NF-AT to enter the nucleus, where it turns on the expression of several lymphocyte growth factors. PP2B is the indirect target of two potent drugs that inhibit the immune rejection of transplanted organs. These drugs—**cyclosporin** and **FK506**—bind two different small proteins: **cyclophilin** and **FK-binding protein.** Both drug-protein complexes bind PP2B and inhibit the phosphatase directly by blocking the active site. This prevents expression of genes regulated by NF-AT. Suppression of the immune response by cyclosporin revolutionized organ transplantation in humans.

PPM Family of Serine/Threonine Phosphates

Members of the large PPM family of serine/threonine phosphatases are found in Bacteria, plants, fungi, and animals. The catalytic domain is incorporated into a variety of polypeptides with additional domains that confer specificity toward substrates such as stress-activated kinases and mitochondrial dehydrogenases. The structures of PPMs and PPPs are unrelated, but both have two metal ions in the active site (Mg^{2+} for PPM), and both catalyze the same phosphomonoester hydrolytic reaction. This is thought to be an example of **convergent evolution** toward similar active sites.

Protein Tyrosine Phosphatases

The human genome contains 107 genes for protein tyrosine phosphatases (PTPs [Table 25-1]), matching the number of tyrosine kinase genes. PTPs participate in many processes, including lymphocyte activation and regulation of the cell cycle by reversing the actions of protein tyrosine kinases. In some cases, dephosphorylation of tyrosine activates the substrate, such as Src tyrosine kinase (Fig. 25-3C) and cyclin-dependent protein kinases (see Fig. 40-14). PTPs are tumor suppressors; somatic mutations that inactivate these enzymes are common in cancer cells. Eleven of these human PTP genes encode proteins that are missing key catalytic residues in the active site, so they do not hydrolyze phosphotyrosine. Perhaps they serve as adapters to bind proteins with phosphotyrosines.

The four families of PTPs represent a remarkable evolutionary tale. Sequence analysis and atomic structures (Fig. 25-5B) show that three of these families arose from different ancestors but have converged to have similar active sites. PTPs and dual-specificity phosphatases derived from a common ancestor and have similar three-dimensional structures, whereas Cdc25 and low-molecular-weight tyrosine phosphatases have different folds. Nevertheless, all bind phosphotyrosine in a narrow but deep pocket, transfer the phosphate to the sulfur atom of a cysteine in the sequence Cys-x-x-x-x-x-Arg, and release the phosphate in the rate-limiting step, when water attacks the phosphocysteine intermediate.

PTPs are said to have more restricted substrate specificity than serine/threonine phosphatases, but some well-characterized PTPs have multiple substrates. Localization contributes additional specificity. For example, a transmembrane segment that anchors a PTP such as CD45 (Fig. 25-6) to the plasma membrane can enhance its access to some substrates and restrict its access to other substrates.

PTP Subfamily

Humans have 38 genes encoding proteins with PTP catalytic domains of about 230 residues in addition to other domains. PTPs favor phosphotyrosine as a substrate by a factor of 10^5 over phosphoserine or phosphothreonine.

Many cytoplasmic PTPs are bound to cellular partners. Adapter domains, such as SH2 domains, bind the phosphatases SHP-1 and SHP-2 to phosphotyrosines. C-terminal hydrophobic residues bind the phosphatase PTP1B to the endoplasmic reticulum. Transient oxidation of the catalytic cysteine by hydrogen peroxide accompanies activation of some signaling pathways that depend on phosphorylation of tyrosines, such as the insulin pathway (see Fig. 27-7).

Other PTPs are transmembrane proteins with a single transmembrane segment linking a variety of extracellular domains to one or two PTP domains in the cytoplasm (Fig. 25-6). The membrane proximal PTP domain has phosphatase activity. In most cases, the second PTP domain is inactive, so it might have regulatory functions. Extracellular domains are attractive candidates as receptors, and some have been implicated in cellular adhesion, but no extracellular ligand has been shown to regulate phosphatase activity.

CD45, the best-characterized transmembrane PTP, constitutes a remarkable 10% of the plasma membrane protein of human white blood cells. CD45 is required for antigens to activate B and T lymphocytes (see Fig. 27-8). Lymphocytes that lack CD45 fail to release intracellular Ca^{2+}, secrete lymphokines, or proliferate in response to antigen stimulation. It is thought that the CD45 phosphatase activates one or more Src-family tyrosine kinases associated with the T-cell receptor by dephosphorylating inhibitory phosphotyrosine residues (Fig. 25-3C).

Dual-Specificity Subfamily

The dual-specificity family of phosphatases prefers phosphotyrosine as a substrate, but owing to the fact that its substrate-binding site is shallower than that of a PTP, it can also dephosphorylate serine and threonine at about 1% of that rate. The most interesting members of this group, the MKPs, inactivate **MAP kinases** by dephosphorylating both phosphotyrosine and phosphothreonine residues (see Fig. 29-5B). Some members of this family, such as the five **PTEN** phosphatases, remove phosphate from lipids, specifically the D-3 position of polyphosphoinositides (see Fig. 26-7).

Cdc25 Subfamily

Cdc25 removes inhibitory phosphates from adjacent threonine and tyrosine residues on the master cell cycle kinases Cdk1 and Cdk2, releasing these enzymes to promote cell cycle progression (see Fig. 43-4). This is an example of a phosphatase having a positive effect on a biological process. Cdc25 itself is activated by serine/threonine phosphorylation during the cell cycle.

Cooperation between Kinases and Phosphatases

Some protein phosphatases are stably associated with their substrate proteins. One example is the dual-specificity MAP kinase phosphatase-3 (MKP-3) bound to MAP kinase (see Fig. 27-6). Following activation by upstream kinases, this MAP kinase is active only transiently, owing to dephosphorylation by the associated phosphatase. These have been called *self-correcting*

signal complexes, but more broadly speaking, this is an example of a biological timer.

Pharmacological Agents for Studying Protein Kinases and Phosphatases

Inhibitors of protein kinases and protein phosphatases (Table 25-1) are widely used to explore the biological functions of these enzymes. Few, if any, of these inhibitors are entirely specific for one protein kinase or phosphatase. Given that these protein families are so large, caution is required in interpreting experiments with these agents. Nevertheless, some inhibitors of tyrosine kinases are successful anticancer drugs. Development of specific inhibitors of protein phosphatases is challenging, owing to the chemistry of the dephosphorylation reactions and the fact that the enzymes have similar active sites.

Guanosine Triphosphate–Binding Proteins

Cells use GTP-binding proteins (called **GTPases** or **G-proteins**) to regulate a host of functions, including protein synthesis, signal transduction from plasma membrane receptors, regulation of the cytoskeleton, membrane traffic, and nuclear transport (Appendix 25-2). These proteins had a common ancestor, share a homologous core domain that binds a guanine nucleotide (Fig. 25-7), and use a common enzymatic cycle of GTP binding, hydrolysis, and product dissociation to switch the protein on and off (Fig. 25-8).

Genes for GTPases are ancient, as all forms of life use GTPases to regulate protein synthesis. Gene duplication and divergence created 10 families of GTPases in eukaryotes. Further molecular evolution produced multiple isoforms within these families to provide more specificity. Tubulin, the microtubule subunit (see Fig. 34-4), also binds and hydrolyzes GTP but has a completely different fold than do the GTPases considered here.

GTPases share a core GTP-binding domain of about 200 residues folded into a β-sheet of six strands sandwiched between five α-helices (Fig. 25-7). The architecture of this domain was maintained during the evolutionary divergence of the GTPases, despite the fact that about 80% of the residues in this core differ between the major classes. GTP binds in a shallow groove formed largely by loops at the ends of elements of secondary structure. A network of hydrogen bonds between the protein and guanine base, ribose, triphosphate, and Mg^{2+} anchor the nucleotide.

The four main classes of GTPases are elongation factors, small GTPases related to Ras, trimeric G-proteins, and dynamin-related GTPases. Small 20-kD GTPases such as Ras (Fig. 25-7A–B) consist simply of a

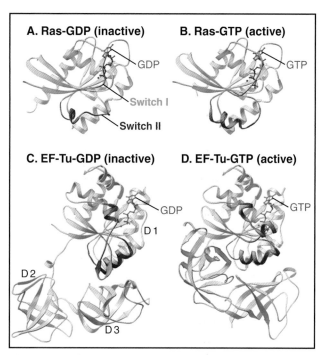

Figure 25-7 GTPase atomic structures. Ribbon models with ball-and-stick models of bound nucleotides. Switch I is *green,* and switch II is *red.* **A,** Ras-GDP. (PDB file: 1Q21.) **B,** Ras-GTP. (PDB file: 121P.) **C,** EF-Tu-GDP. (PDB file: 1TUI.) **D,** EF-Tu-GTP. (PDB file: 1EFT.) GTP hydrolysis and phosphate dissociation cause major changes in the conformations of the switch loops of both proteins and of the orientation of the D2 and D3 domains of EF-Tu.

GTP-binding core domain. The 39- to 45-kD Gα subunits of trimeric G-proteins have an additional domain of α-helices hinged to the core domain by two strands (Fig. 25-9). This helical domain covers the GTP-binding site. Elongation factor EF-Tu (Fig. 25-7C–D) and dynamin (see Fig. 22-11) have additional domains that are required for intermolecular interactions.

All GTPases use the same enzyme cycle. The conformation of a GTPase depends on whether GTP or GDP is bound. The active GTP-bound conformation interacts with effector proteins. The GDP conformation is inactive, because it does not bind effectors. Chapter 4 explains methods that are used to analyze the mechanism (see Figs. 4-6 and 4-7).

The GTPase cycle (Fig. 25-8) consists of four steps: (1) Rapid binding of GTP is coupled to changes in the conformations of three segments of the polypeptide called switch-I, -II, and -III. In the active GTP state, these switch loops form a binding site for downstream target proteins. (2) GTP hydrolysis is slow and irreversible. (3) Dissociation of the γ-phosphate is fast and coupled to the return of the switch loops to the inactive conformation. (4) GTPases tend to accumulate in the inactive GDP-state, because GDP dissociates slowly and GTP cannot bind until GDP dissociates.

GTPases use diverse intrinsic or extrinsic protein modules to regulate the GTPase cycle. Most GTPases

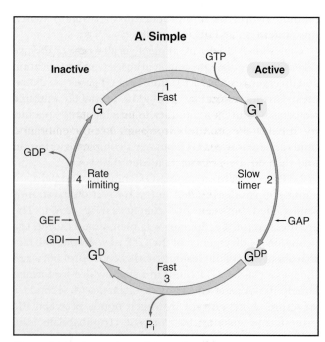

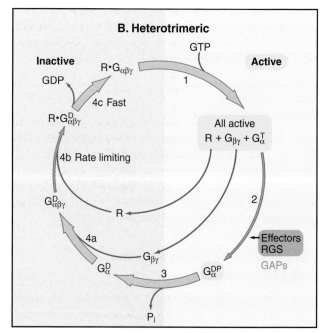

Figure 25-8 Comparison of the GTPase cycles of Ras and a trimeric G-protein. The *size of the arrows* indicates the relative rates of the reactions. **A,** GTPase cycle of Ras. **B,** GTPase cycle and subunit cycle of a trimeric G-protein. R is a seven-helix receptor. Regulators of G-protein signaling (RGS) and some effector proteins stimulate GTP hydrolysis. GAP, GTPase-activating protein; G^D, GTPase with bound GDP; GDI, guanine nucleotide dissociation inhibitor; G^{DP}, GTPase with bound GDP and inorganic phosphate; GEF, guanine nucleotide exchange factor; G^T, GTPase with bound GTP.

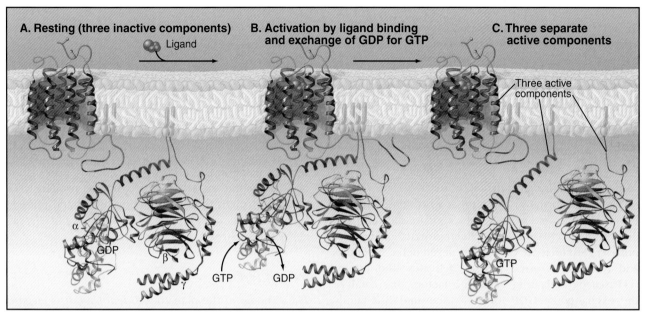

A. Resting (three inactive components)

Ligand

B. Activation by ligand binding and exchange of GDP for GTP

C. Three separate active components

Three active components

α

GDP

β

γ

GTP   GDP

GTP

Figure 25-9 **ATOMIC MODELS OF A SEVEN-HELIX RECEPTOR AND TRIMERIC G-PROTEIN. A,** Resting state lacking a ligand and with the trimeric G-protein in its inactive GDP-Gαβγ state. Both Gα and Gγ are anchored to the lipid bilayer. **B,** Ligand binding activates the receptor, which catalyzes the exchange of GDP for GTP on Gα. **C,** Active Gα and Gβγ dissociate from each other and the receptor and are available to interact with effector proteins.

depend on other proteins, called **guanine nucleotide exchange factors,** to accelerate dissociation of GDP (Appendix 25-2). Although unrelated in structure, guanine nucleotide exchange factors have similar mechanisms. They distort the P loop, the part of the nucleotide binding site that interacts with the β phosphate, allowing GDP to escape, and then bind tightly to the nucleotide-free GTPase. Most small GTPases require extrinsic **GTPase-activating proteins (GAPs)** to stimulate the GTP hydrolysis that turns them off.

Elongation Factors

These GTPases act as timers to ensure the fidelity of protein synthesis (see Fig. 17-10). **Elongation factor Tu (EF-Tu)** has two accessory domains hinged to the GTPase core (Fig. 25-7C–D; see also Fig. 17-10). GTP EF-Tu binds and delivers aminoacyl-tRNAs (transfer RNAs) to the A site of a ribosome. If the tRNA anticodon matches the mRNA codon at the A site, it remains bound long enough for GTP to be hydrolyzed. This releases EF-Tu from the ribosome and allows the correct amino acid to be added to the growing polypeptide chain. The accessory factor EF-Ts is the GDP exchange factor for this system.

Small Guanosine Triphosphatases

The six families of small GTPases consist of a single domain (Fig. 25-7A–B). Three types of small GTPases—Arf, Rab, and Sar—act as switches for intracellular traffic

of membrane vesicles (see Fig. 21-6). The Ran family regulates nuclear transport (see Fig. 14-17) and assembly of the mitotic spindle (see Fig. 44-8). Other chapters explain these processes. This chapter introduces two families of small GTPases, Ras and Rho, that transduce signals from cell surface receptors.

Covalently attached lipids anchor many small GTPases to membrane bilayers. These hydrophobic chains are required for activity. Ras and some Rho and Rab proteins are modified with a C-15 or C-20 prenyl chain on a C-terminal cysteine. Arfs are myristoylated, but other small GTPases, such as Ran, are not modified and are soluble in the cytoplasm. Even membrane-associated GTPases may cycle into the cytoplasm when their lipid tails turn over or when they bind cytoplasmic regulatory proteins such as **Rho-GDI** (Rho-guanine nucleotide dissociation inhibitor [see Fig. 21-11]), Rab, Arf, and Sar GTPases also recycle through the cytoplasm as they direct vesicular traffic from one compartment to another. Membrane association can be regulated either by interactions with accessory proteins (in the case of Rab) or through guanine nucleotide–dependent conformational changes (in the case of Arf and Sar).

Ras is the prototypical small GTPase. Normally, Ras transmits signals from growth factor receptor tyrosine kinases to transcription factors that control genes required for cellular proliferation (see Figs. 27-6 and 27-7). In quiescent cells, Ras accumulates in the inactive GDP form. Stimulation of growth factor receptors attracts SOS, the Ras nucleotide exchange factor, to the membrane, where it activates Ras by exchanging GDP for GTP. Ras-GTP then activates a cascade of protein kinases that ultimately controls gene expression. Ras has low intrinsic GTPase activity (rate = 0.005 s^{-1}; half-time = 140 seconds) that is not stimulated by binding effector proteins. An accessory protein called **Ras-GAP** stimulates GTPase activity 10^5-fold by providing a crucial arginine for the active site. This inactivates Ras until SOS again stimulates dissociation of GDP. Mutations that inhibit GTP hydrolysis predispose to cancer, because without GTP hydrolysis, Ras is continually active and stimulates cellular growth.

The 16 isoforms in the human **Rho** family include Rho itself, Rac, and Cdc42. They regulate the actin and microtubule cytoskeletons, cellular growth, and cellular polarity. Stimulation of certain seven-helix receptors and receptor tyrosine kinases activates Rho family-GTPases by activating exchange factors that catalyze the exchange of GDP for GTP. Activated Rho-family proteins stimulate kinases (such as **p21-activated kinase** and Rho-kinase), which mediate downstream effects on the actin cytoskeleton. For example, Rho-kinase activates myosin-II by phosphorylating the regulatory light chain and inhibiting the light chain phosphatase (see Fig. 39-21). Activated Cdc42 binds **Wiskott-Aldrich syndrome protein** (WASp), a protein that regulates actin filament nucleation (see Figs. 33-17 and 38-8). WASp is defective in Wiskott-Aldrich syndrome, an inherited human disease characterized by a deficiency in blood cell function. Rac stimulates another protein related to WASp that regulates actin filament nucleation.

Trimeric G-Proteins

These GTP-binding proteins transduce signals received from seven-helix receptors for hormones, light, and odors to a variety of effector proteins, including enzymes and ion channels. However, in rare cases, signals that activate trimeric G-proteins can also arise inside the cell independent of transmembrane receptors. The best-characterized examples are G-proteins that regulate asymmetrical cell division.

Trimeric G-proteins have three subunits (Fig. 25-9). Gα subunits have a GTP-binding domain similar to small GTPases plus a helical domain that helps to trap the bound nucleotide. Gβ and Gγ subunits bind tightly to each other and reversibly to Gα. Seven-helix receptors activate trimeric G-proteins by promoting dissociation of GDP bound to an inactive trimeric protein. GTP binding changes the conformation of Gα and releases G$\beta\gamma$. This generates two signals, as both Gα and G$\beta\gamma$ can engage downstream effector proteins.

Subunit Diversity

The genome of the nematode *Caenorhabditis elegans* has genes for 20 Gα, 2 Gβ, and 2 Gγ subunits. Sixteen of the Gα proteins are used in a few chemosensory cells. The others are used by many cell types. Yeasts have genes for just two Gα proteins, one of which participates in responses to sex pheromones. Mammals have genes for 20 Gα, 5 Gβ, and 12 Gγ subunits. Alternative splicing of Gα mRNAs creates additional diversity. If the known subunits were combined in all possible ways, mammals could make more than 1000 different trimeric G-proteins. However, only a limited number of combinations have been detected.

Given more than 1000 genes for seven-helix receptors, many receptors use the same G-proteins to transduce signals. For example, the hundreds of different odorant receptors in the nose all activate G$_{olf}\alpha$ (see Fig. 27-1). Trimeric G-proteins act on a limited variety of downstream effectors, including ion channels, kinases, and enzymes that produce second messengers (Table 25-2).

Table 25-2

RECEPTORS AND EFFECTORS FOR G-PROTEIN ISOFORMS

Family (No. of Human Members)	Receptors	Effectors
G$_i\alpha$ (7)	α-Adrenergic amines, acetylcholine, chemokines, various neurotransmitters, tastants	Inhibit adenylyl cyclase, open potassium channels, close calcium channels
G$_q\alpha$ (5)	α-Adrenergic amines, acetylcholine, various neurotransmitters	Activate phospholipase Cβ to produce IP$_3$, which releases Ca^{2+}
G$_s\alpha$ (3)	β-Adrenergic amines, hormones (corticotropin, glucagon, parathyroid, thyrotropin, others)	Stimulate adenylyl cyclase to produce cAMP, receptor kinase
G$_t\alpha$ (2)	Rhodopsin, which absorbs light	Activate cGMP phosphodiesterase to break down cGMP, receptor kinase
G$_{13}\alpha$ (2)	Thrombin and others	Rho and others
G$_{olf}\alpha$	Odorant receptors	Activate adenylyl cyclase, receptor kinase

Structure of Trimeric G-Proteins

The GTPase core of Gα is linked to a helical domain that covers the GTP-binding site. Gβ is a torus-shaped molecule composed of seven modules, each folded into an antiparallel β-sheet (Fig. 25-9). These so-called **WD repeats** are found in many proteins but are best characterized in Gβ. Loops on one face of the torus interact with Gα, whereas those on the other face interact with Gγ. The small Gγ subunit associates surprisingly tightly with Gβ through an N-terminal helical coiled-coil and other interactions. A C-20 prenyl group on a C-terminal cysteine of most Gγ subunits anchors Gβγ to membrane bilayers. An N-terminal fatty acid, usually myristate, anchors Gα independently to lipid bilayers. Some Gα subunits have an additional palmitic acid anchor on a reactive cysteine. Tight interaction of Gβγ with Gα-GDP blocks effector interaction sites on both partners.

Guanosine Triphosphatase Cycle

Seven-helix receptors activate trimeric G-proteins by catalyzing the exchange of GDP for GTP on the Gα subunit. This dissociates the Gα from Gβγ, allowing each to activate effector proteins (Fig. 25-9). It is convenient to think about this process as two cycles: a GTPase cycle coupled to a subunit cycle (Fig. 25-8B).

The rate of GDP dissociation from trimeric G-proteins is near zero (half-life about 10 to 60 minutes) unless they bind an activated seven-helix receptor. Activated seven-helix receptors are guanine nucleotide exchange factors that increase the rate of GDP dissociation by many orders of magnitude, allowing GTP to exchange for GDP on a millisecond-to-second time scale, fast enough for vision (see Fig. 27-2). Interaction of the receptor with Gα and Gβγ triggers a conformational change that weakens the bonds of GDP to Gα. The cleft between the Gα domains must open transiently to release GDP and accept a GTP from solution.

Gα refolds around GTP in a significantly different conformation than around GDP. This conformational change is the physical manifestation of the transfer of a signal from an activated receptor to Gα. GTP draws the three switch loops together around the γ phosphate in a conformation that favors dissociation of Gβγ and association with effector proteins.

Like all GTPases, the duration of the signal carried by trimeric G-proteins depends on the rate of GTP hydrolysis. The half-time of about 10 to 20 seconds is adequate for prolonged activation of a target protein. Trimeric G-proteins hydrolyze GTP faster than do small GTPases by virtue of a strategically placed arginine (on a linker to the helical domain). Thus, the helical domain acts both as an intrinsic inhibitor of GDP dissociation and as an activator of GTP hydrolysis, similar to two separate regulators of small GTPases (GDI and GAP). When the two

domains are produced separately in the laboratory, the nucleotide-binding core domain binds GTP and activates effectors but does not hydrolyze GTP rapidly unless it is recombined with the separate helical domain containing the critical arginine.

Both effector proteins and extrinsic GTPase activators, called **RGS proteins** (regulators of G-protein signaling), stimulate GTP hydrolysis and terminate the signal. For example, $G_q\alpha$-GTP binds and stimulates phospholipase Cβ, which produces two second messengers: inositol 1,4,5-triphosphate (IP_3) and diacylglycerol (see Fig. 26-12). At the same time, phospholipase Cβ accelerates the GTPase of $G_q\alpha$, providing negative feedback to turn off the signal. G-proteins regulate some physiological processes that require a rapid response, such as the heart rate ($G_i\alpha$) and vision ($G_t\alpha$). In these cases, a family of 20 or more RGS proteins stimulates GTPase activity of G-proteins about 100-fold, yielding half-times of less than 1 second. These RGS proteins work by stabilizing the transition state between GTP and GDP-P_i. Some RGS proteins also have a Rho–guanine nucleotide exchange factor domain, so they may connect seven-helix receptors and trimeric G-proteins to the Rho family of small GTPases.

Subunit Cycle

GTP binding, hydrolysis, and dissociation drive not only the GTPase cycle but also a linked subunit cycle (Fig. 25-8B). Gα cycles on and off both Gβγ and the receptor as it traverses its GTPase cycle. The conformational change in Gα that is induced by GTP binding affects all of its molecular interactions. GTP binding reduces the affinity of Gα for both its receptor and associated Gβγ subunits, so all three molecular partners separate on the cytoplasmic face of the membrane (Fig. 25-9). Once dissociated, the receptor, Gα, and Gβγ are each free to interact with other partners (Table 25-2). The conformation of Gβγ is the same whether bound to Gα or free, so its activation on dissociation from Gβγ is attributable simply to unmasking of effector binding sites. Gβγ is not a passive partner in these linked cycles, as it must be bound to Gα-GDP before activated membrane receptors can trigger dissociation of GDP. In addition to activating membrane targets, such as ion channels, Gβγ provides a membrane anchor to enhance the interaction of cytoplasmic effectors (such as kinases that phosphorylate seven-helix receptors) with membrane targets.

The properties of the linked GTPase and subunit cycles allow activation of a single receptor to generate a large signal. Although most seven-helix receptors are active only briefly (owing to rapid ligand dissociation and rapid inactivation [see Figs. 27-1 and 27-2]), they can turn on multiple G-proteins, each with a longer lifetime. Slow GTP hydrolysis by Gα subunits allows ample time for these G-proteins to activate downstream effector proteins. Because these effectors are typically enzymes or channels, they amplify the signal in a short time.

Mechanisms of Effector Activation

Both Gα and Gβγ subunits participate in signaling by interacting with downstream effector proteins. In some cases, Gα and Gβγ subunits act individually; in other cases, they may act synergistically and even antagonistically. The following two examples, elaborated on in Chapter 27, illustrate how G-proteins activate effector proteins.

In the eye, when the seven-helix photoreceptor rhodopsin absorbs a photon, the G-protein $G_t\alpha$ (also called transducin) relays and amplifies a signal (see Fig. 27-2). Each activated rhodopsin generates about 500 $G_t\alpha$-GTPs, which bind an inhibitory subunit of the enzyme cGMP phosphodiesterase. This stimulates the activity of the phosphodiesterase, which lowers the cytoplasmic concentration of cGMP and closes an ion channel. The signal is transient, because both an RGS protein and the inhibitory subunit itself promote the hydrolysis of GTP bound to $G_t\alpha$. Inactive $G_t\alpha$-GDP dissociates from the inhibitory subunit, terminating the signal that flowed through $G_t\alpha$ to the enzyme.

In the heart, the β-adrenergic receptor activates $G_s\alpha$, releasing both $G_s\alpha$-GTP and Gβγ to bind effector proteins (see Fig. 27-3). During its 10-second lifetime, $G_s\alpha$-GTP binds and stimulates the enzyme adenylyl cyclase to produce the second messenger cAMP. Gβγ assists in receptor inactivation by binding β-ARK, the kinase that phosphorylates and turns off the β-adrenergic receptor, terminating the signal.

GTPases in Disease

Both abnormal activation or inactivation of G-proteins can cause disease (Table 25-3). Mutations that interfere with GTP hydrolysis cause Gα to accumulate in the GTP state and persistently activate downstream effectors. For example, mutations in arginine or glutamine residues of Gα that are crucial for GTP hydrolysis can cause tumors by prolonging the activation of pathways responsible for cell proliferation. Common variants in the sequence of other G-proteins are associated with high blood pressure and other common diseases.

Some bacterial toxins mediate their effects by acting on G-proteins. The cholera bacterium causes diarrhea by enzymatically modifying $G_s\alpha$. **Cholera toxin** is an enzyme that catalyzes the addition of an adenosine diphosphate (ADP)–ribose to the arginine required for GTPase activity. Activated $G_s\alpha$-GTP accumulates, prolonging activation of adenylyl cyclase and producing high levels of cAMP, which causes life-threatening diarrhea by stimulating salt and water secretion into the intestine. **Pertussis toxin** from the whooping cough bacterium secretes an enzyme that adds ADP-ribose to a cysteine residue of $G_i\alpha$ or other Gα subunits. This inhibits the interaction of the trimeric G-protein with activated receptors, so the G-protein accumulates at the inactive GDP state. One consequence is airway irritability. Similarly, *Clostridium botulinus* C3 toxin ADP-ribosylates and inhibits Rho-GTPases, whereas a *Clostridium difficile* toxin uses uridine diphosphate–glucose to glucosylate and turn off the whole class of Rho proteins.

Dynamin-Related GTPases

These large GTPases have an N-terminal GTP-binding domain and a C-terminal GTPase-activating domain that allows self-assembly into spiral polymers (see Fig. 22-11). Dynamin, the prototypical family member, also contains domains that target it to the plasma membrane, where it participates in endocytosis. Other dynamin family members regulate vacuolar trafficking in yeast and the division of mitochondria.

Table 25-3

GUANOSINE TRIPHOSPHATASES AND DISEASE

Disease	GTPase	Mechanism
Excess Signal		
Cholera	$G_s\alpha$	Cholera toxin ADP-ribosylation of R201 inhibits GTP hydrolysis in intestinal epithelium.
Pituitary and thyroid adenomas	$G_s\alpha$	Somatic point mutations of R201 or Q227 inhibit GTP hydrolysis; constitutive activity mimics signal from hormones that stimulate proliferation and secretion by these glands.
Various cancers	Ras	Point mutations inhibit GTP hydrolysis, generating persistent stimulation of signals for cell proliferation.
Deficient Signal		
Whooping cough	$G_i\alpha$	Pertussis toxin ADP-ribosylation of $G_i\alpha$ C347 in the bronchial epithelium blocks receptor activation; connection to coughing not established.
Night blindness	$G_t\alpha$	Germ line point mutation in G38.
Pseudohypoparathyroidism type Ia	$G_s\alpha$	Point mutations result in loss of $G_s\alpha$ or may block its activation by receptors.

C, cysteine; G, glycine; Q, glutamine; R, arginine.
Adapted from Farfel Z, Bourne HR, Iiri T: The expanding spectrum of G protein diseases. N Engl J Med 340:1012–1020, 1999.

Experimental Tools

Mutations, especially those that constitutively activate GTPases (by inhibiting GTP hydrolysis) or inactivate GTPases, have been powerful tools for investigating GTPase functions in live cells. For biochemical experiments, slowly hydrolyzed analogs of GTP, such as GTPγS (with a sulfur substituted for one of the γ-phosphate oxygens), are used to activate GTPases. Similarly, aluminum fluoride and beryllium fluoride bind very tightly in place of the hydrolyzed γ phosphate, keeping Gα in an active GDP-P_i state similar to GTP. The fungal metabolite brefeldin A blocks nucleotide exchange on some Arfs. This disrupts membrane traffic between the Golgi complex and the endoplasmic reticulum (see Fig. 21-14).

Molecular Recognition by Adapter Domains

During the characterization of signaling pathways, several patterns of amino acid sequence appeared repeatedly in different proteins, such as Src (Figs. 25-3C and 25-4B). These turned out to be compactly folded domains (Fig. 25-10) that are incorporated into a variety of proteins (Fig. 25-11), including many unrelated to signaling. These domains mediate interactions of proteins with each other and with membrane lipids (Table 25-4).

The names of adapter domains generally came from the proteins where they were originally recognized. For example, **Src homology (SH)** domains were first recognized in the Src tyrosine kinase (Fig. 25-3E). SH1 is the tyrosine kinase domain; SH2 domain binds phosphotyrosine peptides; and SH3 binds polyproline type II helices. Chapter 27 provides detailed examples of how adapter domains function. This section provides an overview of their structure and ligand-binding properties. The following points apply to adapter proteins in general.

Adapter domains mediate interactions that are required to assemble proteins into multimolecular functional units that typically carry out a series of reactions. To facilitate these interactions, many signaling proteins have more than one adapter domain or bind more than one ligand. In signal transduction, these physical associations make transmission from receptors to effectors more reliable, like a solid-phase machine rather than one that relies solely on diffusion and random associations. Mutations in experimental organisms and roles in various human diseases have verified the importance of adapter domains for many pathways. Interactions mediated by adapter domains complement the organizing activities of anchoring proteins, such as STE5 and AKAPs (see the subsection titled "Targeting" under "Regulation of Protein Kinases," earlier in this chapter).

All members of each family of adapters have similar structures (and common evolutionary origins) but differ in their affinity for a range of similar ligands. For example, all SH2 domains bind peptides with a sequence phosphotyrosine-X-X-hydrophobic residue. All require phosphotyrosine but differ in their affinity for peptides depending on the hydrophobic residue and the intervening residues. This lock-and-key strategy creates specificity with lots of particular combinations, as in real locks and keys. Although lacking in sequence similarity, three of these domains—PH, PTB, and EVH1—have similar folds (Fig. 25-10) and might have had a common ancestor. Nevertheless, their ligands are quite distinct from each other and bind to different sites on the commonly folded domains.

Some interactions depend on reversible covalent modifications of ligands: tyrosine phosphorylation for SH2 and some PTB domains, serine phosphorylation for some 14-3-3 and WW domains, and 3-phosphorylation of inositol for some PH domains. This allows networks that use these adapters to assemble and disassemble in response to signals that modulate phosphorylation.

Many interactions of adapter domains with their ligands are tenuous, so associations are reversible on a time scale of seconds, allowing rapid rearrangements in response to signals. Frequent dissociation is also required for covalent modifications, such as access of phosphatases to their substrates.

Phosphorylation-Sensitive Adapters

SH2 Domains

SH2 domains bind short peptide sequences that begin with a phosphotyrosine. Like a two-pronged plug, these peptides insert into two cavities in the SH2 socket. Phosphotyrosine is one prong. It is the key residue, as it provides most of the binding energy by virtue of an extensive network of hydrogen bonds between the phosphate and its deep binding pocket. A phosphate on the tyrosine increases the affinity of a peptide for its partner SH2 domain by orders of magnitude. This allows reversible phosphorylation to control interactions between SH2 domains and their ligands. This switching mechanism is used in growth factor signaling and lymphocyte activation (see Figs. 27-6 to 27-9). The second prong is a hydrophobic side chain of the third residue C-terminal from phosphotyrosine. It inserts into a hydrophobic cavity on the surface of the SH2 domain. The size of this side chain is a major determinant of binding specificity. Two residues between these plug residues straddle the β-sheet of the SH2 with their side chains exposed to solvent.

SH2 interactions with target peptides and proteins are relatively weak, with K_ds in the range of 0.1 to 1 μM. This allows for rapid exchange of partners and

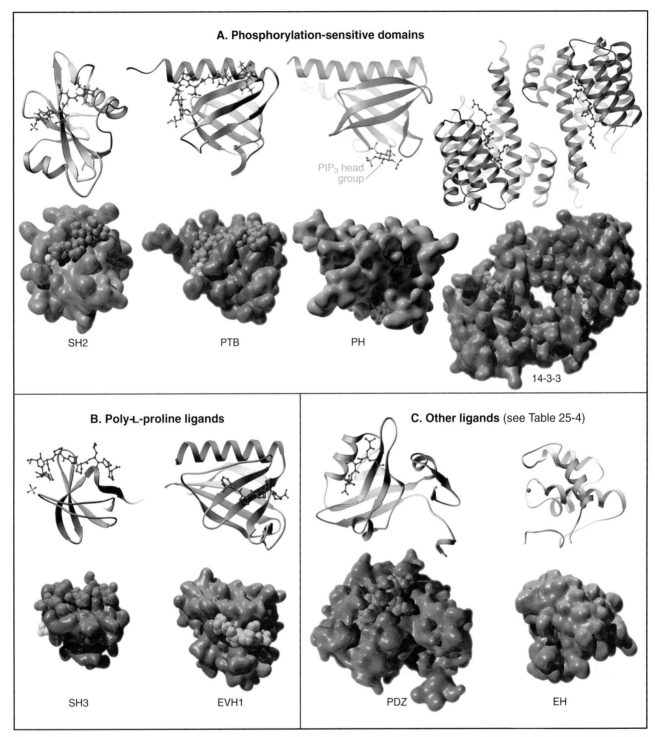

Figure 25-10 ATOMIC MODELS OF ADAPTER PROTEIN DOMAINS. Ribbon diagrams show their architecture, and the surface renderings show how ligands bind. **A,** Domains with phosphorylation-sensitive interactions. **B,** Domains with poly-l-proline ligands. **C,** Domains with other ligands. SH2 (PDB file: 1HCS), PTB (PDB file: 1IRS), PH (PDB file: 1DYN), 14-3-3 (PDB file: 1A38); SH3 (PDB file: 1ABO) and EVH1 (PDB file: 1EVH); PDZ (PDB file: 1BEQ) and EH (PDB file: 1EH2).

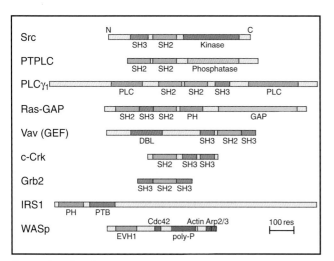

Figure 25-11 SCALE DRAWINGS OF PROTEINS WITH ADAPTER DOMAINS. c-Crk and Grb2, multidomain adapter proteins; DBL, a guanine nucleotide exchange factor domain; GAP, GTPase activating; IRS1, insulin receptor substrate; PH, pleckstrin homology; PLC, phospholipase C; poly-P, polyproline; PTB, protein tyrosine–binding domain; PTPLC, protein tyrosine phosphatase; Ras-GAP, Ras GTPase activating protein; SH, Src-homology; Src, cytoplasmic tyrosine kinase; Vav, a guanine nucleotide exchange protein; WASp, Wiskott-Aldrich syndrome protein. Actin and Arp2/3 indicate binding sites for actin monomers and Arp2/3 complex. Cdc42, a Rho-family GTPase; EVH1, Ena-Vasp homology 1 domain.

dephosphorylation of the phosphotyrosine. Nevertheless, these interactions appear to be specific, the 115 human proteins with SH2 domains engaging a limited number of target phosphoproteins. SH2 domains target several signal transduction enzymes to receptor tyrosine kinases (see Fig. 27-6) as the first step in propagat-

ing signals to effectors, including second messengers and transcription factors. Intramolecular binding of the Src SH2 to a C-terminal phosphotyrosine regulates the catalytic activity of the enzyme (Fig. 25-3C).

Phosphotyrosine-Binding Domains

Most PTB domains require a phosphotyrosine at the C-terminal end of the peptide ligand. Hydrophobic residues preceding phosphotyrosine in the sequence contribute to binding specificity. The bound peptide is hydrogen-bonded onto the edge of a β-sheet, and phosphotyrosine interacts with basic residues. PTB domains target adapter proteins to phosphotyrosines on receptor tyrosine kinases, such as insulin receptor (see Fig. 27-7). In a few cases, PTB domains bind unphosphorylated peptide ligands. Note that the fold of PTB domains and their mode of interaction with ligand peptides have nothing in common with SH2 domains.

14-3-3 Proteins

Vertebrates have at least seven genes for 14-3-3 subunits that assemble into homodimers or heterodimers. Protein ligands with an appropriate sequence and a central phosphoserine bind each subunit with submicromolar affinity. Peptides with two appropriate sequences bind much more tightly. 14-3-3 proteins regulate protein kinases, including the Ras-activated kinase Raf (see Fig. 27-6) and cellular death pathways (see Chapter 46). During interphase or after DNA damage, a 14-3-3 protein inhibits the cell cycle phosphatase Cdc25, when it is phosphorylated on a serine (see Fig. 43-4).

Table 25-4

ADAPTER DOMAINS

Domain Name	Size (Residues)	Consensus Ligands	Example of Proteins with Domain
EH (Eps15 homology)	95	S/T-N-P-F-Φ	Clathrin adapter proteins, synaptojanin I
EVH1 (Ena-VASP homology)	110	D/E-Φ-P-P-P-P	WASp, VASP, Ena
PH (Pleckstrin homology)	100	PIP_2, PIP_3	Kinases, scaffolds, GEFs, GAPs, PLCδ, dynamin
PDZ	100	-x-x-S/T-x-V-COOH -x-x-Φ-x-Φ-COOH	Scaffolds for channels and transduction enzymes
PTB (phosphotyrosine binding)	125	-Φ-x-N-P-x-pY-	IRS1, Shc scaffold proteins
SH2 (Src homology 2)	100	-pY-x-x-Φ-	Transduction enzymes and scaffold proteins
SH3 (Src homology 3)	60	(+) -R/K-x-x-P-x-x-P- (−) -x-P-x-x-P-x-R/K-	Tyrosine kinases, phosphatases, Grb2, PLCγ, spectrin, myosin I
WW	38–40	-P-P-x-Y-	Peptidyl prolyl isomerase, ubiquitin ligase
14-3-3	250	-R-S-X-pS-x-P-	14-3-3 isoforms

Φ, hydrophobic residue; COOH, C-terminus; Ena, enabled gene; GAP, GTPase-activating protein; GEF, guanine nucleotide exchange factor; Grb2, adapter protein; IRS1, insulin receptor substrate 1; PLC, phospholipase C; pS, phosphoserine; pY, phosphotyrosine; Shc, receptor tyrosine kinase substrate; VASP, vasodilator-stimulated phosphoprotein, WASp, Wiskott-Aldrich syndrome protein; (−), minus orientation; (+), plus orientation.

WW Domains

These tiny adapter domains are found in more than 100 proteins. They bind certain phosphoserine or phosphothreonine peptides. These phosphorylation-dependent interactions regulate Cdc25 and ubiquitin-mediated protein destruction (see Chapter 23).

PH Domains

These compact domains of about 100 residues are named for the PH domain that was first recognized in **pleckstrin,** the major substrate for protein kinase C in platelets. PH domains bind **polyphosphoinositides:** PH domains of dynamin and phospholipase Cδ prefer phosphatidylinositol (PI) (4,5) P_2 (PIP$_2$), whereas the PH domain of Bruton's tyrosine kinase (Btk) favors PI(3,4,5)P$_3$ (PIP$_3$). These interactions target proteins with PH domains to membrane bilayers that are rich in PIP$_2$ and PIP$_3$ and make these membrane interactions responsive to the activities of phosphoinositide kinases (see Figs. 26-7 and 38-12). PH-domain proteins include kinases (PKB/Akt, PDK1), signaling scaffolding proteins (insulin receptor substrate 1 [IRS1]; see Fig. 27-7), enzymes (phospholipase Cγ1; see Figs. 26-4 and 26-12), and guanine nucleotide exchange factors. Mutations in the PH domain of the tyrosine kinase, Btk, reduce affinity for PI(3,4,5)P$_3$ and cause a failure of B-lymphocyte development (see Fig. 28-9), resulting in immunodeficiency due to a lack of antibodies.

Adapters with Proline-Rich Ligands

SH3 Domains

SH3 domains found in 253 different human proteins bind to proline-rich sequences of numerous target proteins. These ligands form left-handed, **type II polyproline helices** (see Fig. 29-1) that make hydrophobic interactions with aromatic residues in a shallow groove on the SH3 domain, as well as hydrogen bonds contributed by ligand peptide carbonyl oxygens. Depending on the SH3 domain, the peptide can be oriented in either direction. Residues flanking the central proline helix contribute to binding specificity. Even optimal peptide ligands bind with relatively low affinity (K_ds in the micromolar range), so they exchange rapidly. When incorporated into proteins, type II poly-L-proline helices with appropriate sequences bind somewhat more tightly, owing to secondary interactions.

SH3 domains of the adapter protein Grb2 (Fig. 25-11) link activated growth factor receptors to the nucleotide exchange protein for Ras (see Fig. 27-6). SH3 domains are also found in tyrosine kinases and cytoskeletal proteins, including myosin-I, spectrin, and cortactin.

EVH1 Domains

EVH1 domains (Fig. 25-11) are found in WASp (see Fig. 33-17) and other signaling proteins that regulate actin polymerization. EVH1 domains are folded like PH and PTB domains, but they bind type II proline-rich helices of target protein in a groove. The corresponding groove is occupied by an intrinsic α-helix in some PH domains. This site also differs from that for phosphotyrosine peptides on PTB domains. Thus, a common scaffold has diverged to form three completely different binding sites.

Other Adapter Domains

PDZ Domains

PDZ domains are found in one to seven copies in scaffolding proteins that cluster together ion channels and signal transduction proteins at synapses, in photoreceptors, and in polarized epithelial cells. PDZ domains bind specific sequence motifs, most commonly ones found at the very C-terminus of proteins and less commonly ones found at the end of β hairpin structures. PDZ domains bind their ligands, in a manner reminiscent of PTB domains, by incorporating them through hydrogen bonds as an extra strand in a β-sheet.

EH Domains

EH domains are small and comprise a bundle of four α-helices that bind peptides with the sequence asparagine-proline-phenylalanine. Flanking residues contribute to specificity. The best-characterized EH-mediated interactions are involved with endocytosis (see Chapter 22).

ACKNOWLEDGMENTS

Thanks go to Brad Nolen and Tony Hunter for their suggestions on revisions to this chapter.

SELECTED READINGS

Alonso A, Sasin J, Bottini N, et al: Protein tyrosine phosphatases in the human genome. Cell 117:699–711, 2004.

Aramburu J, Heitman J, Crabtree GR: Calcineurin: A central controller of signalling in eukaryotes. EMBO Rep 5:343–348, 2004.

Barford D, Das AK, Egloff M-P: Structure and mechanism of protein phosphatases: Insights into catalysis and regulation. Annu Rev Biophys Biomol Struct 27:133–164, 1998.

Berwick DC, Tavaré JM: Identifying protein kinase substrates: Hunting for the organ-grinder's monkeys. Trends Biochem Sci 29:227–232, 2004.

Bhattacharyya RP, Reményi A, Yeh BJ, Lim WA: Domains, motifs, and scaffolds: The role of modular interactions in the evolution and wiring of cell signaling circuits. Annu Rev Biochem 75:655–680, 2006.

Bockoch GM: Biology of the p21-activated kinases. Annu Rev Biochem 72:743-781, 2003.

Bourdeau A, Dube N, Tremblay ML: Cytoplasmic protein tyrosine phosphatases, regulation and function: The roles of PTP1B and TC-PTP. Curr Opin Cell Biol 17:203-209, 2005.

Ceulemans H, Bollen M: Functional diversity of protein phosphatase-1, a cellular economizer and reset button. Physiol Rev 84:1-39, 2004.

Cherfils J, Chardin P: GEFs: Structural basis of their activation of small GTP-binding proteins. Trends Biochem Sci 24:306-311, 1999.

Drause DS, VanEtten, RA: Tyrosine kinases as targets for cancer therapy. New Engl J Med 353:172-187, 2005.

Etienne-Manneville S, Hall A: Rho GTPases in cell biology. Nature 420:629-635, 2002.

Farfel Z, Bourne HR, Iiri T: The expanding spectrum of G protein diseases. N Engl J Med 340:1012-1020, 1999.

Ferrell JE: How responses get more switch-like as you move down a protein kinase cascade. Trends Biochem Sci 22:288-289, 1997.

Gallego M, Virshup DM: Protein serine/threonine phosphatases: Life, death, and sleeping. Curr Opin Cell Biol 17:197-202, 2005.

Hampoelz B, Knoblich JA: Heterotrimeric G proteins: New tricks for an old dog. Cell 119:453-456, 2004.

Herrmann C: Ras-effector interactions: After one decade. Curr Opin Struct Biol 13:122-129, 2003.

Hofmann F: The biology of cyclic GMP-dependent protein kinases. J Biol Chem 280:1-4, 2005.

Hubbard SR, Till JH: Protein tyrosine kinase structure and function. Annu Rev Biochem 69:373-398, 2000.

Iiri T, Farfel Z, Bourne HR: G-protein diseases furnish a model for the turn-on switch. Nature 394:35-38, 1998.

Ishii M, Kurachi Y: Physiological actions of regulators of G-protein signaling (RGS) proteins. Life Sci 74:163-171, 2003.

Kim C, Xuong N-H, Taylor SS: Crystal structure of a complex between the catalytic and regulatory (RIa) subunits of PKA. Science 307:690-696, 2005.

Manning G, Plowman GD, Hunter T, Sudarsanam S: Evolution of protein kinase signaling from yeast to man. Trends Biochem Sci 27:514-520, 2002.

Manning G, Whyte DB, Marinez R, et al: The protein kinase complement of the human genome. Science 298:1912-1934, 2002.

Nourry C, Grant SG, Borg JP: PDZ domain proteins: Plug and play! Sci STKE. 2003(179):RE7, 2003.

Parsons SJ, Parsons JT: Src family kinases, key regulators of signal transduction. Oncogene 23:7906-7909, 2004.

Pawson T, Nash P: Assembly of cell regulatory systems through protein interaction domains. Science 300:445-452, 2003.

Pawson T, Scott JD: Protein phosphorylation in signaling: 50 years and counting. Trends Biochem Sci 30:286-290, 2005.

Rossman KL, Der CJ, Sondek J: GEF means go: Turning on RHO GTPases with guanine nucleotide-exchange factors. Nat Rev Mol Cell Biol 6:167-180, 2005.

Siderovski DP, Willard FS: The GAPs, GEFs, and GDIs of heterotrimeric G-protein alpha subunits. Int J Biol Sci 1:51-66, 2005.

Sprang SR: G-protein mechanisms: Insights from structural analysis. Annu Rev Biochem 66:639-678, 1997.

Wong W, Scott JD: AKAP signalling complexes: Focal points in space and time. Nat Rev Mol Cell Biol 5:959-970, 2004.

APPENDIX 25-1

Families of Protein Kinases

Groups	Substrate	Bacterial Genes	Yeast Genes	Human Genes	Examples	Regulation	Targets or Regulated Function
ACC	S, T	0	17	63	PKA	cAMP	Metabolic enzymes, TFs, channels
					PKB	PI3K, PDKs	GSK3/metabolism, survival
					PKC	Ca²⁺, lipids	Receptor tyrosine kinases, channels, TFs
					PKG	cGMP	IP₃R, CFTR, VASP
					RSK	MAPK, PDKs	Ribosome/synthesis of translation machinery
					GRK	G proteins	Seven-helix receptor downregulation
CaMK	S, T	0	16	74	CaMK	Ca²⁺, calmodulin	Synaptic transmission, cytoskeleton, TFs
					AMP-PK	AMP	Fatty acid, cholesterol synthesis
					MLCK	Ca²⁺, calmodulin	Myosin-II/contraction
CK1	S, T, (Y)	0	4	10	CK-I, CK-II		Circadian clocks, Wnt
CMGC	S, T, (Y)	0	21	33	Cdks	Cyclins, phosphorylation	Many/cell cycle
					MAPK	Phosphorylation	TFs/proliferation
					GSK3	PKB	Glycogen metabolism, survival
RGC		0	0	5			
STE	S, T, Y	0	18	47	MAPKK	Phosphorylation	MAP kinase/proliferation
					PAK	Small GTPases	LIM kinase/cytoskeleton
Tyrosine kinase	Y	0	0	90	Receptor tyrosine kinases	Growth factors	PLCγ, Ras, MAP kinase pathway/cell proliferation
					Src family	Phosphorylation	Many/proliferation, lymphocyte activation, cytoskeleton, adhesion
Tyrosine kinase-like	S	0	0	43	Raf	Ras	MAPKK/Proliferation
					TGF-βR	TGF-β	Smads/Differentiation
Other	S, T, Y		38	83	Wee1p	Phosphorylation	Cdks/cell cycle
					Polo-like	Phosphorylation	Several/mitosis, cytokinesis
Atypical	S		0	15	48	ATM, ATR	DNA damage	p53, Chk1/cell cycle arrest
Histidine kinases	H	0 to > 30*	2	?	Tar	Aspartate	Bacterial chemotaxis, gene expression

*Number of histidine kinases in prokaryotes. **Bacteria:** *Bacillus substilis* 37; *Escherichia coli* 7; *Borrelia burgdorferi*—Lyme disease spirochaete 2; *Myobacterium tuberculosis* 14—also has 11 eukaryotic serine/threonine kinase genes, likely derived by lateral gene transfer from eukaryotic hosts. **Archaea:** *Methanococcus jannaschii* 0; *Aquifex aecolicus* 0; *Archaeoglobus fulgidus* 3.

AMP-PK, adenosine monophosphate (AMP)–activated protein kinase; CaMK, calmodulin-activated protein kinase; Cdk, cyclin-dependent kinase; CFTR, cystic fibrosis transmembrane regulator; CK, casein kinase; GF, growth factor; GRK, G protein–coupled receptor kinase; GSK, glycogen synthase kinase; IP₃R, inositol trisphosphate receptor, a Ca²⁺ release channel; MAPK, mitogen-activated protein kinase (also called ERK, for extracellular signal–regulated kinase); MAPKK, MAP kinase kinase; MLCK, myosin light-chain kinase; PAK, p21 (small GTPase)-activated kinase; PDK, 3-phosphoinositide–dependent protein kinase; PKA, cyclic AMP–dependent protein kinase; PKB, protein kinase B (also called Akt); PKC, calcium-dependent protein kinase; PKG, cyclic GMP–dependent protein kinase; polo, a *Drosophila* gene; Raf, cellular homologue of retroviral oncogene; RSK, ribosomal subunit 6 kinase; TFs, transcription factors; VASP, vasodilator-stimulated phosphoprotein; Wee1p, fission yeast kinase.

Parallels among Guanosine Triphosphate-Binding Proteins

Family	Bacterial Genes	Yeast Genes	Worm Genes	Functions	GDP Dissociation Inhibitors	Receptors	GTP Exchange Factors	GTPase-Activating Factors	Direct Effectors
Small GTPases									
Arf	0	6	11	Vesicular formation		Arf-GEFs	Sec-7/ARNO	Arf-GAP	COPI coat proteins
Rab	0	10	24	Vesicle targeting and fusion	Rab-GDI	Rab-GEFs	Rab-GEFs	Rab-GAP	Docking and fusion factors
Ran	0	2	2	Nuclear transport, mitotic spindle			Ran-GDF1, RCC1	RanBP1, RanGAP1	Importin β
Ras	0	4	8	Transduction of growth factor signals		Receptor tyrosine kinases	SOS	Ras-GAP	Raf
Rho	0	7	10	Regulation of actin cytoskeleton	Rho-GDI	Receptor tyrosine kinases, seven-helix receptors	Dbl/PH-GEFs	Rho-GAP	p65 PAK, Rho kinase, WASp
Sar	0	1	3	Vesicular formation		Sec12 GEF	Sec12	Sec23	COPII coat proteins
Trimeric G Proteins									
	0	2	20	Transduction of a wide variety of signals	Gβγ	Seven-helix receptors	Seven-helix receptors	Effector proteins, RGS proteins	Many enzymes, channels
Elongation Factors									
EF-Tu/EF1α	1–2	4	5	Protein synthesis		Ribosome	EF-Ts/EF1β	Ribosome	
EF-G/EF2	1–2	5	4	Protein synthesis		Ribosome	—	Ribosome	
RF1,2/eRF	1–2	1	1–12	Protein synthesis		Ribosome			
Dynamin									
	0	2	1–3	Endocytosis	?		Not required?	Intrinsic GAP domain	Membrane fission factors
Translocation GTPases									
Ffh/SRP54	0	2	?	Translocation of polypeptides into endoplasmic reticulum			Nascent polypeptide chains	SRP receptor	Sec 61 translocon

GEFs, guanine nucleotide exchange factors.

CHAPTER 26

Second Messengers

This chapter considers the remarkable variety of small molecules that carry signals inside living cells. These second messengers are chemically diverse, ranging from hydrophobic lipids confined to membrane bilayers, to an inorganic ion (Ca^{2+}), to nucleotides (cyclic adenosine monophosphate [cAMP] and cyclic guanosine monophosphate [cGMP]), to a gas (nitric oxide). The messages that these molecules carry are encoded by their concentrations. In the simplest case, a rise or fall in the concentration of the second messenger conveys a signal from its source to its target. In other cases, the signal depends on the rate or frequency of the fluctuations in the concentration of the second messenger. The local concentration of a second messenger depends on the rate of production, the rate of diffusion from the site of production, and the rate of removal. Most second messengers are produced by enzymes that can switch on and off rapidly, allowing modulation of the concentration of second messengers on a millisecond time scale. In the case of Ca^{2+}, the cytoplasmic concentration is determined by channels that release the ion from membrane-delimited stores and by pumps that remove it from cytoplasm.

The physical state of second messengers has important consequences. Lipid-derived second messengers reach different targets in the cell depending on whether they are more soluble in the lipid bilayer or in water. Similarly, Ca^{2+} acts only locally in cytoplasm, where a high concentration of binding sites impedes its free diffusion. Cyclic nucleotides diffuse rapidly through cytoplasm, but their concentrations may rise and fall locally, owing to restricted sites of synthesis combined with rapid degradation at particular sites in the cell.

The complexity of the signaling pathways is determined by the number of sources and the number of targets of each second messenger. Generally, multiple signal sources and multiple second messenger targets generate more complexity than one can fully appreciate. This chapter deals with this complexity only in passing. Chapter 27 considers a few model systems in which it is possible to understand how signals are integrated and transduced.

This chapter discusses second messengers in the following four sections: Cyclic Nucleotides, Lipid-Derived Second Messengers, Calcium, and Nitric Oxide. All of these topics are interrelated, as multiple second messengers participate in many signaling systems. For example, nitric oxide controls the production of cGMP, and inositol triphosphate derived from a membrane lipid controls the release of Ca^{2+} into cytoplasm.

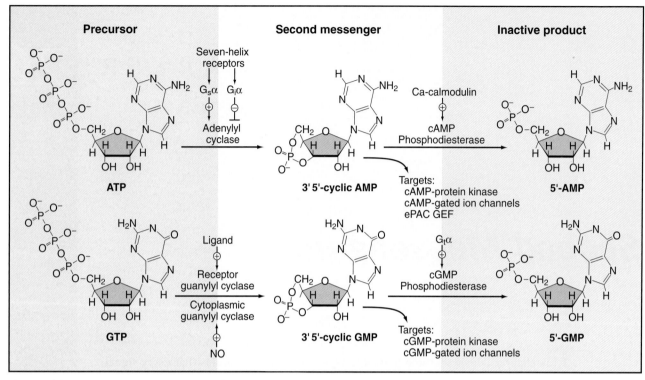

Figure 26-1 CYCLIC NUCLEOTIDE METABOLISM. Synthesis and degradation of cAMP and cGMP, including regulatory inputs and targets. $G_s\alpha$, $G_i\alpha$, and $G_t\alpha$ are trimeric GTPase α subunits (see Fig. 25-9). Ca, calcium; NO, nitric oxide.

Cyclic Nucleotides

Two cyclic nucleoside monophosphates—adenosine 3',5'-cyclic monophosphate **(cAMP)** and guanosine 3',5'-cyclic monophosphate **(cGMP)**—are employed as second messengers (Fig. 26-1). Both act by binding reversibly to specific proteins. Enzymes that produce and degrade cyclic nucleotides determine the concentrations of these messengers available to bind targets. These enzymes turn over substrates rapidly, so they can amplify signals massively on a millisecond time scale, under the control of diverse signaling pathways (see Chapter 27). Cyclases make cyclic nucleotides in a single step from the corresponding nucleoside triphosphate, either adenosine triphosphate (ATP) or guanosine triphosphate (GTP).

Cyclic nucleotides diffuse in the cytoplasm at about the same rate as in free solution, activating a modest repertoire of downstream targets, including **protein kinases** (see Figs. 25-3 and 25-4), **cyclic nucleotide–gated ion channels** (see Fig. 10-10), and, in the case of cAMP, one class of nucleotide exchange factors (Epac) for small GTPases (Rap1 and Rap2). The components of this system are quite ancient, since the protein domains that bind cAMP or cGMP are homologous to the cAMP-binding domain of CAP, a bacterial transcription factor. Enzymes called cyclic nucleotide phosphodiesterases degrade cAMP and cGMP to inactive

nucleoside 5'-monophosphates. Eleven genes encode more than 40 different phosphodiesterases, which vary in their specificities for the two cyclic nucleotides, expression in various tissues, and localization to cellular compartments.

A family (10 human genes) of enzymes called **adenylyl cyclases** synthesize cAMP from ATP. Multiple transmembrane segments anchor most of these enzymes to the plasma membrane. Two homologous catalytic domains reside in the cytoplasm (C_1 and C_2 in Fig. 26-2). These cytoplasmic domains can be produced experimentally as soluble proteins separately from the transmembrane domains and can then be recombined to make a fully active enzyme. Both domains are necessary because the active site lies at the interface of the two domains. One adenylyl cyclase is a soluble enzyme that can concentrate in the nucleus. Generally, the concentration of adenylyl cyclases is very low relative to the trimeric G-proteins that regulate their activity.

Multiple regulatory mechanisms act synergistically to regulate adenylyl cyclases. **GTP-$G_s\alpha$**, the GTPase subunit of a trimeric G-protein, activates many membrane-associated adenylyl cyclases by binding far from the active site (Fig. 26-2) and inducing a conformational change. Ca^{2+}-calmodulin or protein kinase C (PKC) activates some adenylyl cyclases. **GTP-$G_i\alpha$**, the GTPase subunit of another trimeric G-protein, or protein kinase A (PKA) inhibits some cyclases. $G\beta\gamma$ subunits of trimeric

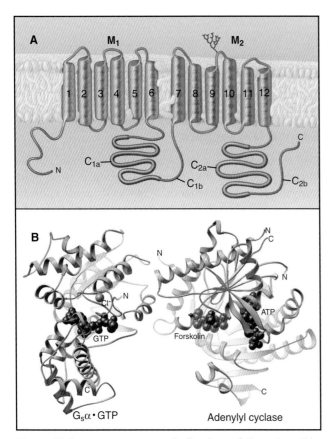

Figure 26-2 ADENYLYL CYCLASE. **A,** Topology of the polypeptide. The C_{1a} and C_{2a} regions fold together to form the active enzyme. **B,** Atomic structure of the catalytic domains of adenylyl cyclase associated with $G_s\alpha$. ATP is bound to the active site. Breaks in the chain are due to disordered regions. (PDB file: 1CJK. Reprinted with permission from Tesmer JJ, Sunahara RK, Gilman AG, Sprang R: Crystal structure of the catalytic domains of adenylyl cyclase in a complex with $G_{s\alpha}$ GTP$_\gamma$S. Science 278:1907–1916, 1997.) Copyright 1997 AAAS.

G-proteins activate some adenylyl cyclases but inhibit others. These diverse regulatory mechanisms allow adenylyl cyclases to integrate a variety of input signals. The diterpene **forskolin** from a *Coleus* plant binds to and activates adenylyl cyclases. Forskolin is useful experimentally for manipulating the cAMP concentration in cells and, on the basis of its ability to bind adenylyl cyclases, was essential in the initial purification of the enzyme by affinity chromatography. Regulation of a soluble form of adenylyl cyclase differs from that of all other isoforms. It is activated by bicarbonate, an essential step in sperm maturation.

In resting cells, the concentration of cAMP is so low, approximately 10^{-8} M, that it does not bind its targets. Stimulation of appropriate receptors (such as the seven-helix β-adrenergic receptor, see Fig. 27-3) increases the cytoplasmic cAMP concentration more than 100-fold, enough to saturate the PKA regulatory subunits (Fig. 26-3). Dissociation of the regulatory (R) subunits frees the active PKA catalytic subunits to phosphorylate cyto-

plasmic and membrane substrates and to move into the nucleus to activate the transcription factor CREB (cyclic nucleotide regulatory element–binding protein) (see Fig. 15-22).

Outside the animal kingdom, cAMP has many functions. In bacteria, cAMP controls gene expression in response to nutritional conditions. The cellular slime mold *Dictyostelium* uses cAMP as an extracellular signal, acting through a seven-helix receptor, for its social interactions (see Fig. 38-12).

Guanylyl cyclases are dimeric enzymes similar to adenylyl cyclases. In fact, mutation of just two amino acid residues can convert a guanylyl cyclase to an adenylyl cyclase. Vertebrates express two types of guanylyl cyclases (see Fig. 24-9). A family of transmembrane receptors with cytoplasmic cyclase domains respond to ligand binding by producing cGMP. Cytoplasmic guany-

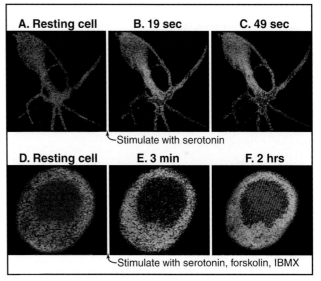

Figure 26-3 Images of cAMP transients in cultured aplysia sensory neurons. Neurons were injected with protein kinase A (PKA) labeled on the catalytic subunit with fluorescein and on the regulatory subunit with rhodamine. Fluorescence energy transfer between the dyes on the two subunits provides an assay for cAMP, which dissociates the subunits and reduces energy transfer. Fluorescent dyes also allow detection of the subunits inside the neuron. **A,** Free cAMP in the resting cell is <50 nM *(blue)*. **B–C,** Stimulation with serotonin activates adenylyl cyclase and increases cytoplasmic cAMP to the micromolar range *(red)*, especially within fine processes with a high surface-to-volume ratio. Images 120 μm wide were taken just inside the cell near the coverslip. **D,** Another resting neuron imaged at the level of the nucleus. At the low resting level of cAMP, <50 nM *(blue)* labeled PKA is excluded from the nucleus. **E,** Stimulation with serotonin plus forskolin (to stimulate adenylyl cyclase) and isobutylmethylxanthine (IBMX) to inhibit phosphodiesterases that catalyze cAMP breakdown, raises the concentration of cAMP around the nucleus *(yellow)*. **F,** Two hours later, the free catalytic subunit of PKA *(pink)* accumulates in the nucleus. (Courtesy of R. Y. Tsien, University of California, San Diego. F, Reprinted with permission from Bacskai BJ, Hochner B, Mahaut-Smith M, et al: Spatially resolved dynamics of cAMP and protein kinase A in *Aplysia* neurons. Science 260:222–226, 1993. Copyright 1993 AAAS.)

lyl cyclases are activated by nitric oxide and carbon monoxide, which bind a heme group in a regulatory domain (see the section titled "Nitric Oxide" later in this chapter).

Lipid-Derived Second Messengers

Phosphoglycerides (see Fig. 7-2) and sphingolipids (see Fig. 7-3) not only form cellular membranes but also participate in a wide range of signaling mechanisms. The long list of intracellular and extracellular second messengers derived from lipids will undoubtedly expand in the future. Three membrane lipids are the primary sources of these signaling molecules (Fig. 26-4):

1. **Phosphatidylinositol** and its various phosphorylated derivatives, discussed later, are minor lipids of the cytoplasmic leaflet of the plasma membrane and some organelle membranes.

2. **Phosphatidylcholine** is a major membrane phosphoglyceride found in both leaflets of the

plasma membrane and organelle membranes (see Fig. 7-2).

3. **Sphingomyelin,** the major membrane sphingolipid, concentrates in the outer leaflet of the plasma membrane (see Fig. 7-3).

Enzyme Reactions That Produce Lipid Second Messengers

Just three kinds of enzymes—phospholipases, lipid kinases, and lipid phosphatases—produce most lipid-derived second messengers. Remarkably, most conceivable products produced by these enzymes from the three parent lipids participate in signaling reactions, either directly or indirectly. The second messengers produced by these reactions partition between the aqueous phase of the cytoplasm (products designated by *italics* in this section) and the hydrophobic phase of the membrane bilayer (products designated by ***bold italics*** in this section). In the following paragraphs, the details of the various enzymatic reactions and the structures of the lipid derivatives are less important than is the broader principle that cells use the full range of chemical diversity in their membrane lipids to create chemical signals to regulate cellular activities.

Three types of enzyme reactions generate lipid second messengers:

1. Different **phospholipases** cleave the four ester bonds of phosphoglycerides (Fig. 26-4). Corresponding enzymes attack the two ester bonds and single amide bond of sphingomyelin. Cells have three main intracellular phospholipases. **Phospholipase A2** (PLA2) removes the C2 fatty acid, yielding a *free fatty acid,* which partitions into the cytoplasm with the aid of fatty acid–binding proteins, and a ***lysophosphoglyceride.*** The corresponding ceramidase removes the fatty acid from sphingomyelin. When **phospholipase C** (PLC) cleaves the phosphorylated head group (such as *inositol 1,4,5-triphosphate [IP$_3$]*) from a phosphoglyceride, it leaves behind ***diacylglycerol (DAG)*** in the membrane bilayer. The corresponding sphingomyelinase leaves behind ***ceramide*** in the membrane bilayer. **Phospholipase D** (PLD) cleaves the polar head group from phosphoglycerides, producing ***phosphatidic acid*** that remains in the bilayer. Production of phosphatidic acid from phosphatidylcholine generates choline, which has no known signaling activity. Note that the phospholipase A1 that cleaves the ester bond linking the fatty acid to the C1 position on the glycerol is not yet known to participate in signaling.

2. **Lipid kinases** add phosphate groups to diacylglycerol to make ***phosphatidic acid*** and to

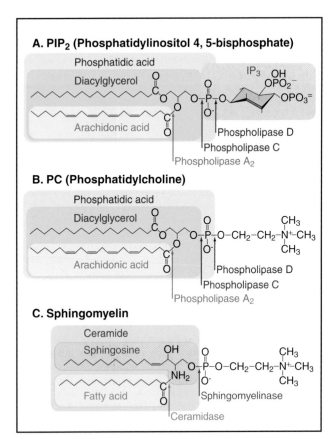

Figure 26-4   **PRODUCTION OF LIPID SECOND MESSENGERS BY ENZYMATIC ATTACKS ON THREE PARENT LIPIDS. A,** PIP$_2$ (phosphatidylinositol 4,5-bisphosphate). **B,** PC (phosphatidylcholine). **C,** Sphingomyelin. Second messengers are named and are surrounded by *colored boxes.*

phosphatidylinositol to make a variety of poly-phosphoinositides, including ***phosphatidylinositol 4-phosphate (PIP), phosphatidylinositol 4,5-bisphosphate (PIP$_2$),*** and ***phosphatidylinositol 3,4,5-trisphosphate (PIP$_3$).*** PIP$_2$ is a substrate for a family of phosphoinositide-specific phospholipase Cs that produce the important signaling molecules ***DAG*** and ***IP$_3$*** (Fig. 26-4A).

3. **Lipid phosphatases** remove phosphate from phosphatidic acid (another way to make ***DAG***) and phosphates from inositol head groups.

Cells also use transferases that add or exchange head groups or fatty acids on membrane phosphoglycerides (see Fig. 7-2). These enzymes are essential for lipid biosynthesis but have not been implicated in signaling. For example, transferases add choline (as the nucleotide conjugate cytidine diphosphate [CDP]–choline) to DAG to make phosphatidylcholine). In the case of phosphatidylinositol, the head group is provided by dephosphorylation of IP$_3$ to inositol, which is recombined enzymatically with a CDP conjugate of DAG to make phosphatidylinositol.

Sequential action of two or more enzymes produces some lipid second messengers. For example, cells can make ***DAG*** in two steps from phosphatidylcholine: PLD first makes phosphatidic acid, which is dephosphorylated by phosphatidic acid phosphatase. PLD followed by PLA2 makes *lysophosphatidic acid* from phosphatidylcholine. PLA2 also initiates the production of a huge family of fatty acid derivatives called *eicosanoids* by cleaving the fatty acid arachidonic acid from phosphatidylcholine. Cyclooxygenases and lipoxygenases then modify arachidonic acid to make *prostaglandins, thromboxanes,* and *leukotrienes* (Figs. 26-9 and 26-10), which leave the cell to interact with cell surface receptors.

Agonists and Receptors

Most signaling pathways have the potential to produce lipid second messengers, depending on the expression of the appropriate enzymes. Some pathways activate enzymes directly; receptor tyrosine kinases bind and activate certain **phosphatidylinositol phospholipase Cs** (PI-PLCs). Seven-helix receptors signal through trimeric G-proteins to activate another PI-PLC. Other pathways are less direct; one leads from G-protein-coupled receptors or receptor tyrosine kinases to DAG and PKC, activating an isoform of phospholipase D.

Targets of Lipid Second Messengers

Downstream targets of the lipid second messengers are diverse but can be generalized to some extent into three categories (Fig. 26-5):

1. Most lipid second messengers derived from phosphoglycerides and retained in the membrane bilayer exert their physiological effects on PKC isozymes (Fig. 26-6). Ceramide is also retained in the bilayer, where it activates another protein kinase and a protein phosphatase (see Fig. 26-11). Phosphatidic acid activates a lipid kinase, PI5 kinase, which phosphorylates phosphatidylinositol (Fig. 26-7).

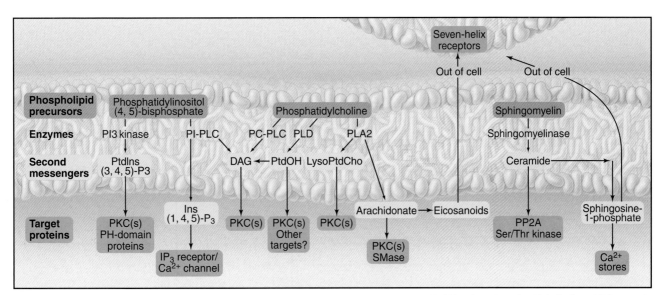

Figure 26-5 GENERATION OF LIPID SECOND MESSENGERS AND THEIR CELLULAR TARGETS. LysoPtdCho, lysophosphatidyl choline; PKC, protein kinase C; PP2A, protein phosphatase 2A; PtdIns (3,4,5)-P$_3$, PIP$_3$; PtdOH, phosphatidic acid; SMase, sphingomyelinase. (Adapted from Liscovitch M, Cantley LC: Lipid second messengers. Cell 77:329–334, 1994.)

2. IP$_3$ and sphingosine-1-phosphate use different mechanisms to release Ca^{2+} from vesicular stores in the cytoplasm (Fig. 26-12).

3. All water-soluble lipid second messengers containing or derived from fatty acids (platelet-activating factor [PAF], lysophosphatidic acid [LPA], eicosanoids) leave the cell and bind to G-protein-coupled, seven-helix receptors on the surface of target cells.

With so much potential for information transfer (multiple agonists, multiple membrane transduction mechanisms, multiple lipid second messengers, and multiple downstream targets), where is the specificity in these systems? Do all cells respond in all possible ways? The answer is no, and the explanation is that the protein hardware required for these reactions is selectively expressed in differentiated cells and carefully localized at particular sites in cells, such as the plasma membrane, nucleus, or cytoskeleton. In addition, targeting of PKC isozymes to particular cellular compartments ensures that only selected substrates are phosphorylated in response to lipid second messenger production. Thus, each cell takes a limited number of items from the lipid second messenger menu and uses them to produce a selective, customized response to each agonist.

Lipid second messengers participate in many processes that are considered elsewhere in the book. For example, regulated secretion (see Chapter 21) in response to an agonist binding a seven-helix or tyrosine kinase receptor requires a transient Ca^{2+} signal in the cytoplasm. The Ca^{2+} is released from the membrane stores by IP$_3$, which is produced by the action of a PI-PLC on PIP$_2$. IP$_3$-mediated Ca^{2+} release from the endoplasmic reticulum also controls smooth muscle contraction (see Fig. 39-21).

Protein Kinase C

Many lipid second messengers, including DAG, PIP$_3$, arachidonic acid, phosphatidic acid, and lysophosphatidylcholine activate one or more of the 10 protein kinase C (PKC) isozymes expressed by vertebrate cells (Fig. 26-6). These multiple PKC isozymes provide a selective response to various lipid second messengers. Some, but not all, PKC isozymes also require Ca^{2+} for activation. Sphingosine may inhibit some PKC isozymes.

PKCs have a protein kinase catalytic domain (see Fig. 25-3) and N-terminal regulatory domains. A **pseudosubstrate sequence** binds intramolecularly to the active site and inhibits activity by blocking substrate binding. Pseudosubstrates have alanine at the phosphorylation site instead of serine as substrates have. During apoptosis, caspases cleave off this regulatory domain (see Fig. 46-10) producing constitutively active PKC isoforms.

Lipid second messengers activate PKC by binding C1 regions and dissociating the pseudosubstrate from the active site. **Phorbol esters,** pharmacological activators of PKC that promote tumor formation, bind PKC in a similar fashion. Binding DAG or phorbol esters also requires phosphoglycerides, such as phosphatidylserine. Ca^{2+}-dependent PKC isozymes have C2 regions that mediate binding to phospholipids in the presence of Ca^{2+}.

Activated PKCs have many potential targets in cells and have been implicated in the regulation of cellular activities ranging from gene expression to cell motility to the generation of lipid second messengers. PKC isozymes differ in their activity toward protein substrates. Localization of various PKC isozymes to different parts of the cell might provide additional specificity. Receptors for activated C kinases bind C2 regions and target PKC isozymes to the plasma membrane, cytoskeleton, or nucleus.

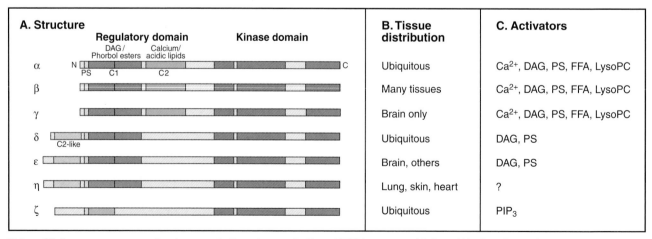

A. Structure		**B. Tissue distribution**	**C. Activators**
α	Ubiquitous	Ca^{2+}, DAG, PS, FFA, LysoPC
β	Many tissues	Ca^{2+}, DAG, PS, FFA, LysoPC
γ	Brain only	Ca^{2+}, DAG, PS, FFA, LysoPC
δ	Ubiquitous	DAG, PS
ε	Brain, others	DAG, PS
η	Lung, skin, heart	?
ζ	Ubiquitous	PIP$_3$

Figure 26-6 PROTEIN KINASE C (PKC) FAMILY. **A,** Domain organization of PKC isozymes with ligand-binding sites. PS indicates the pseudosubstrate sequence that binds to and inhibits the kinase catalytic site. **B,** Tissue distribution. **C,** Activators. DAG, diacylglycerol; FFA, free fatty acid, LysoPC, lysophosphatidylcholine; PIP$_3$ is phosphatidylinositol 3,4,5-trisphosphate; PS, phosphatidylserine.

PKCs can provide either positive or negative feedback to the signaling pathways that turn them on. PKC activates PLD and PLA2 and provides positive feedback, because those enzymes produce more DAG to sustain the activation of PKC. On the other hand, PKC provides negative feedback when it phosphorylates and inhibits both growth factor receptors and PI-PLCγ1. PKC also phosphorylates and inhibits PI-PLCβ, generating negative feedback after activation of seven-helix receptors. Negative feedback makes both of these signaling events transient.

Phosphoinositide Signaling Pathways

Although minor in terms of mass in biological membranes, phosphoinositides are major players in signaling (Fig. 26-7). The parent compound, phosphatidylinositol (PI), is a phosphoglyceride with a cyclohexanol head group called inositol. Specific lipid kinases phosphorylate the 4 and 5 hydroxyl groups of phosphatidylinositol to form PI(4-)P and PI(4,5-)P_2, usually referred to simply as PIP and PIP_2. A specific phosphatase can

remove the D5 phosphate. Inactivation of the single copy of this gene on the X-chromosome causes Lowe's syndrome with cataracts, renal failure, and mental retardation.

PIP_2 is a substrate for a family of receptor-controlled PI-PLCs that cleave off the phosphorylated head group, producing two potent second messengers: IP_3 and DAG. Water-soluble IP_3 activates Ca^{2+} release channels in the endoplasmic reticulum (Fig. 26-12), and lipid-soluble DAG activates PKC. In contrast to Ca^{2+}, which diffuses slowly and acts locally, IP_3 diffuses rapidly through the cytoplasm, triggering Ca^{2+} release. DAG is confined to membranes but diffuses laterally to bind and activate PKC. Enzymes inactivate both IP_3 and DAG. DAG is inactivated by phosphorylation to make phosphatidic acid, a second messenger in its own right but also an intermediate in the resynthesis of phosphoinositides. IP_3 is dephosphorylated to inositol, which is inactive as a second messenger. LiCl inhibits the final step: dephosphorylation of inositol-1-phosphate. Remarkably, Li^+ is clinically useful as a treatment for bipolar disorder, presumably by interfering with phosphoinositide signaling in the brain. In some tissues, IP_3 is inactivated by phosphorylation to inositol 1,3,4,5-tetrakisphosphate (IP_4).

Vertebrates use 10 classes of PI-PLCs to provide tissue-specific coupling of various receptors to the production of IP_3 and DAG. PI-PLCγ1, expressed in the brain, is activated by tyrosine phosphorylation when its SH2 domains bind a tyrosine-phosphorylated receptor tyrosine kinase (Fig. 26-12). The trimeric G-protein $G_q\alpha$ activates another isozyme, PI-PLCβ.

When a PI-PLC hydrolyzes PIP_2, phosphatidylinositol-4 kinase and phosphatidylinositol-5 kinase respond to replace the pool of PIP_2 at the expense of membrane phosphatidylinositol. This generates a transient flux of lipid molecules from phosphatidylinositol to PIP to PIP_2 to DAG. On a longer time scale, phosphatidylinositol is replaced by synthesis from phosphatidic acid and inositol.

Receptor tyrosine kinases activate another family of lipid kinases, **PI-3 kinases,** which phosphorylate the 3-hydroxyl group of PI, PIP, and PIP_2. The products are PI(3-)P, PI(3,4-)P_2, and PI(3,4,5-)P_3. PI(3,4,5-)P_3 is not a substrate for the PI-PLCs that produce IP_3 and DAG, but it activates some PKC isozymes and binds specifically to certain pleckstrin homology domains (see Fig. 25-11), bringing enzymes such as protein kinase B **(PKB/Akt)** to the plasma membrane. Association with the membrane leads to phosphorylation and activation of PKB as part of insulin signaling (see Fig. 27-7). A phosphatase that removes the D3 phosphate from PIP_3 is a tumor suppressor called PTEN (phosphatase and tensin homolog deleted on chromosome 10). Loss of PTEN function in tumors allows PIP_3 to build up, activating PKB and growth promoting downstream

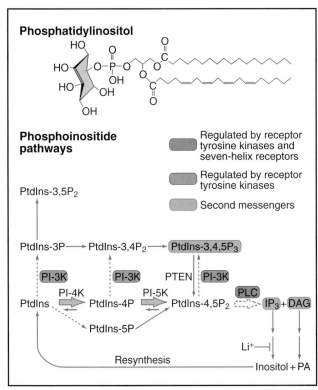

Figure 26-7 SYNTHESIS AND TURNOVER OF PHOSPHOINOSITIDES. Enzymes regulated by receptor tyrosine kinases and seven-helix receptors are *purple.* Enzymes regulated by receptor tyrosine kinases are *blue.* Second messengers are *green.* PA, phosphatidic acid; PI-3k, phosphatidylinositol 3 kinase; PI-4k, phosphatidylinositol 4 kinase; PI-5k, phosphatidylinositol 5 kinase; PtdIns, phosphatidylinositol; PTEN, phosphatase and tensin homolog deleted on chromosome 10 (a tumor suppressor).

pathways in many tumors. A steroid-like molecule called **wortmannin** inhibits PI-3 kinase relatively specifically and is used to investigate the physiological roles of PIP$_3$.

Phosphatidylcholine Signaling Pathways

Phosphatidylcholine is not only a major structural lipid of the plasma membrane but also an important source of DAG and a large family of other signaling molecules (Fig. 26-5). In response to agonist stimulation, cells produce two waves of DAG (Fig. 26-8). Within seconds, PI-PLCs activated by seven-helix or tyrosine kinase receptors produce the first wave of DAG from PIP$_2$. Then, over a period of minutes, a second wave of DAG is derived from phosphatidylcholine, either directly by a PC-PLC or in two steps by PLD (to remove choline) and a phosphatidic acid phosphatase (to remove the phosphate from phosphatidic acid). The first wave of DAG may contribute to the second wave as PKC activates one PLD isoform. Ca^{2+} produced in the first wave may also activate PLD.

Phosphatidylcholine is also the main source of fatty acid–derived second messengers. PLA2 releases **arachidonic acid,** a C20 unsaturated fatty acid that is found predominantly at the C2 position of phosphoglycerides. Arachidonic acid activates some PKC isozymes and, together with DAG, provides positive feedback to PLA2 and PLD to sustain the production of arachidonic acid and DAG.

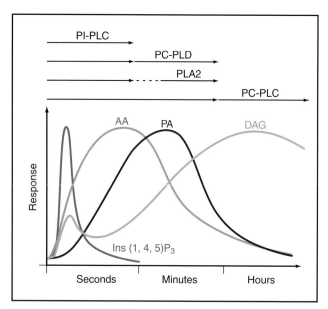

Figure 26-8 TIME COURSE OF LIPID SECOND MESSENGERS PRODUCED BY VARIOUS PHOSPHOLIPASES FOLLOWING ACTIVATION OF RECEPTOR TYROSINE KINASES OR SEVEN-HELIX RECEPTORS. AA, arachidonic acid; DAG, diacylglycerol; PA, phosphatidic acid; PC, phosphatidylcholine; PI, phosphatidylinositol.

Lipid-Derived Second Messengers for Intercellular Communication

Cells produce an amazing array of bioactive compounds from phosphatidylcholine and arachidonic acid, forming second messengers that escape from the cell and mediate their effects by binding to receptors on the surface of the cell of origin or neighboring cells. As such, these compounds are locally active hormones. This sets them apart from classical second messengers, which (with the exception of nitric oxide) act inside the cell of origin. All of the compounds presented here activate target cells by binding G-protein-coupled, seven-helix receptors. Vertebrates make a particularly rich variety of these lipid-derived signaling molecules, but slime molds and algae use some of the same compounds for communication.

Eicosanoids (*eicosa* is Greek for "20") are a diverse family of metabolites derived from the 20-carbon fatty acid arachidonic acid, including **prostaglandins, thromboxanes, leukotrienes,** and **lipoxins** (Figs. 26-9 and 26-10). Depending on the particular receptor and G-protein, eicosanoids selectively activate or inhibit the synthesis of cAMP, release Ca^{2+}, activate PKC, or regulate ion channels. Biological consequences are diverse, depending on the specific eicosanoid and target cell. Eicosanoids are important medically as mediators of inflammation.

Prostaglandins and thromboxanes are synthesized from arachidonic acid by pairs of enzymes, the first being generic and the second being specific for a particular product (Fig. 26-9). Typically, differentiated cells express primarily one second-step enzyme and thus produce just one of these local hormones.

The first enzyme, **prostaglandin H synthetase (cyclooxygenase),** has two active sites that catalyze successive reactions that convert arachidonic acid into prostaglandin G$_2$ and then into prostaglandin H$_2$. Most cells express cyclooxygenase-1 (COX-1) constitutively as a housekeeping enzyme. Inflammatory stimuli induce expression of the closely related enzyme **cyclooxygenase**-2 (COX-2). Cyclooxygenases bind to the cytoplasmic surfaces of the membranes of the endoplasmic reticulum and nuclear envelope. Second-tier enzymes are specific **prostaglandin isomerases** that convert prostaglandin H into various prostaglandin and thromboxane products.

Physiological responses to each eicosanoid depend on selective expression of specific seven-helix receptors. For example, receptors for prostaglandin F$_{2a}$ prepare the uterus, but not other organs of pregnant mammals, for delivery. Receptors for counteracting eicosanoids control the response of platelets to blood vessel damage (see Fig. 30-14). Normally, endothelial cells lining blood vessels produce prostaglandin I$_2$ (prostacyclin), which inhibits interaction of platelets with

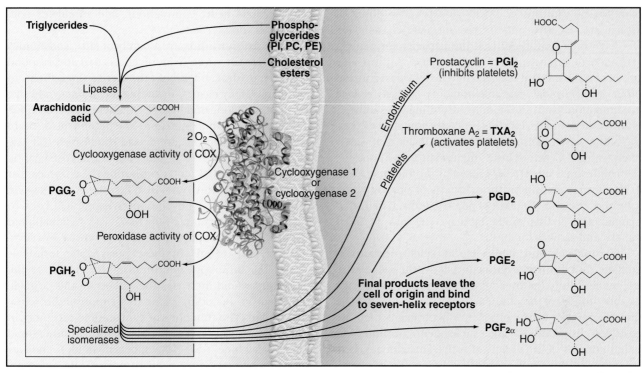

Figure 26-9 PATHWAY OF PROSTAGLANDIN SYNTHESIS. Cyclooxygenase-1 (ribbon diagram) is a homodimer that is bound to the surface of a lipid bilayer by hydrophobic membrane-binding helices. This enzyme has two active sites that convert arachidonic acid to prostaglandin H$_2$. A hydrophobic channel 2.5 nm long leads from the bilayer to the active sites. Nonsteroidal anti-inflammatory drugs compete with arachidonic acid for binding to the cyclooxygenase active site, and aspirin covalently modifies serine 530 in the active site. Specific prostaglandin synthases convert prostaglandin H$_2$ into various products. PC, phosphatidylcholine; PE, phosphatidyl ethanolamine; PI, phosphatidylinositol; TXA$_2$, thromboxane A. (PDB file: 1CQE.)

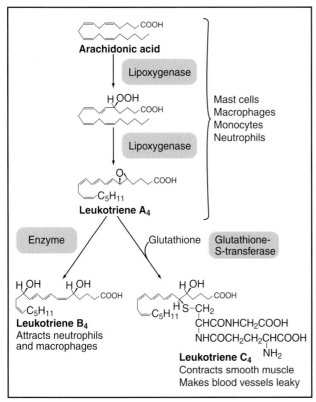

Figure 26-10 PATHWAYS OF LEUKOTRIENE SYNTHESIS.

the vessel wall and promotes blood flow by relaxing smooth muscle cells in the wall of the vessel. In response to damage, the blood-clotting protein thrombin activates platelets to aggregate and plug gaps in the endothelium. Activated platelets produce thromboxane A$_2$, which diffuses locally to promote irreversible platelet aggregation and blood vessel constriction by triggering production of IP$_3$, release of Ca^{2+}, and contraction of smooth muscle (see Fig. 39-21). This secondary response mediated by positive feedback through thromboxane A$_2$ minimizes blood loss but can contribute to pathological formation of clots in vital blood vessels, resulting in heart attacks and strokes. Tissue injury also provokes synthesis of prostaglandins E$_2$ and I$_2$, which mediate inflammation locally by dilating blood vessels, sensitizing pain receptors, and causing fever.

Nonsteroidal anti-inflammatory drugs, including aspirin and ibuprofen, target both cyclooxygenase isozymes. Most of these drugs competitively inhibit arachidonic acid binding to both enzymes, but aspirin covalently and irreversibly acetylates a serine residue in their active sites. Either way, these drugs inhibit the synthesis of all prostaglandins and thromboxanes. Aspirin reduces the incidence of heart attacks and strokes by inhibiting the synthesis of thromboxane A$_2$ by platelets, which reduces platelet aggregation and pathological clotting in blood vessels. Low doses of aspirin are selective and effective for platelets, as platelets have only COX-I and lack the capacity for protein synthesis to replace inactivated enzyme. Aspirin also protects against colon cancer. High doses of aspirin and other nonsteroidal anti-inflammatory drugs reduce inflammation, pain, and fever by inhibiting the synthesis of other eicosanoids, but this is not without side effects, including gastrointestinal bleeding. Drugs that selectively inhibit COX-2 relieve inflammation without the gastrointestinal side effects caused by inhibition of COX-1. However, they inhibit the synthesis of prostaglandin I_2 by endothelium. The lack of prostaglandin I_2 to inhibit platelet aggregation might increase the risk of heart attacks and strokes.

Macrophages and white blood cells produce an enzyme called **5-lipoxygenase** that synthesizes leukotrienes and lipoxins by addition of oxygen to specific double bonds of arachidonic acid (Fig. 26-10). The first biologically active product, leukotriene A_4, can be modified by addition and subsequent trimming of glutathione to yield a variety of active leukotrienes. Leukotrienes mediate inflammatory reactions by constricting blood vessels, allowing plasma to leak from small vessels and attracting white blood cells into connective tissue. These effects, together with constriction of the respiratory tract, contribute to the symptoms of asthma. Drugs that inhibit 5-lipoxygenase and leukotriene receptors are being tested in treatment of asthma and other inflammatory diseases, including atherosclerosis. Lipoxins are another family of mediators that act on blood vessels. They are formed by the addition of oxygen to both the C-5 and C-15 positions of arachidonic acid.

Phosphatidylcholine is also the starting point for production of two other water-soluble, intercellular, second messengers: **lysophosphatidic acid (LPA)** and **platelet-activating factor (PAF)**. Activated platelets and injured fibroblasts produce LPA from phosphatidylcholine by the action of the phospholipases PLD and PLA2 (Fig. 26-4). A variety of cells synthesize PAF in two steps, using PLA2 to remove the C2 fatty acid from phosphatidylcholine molecules with an ether-bonded fatty alcohol (rather than an ester-bonded fatty acid) on the C1 position and a second enzyme to acetylate the C2 hydroxyl group. LPA and PAF escape cells and stimulate target cells by binding to seven-helix receptors. Depending on their signaling hardware, cells respond to LPA in different ways: Activation of the PLC/IP$_3$ pathway releases intracellular Ca^{2+} in some cells; activation of a mitogen-activated protein (MAP) kinase pathway (see Fig. 27-5) stimulates some cells to divide; and activation of Rho-family small GTPases stimulates formation of actin bundles in cultured cells (see Fig. 33-20). As is expected from its name, PAF activates platelets, but it also modifies the behavior of other blood

cells, inhibits heart contractions, and stimulates contraction of the uterus.

Endocannabinoids are a family of fatty acid amides that activate the seven-helix receptors that also respond to Δ^9-tetrahydrocannabinol, the active ingredient in marijuana. Many tissues, including the brain, synthesize the classic endocannabinoid, *N*-arachidonoyl-ethanolamine, from ethanolamine and arachidonic acid. Brain cannabinoid receptors are found exclusively on the axonal side of synapses. Stimulation of the postsynaptic neuron results in Ca^{2+} entry, activating the enzymes that synthesize endocannabinoids. When these lipid second messengers diffuse from the postsynaptic cell back to the presynaptic terminal, they bind class 1 cannabinoid receptors, which suppress transmitter release by blocking Ca^{2+} entry. Some of these presynaptic terminals secrete the inhibitory neurotransmitter GABA, so the endocannabinoid increases the activity of the postsynaptic neuron, including those that suppress the sensation of pain. The functions of cannabinoid receptors in other tissues are less well understood. Another lipid amide, oleamide (*cis*-9,10-octadecenoamide), induces sleep in mammals, most likely through GABA receptors (see Fig. 10-12). An enzyme called fatty acid amide hydrolase degrades all of these signaling molecules.

Sphingomyelin/Ceramide Signaling Pathways

Activation of plasma membrane receptors for **tumor necrosis factor (TNF)** and **interleukin-2 (IL-2)** stimulates formation of the lipid-soluble second messenger *ceramide* from sphingomyelin (Fig. 26-11). Sphingomyelin is concentrated in the external leaflet of the plasma membrane (Fig. 26-4). Ligand binding to TNF or IL-2 receptors activates a plasma membrane **sphingomyelinase** (a specialized PLC) that removes phosphorylcholine from sphingomyelin, producing ceramide. Ceramide flips across the lipid bilayer to the cytoplasmic surface and activates a proline-directed, serine/threonine protein kinase associated with the plasma membrane. Target proteins have the sequence X-Ser/Thr-Pro-X and include epidermal growth factor (EGF) receptor and Raf kinase. Downstream events include activation of MAP kinase, which activates transcription factors and other effectors (see Fig. 27-6). Ceramide also activates a protein phosphatases 1 and 2A.

Sphingosine and *sphingosine-1-phosphate* are produced from sphingomyelin by a succession of enzymatic reactions (Fig. 26-4). Ceramidase removes the fatty acid, and sphingomyelinase removes the phosphorylcholine head group to form sphingosine. Then sphingosine kinase adds phosphate to C1 to make sphingosine-1-phosphate. Growth factor signaling pathways might regulate this lipid kinase. Sphingosine-1-phosphate escapes from cells and activates seven-helix

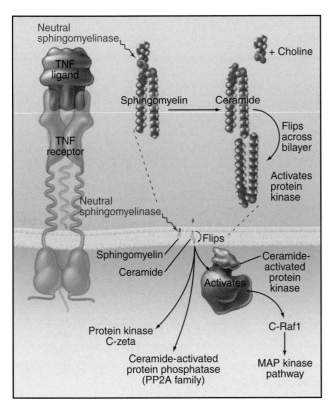

Figure 26-11 SPHINGOMYELIN/CERAMIDE SIGNALING PATHWAY. Stimulation of the tumor necrosis factor (TNF) receptor activates a neutral sphingomyelinase, which cleaves choline from sphingomyelin. Ceramide flips across the bilayer and activates a cytoplasmic kinase as well as PKC-ζ and a protein phosphatase.

receptors on the same or other cells. Cells respond by releasing Ca^{2+}, which influences motility and growth, as well as smooth muscle contraction. The biological effects of sphingosine are incompletely defined but include regulation of PKC.

Cross Talk

Interaction (cross talk) among lipid second messenger pathways is thought to integrate signals from different agonists. Consequently, it is difficult to define distinct linear pathways from an agonist to an individual effector through lipid second messengers. The following are some examples of cross talk using enzymes defined in Figure 26-4:

1. Two pathways may modulate each other. PI-PLCs produce DAG, which activates PKC, which phosphorylates and activates PLA2 and PLD. These activated enzymes produce additional lipid second messengers (arachidonic acid and phosphatidic acid) to amplify and diversify the initial response.

2. Two pathways may converge on the same target. Arachidonic acid (produced by activated PLA2)

and DAG (produced by either a PI-PLC or PLD and phosphatidic acid phosphatase) synergistically activate some PKC isozymes.

3. A messenger from one pathway can be converted to a messenger on a second pathway. DAG and phosphatidic acid are readily interconverted by the appropriate kinase and phosphatase.

Calcium

Overview of Calcium Regulation

Calcium ion, Ca^{2+}, is a versatile second messenger that regulates many processes, including synaptic transmission, fertilization, secretion, muscle contraction, and cytokinesis. All eukaryotes (but not prokaryotes) use Ca^{2+} signals. Nature probably chose Ca^{2+} for signaling by default. Because cells depend on phosphate for energy metabolism (ATP), nucleic acid structure, and many other functions and because calcium phosphate precipitates, early cells evolved mechanisms to extrude Ca^{2+} from cytoplasm. Cells took advantage of the resulting Ca^{2+} gradient between cytoplasm and ocean water (or extracellular space in animals) to drive tiny pulses of Ca^{2+} into cytoplasm for signaling. This movement of Ca^{2+} between compartments via ion channels is very fast.

In contrast to all other second messengers, which are synthesized and metabolized, Ca^{2+} levels are controlled by release into and removal from the cytoplasm (Fig. 26-12). ATP-driven **Ca^{2+} pumps** of the plasma membrane and endoplasmic reticulum keep cytoplasmic Ca^{2+} levels low (about 0.1 μM in resting cells) and generate a 10,000-fold concentration gradient across these membranes. A remarkable variety of stimuli, operating through many different receptors (Table 26-1), open **Ca^{2+} channels** in the plasma membrane or endoplasmic reticulum, allowing a concentrated puff of Ca^{2+}, called a Ca^{2+} transient or "spark," to enter the cytoplasm. Peak cytoplasmic Ca^{2+} concentrations in stimulated cells are in the micromolar range. The durations of Ca^{2+} signals range from milliseconds to minutes depending on the nature of the stimulus, the type of release channel, the rate of Ca^{2+} pumping out of cytoplasm, and the rates of binding and dissociation on target proteins. Ca^{2+} levels can rise and fall locally, flood the whole cytoplasm, or travel in waves across a cell.

Ca^{2+} signals work locally in cytoplasm. Although Ca^{2+} is a small ion with a large diffusion coefficient in water, its diffusion through cytoplasm is very slow, owing to efficient sequestering mechanisms and abundant Ca^{2+}-binding proteins, estimated to be 300 μM. Thus, only about 1 in 100 Ca^{2+} ions is free to diffuse in cytoplasm; the other 99 are bound. At a concentration of 0.1 μM in the cytoplasm of resting cell, the half-time for a free Ca^{2+}

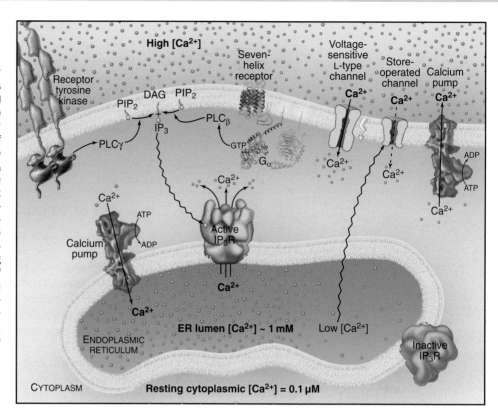

Figure 26-12 Pathways of Ca²⁺ release and uptake. Ca²⁺ pumps in the plasma membrane and endoplasmic reticulum membrane use ATP hydrolysis to pump Ca²⁺ out of the cytoplasm. A variety of receptors activate phospholipase C (PLC) isozymes to produce IP₃ from PIP₂. IP₃ diffuses to the endoplasmic reticulum, where it opens IP₃ receptors (IP₃R), releasing Ca²⁺ from the lumen into cytoplasm. Voltage-sensitive L-type Ca²⁺ channels respond to membrane depolarization by admitting extracellular Ca²⁺. Depletion of Ca²⁺ stored in the endoplasmic reticulum activates plasma membrane Ca²⁺ channels, likely members of the Trp channel family, which admit extracellular Ca²⁺ to replenish stores.

ion is about 30 µs, and its range of diffusion is only about 0.1 µm. Thus, although Ca²⁺ pours through release channels at a rate of 10⁶ ions per second, it does not spread but acts locally. Ca²⁺, when bound to a protein messenger such as **calmodulin,** has a wider range of about 5 µm.

Cellular responses to Ca²⁺ signals depend on the available repertoire of Ca²⁺-sensitive proteins and effector systems (Appendix 26-1). Some Ca²⁺-binding proteins respond directly, such as **Ca²⁺-activated ion channels,** whereas others initiate a cascade of downstream reactions. For example, Ca²⁺ binding to calmodulin has no direct consequence, but Ca²⁺-calmodulin

regulates more than a dozen proteins, including protein kinases and adenylyl cyclase.

The following sections consider each component that regulates Ca²⁺ signals: pumps that clear Ca²⁺ from cytoplasm, Ca²⁺ storage compartments, membrane channels that release Ca²⁺ into cytoplasm, stimuli that open these channels, and effector proteins that mediate the effects of Ca²⁺ signals.

Removal of Ca²⁺ from Cytoplasm

The best-characterized Ca²⁺ storage compartment is the **sarcoplasmic reticulum** of striated muscle (see

Table 26-1

STIMULI FOR CA²⁺ SIGNALS

Stimulus	Receptor Class	Second Messenger	Distribution
Action potentials	Voltage-sensitive Ca²⁺ channels	None	Nerve, muscle
ATP	P2X plasma membrane channels	None	Many cells
	P2Y seven-helix G-protein-coupled receptors	IP₃	Many cells
Peptide growth factors	Receptor tyrosine kinases	IP₃	Many cells
Antigens	T-cell receptor, tyrosine kinases	IP₃	Lymphocytes
Peptide hormones	Seven-helix G-protein-coupled receptors	IP₃	Endocrine cells
Neurotransmitters	Ligand-gated cation channels	None	Neurons
	Seven-helix G-protein-coupled receptors	IP₃	Neurons
Light	Rhodopsin, G-proteins	IP₃	Photoreceptors

Table 26-2

MOLECULAR COMPONENTS OF THE CALCIUM-SEQUESTERING COMPARTMENTS

Cell Type	Ca^{2+} Pump	Sequestering Proteins	Release Channel
Striated muscles	SR calcium ATPase	Calsequestrin	Ryanodine receptor
Smooth muscle	Calcium ATPase	Calreticulin > calsequestrin	IP_3 receptor and ryanodine receptor
Nonmuscle cells	One of five Ca ATPases	Calreticulin > calsequestrin	IP_3 receptor and/or ryanodine receptor

Fig. 39-10), a specialized smooth endoplasmic reticulum with remarkably high concentrations of the SERCA Ca-ATPase pump and ryanodine receptor Ca^{2+} channels (Table 26-2). These proteins give sarcoplasmic reticulum a great capacity to handle the millisecond Ca^{2+} transients that control muscle contraction (see Fig. 39-15). Other cells use similar mechanisms but are endowed more modestly with these Ca^{2+}-handling proteins. Mitochondria sequester Ca^{2+}, using carriers driven by the electrochemical potential across the inner membrane. Although their Ca^{2+} content is high, mitochondria do not participate in signal transduction by regulated release of Ca^{2+} into cytoplasm.

Pumps

ATP-driven Ca^{2+} pumps of the plasma membrane and endoplasmic reticulum remove Ca^{2+} from cytoplasm (see Fig. 8-7). These P-type pumps move Ca^{2+} out of cytoplasm against a concentration gradient of about 10^4, hydrolyzing one ATP for every two Ca^{2+} transferred from the cytoplasm out of the cell or into the endoplasmic reticulum storage compartment. Cytoplasmic Ca^{2+} activates Ca^{2+} pumps until the Ca^{2+} in the cytoplasm falls to about 0.1 μM, the resting level. Three different genes and alternative splicing produce at least five different Ca^{2+}-ATPase pumps. In the heart, the activity of the Ca^{2+}-ATPase is modulated by **phospholamban,** a 6-kD integral membrane protein of the sarcoplasmic reticulum. Phosphorylation by PKA and calmodulin-activated (CaM) kinase dissociates phospholamban from the Ca^{2+} pump, stimulating its activity.

Sequestering Proteins

Proteins in the lumen of the endoplasmic reticulum bind much of the Ca^{2+}, but their low affinity ensures that bound and free Ca^{2+} are in a rapid equilibrium, providing free Ca^{2+} for release when membrane channels open. **Calsequestrin** is a major Ca^{2+}-binding protein of the sarcoplasmic reticulum. In nonmuscle cells, the endoplasmic reticulum lumen sometimes contains calsequestrin, but more commonly, it contains **calreticulin,** a 47-kD protein with a low affinity (K_d = 250 μM) but high capacity (25 moles) for Ca^{2+}. Calreticu-

lin is also a chaperone for protein folding in the endoplasmic reticulum (see Fig. 20-10).

Refilling Endoplasmic Reticulum

Repeated stimulation can deplete Ca^{2+} from intracellular stores, because some released Ca^{2+} is pumped out of the cell by plasma membrane pumps. Endoplasmic reticulum stores can also be depleted experimentally by **thapsigargin,** a lactone isolated from plants that inhibits most known endoplasmic reticulum Ca^{2+} pumps. In either case, cells replenish the stores by admitting extracellular Ca^{2+} through low-conductance channels, most likely but not yet definitely proven to be members of the Trp family (see Fig. 10-9). This is called **store-operated Ca^{2+} entry.** Some Trp channels respond to DAG or arachidonic acid, while others respond to decreased levels of Ca^{2+} in the endoplasmic reticulum, yet the physiological stimuli for refilling the endoplasmic reticulum in most cell types are still unclear.

Calcium-Release Channels

Voltage-gated and agonist-gated channels in the plasma membrane (Table 26-3 and Fig. 26-12) admit Ca^{2+} into the cytoplasm from outside. Chapter 10 explains how the membrane potential or agonists open these channels. Voltage-gated channels are essential for rapid responses in excitable cells such as those of muscles and neurons. Owing to rapid inactivation by negative feedback from the released Ca^{2+}, most of these channels produce brief, self-limited Ca^{2+} pulses.

Two types of agonist-gated channels—called IP_3 receptors and ryanodine receptors—release Ca^{2+} from the endoplasmic reticulum. Skeletal muscle uses ryanodine receptors, whereas smooth muscle and nonmuscle cells have both types of release channels. Each type of channel is regulated in different ways, allowing diverse stimuli to trigger the release of Ca^{2+}. In excitable cells, plasma membrane Ca^{2+} channels trigger ryanodine-receptor channels to release Ca^{2+} from the endoplasmic reticulum. In nonexcitable cells, stimulation of either seven-helix receptors or receptor tyrosine kinases produces IP_3, which triggers IP_3 receptors to release Ca^{2+} from the endoplasmic reticulum.

Table 26-3

CA²⁺-RELEASE CHANNELS

Type	Distribution	Control	Features
Plasma Membrane Ca²⁺ Channels			
ATP-activated channel	Smooth muscle	Extracellular ATP	
cAMP-activated channel	Sperm	Cytoplasmic cAMP	
L-type Ca²⁺-channel	Skeletal and cardiac muscle, brain, other nonmuscle cells	Voltage	Excitation-contraction coupling, defective in muscular dysgenesis. High threshold, dihydropyridine (DHP)-sensitive, regulated by PKA
N-type Ca²⁺-channel	Neurons, endocrine cells	Voltage	Neurotransmitter release, modulated by G-proteins. High threshold, conotoxin-sensitive
P-type Ca²⁺-channel	Purkinje neurons	Voltage	Insensitive to dihydropyridine and conotoxin
T-type Ca²⁺-channel		Voltage	Low threshold
Endoplasmic Reticulum Ca²⁺ Channels			
IP₃ receptors	Most cells including brain and smooth muscle	IP₃, Ca²⁺	Heparin-sensitive
Type I ryanodine receptor	Skeletal muscle	DHP-receptor, Ca²⁺	Ca²⁺ release stimulates contraction
Type II ryanodine receptor	Cardiac muscle, other cells	Ca²⁺, cADP-ribose	Ca²⁺ release stimulates contraction
Type III ryanodine receptor	Smooth muscle, other cells	Ca²⁺, cADP-ribose	Ca²⁺ release stimulates contraction

Inositol 1,4,5-Trisphosphate Receptor Ca²⁺ Channels

Numerous signal transduction pathways generate IP₃ (Fig. 26-7), which activates IP₃ receptors to release Ca²⁺ from the endoplasmic reticulum in animal cells. Plants and fungi appear to lack IP₃ receptors.

IP₃ receptors are tetramers of giant 313-kD polypeptides with multiple domains mostly in the cytoplasm (Fig. 26-13). Six transmembrane segments near the C-terminus form a tetrameric Ca²⁺ channel similar to other cation channels, including a P-loop between segments 5 and 6 facing the lumen of the ER (see Fig. 10-3). The pore is large and nonselective, but Ca²⁺ is the main ion

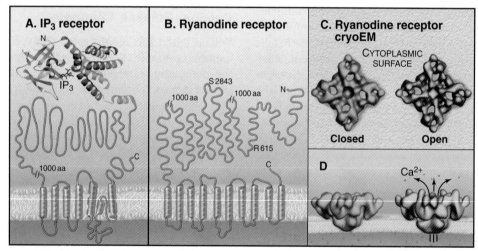

Figure 26-13 CALCIUM RELEASE CHANNELS. **A,** IP₃ receptor–channel domain organization. Residues 225 to 576 form two domains that bind IP₃ in between as shown by the ribbon diagram. The structure of residues 576 to 2350 is not known. Six transmembrane segments starting at about 2350 form the calcium channel with a postulated P-loop facing the lumen of the ER between the last two transmembrane segments. **B,** Ryanodine receptor–channel domain organization. The cytoplasmic domain is far too large to depict to scale in this space, so two segments of 1000 residues are omitted. The number of transmembrane segments is not firmly established. Mutation of R615 causes malignant hyperthermia. S2843 is phosphorylated. **C–D,** Three-dimensional reconstructions of electron micrographs of ryanodine receptors in the closed and open conformations. (A, PDB file: IN4K. Reference: Taylor CW, da Fonseca PCA, Morris EP: IP₃ receptors: The search for structure. Trends Biochem Sci 29:210–219, 2004. B, Reference: Sharma MR, Jeyakumar LH, Fleischer S, Wagenknecht T: Three-dimensional structure of ryanodine receptor isoform three in two conformational states as visualized by cryoelectron microscopy. J Biol Chem 275:9485–9491, 2000.)

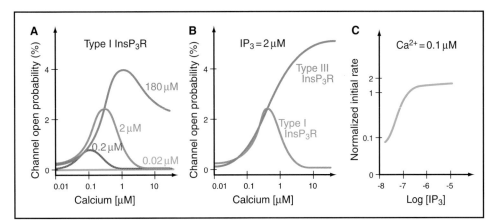

Figure 26-14 Gating of IP$_3$ receptor Ca^{2+} release channels. **A,** Dependence of channel open probability of type I receptors on the concentrations of IP$_3$ (concentrations given next to each curve) and Ca^{2+}. **B,** Comparison of the dependence of open probability of type I and type III receptors on the concentration of Ca^{2+} at a fixed concentration of 2 μM IP$_3$. Note that high concentrations of Ca^{2+} inhibit type I receptors but not type III receptors. **C,** Dependence of open probability of type I receptors on the concentration of IP$_3$ at a fixed concentration of 0.1 μM Ca^{2+}. (A, Based on data from Kaftan EJ, Ehrlich BE, Watras J: InsP$_3$ and Ca^{2+} interact to increase the dynamic range of InsP$_3$ receptor-dependent Ca^{2+} signaling. J Gen Physiol 110:529–538, 1997. B, Based on data from Hagar RE, Burgstahler AD, Nathanson MH, Ehrlich BE: Type III InsP$_3$ receptor channel stays open in the presence of increased calcium. Nature 396:81–84, 1998. C, Based on data from Hirota J, Michikawa T, Miyawaki A, et al: Kinetics of calcium release by IP$_3$ receptor in reconstituted lipid vesicles. J Biol Chem 270:19046–19051, 1995.)

crossing the open channel, owing to its large concentration gradient between the ER lumen and the cytoplasm. IP$_3$ binds with submicromolar affinity between two domains near the N-terminus. Specificity for IP$_3$ is provided by a network of hydrogen bonds between basic residues of the two domains and all three phosphates as well as the hydroxyls of IP$_3$. Ca^{2+} binds to the IP$_3$-binding domains and several other sites along the polypeptide. The organization of the approximately 1500 residues between the IP$_3$ binding domains and the channel domain is not known.

Cytoplasmic IP$_3$ and Ca^{2+} cooperate to open and close these channels, with IP$_3$ setting the sensitivity of the channel to Ca^{2+} (Fig. 26-14). A tetrameric IP$_3$ receptor has four highly selective binding sites for inositol 1,4,5-triphosphate. IP$_3$ must occupy at least two, and perhaps as many as four, of these sites to open the channel. Channels respond rapidly, because binding and dissociation of both ligands occurs quickly ($k_+ = 33$ μM^{-1} s^{-1}, $k_- = 6$ s^{-1} for IP$_3$). High concentrations of Ca^{2+} in the endoplasmic reticulum lumen sensitize receptors to IP$_3$. Phosphorylation by PKA, PKC, and CaM kinase can raise or lower the sensitivity to IP$_3$.

Three human genes and alternative splicing produce a variety of IP$_3$ receptors with different physiological properties for various cell types. Type I and type II IP$_3$ receptors open in response to Ca^{2+} with a bell-shaped concentration dependence. A channel is most likely to be open when the cytoplasmic Ca^{2+} concentration is about 0.3 μM. Below 0.1 μM and above 100 μM Ca^{2+}, the channel is generally closed. When IP$_3$ activates a channel, Ca^{2+} release provides rapid *positive feedback* as its local cytoplasmic concentration rises into the

micromolar range, stimulating channel opening and then slow *negative feedback* as the local Ca^{2+} concentration climbs higher. The result is a short, self-limited pulse of Ca^{2+} release in response to a modest change in IP$_3$ concentration. Calmodulin probably mediates the long-lasting inhibitory effects of high Ca^{2+}. Type III IP$_3$ receptors are different; Ca^{2+} activates them, but high Ca^{2+} concentrations do not compete with IP$_3$ for binding the channel or inhibit Ca^{2+} release. This lack of negative feedback (or very slow feedback) allows cells with type III IP$_3$ receptors to produce a large, global pulse of Ca^{2+} that can ultimately drain Ca^{2+} stores from the endoplasmic reticulum.

Ryanodine Receptor Ca^{2+} Channels

Ryanodine receptors release Ca^{2+} from the endoplasmic reticulum to trigger contraction of striated muscles. The name came from the high affinity of the channel for a plant alkaloid called ryanodine, which can activate or block Ca^{2+} release, depending on its concentration and the target tissue. Ryanodine has no physiological function, but the name has stuck because binding of radioactive ryanodine was the key assay for isolating the protein. Purified protein was reconstituted into phospholipid bilayers and shown to function identically to the Ca^{2+} channels in isolated endoplasmic reticulum.

Ryanodine receptors are homotetramers of 565-kD subunits with a massive cytoplasmic domain and a cation channel domain near the C-terminus (Fig. 26-13B), an architecture similar to that of IP$_3$ receptors. Three ryanodine receptor genes encode proteins that are about 60% identical and expressed in different cells (Table 26-3). Ryanodine receptors are the sole release channels in striated muscles. In smooth muscle and nonmuscle cells, ryanodine receptors augment IP_3 receptor Ca^{2+}-release channels.

The three isoforms respond to different activators: cytoplasmic Ca^{2+}, **cyclic ADP-ribose,** and physical contact with voltage-gated Ca^{2+} channels. Like type I and type II IP_3 receptors, Ca^{2+} activates ryanodine receptors with a bell-shaped concentration dependence. This Ca^{2+}-induced Ca^{2+} release allows a local wave of transient activation to spread from one ryanodine receptor to the next.

Cyclic adenosine diphosphate (cADP)–ribose sets the Ca^{2+} sensitivity of ryanodine receptors, just as IP_3 does for its receptor. At low concentrations of cADP-ribose, high levels of cytoplasmic Ca^{2+} are required to open the channel, whereas at high concentrations of cADP-ribose, even resting Ca^{2+} concentrations open the channel. A single enzymatic step produces cADP-ribose from the metabolite nicotinamide adenine dinucleotide, NAD^+. cGMP regulates **ADP-ribosyl cyclase,** presumably through a cGMP-dependent protein kinase. cADP-ribose has been implicated in the Ca^{2+} transient that triggers secretion of insulin from pancreatic β cells in response to glucose. In fertilization of echinoderm eggs, cADP-ribose releases Ca^{2+} through endoplasmic reticulum ryanodine receptors in parallel with IP_3-mediated Ca^{2+} release. Vertebrate eggs depend entirely on the IP_3 release mechanism (Fig. 26-15).

Physiological and pharmacological agents can stimulate or inhibit ryanodine receptor activity. Phosphorylation by PKA increases ryanodine receptor channel activity and may contribute to the effects of β-adrener-

gic receptor stimulation on the heart (see Fig. 11-12). Caffeine activates Ca^{2+} release by ryanodine receptors and is used to stimulate sperm in fertility tests. Numerous agents suppress the spontaneous release of Ca^{2+} by ryanodine receptors in heart and skeletal muscle: FKBP (the protein that binds the immunosuppressant drug FK506), micromolar ryanodine, the local anesthetic procaine, and calmodulin.

Point mutations in the RyR1 ryanodine receptor gene (expressed in skeletal muscle) cause **malignant hyperthermia** in humans and pigs. The most common human mutation is autosomal dominant with an incidence of about 1 in 50,000. Mutant ryanodine receptors are unusually sensitive to activation by general anesthetics, which trigger Ca^{2+} release, sustained skeletal muscle contraction, and pathological heat generation. If not treated promptly, the fever can be lethal. The pig mutation is autosomal recessive, and stress can trigger lethal attacks.

Other Ca^{2+} Channels

Nicotinic acid adenine dinucleotide phosphate, a metabolic product of β-NADP (nicotinamide-adenine dinucleotide phosphate), also releases Ca^{2+} from internal stores. It is not yet certain whether the receptor is a channel or another protein, so much is still to be learned about its mechanism and physiology. Polycystin 2, a member of the Trp channel family, is another putative intracellular Ca^{2+} release channel that is activated (and inhibited) by Ca^{2+}. This channel is also found in the plasma membrane of primary cilia. Mutations in the polycystin 2 gene cause many cases of human polycystic kidney disease.

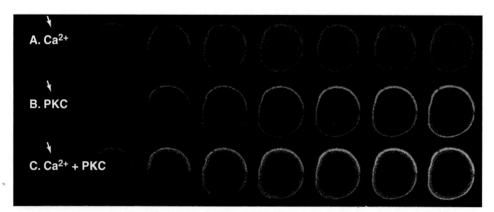

Figure 26-15 Wave of Ca^{2+} release and PKC activation spreading from the site of artificial activation of a *Xenopus* egg. **A,** Ca^{2+} signal. **B,** PKC activation. **C,** Superimposition of the two signals. The egg was injected with calcium *red* (a fluorescent dye sensitive to the concentration of Ca^{2+}) and a fusion protein, consisting of *green* fluorescent protein and PKC, which produces *green* fluorescence when PKC is activated. The egg was activated by a needle prick *(arrows)* and imaged at intervals of 20 seconds. A wave of Ca^{2+} (more intense *red*) precedes a wave of active PKC *(green)* from the site of activation. (Courtesy of Carolyn Larabell, Lawrence Berkeley Laboratory, Berkeley, California.)

Calcium Dynamics in Cells

Methods to visualize Ca^{2+} concentrations inside living cells revealed an amazing temporal and spatial complexity of Ca^{2+} signals. The original experimental Ca^{2+} sensor was a jellyfish protein called **aequorin,** which emits light when it binds Ca^{2+} (see Fig. 39-16). An evolving series of **Ca^{2+}-sensitive fluorescent dyes** (Fura-2, calcium green, calcium red, Fluo-3) have largely replaced aequorin and made possible the observations in the following paragraphs. Ca^{2+} biosensors, constructed by fusing calmodulin to variants of green fluorescent protein, offer advantages, including targeting to particular cellular compartments and the ability to adjust the response range by mutating the Ca^{2+}-binding site.

Voltage-dependent Ca^{2+} channels in excitable cells such as neurons and striated muscles respond rapidly (<1 ms) to an action potential to admit extracellular Ca^{2+}. At chemical synapses, this produces a brief, locally confined Ca^{2+} pulse that triggers the release of synaptic vesicles (see Fig. 11-8). In striated muscles, each action potential causes a transient, global increase in cytoplasmic Ca^{2+} lasting tens of milliseconds (see Fig. 39-15). The details differ in skeletal and cardiac muscle, but the elementary events are similar. Voltage-sensitive Ca^{2+} channels in T tubules (invaginations of the plasma membrane; see Fig. 39-10) activate one or a few ryanodine receptor channels in the adjacent endoplasmic reticulum through direct physical interaction in skeletal muscle and through Ca^{2+} release in the heart. Ca^{2+} released by these ryanodine receptors triggers Ca^{2+} release from nearby ryanodine receptors, generating a local pulse of Ca^{2+} called a **Ca^{2+} spark.** Because T tubules penetrate throughout the muscle cytoplasm, thousands of these sparks are produced simultaneously, yielding a transient global rise in Ca^{2+}. The brief duration of the excitatory signal and the robust Ca^{2+} pumping activity of the endoplasmic reticulum limit the duration of the signal.

Nonexcitable cells generally rely on slower, receptor-mediated production of IP_3 to produce transient changes in cytoplasmic Ca^{2+}. For example, activation of a frog egg at one point by entry of a sperm or artificial activation by pricking with a needle (Fig. 26-15) results in a self-propagating wave of cytoplasmic Ca^{2+} that spreads slowly around the cell. This produces a wave of secretion and activation of downstream effectors, such as PKC.

Many cells with type I and II IP_3 receptors respond to constant agonist stimulation with transient bursts of cytoplasmic Ca^{2+} (Fig. 26-16). The agonist concentration sets the level of cytoplasmic IP_3 (and, possibly, cADP-ribose), which determines the sensitivity of release channels to cytoplasmic Ca^{2+}. A region of a cell with a high density of the most sensitive channels then initiates the release of Ca^{2+} at a focus. The resulting Ca^{2+} transient may spread through the cytoplasm as a planar or spiral wave that is driven locally by Ca^{2+}-induced Ca^{2+} release from either ryanodine receptors or IP_3 receptors. Such transients are self-limited locally, because cytoplasmic Ca^{2+} concentrations exceeding 0.5 μM inhibit both IP_3 receptors and ryanodine receptors. This negative feedback closes release channels and allows Ca^{2+} pumps to clear the cytoplasm of Ca^{2+}. Release channels recover slowly from this negative feedback, creating an interval between Ca^{2+} transients. In this way, the cell decodes the concentration of agonist as a function of the frequency of Ca^{2+} pulses. Colliding waves annihilate each other, owing to negative feedback by high concentrations of Ca^{2+} or local depletion of Ca^{2+} stores.

A different response to continuous agonist stimulation occurs in cells with type III IP_3 receptors, which respond to agonists with a large charge of Ca^{2+} that fills the entire cytoplasm for seconds, owing to their lack of negative feedback by high Ca^{2+}.

Participation of multiple second messengers and channel types can produce complex responses to stimulation. For example, agonists, such as acetylcholine or cholecystokinin, employ Ca^{2+} to stimulate polarized epithelial cells of the pancreas to secrete digestive enzymes. Ca^{2+} transients begin at the apex of these polarized cells, owing to a high concentration of IP_3 receptors. With a strong stimulus, a Ca^{2+} wave spreads from the apex throughout the cell. The frequency of these transients depends on agonist concentration. The pathways downstream from the receptors for these agonists include IP_3, Ca^{2+}, and cADP-ribose and their receptors in the endoplasmic reticulum, which set the sensitivity of the release mechanisms to cytoplasmic Ca^{2+}.

Ca²⁺ Targets

The diversity of targets for Ca^{2+} (Appendix 26-1) emphasizes the widespread and complex effects of this second messenger. The response to a Ca^{2+} signal depends on the available targets, as well as modulating effects of parallel signaling pathways. Some proteins bind Ca^{2+} directly, including Ca^{2+}-activated plasma membrane channels for K^+ and Cl^-, troponin-C in striated muscles, synaptotagmin (a Ca^{2+}-sensing synaptic vesicle protein), and calpain (a Ca^{2+}-activated protease). Parvalbumin and calbindin D28K buffer the cytoplasmic Ca^{2+} concentration. Ca^{2+} activates many proteins indirectly by first binding and activating calmodulin or S100 proteins. Some calmodulin targets, such as CaM kinase II, modify multiple substrate proteins, greatly amplifying the effect of Ca^{2+}. A small protein called "regulator of calmodulin signaling"

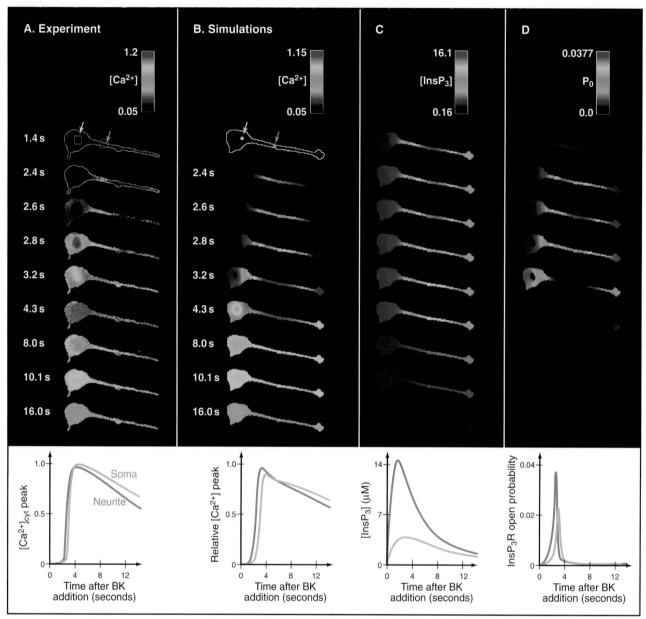

Figure 26-16 Wave of Ca²⁺ released in the cytoplasm of a cultured neuroblastoma cell stimulated at time zero with bradykinin and followed at intervals for 16 seconds. False colors indicate Ca²⁺ concentration or modeled IP₃ concentration or modeled open probability of IP₃ receptor channels. The model was made with Virtual Cell software, taking into account measured local concentrations of IP₃ receptors and their biochemical properties. Graphs show the time course of various parameters in the neurite and cell body. **A,** Experimental data with Ca²⁺ (micromolar) measured with the intracellular indicator calcium *green*. **B,** Model of the local cytoplasmic Ca²⁺ concentration (micromolar). **C,** Model of the local cytoplasmic IP₃ concentration (micromolar). **D,** Model of the open probability of IP₃ receptor channels. InsP3, IP₃. (Courtesy of L. Loew, University of Connecticut, Storrs. Reproduced from Fink CC, Slepchenko B, Moraru II, et al: Morphological control of IP₃-dependent signals. J Cell Biol 147:929–936, 1999, by copyright permssion of The Rockefeller University Press. Reference: Fink CC, Slepchenko B, Moraru II, et al: An image-based model of calcium waves in differentiated neuroblastoma cells. Biophys J 79:163–183, 2000.)

inhibits calmodulin, provided that this regulator is phosphorylated by PKA.

Owing to the oscillatory, transient nature of Ca²⁺ signals, some cellular responses depend on the frequency of Ca²⁺ transients. At least one target protein, CaM kinase II, decodes frequency information into a prolonged adjustment in its level of activity.

Nitric Oxide

The free radical gas nitric oxide (NO•) provides cells with a unique way to transmit signals. It diffuses rapidly through membranes, allowing the signal to spread from cell to cell rather than being confined to the cell of origin like most second messengers. Nitric oxide has long been known as a mildly toxic air pollutant, so it was easy to accept the finding that macrophages produce nitric oxide to the kill microorganisms and tumor cells. On the other hand, it was surprising to learn in the late 1980s that nitric oxide is a diffusible messenger: Endothelial cells lining blood vessels make nitric oxide that relaxes smooth muscle in the walls of arteries, and some neurons in the central and peripheral nervous systems produce nitric oxide as an unconventional neurotransmitter. Carbon monoxide (CO) might be another gaseous intercellular second messenger under some circumstances.

Nitric oxide is not a single chemical species. $NO^{\bullet}$ is only one of several readily interconvertible redox states of nitrogen monoxide, including nitrosonium (NO^{+}) and nitroxyl (NO^{-}) ions. Although nitric oxide is stable in water, it reacts readily with oxygen and has a half-life of only a few seconds in the body. Consequently, nitric oxide must be produced continuously to provide a sustained effect. Much nitric oxide is inactivated by binding to the heme of hemoglobin. Nitric oxide is eventually metabolized to nitrate and nitrite and excreted from the body. Note that the stable anesthetic gas nitrous oxide, N_2O, also known as laughing gas, is not part of this family of nitrogen monoxides.

Enzymes called **nitric oxide synthases** produce nitric oxide by converting L-arginine and molecular oxygen into citrulline and nitric oxide (Fig. 26-17). NADPH provides reducing equivalents for the reaction. Nitric oxide synthase (NOS) is really two enzymes in one. The N-terminal oxidase domain has a heme group that participates directly in oxidation of arginine. The C-terminal reductase domain supplies electrons to the oxidase domain. NOS depends on an extraordinary number of cofactors to handle the electron transfers that are required to produce nitric oxide: heme and tetrahydrobiopterin bound to the oxidase domain, and flavin adenine dinucleotide, flavin mononucleotide, and NADPH in the reductase domain. Some gram-positive bacteria have an NOS with only the N-terminal oxidase domain that is presumably the evolutionary ancestor of eukaryotic NOS. These enzymes catalyze nitration of substrates rather than production of nitric oxide.

Vertebrates express three NOS isozymes selectively in various tissues. NOS1 and NOS3 are synthesized constitutively. Inducible NOS (iNOS or NOS2) is found in macrophages, liver, and fibroblasts. Macrophages produce NOS2 only when stimulated by endotoxin, interferon-γ, or other factors. Endothelial NOS (eNOS or NOS3) is also made by some neurons. NOS3 is targeted to membranes by N-terminal myristoylation and palmitoylation. Neuronal NOS (nNOS or NOS1) is made by about 1% of neurons in the cerebral cortex as well as skeletal muscle and epithelial cells. NOS1 associates with the plasma membrane dystrophin complex in skeletal muscle and is lost from the membrane in patients with muscular dystrophy.

Ca^{2+}-calmodulin and phosphorylation regulate NOS activity independently. Ca^{2+}-calmodulin activates NOS by binding a short regulatory sequence between the two enzyme domains. Ca^{2+} signals activate NOS in most tissues, although macrophage NOS2 binds Ca^{2+}-calmodulin so tightly that it is permanently activated. Protein kinase B/Akt, the kinase activated by PIP_3, phosphorylates and activates NOS3.

The main target for the low concentrations of nitric oxide used for signaling is soluble guanylyl cyclase, the cytoplasmic enzyme that makes cGMP (see Fig. 24-9). Nitric oxide binds reversibly to iron in the heme group of guanylyl cyclase, causing a conformational change that activates the enzyme. Nitric oxide also reacts with cysteine side chains of proteins (S-nitrosylation). This covalent posttranslational modification can modify the activity of sensitive proteins such as NSF (N-ethylmaleimide-sensitive factor), a protein that is required for membrane trafficking (see Fig. 21-12).

Macrophages produce concentrations of nitric oxide that are high enough to kill microorganisms directly. The nitric oxide combines with superoxide anion (O_2^{-}) to form peroxynitrite ($OONO^{-}$), which rapidly breaks down into $OH^{\bullet}$ and $NO_2^{\bullet}$, both very toxic oxidants that kill ingested microorganisms. Plants also produce nitric oxide as part of their defense mechanism against pathogens.

Nitric oxide from three different sources regulates blood flow and blood pressure in response to local physiological demands. During exercise, the repeated release of Ca^{2+} that stimulates skeletal muscle contraction (see Fig. 39-16) also binds calmodulin and activates NOS to produce nitric oxide. Nitric oxide diffuses out of the skeletal muscle and into smooth muscle cells surrounding nearby blood vessels. Nitric oxide relaxes smooth muscle by activating cGMP production and lowering the internal Ca^{2+} level through incompletely understood mechanisms. This increases local blood flow to supply oxygen and nutrients. Endothelial cells lining the inside of blood vessels also use nitric oxide

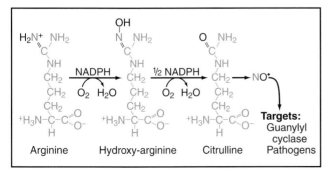

Figure 26-17 SYNTHESIS OF NITRIC OXIDE.

to regulate vascular smooth muscle. Mechanical shear stress from blood flow continuously stimulates endothelial cell phosphatidylinositol-3 kinase to produce PIP_3, which stimulates PKB/Akt to phosphorylate and activate NOS3. This provides a sustained, long-term signal to relax vascular smooth muscle. Acutely, hormones such as acetylcholine and bradykinin can stimulate endothelial cells to produce nitric oxide by causing Ca^{2+} release from endoplasmic reticulum. Mice that lack NOS3 have high blood pressure.

Mono- and di-N^G-methylated arginines strongly inhibit NOS and therefore have been used experimentally to reveal many biological functions of nitric oxide. Inhibition of NOS compromises killing of bacteria by macrophages. Similarly, inhibition of endothelial nitric oxide production causes vascular smooth muscle cells to contract, raising blood pressure and demonstrating a constitutive role for nitric oxide in relaxing these cells. Nitric oxide produced by autonomic nerves causes erection of the penis by stimulating the production of cGMP and relaxing vascular smooth muscle cells. The drug sildenafil (Viagra) is used to treat erectile dysfunction, as it inhibits the phosphodiesterase that breaks down cGMP. Sildenafil and related drugs bind in the active site, excluding cGMP. Other autonomic nerves use nitric oxide to control the smooth muscle cells in the walls of the intestines. Nitric oxide is the active metabolite of nitroglycerin, a drug that is widely used to relieve pain (angina pectoris) associated with compromised blood flow in the heart. It dilates coronary arteries and improves circulation. In addition to regulating cerebral blood flow, nitric oxide produced by nerve cells in the brain may contribute to certain types of learning by reinforcing the release of neurotransmitters (see Fig. 11-10).

ACKNOWLEDGMENTS

Thanks go to Barbara Ehrlich and Paul Insel for their suggestions on revisions to this chapter.

SELECTED READINGS

Baillie, GS, Scott, JD, Houslay, MD: Compartmentalisation of phosphodiesterases and protein kinase A: Opposites attract. FEBS Lett 579:3264-3270, 2005.

Berridge MJ, Lipp P, Bootman MD: The versatility and universality of calcium signaling. Nat Rev Mol Cell Biol 1:11-21, 2000.

Bolotina VM, Csutora P: CIF and other mysteries of the store-operated Ca^{2+}-entry pathway. Trends Biochem Sci 30:378-387, 2005.

Bos JL: EPAC: A new cAMP target and new avenues in cAMP research. Nat Rev Mol Cell Biol 4:733-738, 2003.

Bredt DS: Nitric oxide signaling specificity: The heart of the problem. J Cell Sci 116:9-15, 2003.

De Caterina R, Zampolli A: From asthma to atherosclerosis: 5-lipoxygenase, leukotrienes and inflammation. New Engl J Med 350:4-7, 2004.

Futerman AH, Hannun YA: The complex life of simple sphingolipids. EMBO Rep 5:777-782, 2004.

Garavito RM, Mulichak AM: The structure of mammalian cyclooxygenases. Annu Rev Biophys Biomol Struct 32:183-206, 2003.

Geiger M, Wrulich OA, Jenny M, et al: Defining the human targets of phorbol ester and diacylglycerol. Curr Opin Mol Ther 5:631-641, 2003.

Guatimosim S, Dilly K, Santana LF, et al: Local Ca^{2+} signaling and EC coupling in heart. J Mol Cardiol 34:941-950, 2002.

Guse AH: Second messenger function and the structure-activity relationship of cyclic adenosine diphosphoribose (cADPR). FEBS J 272:4590-4597, 2005.

Ikura M: Calcium binding and conformational response in EF-hand proteins. Trends Biochem Sci 21:14-17, 1996.

McKinney MK, Cravatt BF: Structure and function of fatty acid amide hydrolase. Annu Rev Biochem 74:411-432, 2005.

McLaughlin S, Wang J, Gambhir A, Murray D: PIP_2 and proteins: Interactions, organization, and information flow. Annu Rev Biophys Biomol Struct 31:151-175, 2002.

Meldolesi J, Pozzan T: The endoplasmic reticulum Ca^{2+} store: A view from the lumen. Trends Biochem Sci 23:10-14, 1998.

Niggli E, Egger M: Calcium quarks. Front Biosci 7:1288-1297, 2002.

Patrono C, Garcia Rodriguez LA, Landolfi R, Baigent C: Low-dose aspirin for the prevention of atherthrombosis. New Engl J Med 353:2373-2383, 2005.

Patterson RL, Boehning D, Snyder SH: Inositol 1,4,5-trisphosphate receptors as signal integrators. Annu Rev Biochem 73:437-465, 2004.

Radmark O, Samuelsson B: Regulation of 5-lipoxygenase enzyme activity. Biochem Biophys Res Comm 338:102-110, 2005.

Rhee SG: Regulation of phosphoinositide-specific phospholipase C. Annu Rev Biochem 70:281-312, 2001.

Rosen H, Goetzl EJ: Sphingosine 1-phosphate and its receptors: An autocrine and paracrine network. Nature Rev Immunol 5:560-570, 2005.

Schopfer FJ, Baker PRS, Freeman BA: NO-dependent protein nitration: A cell signaling event or an oxidative inflammatory response? Trends Biochem Sci 28:646-654, 2003.

Sulis ML, Parsons R: PTEN: From pathology to biology. Trends Cell Biol 13:478-483, 2003.

Taylor CW, da Fonseca PCA, Morris EP: IP3 receptors: The search for structure. Trends Biochem Sci 29:210-219, 2004.

Toyoshima C, Inesi G: Structural basis of ion pumping by Ca^{2+}-ATPase of the sarcoplasmic reticulum. Annu Rev Biochem 73: 269-292, 2004.

Vanhaesebroeck B, Leevers SJ, Ahmadi K, et al: Synthesis and function of 3-phosphorylated inositol lipids. Annu Rev Biochem 70:535-602, 2001.

Vetter SW, Leclerc E: Novel aspects of calmodulin target recognition and activation. Eur J Biochem 270:404-414, 2003.

Wehrens SHT, Marks AR: Altered function and regulation of cardiac ryanodine receptors in cardiac disease. Trends Biochem Sci 28:671-678, 2003.

Wilson RI, Nicoll RA: Endocannaboid signaling in the brain. Science 296:678-682, 2002.

Wolfe MM, Lichtenstein DR, Singh G: Gastrointestinal toxicity of nonsteroidal antiinflammatory drugs. N Engl J Med 340:1888-1899, 1999.

Yamasaki M, Churchill GC, Galione A: Calcium signalling by nicotinic acid dinucleotide phosphate (NAADP). FEBS J 272:4598-4906, 2005.

Zaccolo M, Magalhães P, Pozzan T: Compartmentalisation of cAMP and Ca^{2+} signals. Curr. Opin Cell Biol 14:160-166, 2002.

Examples of Ca²⁺ Regulated Proteins

Protein	Binding Site	Function
First-Order Proteins That Bind Ca²⁺ Directly		
Membrane Proteins		
Annexins	Novel	Promote membrane interactions
Ca²⁺-activated Cl⁻ channels	Novel	Participate in secretion
Ca²⁺-activated K⁺ channels	Novel	Control membrane excitability
IP₃ receptor	Novel	Ca²⁺-release channel; activated and inhibited by Ca²⁺
Ryanodine receptor	Novel	Ca²⁺-release channel, activated and inhibited by Ca²⁺
Synaptotagmin	Novel	A synaptic vesicle Ca²⁺ sensor
Enzymes		
Calmodulin-domain protein kinases	ªEF hand	Plant protein kinases
Calpain	EF hand	Ca²⁺-dependent protease
Protein kinase C, some isozymes	C2 domain	Multifunctional protein kinases activated by Ca²⁺
Cytoskeletal Proteins		
α-Actinin (some isoforms)	EF hand	Actin filament cross-linking protein
Centrin/caltractin	EF hand	Ca²⁺-sensitive contractile fibers
Gelsolin, villin	Novel	Actin filament severing and capping proteins
Molluscan myosin light chains	EF hand	Regulate muscle contraction; activated by Ca²⁺
Troponin C	EF hand	Ca²⁺-activated regulator striated muscle contraction
Calcium-Binding Proteins		
Calmodulin	EF hand	Ca²⁺-activated regulator of many proteins
Calbindin-D28K	EF hand	Cytoplasmic Ca²⁺ buffer
Calretinin	EF hand	Activates guanylyl cyclase
Parvalbumin	EF hand	Cytoplasmic Ca²⁺ buffer
S100 proteins (18 human isoforms)	EF hand	Diverse regulatory functions; some isoforms may be secreted
S100 calbindin-D9K	EF hand	Cytoplasmic Ca²⁺ buffer
Recoverin	EF hand	Regulates visual phototransduction
Second-Order Proteins Activated by Ca²⁺-Calmodulin		
Membrane Proteins		
Adenylyl cyclase (some isoforms)		Produces cAMP
Ca²⁺-dependent Na⁺ channels		Na⁺ currents
cGMP-gated cation channels		Phototransduction
Plasma membrane Ca²⁺-ATPase pumps	Clears cytoplasm of Ca²⁺	
Enzymes		
Calcineurin		Protein phosphatase 2B
CaM kinase (several isozymes)		Multifunctional protein kinase
cAMP phosphodiesterase		Degrades cAMP
IP₃ kinase		Phosphorylates IP₃
Myosin light chain kinase		Activates smooth muscle and cytoplasmic myosin
NAD kinase		Phosphorylates NAD
Nitric oxide synthetase		Makes nitric oxide
Phosphorylase kinase		Phosphorylates phosphorylase
Cytoskeletal Proteins		
MARCKS		Actin filament cross-linking protein

ªEF hand is the abbreviation for the Ca²⁺ binding site in calmodulin consisting of α-helices E and F.

CHAPTER 27

Integration of Signals

This chapter summarizes how a variety of well-characterized signal transduction pathways work at the cellular and molecular levels. These examples illustrate diverse mechanisms, but common strategies, for carrying information about changing environmental conditions into cells and for eliciting adaptive responses. Chapters 24 to 26 describe the molecular hardware used in these pathways. Here, the focus is on the flow of information, including examples of branching and converging pathways. For each pathway, the key events are reception of the stimulus, transfer of the stimulus into the cell, amplification of a cytoplasmic signal, modulation of effector systems over time, and adaptation through negative feedback loops. Few signaling pathways operate in isolation; physiological responses usually depend on the integration of pathways.

Although each pathway illustrated here is the best characterized of its kind, none is yet fully understood. Generally, gaps exist in our knowledge about one or more aspects: the full inventory of the components, concentrations of molecules, organization of the system in cells, and rates of reactions that transfer signals. These gaps are expected, as most pathways are complicated and few pathways are amenable to quantitative analysis of their dynamics in live cells. Continued investigations should refine the schemes presented in the following sections, particularly with respect to how each operates as an integrated system.

Signal Transduction by G-Protein-Coupled, Seven-Helix Transmembrane Receptors

The first three signaling pathways use seven-helix receptors coupled to trimeric G-proteins. Two highly specialized sensory systems—olfactory and visual reception—are particularly well characterized because their outputs are electrophysiological events that can be monitored at the level of single cells and single membrane ion channels on a rapid time scale. On a millisecond time scale, these two sensory transducers amplify minute stimuli to produce changes in the membrane potential that initiate a signal to the central nervous system. The response of cells to the hormone epinephrine through the β-adrenergic receptor provides an interesting contrast to these rapidly responding sensory systems. Although many of the protein components are similar, the response is slower and much more global, affecting cellular metabolism and responsiveness as a whole.

Detection of Odors by the Olfactory System

Metazoan sensory systems detect external stimuli with extremely high sensitivity and specificity. The chemosensory processes of smell and taste have evolved into highly specialized biochemical and electrophysiological pathways that connect individuals with their environment. Of these two sensory modalities, olfaction is more sensitive, allowing mammals to detect **odorants** at concentrations of a few parts per trillion in air and to distinguish among more than 10,000 different odorants. Most volatile chemicals with molecular weights of less than 1000 are perceived to have some odor. The olfactory system shares features with many systems that eukaryotes use for communication, including external pheromone signals of yeast and insects as well as internal hormonal signals, such as adrenaline, that circulate in the blood between organs of higher organisms.

Volatile odorant compounds first dissolve in the mucus that bathes the sensory tissue in the nasal cavity. Insects use a family of **odorant-binding proteins** to solubilize odorants in mucus. The role of such proteins is less well established in mammals. Odorant-binding proteins typically have low affinities for their ligands, so odorants exchange rapidly on and off their binding proteins in the mucus. When odorants dissociate, they can interact with receptor proteins located on specialized cilia of the olfactory neurons.

Sensory Neurons

Olfactory sensory neurons located in the nasal epithelium detect specific odorants and respond by sending action potentials to the brain (Fig. 27-1). These neurons have three specialized zones. An apical dendrite extends to the surface of the epithelium and sprouts approximately 12 **sensory cilia** specialized for responding to particular extracellular odorants. The response depends on high concentrations of four proteins in the ciliary membrane: a single type of odorant receptor, the trimeric G-protein G_{olf}, type III adenylyl cyclase, and cyclic nucleotide–gated ion channels. The cell body contains the nucleus, protein-synthesizing machinery, and plasma membrane pumps and channels that set the resting electrical potential of the plasma membrane. An **axon** projects from the base of each neuron to secondary neurons in the **olfactory bulb** at the front of the brain.

Olfactory sensory neurons are unique among adult neurons in their ability to replace themselves from precursor cells in the epithelium within 30 days after they are destroyed. If protected from viruses and environmental toxins, they turn over much more slowly, so the ability of self-renewal appears to be an adaptation to the hazards associated with exposure to the environment.

Loss of olfactory function with age results, in part, from a decreased ability to maintain this neuronal replacement process. The presence of neurons in an epithelium might seem odd, but recall that the entire central nervous system derives from the embryonic ectoderm.

Overview of the Pathway

Extracellular odorants bind to receptors on the cilia of olfactory neurons, depolarize the plasma membrane, and initiate action potentials at the base of the axonal process. The process of reception and transduction of stimuli takes place in five steps:

1. Odorant binding changes the conformation of its plasma membrane receptor.

2. Activated receptor amplifies the signal by catalyzing the exchange of guanosine diphosphate (GDP) for guanosine triphosphate (GTP) on multiple molecules of G_{olf}, causing the dissociation of GTP-$G_{olf}\alpha$ from $G\beta\gamma$.

3. Each GTP-$G_{olf}\alpha$ activates adenylyl cyclase to produce many molecules of cyclic adenosine monophosphate (cAMP). The concentration of cytoplasmic cAMP peaks in less than 100 ms. This is the second stage of amplification.

4. cAMP binds to and opens cyclic nucleotide-gated ion channels, depolarizing the plasma membrane.

5. Membrane depolarization opens voltage-gated ion channels, triggering an action potential (a self-propagating wave of membrane depolarization; see Fig. 11-6) that moves along the axon of the sensory neuron to secondary neurons in the olfactory bulb.

As you can appreciate from everyday experience, olfactory signal transduction is very sensitive but adapts quickly to the continued presence of an odorant. An understanding of each step in the sensory transduction and adaptation pathways helps to explain how animals discriminate among so many different odors.

Odorant Receptors

The olfactory system uses a large family of seven-helix receptors to detect a wide range of ligands present at low concentrations in mucus. These receptors were identified by cloning their complementary DNAs (see Fig. 6-8 for cDNAs) from the olfactory epithelium. Genome sequencing established that mice have about 1000 functional odorant receptor genes (about 4% of total genes!), humans have about 350 functional genes, and fish have 100. Odorants are presumed to bind among the transmembrane helices, the most variable part of

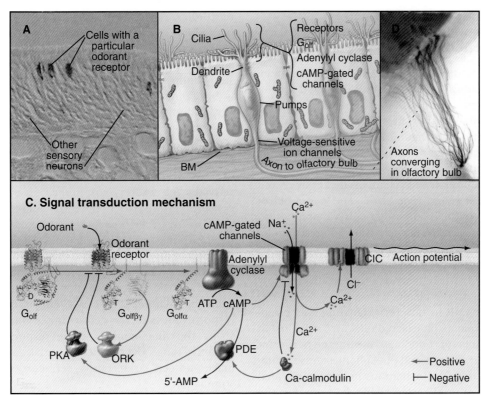

Figure 27-1 OLFACTION. **A,** Light micrograph of a section of sensory epithelium from the nasal passage of a mouse after staining *(purple)* for one olfactory receptor mRNA. Note that only a few cells express this gene. **B,** The sensory epithelium, highlighting one olfactory sensory neuron and the signal-transducing proteins concentrated in three parts of the cell. (BM, basement membrane.) **C,** Signal transduction mechanism. An odorant molecule binds a specific seven-helix plasma membrane receptor and changes its conformation. The activated receptor catalyzes the exchange of GDP for GTP on multiple trimeric G-proteins, causing dissociation of $G_{olf}\alpha$ from $G\beta\gamma$. $G_{olf}\alpha$-GTP activates adenylyl cyclase to produce multiple cAMPs. cAMP binds to and opens cyclic nucleotide–gated ion channels in the plasma membrane, depolarizing the plasma membrane. Ca^{2+} admitted by the cAMP-gated channel opens chloride channels (CIC), which augment membrane depolarization. Membrane depolarization triggers an action potential at the base of the axon that travels along the axon to secondary neurons in the brain. Multiple negative feedback loops *(red)* terminate stimulation. cAMP activates PKA, and $G\beta\gamma$ activates odorant receptor kinase (ORK *[green]*), both of which phosphorylate and inhibit the receptor. Ca^{2+} binds calmodulin, which inhibits the cAMP-gated channel and activates phosphodiesterase (PDE) to break down cAMP. **D,** Light micrograph of the olfactory bulb of a mouse expressing a marker enzyme (beta galactosidase) driven by the promoter for one odorant receptor. A histochemical reaction marks the axons of these cells *blue.* Axons from many olfactory sensory neurons expressing the same receptor converge on the same glomerulus in the olfactory bulb. (A, From Ressler KJ, Sullivan SL, Buck LB: A zonal organization of odorant receptor gene expression in the olfactory epithelium. Cell 73:597–609, 1993. D, Courtesy of Charles Greer, Yale University, New Haven, Connecticut. Reference: Zou D-J, Feinstein P, Rivers AL, et al: Postnatal refinement of peripheral olfactory projections. Science 304:1976–1979, 2004.)

these proteins. Each sensory neuron typically expresses a single type of odorant receptor (Fig. 27-1A), using negative feedback from the receptor itself to suppress the expression of other types of odorant receptors. The 1000 cells that express each receptor are scattered in zones throughout the olfactory epithelium.

G-Protein Relay

Odorant binding changes the conformation of the receptor, allowing it to catalyze the exchange of nucleotide on G_{olf} on the cytoplasmic face of the plasma membrane. In less than 100 ms, an activated receptor can produce 10 to 100 activated GTP-$G_{olf}\alpha$ molecules, which then dissociate from their $G\beta\gamma$ subunits.

Production of cAMP

In the third step, GTP-$G_{olf}\alpha$ binds to and activates a specialized olfactory isozyme of **adenylyl cyclase.** While active, each enzyme generates nearly 100 cAMP molecules. By 75 ms after stimulation, the concentration of cAMP inside the cilium peaks at >10 µM, returning to baseline within 500 ms. This dramatic fluctuation in cAMP concentration is made possible by the high surface-to-volume ratio of cilia, which ensures that membrane-associated signaling components interact rapidly and confines the cAMP within a small volume. The cAMP transient is short-lived, owing to hydrolysis by a **phosphodiesterase** with a high turnover rate but a relatively low affinity for cAMP.

Cyclic Nucleotide–Gated Channels Depolarize the Plasma Membrane and Trigger an Action Potential

The fast cAMP transient depolarizes the plasma membrane by activating **cyclic nucleotide**–gated cation channels. The concentration of these channels in ciliary membranes ($>2000/\mu m^2$) is much higher than that in the cell body ($6/\mu m^2$). Binding of at least two cAMP molecules increases the probability that the channel is open from near 0 to about 0.65. Because the probability is not 1.0, individual activated channels flicker open and closed on a millisecond time scale. The ensemble of many activated channels admits enough Na^+ and Ca^{2+} to depolarize the membrane. Ca^{2+}-activated chloride channels carry additional current. The lag of 200 to 500 ms between binding of the odorant and peak membrane depolarization is attributable to the relatively slow binding of cAMP to the channel.

The role of cAMP in olfactory signaling was established by experiments on isolated olfactory neurons, in which the effects of odorants, membrane-permeant cyclic nucleotide analogs, and phosphodiesterase inhibitors were explored. Null mutations in mice confirmed the importance of cAMP-gated channels. Note that the role of cAMP in olfaction is distinctly different from its role in most other tissues, where the main target of cAMP is protein kinase A (PKA [see Fig. 25-3]).

Depolarization of the ciliary membrane initiates an action potential (see Fig. 11-6) by activating voltage-gated sodium channels (see Fig. 10-2) in the cell body. The action potential propagates along the axon to a chemical synapse with the second neuron in the olfactory bulb of the brain. The two stages of amplification downstream of the receptor allow a few active receptors to produce an action potential.

Adaptation

Desensitization—the waning of perceived odorant intensity despite its continued presence—results from a combination of central and peripheral processes. Peripheral processes that contribute to adaptation include modulation of each step in the signaling pathway following odorant binding (Fig. 27-1C). At the molecular level, this adaptation is reflected in the transient nature of G-protein activation, the self-limited increase in cAMP, and the limited duration of the membrane depolarization, all of which occur with constant exposure to odorant. Importantly, the sequential nature of many of these feedback circuits implies that they have intrinsic delays and therefore serve not only to alter the magnitude of the response but also to shape its time course.

G-protein-coupled receptors are desensitized by protein kinases that phosphorylate the receptor and by proteins called **arrestins** that bind phosphorylated receptors (see Fig. 24-3). These modifications inhibit the interaction of activated receptors with G-proteins and provide negative feedback at the first stage of signal amplification. Negative feedback is coupled to receptor stimulation, because the **olfactory receptor kinase** is brought to the plasma membrane by binding the G$\beta\gamma$ subunits released by receptor-induced G-protein dissociation.

Ca^{2+} entering the cell through cyclic nucleotide–gated channels binds calmodulin, and the complex provides negative feedback at two levels. Calcium-calmodulin activates the cAMP phosphodiesterase, which rapidly converts cAMP to $5'$-AMP. Calcium-calmodulin also binds to the cyclic nucleotide–activated channel, reducing its affinity for cAMP by 10-fold. This change reduces the probability of the channel's opening at less than saturating cyclic nucleotide concentrations and might accelerate the otherwise slow dissociation of cAMP from the channel. These two effects of Ca^{2+} alter the responsiveness of the cell to initial odorant exposure, shape the time course of the response, extend the dynamic range over which the cell can respond, and make a cell transiently refractory to additional stimulation.

Processing in the Central Nervous System

Mammals discriminate many more odorants than the number of available receptors by combining information from multiple types of receptors in their central nervous systems. While the sensory neurons that express any single odor receptor are broadly distributed across the olfactory epithelium, the axons from this family of like sensory neurons converge on only two to three targets in the olfactory bulb. The target, a glomerulus, is a dense area with synapses between axons of olfactory sensory neurons and dendrites of the second neurons in the pathway. Because each glomerulus receives input only from axons that express the same odor receptor, the molecular specificity established in the olfactory epithelium is preserved. Given approximately 1000 odor receptors in the mouse, each mouse olfactory bulb has approximately 2000 glomeruli (Fig. 27-1D). Of special interest, the odor receptor itself is an important determinant of axon targeting to the glomeruli. Substitution of odor receptors results in the axons selecting new glomerular targets. About 50 secondary neurons receive synaptic input within a glomerulus. Most of these neurons send their axons to higher levels, where they terminate in a combinatorial manner on cortical neurons.

The discrimination of a particular odorant is achieved in two stages: At the first stage, each odorant activates several different receptors, and each receptor can bind a group of related odorants. Therefore, each odorant

Animals use olfaction to find their mates, identify their offspring, and mark their territories. Some of the odorants that are used for these social interactions are volatile chemicals that stimulate the main olfactory system. A second accessory olfactory system detects other social odorants. Some are volatile chemicals found in urine; others are not volatile, including MHC class II peptide complexes that are shed from the surfaces of cells into the urine and other secretions. Accessory sensory neurons are located in a special part of the epithelium lining nasal cavity called the vomeronasal organ. Each of these neurons expresses one of about 300 seven-helix receptors from a different family than the main odorant receptors. Odorant binding activates a signal transduction pathway distinct from main olfactory neurons, dependent on a Trp channel (see Fig. 10-9) rather than a cyclic nucleotide–gated channel. The axons project to the accessory olfactory bulb in the brain.

activates a particular pattern of olfactory sensory neurons and their coupled glomeruli. At the next level, neurons in the cerebral cortex receive information from a combination of glomeruli, leading to eventual discrimination of many different smells at higher levels of the brain. See Box 27-1 for information on our second olfactory system.

Photon Detection by the Vertebrate Retina

Overview of Visual Signal Processing

Photons are energetic but unconventional agonists. They are tiny, move very fast, and penetrate most biochemical materials. These properties create a formidable challenge for detecting photons and transducing their properties (intensity and wavelength) into a signal that can be transmitted to the brain. Nevertheless, vertebrate photoreceptor cells capture single photons and convert this energy into a highly amplified electrical response (Fig. 27-2). Phototransduction is the best-understood eukaryotic sensory process because the system is amenable to sophisticated biophysical, biochemical, and physiological analysis. Single-cell organisms use similar mechanisms to respond to light (see Fig. 38-19).

Vertebrate **photoreceptor cells** are neurons located in a two-dimensional array in the retina, an epithelium inside the eye. The cornea and lens of the eye form an inverted real image of the outside world on the retina, so the intensity of the light across the field of view is encoded by the array of geographically separate photoreceptor cells. Photoreceptor cells lie at the base of a complex neural processing system. Having detected the rate of photon stimulation at a particular place in the visual field, photoreceptor neurons communicate this information to higher levels of the visual system. Initial processing of the information takes place in the retina, where secondary and tertiary neurons take input from multiple photoreceptors to derive local information regarding image contrast, as well as color and intensity. Neuroscience texts present more detailed information on higher levels of visual processing in the retina and brain.

The response of photoreceptor cells depends on the intensity of the light, that is, the flux of photons. Vertebrate retinas detect light with intensities that range over 10 orders of magnitude. **Rod photoreceptors** (Fig. 27-2A) detect low levels of light from about 0.01 photon per μm^2 per second (dim stars) to 10 photons per μm^2 per second but do not discriminate light of different colors. **Cone photoreceptors** (cones) respond to more intense light, up to about 10^9 photons per μm^2 per second (full sunlight). Three classes of cones with chromophores that are sensitive to different wavelengths of light allow humans to encode wavelength and color vision to operate (Box 27-2).

Rods and cones have three specialized regions with different molecular components and functions. The nucleus and the organelles in the **inner segment** maintain the cell's structure and metabolism. A vestigial cilium connects the inner segment to the **outer segment,** which consists of a stack of internal membrane **disks** containing the photoreceptor protein, rhodopsin in the case of rods, surrounded by the plasma membrane. Disks form by invagination and pinching off of flattened sacks of plasma membrane. Rhodopsin synthesized in the cell body is transported to the plasma membrane along the secretory pathway and segregated into disk membranes. The lumen of the disks corresponds topologically to the lumen of the endoplasmic reticulum or the extracellular space.

Absorption of a photon activates rhodopsin and initiates a signaling cascade (Fig. 27-2) involving a trimeric G-protein and a cGMP phosphodiesterase, both attached to the cytoplasmic face of the disk membrane by covalent lipid groups. Active phosphodiesterase lowers the cytoplasmic concentration of cGMP and closes cGMP-gated channels in the plasma membrane. Closing these channels reduces the release of glutamate at the synapse with the next neuron in the visual circuit. Signals flow through the system as follows:

1. A chromophore bound to a seven-helix receptor absorbs light and changes the conformation of the receptor.

2. Active receptor catalyzes the exchange of GDP for GTP on a trimeric G-protein.

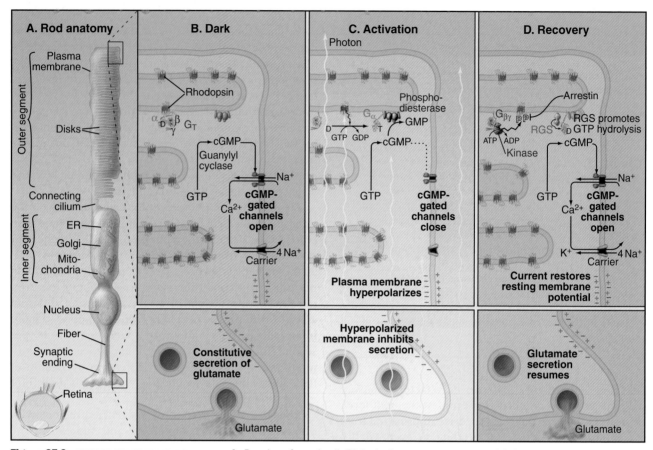

Figure 27-2   VERTEBRATE VISUAL TRANSDUCTION. **A,** Drawing of a rod cell. Disks in the outer segment are rich in rhodopsin. **B–D,** Drawings of small portions of an outer segment (*upper panels*) and the synaptic terminal of a rod cell (*lower panels*) in three physiological states. Active components are highlighted by bright colors. **B,** Resting cell in the dark. Constitutive production of cGMP keeps a subset of the plasma membrane cGMP-gated channels open most of the time, allowing an influx of Na^+ and Ca^{2+}. At the resting membrane potential, the synaptic terminal constitutively secretes the neurotransmitter glutamate. Ca^{2+} leaves the outer segment via a sodium/calcium exchange carrier in the outer segment, whereas Na^+ leaves the cell via a sodium pump in the plasma membrane of the inner segment. **C,** Absorption of a photon activates one rhodopsin, allowing it to catalyze the exchange of GTP for GDP bound on many molecules of transducin (G_T). This dissociates $G_T\alpha$ from $G\beta\gamma$. Each $G_T\alpha$-GTP binds and activates one molecule of phosphodiesterase (attached to the disk membrane by N-terminal isoprenyl groups), which rapidly converts cGMP to GMP. As the concentration of free cGMP declines, the cGMP-gated channels close, leading to hyperpolarization of the plasma membrane and inhibition of glutamate secretion at the synaptic body. **D,** Recovery is initiated when rhodopsin kinase phosphorylates activated rhodopsin. Binding of arrestin to phosphorylated rhodopsin prevents further activation of G_T. Phosphodiesterase and an RGS protein cooperate to stimulate hydrolysis of GTP bound to G_T, returning G_T to the inactive $G_T\alpha$-GDP state. Synthesis of cGMP by guanylyl cyclase returns the cytoplasmic concentration of cGMP to resting levels and opens the cGMP-gated channels. Constitutive secretion of glutamate resumes.

BOX 27-2
Color Vision

Three types of cones are responsible for our ability to discriminate colors. Cones are organized much like rods but express one of three different seven-helix photoreceptors, each with a distinct visual pigment. The absorption spectra of the photoreceptors overlap, so the central nervous system can perceive colors from deep purple to deep red by comparing the relative activation of the three types of cones at each point in the visual field. As in rods, signal transduction in cones depends on degradation of cGMP and closure of cGMP-gated channels. Activation of cones requires much more intense light, but cones respond faster than rods.

3. G-proteins activate an enzyme, cGMP phosphodiesterase.

4. Phosphodiesterase rapidly reduces the cytoplasmic concentration of cGMP.

5. The reduction in cytoplasmic cGMP closes cGMP-gated cation channels, hyperpolarizing the plasma membrane.

6. The change in membrane potential reduces the rate of transmitter release at the synapse between the photoreceptor cell and the next neuron in the visual circuit.

Feedback loops operate at every level in this signal transduction pathway, turning off the response to a flash of light. The following sections explain how these reactions achieve their spectacular sensitivity in rods.

Rhodopsin

Rhodopsin, the photoreceptor protein of rods, is a seven-helix, G-protein-coupled receptor with a light-absorbing chromophore, **11-*cis* retinal,** covalently attached to lysine 296 through a protonated Schiff base (see Fig. 24-2B). Although 11-*cis* retinal is bound to a site in the bundle of transmembrane helices similar to sites where ligands bind other seven-helix receptors, this form of rhodopsin is inactive with respect to catalyzing nucleotide exchange on its trimeric G-protein. Thus, rhodopsin is a seven-helix receptor with a covalently attached, but inactive, ligand.

The ability of rods to detect single photons depends on two favorable properties. First, the noise level is very low, owing to the stability of the 11-*cis* retinal. In vertebrate rods, fewer than one molecule in 4×10^{10} isomerizes spontaneously every second, so the background level of activated rhodopsin is very low, even with more than 10^8 molecules of rhodopsin per cell. Thus, one does not see spots of light in the dark. Second, rods absorb photons very efficiently by virtue of the high concentration of rhodopsin in disks (~25,000 rhodopsins/μm^2) and stacking thousands of disks on top of each other in the direction of incoming photons. Rhodopsin constitutes 90% of the disk membrane protein and 45% of the disk membrane mass. About half of the photons that traverse the outer segment are absorbed, and about two thirds of absorbed photons produce an electrical change in the plasma membrane.

Absorption of light initiates the signal transduction pathway. Picoseconds after the 11-*cis* retinal chromophore absorbs a photon, the energy isomerizes it to **all-*trans* retinal.** This change initiates a cascade of intramolecular reactions that activates rhodopsin by changing its conformation. **Metarhodopsin II,** the stable active conformation, has rearranged cytoplasmic loops that catalyze nucleotide exchange on **transducin,** its trimeric G-protein partner (see Fig. 25-9). The signal initiated by absorption of light is amplified by two successive enzymatic reactions and by closing ion channels. Following activation, rhodopsin is inactivated by hydrolysis of the Schiff base linking all-*trans* retinal to the protein and dissociation of the chromophore. Rhodopsin is regenerated by binding a fresh molecule of 11-*cis* retinal, derived from vitamin A.

The Positive Arm of the Signal Cascade

Metarhodopsin II catalyzes the exchange of GDP for GTP on the α subunit of transducin, which then dissociates its $\beta\gamma$ subunits. Each metarhodopsin II produces hundreds of activated transducins in a fraction of a second, nearly as fast as the molecules collide while they diffuse in the plane of the very crowded disk bilayer. Nucleotide exchange on transducin is rate-limiting in the whole transduction cascade, even with a 10^7 acceleration by metarhodopsin II.

Transducin α-GTP activates **phosphodiesterase** by binding its two inhibitory γ subunits. This binding reaction does not amplify the signal but frees the catalytic α and β subunits of phosphodiesterase to break down cGMP to GMP at a high rate. The cytoplasmic concentration of cGMP depends largely on its rate of destruction by light-activated phosphodiesterase, as it is made continuously by **guanylyl cyclase.**

As the concentration of cGMP falls, **cGMP-gated cation channels** in the plasma membrane close. These channels (see Fig. 10-10) are very sensitive to the concentration of cGMP. Binding of four cGMPs opens a channel, whereas the loss of one cGMP closes a channel. Amplification in this pathway is spectacular. Within 1 second after absorption of a single photon, rhodopsin activates 1000 transducins and a similar number of phosphodiesterases, which break down 50,000 cGMPs. This change in concentration closes hundreds of cGMP-gated channels, each of which blocks the entry of more than 10,000 cations. Box 27-3 provides more details about the electrical circuit in the rod cell.

Closure of cGMP-gated channels hyperpolarizes the membrane and inhibits glutamate release at the synapse. This light-induced decline in glutamate release has opposite effects on the two types of "bipolar neurons" connected to rods: It stimulates "on-type" bipolar neurons to fire action potentials and hyperpolarizes the "off-type" bipolar neurons. This combination of responses is the first step in the discrimination of contrast in our visual world.

Recovery and Adaptation

After a dim flash of light, the reduced cytoplasmic cGMP concentration and the plasma membrane hyperpolarization are short-lived, on the order of 2 seconds in rods, briefer in cones. Rods reset the signaling pathway by inhibiting metarhodopsin II, inactivating transducin α-GTP, and activating the synthesis of cGMP.

Rhodopsin kinase (now called GRK1 for G-protein-coupled receptor kinase 1), associated with the disk membrane by a C-terminal farnesyl group, phosphorylates several residues near the C-terminus of metarhodopsin II. Like other seven-helix receptor kinases, rhodopsin kinase is active only toward the active form of the receptor. Phosphorylation of rhodopsin reduces its ability to activate transducin. Binding of a second protein, **arrestin,** to phosphorylated rhodopsin prevents further production of transducin α-GTP.

GTP hydrolysis dissipates the light-activated burst in transducin α-GTP. The low GTPase activity of transducin is activated by association with phosphodiesterase and by an **RGS protein** (regulator of G-protein signaling; see Fig. 25-8), inactivating transducin in less than 1 second. Humans with mutations that disable the retinal RGS protein cannot adapt to rapid changes in light, so they are blinded for several seconds when they step out of a dark room into full sunlight. Dissociation of transducin α-GDP from phosphodiesterase inhibitory subunits terminates cGMP breakdown.

The reduction in cytoplasmic Ca^{2+} that accompanies closure of cGMP-gated cation channels stimulates the guanylyl cyclase that rapidly restores the cGMP concentration. This change opens the cation channels and returns the membrane potential to the resting level. See Box 27-4 for information on our second visual system.

BOX 27-3
Electrical Circuits in the Photoreceptor

Absorption of light changes currents flowing through electrical circuits in photoreceptor cells. In the dark, the resting cGMP concentration in the outer segment keeps open 1% of the cGMP-gated channels. These open channels produce an inward "dark current" of Na^+ and Ca^{2+}, which is balanced by an outward current of K^+ through channels in the inner segment. Sodium-potassium ATPase pumps in the inner segment compensate for the accumulation of Na^+ and the depletion of K^+. Ca^{2+} entering the outer segment is exported by a carrier in the plasma membrane of the outer segment that exchanges Ca^{2+} and K^+ for Na^+.

Following absorption of a photon, both the cGMP concentration and the probability of the cGMP-gated channels being open declines on a millisecond time scale. In parallel, the cation current into the outer segment falls, hyperpolarizing the plasma membrane. The cytoplasmic Ca^{2+} concentration also declines from about 300 nM to 50 nM. The magnitudes of these responses depend on the number of photons absorbed and the size of the amplified signal.

Two useful properties emerge from the fact that the extracellular concentration of Ca^{2+} largely blocks open photoreceptor channels, similar to the cyclic nucleotide–gated channel of olfactory neurons. First, it reduces the burden on the pumps that maintain the ionic gradients in the cell. Second, using multiple channels with low ionic conductance improves the signal-to-noise ratio. For example, if only two channels carried the dark current, the statistical opening or closing of one channel would create large fluctuations in the current. If 100 partially blocked channels carried the same current, then opening or closing single channels has a modest effect on total current.

BOX 27-4
Second Visual System to Set Circadian Clocks

Many organisms, including humans, use the regular variation in light during the day and night to entrain a network of transcription factors that control a 24-hour circadian cycle of metabolic activities throughout the body. For example, mice that are kept in complete darkness will continue to run (searching for food) during the hours corresponding to night and will sleep during the hours corresponding to day. Without light input, they gradually drift from a precise 24-hour cycle. Reception of the light that synchronizes the internal cycle with the 24-hour day does not require either rods or cones. Instead, a subset of retinal ganglion cells absorbs the light and sends signals to the hypothalamic region of the brain. At least two different photoproteins absorb the light: melanopsin, an opsin family member; and cryptochromes, proteins with a flavin chromophore. So the eye is two photodetectors in one.

Regulation of Metabolism through the β-Adrenergic Receptor

Epinephrine, a catecholamine that is also called *adrenaline* (Fig. 27-3), is secreted by the neuroendocrine cells of the adrenal gland and other tissues when an animal is startled, is stressed, or otherwise needs to respond vigorously. **Norepinephrine,** a closely related catecholamine, is secreted by sympathetic neurons, including those that regulate the contractility of the heart. These hormones flow through the blood and stimulate cells of many types throughout the body to heighten their metabolic activity. Skeletal muscle and liver cells respond by breaking down glycogen to glucose to provide energy. Smooth muscle cells of arteries relax to facilitate blood flow. Norepinephrine stimulates heart cells to contract more frequently and with greater force (see Fig. 11-12) and stimulates brown fat cells to dissipate energy as heat (see Fig. 28-6). The variety of physiological responses depends on selective expression of a family of nine **adrenergic receptors** and their associated signaling hardware in particular differentiated cells (Table 27-1).

Epinephrine binding to the β-adrenergic receptor is the classic example of a pathway utilizing a seven-helix receptor (see Fig. 24-2), a trimeric G-protein (see Fig. 25-9), and adenylyl cyclase (see Fig. 26-2) to produce cAMP. This second messenger mediates a wide variety of cellular responses by activating protein kinase A (PKA; see Fig. 25-3), which changes the activity of many different cellular proteins by phosphorylation. Differentiated cells vary in their responses to epinephrine and norepinephrine, because they express different targets

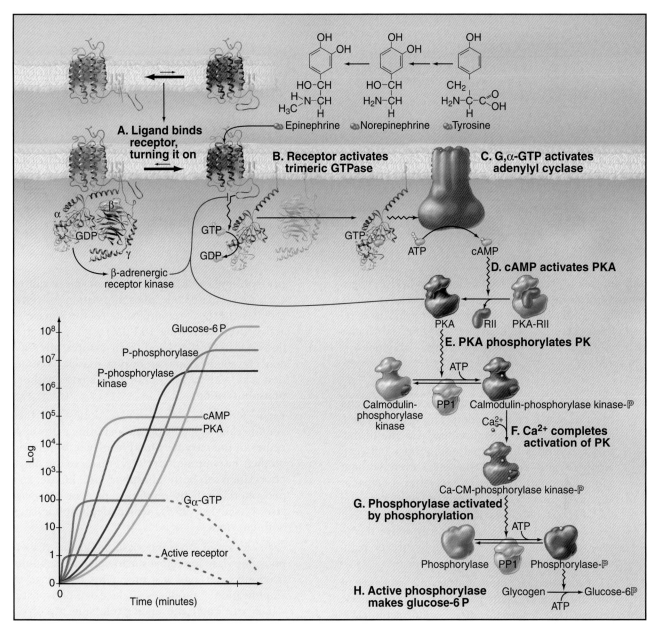

Figure 27-3 β-ADRENERGIC SIGNALING MECHANISM. Active components are shown in bright colors. **Upper right,** Pathway of epinephrine synthesis. **Lower left,** Time course of the amplification of the signal by the catalytic cascade of signal-transducing enzymes. **A,** Epinephrine binds the seven-helix β-adrenergic receptor, shifting its equilibrium to the active conformation. **B,** Active receptor catalyzes the exchange of GDP for GTP on $G_s\alpha$, dissociating $G_s\alpha$-GTP from Gβγ. **C,** $G_s\alpha$-GTP activates adenylyl cyclase, which produces multiple cAMPs. **D,** cAMP activates protein kinase A (PKA) by dissociating the regulatory subunit, RII (not shown to scale). **E,** PKA phosphorylates and partially activates multiple molecules of phosphorylase kinase (PK). **F,** Ca^{2+} binds to calmodulin (CM) associated with phosphorylase kinase, completing activation. **G,** Phosphorylase kinase phosphorylates and activates phosphorylase. **H,** Phosphorylase catalyzes the conversion of glycogen to glucose-6 phosphate. Negative feedback loops *(red)* terminate stimulation. cAMP activates PKA and Gβγ activates β-adrenergic receptor kinase, both of which phosphorylate and inhibit the receptor from catalyzing nucleotide exchange. PP1, protein phosphatase 1.

for PKA. In the heart, PKA phosphorylates voltage-gated Ca-channels, increasing Ca^{2+} release, and phospholamban, a small membrane protein that stimulates the Ca^{2+} pump of the smooth endoplasmic reticulum to clear Ca^{2+} from the cytoplasm (see Fig. 39-15). These changes strengthen contraction. Smooth muscle PKA phosphorylates and inhibits myosin light chain kinase, preventing

it from initiating contraction and increasing blood flow (see Fig. 39-21). Liver PKA activates enzymes that break down glycogen, releasing glucose into the circulation.

This section explains how β-adrenergic receptors regulate the production of glucose-6 phosphate from glycogen (Fig. 27-3). As with vision and olfaction, the response to epinephrine is sensitive, highly amplified,

Table 27-1

FOUR EXAMPLES OF ADRENERGIC RECEPTORS AND PHYSIOLOGICAL RESPONSES

Receptor	Tissue	Signaling Pathway	Responses
α_1	Smooth muscle, blood vessels	G_q, PLC-β, IP_3, Ca^{2+}, MLCK	Contraction
	Smooth muscle, GI tract	G_q	Relaxation
	Liver	G_q	Glycogenolysis
α_2	Smooth muscle, blood vessels	G_i, Ca^{2+}	Contraction
	Pancreatic islets	G_i, inhibit A-cyclase, K^+ channel open	Secretion inhibition
β_1	Heart	G_s, A-cyclase, cAMP, PKA, phospholamban	Increased contraction
β_2	Liver	G_s, A-cyclase, cAMP, PKA, phosphorylase	Glycogenolysis
	Skeletal muscle	G_s, A-cyclase, cAMP, PKA, phosphorylase	Glycogenolysis

GI, gastrointestinal; MLCK, myosin light-chain kinase; PLC-β, phospholipase C-β.

and subject to negative feedback control. Five stages of amplification along the seven-step pathway allow binding of a single molecule of epinephrine to a receptor to activate millions of enzyme molecules that produce many million molecules of glucose-6 phosphate:

1. Epinephrine binds to a β-adrenergic receptor and traps its active conformation. The resting system is on the verge of activation, because the ligand-free receptor is in a rapid equilibrium between activated and unactivated states. Even without agonist, a small fraction of receptors is active at any given time. Thus, experimentally increasing the total concentration of receptors (and therefore the concentration of spontaneously active receptors) can maximally activate downstream pathways, even in the absence of agonists.

2. Each activated receptor catalyzes the exchange of GDP for GTP on many molecules of the trimeric protein G_s, causing the dissociation of the GTP-$G_s\alpha$ from the $G\beta\gamma$ subunits and amplifying the signal up to 100-fold. The G-protein subunits remain attached to the membrane by their lipid anchors but go their separate ways to activate different targets. This is the first branch point in the pathway.

3. The GTP-$G_s\alpha$ binds and activates **adenylyl cyclase,** an integral membrane protein (see Fig. 26-2), which produces many molecules of cAMP. This is the second stage of amplification.

4. cAMP activates **PKA** by binding and dissociating the inhibitory RII subunit (see Fig. 25-3). Activation of PKA mediates most effects of cAMP, but cAMP also activates cyclic nucleotide–gated ion channels in some cells.

5. Each activated PKA amplifies the signal by phosphorylating many substrate molecules, including

phosphorylase kinase. This enzyme requires Ca^{2+} for activity, but phosphorylation by PKA reduces the Ca^{2+} requirement, so the kinase is active even at resting (0.1 μM) Ca^{2+} concentrations. On the other hand, high cytoplasmic Ca^{2+} concentrations alone, as during muscle contraction, can activate phosphorylase kinase without phosphorylation.

6. Each activated phosphorylase kinase further amplifies the signal by phosphorylating many molecules of the enzyme **phosphorylase b,** turning on their enzyme activity. PKA enhances the phosphorylation of both phosphorylase kinase and phosphorylase b by inhibiting protein phosphatase 1 (see Fig. 25-5), which dephosphorylates both enzymes.

7. Each activated phosphorylase molecule (called phosphorylase a) removes many glucose subunits from glycogen, one at a time. This fifth stage of amplification produces glucose-6-phosphate, which can enter the energy-releasing glycolytic pathway of the cell (see Fig. 19-4) or, in the case of liver, can be dephosphorylated and released into the bloodstream to provide an energy source for other cells in the body.

The positive response to epinephrine is transient, owing to reactions that counterbalance the positive arm of the pathway, even in the continued presence of epinephrine. First, each activating reaction is reversible, either spontaneously or after being catalyzed by specific enzymes. Second, the system has several negative feedback loops.

Activating steps are reversed in several different ways. Epinephrine dissociates rapidly from receptors, so if the plasma concentration of epinephrine declines, the β-receptor equilibrium shifts promptly toward the inactive state. Activated GTP-$G_s\alpha$ hydrolyzes its bound nucleotide slowly, at a rate of about 0.05 s^{-1}.

GDP-G$_s$α then rebinds Gβγ, returning the complex to its inactive state. cAMP is degraded to 5′AMP by a phosphodiesterase, an enzyme activated by Ca^{2+}-calmodulin. This convergence allows signaling pathways that release Ca^{2+} (see Fig. 26-12) to modulate the β-adrenergic pathway.

The negative feedback loops operate on a range of time scales. Gγ is anchored to the membrane lipid bilayer by a C-terminal C-20 geranylgeranyl group, so Gβγ subunits released from G$_s$α provide a membrane-binding site for cytoplasmic **β-adrenergic receptor kinase** (now called GRK2). Over seconds to minutes, membrane-associated GRK2 phosphorylates serines in the C-terminal cytoplasmic tail of active receptors. **β-arrestin** binding to phosphorylated receptors has three negative effects: It blocks interactions of the active receptor with G-proteins, attracts cAMP phosphodiesterase to the membrane, and on a time scale of many minutes, its interactions with β-arrestin, clathrin, and adapter proteins (see Fig. 22-10) mediates removal of receptors from the cell surface by endocytosis. Prolonged stimulation results in receptor ubiquitination (see Fig. 23-2), endocytosis, and degradation. Active PKA produced by the pathway independently phosphorylates the receptor with the same negative consequences as phosphorylation by GRK2.

In addition to these effects on glucose metabolism, active β-adrenergic receptors produce at least two other signals. Gβγ subunits activate calcium channels in some cells. This Ca^{2+} can augment glycogen breakdown at the phosphorylase kinase step. In addition to its negative effects, β-arrestin binding to phosphorylated receptors can initiate a positive signal: activation of the mitogen-activated protein (MAP) kinase pathway (see Fig. 27-6). β-arrestin serves as a membrane-anchoring site for the cytoplasmic tyrosine kinase, c-Src, which initiates signaling to the MAP kinase cascade.

Signaling Pathways Influencing Gene Expression

Many extracellular ligands influence gene expression, all through just three kinds of generic pathways (Fig. 27-4). The ligands for the first generic pathway are small and hydrophobic, such as steroids, vitamin A, and thyroid hormone. These ligands penetrate the plasma membrane and bind nuclear receptors in the cytoplasm. The ligands for the other two generic pathways include small charged molecules, peptides, and proteins that cannot penetrate the plasma membrane. Therefore, they must bind receptors on the cell surface to initiate pathways that activate transcription factors. In all cases, activated transcription factors cooperate with other nuclear proteins to regulate the expression of specific genes:

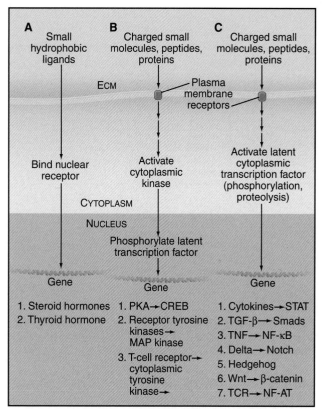

Figure 27-4 THE THREE SIGNALING PATHWAYS BY WHICH EXTRACELLU-LAR LIGANDS INFLUENCE GENE EXPRESSION. **A,** Nuclear receptor pathway for small hydrophobic ligands that penetrate the plasma membrane (see Fig. 15-22A for an example). **B,** Pathways employing a plasma membrane receptor and a cytoplasmic protein kinase that enters the nucleus to activate a latent transcription factor. (See Fig. 15-22 for the PKA pathway, Fig. 27-6 for a receptor tyrosine kinase pathway, and Fig. 27-8 for a cytoplasmic tyrosine kinase pathway.) **C,** Pathways employing a plasma membrane receptor and activating a latent transcription factor in the cytoplasm. The list includes six known pathways of this type. (See Fig. 27-8 for NF-AT, Fig. 27-9 for a STAT pathway, Fig. 27-10 for a Smad pathway, Fig. 15-22 for the NF-κB pathway, Chapter 24 for the Notch and Hedgehog pathways, and Fig. 30-8 for the β-catenin pathway.) CREB, cAMP response element–binding protein; ECM, extracellular matrix; TCR, T-cell receptor; TNF, tumor necrosis factor.

1. *Nuclear receptor pathways:* Ligands such as steroid hormones cross the plasma membrane into the cytoplasm, where they bind latent transcription factors called **nuclear receptors.** Ligand-bound receptors move from the cytoplasm into the nucleus and, in combination with other proteins, activate transcription of specific genes (see Fig. 15-22A).

2. *Pathways activating mobile kinases in the cytoplasm:* Some plasma membrane receptors turn on pathways to activate cytoplasmic protein kinases, which enter the nucleus, where they phosphorylate latent transcription factors. These **mobile kinases** include PKA (see Fig. 15-22B) and several MAP kinases (Figs. 27-5 through 27-8).

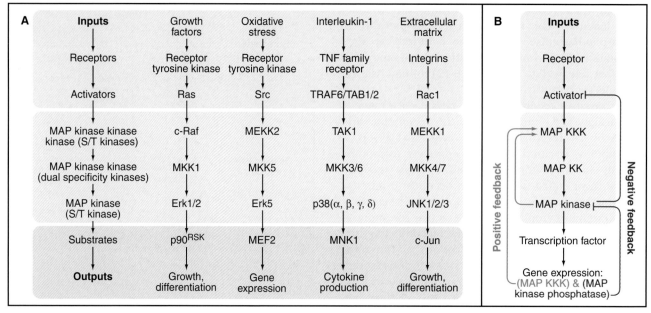

Figure 27-5   A, Four MAP kinase pathways. The pathways are arranged vertically. The levels of the pathways are arranged horizontally. Dual-specificity protein kinases phosphorylate S/T and Y residues. **B,** Positive and negative feedback loops along a generic MAP kinase pathway. K, kinase.

3. *Pathways activating latent transcription factors in the cytoplasm:* Other plasma membrane receptors activate latent transcription factors in the cytoplasm, generally by phosphorylation or proteolysis. These activated transcription factors then enter the nucleus. The seven known pathways use **mobile transcription factors** called NF-AT (Fig. 27-8), STATs (Fig. 27-9), Smads (Fig. 27-10), NF-κB (see Fig. 15-22C), Notch (see Chapter 24), Hedgehog (see Chapter 24), and β-catenin (see Fig. 30-8).

MAP Kinase Pathways to the Nucleus

Cascades of three protein kinases terminating in a **MAP kinase** (mitogen-activated protein kinase) relay signals from diverse stimuli and receptors to the nucleus (Fig. 27-5). The first kinase activates the second kinase by phosphorylating serine residues. The second kinase activates MAP kinase by phosphorylating both a tyrosine and a serine residue in the activation loop (see Fig. 25-3E). Active MAP kinase enters the nucleus and phosphorylates transcription factors, which regulate gene expression. Key targets include genes that advance or restrain the cell cycle, depending on the system. MAP kinases also regulate the synthesis of nucleotides required for making RNA and DNA.

A variety of cell surface receptors initiate pathways that activate MAP kinase cascades. Many of these path-

ways pass through the small guanosine triphosphatase (GTPase) **Ras,** allowing cells to integrate diverse growth-promoting signals to control the cell cycle (see Fig. 41-8). Receptor tyrosine kinases for growth factors (Fig. 27-6) and insulin (Fig. 27-7) send signals through Ras. Other receptors use nonreceptor tyrosine kinases coupled to Ras and MAP kinase, such as T-lymphocyte receptors via zeta-associated protein kinase (ZAP-kinase) (Fig. 27-8). Seven-helix receptors can also activate MAP kinase pathways. For example, β-arrestin not only inactivates β-adrenergic receptors but also couples them to a MAP kinase pathway. Budding yeast activates MAP kinase pathways in two ways. Mating pheromones bind seven-helix receptors that release Gβγ subunits of trimeric G-proteins, which activate the first kinase in the cascade. On the other hand, osmotic shock activates a two-component receptor (Fig. 27-11) upstream of another MAP kinase pathway that regulates the synthesis of glycerol, which is used to adjust cytoplasmic osmolarity.

Animal cells have multiple MAP kinase cascades with particular isoforms of the three kinases linked in series and leading to different effectors (Fig. 27-5). The kinases that make up these pathways are expressed selectively in various cells and tissues. However, deletion of single MAP kinases in mice is generally not lethal, so cross talk between pathways is likely to be extensive.

A cascade of kinases provides opportunities to integrate inputs from converging pathways and to amplify signals. Amplification can be so strong that a MAP kinase cascade acts like an all-or-nothing switch. For example, frog oocytes that are arrested in the G2 stage of the cell cycle react to the hormone progesterone by either remaining arrested or entering the cell cycle. Progesterone activates a MAP kinase cascade consisting of Mos, MEK1, and the p42 MAP kinase. In individual cells, the MAP kinase is either unphosphorylated and inactive or doubly phosphorylated and fully active. This switch-like response depends in part on the fact that both MEK1 and MAP kinase require two independent phosphorylation events for activation. In addition, active MAP kinase provides two types of positive feedback (Fig. 27-5B). MAP kinase not only activates Mos by phosphorylation but also drives Mos expression. Consequently, a marginal stimulus turns some cells on strongly and others not at all rather than producing a graded response in all of the cells.

On the other hand, both yeast and mammals anchor two or three of the kinases in certain MAP kinase pathways to a common **scaffold protein.** Physical association of the enzymes insulates these pathways from parallel pathways but precludes amplification.

Growth Factor Receptor Tyrosine Kinase Pathway through Ras to Map Kinase

Protein and polypeptide growth factors control the expression of genes required for growth and development. For example, the protein **epidermal growth factor** (EGF) controls proliferation and differentiation of epithelial cells in vertebrates. **Platelet-derived growth factor** (PDGF) stimulates the proliferation of connective tissue cells required to heal wounds (see Fig. 32-11). Similar proteins specify the differentiation of cells in fly eyes and the reproductive tract of nematode worms.

Growth factor signaling pathways transfer information from the cell surface through at least eight different protein molecules to the nucleus (Fig. 27-6). Conservation of the main features of the mechanism in vertebrates, worms, and flies made it possible to piece together this complex pathway by pooling information from different systems. Genetic tests identified the components and established the order of their interactions. Many components were identified independently as **oncogenes** and by biochemical isolation and reconstitution of individual steps.

Information flows from growth factors to the nucleus as follows:

1. Growth factors such as EGF bind to the extracellular domain of their receptors. A conformational change induced by EGF binding allows two receptors to bind together.

2. Dimerization of receptors brings together their tyrosine kinase domains inside the cell. The juxtaposed kinases activate each other and **transphosphorylate** tyrosine residues on the **activation loop** of their partner (see Fig. 25-3E). Phosphorylation increases the kinase activity and leads to phosphorylation of other tyrosines on cytoplasmic domains of the receptor.

3. The newly created **phosphotyrosines** are specific binding sites for SH2 domains of several downstream effectors, including **phospholipase Cγ1, phosphatidylinositol 3-kinase** (PI-3 kinase) and a preformed complex of the adapter protein **Grb2** with **SOS.** Amino acids flanking each phosphotyrosine create specific binding sites for the various SH2 domains.

4. Grb2 and SOS continue the signaling pathways to the nucleus. Grb2 consists of three Src homology domains: SH3/SH2/SH3 (see Fig. 25-11). The SH2 domain binds tyrosine-phosphorylated growth factor receptors. The SH3 domains anchor proline-rich sequences (PPPVPPRR) of SOS, a guanine nucleotide exchange factor for the small GTPase **Ras** (see Fig. 4-6). Association of Grb2-SOS with the receptor raises its local concentration near Ras, which is anchored to the bilayer by farnesyl and palmitoyl groups. Proximity appears to be all that is required for SOS to activate Ras, by exchanging GDP for GTP, as experimental targeting of SOS to the plasma membrane by other means also activates Ras. Ras-GTP sustains an activating signal for some time, as its intrinsic rate of GTP hydrolysis is very low ($0.005 \, s^{-1}$). Two mechanisms normally inactivate Ras-GTP: a GTPase-activating protein (**Ras-GAP**) binds to the receptor and stimulates GTP hydrolysis; and removal of the palmitate releases Ras from the plasma membrane.

5. Ras-GTP triggers a MAP-kinase cascade by providing a binding site on the membrane for **Raf-1,** a serine/threonine kinase (a MAP kinase kinase kinase). Interaction with Ras-GTP, and possibly other factors, activates Raf-1.

6. Active Raf-1 phosphorylates and activates the dual-function protein kinase **MEK** (also called MAP kinase kinase or MKK1).

7. MEK activates MAP kinase by phosphorylating both threonine and tyrosine residues on the activation loop.

8. Some of the active MAP kinase acts on cytoplasmic substrates, and some enters the nucleus to phosphorylate and activate transcription factors already bound to DNA (Fig. 27-5). These transcrip-

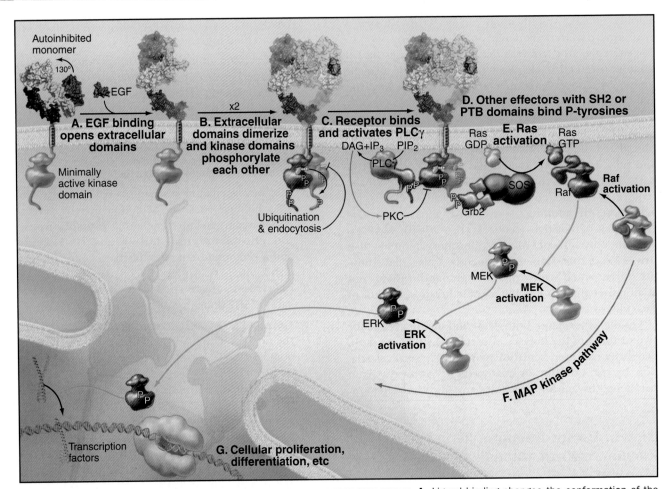

Figure 27-6 EGF RECEPTOR TYROSINE KINASE SIGNALING PATHWAY THROUGH MAP KINASE. **A,** Ligand binding changes the conformation of the extracellular domains of the receptor. **B,** Extracellular domains dimerize, bringing together the tyrosine kinase domains of two receptor subunits in the cytoplasm. Direct interactions and transphosphorylation activate the kinases and create specific docking sites for effector proteins with SH2 domains. **C,** Phospholipase Cγ (PLCγ) binds one phosphotyrosine and is activated by phosphorylation to break down phosphatidyl 4,5-bisphosphate-(PIP_2) into diacylglycerol and IP_3. **D,** A complex of the adapter protein Grb2 and the nucleotide exchange factor SOS binds another phosphotyrosine. (The gene for SOS protein got its name—"son of sevenless"—as a downstream component of the *sevenless* growth factor receptor gene required for the development of photoreceptor cell number seven in the fly eye.) SOS catalyzes the exchange of GDP for GTP on the membrane-associated small GTPase Ras. Ras-GTP attracts the cytoplasmic serine/threonine kinase Raf to the plasma membrane. **E,** Raf phosphorylates and activates the dual-function kinase MEK. **F,** MEK phosphorylates and activates MAP kinase. **G,** MAP kinase enters the nucleus and activates latent transcription factors. (Receptor drawings based on originals by Daniel J. Leahy, Johns Hopkins University, Baltimore, Maryland. Unliganded receptor PDB file: 2AHX. Reference: Bouyain S, Longo PA, Li S, et al: The extracellular region of ErbB4 adopts a tethered conformation in the absence of ligand. Proc Natl Acad Sci U S A 102:15024–15029, 2005.)

tion factors control the expression of genes for proteins that drive the cell cycle (see Fig. 41-8), as well as phosphatases that generate negative feedback by inactivating the kinases along these pathways (Fig. 27-5B).

The routes from the cell surface through Ras and MAP kinase to nuclear transcription factors are not simple linear pathways. The signal is amplified at some steps and influenced by both positive and negative feedback loops at multiple levels. For example, pathways through phospholipase Cγ1 and phosphatidylinositol-3

kinase produce Ca^{2+} and lipid second messengers that activate PKC isoforms (see Fig. 26-6), which provide negative feedback by phosphorylating growth factor receptors. Active receptors are also modified by addition of a single ubiquitin, a signal for inactivation by endocytosis (see Fig. 23-2).

Growth factor pathways are double-edged swords. They are essential for normal growth and development, but malfunctions cause disease by inappropriate cellular proliferation. One example is the release of PDGF at the sites of blood vessel injury. Normally, PDGF stimulates wound repair (see Fig. 32-11), but excess stimula-

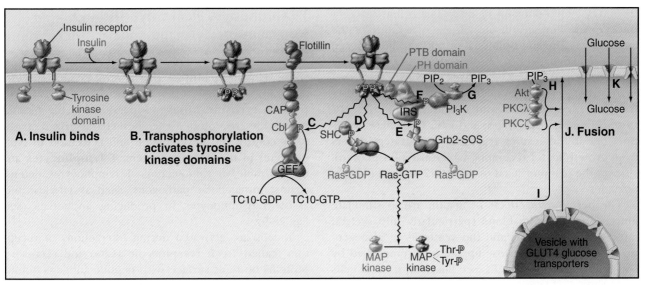

Figure 27-7   **INSULIN SIGNALING PATHWAYS IN AN ADIPOSE CELL.** Active components are shown in bright colors. **A,** Insulin binds the preformed dimeric receptor, bringing together the tyrosine kinase domains in the cytoplasm. **B,** The tyrosine kinase domains activate each other by transphosphorylation of activation loops (Fig. 27-3F). Receptor kinases then phosphorylate a variety of downstream targets: the adapter protein Cbl, which activates a nucleotide exchange protein (GEF), which activates the small GTPase TC10 **(C)**; the adapter protein SHC, which binds Grb2-SOS and slowly initiates the MAP kinase pathway **(D)**; the adapter protein IRS, which binds Grb2-SOS and rapidly initiates the MAP kinase pathway **(E)**; and another IRS phosphotyrosine, which binds phosphatidylinositol 3-kinase (PI3K) **(F)**. **G,** PI3K phosphorylates PIP_2 to make PIP_3. **H,** PIP_3 binds and activates several protein kinases: Akt (PKB), PKCλ, and PKCζ. **I,** These kinases, together with activated TC10, stimulate fusion **(J)** of vesicles carrying the glucose transporter GLUT4 with the plasma membrane. **K,** GLUT4 transports glucose into the cell. CAP binds Cbl to the plasma membrane protein flotillin. The PTB domain of IRS binds phosphotyrosine and the PH domain binds PIP_3.

tion of the proliferation of smooth muscle cells in the walls of injured blood vessels is an early event in the development of **arteriosclerosis.**

Many components of growth factor signaling pathways were discovered during the search for genes that cause cancer. As Jean Marx put it, "growth pathways are liberally paved with oncogene products."* Several of the genes were identified in cancer-causing viruses as oncogenes that are capable of transforming cells in tissue culture. Oncogenes include *sis,* a retroviral homolog of PDGF; *erbB,* a homolog of the EGF receptor; and *raf* kinase. Subsequently, the normal homologs of these genes were found to have mutations in human cancers. Cancer-causing mutations typically make the protein constitutively active, producing a positive signal for growth in the absence of external stimuli (see Fig. 41-10).

For example, two types of mutations can increase the concentration of active Ras. Point mutations (such as substitution of valine for glycine-12) can constitutively activate Ras by reducing its GTPase activity. Alternatively, mutations that inactivate GAPs, such as NF1 (the

gene causing neurofibromatosis, the so-called elephant man disease), reduce the rate that Ras hydrolyzes GTP. In both cases, the high concentration of active Ras-GTP transmits positive signals for growth in the absence of external stimuli, predisposing individuals to malignant disease.

Insulin Pathways to GLUT4 and MAP Kinase

The **insulin receptor tyrosine kinase** not only stimulates the MAP kinase cascade but also triggers the acute response of muscle and adipose cells to the elevation of blood glucose following a meal (Fig. 27-7). High blood glucose levels stimulate β cells in the islets of Langerhans in the pancreas to secrete insulin, a small protein hormone. Insulin receptors are found on many cells, particularly muscle and fat cells. The insulin receptor is a stable dimer of two identical subunits, each consisting of two polypeptides covalently linked by a disulfide bond. One polypeptide forms the insulin-binding extracellular domain. The other has a single transmembrane helix connected to a cytoplasmic tyrosine kinase domain. Insulin binding changes the conformation of

*Marx J: Forging a path to the nucleus. Science 260:1588–1590, 1993.

the extracellular domains in a way that brings together the tyrosine kinase domains on the other side of the membrane. Transphosphorylation of the juxtaposed kinase domains (see Fig. 25-3E) stimulates their kinase activities (Fig. 27-7D). The kinases propagate the signal by phosphorylating adapter proteins including **IRS (insulin receptor substrates,** isoforms 1 to 4), **SHC** (for SH2 and collagen-like), and **Cbl.** Each plays a distinct role in the ensuing response. This strategy differs from growth factor receptors, which use phosphotyrosine on the receptor itself to dock SH2-domain effector enzymes.

The best-known effects of insulin are to stimulate glucose uptake from blood (particularly into skeletal muscle and white fat) and the synthesis of glycogen, protein, and lipid. Glucose uptake is accomplished by the glucose carrier, **GLUT4** (see Fig. 9-5). Resting cells store the GLUT4 uniporter in the membranes of cytoplasmic vesicles. Insulin stimulates fusion of these vesicles with the plasma membrane, making GLUT4 available to transport glucose into the cell. This membrane fusion event requires two separate signals, both of which are downstream from the insulin receptor. Binding of PI-3 kinase to a particular phosphotyrosine on IRS initiates one signal. PI-3 kinase synthesizes PIP_3, which activates the protein kinases PKB/Akt, PKCγ, and PKCζ. Phosphorylation of the adapter protein Cbl initiates the second signal. Cbl activates a nucleotide exchange protein (**guanine nucleotide exchange factor** [GEF]), which activates the small GTPase **TC10.** Within minutes of insulin stimulation, the three kinases and TC10-GTP cooperate to release GLUT4 vesicles from intracellular tethers and promote their fusion with the plasma membrane. PKB also stimulates the conversion of the newly acquired glucose to its storage form, glycogen, by releasing **glycogen synthase** (the enzyme that makes glycogen) from inhibition by glycogen synthase kinase (GSK) 3. The importance of PKB in the response to insulin was verified by the discovery that an inactivating mutation of PKB causes a rare form of diabetes.

Insulin is also a growth factor for some cells, acting through the Ras/MAP kinase pathway to nuclear transcription factors. The signaling circuit to Ras has two arms that operate on different time scales. The fast pathway, acting within seconds, is through tyrosine phosphorylation of IRS, which binds Grb2-SOS and initiates the MAP kinase pathway. The slow arm, acting over a period of minutes, is through phosphorylation of SHC, which binds larger quantities of Grb2-SOS and slowly initiates a sustained response of the MAP kinase pathway. Normal growth and tissue differentiation of many animals depend on insulin-like growth factors, which act on receptors similar to insulin receptor and use IRS1 to channel growth-promoting signals to the nucleus.

T-Lymphocyte Pathways through Nonreceptor Tyrosine Kinases

Some signaling pathways that control cellular growth and differentiation operate through **cytoplasmic protein tyrosine kinases** separate from the plasma membrane receptors. The best-characterized pathways control the development and activation of lymphocytes in the immune system. **T lymphocytes** are the example in this section. T lymphocytes defend against intracellular pathogens, such as viruses, and assist B lymphocytes in producing antibodies (see Fig. 28-9).

T cells are activated during interactions of receptors (called T-cell receptors or TCRs) and accessory proteins on their surface with peptide antigens bound to histocompatibility proteins on the surface of an antigen-presenting cell (Fig. 27-8). Some interactions of T cells with the antigen-presenting cells are generic; others are specific. These interactions on the surface of the T lymphocyte trigger a network of interactions among protein tyrosine kinases, adapter proteins, and effector proteins on the inner surface of the plasma membrane. Tyrosine phosphorylation of multiple membrane and cytoplasmic proteins activates three separate pathways to the nucleus. Two activate cytoplasmic transcription factors; the third uses the Ras/MAP kinase pathway to activate transcription factors in the nucleus.

The **T-cell antigen receptor** is a complex of eight transmembrane polypeptides (Fig. 27-8A). The α and β chains, each with two extracellular immunoglobulin-like domains, provide antigen-binding specificity. Similar to antibodies, one of these immunoglobulin domains is constant and one is variable in sequence. The genes for T-cell receptors are assembled from separate parts, similar to the rearrangement of antibody genes (see Fig. 28-10). Genomic sequences for variable domains are spliced together randomly in developing lymphocytes from a panel of sequences, each encoding a small part of the protein. This combinatorial strategy creates a diversity of T-cell antigen receptors, with one type expressed on any given T cell. Variable sequences of α and β chains provide binding sites for a wide range of different peptide antigens bound to proteins, collectively termed the **major histocompatibility complex (MHC)** antigens, and presented on the surface of cells (Fig. 27-8D). These peptides are fragments of viral proteins or other foreign matter that have been degraded inside the cell, inserted into compatible MHC molecules during their assembly in the endoplasmic reticulum, and transported to the cell surface. Assembly of T-cell receptors in the endoplasmic reticulum requires six additional transmembrane polypeptides, each with one or more short sequence motifs,

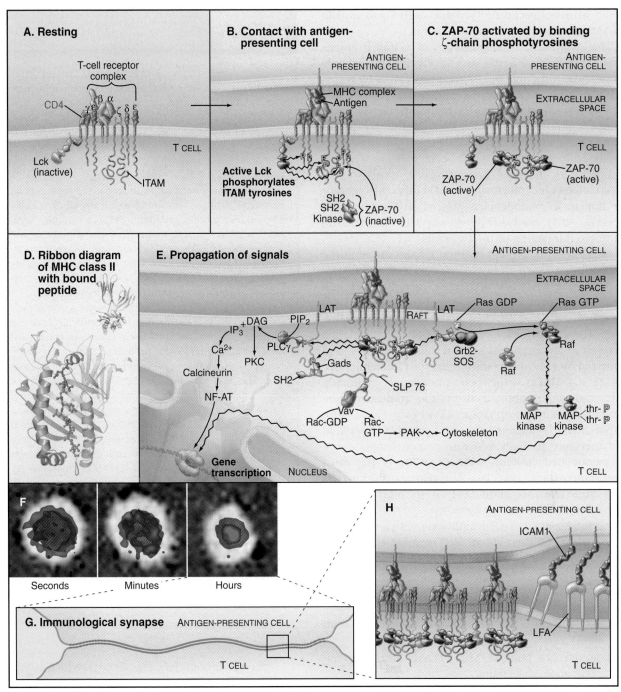

Figure 27-8 **T-LYMPHOCYTE ACTIVATION. A,** Resting T cell with inactive nonreceptor tyrosine kinase Lck and the T-cell receptor complex (TCR) with unphosphorylated cytoplasmic phosphorylation sites (ITAMs). **B,** An encounter with an antigen-presenting cell with an MHC-antigenic peptide complex complementary to the particular TCR initiates signaling. Active Lck phosphorylates various ITAMs. **C,** The nonreceptor tyrosine kinase ZAP-70 is activated by binding via its two SH2 domains to phosphorylated ITAMs on the zeta chains. **D,** Ribbon diagrams of MHC II *(green)* with bound peptide from moth cytochrome c *(orange).* The main model is reduced in size and tilted 90 degrees forward in the view in the *upper right corner,* the same orientation as in the panels **B, C, E,** and **H. E,** Active ZAP-70 phosphorylates various targets, including the transmembrane protein LAT and the adapter protein SLP76, which then propagate the signal. Phospholipase Cγ binds a LAT phosphotyrosine and produces IP$_3$ and DAG. IP$_3$ releases Ca^{2+} from vesicular stores. Ca^{2+} activates calcineurin (protein phosphatase 2B), which activates the latent transcription factor NF-AT. Vav, the nucleotide exchange factor of the small GTPase Rac, is activated by binding to SLP76. Grb2-SOS binds another phosphorylated ITAM and initiates the MAP kinase cascade. **F,** Micrographs of the time course of the interaction of a T cell with an artificial membrane mimicking a specific antigen-presenting cell. Each image comprises a superimposition interference reflection micrograph, showing the closeness of contact as shades of *gray* (with *white* being closest apposition), and a fluorescence micrograph, showing TCRs *(green)* and ICAM1 *(red).* The stable arrangement of ICAM1 around concentrated TCRs is called an immunologic synapse. **G–H,** Immunologic synapse with a central zone of TCRs bound to MHC complexes and peripheral ICAM1 bound to the integrin LFA. Gads is an adapter protein; RAFT is a lipid raft. (D, PDB file: 1KT2. Reference: Fremont DH, Dai S, Chiang H, et al: Structural basis of cytochrome c presentation by IE^k. J Exp Med 195:1043–1052, 2002. F, Courtesy of M. Dustin, New York University, New York.)

called **immunoreceptor tyrosine activation motifs (ITAMs),** in their cytoplasmic domains.

The expression of single types of α and β chains provides individual T cells with specificity for a particular peptide. Although T-cell antigen receptors bind specifically, their affinity for the complex of peptide and MHC is low (K_d in the range of 10 μM). Given the small number (hundreds) of unique MHC-peptide complexes found on the target cell surface, this low affinity would not be sufficient for a lymphocyte to form a stable complex with an antigen-presenting cell. Accessory proteins called coreceptors, such as **CD4** (also the receptor for human immunodeficiency virus [HIV]) and **CD8** (see Fig. 30-3), bind directly to any MHC protein and reinforce interaction of the two cells.

Two classes of protein tyrosine kinases are required to transmit a signal from the engaged TCR to effector systems. The first class of kinases, including **Lck** and **Fyn,** are relatives of the product of the Src gene (see Fig. 25-3C), the first oncogene to be characterized (Box 27-5). These tyrosine kinases are anchored to the plasma membrane by myristolated N-terminal glycines and inhibited by a phosphotyrosine near the C-terminus (see Fig. 25-3C). This tyrosine is phosphorylated by a kinase, Csk, and dephosphorylated by the transmembrane protein tyrosine phosphatase, **CD45** (see Fig. 25-6B). Apparently, CD45 keeps Lck partially dephosphorylated and therefore partially active in resting lymphocytes. Zeta-associated protein–70 kD **(ZAP-70)** is the most important of the second class of protein tyrosine kinases. Two SH2 domains allow ZAP-70 to bind tyrosine-phosphorylated ITAMs on ζ chains.

Physical contact of a T lymphocyte with an **antigen-presenting** cell carrying an MHC-peptide specific for its T-cell receptor generates multiple signals as follows:

1. Engagement of TCRs leads to activation of Lck by dephosphorylation of the inhibitory C-terminal tyrosine and phosphorylation of its activation loop.

2. Active Lck phosphorylates ITAMs on the several TCR accessory chains.

3. ZAP-70 is activated by binding phosphorylated ITAMs and phosphorylation of its activation loop by Lck.

4. Active ZAP-70 phosphorylates various targets, including the transmembrane protein LAT and the adapter protein SLP76, which then propagate the signal along several branches.

5. Signals reach the nucleus by three pathways. First, phospholipase Cγ1 is activated by binding a phosphotyrosine on LAT and by tyrosine phosphorylation. Active phospholipase Cγ1 produces IP$_3$ and diacylglycerol. Release of Ca^{2+} from vesicular stores by IP$_3$ activates **calcineurin** (protein

---

BOX 27-5
Src Family of Protein Tyrosine Kinases

The founding member of the Src family of protein tyrosine kinases has a prominent place in modern biology. During the 1920s, Peyton Rous discovered the first cancer-causing virus in a mesodermal cancer of chickens called a sarcoma. Later, the Rous sarcoma virus was found to be a retrovirus with an RNA genome. By comparing similar viruses that did not cause cancer, investigators learned that one gene, named *src*, is responsible for transforming cells into cancer cells. Finally, a gene very similar to *src* was found in normal chicken cells. The cellular protein product, c-Src, is a carefully regulated protein tyrosine kinase that participates in the control of cellular proliferation and differentiation. Mutations in the gene for viral *src, v-src,* activate its protein product constitutively, driving cells to proliferate and contributing to the development of cancer.

The family of Src-like proteins shares a common structure (see Fig. 25-3C). Five functionally distinct segments are recognized in the sequences. An N-terminal myristic acid anchors the protein to the plasma membrane. Without this modification, the protein is inactive. The next domains are the founding examples of Src homology domains SH3, which bind proline-rich peptides, and SH2, which bind peptides containing a phosphorylated tyrosine (Fig. 25-10). The kinase domain is followed by a tyrosine near the C-terminus. Phosphorylation of this tyrosine and its intramolecular binding to the SH2 domain lock the kinase in an inactive conformation. Dephosphorylation of the C-terminal tyrosine and phosphorylation of the activation loop activate the kinase.

Expression of c-Src is highest in brain and platelets, but a null mutation in mice produces relatively few defects, except in bones, where a failure of osteoclasts to remodel bone leads to overgrowth, a condition called osteopetrosis (see Fig. 32-6).

---

phosphatase 2B [see Fig. 25-6A]), which activates the latent transcription factor **NF-AT.** Second, Grb2-SOS binds another phosphotyrosine on LAT and initiates the MAP kinase cascade by activating Ras. Third, Vav, the nucleotide exchange factor of the small GTPases, is anchored indirectly to LAT and initiates a pathway that degrades IκB, freeing NF-κB (see Fig. 15-22) to enter the nucleus. These events appear to take place in lipid rafts.

6. The signal reaches the cytoskeleton via Vav, which is activated by binding a phosphotyrosine on the adapter protein SLP76. Vav catalyzes the exchange of GTP for GDP on the Rho-family GTPase Rac, which stimulates assembly of actin filaments.

When a T cell recognizes an antigen-presenting cell with an appropriate peptide bound to MHC on its surface, the TCRs and adhesion proteins in the interface between the cells rearrange to form an "**immunologic synapse**" (Fig. 27-8F). TCRs initially gather around a region of contact between integrins (LFA) on the T cell and immunoglobulin-cellular adhesion molecules (ICAMs) on the antigen-presenting cell. With time, these zones reverse positions, yielding a stable immunologic synapse, with a ring of adhesion molecules (Fig. 27-8G–H) around a central region with concentrated MHCs and TCRs. In this crowded central region, even a few specific MHC-peptides can activate multiple TCRs in serial fashion. Each active TCR generates a signal to the nucleus and is then internalized and degraded.

The best available **immunosuppressive drugs** used in human organ transplantation block lymphocyte proliferation by inhibiting calcineurin, the phosphatase that activates NF-AT. When given within 1 hour of the stimulus, these drugs completely block T-cell activation, but they have little effect after several hours once the genetic program has been initiated. **Cyclosporin** and FK506 bind to separate cytoplasmic proteins, cyclophilin, and FK-binding protein. Both of these drug-protein complexes bind calcineurin and inhibit phosphatase activity. Considering that many cells express calcineurin, the effects of these drugs on lymphocytes is amazingly specific, with relatively few side effects. Specificity arises from the low concentration of calcineurin in lymphocytes: only 10,000 molecules in T cells compared with 300,000 in other cells. Hence, low concentrations

of inhibitor can selectively block calcineurin in T lymphocytes. Cyclosporin made human heart and liver transplantation feasible.

The response to T cell receptor activation depends on the particular state of differentiation of the T cell that encounters its partner antigenic peptide. Stimulation causes some T cells to secrete toxic peptides that kill the antigen-presenting cell, others to synthesize and secrete lymphokines (immune system hormones), others to proliferate and differentiate, and yet others to commit to apoptosis (see Fig. 46-8).

Cytokine Receptor, JAK/STAT Pathways

Many polypeptide hormones and growth factors (collectively called **cytokines**; see Fig. 24-6) regulate gene expression through a three-protein relay without a second messenger—the most direct signal transduction pathway from extracellular ligands to the nucleus (Fig. 27-9). Growth hormone uses this mechanism to drive overall growth of the body, erythropoietin directs the proliferation and maturation of red blood cell precursors, and several interferons and interleukins mediate antiviral and immune responses. Slime molds and animals use these pathways, but these proteins are not present in fungi or plants.

The three components in these pathways are a plasma membrane receptor that lacks intrinsic enzymatic activity, an associated tyrosine kinase (**JAK**), and a

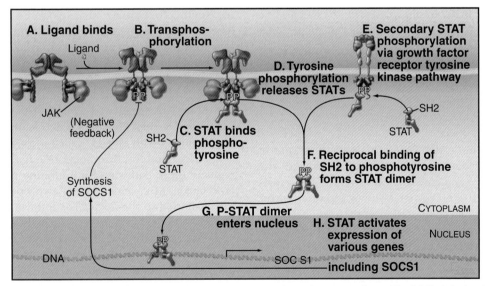

Figure 27-9 CYTOKINE JAK/STAT SIGNALING PATHWAY. **A,** Cytokine binds a preformed receptor dimer (Fig. 24-7), bringing together the cytoplasmic domains with a bound tyrosine kinase, JAK. **B,** JAKs activate each other by transphosphorylation and then phosphorylate other tyrosines on the receptor. **C,** The SH2 domain of the latent transcription factor STAT binds a receptor phosphotyrosine. **D,** JAK phosphorylates the STATs, which then dissociate from the receptor. **E,** Growth factor receptor tyrosine kinases can also activate STATs. **F,** The STATs form an active dimer by reciprocal SH2-phosphotyrosine interactions. **G,** The STAT dimer enters the nucleus. **H,** The STAT dimer activates the expression of various genes. One of these genes encodes SOCS1, which creates negative feedback by inhibiting further STAT activation.

latent, cytoplasmic transcription factor called a **STAT** (signal transducer and activator of transcription). Crystal structures of the extracellular domain of the human erythropoietin receptor (see Fig. 24-6) suggest that the inactive receptor is preformed dimer in the membrane. Most of these receptors use two fibronectin III domains to bind their ligands.

JAKs were originally given the lighthearted name "just another kinase." In view of their role between diverse receptors and transcription factors, the revisionist name "Janus kinase" (for the Greek god who opens doors) has been suggested. The tyrosine kinase domain is located near the C-terminus next to an inactive kinase-like domain. The N-terminal half of these proteins and kinase-like domain mediate the association of JAKs with receptors. Some cytokine receptors bind and activate a single type of JAK; others are promiscuous (see Fig. 24-6).

JAKs activate STATs by tyrosine phosphorylation, which promotes the formation of active dimers. These dimers enter the nucleus and bind to specific promoter sequences. The signal moves from the cytokine receptor to JAK to STAT to the nucleus as follows:

1. Ligand binding to the extracellular domain of a cytokine receptor rearranges the extracellular domains and brings together the cytoplasmic domains with the associated JAKs.

2. Juxtaposition allows the JAKs to activate each other by transphosphorylation. JAKs also phosphorylate tyrosines on the cytoplasmic tails of the receptors, creating docking sites for STATs.

3. An SH2 domain targets a STAT to a particular phosphotyrosine binding site on the receptor, where the JAK can phosphorylate the STAT.

4. Phosphorylated STAT dissociates from the receptor and forms an active dimer by reciprocal interactions between the SH2 domain of one partner and a phosphotyrosine of the other partner.

5. Active STAT dimers enter the nucleus and activate expression of various genes.

Three different mechanisms turn down the response to cytokine activation. Phosphatases inactivate the receptor, kinase, and intranuclear STATs. Endocytosis also turns off active receptors. A slowly acting, negative feedback loop limits the duration of the response. One of the genes expressed in response to STAT encodes SOCS1. Once synthesized, the SOCS1 protein inhibits further STAT activation by interaction with the cytokine receptor.

Selective expression of specific cytokine receptors, four JAKs, and seven STATs prepares differentiated mammalian cells to respond specifically to various cytokines. Active STAT dimers are either homodimers or heterodimers of two different STATs. A variety of STATs,

with some unique and some common subunits, bind regulatory sites for the family of genes required to activate the target cells. The products of genes controlled by STATs not only contribute to differentiated cellular functions; some also drive proliferation. Accordingly, loss of JAK function causes certain immune deficiencies, while patients with mutations in STAT5b are resistance to growth hormone and fail to grow. The opposite effect follows from a mutation that renders JAK2 constitutively active: Red blood cells proliferate out of control, independent of stimulation by erythropoietin.

The three-protein pathway from a cytokine receptor to JAK to activated STAT is appealing in its simplicity, but in reality, these pathways do not operate in isolation. On one hand, converging signals from EGF- and PDGF-receptors can phosphorylate and activate STATs, a second input to STAT-responsive genes. On the other hand, some cytokine receptors can regulated gene expression through Shc and Grb2-SOS to Ras and MAP kinases and other pathways.

Serine/Threonine Kinase Receptor Pathways through Smads

Metazoans use a family of dimeric polypeptide growth factors related to **transforming growth factor-β (TGF-β** [see Fig. 24-8]) to specify developmental fates during embryogenesis and to control cellular differentiation in adults. More than 40 genes in this family are divided into two classes: (i) those related to TGF-β and **activins** and (ii) a large family of **bone morphogenetic proteins.** All activate a short pathway consisting of **receptor serine/threonine kinases** and a family of eight mobile transcription factors called **Smads.** The receptors consist of two types of subunits called RI and RII.

Ligand binding brings together two RI and two RII receptors, allowing the RII receptors to activate the RI receptors by transphosphorylation. Active RI receptors phosphorylate "regulated Smads" (R-Smads), such as Smad2 and Smad3. Phosphorylated R-Smads form active heterodimers with Smad4, called a co-Smad, because it is not subjected to phosphorylation itself. Other Smads regulate these pathways by inhibiting phosphorylation of R-Smads. After activation of a receptor, information is transmitted to the nucleus as follows (Fig. 27-10):

1. An autoinhibited R-Smad binds an activated RI receptor in a complex with an adapter protein called SARA (Smad anchor for receptor activation).

2. Active RI receptor kinase phosphorylates the R-Smad.

3. Phosphorylated R-Smad dissociates from RI and binds co-Smad4.

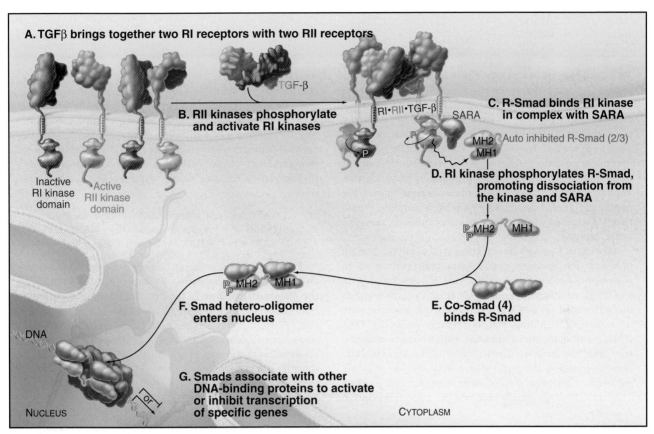

A. TGFβ brings together two RI receptors with two RII receptors

Inactive RI kinase domain

Active RII kinase domain

B. RII kinases phosphorylate and activate RI kinases

TGF-β

RI·RII·TGF-β   SARA

C. R-Smad binds RI kinase in complex with SARA

Auto inhibited R-Smad (2/3)

MH2
MH1

D. RI kinase phosphorylates R-Smad, promoting dissociation from the kinase and SARA

P P MH2   MH1

P P MH2   MH1

F. Smad hetero-oligomer enters nucleus

E. Co-Smad (4) binds R-Smad

DNA

or

NUCLEUS

G. Smads associate with other DNA-binding proteins to activate or inhibit transcription of specific genes

CYTOPLASM

Figure 27-10   TGF-β/Smad signaling pathway. **A,** TGF-β binding assembles a complex consisting of two RII receptors and two RI receptors. **B,** RII phosphorylates and activates RI. **C,** An autoinhibited R-Smad binds RI in a complex with the adapter SARA. **D,** RI kinase phosphorylates R-Smad, which promotes dissociation. **E,** Co-Smad binds to R-Smad. **F,** The Smad heterodimer enters the nucleus. **G,** The Smad heterodimer associates with other DNA-binding proteins to activate or inhibit transcription of specific genes.

4. The R-Smad/co-Smad heterodimer enters the nucleus and associates with other DNA binding proteins to activate or inhibit transcription of specific genes.

The Smad pathway activated by TGF-β regulates cellular proliferation and differentiation of many cell types, including epithelial and hematopoietic cells. Although its name implies that it should drive transformation, TGF-β actually stops the cell cycle in G1 by promoting expression of negative regulators of cyclin-dependent kinases (see Fig. 41-3).

In accord with the ability of TGF-β pathways to inhibit cellular growth, many human tumors have loss of function mutations in the genes for TGF-β receptors or Smads. Mutations in an accessory receptor for TGF-β cause malformed blood vessels in the human disease hereditary hemorrhagic telangiectasia. Mice with homozygous loss of function mutations in genes for the components of the TGF pathway die during embryonic development.

Like other signaling pathways, these receptors and Smads do not operate in isolation. MAP kinases and cyclin dependent kinases can phosphorylate Smads, and active RI receptors can activate MAP kinase pathways.

Two-Component Phosphotransfer Systems

Prokaryotes, fungi, and plants transduce stimuli ranging from nutrients to osmotic pressure using signaling systems consisting of as few as two proteins, a receptor-linked histidine kinase, and a "response regulator" activated by phosphorylation of an aspartic acid (Box 27-6 and Fig. 27-11). Such "two-component" systems from bacteria are one of the few signaling pathways in which the dynamics of information transfer are well understood. Extensive collections of mutants in these pathways and sensitive single-cell assays for responses, such as flagellar rotation, provide tools for rigorous tests of concepts and mathematical models derived from biochemical experiments on isolated components.

For years, two-component systems appeared to be restricted to prokaryotes, but response regulators eventually were discovered in yeast and plants. Bacteria

BOX 27-6
Two-Component Signaling

Two-component receptors either may include a cytoplasmic histidine kinase domain (Fig. 27-11C) or may bind a separate histidine kinase, such as the aspartate chemotactic receptor **Tar** (Fig. 27-11B). Tar consists of two identical subunits. Three of these dimers are thought to be anchored at their bases in the cytoplasm (Fig. 27-11B). Binding of aspartic acid between the extracellular domains of two subunits changes their orientation by a few degrees. Transmission of this conformational change across the membrane alters the activity of **CheA,** a histidine kinase that is associated with the most distal cytoplasmic domains of the receptor.

Histidine kinases have a conserved catalytic domain of about 350 residues that is structurally unrelated to eukaryotic serine/threonine/tyrosine kinases (shown in Fig. 25-3). Another domain allows them to form homodimers. Histidine kinases are incorporated into a wide variety of proteins, including transmembrane receptors (Fig. 27-11C) and cytoplasmic proteins with a variety of accessory domains such as CheA (Fig. 27-11B). The catalytic domain transfers the γ-phosphate from ATP to just one substrate, a histidine residue of its homodimeric partner. This histidine is usually located in the dimerization domain.

All **response regulators** have a domain of about 120 residues folded like **CheY** (Fig 27-11B; also see Fig. 3-7). Transfer of phosphate from the phosphohistidine of a kinase to an invariant aspartic acid changes the conformation of the response regulator. Most response regulators such as CheB (Fig. 27-11B) and OmpR (Fig. 27-11C) are larger than CheY, having C-terminal effector domains. Many effector domains, including OmpR, bind DNA and regulate transcription of specific genes when the response regulator is activated by aspartate phosphorylation. Other response regulators are included as a domain of the histidine kinase itself.

Reversible phosphorylation transfers information through two-component systems. The mechanism differs fundamentally from eukaryotic kinase cascades, which transfer phosphate from ATP to serine, threonine, or tyrosine, forming phosphoesters at every step. By contrast, two-component systems first transfer a phosphate from ATP to a nitrogen of a histidine of the kinase, the first of the two protein components. The high-energy his~P phosphoramidate bond is unstable, so the phosphate is readily transferred to the side chain of an aspartic acid of the response regulator (RR):

$$\text{ATP} + \text{kinase-his} \rightleftharpoons \text{ADP} + \text{kinase-his~P}$$
$$\text{kinase-his~P} + \text{RR-asp} \rightleftharpoons \text{kinase-his} + \text{RR*-asp~P}$$
$$\text{RR*-asp~P} + \text{H}_2\text{O} \rightleftharpoons \text{RR-asp} + \text{phosphate}$$

Phosphorylation activates response regulators (RR*) by changing their conformation. Details differ depending on the response regulator. In the case of OmpR, phosphorylation relieves autoinhibition of the DNA-binding domain (Fig. 27-11C). Phosphorylation of CheY reveals a binding site for the flagellar rotor. The signal dissipates by dephosphorylation of the response regulator, either by autocatalysis or by stimulation by accessory proteins. Lifetimes of the high-energy aspartic acylphosphate vary from seconds to hours.

A minimal two-component system, such as a bacterial osmoregulatory pathway (Fig. 27-11C), consists of a dimeric plasma membrane receptor with a cytoplasmic histidine kinase domain and a cytoplasmic response regulator protein. Signal transduction is carried out in four steps. A change in osmolarity alters the conformation of the receptor, activating the kinase activity of its cytoplasmic domain. The kinase phosphorylates a histidine residue on the other subunit of the dimeric receptor. This phosphate is transferred from the receptor to an aspartic acid side chain of the response regulator protein OmpR. Phosphorylation changes the conformation of the response regulator domain of OmpR, allowing its DNA-binding domain to activate the expression of certain genes.

---

have genes for up to 70 response regulators, with 32 response regulators and 30 histidine kinases in *Escherichia coli*. Archaea have genes for up to 24 response regulators. The slime mold *Dictyostelium* has more than 10 histidine kinases, whereas fungi have just one or two of these systems. Plants use a two-component system to regulate fruit ripening in response to the gas ethylene.

Bacterial Chemotaxis

The two-component system regulating bacterial chemotaxis (Fig. 27-12) is the best-understood signaling pathway of any kind. *E. coli* cells use five types of plasma membrane receptors to sense a variety of different chemicals. These receptors are also called methyl-accepting chemotaxis proteins, as they are regulated by methylation. The most abundant, with about 2000 copies per cell, is Tar (Fig. 27-11A–B), the receptor for the nutrients aspartic acid (Tar-D) and maltose, protons (as part of pH sensing), temperature, and the repellent nickel. A few thousand Tar molecules are concentrated at one end of the cell (Fig. 27-12A). Clustering facilitates interactions between receptor molecules, but this polarized distribution has nothing to do with sensing the direction of chemical gradients.

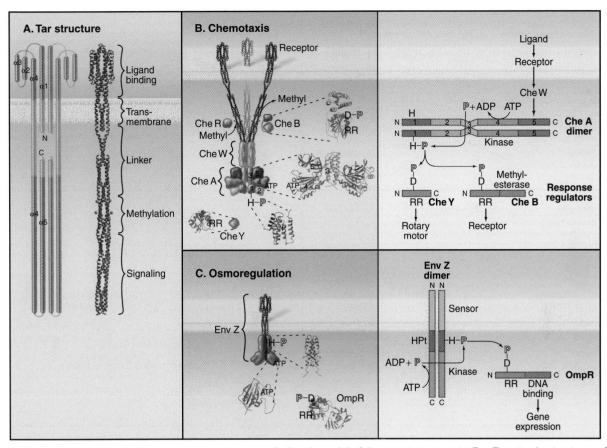

Figure 27-11 TWO-COMPONENT BACTERIAL SIGNALING SYSTEMS. **A,** Atomic model of the aspartate receptor Tar. The atomic structures of the extracellular and cytoplasmic domains were determined by X-ray crystallography. The transmembrane α-helices are models based on the primary structure. The two polypeptides are shown in *red* and *blue*. Each polypeptide starts in the cytoplasm and passes twice through the lipid bilayer. **B,** Bacterial chemotaxis signaling proteins. Scale models of the molecular components and pathway of information transfer. The domains shown on the *right* are color coded in the molecular models on the *left*. An accessory protein, CheW, facilitates binding of the histidine kinase CheA to the aspartate receptor Tar. CheY and CheB are response regulators. CheR is a methyl transferase. **C,** Bacterial osmoregulation. The histidine kinase forms the cytoplasmic domain of the receptor. OmpR is the response regulator with a DNA-binding domain. Scale models of the molecules *(left)* and pathway of information transfer *(right)*. (A, Modified from material provided courtesy of S. H. Kim, University of California, Berkeley. Reference: Kim KK, Yokata H, Kim SH: Four helical-bundle structure of the cytoplasmic domain of a serine chemotaxis receptor. Nature 400:787–792, 1999. PDB file: 1QU7. B–C, Based on material provided courtesy of A. M. Stock, Howard Hughes Medical Institute, and Robert Wood Johnson Medical School. Reference: Stock AM, Robinson WL, Goudreau PN: Two-component signal transduction. Annu Rev Biochem 69:183–215, 2000.)

The chemotactic signaling system guides swimming bacteria toward attractive chemicals and away from repellents in a biased random walk. Environmental chemicals influence the behavior of the cell by biasing the direction that the rotary flagellar motor turns (see Figs. 38-23 and 38-24 for details on the motor itself). In its default mode, the motor turns counterclockwise, and the bacterium swims smoothly in a more or less linear path. When the flagella turn the other way, the bacterium tumbles about in one place. A **tumble** allows a bacterium to reorient its direction randomly, so when it resumes **smooth swimming,** it usually heads off in a new direction. In the absence of chemoattractants, bacteria swim for about 0.9 s and then tumble for about 0.1 s, allowing for random reorientations every second.

A gradient of chemical attractant promotes the length of runs up the gradient by suppressing tumbling if the concentration of attractant increases over time (Fig. 27-12D). A two-component signaling pathway senses the attractant and controls the frequency of tumbling. The degree of saturation of the flagellar motor with the response regulator **CheY** determines which way it rotates.

Ligand-free Tar stimulates the phosphorylation of the associated histidine kinase **CheA**. ("Che" refers to a gene required for chemotaxis, as most of these components were discovered by mutagenesis. A lowercase "p"

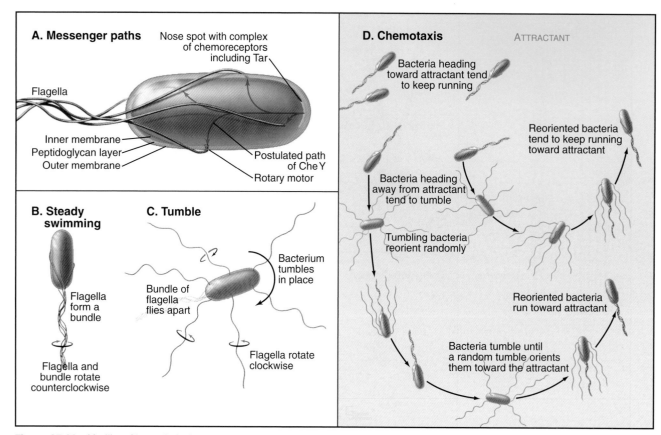

Figure 27-12   Motility of bacteria is determined by the direction of rotation of their flagella. **A,** Arrangement of signal transduction components and flagella in *Escherichia coli*. **B,** Flagella that are rotating counterclockwise (viewed from the tip of the flagella) form a bundle that pushes the cell smoothly forward. **C,** When flagella rotate clockwise, the bundle flies apart, and the cell tumbles in place. **D,** An attractive chemical biases movement toward its source by modulating the frequency of runs and tumbles. (A, Reference: Parkinson JS, Blair DF: Does *E. coli* have a nose? Science 259:1701–1702, 1993.)

represents the shorthand for phosphorylation in these bacterial systems.) CheAp activates the response regulator, CheY, by transferring phosphate from histidine to D57 of CheY. CheYp has a higher affinity for the flagellar motor than CheY, and ligand-free receptor maintains an equilibrium with the rotors partially saturated with CheYp. With several bound CheYps, the motor reverses from its free-running, counterclockwise state about 10% of the time, inducing a brief tumble about once per second.

Information about aspartate in the environment flows rapidly through the pathway as changes in the *concentrations* of the phosphorylated species CheAp and CheYp. A key point is that Tar with bound aspartate, Tar-D, does not activate histidine phosphorylation of CheA. Hence aspartate binding to Tar reduces the saturation of the flagellar motors with CheYp and the frequency of tumbles.

For the cell to respond to aspartate on a subsecond time scale, an accessory protein, **CheZ,** is required to increase the rate of CheYp dephosphorylation more than 100-fold from its slow spontaneous rate of 0.03 s^{-1}. Given this fast dissipation of CheYp, maintenance of a

tumbling rate of about 1 s^{-1}, in the absence of an attractant, requires constant flow of phosphate from ATP to CheAp to CheYp (Fig. 27-13A). (In most other two-component pathways, dephosphorylation of the response regulator is much slower, allowing responses over a period of minutes rather than milliseconds.) The following sections examine chemotaxis on the system level, starting with the response to a rapid change in concentration of aspartate.

Temporal Sensing of Gradients

Bacteria are too small and move too fast to detect a spatial gradient directly. Instead, they sense the gradient as a change in concentration of attractant or repellent as a function of time. When a bacterium swims up a gradient of chemoattractant, the concentration of attractant increases with time, and the signaling mechanism suppresses tumbling. Fewer tumbles bias movement toward the attractant. When a cell swims down the gradient, tumbling is more frequent, allowing for reorientation.

A sudden increase in the concentration of aspartate yields a smooth swimming response within 200 ms due

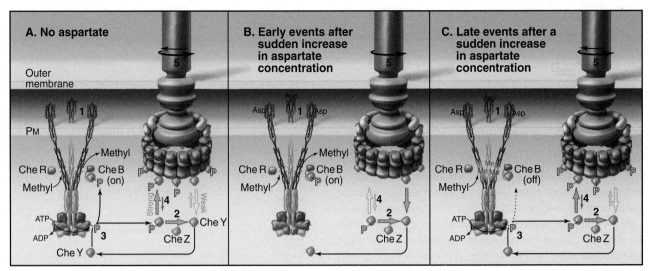

Figure 27-13 SIGNALING DURING BACTERIAL CHEMOTAXIS. **A,** Absence of aspartate. Ligand-free Tar (1) allows CheA to phosphorylate CheY and CheB (3). Constant dephosphorylation of CheYp drives a cycle of phosphorylation (2). The steady-state concentration of CheYp keeps the motor partially saturated (4). The partially saturated motor turns counterclockwise 90% of the time (runs [thick arrow]) and clockwise 10% of the time (tumbles [thin arrow]) (5). **B,** Rapid response to the presence of aspartate. Aspartate binding turns off Tar (1). Constant dephosphorylation depletes CheYp on a time scale of tens of milliseconds (2). CheYp dissociates from the motor (4). The motor, without CheYp, rotates counterclockwise, so the bacterium runs continuously (5). **C,** Slower, adaptive response to the presence of aspartate. Inactive CheA stops phosphorylating CheB, allowing dephosphorylation of CheBp on a time scale of seconds; this inactivation of CheB allows net methylation of Tar by CheR (1). Even with bound aspartate, methylated Tar is partially active, allowing phosphorylation of CheA (2). CheY is phosphorylated (3). CheYp rebinds the motor (4). The flagella turn clockwise part of the time, causing occasional tumbles (5).

to rapid reequilibration of the concentrations of all of the cytoplasmic signaling components (Fig. 27-13B). Aspartate binds Tar and inhibits autophosphorylation of CheA. Because CheYp has a half-life less than 100 ms, the concentrations of CheAp and CheYp decrease rapidly. CheYp dissociates from the flagellar motor and the motor persists in the counterclockwise, smooth swimming direction. If the concentration change with time is due to a gradient of aspartate, the bacterium tends to swim steadily up the gradient toward the source.

The opposite sequence of events takes place if a bacterium swims down a gradient of aspartate. The fraction of Tar with bound aspartate declines, CheAp and CheYp concentrations rise, and tumbling is more frequent, providing opportunities to reorient and swim back up the gradient.

Adaptation

After a step change in aspartate, bacteria respond quickly with smooth swimming, but within tens of seconds to minutes, they return to their normal pattern of intermittent tumbling. In fact, the steady-state tumbling frequency is independent of the concentration of aspartate. This remarkable capacity to adapt is accomplished by a negative feedback loop provided by reversible **methylation** of the receptor (Fig. 27-13C). Methylated Tar has a somewhat lower affinity for aspartate than unmethylated Tar, but Me-Tar with bound aspartate is more effective at stimulating CheA phosphorylation than Tar with bound aspartate.

Two relatively slow enzymes determine the level of Tar methylation (Fig. 27-11B). **CheR** adds methyls to four glutamic acid residues on each receptor polypeptide, whereas **CheB** removes them. CheR is constitutively active but sensitive to the overall metabolic state of the cell, as it depends on the concentration of *S*-adenosyl methionine, a methyl donor that is used in many metabolic reactions.

A variable rate of demethylation determines the level of Tar methylation. CheB methylesterase is a response regulator that is activated by phosphorylation by CheAp. CheB is autoinhibited by its response regulator domain blocking the active site. Phosphorylation displaces the response regulator domain from the active site, making CheBp much more active than CheB.

Adaptation occurs because aspartate binding to Tar activates two different pathways on different time scales. On a *millisecond* time scale, the concentrations of both CheAp and CheYp decline, CheYp dissociates from the motor, and the cell swims smoothly. The rapid reduction in CheAp also reduces the concentration of CheBp, but on a *second* time scale, as the rate of CheBp dephosphorylation is only $0.1 \ s^{-1}$. The slow decline in CheBp gradually reduces methylesterase activity and results in a higher level of Tar methylation. This, in turn, allows the receptor, still saturated with aspartate, to reactivate CheA phosphorylation. Remarkably, the cell returns exactly to its prestimulus frequencies of runs and tumbles. This **robust adaptation** mechanism is an integral feedback system, just like a thermostat on a heater. Both methylation and demethylation are sensitive to the conformation of the receptor, so another level of complexity contributes to the capacity of the system to adapt.

Extended Range of Response

An amazing feature of this system is its ability to respond with fast changes in flagellar rotation and slow adaptation to changes of *just a few percentage points* in aspartate concentration over a range of five orders of magnitude. Clearly, a simple bimolecular reaction of aspartate with Tar cannot change the fractional saturation of Tar over such an extended range of concentrations. This extended range of sensitivity is valuable for the survival of the bacterium and must depend on some sort of amplification at the level of the receptor. A likely mechanism is that aspartate binding to one Tar activates many surrounding Tars in the receptor clusters at the end of the cell.

Bacterial chemotaxis illustrates some of the classical features of signaling pathways, including high sensitivity due to amplification at the level of CheA phosphorylation, negative feedback through methylation of Tar, and branching networks that respond on different time scales to the same stimulus. The mechanism has been tested thoroughly by mutating all of the signaling components and observing the consequences. For example, loss of either CheA or CheY results in smooth-running bacteria. Cells without CheZ respond slowly to a change in aspartate. Loss of CheR and CheB results in bacteria that respond to signals over a limited range of concentrations but are unable to adapt to them.

SELECTED READINGS

Aaronson DS, Horvath CM: A road map for those who don't know JAK-STAT. Science 296:1653–1655, 2002.

American Association for the Advancement of Science: Signal Transduction Knowledge Environment. Available at http:/stke.sciencemag.org.

Armitage JP: Bacterial tactic responses. Adv Microb Physiol 41:229–289, 1999.

Attisano L, Wrana JL: Signal transduction by the TGF-β superfamily. Science 296:1646–1647, 2002.

Bray D, Duke T: Conformational spread: The propagation of allosteric states in large multiprotein complexes. Annu Rev Biophys Biomol Struct 33:53–73, 2004.

Call ME, Wucherpfennig KW: The T cell receptor: Critical role of the membrane environment in receptor assembly and function. Annu Rev Immunol 23:101–125, 2005.

Chang L, Karin M: Mammalian MAP kinase signalling cascades. Nature 410:37–40, 2001.

Davis M, Krogsgaard M, Huppa JB, et al: Dynamics of cell surface molecules during T-cell recognition. Annu Rev Biochem 72:717–742, 2003.

Derynck R, Zhang YE: Smad-dependent and Smad-independent pathways in TGF-β signalling. Nature 425:577–584, 2003.

Ferrell JE Jr: Self-perpetuating states in signal transduction: Positive feedback, double-negative feedback and bistability. Curr Opin Cell Biol 14:140–148, 2002.

Ihle JN: The Stat family in cytokine signaling. Curr Opin Cell Biol 13:211–217, 2001.

Johnson GL, Lapadat R: Mitogen-activated protein kinase pathways mediated by ERK, JNK and p38 protein kinases. Science 298:1911–1912, 2002.

Lefkowitz RJ, Shenoy SK: Transduction of receptor signals by β-arrestins. Science 308:512–517, 2005.

Mombaerts P: Seven-transmembrane proteins as odorant and chemosensory receptors. Science 286:707–711, 1999. [See also related articles in same issue.]

Mombaerts P: Genes and ligands for odorant, vomeronasal and taste receptors. Nat Rev Neurosci 5:263–278, 2004.

Ottensmeyer FP, Beniac DR, Luo R Z-T, Yip C: Mechanism of transmembrane signaling: Insulin binding and the insulin receptor. Biochemistry 39:12103–12112, 2000.

Ptashne M, Gann A: Imposing specificity on kinases [MAP kinase cascades]. Science 299:1025–1027, 2003.

Rana BK, Shiina T, Insel PA: Genetic variations and polymorphisms of G protein-coupled receptors: Functional and therapeutic implications. Annu Rev Pharmacol Toxicol 41:593–624, 2001.

Ridge KD, Abdulaev NG, Sousa M, Palczewski K: Phototransduction: Crystal clear. Trends Biochem Sci 28:479–487, 2003.

Rieke F, Baylor DA: Single photon detection by rod cells of the retina. Rev Mod Phys 70:1027–1036, 1998.

Saltiel AR, Kahn R: Insulin signalling and the regulation of glucose and lipid metabolism. Nature 414:799–806, 2001.

Shi Y, Massague J: Mechanisms of TGF-β signaling from cell membranes to the nucleus. Cell 113:685–700, 2003.

Shimizu TS, Aksenov AV, Bray D: A spatially extended stochastic model of the bacterial chemotaxis signalling pathway. J Molec Biol 329:291–309, 2003.

Stock AM, Robinson VL, Goudreau PN: Two-component signal transduction. Annu Rev Biochem 69:183–215, 2000.

ten Dijke P, Hill CS: New insights into TGF-Smad signalling. Trends Biochem Sci 29:265–273, 2004.

Wadhams GH, Armitage JP: Making sense of it all: Bacterial chemotaxis. Nat Rev Mol Cell Biol 5:1024–1037, 2004.

Whitehead JP, Clark SF, Urso B, James DE: Signalling through the insulin receptor. Curr Opin Cell Biol 12:222–228, 2000.

Wiley HS, Shvartsman SY, Lauffenburger DA: Computational modeling of the EGF-receptor system: A paradigm for systems biology. Trends Cell Biol 13:43–50, 2003.

Cellular Adhesion and the Extracellular Matrix

SECTION **VIII** OVERVIEW

This section covers the variety of extracellular matrices that provide mechanical support for the tissues of multicellular organisms. After their divergence about 1 billion years ago, animals and plants evolved completely different macromolecules to construct their extracellular matrices. The main biopolymer in animals is the protein collagen, whereas plants depend on the polysaccharide cellulose. Both can make impressively strong structures, including cartilage and bone in animals and the wood that supports giant trees. This section also explains the mechanisms that cells of all sorts use to adhere to each other and the objects in their environments, including the extracellular matrix. Cell surface adhesion proteins enable cells to establish intimate relationships with each other and macromolecules in the extracellular matrix. These interactions are essential for tissue integrity and intercellular communication in complex tissues, including the brain, heart, and other organs.

Chapter 28 describes the cells that are found in the **extracellular matrix** of animals. **Fibroblasts** synthesize and secrete the macromolecules that form the extracellular matrix. Fat cells store high-energy lipid molecules. Specialized **phagocytic cells** and immune system cells patrol the extracellular matrix of connective tissues, seeking to find and destroy foreign cells and molecules throughout the body.

Chapter 29 describes the biosynthesis of the macromolecules that form the extracellular matrices of animals. In connective tissue, fibroblasts secrete the protein subunits of **collagen fibrils** and **elastic fibers** as well as adhesion proteins and complex polysaccharides that reinforce the protein fibers in the extracellular matrix. The proportions of these macromolecules vary considerably. Tendons, ligaments, and some layers of the intestinal wall are composed largely of massive collagen fibrils with relatively few cells. The vitreous body of the eye is composed mostly of gelatinous polysaccharides with few fibers. The simplest type of extracellular matrix is the **basal lamina,** a thin layer of matrix that is secreted as rug beneath epithelial cells and a sheath around muscle cells, and neurons.

Remarkably, just four families of adhesion proteins, **IgCAMs, cadherins, integrins,** and **selectins,** account for much of cellular adhesion. Chapter 30 introduces these adhesion proteins and explains some of their diversity. IgCAMs and cadherins make specific interactions with complementary proteins on the surface of

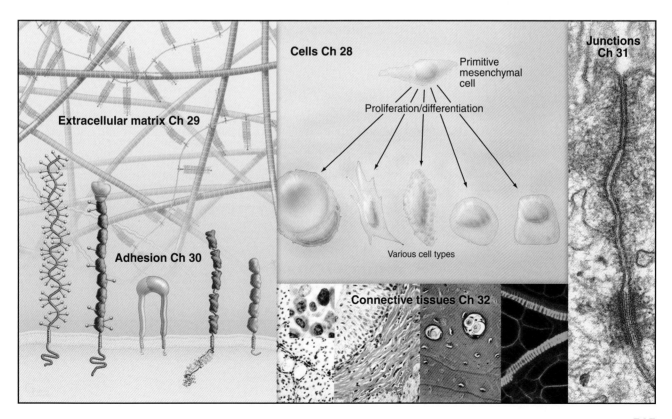

515

partner cells. Most integrins bind to extracellular matrix molecules, but some engage adhesion proteins on other cells. Selectins interact with glycoproteins called mucins on the surfaces of other cells. Expression of a limited repertoire of adhesion protein isoforms allows cells of multicellular organisms to establish specific interactions with appropriate partner cells while avoiding inappropriate interactions. The specificity provided by these adhesion molecules is required for the formation of epithelia during embryonic development, assembly of specialized connective tissues (Chapter 32), wound healing, and transmission of the force of muscle contraction to the extracellular matrix. Chapter 30 features two examples of dynamic, selective adhesion: adhesion of platelets to each other during the repair of damage to small blood vessels and blood clotting and adhesion of white blood cells to the endothelial cells lining blood vessels of inflamed tissues. Even unicellular organisms require molecular mechanisms so that they can adhere to other cells and objects that they encounter in their environments. For example, unicellular algae and yeast adhere to each other during mating, and slime mold amoebas adhere to each other as they develop into fruiting bodies.

Multicellular organisms use specialized intercellular junctions to interact with each other (Chapter 31). **Tight junctions** allow a sheet of epithelial cells to create semipermeable barriers between compartments such as the lumen and the wall of the intestine. Such barriers allow epithelia to concentrate materials on one side or the other. **Gap junctions** are composed of nonselective ion channels that connect the cytoplasms of two cells. These channels enable action potentials to spread directly from one cell to the next, as in the heart. Gap junction channels also allow solutes that are less than 1000 D in molecular weight to move between the coupled cells. Cadherins connect adjacent cells to the cytoskeleton at two types of adhesive junctions. The cadherins are anchored to cytoplasmic actin filaments at **adherens junctions** and to intermediate filaments at **desmosomes.**

The abundance, organization, and proportions of macromolecular components determine the mechanical properties of the extracellular matrix (Chapter 32). Plant cells secrete cellulose, a polymer of glucose units, and a mixture of other polysaccharides, glycoproteins, and organic molecules to make a delicate wall around each cell. These cell walls form materials ranging from soft cotton fibers to the wood that supports large trees. Connective tissues of animals also exhibit striking variety, owing to their particular mixtures of matrix molecules. Skin and blood vessels are resilient because of numerous elastic fibers. Tendons have great tensile strength, owing to the high density of collagen fibrils. Bone is incompressible and rigid because of its calcified collagen matrix. On the level of gross anatomy, cells and fibers form fascia, tendons, cartilage, and bones that support the organs of the body. Connective tissue also provides avenues for communication and supply within the body. Both the circulatory system and the peripheral nervous system run through connective tissue compartments of each organ. The vascular system transports phagocytic and immune system cells to sites where they are needed for defense.

CHAPTER 28

Cells of the Extracellular Matrix and Immune System

A remarkable variety of specialized cells populate the connective tissues of animals. These cells manufacture extracellular matrix, defend against infection, and maintain energy stores in the form of lipid (Fig. 28-1). Some of these cells arise in connective tissue and remain there. These **indigenous cells** are specialized: Fibroblasts make the collagen, elastic fibers, and proteoglycans of the extracellular matrix; chondrocytes secrete the matrix for cartilage; and osteoblasts manufacture the calcified matrix of bone. Fat cells store lipids, and mast cells secrete histamine and other mediators of inflammation. The remaining cells arise elsewhere, travel through blood and lymph, and enter connective tissue as needed, so they are known as **immigrant cells**. These visitors are part of the immune system, which defends against microorganisms. This chapter introduces all of these cells.

Indigenous Connective Tissue Cells

Primitive Mesenchymal Cells

Primitive mesenchymal cells are undifferentiated, multipotential stem cells (see Box 41-1) that proliferate and differentiate (Fig. 28-1) to give rise to all the indigenous cells of connective tissue (fibroblasts, fat cells, mast cells, chondrocytes, and osteoblasts). Small numbers of these inconspicuous precursor cells hide along the small blood vessels but cannot be identified by light microscopy. By electron microscopy (Fig. 28-2), mesenchymal cells resemble fibroblasts but with fewer organelles of the secretory pathway.

Fibroblasts

Fibroblasts are the connective tissue workhorses, synthesizing and secreting most of the macromolecules of the extracellular matrix (Fig. 28-2). Chapter 29 considers the synthesis of these matrix molecules in detail. Accordingly, mature fibroblasts have abundant rough endoplasmic reticulum and a large Golgi apparatus. They are generally spindle-shaped, with an oval, flattened nucleus, but can assume many other shapes depending on the mechanical forces in the surrounding matrix. The migratory patterns

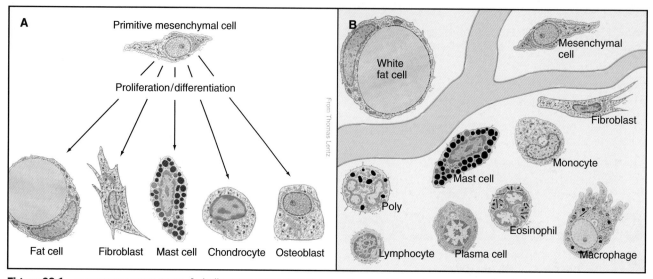

Figure 28-1 **CONNECTIVE TISSUE CELLS. A,** Indigenous connective tissue cells all originate from a stem cell called a primitive mesenchymal cell. **B,** Connective tissue near a small blood vessel showing indigenous cells in *pink* and immigrant cells in *green.* Poly, polymorphonuclear leukocyte.

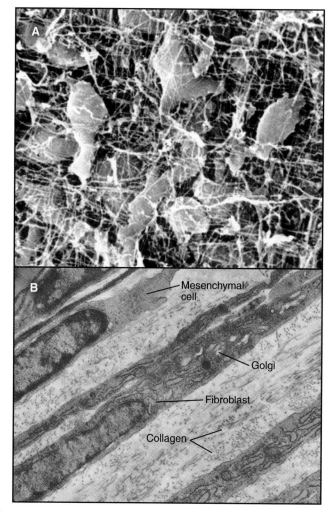

Figure 28-2 **FIBROBLASTS. A,** Scanning electron micrograph of fibroblasts migrating through collagen fibrils. **B,** Transmission electron micrograph of a thin section of a fibroblast illustrating the abundant organelles of the secretory pathway (endoplasmic reticulum and Golgi apparatus) and extracellular collagen fibrils. A primitive mesenchymal cell is shown in the *upper left.* (A, Courtesy of E. D. Hay, Harvard Medical School, Boston, Massachusetts. B, Courtesy of D. W. Fawcett, Harvard Medical School, Boston, Massachusetts.)

of the fibroblasts determine the patterns of collagen fibrils in tissues. In response to tissue damage, fibroblasts proliferate and migrate into the wound, where they synthesize new matrix to restore the integrity of the tissue (see Fig. 32-11).

Mast Cells

Mast cells are secretory cells that mediate "immediate hypersensitivity" reactions by secreting the contents of histamine-containing granules in response to insect bites or exposure to allergens, as in hay fever. Mast cells distribute along blood vessels in connective tissue (Fig. 28-3). The large, abundant **granules** contain, by mass, 30% heparin–basic protein complex, 10% **histamine,** and 35% basic proteins, including proteases. A variety of stimuli can induce secretion of the granule contents. The most specific stimulus operates through plasma membrane receptors for immunoglobulins of the **immunoglobulin E (IgE)** class. These receptors bind a random selection of soluble IgEs that the immune system makes in response to exposure to allergens. When the corresponding antigen binds to IgE on the surface of a mast cell, the receptors aggregate, triggering a cytoplasmic Ca^{2+} pulse (see Chapter 26) and fusion of granules with the plasma membrane (see Fig. 21-12). Mechanical trauma, radiant energy (heat, X-rays), and toxins or venoms are less specific stimuli but can also trigger secretion. Outside the cell, the carrier proteins release heparin and histamine. Histamine binds to cellular receptors, causing blood vessels to leak plasma, smooth muscle to contract, and itching sensations to occur. This results in the congestion and constriction of the respiratory tract in allergic reactions and swelling of the skin after an insect bite. Secreted fibrinolysin and heparin inhibit blood clotting. Stimulated mast cells also secrete tumor necrosis factor-α and eicosanoids, contributing to the activation of other inflammatory cells in chronic conditions including asthma and arthritis.

White Fat Cells

Fat cells **(adipocytes)** distributed in the connective tissue beneath the skin and in the abdominal mesentery of vertebrates store lipids as a readily accessible reserve of energy. These round cells vary in diameter depending on the size of their single, large, **lipid droplet** (Fig. 28-4) containing **triglycerides,** neutral lipids with a fatty acid esterified to all three carbons of glycerol (see Fig. 7-2 for the structures of glycerol and fatty acids). Intermediate filaments and endoplasmic reticulum separate the lipid droplet from the thin rim of cytoplasm. After a meal, fat cells take up fatty acids and glycerol from blood and synthesize triglycerides for storage. During fasting or when the body requires energy, enzymes called lipases hydrolyze fatty acids from triglycerides for release back into the blood for use by other organs. Hormones including epinephrine (see Fig. 27-3) regulate these metabolic reactions.

Fat cells also secrete a polypeptide hormone called **leptin** that binds receptors on neurons in the brain. These neurons respond by secreting other polypeptide hormones that regulate appetite. The congenital absence of leptin or defects in its receptor lead to massive obesity.

Mutations in four different genes cause inherited lipodystrophies, human conditions with loss of fat tissue. Loss of function of an enzyme required to synthesize triglycerides or a nuclear receptor that stimulates differentiation of fat cells make sense. It is less clear why mutations in the gene for nuclear lamins A and C (see Fig. 14-9) or a protease that processes lamin A should cause loss of fat.

Brown Fat Cells

Brown fat cells derive their color from numerous mitochondria, which they use to generate heat in response

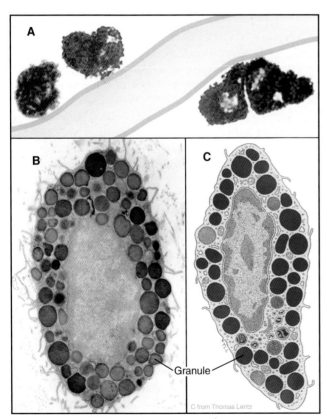

Figure 28-3 **MAST CELLS. A,** Light micrograph of loose connective tissue, stained with toluidine *blue,* illustrating mast cells scattered along a blood vessel (drawn in to enhance the contrast). Large mast cell granules stain intensely *purple* with basic thiazine dyes such as toluidine *blue.* **B,** Transmission electron micrograph of a thin section of a mast cell. **C,** Drawing of a mast cell. (A–B, Courtesy of D. W. Fawcett, Harvard Medical School, Boston, Massachusetts. C, Modified from T. Lentz, Yale Medical School, New Haven, Connecticut.)

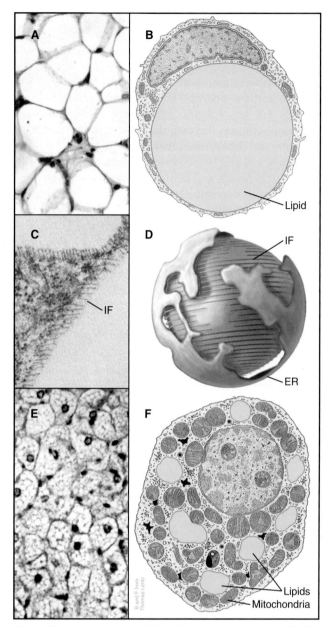

humans have more brown fat than do adults in order to generate heat during the adjustment to a new environment after birth. Hibernating animals use brown fat to raise their temperatures when emerging from hibernation.

Brown fat cells generate heat by short-circuiting the proton gradient that is usually used to generate adenosine triphosphate (ATP) in mitochondria (see Fig. 19-5). Sympathetic nerves acting through β-adrenergic receptors (see Fig. 27-3) and protein kinase A stimulate brown fat cells to express an "uncoupling protein" and to break down lipids to provide fatty acids for oxidation by mitochondria. Uncoupling protein inserts into the inner mitochondrial membrane and dissipates the proton electrochemical gradient across the inner membrane. Energy is lost as heat rather than being used to synthesize ATP. **Thermogenesis** may be an "energy buffer" that, when defective in animals, can contribute to obesity.

Origin and Development of Blood Cells

The blood of vertebrates contains a variety of cells, each with a specialized function (Fig. 28-5; Table 28-1). Red blood cells transport oxygen, platelets repair damage to blood vessels, and various types of white blood cells defend against infections. All blood cells derive ultimately from **pluripotential stem cells** (Fig. 28-5B; also see Box 41-1). After purification, these stem cells can restore the production of all blood cells in mice that have been irradiated to destroy their own blood cell precursors. Destruction of stem cells (e.g., by drugs such as chloramphenicol) leads to **aplastic anemia,** a condition in which few blood cells are produced, owing to a lack of precursors. These stem cells are also responsible for restoring blood cell production following human bone marrow transplantation.

Proliferation and differentiation of the progeny of pluripotential stem cells produce mature blood cells. At several stages in each line of cells, precursors undergo irreversible differentiation that commits them to a particular lineage. The first branch in the pathway of differentiation separates the precursors of lymphocytes from the precursors of the other blood cells called myeloid stem cells. Next, the myeloid stem cell differentiates into three different committed stem cells. One gives rise to red blood cells; another gives rise to megakaryocytes and platelets. Monocytes and the three types of granulocytes (neutrophils, eosinophils, and basophils) originate from a common committed stem cell in bone marrow and share a number of physiological features. Through differentiation, each also acquires unique functions. Platelets, red cells, granulocytes, and monocytes develop in bone marrow. Lymphocytes develop in

Figure 28-4 FAT CELLS. **A,** Light micrograph of a section of white fat cells stained with hematoxylin and eosin. **B,** Drawing of a white adipose cell. **C,** Transmission electron micrograph of a thin section of the edge of a lipid droplet showing the circumferential sheath of vimentin intermediate filaments (IF [see Chapter 35]). **D,** Interpretive drawing of a lipid droplet with its associated filaments and endoplasmic reticulum (ER). **E,** Light micrograph of a section of brown fat. **F,** Drawing of a brown fat cell. (A, C, and E, Courtesy of D. W. Fawcett, Harvard Medical School, Boston, Massachusetts. B and F, Modified from T. Lentz, Yale Medical School, New Haven, Connecticut. D, Modified from Werner Franke, University of Heidelberg, Germany.)

to cold or (in lean rodents) to excess food intake. Cytochromes make mitochondria brown. Fat is stored in multiple, small droplets (Fig. 28-4F). Brown fat is less abundant than white fat, being concentrated in connective tissue between the scapulae in mammals. Newborn

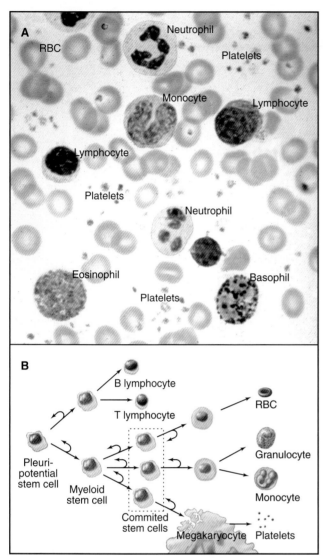

Figure 28-5 BLOOD CELLS. **A,** Light micrograph of a dried blood smear prepared with Wright's stain. **B,** Family tree of blood cells showing the developmental relationships of the various lineages. *Looping-back arrows* indicate renewal of the cell type. *Forward-oriented arrows* indicate differentiation and proliferation. RBC, red blood cell. (A, Courtesy of J.-P. Revel, California Institute of Technology, Pasadena.)

residue, marking it for ubiquitination and destruction (see Fig. 23-8), turning down the expression of erythropoietin. When kidney cells lack oxygen (owing to low levels of red blood cells, poor blood circulation in the kidney, or high altitude) HIF-1α/HIF-1β accumulates, and erythropoietin is expressed and secreted to stimulate red blood cell production by bone marrow. The reciprocal relationship between oxygen and erythropoietin that is achieved by this feedback mechanism sets red blood cell production at a level required to deliver oxygen to the tissues. Many other cells use the HIF-1α/HIF-1β system to adjust gene expression to local oxygen levels.

Mutations altering the growth control (see Fig. 41-10) of a stem cell can give rise to monoclonal proliferative disorders, such as **leukemia.** In chronic myelogenous leukemia, a chromosomal rearrangement in a single white blood cell precursor creates a fusion between the genes for BCR (breakpoint cluster region) and ABL (a Src family cytoplasmic tyrosine kinase; see Fig. 25-3 and Box 27-1). The BCR-ABL protein is constitutively active and drives the proliferation of a clone of immature white blood cells that crowd out and inhibit the production of other blood cells, leading to anemia and platelet deficiency. Affected individuals are prone to infection because the immature white blood cells are ineffective phagocytes. Fortunately, a small-molecule inhibitor of the kinase activity of BCR-ABL suppresses this clone in many patients. Uncontrolled proliferation of a clone of red blood cell precursors causes a similar condition, characterized by excess red cells, called **polycythemia vera.**

Cells Confined to the Blood

Erythrocytes (Red Blood Cells)

Red blood cells (Fig. 28-5; also see Fig. 7-6) contain more than 300 mg/mL of hemoglobin to carry oxygen from the lungs to tissues and carbon dioxide from tissues to the lungs. These highly specialized cells discard their nuclei and organelles late in their development. A resilient, spectrin-actin membrane cytoskeleton (see Fig. 7-10) maintains the biconcave shape even after the cell is heavily distorted each time it passes through a small capillary. The elasticity of the membrane skeleton allows it to regain its shape. After circulating in blood for 120 days, erythrocytes abruptly become senescent, and phagocytes in the spleen, liver, and bone marrow remove them from the blood. The biochemical basis of this precise cellular aging and clearance process is still being investigated.

In **hereditary spherocytosis** (and other hemolytic anemias), the membrane cytoskeleton loses its resiliency as a result of mutations, causing deficiencies or

bone marrow as well as in lymphoid tissues (thymus, spleen, and lymph nodes).

Minute quantities of specific glycoprotein **growth factors** control the balance between self-renewal and proliferation at each stage of development, starting with pluripotential stem cells. Feedback mechanisms control production of these growth factors. For example, the oxygen level in the kidney controls the synthesis of **erythropoietin,** the growth factor for the red blood cell series. (See Fig. 27-9 for the erythropoietin signaling pathway.) A dimeric transcription factor called HIF-1α/HIF-1β regulates the expression of erythropoietin. When oxygen is abundant, HIF-1α is hydroxylated on a proline

Table 28-1

BLOOD CELLS (AS SEEN ON A STAINED SMEAR OF BLOOD)

Type	Concentration	Features
Platelets	300,000/µL	Anucleate; 2–3 µm wide; purple granules
Erythrocytes	~5 × 10^6/µL	7-µm; diameter biconcave disks; no nucleus; pink cytoplasm
Neutrophils	~60% of total WBCs	10–12 µm wide; multilobed nucleus; many unstained granules; few azurophilic granules
Eosinophils	~2% of total WBCs	Bilobed nucleus; numerous, large, refractile, pink-stained granules; ~12 µm wide
Basophils	~0.5% of total WBCs	Lobed nucleus; large, blue-stained granules; ~10 µm wide
Lymphocytes	~30% of total WBCs	Small, round, intensely stained nucleus; some small azurophilic granules; variable amount of clear blue cytoplasm, so they may be classified as either small (~7–8 µm wide), medium, or large
Monocytes	~5% of total WBCs	Up to 17 µm wide; large, indented nucleus and gray-blue cytoplasm with a few azurophilic granules

WBCs, white blood cells.

molecular defects of spectrin or other component proteins. These defective cells are easily damaged and eventually become smaller and rounder than normal. Many different mutations of the globin genes decrease the stability or oxygen-carrying capacity of hemoglobin. In **sickle-cell disease,** hemoglobin S is prone to assemble into tubular polymers that distort the cell and clog up the circulation.

Platelets

Platelets, small anucleate cellular fragments derived from megakaryocytes, contribute to both blood clotting and the repair of minor defects in the sheet of endothelial cells that lines blood vessels. A long, coiled microtubule presses out against the plasma membrane, like a spring, to maintain the platelet's disk shape (Fig. 28-6). The most prominent organelles are two types of membrane-bound granules. Dense granules contain adenosine diphosphate (ADP) and serotonin. Alpha granules contain stores of adhesive glycoproteins including fibrinogen, fibronectin (see Fig. 29-15) and thrombospondin as well as the potent protein hormone called **platelet-derived growth factor.** Platelet-derived growth factor has a role in wound healing (see Fig. 32-11) but also contributes to atherosclerosis by stimulating the

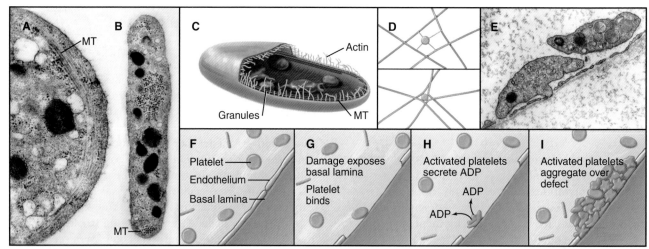

Figure 28-6 **PLATELETS AND THEIR ROLE IN HEMOSTASIS. A–B,** Transmission electron micrographs of thin sections of platelets. **C,** Interpretive drawing showing the circumferential band of microtubules (MT), actin filaments in the cortex, and granules in the cytoplasm. **D,** Role of platelets in blood clot retraction. Filopodia grasp strands of fibrin in a blood clot *(upper panel)* and pull them together *(lower panel).* **E,** Electron micrograph of a thin section showing platelets adhering to the basal lamina through a small defect in the endothelium and to a second platelet in the lumen. **F–I,** Stages in the repair of a defect in the endothelial lining of a blood vessel. **F,** Circulating platelets do not bind to normal endothelial cells. **G,** Damage to the endothelium exposes the basal lamina, and a platelet binds to the collagen. **H,** Collagen activates the platelet to secrete ADP, which activates passing platelets. **I,** Activated platelets bind together, covering the defect in the endothelium. (A–B, Courtesy of O. Behnke, University of Copenhagen, Denmark.)

abnormal proliferation of smooth muscle cells in the walls of damaged arteries.

Platelets that contain a full complement of organelles bud from the tips of protrusions on the surface precursor cells—giant polyploid **megakaryocytes** in the bone marrow. **Thrombopoietin,** a protein hormone related to erythropoietin, is the major factor controlling platelet production. Liver and kidney cells secrete thrombopoietin at a constant rate. Receptors on circulating platelets bind part of the thrombopoietin. Consequently, the blood concentration of thrombopoietin available to stimulate megakaryocyte maturation and platelet formation is inversely related to the total number of platelets. This feedback loop stimulates platelet production if the platelet supply is low.

Like red blood cells, platelets are confined to the blood. Two pools of platelets freely exchange with each other: About two thirds of the total platelets circulate, whereas one third of the platelets are stored in the blood vessels of the spleen. The stored pool may increase when the spleen is enlarged, decreasing the platelet count in the blood.

Platelets control bleeding in three ways. First, they adhere and change shape to cover damaged vascular surfaces. Second, platelets stimulate **blood clotting.** Activated platelets express a specialized surface protein, which stimulates a cascade of proteolytic reactions that culminate in the cleavage of plasma fibrinogen to form fibrin, which polymerizes to clot blood. The fibrin gel stops the flow of blood from damaged blood vessels. Third, platelets also bind to fibrin strands forming the clot and cause the clot to contract. This may help to close the defect in a damaged blood vessel.

Platelets repair defects in the endothelial cell lining of blood vessels that are produced by the mild trauma of daily existence. Platelets bind to von Willebrand factor and collagen in the basal lamina when it is exposed by damage to the endothelium. This triggers one of the best-understood examples of regulated cellular adhesion (for more detail, see Fig. 30-14). Activated platelets aggregate, extend actin-containing filopodia, and secrete the contents of their granules. The secreted ADP sets up a positive feedback loop, activating more platelets that form a cluster to fill the defect in the endothelium. Patients with defective platelets or reduced circulating platelets (a complication of bone marrow disease and cancer chemotherapy) bruise easily, owing to unrepaired damage in small blood vessels, and may even bleed spontaneously. Conversely, hyperactive platelets may initiate pathological clots in the blood vessels of the heart, causing heart attacks or thrombosis in the veins of the legs.

Human platelets circulate in the blood for about seven days. During this time, some are utilized to repair vascular defects, while phagocytic cells in the liver and spleen remove others. Exposure of platelets to temperatures below 37°C promotes aggregation of a major plasma membrane glycoprotein called GPIb$_\alpha$, a component of the von Willebrand factor receptor, priming chilled platelets to be recognized and removed by liver phagocytes. This has presented a problem for blood banks that store platelets for transfusing into patients who are deficient in platelets, but this rapid clearance of chilled platelets can be overcome by glycosylation of GPIb$_\alpha$.

Cells Responsible for Innate and Adaptive Immunity

All multicellular animals use two forms of **innate immunity** to defend themselves against infection by microorganisms. Phagocytic cells similar to unicellular amoebas track down, ingest, and kill bacteria and fungi (see Fig. 22-3). The main mammalian phagocytes are macrophages and neutrophils. A second line of defense is secretion of cytokines and small antimicrobial proteins by white blood cells and epithelial cells of the skin and intestine. These cells are alerted to the presence of microorganism by "pattern recognition receptors," the best known of which are Toll-like receptors (see Fig. 24-12). These receptors bind macromolecular products that are essential for the microorganisms, such as bacterial flagella and viral single-stranded RNA. Toll-like receptors regulate gene expression through transcription factors, including NF-κB. Secreted tumor necrosis factor and other cytokines attract cells of the innate immune system (see Fig. 26-11). Antimicrobial peptides such as defensins and cathelicidins not only kill pathogens by interacting with their membranes but also attract and activate cells of both the innate and the adaptive immune systems. These elements of the innate immune system are programmed genetically, so they respond without prior exposure to the pathogen. In spite of their generic nature, these innate responses work remarkably well, defending all metazoans against infection. In addition to phagocytes, mammals have special lymphocytes called **natural killer cells** that express a variety of receptors to detect infected cells.

Later during evolution, starting with cartilaginous fish, our ancestors developed a more sophisticated **adaptive immune system.** The response is slower than innate immunity, because it depends on the selection and multiplication of lymphocytes that produce soluble antibodies or cell surface receptors precisely targeted to foreign molecules. This response depends on rearrangement and mutation of genes to produce highly selective antibodies and receptor proteins. Although this adaptive response takes about a week to mobilize, it has the advantage that some of the specialized lymphocytes survive for years, providing the host with a faster adaptive response if the host is exposed to the pathogen a second time.

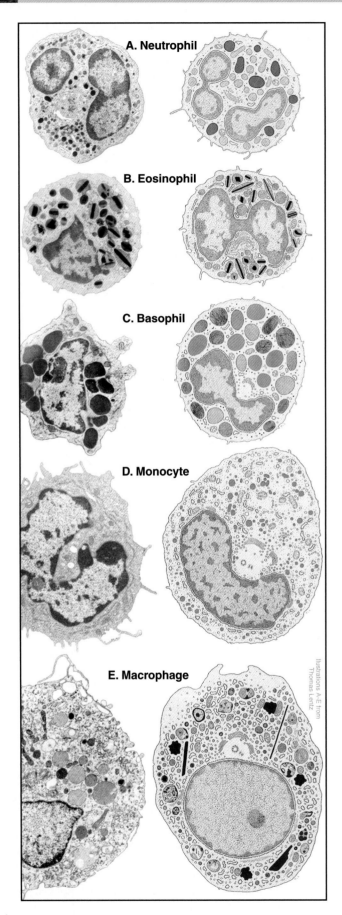

A. Neutrophil

B. Eosinophil

C. Basophil

D. Monocyte

E. Macrophage

Illustrations A-E from Thomas Lentz

Cellular Basis of Innate Immunity

The phagocytes in the blood and tissues originate in bone marrow from a common committed stem cell (Fig. 28-5) and acquire unique functions as they differentiate. All of these motile cells are attracted to sites of infection or inflammation by (in humans) a family of about 40 small proteins called **chemokines.** Tissue cells and leukocytes secrete chemokines at sites of infection or inflammation. Chemokines with many unrelated names (IL-8, RANTES, eotaxin, MCP-1, etc.) have similar structures and bind to a family of 14 different **chemokine receptors** expressed selectively by lymphocytes, monocytes, and granulocytes. These seven-helix receptors are coupled to trimeric G-proteins (see Fig. 24-3) that mediate chemotaxis (see Fig. 38-12) toward the source of the chemokine.

Neutrophils

Neutrophils, also known as polymorphonuclear leukocytes or "polys," are the main phagocytes circulating in blood on their way to connective tissues. They are distinguished by a multilobed nucleus and two types of granules (Fig. 28-7). The more abundant specific granules contain lysozyme (an enzyme that digests bacterial cell walls) and alkaline phosphatase. These granules do not stain with either the basic or acidic dyes used for blood smears, so these cells are called neutrophils. Azurophilic granules are true lysosomes containing hydrolytic enzymes bound to acidic proteoglycans (see Fig. 21-17). Neutrophils have copious glycogen but few mitochondria, so they rely on glycolysis for ATP synthesis in poorly oxygenated wounds. They are among the most motile cells in the body.

Human bone marrow produces about 80 g of neutrophils each day. In response to infection or injury, a circulating factor releases neutrophils from the bone marrow into the blood. Neutrophils spend about 10 hours in blood, alternating between a circulating pool and a so-called marginated pool adherent to endothelial cells, chiefly in the lung. Exercise and epinephrine release marginated neutrophils into the circulating

Figure 28-7 WHITE BLOOD CELLS. Transmission electron micrographs of thin sections of each cell and interpretive drawings with lysosomes shown in *brown*. **A,** A neutrophil showing the multilobed nucleus (the connections between lobes are in other sections) and the two classes of granules. **B,** An eosinophil showing the bilobed nucleus and the large, specific granules containing a darkly stained crystalloid. **C,** Basophil with large specific granules colored *blue*. **D,** Blood monocyte. **E,** Macrophage grown in tissue culture. (Micrographs courtesy of D. W. Fawcett, Harvard Medical School, Boston, Massachusetts. Drawings modified from T. Lentz, Yale Medical School, New Haven, Connecticut.)

pool; smoking increases the marginated pool. Neutrophils leave the blood by receptor-mediated attachment to endothelial cells and then crawl between endothelial cells into the connective tissue (see Fig. 30-13), where they perish after a day or two of phagocytosis.

Neutrophils are humans' first line of defense against bacterial infection, as they are highly specialized for finding and destroying bacteria. Provided that the concentration of neutrophils is high enough (about 10 million cells per milliliter), these motile phagocytes can find and destroy bacteria faster than the invaders can reproduce. Bacterial products, especially *N*-formylated peptides, attract neutrophils by binding plasma membrane receptors and stimulating locomotion, similar to chemotaxis by other cells (see Fig. 38-12). Neutrophils bind and ingest bacteria by phagocytosis (see Fig. 22-3). Both types of granules fuse with phagosomes, delivering antibacterial proteins and proteolytic enzymes that kill the ingested bacteria. Some granules fuse with the plasma membrane, releasing antibacterial proteins outside the cell. Phagosome membranes produce millimolar concentrations of superoxide (O_2^-) radicals and other reactive oxygen species that help to disperse the granule enzymes and contribute to killing bacteria. These toxic oxygen species may also cause collateral damage to the neutrophil. Genetic defects in the enzymes that produce superoxide cause chronic granulomatous disease, a serious human disease, because neutrophils cannot kill ingested bacteria and fungi.

Monocytes and Macrophages

Monocytes in the blood are precursors of tissue macrophages. Monocytes are large cells with an indented nucleus and a small number of azurophilic granules (Figs. 28-5 and 28-7D). After circulating in the blood for about three days, monocytes enter tissues and differentiate into macrophages under the influence of local growth factors, including lymphokines secreted by lymphocytes (Fig. 28-8). They enlarge and amplify their machinery for locomotion, phagocytosis, and killing microorganisms and tumor cells.

Macrophages are professional phagocytes, which generally follow neutrophils to wounds or infections to clean up debris, including cellular debris and foreign material. Plasma membrane receptors for antibodies allow macrophages to recognize foreign matter marked with antibodies and to facilitate its ingestion. Primary lysosomes fuse with phagosomes to degrade the contents. Eventually, the cytoplasm fills with residual bodies containing the remains of ingested material (see Fig. 23-3). These "professional phagocytes" may divide and survive for months in tissues, where they ingest foreign material, participate in immune responses, and secrete growth factors that influence other cells. When con-

fronted with large foreign bodies, macrophages can fuse together to form **giant cells.** No challenge is too great. Giant multinucleated microphages will even try to ingest a Petri dish if it is coated with antibody. Local growth factors in bone stimulate monocytes to fuse and differentiate into multinucleated **osteoclasts** that degrade bone matrix during bone remodeling (see Fig. 32-6).

Macrophages participate in the immune response by degrading ingested protein antigens and presenting fragments on their surface bound to MHC class II proteins (Fig. 28-8). This complex activates helper T lymphocytes carrying the appropriate T-cell receptors (see Fig. 27-8). Activated T cells proliferate and secrete growth factors that stimulate B lymphocytes to produce antibody. Macrophages also secrete a variety of factors involved with host defense and inflammation. Interleukin-1, transforming growth factor-α, transforming growth factor-β, and platelet-derived growth factor stimulate the proliferation and differentiation of the cells required to heal wounds (see Fig. 32-11). Chemokines attract cells of the immune system to sites of inflammation.

Eosinophils

Eosinophils are identified in blood smears as cells with a bilobed nucleus and large specific granules that stain brightly with eosin (Fig. 28-7B). Specific granules contain a cationic protein, a ribonuclease and peroxidase, in addition to a crystalloid of a basic protein. Like neutrophils, eosinophils pass briefly through the blood on their way to connective tissue, where they survive for about two weeks. Chemotactic factors generated by the complement system, basophils, some tumors, parasites, and bacteria all attract eosinophils. Many of the same factors attract other leukocytes, but particular chemokines are specialized for eosinophils. Eosinophils accumulate in blood and tissues in response to parasitic infections. Eosinophils bind parasites and lyse them, like killer lymphocytes (see later discussion), by secreting a cationic protein that forms pores in their membrane. Production of superoxide, hydrogen peroxide, and antimicrobial peptides also contributes to killing. Activated eosinophils contribute to inflammation in some allergic disorders such as asthma.

Basophils

Basophils are the least abundant and least understood granulocytes. They look much like neutrophils but have a bilobed nucleus and large, basophilic, specific granules containing heparin, serotonin, and all of the blood histamine (Fig. 28-7C). Basophils are weak phagocytes. Like mast cells, they have cell surface receptors that bind IgE and release the vasoactive agents stored in

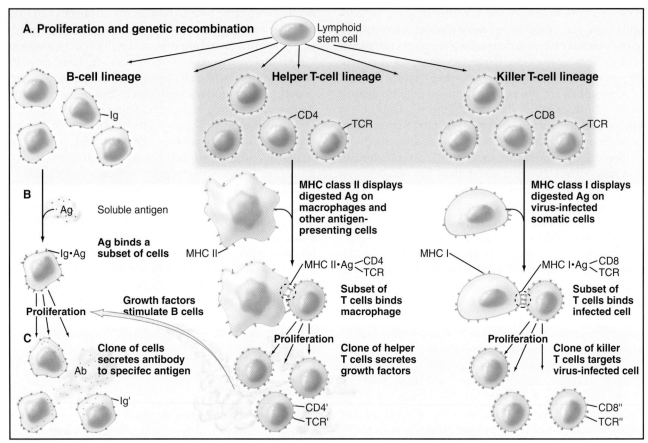

Figure 28-8   THE IMMUNE RESPONSE BY THREE CLASSES OF LYMPHOCYTES THROUGH THREE PARALLEL STEPS. **A,** Genetic recombination produces populations of cells with a wide variety of antigen specificities provided by cell surface immunoglobulins (Ig) or T-cell receptors (TCR). **B,** The binding of specific antigens (Ag) to surface immunoglobulins or T-cell receptors selects a subset of the cells. **C,** Proliferation of clones of the selected cells yields many cells specialized to produce antibody (Ab) to soluble antigens, secretion of growth factors by helper T cells in response to ingested and degraded antigens, or killing of virus-infected cells identifiable by the viral peptides on their surface. The helper and killer T cells use a common set of T-cell receptors and are guided to the appropriate target cells by the CD4 and CD8 accessory molecules. See Figures 27-8 and 46-8 for details on T-lymphocyte activation and selection, respectively.

their granules when antigens bind to these bound immunoglobulins.

Basophils and mast cells have much in common, but they appear to have different origins. Basophils arise from bone marrow stem cells, whereas mast cells are derived from connective tissue mesenchymal cells. Humans have both circulating basophils and tissue mast cells, but this is not universal. Mice have mast cells but no basophils. Turtles have basophils but no mast cells.

Cellular Basis of Adaptive Immunity

In response to infection, lymphocytes of the immune systems of vertebrates produce two kinds of adaptive responses: humoral (in the body fluids) and cellular. **B lymphocytes** produce the humoral response by secreting **antibodies (immunoglobulins),** soluble proteins that diffuse in the blood and tissue fluids. Two types of T lymphocytes mediate the cellular arm of the adaptive immune response. **Cytotoxic T lymphocytes**

(killer T cells) destroy cells infected with viruses, whereas **helper T cells** regulate other lymphocytes. These responses protect against infection but fail in acquired immunodeficiency syndrome (AIDS) when the human immunodeficiency virus (HIV) kills helper T cells. A blood smear reveals lymphocytes of various sizes and shapes (Fig. 28-5) but not their remarkable heterogeneity at the molecular level (Fig. 28-8).

Antibodies produced by B cells provide a chemical defense against viruses, bacteria, fungi, and toxins. Antibodies, or immunoglobulins, are an incredibly diverse family of proteins, each with a binding site that accommodates one of millions of different ligands termed **antigens.** Antigens include proteins, polysaccharides, nucleic acids, lipids, and small organic molecules produced biologically or chemically. Antibody binding can mark an antigen for phagocytosis or neutralize its toxicity.

The huge repertoire of antigen-binding sites present in the collection of antibodies that circulate in a single individual arises through **rearrangement** and **somatic**

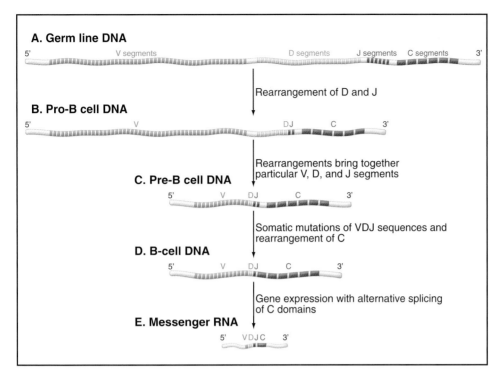

A. Germ line DNA

5'   V segments   D segments   J segments   C segments   3'

Rearrangement of D and J

B. Pro-B cell DNA

5'   V   DJ   C   3'

Rearrangements bring together
particular V, D, and J segments

C. Pre-B cell DNA

5'   V   DJ   C   3'

Somatic mutations of VDJ sequences and
rearrangement of C

D. B-cell DNA

5'   V   DJ   C   3'

Gene expression with alternative splicing
of C domains

E. Messenger RNA

5'   VDJC   3'

Figure 28-9 ASSEMBLY OF IMMU-
NOGLOBULIN GENES BY REARRANGE-
MENT OF GENE SEGMENTS. **A,** Region
of germ line DNA with multiple,
tandem V, D, J, and C segments
for assembling an immunoglobulin heavy chain, **B,** Same region
after rearrangement of D and J
segments in a Pro-B cell. **C,** After
rearrangement of V in a Pre-B
cell. **D,** B-cell. **E,** Immunoglobulin
mRNA produced by a B-cell.
(Based on a drawing in Chiorazzi
N, Rai KR, Ferrarini M: Chronic
lymphocytic leukemia. New Engl J
Med 352:804–815, 2005.)

mutations of immunoglobulin genes (Fig. 28-9). This remarkable process was exploited during evolution specifically for the use of the immune system. Each mammalian immunoglobulin is composed of four polypeptide chains—two identical heavy chains and two identical light chains—each encoded by different genes (see Fig. 3-13). Light chains and heavy chains both contribute to the antigen-binding site. In vertebrate genomes, immunoglobulin genes exist in segments aligned along a chromosome. Several of these gene segments must be combined in the proper order to make a full-length functional antibody gene. Some of these gene segments encode the framework of the antibody protein, which is essentially identical within each class of antibodies. Other gene segments, present in many variations, encode the part of the polypeptide chain that forms the antigen-binding site.

During maturation of a particular B cell, **recombination enzymes** (RAG1 and RAG2) assemble immunoglobulin gene segments into one unique full-length gene for a heavy chain and one for a light chain. As a result of random gene arrangements, each B cell assembles and expresses novel immunoglobulin genes. The process is precise in that the right number of segments is always chosen to make a heavy chain or a light chain, but it is also random in that any one of the variable segments may be chosen. The resulting antibody contains two identical but unique antigen-binding sites. The gene segments can be assembled in many different combinations, and most heavy chains can assemble with most light chains. The diversity arising from the combinato-

rial process is expanded further in two ways. First, the recombination process inserts a variable number of nucleotides between the gene segments. Second, pre-B cells use enzymes to mutate codons for amino acids in the antigen-binding site, creating variations in the antigen-binding specificity in different cells. In principle, about 3000 different light chains and 60,000 heavy chains can combine to produce about 100 million different antibodies even without taking mutations into account. Accordingly, it is possible experimentally to induce a mouse to make an antibody that is specific for almost any naturally occurring or synthetic chemical.

Infection by a pathogen results in the production of antibodies that bind to the pathogen but not to any of the individual's own molecules. This response comes from activation and proliferation of preexisting B cells that have the capacity to make antibodies to molecules of the pathogen. Activation requires a chance encounter of particular B cells with the pathogen and stimulates the cell to mature into a factory for secreting antibodies. Alternate splicing of messenger RNA (mRNA [see Fig. 16-6]) selects domains required to direct the same antibody to either the plasma membrane or the secretory pathway.

Cells that are activated by antigen binding to a surface immunoglobulin divide to increase their numbers. This process, called **clonal expansion,** amplifies the production of antibody specific for the antigen. The mature cellular product of the B-cell response is a **plasma cell,** which is highly specialized to secrete one specific antibody. Other B cells that are activated by the antigen become **memory cells.** These long-lived cells display the specific antibody on their surface and stand poised to mount an amplified response on subsequent exposure to the same antigen. This immunologic memory explains why exposure to a particular pathogen or vaccination against a pathogen results in protection, in the form of antibodies, for many years.

Specialized B lymphocytes and plasma cells secrete different antibody isoforms or isotypes. Formation of immunoglobulins with the various isotypes requires further recombination events to join the variable region with the antigen-binding site to the isotype constant domain. **IgG** isotypes, produced in lymph nodes and spleen, circulate in blood and tissue fluids. **IgA** isotypes, produced by lymphoid nodules in the respiratory and gastrointestinal tracts and by mammary glands, are first taken up and then secreted by epithelial cells of these organs (transcytosis [see Fig. 22-6]). **IgE** isotypes bind to receptors on the surface of mast cells and basophils (see earlier discussion).

T lymphocytes provide cellular responses to pathogens. Cytotoxic T cells execute tumor cells and virus-infected cells. Helper T cells stimulate antibody production by B cells. The specificity of these responses is provided by variable cell surface receptors called **T-cell receptors** (see Fig. 27-8). A set of segmented genes analogous to immunoglobulin genes encode T-cell receptors. In contrast to antibodies, T-cell receptors do not bind free antigens but rather recognize peptide antigens displayed on the surface of target cells complexed to proteins called **major histocompatibility complex (MHC)** antigens (see Fig. 27-8). These highly variable MHC proteins are responsible for the rejection of tissue grafts from nonidentical individuals.

The two types of MHC proteins—class I and class II—acquire their antigenic peptides differently. All somatic cells produce class I MHC proteins. In cells that have been infected by a virus, cytoplasmic immunoproteasomes degrade some viral proteins to peptides (see Chapter 23), which ABC transporters (TAP1, 2) move from the cytoplasm (see Fig. 8-9) into the endoplasmic reticulum. In the lumen of the ER, peptides insert into the binding site of compatible class I molecules and the complex moves to the plasma membrane. In contrast, macrophages and other **antigen-presenting cells,** such as **dendritic cells,** ingest foreign matter and degrade it in endosomes and lysosomes. Peptide fragments bind to class II proteins in endosomes and thence move to the cell surface of these antigen-presenting cells.

T lymphocytes patrol the body, inspecting the surfaces of other cells. A chance encounter with a cell displaying a peptide-MHC complex complementary to its T-cell receptor stimulates the T cell (see Fig. 27-8). The response is proliferation and expansion of a clone of identical T cells. Accessory membrane proteins CD4 and CD8 on the T-cell surface cooperate with T-cell recep-

tors to direct the two types of T cells to target cells with the appropriate MHC proteins. T-cell receptors provide antigen specificity. Immature T-cells express both CD4 and CD8 but lose one of them as they mature into cytotoxic (CD8$^+$) or helper (CD4$^+$) T cells.

CD8-positive cytotoxic T cells are specialized to kill cells infected with viruses. The presence of virus inside is revealed by MHC class I proteins displaying vital peptides on the surface of the infected cell. CD8 binds to a constant region of MHC class I proteins carrying viral peptides. During its intimate encounters with the target cell, a cytotoxic T cell uses three weapons to kill the target: First, T cells carry a ligand for the Fas receptor on the target, which stimulates apoptosis of the target cell (see Fig. 46-17). Second, activated T cells secrete **perforin,** a protein that inserts into the plasma membrane of the target cell, forming large (10 nm) pores that leak cytoplasmic contents and ultimately lyse the cell. Third, T cells secrete toxic enzymes that enter target cells through the plasma membrane pores.

CD4 binds a constant part of the MHC class II protein and targets helper T cells to cells presenting ingested antigens. The progeny of stimulated helper T cells secrete growth factors (lymphokines or interleukins) in the vicinity of B cells with the foreign antigen bound to immunoglobulins on their surface. Helper T cells are required for B cells to make antibodies against most antigens. This explains how **HIV** causes AIDS. The virus uses CD4 as a receptor to infect and eventually kill helper T cells. Loss of helper T cells severely limits the capacity of B cells and cytotoxic T cells (which also require T-cell help) to mount antibody and cellular responses to microorganisms. Infections that the immune system normally dispatches with ease then become life-threatening.

Genetic defects cause a wide variety of **immunodeficiency diseases.** For example, defects in Bruton tyrosine kinase result in failure to produce B cells. Remarkably, humans who lack function of the enzyme adenosine deaminase have no B cells or T cells but are otherwise normal. Deficiencies of many specialized lymphocyte proteins (cytokine receptors, interleukin receptors, Lck tyrosine kinase, ZAP-70 tyrosine kinase, RAG1 or RAG2, TAP1 or TAP2) also lead to immunodeficiencies.

ACKNOWLEDGMENTS

Thanks go to John Hartwig and Sam Silverstein for their suggestions on revisions to this chapter.

SELECTED READINGS

Beutler B: Inferences, questions and possibilities in Toll-like receptor signalling. Nature 430:257–263, 2004.

Boes M, Ploegh HL: Translating cell biology in vitro into immunity in vivo. Nature 430:264–270, 2004.

Buckley RH: Primary immunodeficiency diseases due to defects in lymphocytes. New Engl J Med 343:1313-1324, 2000.

Call ME, Wucherpfennig KW: The T cell receptor: Critical role of the membrane environment in receptor assembly and function. Annu Rev Immunol 23:101-125, 2005.

Cannon B, Nedergaard J: Brown adipose tissue: Function and physiological significance. Physiol Rev 84:277-359, 2004.

Delves PJ, Roitt IM: The immune system. New Engl J Med 343:37-49, 108-117, 2000.

Galli SJ, Kalesnikoff J, Grimbaldeston MA,et al: Mast cells as "tunable" effector and immunoregulatory cells. Annu Rev Immunol 23:749-786, 2005.

Garg A: Acquired and inherited lipodystrophies. New Engl J Med 350:1120-1134, 2004.

Grinnell F: Fibroblast biology in three-dimensional collagen matrices. Trends Cell Biol 13:264-269, 2003.

Hargreaves DC, Medzhitov R: Innate sensors of microbial infection. J Clin Immunol 25:503-510, 2005.

Hartwig J, Italiano J Jr: The birth of the platelet. J Thromb Haemost 1:1580-1586, 2003.

Janeway CA Jr., Medzhitov R: Innate immune recognition. Annu Rev Immunol 20:197-216, 2002.

Kaufmann SHE: Cell-mediated immunity: Dealing a blow to pathogens. Curr Biol 9:R97-R99, 1999.

Kaushansky K: Thrombopoietin. N Engl J Med 339:746-754, 1998.

Klein J, Sato A: The HLA system. New Engl J Med 343:702-709, 782-786, 2000.

Lanzavecchia A, Sallusto F: Dynamics of T lymphocyte responses: Intermediates, effectors and memory cells. Science 290:92-97, 2000.

Lekstrom-Himes JA, Gallin JI: Immunodeficiency diseases caused by defects in phagocytes. New Engl J Med 343:1703-1714, 2000.

Marx J: How cells endure low oxygen. Science 303:1454-1456, 2004.

Rot A, von Adrian UH: Chemokines in innate and adaptive host defense: Basic chemokinese grammar for immune cells. Annu Rev Immunol 22:891-928 , 2004.

Segal AW: How neutrophils kill microbes. Annu Rev Immunol 23:197-223, 2005.

Takeda K, Kaisho T, Akira S: Toll-like receptors. Annu Rev Immunol 21:335-376, 2003.

Trombetta ES, Mellman I: Cell biology of antigen processing in vitro and in vivo. Annu Rev Immunol 23:975-1028, 2005.

van Andrian UH, Mackay CR: T-cell function and migration. New Engl J Med 343:1020-1034, 2000.

Verfaillie CM: Adult stem cells: Assessing the case for pluripotency. Trends Cell Biol 12:502-508, 2002.

Yang D, Biragyn A, Hoover DM, et al: Multiple roles of antimicrobial defensins, cathelicidins, and eosinophil-derived neurotoxin in host defense. Annu Rev Immunol 22:181-215, 2004.

Yokoyama WM, Kim S, French AR: The dynamic life of natural killer cells. Annu Rev Immunol 22:405-429, 2004.

CHAPTER 29

Extracellular Matrix Molecules

Although the extracellular matrix is composed of only five classes of macromolecules—collagens, elastin, proteoglycans, hyaluronan, and adhesive glycoproteins—it can take on a rich variety of different forms with vastly different mechanical properties. This is possible for two reasons. First, each of these classes of macromolecule comes in a number of variants (encoded by different genes or produced by alternative splicing), each with distinctive properties. Second, the cells that constitute the extracellular matrix are versatile with respect to secreting different proportions of these isoforms in different geometrical arrangements. As a result, the extracellular matrix in different tissues is adapted to particular functional requirements, which vary as widely as tendons, blood vessel walls, cartilage, bone, the vitreous body of the eye, and subcutaneous fat. Beyond providing mechanical support, the extracellular matrix also strongly influences embryonic development, provides pathways for cellular migration, provides essential survival signals, and sequesters important growth factors. This chapter introduces the macromolecules of the extracellular matrix.

Collagen

The collagen family is the most abundant class of proteins in the human body. It is also one of the most versatile. Collagens form a wide range of different structures with remarkable mechanical properties. Weight for weight, fibrous collagens are as strong as steel. Their name, which comes from the Greek words for "glue" and "birth," reflects the long-known adhesive properties of denatured collagen extracted from animal tissues.

The defining feature of collagens is a rod-shaped domain composed of a **triple helix** of polypeptides (Fig. 29-1). Each polypeptide folds into a left-handed helix that repeats every third residue with the side chains on the outside. Three of these helices associate to form a triple helix that may be up to 420 nm long. The triple helical domains have a repeating amino acid sequence: glycine-X-Y, where X is most often proline and Y is most often hydroxyproline. The small glycine residues allow tight contact between the polypeptides in the core of the triple helix. Larger residues, even alanine, interfere with packing. Poly-L-proline has a strong tendency to form a left-handed helix like individual collagen chains but does not form a triple helix, owing to steric interference. The triple helix is most stable if all X residues are proline and all Y residues are hydroxyproline, but

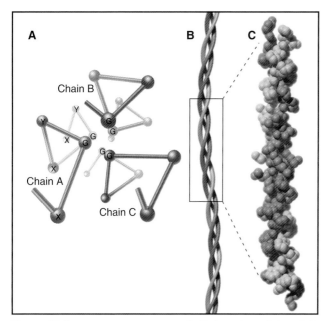

Figure 29-1   COLLAGEN TRIPLE HELIX. **A,** End-on view of three left-handed polyproline type II helices with glycines (G) in the core. **B,** Longitudinal view of the strands of a triple helix. **C,** Space-filling model of the structure of a short collagen triple helix. (A, Redrawn from van der Rest M, Garrone A: Collagen family of proteins. FASEB J 5:2814–2823, 1991. C, PDB file: 1BKV.)

other residues at some of these positions are essential for collagen to assemble higher-order structures. (Despite their name, α-chains, the collagen polypeptides do not form α-helices.)

The collagen family is remarkably diverse. Humans have about 100 genes with collagen triple repeats, and more than 20 specialized collagen proteins have been characterized (Fig. 29-2 and Appendix 29-1).

Other proteins, including the extracellular enzyme acetylcholine esterase (see Fig. 11-8) and some cell surface receptors, have similar triple helical domains but are not classified as collagens. To be a collagen, a protein must also form fibrils or other assemblies in the extracellular matrix. Nematodes, which lack connective tissue, seem to have lost the genes for fibrillar collagens but have elaborated a family of 160 genes for collagens that form their cuticle.

Collagen biochemistry is challenging because many tissue collagens are insoluble, owing to covalent cross-linking between proteins. Historic purification protocols began with proteolytic digestion to liberate protease-resistant triple helical fragments. A newer approach has been to isolate intact collagens produced by cells in tissue culture.

The size and shape of collagens vary according to function. Collagens are named numerically (type I, type II, etc.) in the order of their discovery, a nomenclature that bears no relationship to their function. Appendix 29-1 groups collagens according to function. Polypeptides are called **α-chains,** and Roman numerals in their names correspond to their type number. Some collagens are homotrimers of three identical α-chains. Others are heterotrimers of two or three different α-chains. Some chains (e.g., [α1(II)]) are used in more than one type of collagen.

Fibrillar Collagens

Triple helical rod-shaped collagen molecules about 300 nm long self-associate to form banded fibrils (Fig. 29-2). Collagen fibrils provide tensile strength to tendons, ligaments, bones, and dense connective tissue, thus reinforcing most organs. They also form the scaffolding for cartilage and the vitreous body in the eye. Fibrillar collagens are widespread in nature and have been highly conserved during evolution, so the homologs from sponges to vertebrates are similar. Each fibrillar collagen can form homopolymers in vitro; but in vivo, most form heteropolymers with at least one other type of fibrillar collagen (Appendix 29-1). This mix of the fibrillar collagen subunits is one factor that regulates the size of collagen fibers. Proteoglycans also participate (Appendix 29-2).

The biosynthesis and assembly of fibrillar collagens involve a remarkable number of posttranslational modifications, including several rounds of precise proteolytic cleavage, glycosylation, catalyzed folding, and chemical cross-linking (Fig. 29-4). The final product is a smooth fibril with staggered molecules that are cross-linked to their neighbors. These strong but flexible collagen fibrils reinforce all the tissues of the body, where they form a variety of higher-order structures. Loose connective tissue (see Fig. 32-1A) has an open network of individual fibrils or small bundles of fibrils that support the cells. In many tissues, the fibrils of type I and associated collagens aggregate to form the so-called collagen *fibers* that are visible by light microscopy (Fig. 29-3A). In extreme cases, such as in tendons, the extracellular matrix consists almost exclusively of tightly packed, parallel bundles of collagen fibers (see Fig. 32-1B). Layers of orthogonal collagen fibers make the transparent cornea through which one sees (Fig. 29-3C). In bone, type I collagen fibrils form regular layers reinforced by calcium phosphate crystals (see Fig. 32-5). In cartilage and the vitreous body of the eye, type II collagen fibrils trap glycosaminoglycans and proteoglycans, which retain enough water for the matrix to resist compression (see Fig. 32-3) and, in the case of the eye, to provide an optically clear path for light.

Biosynthesis and Assembly of Fibrillar Collagens

All fibrillar collagens are most likely to be produced by similar mechanisms, but type I collagen has been studied the most extensively. Type I collagen is synthesized and

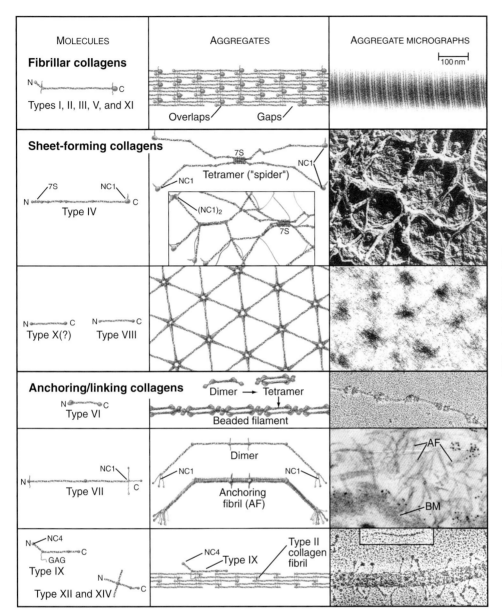

Figure 29-2 COMPARISON OF MAJOR COLLAGEN FAMILIES. Scale drawings and micrographs of collagen molecules and their assembly into higher-order structures. AF, anchoring fibrils; BM, basement membrane. (Redrawn from van der Rest M, Garrone A: Collagen family of proteins. FASEB J 5:2814–2823, 1991.)

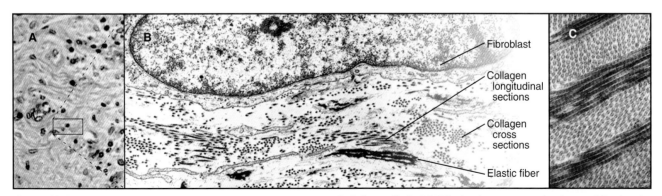

Figure 29-3 MICROGRAPHS OF COLLAGEN FIBRILS IN CONNECTIVE TISSUES. **A,** Collagen fibrils *(pink)* in the dense connective tissue of the dermis. **B,** Electron micrograph of a thin section of a fibroblast, collagen fibrils, and elastic fibers. **C,** Orthogonal layers of collagen fibrils in the cornea of the eye. (A, Courtesy of D. W. Fawcett, Harvard Medical School, Boston, Massachusetts. B, Courtesy of J. Rosenbloom, University of Pennsylvania, Philadelphia. C, Courtesy of E. D. Hay, Harvard Medical School, Boston, Massachusetts.)

secreted by fibroblasts, using the exocytic pathway that is employed for other secretory proteins (see Chapter 21), but the biosynthesis of collagen is noteworthy for the extensive number of processing steps required to prepare the protein for assembly in the extracellular matrix.

Large genes with 42 exons encode the α-chains of type I collagen. All the exons for the triple helical domain are derived by duplication and divergence from a primordial exon of 54 base pair (bp) coding for 18 amino acids or six turns of polyproline helix. About half of the exons consist of 54 bp; a few with 45 bp have lost one Gly-X-Y; and the rest are 108 (2 × 54) or 162 (3 × 54) bp. Distinctive exons encode the N- and C-terminal globular domains.

The initial transcript, referred to as **preprocollagen,** translocates into the lumen of the rough endoplasmic reticulum, where intracellular processing begins (Fig. 29-4). First, removal of the N-terminal signal sequence yields **procollagen** with unfolded α-chains with N- and C-terminal nonhelical propeptides. Second, enzymes hydroxylate some prolines and lysines. Third, enzymes add sugars (gal-glu or gal) to the delta-carbon of some *lysines,* by a mechanism distinct from the typical glycosylation of asparagine or serine.

A novel mechanism initiates the folding of collagen in the endoplasmic reticulum: the **C-terminal propeptides** of three α-chains form a globular structure stabilized by cysteines linked in disulfide bonds. An enzyme, **protein disulfide isomerase,** catalyzes the formation of these disulfides. Formation of this globular domain has three important consequences. First, it ensures the correct selection of α-chains (two α1-chains and one α2-chain in the case of type I collagen). Second, it aligns the three polypeptides with their C-terminal Gly-X-Y repeats in register, ensuring that the triple helix forms with all three chains in phase. Third, the globular propeptides prevent assembly of procollagen into fibrils during transit through the secretory pathway. Given their repeating Gly-X-Y structure, separated collagen chains without propeptides associate indiscriminately and out of register with other chains. For example, gelatin is simply a mixture of collagen chains without propeptides. Boiling dissociates the chains from each other. When cooled, the chains randomly associate *out of register* at random positions along their lengths, forming a branching network that solidifies into the gel that is used in food preparation.

Following selection and registration of the three α-chains, the helical rod domains zip together, beginning at the C-terminus. Correct folding of the triple helix requires all-*trans* peptide bonds. Because proline forms *cis* and *trans* peptide bonds randomly, the slow isomerization of *cis* prolyl-peptide bonds to *trans* limits the rate of triple helix folding in vitro. The enzyme **prolyl-peptide isomerase** catalyzes the interconversion of these prolyl-peptide bonds and rapid folding of the triple helix in vivo. The resulting rod-shaped, triple-helix glycoprotein is called procollagen.

Procollagen passes through the Golgi apparatus and moves in vesicles to the cell surface, where it is secreted. Some cells have specialized collagen assembly sites (Fig. 29-4). Like ships laying down communication cables on the ocean floor, fibroblasts help to determine the arrangement of collagen fibrils as they move through tissues (Fig. 29-3C).

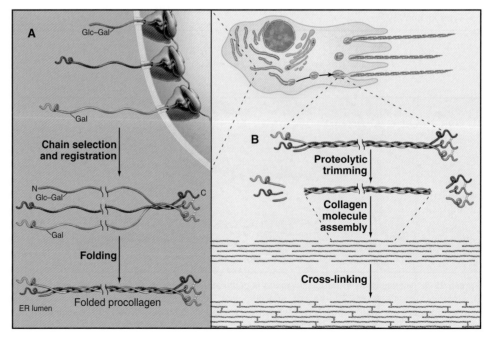

Figure 29-4 BIOSYNTHESIS AND ASSEMBLY OF FIBRILLAR COLLAGEN ILLUSTRATING DETAILS COVERED IN THE TEXT. **A,** Translation of α-chains, chain registration, and folding. **B,** Secretion, assembly, and cross-linking. (Redrawn from Prokop DJ: Mutations in collagen genes as a cause of connective tissue diseases. N Engl J Med 326:540–546, 1992. Copyright © 1992 Massachusetts Medical Society. All rights reserved.)

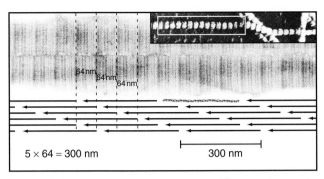

Figure 29-5 STRUCTURE OF COLLAGEN FIBRILS. Electron micrographs and drawing of molecular packing. (Micrographs courtesy of Alan Hodges, Marine Biological Laboratory, Woods Hole, Massachusetts.)

Outside the cell, proteolytic enzymes—procollagen proteases—cleave the propeptides from the triple helical domain, forming the mature collagen molecule (formerly called tropocollagen). Relieved of its inhibitory propeptides, collagen self-assembles into fibrils by a classical entropy-driven process (Fig. 29-5). Adjacent collagen molecules are staggered by 67 nm, so a 35-nm gap is required between the ends of the collagen molecules (five staggers at 67 nm = 335 nm = one molecular length of 300 nm + a 35-nm gap).

Weak, noncovalent bonds between collagen molecules specify the self-assembly of fibrils but provide little tensile strength, so **covalent cross-linking** is required for reinforcement. For most fibrillar collagens, the enzyme **lysyl oxidase** catalyzes the formation of covalent bonds between the ends of collagen molecules (Figs. 29-4 and 29-6). The enzyme oxidizes the ε amino groups of selected lysines and hydroxylysines to aldehydes. These aldehydes react spontaneously with nearby lysine and hydroxylysine side chains to form a variety of covalent cross-links between two or three polypeptides. Disulfide bonds, rather than modified lysine side chains, cross-link type III collagen fibrils. Covalent

bonds between the inextensible triple helices give mature collagen fibrils their great tensile strength.

Point mutations or deletions in collagen genes or lack of function of one of the enzymes that processes collagen (lysyl hydroxylase, lysyl oxidase, or procollagen proteases) can each cause defective collagen fibrils (Appendix 29-1). These defects cause a remarkable variety of deforming and even lethal human diseases: brittle bones (osteogenesis imperfecta), fragile cartilage (several forms of dwarfism), and weak connective tissue (Ehlers-Danlos syndrome). Chapter 34 covers these diseases in more detail.

Sheet-Forming Collagens

A second group of collagens polymerizes into sheets rather than fibrils (Fig. 29-2). These sheets surround organs, epithelia, or even whole animals. Six different human genes for type IV collagen encode proteins that form net-like polymers that assemble into the **basal lamina** beneath epithelia (Fig. 29-7) and around muscle and nerve cells. The concluding section of this chapter provides details about basal lamina structure, function, and diseases. Hexagonal nets of type VIII collagen form a special basement membrane (Descemet's membrane) under the endothelium of the cornea. Related collagens form the cuticle of earthworms and the organic skeleton of sponges.

Linking Collagens

Connecting and anchoring collagens link fibrillar and sheet-forming collagens to other structures (Fig. 29-2). The type VII collagen homotrimer has an exceptionally long triple-helix domain with nonhelical domains at the N-terminus of each chain. Type VII molecules self-associate tail to tail to form antiparallel dimers. In the process, proteases remove the C-terminal globular domain. Several dimers associate laterally to form so-called **anchoring fibrils** that link type IV collagen of

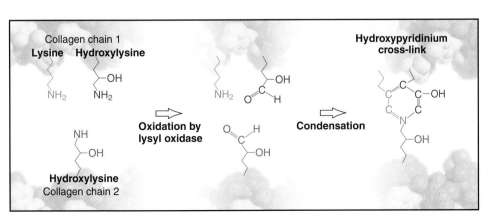

Figure 29-6 COVALENT CROSS-LINKING OF COLLAGEN MOLECULES. After lysyl oxidase oxidizes hydroxylysine side chains, the aldehydes condense with each other and a lysine to form two- and three-membered (shown) cross-links between adjacent collagen molecules.

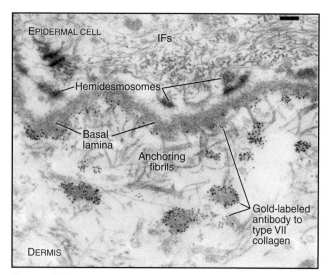

Figure 29-7 ANCHORING FIBRILS OF TYPE VII COLLAGEN. Electron micrograph of a thin section of human skin reacted with a gold-labeled antibody to the C-terminal domain of type VII collagen. **Top to bottom,** Basal epithelial cell with keratin intermediate filaments (IFs) attached to hemidesmosomes, which link to the basal lamina. Short fibrils of type VII collagen link the basal lamina to plaques in the dermis. Both ends of these bipolar fibrils (Fig. 29-2) are labeled with gold. Bar is 0.1 μm. (Courtesy of D. R. Keene, Portland Shriners Hospital, Oregon.)

the basal lamina of stratified epithelia to plaques in the underlying connective tissue (Fig. 29-7). Mutations in type VII collagen cause both the dominant and recessive forms of a severe blistering disease, dystrophic **epidermolysis bullosa.** In heterozygotes, mutated chains interfere with the assembly of anchoring fibrils by normal type VII collagen chains. Without anchoring fibrils, the basal lamina adheres weakly to the connective tissue matrix. Even mild physical trauma to the skin causes the epithelium to pull away from the connective tissue, forming a blister. Related diseases are caused by mutations in intermediate filaments (see Fig. 35-6).

Type IX collagen links glycosaminoglycans to type II collagen fibrils (Fig. 29-2). This collagen heterotrimer has a serine modified with a glycosaminoglycan chain of variable length. Type IX collagens do not polymerize, but they associate laterally with type II collagen fibrils. The N-terminal helical segment and associated glycosaminoglycan project from the surface of the type II collagen fibril. In the vitreous body of the eye, these polysaccharides fill most of the extracellular space.

Elastic Fibers

In contrast to inextensible collagen fibrils, elastic fibers are similar to rubber. They are found throughout the body but are prominent in the connective tissue of skin,

the walls of arteries (Fig. 29-8), and the lung. They recoil passively after tissues are stretched. Every time the heart beats, pressurized blood flows into and stretches the large arteries. Energy stored in elastic fibers pushes blood through the circulation between heartbeats.

Elastic fibers are a composite material: A network of **fibrillin microfibrils** is embedded in an amorphous core of cross-linked **elastin,** which makes up 90% of the organic mass (Fig. 29-9). Fibroblasts produce both components. Loose bundles of microfibrils initiate

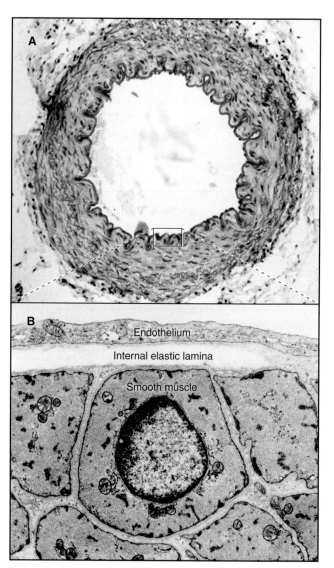

Figure 29-8 ELASTIC FIBERS IN THE WALL OF A SMALL ARTERY. **A,** Light micrograph of a cross section prepared with a special red stain to visualize elastic fibers. The boxed area includes the internal elastic lamina between the endothelial cells lining the lumen and the underlying smooth muscle cells. **B,** Electron micrograph of a longitudinal thin section illustrating the internal elastic lamina. In such standard preparations, elastic fibers stain poorly and appear amorphous except for occasional 10-nm microfibrils on the surface. (Courtesy of Don W. Fawcett, Harvard Medical School, Boston, Massachusetts.)

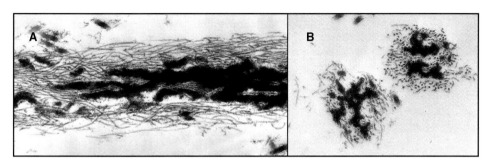

Figure 29-9 ELECTRON MICRO-GRAPHS OF DEVELOPING ELASTIC FIBERS FROM A FETAL CALF. **A,** Longitudinal section. **B,** Cross section. Fibrillin microfibrils form a scaffolding for elastin, which stains darkly in this preparation. (Courtesy of J. Rosenbloom, University of Pennsylvania, Philadelphia.)

assembly. A third protein, called fibulin, is required for elastin subunits to assemble between the microfibrils.

Fibrillin is the primordial component of elastic fibers, having arisen in Cnidarians (see Fig. 2-9). It is a long, floppy protein consisting of a tandem array of domains (Fig. 29-10). Humans have two fibrillin genes, and both fibrillin-1 and fibrillin-2 are components of 10-nm microfibrils, along with several glycoproteins. In microfibrils, fibrillin molecules interact head to tail with a reinforcing disulfide bond, but their arrangement is still being investigated. Microfibrils are about 100 times stiffer than elastin, and they stretch by rearrangement of molecules and domains rather than unfolding.

Elastin subunits are a family of closely related 60-kD proteins called **tropoelastins,** the products of alternative splicing from a single elastin gene. They have long sequences that are rich in hydrophobic residues interrupted by short sequences with pairs of lysines separated by two or three small amino acids (Fig. 29-11). Lysine-rich sequences are thought to form α-helices with pairs of lysines adjacent on the surface.

As tropoelastin assembles on the surface of elastic fibers, lysyl oxidase oxidizes paired lysines of tropoelastin to aldehydes. Oxidized lysines condense into a **desmosine** ring that covalently cross-links tropoelastin molecules to each other (Fig. 29-11). The four-way cross-links, involving pairs of lysines from two tropoelastin molecules, are unique to elastin. The same enzyme catalyzes the cross-linking of collagen, but it forms only two- and three-way cross-links.

Elastic fibers are similar to rubber except that elastic fibers require water as a lubricant. Hydrophobic segments between the cross-links are thought to form extensible random coils that account for the elastic properties of the fibril (Fig. 29-12). A difference in entropy of the polypeptide in the contracted and stretched states is thought to be the physical basis for the elasticity. The birefringence of elastic fibers increases when they are stretched, presumably as a result of alignment of polypeptide chains. Stretched fibers store energy, owing to ordering (low entropy) of the polypeptide chains. Fibers shorten when the resistance is reduced, because the polypeptide chains return to their disordered, lower-energy, higher-entropy state. Unfolding of fibrillin domains may contribute to the elasticity similar to titin in muscle cells (see Fig. 39-7), but this has not been studied.

Only embryonic and juvenile fibroblasts synthesize elastic fibers, which turn over slowly, if at all, in adults. Consequently, adults must make do with the elastic fibers that are formed during adolescence. Fortunately, these fibers are amazingly resilient. Arterial elastic fibers withstand more than 2 billion cycles of stretching and recoil during a human life. Many tissues become less elastic with age, particularly the skin, which is subjected to damage from ultraviolet irradiation. Compare, for example, how readily the skin of a baby recoils from stretching compared with that of an aged person. The loss of elastic fibers in skin is responsible for wrinkles.

Collagens are found across the phylogenetic tree, but only vertebrates are known to produce elastin. Inverte-

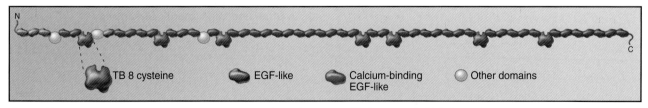

N   TB 8 cysteine   EGF-like   Calcium-binding EGF-like   Other domains   C

Figure 29-10   DOMAIN ORGANIZATION OF HUMAN FIBRILLIN. A tandem array of independently folded domains, including 47 epidermal growth factor–like (EGF-like) domains, forms a linear molecule. (Redrawn from Rosenbloom J, Abrams WR, Mecham R: Extracellular matrix 4: The elastic fiber. FASEB J 7:1208–1218, 1993.)

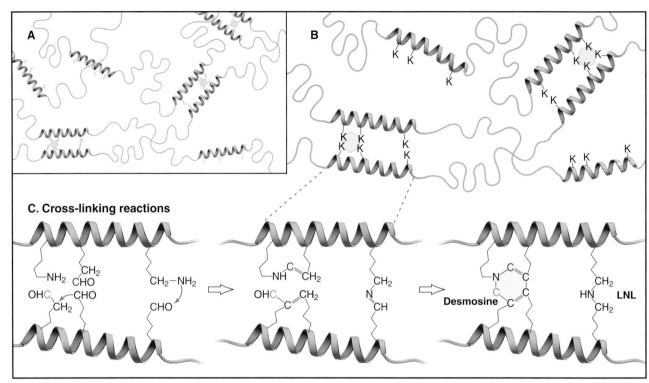

Figure 29-11 ELASTIN POLYPEPTIDES AND CROSS-LINKING REACTIONS. **A,** Lysine-rich helical domains separate random chains rich in hydrophobic residues. **B–C,** Lysyl oxidase converts lysine amino groups to aldehydes, which react with other lysines to form simple linear cross-links or six-membered rings linking two polypeptides. If the peptide bonds are hydrolyzed experimentally (not shown here), the linear cross-link is released as leucyl-norleucine (LNL) and the six-membered cross-link is released as the amino acid desmosine. (Redrawn from Rosenbloom J, Abrams WR, Mecham R: Extracellular matrix 4: The elastic fiber. FASEB J 7:1208–1218, 1993.)

Figure 29-12 PHYSICAL MODEL OF ELASTIN ELASTICITY. **A,** Contracted state with low-energy disordered chains having high entropy. **B,** Stretched state with high-energy ordered chains having low entropy. Elastin polypeptides form a continuous, covalently bonded network. Application of force stretches the chains between the cross-links. This is a low-entropy, high-energy state. Reduced force allows the chains to contract into a more disordered, higher-entropy state with lower energy. (Redrawn from Rosenbloom J, Abrams WR, Mecham R: Extracellular matrix 4: The elastic fiber. FASEB J 7:1208–1218, 1993.)

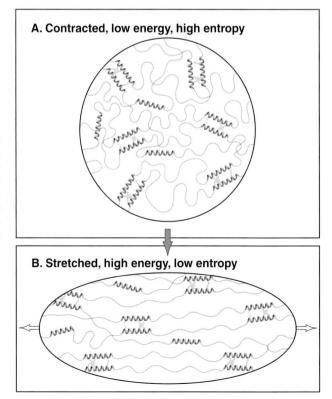

brates evolved two completely different elastic proteins. Mollusks have elastic fibers composed of the protein abductin. Insects use another protein, called resilin, to make elastic fibers.

Marfan syndrome, the disease caused by dominant mutations in the fibrillin-1 gene, illustrates the physiological functions of elastic fibers. Elastic fibers of patients with Marfan syndrome are poorly formed, accounting for most of the pathological changes that are observed. Most dangerously, weakness of elastic fibers in the aorta leads to an enlargement of the vessel, called an aneurysm, which is prone to rupture, with fatal consequences. Prophylactic replacement of the aorta with a synthetic graft and medical treatment with drugs that block β-adrenergic receptors (see Fig. 27-3) allow patients a nearly normal life span. In some patients, a floppy mitral valve in the heart causes regurgitation of blood from the left ventricle back into the left atrium. Weak elastic fibers that suspend the lens of the eye result in dislocation of the lens and impaired vision. Weak elastic fibers result in lax joints and curvature of the spine. Most affected patients are tall, with long limbs and fingers, but the connection of these features to fibrillin is not known. The manifestations of the disease are quite variable, even within one family, for reasons that are not understood. Mutations in fibrillin-2 cause congenital contractural arachnodactyly, a disease characterized by joint stiffness. New fibrillin mutations arise spontaneously, and most families that are tested have different mutations, including both point mutations and deletions. All patients are heterozygotes. Most of the known fibrillin-1 mutations make the protein unstable and susceptible to proteolysis. Other point mutations interfere with folding.

Dominant mutations in the elastin gene cause a human disease called cutis laxa. The skin and other tissues of patients with this disease lack resilience.

Glycosaminoglycans and Proteoglycans

Glycosaminoglycans (GAGs, formerly called mucopolysaccharides) are long polysaccharides made up of repeating disaccharide units, usually a hexuronic acid and a hexosamine (Fig. 29-13). With one important exception—hyaluronan—GAGs are synthesized as covalent, posttranslational modifications of a large family of proteins called proteoglycans. These proteins vary in structure and function, but their associated GAGs confer some common features.

Many cells, including all vertebrate cells, synthesize proteoglycans. Most are secreted into the extracellular matrix, where they are major constituents of cartilage, loose connective tissue, and basement membranes. Mast cells package the proteoglycan serglycin, along with other molecules in secretory granules. A few proteoglycans, including syndecan and CD44, are plasma membrane proteins with their GAGs exposed on the cell surface.

Of the known GAGs, **hyaluronan** (formerly called hyaluronic acid) is exceptional in two regards. First, enzymes on the cell surface synthesize the alternating polymer of [D-glucuronic acid β $(1 \rightarrow 3)$ D-N-acetyl glucosamine β $(1 \rightarrow 4)]_n$ (Fig. 29-13). Other GAGs are synthesized as posttranslational modifications of a core protein. Second, hyaluronan is not modified postsynthetically, as are all other GAGs. The linear polymer, often exceeding 20,000 disaccharide repeats (a length >20 μm) is released into the extracellular space.

In contrast to proteins, nucleic acids, and even N-linked oligosaccharides, which are precisely determined macromolecular structures, the GAG chains of proteoglycans appear to vary both in length and the sequence of the sugar groups. The four-step synthesis of GAGs (Fig. 29-13) explains this variability:

1. Ribosomes associated with endoplasmic reticulum synthesize the **core protein,** which enters the secretory pathway.

2. In compartments between the endoplasmic reticulum and the *trans*-Golgi apparatus, **glycosyltransferases** initiate GAG synthesis by adding one of three different, short, *link oligosaccharides* to serine or asparagine residues of the core proteins (Fig. 29-13A–B). The structural clues identifying these sites are not understood, as they do not have a common sequence motif. A tetrasaccharide attached to serine anchors dermatan sulfate, chondroitin sulfate, and heparan sulfate. Branched oligosaccharides anchor keratan sulfate to serine or asparagine.

3. In the *trans*-Golgi network, other glycosyltransferases elongate the polysaccharide by adding, sequentially, *two alternating sugars* to the growing chain (Fig. 29-13D–F). The three primary products are homogeneous, linear polymers, each with one pair of alternating sugars.

4. Enzymes modify some but not all of the residues along these alternating sugar polymers by adding sulfate to hydroxyl or amino groups, or by isomerizing certain carbons to convert D-glucuronic acid to its epimer L-iduronic acid (Fig. 29-13D–F). The result is a heterogeneous polymer. The mechanisms that select sites for modification are not understood.

The nomenclature for proteoglycans is in flux, so specific proteoglycans may have multiple names. The old nomenclature was based on the identity of the

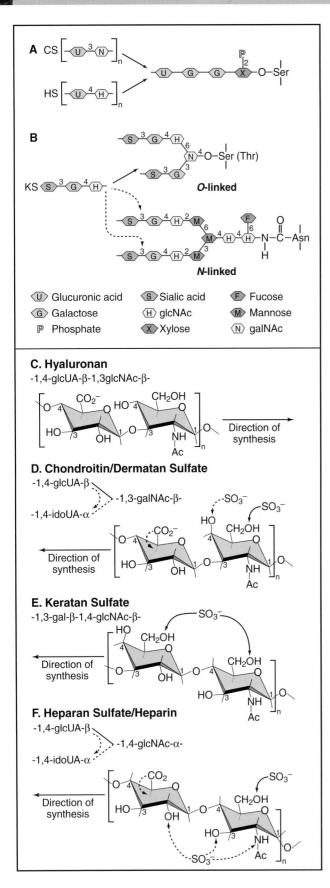

C. Hyaluronan
-1,4-glcUA-β-1,3glcNAc-β-

D. Chondroitin/Dermatan Sulfate
-1,4-glcUA-β
-1,3-galNAc-β-
-1,4-idoUA-α

E. Keratan Sulfate
-1,3-gal-β-1,4-glcNAc-β-

F. Heparan Sulfate/Heparin
-1,4-glcUA-β
-1,4-glcNAc-α-
-1,4-idoUA-α

GAGs that are bound to the protein. For example, the major proteoglycan of basement membranes was called heparan sulfate proteoglycan. This nomenclature is imprecise, as more than one type of proteoglycan carries heparan sulfate. Once the core proteins were characterized, it was reasonable to develop a nomenclature based on these core proteins. Consequently, the basement membrane proteoglycan is now known as *perlecan,* the name of its core protein. The weakness of this system is that the protein name reveals nothing about the associated GAGs. This information is important because various cells add different GAGs to the same core protein or can modify the same GAG in different ways.

Cells secrete many proteoglycans into the extracellular matrix, but they retain some types on the plasma membrane through transmembrane polypeptides or a glycosylphosphatidylinositol anchor (Appendix 29-2 and Fig. 29-14). The core proteins vary in size from 100 to 4000 amino acids. Many are modular, consisting of familiar structural domains: EGF, complement regulatory protein, leucine-rich repeats, or lectin. Three collagens carry GAG side chains: Types IX and XII have chondroitin sulfate chains, and type XVII has heparin sulfate chains.

The number of GAGs attached to the core protein varies from one (decorin) to more than 200 (aggrecan) (Fig. 29-14). A particular core protein can have identical (fibroglycan, glypican, versican) or different (aggrecan, serglycin, syndecan) types of GAGs. Some cell types can add different GAGs to the same core protein or secrete a core protein without GAGs.

Figure 29-13 SYNTHESIS OF GLYCOSAMINOGLYCANS. **A–B, Three short oligosaccharides link GAGs (left) to proteoglycan core proteins (right). A,** A tetrasaccharide anchors chondroitin sulfate (CS), dermatan sulfate, and heparan sulfate (HS) to serine residues. **B,** Two different, branched oligosaccharides link keratan sulfate (KS) to either serine or asparagine. **C–F, Four parent polymers and postsynthetic modifications. C,** Hyaluronan [D-glucuronic acid β (1 → 3) D-N-acetylglucosamine β (1 → 4)]$_n$ (n ≥ 25,000) is not modified postsynthetically. **D,** Chondroitin sulfate and dermatan sulfate are synthesized as [D-glucuronic acid β (1 → 3) D-N-acetylgalactosamine β (1 → 4)]$_n$ (n usually <250) and then modified. Some N-acetylgalactosamines are sulfated. In dermatan sulfate, D-glucuronic acids are epimerized to L-iduronic acid. **E,** Keratan sulfate is synthesized as [D-galactose β (1 → 4) D-N-acetylglucosamine β (1 → 3)]$_n$ (n usually = 20–40) and then modified by sulfation. **F,** Heparan sulfate/heparin is synthesized as [D-glucuronic acid β (1 → 4) D-N-acetylglucosamine α (1 → 4)]$_n$ (n usually <100) and then modified by sulfation and by epimerization of D-glucuronic acid to L-iduronic acid. galNAc, N-acetylgalactosamine; glcNAc, N-acetylglucosamine. (Redrawn from Wright TN, Heinegard DK, Hascall VC: Proteoglycans, structure and function. In Hay ED [ed]: Cell Biology of the Extracellular Matrix, 2nd ed. New York, Plenum Press, 1991, pp 45–78. With the kind permission of Springer Science and Business Media.)

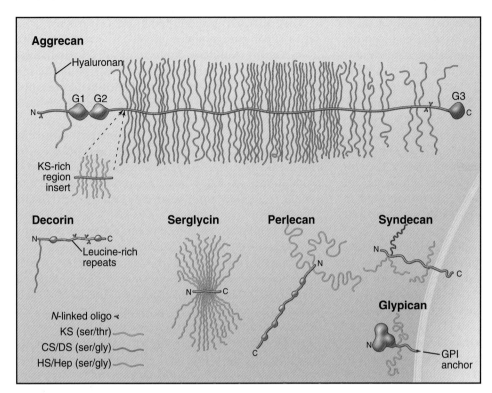

Figure 29-14 SCALE DRAWINGS OF A VARIETY OF PROTEOGLYCANS. Core proteins are *purple* and *pink,* and the glycosaminoglycans are color-coded. Proteins were named according to the following: aggrecan aggregates along hyaluronan; decorin decorates collagen fibrils; perlecan resembles a string of pearls; serglycin has 24 ser-gly repeats; syndecan (syndein = link) links cells to the matrix; glypican has a glycosylphosphatidylinositol (GPI) membrane anchor. CS, chondroitin sulfate; DS, dermatan sulfate; Hep, heparin; HS, heparan sulfate; KS, keratan sulfate. (Redrawn from Wright TN, Heinegard DK, Hascall VC: Proteoglycans, structure and function. In Hay ED [ed]: Cell Biology of the Extracellular Matrix, 2nd ed. New York, Plenum Press, 1991, pp 45–78. With the kind permission of Springer Science and Business Media.)

Given their physical properties and distribution among the fibrous elements of the extracellular matrix, proteoglycans and hyaluronan are thought to be elastic space-fillers. Each hydrophilic disaccharide unit bears a carboxyl or sulfate group or both, so GAGs are highly charged polyanions that extend themselves by electrostatic repulsion in solution and attract up to 50 g of water per gram of proteoglycan. Hyaluronan, the largest GAG, occupies a vast volume. A single hydrated molecule of 25,000 kD occupies a volume similar to that of a small organelle with a diameter of 200 nm. Retention of water by hyaluronan and **aggrecan**-keratan sulfate/chondroitin sulfate proteoglycan is essential in cartilage (see Fig. 32-3). In the extracellular matrix of other tissues, networks of densely charged hyaluronan restrict water flow, limit diffusion of solutes (especially macromolecules), and impede the passage of microorganisms. Hyaluronan and proteoglycans also act as lubricants in joint cavities and as an optically transparent, space-filling medium in the vitreous body of the eye.

Beyond these mechanical functions, proteoglycans influence cellular behavior such as adhesion or motility. Transmembrane proteoglycans can link cells to fibronectin and connective tissue collagens. **Syndecan** provides a particularly clear example. Lymphocytes express syndecan twice: early in their maturation, when they adhere to matrix fibers in the bone marrow, and later, when, as mature plasma cells, they adhere to the matrix of lymph nodes. In between, syndecan expression is lower while the lymphocytes circulate in the blood.

Carefully regulated expression allows proteoglycans to influence embryonic development and wound healing in at least three different ways. First, both decorin and fibromodulin regulate assembly of collagen fibrils. Second, membrane-bound proteoglycans, including syndecan and glypican, act as coreceptors for growth factors. Third, many polypeptide growth factors (including platelet-derived growth factor and transforming growth factor-β) bind to proteoglycans in the extracellular matrix. This allows the matrix to concentrate circulating growth factors at specific locations and to release them locally over a period of time.

The well-known anticoagulant effects of heparin and heparan sulfate are attributable to their ability to bind both thrombin (the proteolytic enzyme that converts fibrinogen to fibrin) and a thrombin inhibitory protein. This promotes interaction of the inhibitor with thrombin and inactivates the clotting cascade. A short sequence of five modified sugars has the anticoagulant activity.

Adhesive Glycoproteins

In principle, the macromolecules of the extracellular matrix and the constituent cells might interact relatively nonspecifically, but the evidence suggests that specific molecular interactions mediate virtually all of the interactions that organize the matrix and the associated cells. Most interactions are between proteins. Some are between proteins and sugars. Although some of these interactions are direct (with some cell surface receptors binding collagen directly), adapters called adhesive glycoproteins mediate many of the interactions (Appendix 29-3).

Adhesive glycoproteins were discovered by using biochemical assays for factors that favor particular interactions, such as adherence of cells to a matrix component. Further work revealed that adhesive glycoproteins are more than molecular glue; they also provide cells with signals required for the development and repair of tissues. Cells receive these signals when they bind to the matrix components. Chapter 30 focuses on their receptors.

Adhesive glycoproteins provide specific molecular interactions in the matrix by binding to cells, matrix macromolecules, or both. Adhesive proteins with multiple binding sites for cell surface receptors link cells together. For example, fibrinogen aggregates platelets during blood clotting (see Fig. 30-14). Other adhesive proteins link cells to the extracellular matrix. For instance, fibronectin mediates the attachment of cells to fibrin and collagen (Fig. 29-15). A third group of adhesive proteins link matrix macromolecules together. For example, nidogen attaches laminin to collagen and link protein attaches aggrecan-proteoglycan to hyaluronan.

The variety of tasks requires numerous adhesive proteins. In fact, the diversity exists beyond the named proteins (Appendix 29-3), as multiple genes or, more commonly, alternative splicing of the product of a single gene (see Fig. 16-6), generate multiple, functionally distinct isoforms of most of the named proteins. Particular isoforms are often expressed in specific tissues at predictable times during development.

Most adhesive glycoproteins are constructed of a series of compact modules (see Fig. 3-13 and Appendix 29-3). During evolution, duplication and recombination of the coding sequences for the domains produced the genes for these large proteins. In addition to the domains, each of these proteins also contains a significant fraction of unique sequences.

Most adhesive glycoproteins that interact with cells bind to heterodimeric transmembrane receptors called **integrins** (see Fig. 30-9). Remarkably, the integrin-binding sites of many adhesive proteins include the simple tripeptide arginine-glycine-aspartic acid (RGD [Fig. 29-15]).

Establishing the biological functions of adhesive glycoproteins is challenging because of overlapping functions and the large size of matrix macromolecules. Initial hypotheses were based on the identification of binding partners and the time and place of expression of each protein. Later, antibodies or peptides were used to disrupt specific molecular interactions in live organisms. Disruption of the gene for each protein or its receptors provides the most definitive data, and the consequences can be surprising. Some phenotypes are milder than expected from earlier studies. These results argue that the adhesive glycoproteins function as a complementary system with partially overlapping functions. Two examples illustrate what we know about adhesive glycoproteins.

Fibronectin

Fibronectins are large proteins that consist of two polypeptides of about 235 kD linked by disulfide bonds near their C-termini (Fig. 29-15). In electron micrographs, fibronectin appears as a V-shaped pair of long, flexible

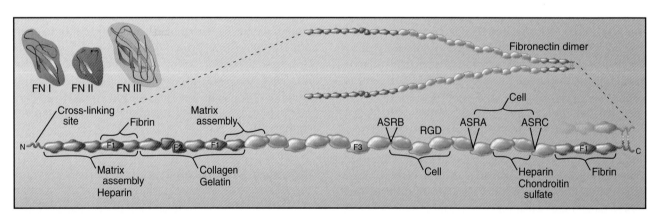

Figure 29-15 **DOMAIN ORGANIZATION OF FIBRONECTIN.** A linear array of FN-I (45 residues), FN-II (45 residues), and FN-III (90 residues) domains forms a rod-shaped subunit. Disulfide bonds near the C-termini covalently link two identical subunits in the dimeric molecule. Ligand-binding sites are indicated. The FN-III domain 10 contains the RGD sequence that binds cell surface integrins. Binding sites for fibrin, collagen, and glycosaminoglycans are indicated. Alternative splicing at sites ASRB, ASRA, and ASRC creates different isoforms. (Reference: Potts JR, Campbell ID: Fibronectin structure and assembly. Curr Opin Cell Biol 6:648–655, 1994. PDB files: FN7, 1PDC, 1FNA.)

rods connected at one end. In solution, the molecule is probably more compact. Each polypeptide is a linear array of three types of domains called FN-I, FN-II, and FN-III. All three types of fibronectin domains consist of antiparallel β strands with conserved residues in their hydrophobic cores. Two disulfide bonds stabilize FN-I and FN-II domains, whereas FN-III domains have no disulfide bonds. FN-I and FN-II domains consist of about 45 residues; FN-III domains are twice as large. FN-I and FN-II domains are present in a few other proteins, whereas the human genome contains about 170 genes with FN-III domains, including proteins in the extracellular matrix (Appendix 29-3), on the cell surface (human growth hormone receptor; see Fig. 24-6), and inside cells (titin; see Fig. 39-7).

Fibronectin binds a variety of ligands, including cell surface receptors, collagen, proteoglycans, and fibrin (another adhesive protein). Thus, it contributes to adhesion of cells to the extracellular matrix and may also cross-link matrix molecules. Ligand-binding sites in the various domains were identified by isolating proteolytic fragments and by expressing fibronectin fragments (Fig. 29-15). Some of these binding sites are cryptic and are exposed only when the protein is stretched. The RGD sequence that contributes to the integrin-binding site of fibronectin is located on an exposed loop of FN-III domain 10. The variably spliced V domain included in plasma fibronectin has a second integrin-binding site. Chapter 30 provides additional details on integrins.

Two pools of fibronectin have different distributions and solubility properties. *Tissue fibronectin* forms insoluble fibrils in connective tissues throughout the body, especially in embryos and healing wounds. Fibroblasts use an integrin-dependent process to assemble fibronectin dimers into fibrillar aggregates large enough to visualize by light microscopy (Fig. 29-16). The structure of these microscopic fibrils is not known. Denaturing agents and disulfide reduction are required to solubilize these fibrils. Disulfide bonds between the two subunits of fibronectin are also essential to form this continuous protein network, so fibronectin with deletions from the C-terminus cannot assemble into fibrils. Although difficult to study because of their large size and insolubility, fibronectin fibrils seem to bind cells more efficiently than soluble fibronectin, and may have additional activities important for biological functions.

Soluble *plasma fibronectin* dimers circulate in the body fluids. The protein differs from tissue fibronectin as a result of alternate splicing of the mRNA. In blood clots, the enzyme transglutaminase covalently couples plasma fibronectin to fibrin, forming a provisional matrix for wound repair (see Fig. 32-11).

Given its ligand-binding and assembly properties, together with its expression in vertebrate embryos even before their implantation in the uterus, fibronectin appears to contribute to the extracellular matrix in early

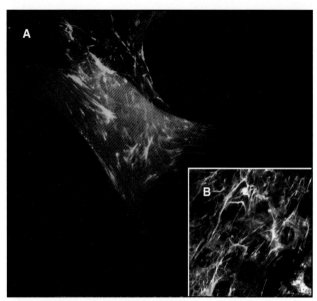

Figure 29-16 FLUORESCENCE MICROGRAPHS OF FIBRONECTIN NETWORKS IN TISSUE CULTURE. **A,** This fibroblast expressed fibronectin-YFP (fibronectin fused to yellow fluorescent protein, appearing *yellow-green*) and moesin-CFP (moesin fused to cyan fluorescent protein, appearing *red*). The fibronectin assembled an extracellular network. Moesin is associated with actin filaments in stress fibers. **B,** Lower magnification of a fibronectin network. (Courtesy of T. Ohashi and H. P. Erickson, Duke University, Durham, North Carolina.)

embryos. A collagen-based matrix replaces this primordial matrix as the embryo matures. Furthermore, embryonic cells, such as neural crest cells (precursors of pigment cells, sympathetic neurons, and adrenal medullary cells), migrate along tracks in the extracellular, fibronectin-rich matrix. Antibodies or fibronectin fragments that interfere with the adhesion of cells to fibronectin inhibit neural crest cell migration, gastrulation, and the formation of many embryonic structures derived from mesenchymal cells. Consequently, it was thought that fibronectin might provide cellular adhesion sites required for these movements.

Thus, it was predicted that deletion of the single fibronectin gene in mice would be lethal, owing to devastating effects very early in embryogenesis. It is true that homozygous null mutant mice die during embryogenesis as a result of failure to form mesodermal structures, including the notochord, muscles, heart, and blood vessels. However, the surprise was how far the embryos developed without fibronectin. In fact, up to about day 8 (when the basic body plan is already determined), the embryos appeared to be almost normal. (Mice with null mutations in the main fibronectin receptor, integrin $\alpha 5$, have similar but slightly milder defects.) One interpretation is that fibronectin and its receptor are less important for early development than was anticipated. Changes in the expression of other adhesive glycoproteins or receptors may compensate for the fibronectin defects during the first few days of development.

Tenascin

Tenascins are a family of giant proteins with six arms (Fig. 29-17), found in the extracellular matrix of many embryonic tissues, wounds, and tumors. The N-terminal ends of three subunits self-associate through a triple helical coiled-coil. Disulfides covalently link two of these three-chain units to make the hexameric molecule. The arms of the four isoforms consist of different numbers of EGF and FN-III domains, terminated by three similar FN-III domains and the fibrinogen-like domains.

All vertebrates express tenascin, but it has yet to be found in an invertebrate. Vertebrates have maintained the tenascin genes over hundreds of millions of years, and each isoform is expressed selectively in particular embryonic tissues, so it was surprising that mice with a disrupted tenascin-C gene appear normal. The expression of tenascin-R, tenascin-X, and tenascin-Y hardly overlaps with tenascin-C, but one of these isoforms may compensate for the loss of tenascin-C. On the other hand, genetic deficiency of tenascin-X is one cause of Ehlers-Danlos syndrome, a human condition with hyperextensible skin and lax joints, most often caused by mutations in collagen type V gene.

Tenascins bind to integrins, proteoglycans, and immunoglobulin-superfamily receptors on the cell surface, but the significance of these interactions is unclear. Depending on the cell and the experimental situation, tenascin can promote or inhibit adhesion of cells to culture dishes. Further experimentation is required to understand the selective advantage provided by tenascins.

The Basal Lamina

The basal lamina, a thin, planar assembly of extracellular matrix proteins, supports all epithelia, muscle cells, and nerve cells outside the central nervous system (Fig. 29-18). This two-dimensional network of protein polymers forms a continuous rug under epithelia and a sleeve around muscle and nerve cells. In addition, basal laminae are semipermeable filters for macromolecules, a particularly important role that they play in the conversion of blood plasma into urine in the kidney. The genes for basal lamina components are very ancient, having arisen in early metazoans.

In electron micrographs of thin sections of tissues prepared by chemical fixation, the basal lamina is a homogenous, finely fibrillar material that is separated from the adjacent cell by a clear gap (Fig. 29-18D). This gap is not present when the tissue is prepared by rapid freezing, so it might be an artifact. This would reconcile biochemical evidence that plasma membrane proteins connect cells directly to the basal lamina. In some tissues, fine type VII collagen fibrils connect the lamina

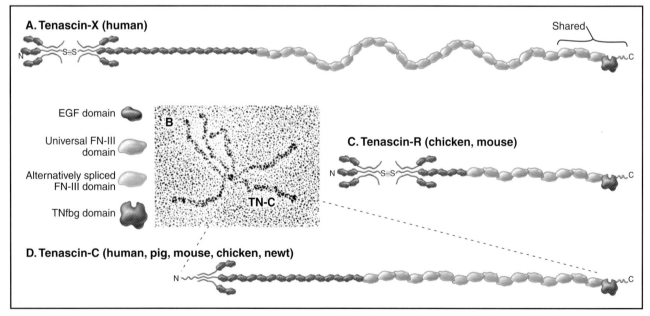

Figure 29-17 **DOMAIN ORGANIZATION OF THE THREE ISOFORMS OF TENASCIN.** TNFbg, fibrinogen-like domain. **A,** Tenascin-X. **B,** Electron micrograph of tenascin-C. **C,** Tenascin-R. **D,** Tenascin-C. Each of these tenascin molecules has six identical chains. One is shown in its entirety. Five chains are represented only by two of their N-terminal EGF domains (**A** and **C**) or just two of the other five chains (**D**). (Courtesy of H. P. Erickson, Duke University, Durham, North Carolina.)

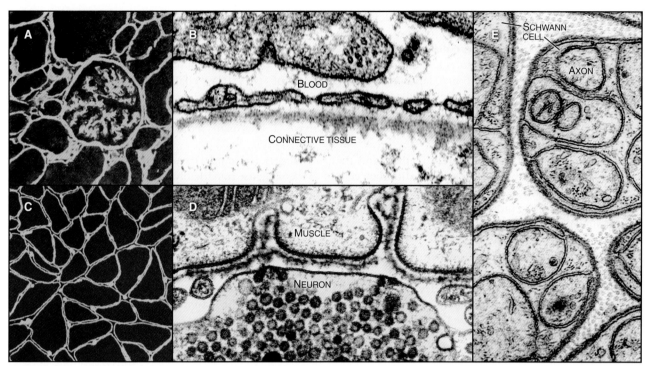

Figure 29-18 MICROGRAPHS OF THE BASAL LAMINA. **A** and **C,** Fluorescence micrographs of tissue sections stained with fluorescent antibodies to type IV collagen, a major component of basal laminae. **A,** Kidney with basal laminae around the tubules and blood vessels, including those of the glomerulus in the center. **C,** Skeletal muscle with basal laminae around the muscle cells. **B, D,** and **E,** Electron micrographs of thin sections showing basal laminae (colored *pink*). **B,** Endothelial cell lining a blood vessel with a platelet in the lumen. **D,** Neuromuscular junction. **E,** Unmyelinated nerve with numerous axons *(yellow)* surrounded by invaginations of Schwann cells *(blue).* (A and C, From Odermatt BF, Lang AB, Ruttner JR, et al: Monoclonal antibody to human type IV collagen. Proc Natl Acad Sci U S A 81:7343–7347, 1984. B and E, Courtesy of Don W. Fawcett, Harvard Medical School, Boston, Massachusetts. D, Courtesy of J. Heuser, Washington University, St. Louis, Missouri.)

to underlying connective tissue. The basal lamina and associated collagen fibrils form the "basement membrane" that is observed in histologic preparations of epithelia. A basal lamina alone cannot be seen by light microscopy without special labels, such as those used in Figure 29-18A and C.

Although many proteins contribute to the stability of the basal lamina (Fig. 29-19), only the adhesive glycoprotein **laminin** is essential for the initial assembly of basal laminae during embryogenesis. The C-terminal end of the cross-shaped laminin molecule binds to cell surface receptors (integrins, **dystroglycan;** see Fig. 39-7). Laminins self-assemble into continuous, two-dimensional networks through noncovalent interactions of their short arms. Mouse embryos that lack dystroglycan or laminin die early in development, owing to failure to make basal laminae.

The subsequent addition of other proteins reinforces the laminin network. A two-dimensional network of **collagen IV** self-assembles through head-to-head interactions of the N-termini of four molecules and tail-to-tail interactions of the C-terminal NC1 domains of two molecules (Fig. 29-2). Mouse embryos that lack collagen IV make nascent basal laminae composed of laminin but eventually die from defects in basal lamina.

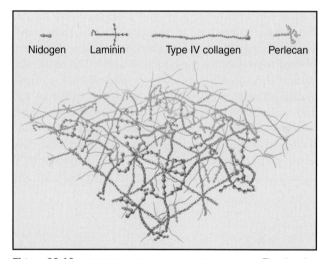

Figure 29-19 MOLECULAR MODEL OF THE BASAL LAMINA. The drawing shows the sizes and shapes of the component molecules and their postulated three-dimensional arrangement in the basal lamina. (Reproduced from Yurchenco P, Cheng YS, Colognato H: Laminin forms an independent network in basement membranes. J Cell Biol 117:1119–1133, 1992, by copyright permission of The Rockefeller University Press.)

Other proteins reinforce the collagen IV and laminin in basal laminae. The rod-shaped protein **nidogen** cross-links laminin to type IV collagen. **Perlecan,** a heparan sulfate proteoglycan, provides additional cross-links, as it binds to itself in addition to laminin, nidogen, and collagen IV. These cross-links help to determine the porosity of basal lamina and thus the size of molecules that can filter through it. Fibrillin and an associated protein, fibulin, are also present.

Epithelial and muscle cells secrete laminin and the other components of basal lamina. Two different cells can cooperate to produce a basal lamina between two tissues. For example, epithelial cells make laminin, and mesenchymal cells make nidogen for the same basal lamina.

The interwoven network of protein fibers provides the physical basis for the two main functions of the basal lamina: physical support and selective permeability. The basal lamina is a physical scaffold to anchor epithelial, muscle, and nerve cells. In epithelia, all of the basal cells attach to the underlying basal lamina. The basal lamina, in turn, is anchored to the underlying connective tissue. Thus, force applied to an exposed epithelial surface, such as skin, is transmitted through the basal lamina to the connective tissue. Similarly, all epithelial cells in tubular structures, such as blood vessels and glands, adhere to a cylindrical basal lamina that contributes to the integrity of the tube. In muscle, the basal lamina around each cell transmits the contractile forces between cells and to tendons.

The fibrous network in the basal lamina also acts as a filter for macromolecules and a permeability barrier for cellular migration. In kidney, a basal lamina sandwiched between two epithelial cells filters the blood plasma to initiate the formation of urine. The molecular weight threshold for the filter is about 60 kD, so most serum proteins are retained in the blood, whereas salt and water pass into the excretory tubules. The high charge of basal lamina proteoglycans contributes to filtering by electrostatic repulsion. Basal laminae also confine epithelial cells to their natural compartment. If neoplastic transformation occurs in an epithelium, the basal lamina prevents the spread of the tumor until matrix metalloproteinases (see the next section) break down the basal lamina.

The major basement membrane type IV collagen consists of two α1(IV) chains and one α2(IV) chain. No human mutations in the two major type IV collagen genes have been observed, presumably because they have a dominant lethal phenotype, as observed in *Drosophila.*

Restricted human tissues express four additional type IV collagens; remarkably, each has been implicated in human disease (Table 29-1). Patients with Alport's X-linked familial nephritis all have mutations in the α5(IV) collagen gene. More than 200 different point mutations and deletions are known. Other patients with autosomally inherited Alport's syndrome have mutations in their α3(IV) or α4(IV) collagen genes. These mutations generally interfere with folding of the collagen molecule and disrupt the basement membranes that form the blood filtration barrier in the glomerulus of the kidney, causing progressive kidney failure that is usually fatal in males. These mutations also cause defects in the eye and ear, other places where the α5(IV) collagen gene is expressed. In Goodpasture's syndrome, the immune system produces autoantibodies to the C-terminal NC1 domain of α3(IV) collagen. The protein sequences that elicit autoantibody production are buried in the NC1 domain, so they may be exposed by bacterial infections or organic solvents, predisposing events in the syndrome. Antibodies bound to basement membranes in the kidney and lung cause inflammation that leads to kidney failure and bleeding in the lungs.

Matrix Metalloproteinases

Many physiological processes depend on the controlled degradation of the extracellular matrix. Examples include tissue remodeling during embryogenesis (e.g., resorption of a tadpole tail), wound healing, involution (massive shrinkage secondary to loss of cells and extracellular matrix) of the uterus after childbirth, shedding

---

Table 29-1

INHERITED DISEASES OR MUTANT PHENOTYPES OF BASAL LAMINA COMPONENTS

Protein Subunit	Distribution	Disease or Mutant Phenotype
Collagen α3IV	Many tissues	Human autoantibodies cause Goodpasture's syndrome of renal failure.
Collagen α5IV	Kidney, muscle	Human mutation causes Alport's syndrome of renal failure.
Laminin α1	Many tissues	Fly null mutation is lethal during embryogenesis.
Laminin α2	Muscle, heart	Mouse dy mutation causes muscular dystrophy.
Laminin γ2	Epidermis	Human mutation causes Herlitz's junctional epidermolysis bullosa.
Perlecan	Many tissues	Worm unc-52 mutation disrupts myofilament attachment to membrane.

of the uterine endometrium during menstruation, and invasion of the uterine wall by the embryonic tropho-blast during implantation. Conversely, uncontrolled destruction of extracellular matrix contributes to degenerative diseases, such as emphysema and arthritis. In addition to their roles in remodeling, many of these enzymes cleave and release biologically active fragments from matrix or membrane proteins. Three classes of Zn-depended proteases account for both the physiological and pathological degradation of diverse extracellular matrix and cell surface proteins.

The first class is called **matrix metalloproteinases (MMPs).** These 24 homologous enzymes share a zinc-protease domain (Fig. 29-20) similar to bacterial thermolysin. Gelatinases have three FN-II domains inserted into the sequence of the catalytic domain. All have an N-terminal signal sequence and are processed through the secretory pathway. Between the signal sequence and catalytic domain, all MMPs have an **autoinhibitory propeptide,** including a conserved cysteine that binds

to the zinc ion in the catalytic site. A C-terminal trans-membrane domain anchors several MMPs to the plasma membrane. All other MMPs are secreted. Most MMPs have a C-terminal regulatory domain that influences the substrate specificity of the catalytic domain. After secretion, inactive pro-MMPs bind directly or indirectly to cell surface receptors.

MMP activity is carefully regulated at three levels, normally restricting proteolysis to sites of tissue remodeling or physiological breakdown, such as the involuting uterus. First, only particular connective tissue, inflammatory, and epithelial cells are genetically programmed to express MMP genes and to respond to growth factors and cytokines to increase production under appropriate circumstances. Second, autoinhibited MMPs on the cell surface require propeptide cleavage for activation. Proteolytic cleavage and dissociation of the propeptide activate the enzyme. Then the cellular movements deliver the active protease to specific substrates. For example, membrane-anchored MMP-14 directly activates MMP-2, which then degrades basement membrane collagen and other substrates. Third, secreted proteins called **tissue inhibitors of metalloproteinases (TIMPs)** and the plasma protein α2-macroglobulin bind to the active site of MMPs, keeping their activity in check.

Each MMP is selective for targets in the extracellular matrix. In some cases, proteolysis disrupts the mechanical integrity of the matrix. In others, cleavage of a collagen isoform or other matrix protein releases a fragment that favors or inhibits the formation of blood vessels. For example, the N-terminal domain cleaved from collagen XVIII is an inhibitor of angiogenesis that has been called endostatin. Mice survive null mutations in any one of several MMPs tested, but the loss of an MMP may alter the susceptibility to disease dramatically. Mice without MMP-12 (macrophage elastase) are resistant to cigarette smoke, which causes emphysema in normal mice. Without MMP-12, smoke fails to stimulate elastin degeneration, which weakens lung tissue and mediates inflammation. MMPs contribute to the spread of tumors in mice, but disappointingly small-molecule inhibitors of MMPs have not proven useful for treatment of advanced tumors in humans.

The second class of Zn-dependent proteases consists of about 35 proteases called **ADAMs** (a disintegrin and metalloproteinase). These enzymes are anchored to the plasma membrane by a single transmembrane sequence. Like other metalloproteinases, they are inhibited by TIMPs. ADAMs cleave and release extracellular domains of cell surface proteins, some of which are important informational molecules (e.g., tumor necrosis factor [TNF]-α; transforming growth factor [TGF]-α). ADAM-17 null mutations are lethal during embryogenesis, owing to a lack of TGF-α or other ligands for EGF receptors. A polymorphism in the ADAM-33 gene is strongly

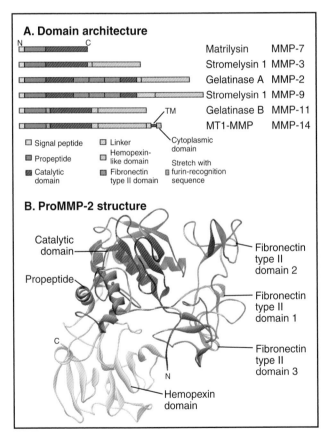

A. Domain architecture

Matrilysin	MMP-7
Stromelysin 1	MMP-3
Gelatinase A	MMP-2
Stromelysin 1	MMP-9
Gelatinase B	MMP-11
MT1-MMP	MMP-14

□ Signal peptide
■ Propeptide
■ Catalytic domain
□ Linker
□ Hemopexin-like domain
■ Fibronectin type II domain
Cytoplasmic domain
◨ Stretch with furin-recognition sequence

B. ProMMP-2 structure

Catalytic domain
Propeptide
Fibronectin type II domain 2
Fibronectin type II domain 1
Fibronectin type II domain 3
Hemopexin domain

Figure 29-20 MATRIX METALLOPROTEINASE STRUCTURES. **A,** Domain organization of MMP isoforms. All have an N-terminal cleaved signal sequence, a propeptide that binds to the active site and inhibits the protease activity, and a catalytic domain. Gelatinases have FN-II domains inserted in the catalytic domain. Matrilysin lacks the C-terminal domain. MMP-14 has a transmembrane segment near its C-terminus. **B,** Atomic structure of MMP-2 showing the arrangement of the domains and the propeptide occupying the active site. (PDB file: 1CK7.)

associated with human asthma, although the mechanism is not yet understood.

A third class of Zn-dependent proteases is called **ADAMTS,** ADAMs with a thrombospondin domain. These secreted proteases cleave specific matrix substrates, such as the cartilage proteoglycan aggrecan. Experiments with mice show that inactivation of the protease domain of ADAMTS5 reduces the development of a common joint disease called osteoarthritis.

ACKNOWLEDGMENTS

Thanks go to Robert Linhardt for his suggestions on revisions to this chapter.

SELECTED READINGS

Baum J, Brodsky B: Folding of peptide models of collagen and misfolding in disease. Curr Opin Struct Biol 9:122–128, 1999.

Burgeson RE, Christiano AM: The dermal-epidermal junction. Curr Opin Cell Biol 9:651–658, 1997.

Capila I, Linhardt RJ: Heparin-protein interactions. Angewandte Chemie Int Ed 41:390–412, 2002.

Hacker U, Nybakken K, Perrimon N: Heparan sulphate proteoglycans: The sweet side of development. Nat Rev Mol Cell Biol 6:530–541, 2005.

Hudson BG, Tryggvason K, Sundraamoorthy M, Neilson EG: Alport's syndrome, Goodpasture's syndrome and Type IV collagen. New Engl J Med 348:2543–2556, 2003.

Hutter H, Vogel BE, Plenefisch JD, et al: Conservation and novelty in the evolution of cell adhesion and extracellular matrix genes. Science 287:989–994, 2000.

Iozzo RV: Basement membrane proteoglycans: From cellar to ceiling. Nat Rev Mol Cell Biol 6:646–656, 2005.

Kielty CM, Sherrat MJ, Marson A, Baldock C: Fibrillin microfibrils. Adv Protein Chem 70:405–436, 2005.

Kreis T, Vale R (eds): Guidebook to the Extracellular Matrix and Adhesion Proteins, 2nd ed. Oxford, UK, Oxford University Press, 1999.

Mao Y, Schwarzbauer JE: Fibronectin fibrillogenesis: A cell-mediated matrix assembly process. Matrix Biol 24:389–399, 2005.

Mithieux SM, Weiss AS: Elastin. Adv Prot Chem 70:437–461, 2005.

Mott JD, Werb Z: Regulation of matrix biology by matrix metalloproteinases. Curr Opin Cell Biol 16:558–564, 2004.

Ricard-Blum S, Dublet B, van der Rest M: Unconventional Collagens Types VI, VII, VIII, IX, XIV, XVI and XIX. Oxford, UK, Oxford University Press, 2000.

Rosenbloom J, Abrams WR, Mecham R: Extracellular matrix 4: The elastic fiber. FASEB J 7:1208–1218, 1993.

Schenk S, Quaranta V: Tales from the crypt[ic] sites of the extracellular matrix. Trends Cell Biol 13:366–375, 2003.

Sugahara K, Mikami T, Uyama T, et al: Recent advances in the structural biology of chondroitin sulfate and dermatan sulfate. Curr Opin Struct Biol 13:612–620, 2003.

Taylor KR, Gallo RL: Glycosaminoglycans and their proteoglycans: Host-associated molecular patterns for initiation and modulation of inflammation. FASEB J 20:9–22, 2005.

Timpl R, Sasaki T, Kostka G, Chu ML: Fibulins: A versatile family of extracellular matrix proteins. Nat Rev Mol Cell Biol 4:479–489, 2003.

White JM: ADAMs: Modulators of cell-cell and cell-matrix interactions. Curr Opin Cell Biol 15:598–606, 2003.

Yurchenco PD, Wadsworth WG: Assembly and tissue functions of early embryonic laminins and netrins. Curr Opin Cell Biol 16:572–579, 2004.

APPENDIX 29-1

Collagen Families

Type	Chains	Assembly	Interactions	Distribution	Diseases
Fibrillar Collagens					
I	α1.α1.α2(I)	Fibrils	Self; types III and V collagen; types XII and XIV collagen	Bone, tendons, ligaments, skin, dentin	Mutated in osteogenesis imperfecta; mutated in Ehlers-Danlos syndrome type VII Kniest dysplasia, Stickler's syndrome
II	[α1(II)]3	Fibrils	Self; type IX and XI collagen	Hyaline cartilage, vitreous body	Mutated in spondyloepiphyseal dysplasia, hypochondrogenesis, achondrogenesis, Kniest dysplasia, Stickler's syndrome
III	[α1(III)]3	Fibrils	Self; type I collagen	Skin, blood vessels	Mutated in Ehlers-Danlos syndrome type IV
V	α1.α1.α2(V) α1.α2.α3(V)	Fibrils	Self; type I collagen	Fetal membranes, skin, bone, placenta, synovial membranes	
XI	α1(XI)α2(XI)α1(II)	Fibrils	Self; type II collagen	Hyaline cartilage	Mutated in some Stickler's syndrome
Sheet-Forming Collagens					
IV	α1.α1.α2(IV) α3.α4.α5(IV) α5.α5.α6(IV)	Nets	Self; perlecan laminin, nidogen, integrins	Basement membranes	Autoantigen in Goodpasture's syndrome; mutated in Alport's nephritis & in porencephaly
VIII	[α1(VIII)]? [α2(VIII)]?	Hexagonal net	Self	Descemet's membrane (cornea)	
X	[α1(X)]3	?	?	Hypertrophic cartilage	Mutated in Schmid metaphyseal chondrodysplasia
Connecting and Anchoring Collagens					
VI	α1.α2.α3(VI)	Beaded fibrils	Self; type IV collagen	Vessels, skin, intervertebral disk	Mutated in Bethlem myopathy
VII	[α1(VII)]3	Anchoring fibril	Self; type IV collagen	Epidermal-dermal junction	Mutated in dystrophic epidermolysis bullosa
IX	α1.α2.α3(IX)	Linker	Covalent GAG; type II collagen	Hyaline cartilage, vitreous body	Mutated in multiple epiphyseal dysplasia
XII	[α1(XII)]3	? Linker	GAG; ? type I collagen	Embryonic tendon, skin	
XIV	[α1(XIV)]3	? Linker	GAG; ? type I collagen	Fetal tendon, skin	
XVIII	[α1(XVIII)]3	? Linker	GAG	Basal lamina	
Transmembrane					
XIII	[α1(XIII)]3	Transmembrane			
XVII	[α1(XVII)]3	Transmembrane	Hemidesmosomes, basal lamina	Epidermal-dermal junction	Mutated in blistering conditions; antigen in bullous pemphigoid

APPENDIX 29-2

Proteoglycans

Name	Core Protein	Glycosaminoglycans	Expression	Functions
Secreted Proteoglycans				
Aggrecan	One-gene, 250-kD protein with link protein, EGF, lectin & complement regulatory domains	100–150 keratin sulfate chains >150 chondroitin sulfate chains	Cartilage	Binds hyaluronan and link protein; hydrates and fills the ECM; no known diseases
Biglycan	One-gene, 38-kD protein	2 chondroitin sulfate or dermatan sulfate chains	Developing muscle, bone, cartilage and epithelia	Associated with cell surfaces; no known ligands or functions
Decorin	One-gene, 38-kD protein	1 chondroitin sulfate or dermatan sulfate chain	Connective tissue fibroblasts	Binds collagen fibrils and modifies their assembly
Fibromodulin	One-gene, 43-kD protein	4 asparagine-linked keratin sulfate chains	Cartilage, skin, tendon	Binds collagen I and II; limits size of collagen fibrils
Perlecan	One-gene, 400-kD protein	3 heparan sulfate chains of 30–60 kD	All cells making basement membranes (epithelia, muscle, peripheral nerve)	Self-associates; binds laminin in basal lamina; binds basic fibroblast growth factor
Serglycin	One-gene, 12-kD protein; 24 serine-glycine repeats	Heparin or chondroitin sulfate	White blood cells, Mast cells	Binds histamine in secretory granules
Versican	One-gene, 260-kD protein with link-protein, GAG attachment, 2 EGF, lectin & complement regulatory domains	12–15 chondroitin sulfate chains *N*- and *O*-linked oligosaccharides	Fibroblasts; ? other cells	May bind hyaluronan; functions unknown
Membrane-Associated Proteoglycans				
Fibroglycan	One-gene, integral membrane protein of 20 kD	Heparan sulfate chains	Fibroblasts	Binds collagen I and fibronectin; cell adhesion to ECM
Glypican	62-kD protein with glycosylphosphatidylinositol anchor to membrane on C-terminus	4 heparan sulfate chains	Lung, skin, epithelia, endothelium, smooth muscle	Binds fibronectin, collagen I, and antithrombin III; cell adhesion to ECM
Syndecan	One-gene, integral membrane protein of 33 kD	Variable number of heparan sulfate and chondroitin sulfate chains	Embryonic epithelia and mesenchyme, developmentally regulated in adult lymphocytes	Binds fibronectin; collagen I, III, and V; thrombospondin; basic fibroblast growth factor; cell adhesion to ECM

ECM, extracellular matrix.

A P P E N D I X **29-3**

Adhesive Glycoproteins

Name(s)	Composition	Expression	Ligands	Functions and Diseases
Agrin	One-gene, 205-kD protein with cysteine-rich, EGF, and Kazal protease inhibitor domains	Motor neurons secrete into basal lamina of neuromuscular junction	? Acetylcholine receptor	Aggregates acetylcholine receptors
Fibrinogen	2 × 67 kD Aα chains, 2 × 56 kD Bβ chains, 2 × 47 kD γ chains, joined by disulfide bonds; N-linked CHO on Bβ & γ chains	Hepatocytes secrete into blood	Platelet integrin GPIIb/GPIIIa	Thrombin cleavage releases fibrin, which polymerizes into fibrils stabilized by covalent cross-linking by transglutaminase; deficiency or defects cause bleeding
Fibronectin	One gene; RNA splicing isoforms of 235–270 kD; dimers disulfide-bonded; 12 FN-I, 2 FN-II and 15–17 FN-III domains; N- and O-linked CHO	Many tissues; increased with wounding	Fibrin, heparin, cells via integrins, collagen	Assembles fibrils in ECM; promotes cellular adhesion to ECM and migration
Fibulin	One gene; RNA splicing generates monomeric isoforms of 566, 601 and 683 residues with 9 EGF and 3 complement-like domains; N- and O-linked CHO	Fibroblasts; present in plasma and some basement membranes	Ca^{2+}, fibronectin, fibrinogen	Required for elastin assembly; mutated in some patients with macular degeneration
HB-GAM (heparin-binding, growth-associated molecule)	136 residues, 5 internal disulfide bonds	Brain, uterus, intestine, kidney, muscle, lung, skin	Heparin	? Neuronal differentiation
Laminin	1 × 200–400 kD A chain, 1 × 200 kD B1 chain, 1 × 200 kD B2 chain, several isoforms of each; poly-N-acetyl galactosamine	Epithelium, endothelium, smooth & striated muscle, peripheral nerve, myotendinous junction	Nidogen, 6 integrins perlecan, collagen IV, α-dystroglycan	Self-associates into network in basement membrane linked to collagen IV network by nidogen; promotes cell adhesion and migration
Laminin-binding protein (Mac-2)	Soluble S-type monomeric lectin of 29–35 kD	Macrophages, epithelia, fibroblast, trophoblast, cancer cells	Poly-N-acetyl galactosamine on laminin	?
Link protein	One gene; alternative splicing generates isoforms of 41, 46, & 51 kD with two 4-cysteine & one immunoglobulin domains; CHO content variable	Cartilage	Aggrecan and hyaluronan	Links aggrecan to hyaluronan
Mucins	Heterogeneous secreted & transmembrane glycoproteins	GI tract, salivary glands	Selectins	Lubricates mucous membranes
Nidogen (entactin)	One-gene, 148-kD monomeric protein with 8 EGF & 2 EF hand domains; N- & O-linked CHO	Basement membranes of epithelia, muscles, and nerves	Laminin, collagen IV, Ca^{2+}	Links collagen IV to laminin in basement membrane
Osteopontin (secreted phosphoprotein)	Monomer of ~300 residues, phosphorylated, N- & O-linked CHO, including sialic acid	Bone, milk, kidney, uterus, ovary	? Vitronectin receptor; ? hydroxyapatite	Promotes cell adhesion to ECM, including osteoclasts to bone

CHO, oligosaccharide chains; EF, hand calcium binding motif of calmodulin family.

Continued

Name(s)	Composition	Expression	Ligands	Functions and Diseases
Restrictin	3 × 180 kD chains linked by disulfide bonds; each has 1 cysteine-rich, EGF, 9 FN-III and 1 fibrinogen-like domains	A limited number of neurons in embryonic nervous systems	Cells, receptor unknown	? Cell adhesion
SPARC (secreted protein rich in cysteine); osteonectin	One-gene; 32-kD monomer	Bone, skin, connective tissue	Collagens III and V, Ca^{2+}, hydroxyapatite, cells	? Wound healing, development
Tenascin (cytotactin)	Four genes (C, R, X, Y) and alternate splicing; EGF, FN-III, and fibrinogen-like domains; chains linked by disulfides	Embryonic mesenchyme; adult perichondrium, periosteum, tendon, ligament, myotendinous junction, wounds	Integrins, Ig-CAMs, proteoglycans	Tenascin-X mutated in some patients with Ehlers-Danlos syndrome; mice with tenascin-C null mutation develop normally
Thromobospondin	420-kD protein with procollagen, EGF, and complement-like domains	Platelets, fibroblasts, embryonic heart, muscle, bone, brain	Integrin αvβ3, CD36 cell surface receptor, syndecan, Ca^{2+}	Platelet aggregation; stimulates proliferation of smooth muscle; inhibits proliferation of endothelium
Vitronectin	One-gene, 75-kD protein with N-linked CHO, phosphorylated, sulfated Secreted by liver into blood	Integrin αVβ3, heparin, glass, plastic	Promotes cell adhesion, inactivates heparin, stabilizes plasminogen activator inhibitor	
von Willebrand's factor	One-gene, 2050-residue protein that forms head to head and tail to tail disulfide-linked oligomers, N- & O-linked CHO	Endothelium, platelets	Factor VIII, heparin, collagen, platelet integrin GPIIb/ GPIIIa	Promotes adhesion of platelets to collagen and each other; required to control bleeding; deficiency causes most common congenital blood clotting abnormality

Cellular Adhesion

$\mathbf{A}$ll cells interact with molecules in their environment, in many cases relying on cell surface adhesion proteins to bind these molecules. Multicellular organisms are particularly dependent on adhesion of cells to each other and the extracellular matrix (ECM). During development, carefully regulated genetic programs specify cell-cell and cell-matrix interactions that determine the architecture of each tissue and organ. Some adhesive interactions are stable. Muscle cells must adhere firmly to each other and to the connective tissue of tendons to transmit force to the skeleton (see Chapter 39). Skin cells must also bind tightly to each other and the underlying connective tissue to resist abrasion (see Fig. 35-6). On the other hand, many cellular interactions are transient and delicate. At sites of inflammation, leukocytes bind transiently to endothelial cells lining small blood vessels and then use transient interactions with the ECM to migrate through connective tissue (look ahead to Figs. 30-13 and 30-14).

Cells use a relatively small repertoire of adhesion mechanisms to interact with matrix molecules and each other. This conceptual breakthrough came when comparisons of amino acid sequences showed that most adhesion proteins fall into five large families (Fig. 30-1). Within each of these distinctive families, ancestral genes duplicated and diverged during evolution, giving rise to adhesion proteins with the many different specificities that are required for embryonic development, maintenance of organ structure, and migrations of cells of our defense systems. Common properties within each family allowed the appreciation of general mechanisms to emerge from characterizing a few examples. Several important adhesion proteins fall outside the five major families, and additional families may emerge from continued research.

Many adhesion proteins were named before they were classified into families. Tables 30-1 through 30-5 are designed to help the reader with the nomenclature. Many adhesion proteins are named "CD" followed by a number. This stands for "clusters of differentiation," a term that is used to classify cell surface antigens recognized by monoclonal antibodies, independent of any knowledge about the structure or function of the antigen. Hence, members of the four major families of adhesion proteins have CD numbers.

This chapter first highlights some general features of adhesion proteins and then introduces four major families: immunoglobulin–cell adhesion molecules (**Ig-CAMs**), **cadherins, integrins,** and **selectins.** While learning about each family, the reader should not lose track of an important point: These receptors rarely act alone. Rather, they usually function as parts of multicomponent systems. Two examples at the end of the chapter illustrate the cooperation that is required for leukocytes to respond to inflammation and for platelets to repair damage to blood vessels. Chapter 31 on intercellular junctions, Chapter 32 on specialized connective tissues, and Chapter 38 on

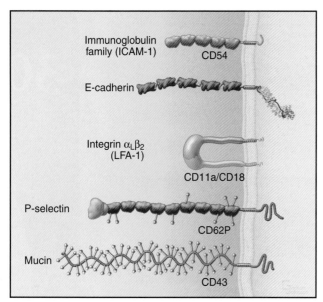

Figure 30-1 THE MAJOR CLASSES OF ADHESION PROTEINS. Ig-CAMs have one or more extracellular domains folded like an immunoglobulin domain (orange). Cadherins have five or more extracellular CAD domains (maroon) that typically bind the same class of cadherin on a neighboring cell. Ca^{2+} stabilizes the interaction of neighboring CAD domains. Their cytoplasmic tails bind β-catenin (blue) and other adapter proteins. Integrins are heterodimers of α and β subunits that establish a wide range of specificities for matrix molecules by pairwise combinations of 1 of 16 α-chains and 1 of 8 β-chains. Selectins have a Ca^{2+}-dependent lectin (carbohydrate-binding) domain (green), an EGF-like domain (blue), and a variable number of complement regulatory domains (red). Mucins display multiple carbohydrates for interactions with other cells. CD numbers refer to the names of representative adhesion molecules based on the "clusters of differentiation" nomenclature (see the text). Single transmembrane segments attach all of these receptors to the plasma membrane. Adapter proteins link the cytoplasmic tails of most adhesion proteins to the actin cytoskeleton or, in the case of specialized cadherins and integrins, to intermediate filaments. (Redrawn from van der Merwe PA, Barclay AN: Transient intercellular adhesion: The importance of weak protein-protein interactions. Trends Cell Biol 19:354–358, 1994.)

General Principles of Cellular Adhesion

First Principle of Adhesion

Cells define their capacity for adhesive interactions by selectively expressing plasma membrane receptors (cell adhesion molecules, or CAMs) with limited ligand-binding activity. Generally, expression of the proper mix of receptors is part of a genetic program for the differentiation of the cell. In some cases, extracellular stimuli control expression of adhesion recep-

tors. For example, endothelial cells produce E-selectin only when stimulated by inflammatory hormones or endotoxin.

Second Principle of Adhesion

Many adhesion proteins bind one main ligand, and many ligands bind a single type of receptor (refer to Tables 30-1 through 30-5). If this one-to-one pairing were the rule, adhesion would be simple indeed. However, many exceptions exist, particularly in the integrin family of receptors (Table 30-3). These receptors generally bind more than one ligand, and some ligands, such as fibronectin, bind more than one integrin. One can generalize about the ligands for the several families of cell adhesion molecules:

- Most cadherins prefer to bind themselves, so they promote the adhesion of like cells. These **homophilic interactions** (association of like receptors on two cells) require Ca^{2+}.
- Selectins bind anionic polysaccharides like those on **mucins.** Generally, such interactions bind together two different types of cells.
- Most Ig-CAMs bind other cell surface adhesion proteins. These **heterophilic interactions** (association of unlike receptors on two cells) may occur between the same or different cell types.
- Integrins stand apart because they bind a variety of ligands: matrix macromolecules, such as fibronectin (see Fig. 29-15) and laminin (see Fig. 39-9); soluble proteins, such as fibrinogen in blood; and adhesion proteins on the surface of other cells, including Ig-CAMs and one cadherin.

Third Principle of Adhesion

Cells modulate adhesion by controlling the surface density, state of aggregation, and state of activation of their adhesion receptors. Surface density reflects not only the level of synthesis but also the partitioning of adhesion molecules between the plasma membrane and intracellular storage compartments. For example, endothelial cells express P-selectin constitutively but store it internally in membranes of cytoplasmic vesicles. When inflammatory cytokines activate endothelial cells, these vesicles fuse with the plasma membrane, exposing P-selectin on the cell surface, where it binds white blood cells (Fig. 30-13). The importance of surface density is illustrated by an experiment in which cells that express different levels of the same cadherin are mixed together. Over time, they sort out from each other, the more adherent cells forming a cluster surrounded by the less adherent cells (Fig. 30-2). Such differential expression

cellular motility provide more examples of cellular adhesion.

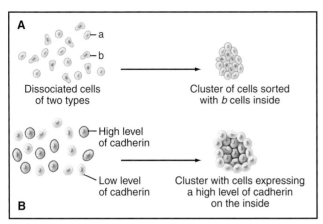

Figure 30-2 TWO EXPERIMENTS ON SORTING OF EMBRYONIC CELLS. **A,** When cells from different tissues are dissociated and mixed together, they spontaneously sort themselves into two layers, with the more adherent cells inside the less adherent cells. **B,** Cells with high concentrations of cadherin sort inside less adherent cells. (Based on the work of M. Steinberg, Princeton University, Princeton, New Jersey.)

of cadherin determines the position of the oocyte in *Drosophila* egg follicles. Intracellular signals control the extracellular binding activity of integrins and cadherins. A variety of extracellular stimuli activate intracellular signaling pathways in lymphocytes, platelets, and other cells, which enhance or inhibit the ligand-binding activity of integrins already located on the cell surface. Integrin activation also regulates cellular interactions during development.

Fourth Principle of Adhesion

The rates of ligand binding and dissociation are important determinants of cellular adhesion. Many cell surface adhesion proteins (including members of the Ig-CAM, cadherin, integrin, and selectin families) bind their ligands weakly in comparison with other specific macromolecular interactions, such as the interaction of antigens and antibodies, hormones and receptors, or transcription factors and DNA. The measured dissociation equilibrium constants for these adhesion receptors are in the range of 1 to 100 μM, reflecting high rate constants (>1 s^{-1}) for dissociation of ligand. In some cases, this makes good biological sense. Rapidly reversible interactions allow white blood cells to roll along the endothelium of blood vessels (Fig. 30-13). Transient adhesion also allows fibroblasts to migrate through connective tissue. On the other hand, the interactions of cells in epithelia and muscle appear to be more stable, perhaps owing to multiple weak interactions between clustered adhesion proteins cooperating to stabilize adherens junctions and desmosomes (Fig. 31-7). The combined strength of these bonds is said to increase the "avidity" of the interaction.

Fifth Principle of Adhesion

Many adhesion receptors interact with the cytoskeleton inside the cell. Adapter proteins link cadherins and integrins to actin filaments or intermediate filaments. These interactions provide mechanical continuity from cell to cell in muscles and epithelia, allowing them to transmit forces and resist mechanical disruption.

Sixth Principle of Adhesion

Association of ligands with adhesion receptors can activate intracellular signal transduction pathways, leading to changes in gene expression, cellular differentiation, secretion, motility, receptor activation, and cell division. Signaling through adhesion receptors allows cells to respond appropriately to physical interactions with the surrounding matrix or cells.

Identification and Characterization of Adhesion Receptors

The ability of mixed populations of cells to sort into homogeneous aggregates revealed that cells have mechanisms that are designed to bind like cells together. Similar assays showed that cells also bind matrix macromolecules, such as fibronectin, laminin, collagen, and proteoglycans. Biochemical isolation of the responsible adhesion proteins was challenging, but it progressed rapidly once it was possible to produce monoclonal antibodies that inhibit adhesion. These antibodies provided assays for purification of adhesion proteins and cloning of their cDNAs. With representatives from each family in hand, the cloning of cDNAs for related proteins was straightforward.

The modular construction of adhesion receptors makes it possible to isolate proteolytic fragments or to express one or more domains of recombinant protein suitable for structural analysis. Given sequence homologies within each family, the structures of many extracellular domains can be approximated from crystal structures of other family members.

Insights about the functions of adhesion receptors have usually come in several steps. Localization of a protein on specific cells frequently provides the first clues. Typically, the expression of each protein is restricted to a subset of cells or to a specific time during embryonic development or both. Next, investigators use specific antibodies to test for the participation of the adhesion protein in cellular interactions in vitro or in tissues. Blistering skin diseases called pemphigus illustrate the serious consequences when pathological autoantibodies disrupt adhesion between skin cells expressing the antigen (see the sections "Desmosomes" and "Adhesion to the Extracellular Matrix" in Chapter 31). Both human genetic diseases and experimental genetic knockouts in mice and other organisms produce defects caused by the absence of adhesion proteins. In leukocyte adhesion deficiency, white blood cells lack the β₂ integrin that is required to bind the endothelial cells that line blood vessels. These defective white blood cells fail to bind to blood vessel walls or to migrate into connective tissue at sites of infection. Similarly, patients with a bleeding disorder called Bernard-Soulier syndrome lack one of the adhesion receptors for von Willebrand factor, a protein that promotes platelet aggregation. Loss of cadherins contributes to the spread of some cancer cells.

Immunoglobulin Family of Cell Adhesion Molecules

The Ig-CAM family contains hundreds of adhesion proteins, each with one to seven extracellular domains, similar to immunoglobulin domains, anchored to the plasma membrane by a single transmembrane helix (Fig. 30-3 and Table 30-1). Crystal structures established the antibody-like fold of the extracellular domains of several Ig-CAMS. These compact Ig domains consist of 90 to 115 residues folded into seven to nine β-strands in two

sheets, usually stabilized by an intramolecular disulfide bond. The N- and C-termini are at opposite ends of these domains, allowing the formation of linear arrays of immunoglobulin domains.

Some Ig-CAMs consist of a single polypeptide, but others are multimeric, with two (CD8) or four (see Fig. 27-8 for the T-cell receptor) subunits. Some nervous system Ig-CAMs have three or four fibronectin III (FN-III) domains between the immunoglobulin domains and the membrane anchor. The C-terminal cytoplasmic tails of these receptors vary in sequence and binding sites. The cytoplasmic domains of the lymphocyte accessory receptors CD4 and CD8 bind protein tyrosine kinases required for cellular activation (see Fig. 27-8). The cytoplasmic domains of neuronal Ig-CAMs bind PDZ domain proteins or membrane skeleton (see Fig. 7-10).

Differentiated metazoan cells express Ig-CAMs selectively, especially during embryonic development, when they may contribute to the specificity of cellular interactions required to form the organs. Neurons and glial cells express specific Ig-CAMs that guide the growth of neurites, mediate synapse formation and promote the formation of myelin sheaths. In adults, interaction of endothelial cell ICAM-1 with a white blood cell integrin is essential for adhesion and movement of the leukocytes into the connective tissue at sites of inflammation (Fig. 30-13).

Like other cell adhesion proteins, Ig-CAMs participate in signaling processes. Best understood are interactions of lymphocytes with antigen-presenting cells during immune responses. Ig-CAMs reinforce the interaction of antigen-specific T-cell receptors with major histocompatibility complex molecules carrying appropriate antigens on other cells (see Fig. 27-8). Although individual interactions are weak, the combination of specific (T-cell receptor) and nonspecific (CD2 and CD4) interactions with the target cell is sufficient to initiate signaling.

Cadherin Family of Adhesion Receptors

The complex architecture of organs in vertebrates depends on Ca²⁺-dependent associations between the cells mediated by more than 80 cadherins (Table 30-2). Their name derives from "calcium-dependent adhesion" protein. Genes for cadherin domains appeared in unicellular precursors of sponges, an early step toward the evolution of metazoan organisms.

Cadherins generally interact with like cadherins on the surfaces of other cells in a calcium-dependent fashion, but research is uncovering a growing list of examples of heterophilic interactions. Homophilic interactions of cadherins link epithelial and muscle cells to their neighbors, especially at specialized adhesive junc-

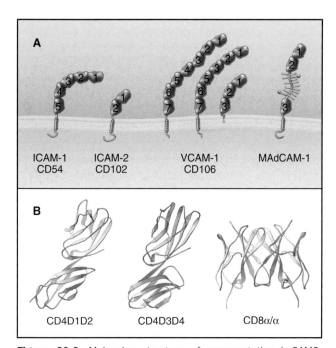

Figure 30-3 Molecular structure of representative Ig-CAMS. **A,** Domain maps of examples with their common names and CD numbers. **B,** Ribbon diagrams of the lymphocyte coreceptors CD4 (domains 1 and 2 on the *left* and domains 3 and 4 on the *right*) and CD8. (A, Reference: Springer T: Traffic signals for lymphocyte and leukocyte emigration: The multi-step paradigm. Cell 76:301–314, 1994. PDB files: 3CD4, 1CID, and 1CD8.)

Table 30-1

CELL ADHESION MOLECULES: IMMUNOGLOBULIN FAMILY*

Examples	Structure	Extracellular Ligands	Intracellular Ligands	Expression	Functions
CD2[†]	2Ig-1TM	LFA-3 (CD58)		T cells	T-cell activation
CD4[†]	4Ig-1TM	Class II MHC	Lck	T cells, macrophages	T-cell coreceptor
CD8[†]	Dimer: 1Ig-1TM	Class I MHC	Lck	Cytotoxic; other T cells	T-cell coreceptor
C-CAM	4Ig-1TM	Self		Liver, intestine, WBCs	Cell adhesion
F11 (contactin)	6Ig-4FN-II-1TM			Neurons	Neurite fasciculation
ICAM-1[†]	5Ig-1TM	LFA-1, MAC-1		Epithelia, WBCs	WBC adhesion
ICAM-2	2Ig-1TM			Endothelium, WBCs	
L1 (Ng-CAM) [mouse]	6Ig-3FN-III-1TM	Self	Ankyrin	Neurons, Schwann cells	Adhesion
LFA-3 (CD58)	2Ig-1TM or GPI anchor	CD2		WBCs, epithelia, fibroblasts	Adhesion
MAG	5Ig-1TM	Neurons		Glial cells	Myelin formation
NCAM	5Ig-3FN-III-1TM	Self		Neurons, other cells	Adhesion
Neurofascin [chick]	6Ig-4FN-III-1TM	? Self	Ankyrin	Neurites	Bundling neurites
PECAM-1 (CD31)	6Ig-1TM	Self		Platelets, endothelium, myeloid cells	Adhesion
TAG-1	6Ig-4FN-III-GPI anchor	? Self		Neurons	Neuron migration
VCAM-1	7Ig-1TM	WBC α_4 integrin		Endothelium (regulated)	WBC/endothelium adhesion

*Hundreds are known.
[†]Partial atomic structure.
CAM, cell adhesion molecule; CD, cellular differentiation antigen; FNIII, fibronectin-III domain; GPI, glycosylphosphatidylinositol; ICAM, intercellular adhesion molecule; Ig, immunoglobulin domain; Lck, nonreceptor tyrosine kinase; LFA, lymphocyte function associated antigen; MAG, myelin associated glycoprotein; MHC, major histocompatibility complex; NCAM, neural cell adhesion molecule; PECAM, platelet/endothelial cell adhesion molecule; TAG, transient axonal glycoprotein; TM, transmembrane domain; VCAM, vascular cell adhesion molecule; WBC, white blood cells.

Table 30-2

EXAMPLES OF CELL ADHESION MOLECULES: CADHERIN FAMILY*

Type (Examples)	Extracellular Ligands	Intracellular Ligands	Expression	Functions
Classic Cadherins				
E-cadherin	Self	Catenins [actin]	Epithelia, others	Adherens junctions
N-cadherin	Self	Catenins [actin]	Neurons, muscle, endothelium	Adhesion
R-cadherin	Self	Catenins [actin]	Retina, neurons	Adhesion
Desmosomal Cadherins				
Desmocollins	Self, desmogleins	Plakoglobulin [desmoplakin, lackophilin, IF]	Epithelia	Desmosomes
Desmogleins	Self, desmocolins	Plakoglobulin [desmoplakin, lackophilin, IF]	Epithelia, heart	Desmosomes
Atypical Cadherins				
T-cadherin	Self	None (GPI anchor)	Early embryos, neurons	Intercellular adhesion
Protocadherins				
α-, β-, and γ-Protocadherins	Self	Fyn tyrosine kinase (some)	Vertebrate neurons, other cells	Synapse formation
Signaling Cadherins				
RET protooncogene	Self	None	Endocrine glands, neurons	Intercellular adhesion

*More than 80 are known. Plakoglobulin is also known as γ-catenin.
GPI, glycosylphosphatidylinositol; IF, intermediate filament.

tions called **adherens junctions** and **desmosomes** (Fig. 30-4; also see Fig. 31-7). The cytoplasmic domains of cadherins interact with actin filaments or intermediate filaments to reinforce these junctions and maintain the physical integrity of tissues. Contacts mediated by cadherins also influence cellular growth and migration, including suppression of growth and invasion of tumors, as well as formation of synapses in the nervous system.

The structural hallmark of the cadherin family is the **CAD domain** (Figs. 30-5 and 30-6). CAD domains consist of about 110 residues folded into a sandwich of seven β-strands. This fold is similar to immunoglobulin and FN-III domains, but the limited sequence homology suggests independent origins and convergent evolution. N- and C-termini are on opposite ends of CAD domains. Ca^{2+} bound to three sites between adjacent CAD domains links them together into rigid rods. Without Ca^{2+}, the domains rotate freely around their linker peptides.

Many cadherins have five extracellular CAD domains. A single α-helix links classic cadherins and desmosomal cadherins to the plasma membrane, but T-cadherin has a glycosylphosphatidylinositol (GPI) anchor (see Fig. 7-9). Cytoplasmic domains vary in size, sequence, and binding sites for associated proteins. The proto-oncogene RET is a cadherin with a cytoplasmic tyrosine kinase domain.

Crystals of cadherins revealed how N-terminal CAD1 domains interact (Fig. 30-6A). A flexible strand located

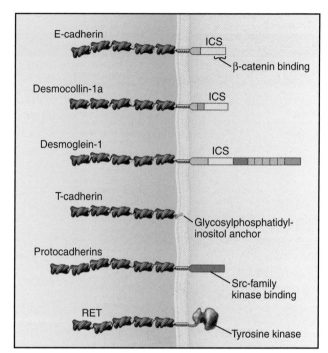

Figure 30-5 DOMAIN MAPS OF A VARIETY OF CADHERINS, ALL WITH EXTRACELLULAR CAD DOMAINS *(MAROON)* BUT DIFFERING IN THEIR MEMBRANE ANCHORS OR CYTOPLASMIC DOMAINS. Five are anchored by a single transmembrane segment; T-cadherin is anchored by a GPI tail. One has a cytoplasmic tyrosine kinase domain; three have cytoplasmic ICS domains that interact with actin filaments (E-cadherin) or intermediate filaments (desmocollin and desmoglein) via catenin adapters. Protocadherins bind Src family cytoplasmic tyrosine kinases.

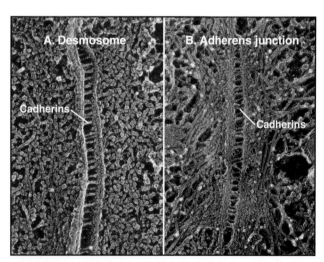

Figure 30-4 ELECTRON MICROGRAPHS OF ROD-LIKE CADHERINS CONNECTING THE PLASMA MEMBRANES OF ADJACENT CELLS. Intestinal epithelial cells were prepared by rapid freezing, freeze-fracture, deep etching, and rotary shadowing. **A,** Desmosome with associated intermediate filaments in the cytoplasm. **B,** Adherens junction with associated actin filaments. (Courtesy of N. Hirokawa, University of Tokyo, Japan. Reproduced from Hirokawa N, Heuser J: Quick-freeze, deep-etch visualization of the cytoskeleton beneath surface differentiations of intestinal epithelial cells. J Cell Biol 91:399–409, 1981, by copyright permission of The Rockefeller University Press.)

at the N-terminus of each CAD1 domain interacts with the CAD1 domain of its partner. A conserved tryptophan fits into a hydrophobic pocket of the partner CAD1 domain, forming the reciprocal interactions that link the partners together head to head. In crystals of C-cadherin, the CAD1 domains are antiparallel, suitable for a "*trans*-interaction" with a partner on another cell. In crystals of N-cadherin, this same exchange of N-terminal strands links parallel cadherins suitable for a "*cis*-interaction" with a cadherin on the same membrane. Three-dimensional reconstructions of electron micrographs of desmosomes show *trans*- and *cis*-interactions (Fig. 30-6B). Cadherins are synthesized with a small domain before the interaction strand, which must be removed by proteolysis to allow binding to another cadherin.

Cytoplasmic associations of cadherins with the cytoskeleton and adapter proteins contribute to adhesion by stabilizing the physical links between cells (Fig. 30-6C). The cytoplasmic tails of classic cadherins bind along the entire length of the adapter protein β-**catenin** (catenin is "link" in Greek), a long, twisted coil of 36 short α-helices (see Fig. 7-9F). α-**Catenin** binds both β-catenin

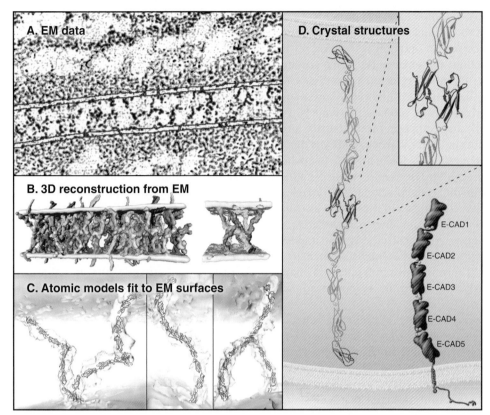

Figure 30-6 ADHESION MECHANISM OF CADHERINS. **A,** Electron micrograph of a thin section of a desmosome, colorized to emphasize the plasma membrane *(red)* and extracellular domains of the cadherins *(blue).* **B,** Three-dimensional reconstructions of the plasma membrane and the extracellular domains of the cadherins. **C,** Crystal structure of the C-cadherin extracellular domains fit into electron microscopic reconstructions of intercellular links between the cells. **D,** Ribbon diagrams of the crystal structure of a dimer of C-cadherin extracellular domains compared with the book icon for cadherins. The *inset* highlights the antiparallel intermolecular interaction of the two CAD1 domains mediated by flexible N-terminal peptides. Calcium ions *(blue)* stabilize intramolecular interactions between CAD domains. (A–C, Reprinted with permission from He W, Cowin P, Stokes DL: Untangling desmosomal knots with electron tomography. Science 302:109–113, 2003. Copyright 2003 AAAS. D, PDB file: 1L3W. Reference: Boggen TJ, Murray J, Chappuis-Flament S, et al: C-Cadherin ectodomain structure and implications for cell adhesion mechanisms. Science 296:1308–1313, 2002.)

and actin filaments, but these interactions appear to be mutually exclusive, so other proteins must help to link cadherins to actin. The more complicated cytoplasmic domains of desmosomal cadherins (desmocollins and desmogleins) interact with **γ-catenin** (a relative of β-catenin called plakoglobin) and desmoplakin. Desmoplakin links these cadherins to keratin intermediate filaments (see Fig. 31-7). The tails of some cadherins interact with formins, proteins that nucleate and elongate actin filaments (see Fig. 33-12).

Differential expression and regulation of cadherins help to guide organ formation during embryonic development (Fig. 30-7). Cells with matching cadherins bind together and exclude cells that do not share those cadherins (or other appropriate adhesion receptors), although the mechanism is more complicated than differential affinities of cadherins for each other. For example, cadherins can be activated or inactivated from inside the cell by signaling pathways that are responsive

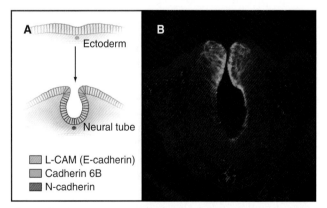

Figure 30-7 RESTRICTED EXPRESSION OF CADHERINS DURING EMBRYONIC FORMATION OF THE NEURAL TUBE. **A,** Distribution of three cadherins before and after the neural tube forms. **B,** Fluorescent antibody staining reveals the selective expression of cadherin 6B *(green)* and N-cadherin *(red)* in the neural tube of a developing chick embryo. (Courtesy of M. Takeichi, Kyoto University, Japan.)

to growth factors or other adhesion proteins. In other situations, Ig-CAMs facilitate the assembly of cadherins in adhesive junctions. In addition to helping with the mechanical sorting of embryonic cells, cadherins produce signals that influence cellular proliferation and differentiation. All cells of early embryos express several different cadherins, but as soon as the embryo forms three germ layers, the ectoderm on the outside surface expresses E-cadherin. In its absence, embryos die. Subsequently, when ectoderm folds inward to form the neural tube, the cells switch to expressing N-cadherin. Later in development, cells in specialized organs typically express characteristic cadherins, such as those in osteoblasts (OB-cadherin), kidney (K-cadherin), and muscle (M-cadherin). A giant-sized cadherin appears to form links between sensory stereocilia on the hair cells in the inner ear. These tip links pull open ion channels when the stereocilia move in response to sound waves.

Cells in the nervous system express not only classic N-cadherin but also a large family of more than 50 protocadherins. Each protocadherin has a unique extracellular domain consisting of six CAD domains encoded by a single exon. These novel regions are spliced to one of three common cytoplasmic domains that bind signaling molecules, such as the cytoplasmic tyrosine kinase Fyn, rather than catenins. Selective expression of protocadherins, alone or with N-cadherin, is thought to contribute to the specificity of synaptic connections in the central nervous system. A point mutation in one protocadherin gene is a common cause of human deafness and blindness.

Cadherins and catenins also participate in transduction of extracellular signals that control cell proliferation, migration, and differentiation. Cadherins contribute to the signal for "**contact inhibition**" of growth and motility produced when epithelial cells interact. Within a few seconds after epithelial cells contact each other, adherens junctions form. Signals originating from cadherins suppress proliferation of normal cells and inhibit the spread of cancer cells that arise due to somatic mutations. Loss of E-cadherin can contribute to the transition from benign to invasive malignant tumors. Expression of E-cadherin can correct this adhesion defect in tissue culture cells. Genetic defects in E-cadherin predispose people to stomach cancer. The oncogenic tyrosine kinase Src (see Box 27-1) phosphorylates both E-cadherin and β-catenin. This is associated with loss of adhesion of epithelial cells, suggesting one way in which transformation might alter cellular adhesion.

The **RET proto-oncogene** signals through its cytoplasmic tyrosine kinase domain (Fig. 30-5). Point mutations in the segment between the CAD domains and the plasma membrane or tyrosine kinase of RET cause dominantly inherited cancers of endocrine glands. These mutations cause constitutive dimerization of the receptor or activation of the tyrosine kinase or both, leading to neoplastic transformation. On the other hand, mutations that disable RET cause **Hirschsprung's disease.** Autonomic nerves in the wall of the intestines fail to develop, causing severe dysfunction.

β-Catenin participates in a signal transduction pathway that regulates gene expression during embryonic development (Fig. 30-8). The pathway was discovered in *Drosophila* as part of the mechanism that determines the polarity of segments in early embryos. Vertebrates have a similar pathway. Most β-catenin is bound to cadherins, but a second pool exchanges between a cytoplasmic protein complex and the nucleus. Nuclear β-catenin recruits transcription factors to regulate the expression of genes that regulate cellular proliferation and tissue differentiation. In resting cells, cytoplasmic β-catenin turns over rapidly, so little enters the nucleus. Degradation is controlled by a cytoplasmic complex that includes the product of the **APC** gene (defective in patients with familial adenomatous polyposis coli, giving rise to multiple precancerous polyps in the large intestine) and glycogen synthase kinase (GSK), a protein kinase that phosphorylates β-catenin. Phosphorylated β-catenin is ubiquinated and degraded by proteasomes. Loss of APC or mutations in the phosphorylation site on β-catenin result in excess free β-catenin that enters the nucleus and stimulates proliferation. A family of extracellular signaling proteins (19 in humans) called **Wnts** (from the original *Drosophila* gene *Wingless* and the mouse proto-oncogene *Int-1*) activate the β-catenin gene expression pathway. Wnts bind to a large extracellular domain of seven-helix receptors and another class of receptors in the plasma membrane. Several steps downstream in an incompletely characterized pathway, the Wnt signal inhibits GSK. Inhibition of GSK stops β-catenin proteolysis and raises the concentration of β-catenin that is free to enter the nucleus. Stem cell proliferation is one of many developmental events influenced by Wnt signaling and adhesion by cadherins (see Box 41-1).

Integrin Family of Adhesion Receptors

Integrins are the main cellular receptors for the ECM (Table 30-3). Certain integrins bind adhesion molecules on other cells or protein growth factors. These interactions generate signals that control cell growth and structure. Fibroblasts and white blood cells use integrins to adhere to fibronectin and collagen as they move through the ECM. Integrins bind epithelial and muscle cells to laminin in the basal lamina, providing the physical attachments necessary to transmit internal forces to the

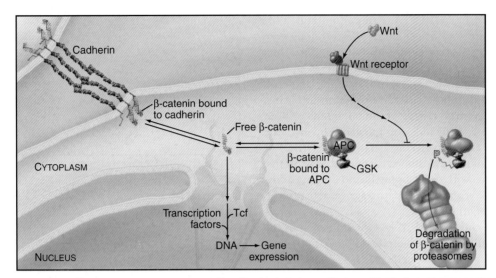

Figure 30-8 PARTICIPATION OF β-CATENIN IN GENE EXPRESSION. Free β-catenin is in equilibrium with binding sites on cadherins and APC and may also enter the nucleus, where it combines with Tcf/LEF-1 transcription factors. In the absence of β-catenin, Tcf/LEF-1 represses gene expression, but in its presence, the complex activates the expression of genes that regulate cellular growth and differentiation. The concentration of free β-catenin is determined by its rate of degradation: GSK phosphorylates β-catenin bound to APC, triggering its degradation. Extracellular Wnt acts through a seven-helix receptor and another class of receptors to promote gene expression by blocking the degradation of β-catenin through inhibition of GSK.

matrix and to resist external forces. When defects in small blood vessels need repair, integrins allow platelets to adhere to basement membrane collagen and to each other via plasma fibrinogen. Mouse sperm bind integrins on the egg membrane during fertilization. Other integrins cooperate with adhesion receptors of the Ig-CAM, mucin, and selectin families to facilitate the adhesion of white blood cells to endothelial cells at sites of inflammation. Some cells supplement integrins with structurally distinct matrix adhesion proteins, such as muscle dystroglycans and platelet GPIb-IX-V. Together, these interactions are essential for tissue development and integrity in multicellular organisms. Genetic losses of integrin function result in several human diseases.

Table 30-3

CELL ADHESION MOLECULES: INTEGRIN FAMILY*

Examples	Structure	Extracellular Ligands	Me²⁺	Intracellulars Ligands	Expression	Function
Fibronectin receptors	$\alpha_5\beta_1$, others	Fibronectin	Ca	Talin, paxillin	Fibroblasts, other cells	Cell-matrix adhesion
GPIIb/GPIIIa	$\alpha IIb\beta_3$	Fibrinogen, von Willebrand	Ca	Talin, paxillin	Platelets	Platelet aggregation
Laminin receptor	$\alpha_6\beta_1$, $\alpha_7\beta_1$	Laminin	Yes	Talin, paxillin	Epithelia, muscle	Cell-matrix adhesion
LFA-1[†] (CD11/CD18)	$\alpha L\beta_2$	Ig-CAM-1, -2, -3	Mg	Talin, paxillin	All WBCs	WBC/endothelium adhesion
MAC-1[†]	$\alpha M\beta_2$	Ig-CAM-1, fibrinogen	Yes	Talin, paxillin	WBCs except lymphocytes	WBC/endothelium adhesion
Vitronectin receptor[†]	$\alpha V\beta_3$	Vitronectin, fibronectin	Ca	Talin, paxillin	Endothelium, smooth muscle, others	
VLA-4[†]	$\alpha_2\beta_1$	Collagen, laminin	Mg	Talin, paxillin	WBCs, epithelium, endothelium	WBC/matrix adhesion

*24 are known.

[†]Partial atomic structure.

CD, cellular differentiation antigen; GP, glycoprotein; ICAM, intercellular adhesion molecule; LFA, lymphocyte function associated antigen; Me²⁺, divalent cation dependence; VLA, very late antigen; WBC, white blood cell.

Integrins tend to be more promiscuous than most adhesion receptors, as some bind to several protein ligands, and many matrix molecules bind to more than one integrin. For example, fibronectin binds to at least nine different integrins, and both laminin and von Willebrand's factor bind at least five different integrins. This promiscuity may reflect common motifs. About one third of matrix ligands for integrins involve the sequence motif arginine-glycine-aspartic acid (RGD) or other simple sequences in otherwise unrelated proteins. Multiple integrins with overlapping ligand-binding activity provide cells with diverse pathways to activate different signaling pathways.

Integrins are heterodimers of two transmembrane polypeptides called α- and β-chains, which both contribute to ligand-binding specificity (Fig. 30-9). Vertebrate cells use a combinatorial strategy to establish their integrin repertoire by selectively expressing a subset of 18 different α-chains and 8 β-chains. These chains combine to form at least 24 different kinds of dimers, each with different ligand-binding specificity. Alternative mRNA splicing (see Fig. 16-6) also adds to the diversity of integrin isoforms.

With the exception of red blood cells, integrins are present in the plasma membranes of most animal cells, including sponges and corals from phyla that branched early in evolution (see Fig. 2-9). Many vertebrate cells express β_1 and β_3 integrins for adhesion to the ECM. Only white blood cells express β_2 integrins, which they use to bind endothelial cells lining the walls of blood vessels. Only platelets express α_{IIb} integrins, important receptors for soluble adhesive ligands in plasma, such as fibrinogen.

The ligand-binding domains of the α- and β-chains form a globular head connected to the plasma membrane by 16-nm legs (Fig. 30-9). All integrin β-chains and a subset of integrin α-chains have an I-domain (inserted domain) with a bound divalent cation that interacts with acidic residues of ligands. All α-chains have an N-terminal β-propeller domain similar to a Gβ subunit of a trimeric G protein (see Fig. 25-9). Interaction of the α-chain propeller domain with the β-chain I-domain holds the integrin dimer together, remarkably like the interaction between Gα and Gβ subunits of trimeric G-proteins. Ligands bind to both the I-domains and the β-propeller. Single transmembrane segments anchor both integrin chains to the cell. Short (α ≤ 77 residues; β = 40 to 60 residues, except β_4 = 1000 residues) C-terminal cytoplasmic tails contribute to efficient heterodimer assembly. Tail sequences of homologous chains are conserved between species, and several have important roles in signal transduction.

Both α- and β-chains participate in binding at least two sites on ligands. Integrin $\alpha_5\beta_1$ binds two sites on

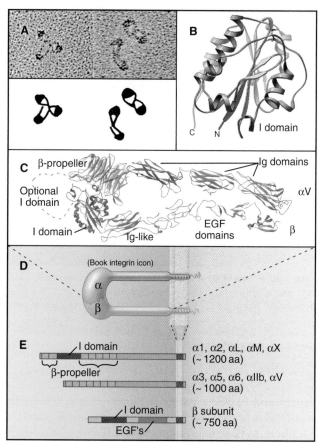

Figure 30-9 INTEGRIN ARCHITECTURE. **A,** Electron micrographs and interpretative drawings of isolated integrin molecules. **B,** Ribbon model of the I-domain from integrin α_L with the bound divalent cation (manganese in this experiment, shown in *red*) at the top. The incomplete coordination shell of this divalent cation is completed by oxygens from the side chains of ligands, such as the aspartic acid in RGD peptides. **C,** Model of integrin $\alpha_V\beta_3$ based on an atomic structure of the extracellular domain. The I-domain is inserted into the sequence of an immunoglobulin-like domain. **D,** Integrin icon used throughout this book. **E,** Domain models of integrin polypeptides. Both α-chains and β-chains have single transmembrane segments and cytoplasmic tails that vary in length. All β-chains and some α-chains have an I-domain *(red)* that binds a divalent cation and participates in ligand binding. The seven blades of the α-chain beta-propeller domains are shown in *orange*. The α-chain I-domain, if present, is inserted between the second and third of the seven blades of its propeller domain. (A, From Nermut MV, Green NM, Eason P, et al: Electron microscopy and structural model of human fibronectin receptor. EMBO J 7:4093–4099, 1988. B, Courtesy of D. Leahy, Johns Hopkins Medical School, Baltimore, Maryland. PDB file: 1LFA. C, Based on an atomic model. PDB file: 1JV2. Reference: Xiong JP, Stehle T, Diefenbach B, et al: Crystal structure of the extracellular segment of integrin $\alpha_V\beta_3$. Science 294:339–345, 2001. E, Redrawn from Kuhn K, Eble J: The structural basis of integrin-ligand interactions. Trends Cell Biol 4:256–261, 1994.)

fibronectin: an RGD sequence on a surface loop of FN-III domain 10 and a secondary site on the adjacent FN-III domain 9 (see Fig. 29-15). Neither site is sufficient for binding, so simple RGD peptides can dissociate fibronectin. Integrin binding sites of some ligands are on

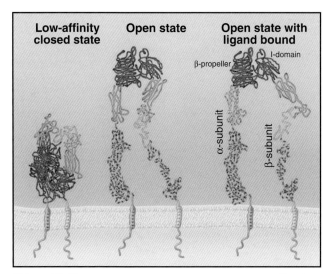

Low-affinity closed state **Open state** **Open state with ligand bound**

Figure 30-10 CONFORMATIONAL STATES OF INTEGRINS. Drawings based on atomic models derived from crystal structures and electron microscopy. Binding of either an extracellular ligand to the head or activated signal transduction proteins to the cytoplasmic domains can favor the open state. (Redrawn by permission from Macmillan Publishers Ltd. from Xiao T, Takagi J, Coller BS, et al: Structural basis for allostery in integrins and binding to fibrinogen-mimetic therapeutics. Nature 432:59–67, 2004, copyright 2004.)

separate polypeptide chains. The RDD binding site for integrin $\alpha_1\beta_1$ is on three different polypeptide chains of the type IV collagen triple helix.

Ligands on both sides of the plasma membrane influence the conformations of integrins (Fig. 30-10). The open state has the highest affinity for extracellular ligands, with the head held above the membrane by extended, widely placed legs. The closed state has a low affinity for extracellular ligands, with the head bent over on closely spaced legs. Binding of extracellular ligands stabilizes the open state, and the wide spacing of the cytoplasmic domains presumably influences the activities of signal transduction proteins associated with the cytoplasmic domains. Operating in the opposite direction, "inside-out signals" can influence the affinity of integrins for extracellular ligands by favoring the open state.

Even in the open state, integrins generally have a low affinity for extracellular ligands. For example, the micromolar K_d for integrin $\alpha_5\beta_1$ binding fibronectin results in rapid association and dissociation, allowing cells to adjust their grip on fibronectin in the matrix as they move through connective tissue. Nonadhesive RGD proteins, such as tenascin (see Fig. 29-17), may modulate these interactions by competing with fibronectin and other ligands for binding integrins.

Cytoplasmic tails of integrins interact directly or indirectly with a remarkable variety of signaling and structural proteins (Fig. 30-11). These interactions are best

understood at **focal contacts,** specialized sites where integrins cluster together to transduce transmembrane signals and link actin filaments to the ECM. The adapter proteins **talin** and **vinculin** link the cytoplasmic domains of β integrins to actin filaments at the ends of stress fibers. Talin transmits signals that activate integrins from the cytoplasm. **Paxillin** links integrins to signaling proteins, forming a scaffold for Src family tyrosine kinases (see Fig. 25-3) and **focal adhesion kinase** (a novel tyrosine kinase lacking SH2 and SH3 domains).

Integrin binding to matrix ligands initiates signals that modify cellular adhesion, locomotion, and gene expression. The responses depend on the particular integrin and cell but include the following:

1. Within seconds, cytoplasmic tyrosine kinases phosphorylate several focal adhesion proteins, including paxillin, tensin, and focal adhesion kinase.

2. Within a minute, some cells raise their cytoplasmic Ca^{2+} concentration high enough to initiate many calcium-dependent processes (see Chapter 26).

3. Over a period of minutes, cells in culture spread out on ligand-coated surfaces rearrange their cytoskeleton, and begin to move (see Fig. 38-7). Integrins cluster together in small "focal complexes" at the leading edge and grow into mature focal contacts (Fig. 30-11A), also called *focal adhesions,* which anchor actin filament stress fibers to the cell membrane. Contraction of stress fibers applies tension to the focal contacts, which remain stationary as the cell advances past them. A Ca^{2+}-mediated signal inactivates obsolete attachments at the rear of the cell. The adhesiveness of a cell for its substrate (a function of integrin density on the cell, ligand density on the substratum, and their affinity) determines the rate of movement. The maximum rate occurs at intermediate adhesiveness. Rapid association and dissociation of integrins on matrix ligands allow cells to rearrange their hold on the matrix as they move. Rho-family GTPases regulating actin assembly and contraction (see Fig. 33-20) coordinate protrusion of the leading edge and withdrawal of the tail.

4. In an hour, the pH of the cytoplasm rises, owing to the activation of an Na^+/H^+ antiporter (see Chapter 9).

5. After several hours, activation of the Ras/mitogen-activated protein kinase pathway (see Fig. 27-6) turns on the expression of selected genes. In the long term, these changes in gene expression contribute to cellular differentiation during development. Other stimuli operating through different

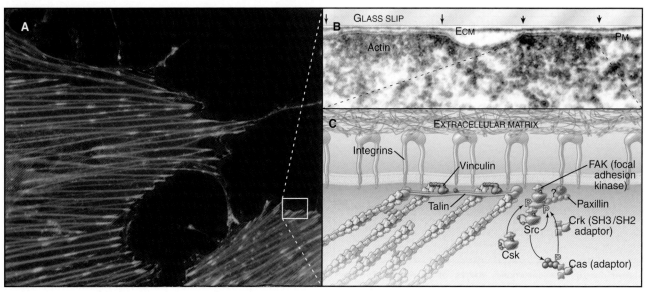

Figure 30-11 FOCAL CONTACTS OF EPITHELIAL CELLS WITH THE EXTRACELLULAR MATRIX. **A,** Fluorescence micrograph of parts of two vertebrate tissue culture cells with focal contacts labeled with a fluorescent antibody to phosphotyrosine *(orange)*. Actin filament stress fibers are stained *green* with phalloidin. **B,** Electron micrograph of a thin section of two focal contacts showing fine connections to the ECM deposited on the surface of the glass coverslip and cross sections of actin filaments in the cytoplasm. This HeLa cell was grown on a glass coverslip, fixed, and cut perpendicular to the substrate. **C,** Drawing of the interactions of some of the proteins concentrated on the cytoplasmic face of the membrane at focal contacts. For clarity, the actin filament interactions *(left)* are shown separately from some signaling proteins *(right)*. The short cytoplasmic domains of β-integrins interact with multiple sites on the dimeric protein talin. Vinculin interacts with membrane phospholipids, actin filaments, and talin. An unidentified protein (the question mark) links the adapter protein paxillin to integrins. Paxillin anchors tyrosine kinases (FAK and Src) and, after phosphorylation, the adapter proteins Crk and Cas. (A, Courtesy of K. Burridge, University of North Carolina, Chapel Hill. B, Courtesy of Pamela Maupin, Johns Hopkins University, Baltimore, Maryland. Reproduced from Maupin P, Pollard TD: Improved preservation and staining of HeLa cell actin filaments. J Cell Biol 96:51–62, 1983. Copyright 1983 The Rockefeller University Press. C, References: Turner C: Paxillin and focal adhesion signaling. Nature Cell Biol 2:E231–E236, 2000; Critchley DR: Focal adhesions—the cytoskeletal connection. Curr Opin Cell Biol 12:133–139, 2000.)

receptors can activate most of these cellular responses. Integrins allow cells to include the ECM as an input that affects their behavior.

As in other signaling systems (see Chapters 24 and 27), conformational changes (Fig. 30-10) or physical aggregation of integrins may activate focal adhesion kinase and other associated kinases by bringing them close enough together to transphosphorylate each other. Aggregation of integrins by multivalent extracellular ligands or force on the integrins promotes interaction of integrin cytoplasmic domains with the dimeric protein talin. Talin in turn interacts with actin filaments, as well as with multiple signal transduction proteins (Fig. 30-11C). Ligand binding to integrins also activates Rho-family GTPases. Focal adhesion kinase has a central role in transducing these signals. Mouse mutants that lack focal adhesion kinase die during development, but surprisingly, their cells assemble focal contacts with high levels of tyrosine-phosphorylated proteins.

Several types of integrins associate laterally, in the plane of the bilayer, with other transmembrane proteins. The best characterized of the latter is CD47 (integrin-associated protein), an Ig-CAM with five transmembrane segments. Binding of the adhesive glycoprotein, thrombospondin, to the extracellular immunoglobulin-like domain of CD47 generates a transmembrane signal through trimeric G-proteins that contributes to neutrophil and platelet activation.

Integrins also participate in the decision of cells to undergo apoptosis, programmed cell death (see Chapter 46). Normal epithelial cells require anchorage to the basal lamina by β4 integrins to grow and divide. When forced to live in suspension or when dissociated from the matrix by RGD peptides, these cells arrest in the G1 phase of the cell cycle (see Chapter 41) and eventually undergo apoptosis. Anchorage by other adhesion proteins will not substitute for integrins. Loss of contact with the basal lamina may contribute to the terminal differentiation and death of cells in the upper levels of stratified epithelia, such as skin (see Figs. 35-6 and 40-1). Epithelial cancers typically lose this integrin-mediated, anchorage dependence for growth, one of the normal limitations on uncontrolled proliferation in inappropriate locations.

Integrins not only participate in signal transduction but are also controlled by three different mechanisms, operating in different time domains.

1. Cells fine-tune their interactions with the matrix on a fast time scale by regulating the activity of cell surface integrins. Integrins on white blood cells (Fig. 30-13) and platelets (Fig. 30-14) require "inside-out" activation by an intracellular signal before binding their ligands.

2. In minutes, some cells mobilize a reserve pool of integrins stored in cytoplasmic vesicles. For example, chemoattractants stimulate white blood cells to fuse storage vesicles containing integrins with the plasma membrane (Fig. 30-13).

3. Over hours or days, developmental programs establish the basic integrin repertoire. Growth factors such as transforming growth factor-β (TGF-β [see Fig. 24-8]) also influence integrin expression by differentiated cells.

Experiments with neutralizing antibodies and competitive peptides provided initial clues about the functions of integrins, but genetic diseases and experimental gene disruptions provide more definitive answers. For example, RGD peptides and integrin antibodies inhibit cell migration and embryonic development by competing with fibronectin. Like null mutations in fibronectin (see Fig. 29-15), homozygous disruption of the integrin α_4 or α_5 genes is lethal during development. Cells that lack these integrins can form focal contacts in vitro, but fibronectin receptors using other α subunits cannot substitute for α_5 in vivo. Dysfunction of β_2 integrins is not lethal, but patients are highly susceptible to infections, owing to defects in the emigration of white blood cells from the blood at sites of infection (Fig. 30-13).

Snake venoms contain small, monomeric RGD proteins that inhibit blood clotting by competing with fibrinogen for binding the integrins that activated platelets use for aggregation. These "disintegrins" are potential inhibitors of the pathological thrombosis that contributes to heart attacks and strokes. Both small-molecule and antibody antagonists for integrins are now used as clinical treatments for heart attacks and stroke.

Selectin Family of Adhesion Receptors

White blood cells and platelets use selectins to interact with vascular endothelial cells. In lymph nodes or at sites of inflammation, selectins snare circulating white blood cells, allowing them to roll over the surface of endothelial cells and eventually to exit the blood (Fig. 30-13). Selectins (Table 30-4) contribute to adhesion in other systems, including the initial binding of early mammalian embryos to the wall of the mother's uterus.

The defining feature of selectins is a calcium-dependent lectin domain (Fig. 30-12) that binds O-linked sulfated oligosaccharides containing sialic acid and fucose. The lectin domain sits at the end of a rod-shaped projection that is anchored to the plasma membrane by a single transmembrane sequence.

Natural ligands for selectins are mucin-like glycoproteins expressed on endothelial and white blood cells. Selective binding to mucins requires selectins to interact with both the oligosaccharide and mucin protein. The lectin domains bind mucin oligosaccharides, but the affinity is low (millimolar K_ds), and they do not discriminate among oligosaccharides. Interaction with the mucin protein is less well understood, but one or more sulfated tyrosine residues on the leukocyte mucin called PSGL-1 participate in binding P-selectin.

Bonds between selectins and their mucin ligands have high tensile strength (withstanding forces over 100 pN) but form and dissociate rapidly, on a second time scale. Low forces on these bonds prolong their lifetimes modestly, whereas high forces promote dissociation. Consequently, few selectin-mucin bonds are required to tether white blood cells to the endothelium, whereas the brief lifetime of the bonds allows blood flow to propel the cells with a rolling motion over the surface of the endothelium (Fig. 30-13).

Inflammatory mediators regulate selectins in several different ways. Activation of endothelial cells with histamine or platelets with thrombin causes vesicles storing

Table 30-4

CELL ADHESION MOLECULES: SELECTIN FAMILY (LEC-CAM)

Examples	Structure	Extracellular Ligands	Me²⁺	Expression	Functions
E-selectin* (CD62E, ELA)	Lectin-EGF-6CR-1TM	L-selectin	Ca	Endothelium (regulated)	WBC-endothelium adhesion
L-selectin (CD62L, gp90M)	Lectin-EGF-2CR-1TM	E-selectin, mucins	Ca	Lymphocytes, other WBCs	WBC-endothelium adhesion
P-selectin (CD62P, GMP-14)	Lectin-EGF-9CR-1TM	Mucins	Ca	Endothelium, platelets	WBC-endothelium adhesion

*Partial atomic structure.

CD, cellular differentiation antigen; CR, complement regulatory domain; EGF, epidermal growth factor; Me²⁺, divalent cation dependence; TM, transmembrane domain; WBC, white blood cell.

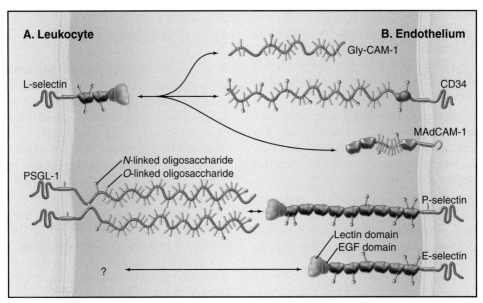

Figure 30-12 STRUCTURE OF SELECTINS AND THEIR MUCIN LIGANDS. Domain architecture of selectins and mucins exposed on the surfaces of leukocytes **(A)** and endothelial cells **(B).** Complement regulatory domains of the selectins are shown in *red*. (Redrawn and modified from Rosen SD, Bertozzi CR: The selectins and their ligands. Curr Opin Cell Biol 6:663–673, 1994.)

P-selectin to fuse with the plasma membrane, exposing the selectin on the cell surface. Various inflammatory agents stimulate endothelial cells to synthesize E-selectin and P-selectin. Activation of white blood cells increases the affinity of L-selectin for mucins and later leads to its proteolytic release from the cell surface. Furthermore, selectin binding to mucins initiates intracellular signals that result in Ca^{2+} release inside the cell.

Other Adhesion Receptors

Table 30-5 lists a variety of adhesion receptors that fall outside the four main families. See Chapter 25 for CD45 and Chapter 31 for connexins.

Mucins

The extracellular segments of mucins are rich in serine and threonine, which are heavily modified with acidic oligosaccharide chains (Fig. 30-12). Because of their strong negative charge, these proteins extend like rods up to 50 nm from the cell surface. Mucins on endothelial cells or white blood cells interact with complementary selectins on the other cell type. Endothelial mucin CD34 interacts with white blood cell L-selectin, whereas endothelial P-selectin interacts with white blood cell PSGL-1 mucin. This interaction depends on anchoring of the cytoplasmic domain of PSGL-1 to the actin cyto-

skeleton. Other mucins are displayed on the surface of or secreted by epithelia lining the respiratory and gastrointestinal tracks.

Galactosyltransferase

One enzyme, galactosyltransferase, is also an adhesion receptor. This enzyme is usually considered in another context: protein glycosylation in the Golgi apparatus (see Chapter 21). However, the messenger RNA (mRNA) for galactosyltransferase has two alternative initiation sites, one of which adds 13 amino acids to the cytoplasmic, N-terminus of this transmembrane protein. The longer enzyme moves to the cell surface rather than being retained in the Golgi apparatus. On the cell surface, the enzyme can bind oligosaccharides that terminate in *N*-acetylglucosamine. These ligands are found on both cell surface and matrix proteins. The complex of transferase and ligand oligosaccharide is stable, because the galactose-nucleotide substrate added to the oligosaccharide in the Golgi apparatus is not available outside the cell to complete the reaction. During fertilization, a surface galactosyltransferase mediates the initial contact of mouse sperm with the matrix surrounding the egg (called the zona pellucida). This association induces secretion of the contents of the sperm acrosomal vesicle, including an enzyme that destroys the transferase binding site on the matrix so that the sperm can proceed through the zona to fuse with the egg. The enzyme is present on the

Table 30-5

OTHER CELL ADHESION MOLECULES

Examples	Structure	Extracellular Ligands	Me^{2+}	Intracellular Ligands	Expression	Functions
CD44	Link protein-1TM	Hyaluronan		Ankyrin	Lymphocytes	Adhesion to endothelium
CD44E	Link protein-HS/CS-1TM	Fibronectin, hyaluronan	No		Many epithelial cells	Adhesion to matrix
Connexin	Multispan, hexamer	Self	No		Epithelia, muscle, nerve	Gap junctions
Dystroglycans	Multi-subunit, TM	Laminin, agrin	Ca	Dystrophin	Muscle	Adhesion, synapse format
Galactosyl-transferase	Galactose transferase-1TM	*N*-acetylglucosamine	No	? Actin filaments	Many cells, including sperm	Adhesion to cells and matrix
Glypican	4HS-GPI anchor	Fibronectin, collagen I	No	None	Endothelium, small muscle, epithelium	Adhesion to matrix
GPIB-IX	7 leucine-rich-1TM	von Willebrand factor		Filamin, actin	Platelets, endothelium	Adhesion
LCA (CD45)	50kD-1TM-tyrosine phosphatase				WBCs	Tyrosine phosphatase
Mucins (CD34, CD43)	Sialylated oligosaccharide-1TM	Selectins	No		Epithelia, leukocytes	Intercellular adhesion

CD, cellular differentiation antigen; CS, chondroitin sulfate; GPI, glycosylphosphatidylinositol; HS, heparan sulfate; LCA, leukocyte common antigen; Me^{2+}, divalent cation dependence; TM, transmembrane domain; WBC, white blood cell.

surface of many cells that migrate during embryogenesis and may contribute to their interactions with the matrix.

Adhesion Receptors with Leucine-Rich Repeats (GPIb-IX-V)

The platelet receptor for the adhesive glycoprotein called von Willebrand factor (Fig. 30-14) is a disulfide-bonded complex of four transmembrane polypeptides: GPIbα GPIbβ, GPIX, and GPV. Leucine-rich repeats at the end of a long stalk bind von Willebrand factor (see Fig. 24-12 for another example of receptors with leucine-rich repeats). Platelets bind to von Willebrand factor to initiate the repair of damaged blood vessels. This interaction also generates an intracellular signal that enhances affinity of integrin α$_{IIb}$β$_3$ for fibrinogen and reorganizes the cytoskeleton.

Dystroglycan/Sarcoglycan Complex

In muscles, a complex of transmembrane glycoproteins links a network of dystrophin and actin filaments on the inside of the plasma membrane to two proteins of the extracellular basal lamina, α2 laminin and agrin (see Fig. 39-9 and Table 39-2). These protein associations stabilize the muscle plasma membrane from inside and

outside. This muscle membrane skeleton resembles in concept and function the actin-spectrin network of red blood cells (see Fig. 7-10). Genetic defects or deficiencies in dystrophin, transmembrane linker proteins of the dystroglycan/sarcoglycan complex, or α2 laminin cause muscular dystrophy in humans, most likely owing to the mechanical instability of the membrane, leading to cellular damage and eventual atrophy of the muscle. Chapter 39 provides details on their role in muscle function and disease. In other tissues, nonmuscle cells express many of these proteins (or their homologs), where they may contribute to adhesion to the ECM. Some pathogens use the dystroglycan complex to bind their cellular targets. Arenavirus, the cause of Lassa fever, binds directly to α-dystroglycan, and the leprosy bacterium binds laminin-2.

Examples of Dynamic Adhesion

Cellular Adhesion between Leukocytes and Endothelial Cells in Response to Inflammation

Movement of white blood cells from blood to sites of inflammation in connective tissue illustrates how cells integrate the activities of selectins, mucins, integrins, Ig-CAMs, and chemoattractant receptors. Infection or

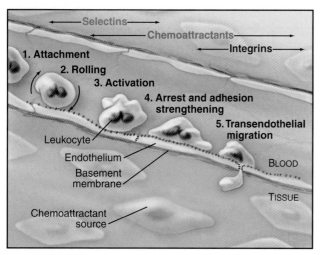

Figure 30-13 FIVE STEPS IN THE MIGRATION OF A NEUTROPHIL FROM THE BLOOD TO THE CONNECTIVE TISSUE. Endothelial cells exposed to inflammatory agents like histamine expose selectins on their surface and snare mucins on neutrophils flowing in the bloodstream (1). As a neutrophil rolls along the surface (2), chemotactic factors activate their integrins (3), causing the neutrophil to bind tightly to Ig-CAMs on the endothelium (4). The neutrophil then migrates between the endothelial cells into the connective tissue (5). (Reference: Springer T: Traffic signals for lymphocyte and leukocyte emigration: The multi-step paradigm. Cell 76:301–314, 1994.)

inflammation in connective tissue attracts lymphocytes as well as neutrophils and monocytes, the main phagocytes circulating in blood (see Fig. 28-7).

In the absence of inflammation, neutrophils flow rapidly over the surface of endothelial cells but do not bind to them because the appropriate pairs of adhesion molecules are not exposed or activated or both. Infection or other inflammation in nearby tissues causes neutrophils to bind to the vascular endothelium and to move out of the blood into the tissue. Neutrophils adhere to the endothelium in three sequential but overlapping steps (Fig. 30-13):

1. Locally generated inflammatory chemicals, including histamine (secreted by mast cells), bind to seven-helix receptors on endothelial cells and stimulate fusion of cytoplasmic vesicles (called Weibel-Palade bodies) with the plasma membrane. This exposes P-selectin, formerly stored in the vesicle membranes, on the cell surface facing the blood. Selectins bind mucins that are constitutively exposed on the surface of neutrophils, tethering them to the surface in less than 1 ms. The bonds form and break rapidly, allowing the neutrophil to roll along the surface of the endothelium at rates greater than 10 µm/s as the blood flow pushes them along.

2. Chemotactic factors bind seven-helix receptors on the surface of the leukocyte and activate integrins

from inside the cell (Fig. 30-10). A signal transduction pathway downstream of trimeric G-proteins activates about 10% of the neutrophil integrins, increasing their affinity for their ligand by 200-fold. This makes the third step possible.

3. Activated integrins bind tightly to Ig-CAMs on the surface of endothelial cells, immobilizing the leukocyte despite the force of the blood flow. Within 2 minutes, the leukocyte crawls between endothelial cells into connective tissue toward the source of the chemoattractant. The leukocyte and endothelial cells interact closely during this passage because they share a self-associating Ig-CAM called PECAM.

Defects in either the weak or strong interactions compromise the movement of leukocytes into connective tissue, increasing the risk of acute and chronic infections. One type of human leukocyte adhesion deficiency is caused by a genetic defect in fucose metabolism that interferes with the synthesis of a carbohydrate ligand on leukocytes that binds endothelial selectins. Cells cannot roll, so they fail to initiate the emigration process. A genetic deficiency of β_2 integrins causes a second type of leukocyte adhesion deficiency. White blood cells that lack β_2 integrins roll on the endothelium through the selectin mechanism but do not bind tightly enough to migrate out of the circulation. Consequently, these individuals are susceptible to bacterial infections.

On the other hand, neutrophils are double-edged swords because they also generate reactive oxygen species that can damage tissues at sites of inflammation or at sites that are temporarily deprived of oxygen. Thus, movement of white blood cells into tissues contributes to damage that occurs when blood flow is restored to an ischemic tissue. In the future, drugs or monoclonal antibodies targeted to adhesion proteins might be therapeutically useful to mitigate damage after heart attacks or severe frostbite.

A similar mechanism and a partially overlapping set of receptors attract blood monocytes and eosinophils to sites of inflammation. Once they are in connective tissue, interactions of monocyte integrins with matrix molecules trigger the expression of genes required for differentiation into macrophages (see Chapter 28).

Lymphocytes (see Fig. 28-9) patrol the body, circulating from the blood through organs to lymphoid tissues and through the lymphatic circulation back to the blood. This "recirculation" requires lymphocytes to recognize endothelial cells in organs and specific lymphoid tissues where they exit from the blood. Lymphocytes use L-selectin, three different mucin-like proteins, and $\alpha_4\beta_2$ integrins to bind to these target endothelial cells. Lymphocytes from mice that lack L-selectin do not roll on endothelial cells or accumulate in lymph nodes.

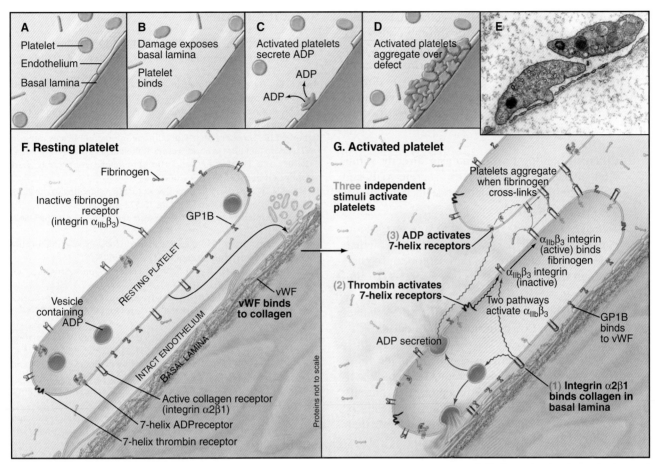

Figure 30-14 PLATELET ACTIVATION AND AGGREGATION AT THE SITE OF A DEFECT IN THE ENDOTHELIUM. **A–D,** Steps in platelet activation and aggregation. **E,** Electron micrograph of a thin section of a platelet adhering to the basal lamina through a tiny defect in the endothelium. **F,** Resting platelets circulate in the blood without interacting with the intact endothelium lining the vessel. **G,** Platelets are activated in three ways: Binding of $\alpha_2\beta_1$ integrins to collagen results in firm adhesion *(1)*. Where the basal lamina is exposed, von Willebrand factor (vWF) binds the collagen; platelet GP1B-IX binds weakly to von Willebrand factor, allowing platelets to adhere to the exposed matrix *(2)*. Thrombin activates seven-helix receptors *(3)*. These interactions stimulate secretion of ADP, which binds seven-helix receptors and activates the $\alpha_{IIb}\beta_3$ integrins; then $\alpha_{IIb}\beta_3$ integrins bind dimeric fibrinogen and aggregate platelets together. Platelet proteins are not to scale.

Antibodies that block α_4 integrins mitigate inflammation in the autoimmune disease multiple sclerosis by interfering with movement of lymphocytes into the brain, although side effects have limited their widespread use.

Platelet Activation and Adhesion

Platelets aggregate at sites where damage to vascular endothelial cells exposes the underlying basal lamina (Fig. 30-14). This process requires the coordinated activity of a variety of receptors, including integrins, leucine-rich repeat adhesion proteins, and seven-helix receptors. These reactions prevent bleeding and bruising, but inappropriate activation of platelets produces clots in blood vessels, causing heart attacks and strokes. To understand the good effects and avert the bad, investigators have studied platelet activation and adhesion in great detail.

Resting platelets have a low tendency to aggregate, even though they circulate in a sea of ligands, including fibrinogen and the adhesive glycoprotein von Willebrand factor. Multiple mechanisms limit the reactivity of resting platelets, where the major integrin, $\alpha_{IIb}\beta_3$, has a low affinity ($K_d \gg \mu M$) for its plasma ligand, fibrinogen. Similarly, the GPIb-IX-V complex has a low affinity for the soluble von Willebrand factor. Third, the endothelium masks potential ligands, collagen, and von Willebrand factor in the basal lamina. The concentrations of soluble activators, such as adenosine diphosphate (ADP) and thrombin, are low under physiological conditions.

Damage to the endothelium usually initiates platelet activation by exposing platelets to von Willebrand factor and collagen in the basal lamina. Under conditions of high shear, GPIb-IX-V interacts strongly with von Willebrand factor bound to basal lamina collagen. This interaction transiently tethers platelets to the basal lamina and favors binding of integrin $\alpha_2\beta_1$ to collagen. Exposure to soluble agonists such as ADP or thrombin also activates platelets and promotes their aggregation. Within seconds of activation, platelet $\alpha_{IIb}\beta_3$ integrins convert to a high-affinity state ($K_d < \mu$M) and bind tightly to fibrinogen. Dimeric fibrinogen links platelets into aggregates.

Agonists activate platelet $\alpha_{IIb}\beta_3$ integrins through three different pathways:

1. Collagen binding to $\alpha_2\beta_1$ integrin directly stimulates platelets to activate $\alpha_{IIb}\beta_3$, secrete ADP, and synthesize the lipid second messenger thromboxane A_2 (see Fig. 26-9).

2. Damage to blood vessels activates the blood-clotting proteolytic enzyme thrombin, which binds two related seven-helix receptors and signals through trimeric G-proteins (see Fig. 25-9) to activate $\alpha_{IIb}\beta_3$.

3. von Willebrand factor binding to the platelet receptor GPIb-IX-V activates $\alpha_{IIb}\beta_3$ integrins.

Two additional mechanisms augment all of these responses. Activated platelets secrete ADP, which activates two types of seven-helix receptors that amplify the response to thrombin. Aggregation of platelets by binding dimeric fibrinogen further stimulates their response to ADP and thrombin.

Platelet aggregation is disadvantageous in the normal circulation, so several mechanisms actively inhibit platelet activation. Endothelial cells produce both nitric oxide and an eicosanoid, prostacyclin (PGI_2), which inhibit platelet activation (see Fig. 26-9). Nitric oxide acts through cyclic guanosine monophosphate (cGMP), and prostacyclin acts through cyclic adenosine monophosphate (cAMP; see Fig. 26-1). Drugs that inhibit $\alpha_{IIb}\beta_3$ are being tested to treat heart attacks.

The most common human bleeding disorder is von Willebrand disease, caused by mutations in von Willebrand factor or its receptor, the GPIbα subunit of GPIb-IX-V. Some mutations reduce the concentration of the factor in blood or reduce the affinity of the factor for its receptor. Remarkably, mutations in either the factor or receptor that increase their affinity for each other also cause bleeding. These high-affinity interactions cause platelets to aggregate and be removed from the blood. Loss-of-function mutations in GPIbα cause the human bleeding disorder called Bernard-Soulier syndrome. Individuals with Glanzmann's thrombasthenia bleed abnormally because $\alpha_{IIb}\beta_3$ integrin is absent or defective, and their platelets do not aggregate.

ACKNOWLEDGMENTS

Thanks go to Barry Gumbiner for his suggestions on revisions to this chapter.

SELECTED READINGS

Arnaout MA, Mahalingam B, Xiong J-P: Integrin structure, allostery and bidirectional signaling. Annu Rev Cell Dev Biol 21:381–410, 2005.

Brown EJ, Fraizer WA: Integrin-associated protein (CD47) and its ligands. Trends Cell Biol 11:130–135, 2001.

Burridge K, Chrzanowska-Wodnicka M: Focal adhesions, contractility and signaling. Annu Rev Cell Dev Biol 12:463–519, 1996.

Campbell ID, Ginsberg MH: The talin-tail interaction places integrin activation on FERM ground. Trends Biochem Sci 29:429–435, 2004.

Critchley DR: Focal adhesions: The cytoskeletal connection. Curr Opin Cell Biol 12:133–139, 2000.

DeMali KA, Wennerberg K, Burridge K: Integrin signaling to the actin cytoskeleton. Curr Opin Cell Biol 15:572–582, 2003.

Frank M, Kemler R: Protocadherins. Curr Opin Cell Biol 14:557–562, 2002.

Gumbiner BM: Regulation of cadherin-mediated adhesion in morphogenesis. Nat Rev MolCell Biol 6:622–634, 2005.

Harwood A, Coates JC: A prehistory of cell adhesion. Curr Opin Cell Biol 16:470–476, 2004.

Henry MD, Campbell KP: Dystroglycan: An extracellular matrix receptor linked to the cytoskeleton. Curr Opin Cell Biol 8:625–631, 1996.

Kalderon D: Similarities between the Hedgehog and Wnt signaling pathways. Trends Cell Biol 12:523–531, 2002.

Logan CY, Nusse R: The Wnt signaling pathway in development and disease. Annu Rev Cell Dev Biol 20:781–810, 2004.

McEver RP: Selectins: Lectins that initiate cell adhesion under flow. Curr Opin Cell Biol 14:581–586, 2002.

Mould AP, Humphries MJ: Regulation of integrin function through conformational complexity: Not simply a knee-jerk reaction? Curr Opin Cell Biol 16:544–551, 2004.

Nayal A, Webb DJ, Horwitz AF: Talin: An emerging focal point of adhesion dynamics. Curr Opin Cell Biol 16:94–98, 2004.

Nelson WJ, Nusse, R: Convergence of Wnt, β-catenin and cadherin pathways. Science 303:1483–1487, 2004.

Patel SD, Chen CP, Bahna F, et al: Cadherin-mediated cell-cell adhesion: Sticking together as a family. Curr Opin Struct Biol 13:690–698, 2003.

Reya T, Clevers H: Wnt signalling in stem cells and cancer. Nature 434:843–850, 2005.

Rosen SD: Ligands for L-selectin: Homing, inflammation, and beyond. Annu Rev Immunol 22:129–156, 2004.

Ruoslahti E: RGD and other recognition sequences for integrins. Annu Rev Cell Dev Biol 12:697–715, 1996.

Seto ES, Bellen HJ: The ins and outs of Wingless signaling. Trends Cell Biol 14:45–53, 2004.

Shapiro L, Colman DR: The diversity of cadherins and implications for a synaptic adhesive code in the CNS. Neuron 23:427–430, 1999.

Springer TA: Traffic signals for lymphocyte and leukocyte emigration: The multi-step paradigm. Cell 76:301–314, 1994.

Turner CE: Paxillin and focal adhesion signaling. Nat Cell Biol 2:E231–E236, 2000.

van der Merwe PA, Barclay AN: Transient intercellular adhesion: The importance of weak protein-protein interactions. Trends Cell Biol 19:354–358, 1994.

Vestweber D: Regulation of endothelial cell contacts during leukocyte extravasation. Curr Opin Cell Biol 14:587–593, 2002.

Webb DJ, Brown CM, Horwitz AF: Illuminating adhesion complexes in migrating cells: Moving toward a bright future. Curr Opin Cell Biol 15:614–620, 2003.

Wheelock MJ, Johnson KR: Cadherins as modulators of cellular phenotype. Annu Rev Cell Dev Biol 19:207–235, 2003.

Xiao T, Takagi J, Coller BS, et al: Structural basis for allostery in integrins and binding to fibrinogen-mimetic therapeutics. Nature 432:59–67, 2004.

CHAPTER 31

Intercellular Junctions

The mechanical integrity of animal tissues such as epithelia, nerves, and muscles depends on the ability of the cells to interact with each other and the extracellular matrix. Plasma membrane specializations, called cellular junctions, mediate these interactions. Physical connections from the extracellular matrix or adjacent cells through these junctions and the associated cytoskeletal filaments inside cells impart mechanical strength to tissues.

Investigation of junctions began when microscopists and physiologists recognized that epithelial and muscle cells adhere to each other and the underlying extracellular matrix. They also discovered that some epithelia form a tight barrier between the luminal surface and the underlying tissue spaces. The physical basis of these interactions became clear during the 1960s, when electron micrographs of thin sections of vertebrate tissues revealed four types of intercellular junctions that connect the plasma membranes of adjacent cells (Table 31-1 and Fig. 31-1) and two types of junctions to bind to the extracellular matrix. Subsequent research established the molecular architecture of these junctions, each based on a different transmembrane protein:

Adherens junctions: Transmembrane proteins called cadherins (see Fig. 30-5) link neighboring cells and connect to actin filaments in the cytoplasm.

Desmosomes: Another type of cadherin links cells together and connects to cytoplasmic intermediate filaments.

Tight junctions: Transmembrane proteins called claudins not only join the plasma membranes of two cells together but also limit diffusion of ions and solutes between the cells and lipids and proteins in the plane of the plasma membrane. This barrier allows epithelial cells to maintain apical and basolateral membrane domains with different biochemical compositions.

Gap junctions: Transmembrane channel proteins link cells together, but their main function is to provide channels for small molecules to move from the cytoplasm of one cell into the cytoplasm of the neighboring cell.

Hemidesmosomes: Integrins (see Fig. 30-9) connect cytoplasmic intermediate filaments to the basal lamina across the plasma membrane.

Focal adhesions: Integrins associated with actin filaments adhere to the extracellular matrix.

Vertebrates use a selection of junctions that are suited to the physiological functions of each tissue. Columnar epithelial cells in the intestine interact with their neighbors

Table 31-1

MOLECULAR COMPONENTS OF CELL-CELL AND CELL-MATRIX JUNCTIONS

Junction	Target Molecule	Adhesive Protein	Cytoplasmic Proteins	Cytoskeletal Filaments
Sealing of the Extracellular Space				
Tight junction	Occludin Claudin	Occludin Claudin	ZO-1, ZO-2, cingulin, spectrin	Actin
Communication between Cells				
Gap junction	Connexin	Connexin	ZO-1, drebrin	Actin
Adhesion to Other Cells				
Zonula adherens	Cadherin	Cadherin	Catenins, plakoglobin	Actin
Desmosome	Desmoglein Desmocollin	Desmoglein Desmocollin	Plakoglobin, desmoplakin Plakoglobin, desmoplakin	Intermediate Intermediate
Adhesion to the Extracellular Matrix				
Hemidesmosome	Laminin	Integrin	Plectin, BP 180	Intermediate
Focal contact	Fibronectin	Integrin	Talin, vinculin, α-actinin	Actin

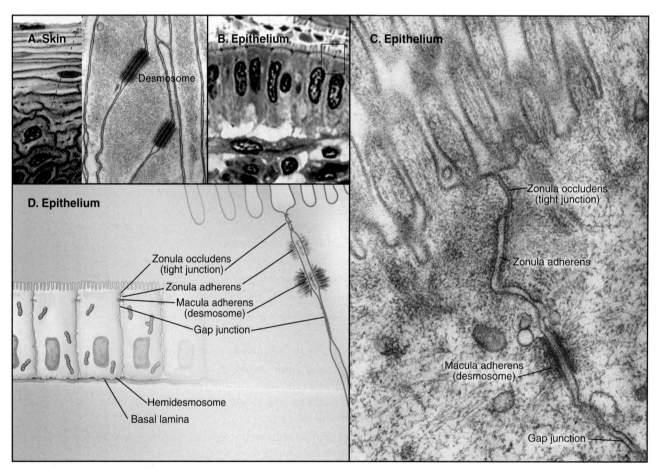

Figure 31-1 **LIGHT AND ELECTRON MICROGRAPHS OF JUNCTIONS. A,** Desmosomes. **Left,** Light micrograph of a section of skin showing numerous desmosomes as *pink dots* between the cells. **Right,** Electron micrograph of a thin section of skin showing desmosomes. **B,** Light micrograph of a section of intestinal epithelium stained with hematoxylin-eosin, showing the junctional complex (also called "terminal bars") as *bright pink dots* between the cells near their apex, just below the microvilli of the brush border. **C,** Electron micrograph of a thin section of intestinal epithelial cells, showing the junctional complex consisting of a belt-like tight junction (also called the zonula occludens), a belt-like adherens junction (also called the zonula adherens), and desmosomes (also called the macula adherens), all in their characteristic relation to each other. The circumferential tight junction seals the extracellular space. The zonula adherens is anchored to the actin cytoskeleton. Desmosomes are attached to cytoplasmic intermediate filaments. **D,** Drawing showing the position of the junctional complex in the cell and the locations of gap junctions, basal lamina, and hemidesmosomes. (A, Courtesy of Don W. Fawcett, Harvard Medical School, Boston, Massachusetts. C, Courtesy of Marilyn Farquhar, University of California, San Diego.)

using all four types of intercellular junctions (Fig. 31-1B–D). Belt-like tight junctions and adherens junctions encircle the apex of the cell. Desmosomes and gap junctions form patch-like lateral connections between the cells. Hemidesmosomes anchor the cells to the basal lamina. Stratified epithelial cells in the skin (Fig. 31-1A) emphasize desmosomes and intermediate filaments (Fig. 31-1B) to resist mechanical forces but also interact via claudins and adherens junctions. Desmosomes and adherens junctions link muscle cells to the surrounding basal lamina (see Fig. 29-18C). Gap junctions connect heart and smooth muscle cells but not skeletal muscle cells. Most nerve cells communicate chemically, but some use gap junctions for electrical communication.

Invertebrate animals assemble junctions from homologous proteins but with different organization than the junctional complex of vertebrate epithelia. Insect epithelia have apical adherens junctions and more basal "septate junctions" built from claudins and cytoplasmic proteins with sequence homology to the tight junction proteins ZO-1 and ZO-2. Nematode epithelia have one junction with adherens functions and claudins.

Tight Junctions

Tight junctions, also called zonula occludens, occlude the extracellular space between epithelial cells, forming a tight, belt-like adhesive seal that selectively limits the diffusion of water, ions, and larger solutes as well as migration of cells (Fig. 31-2). Thus, they separate the interior of the body from the external world. Tight junctions also define the boundary between the biochemically distinct **apical** and **basolateral domains** of the plasma membrane of polarized epithelial cells. Many physiological processes (see Figs. 11-2 through 11-4) depend on the selective permeability of the two pathways across an epithelium: passive "paracellular" diffusion through tight junctions and transcellular movement made possible by the action of pumps, carriers, and channels located selectively in the apical and basolateral domains of the plasma membrane.

In electron micrographs of thin sections of tight junctions, the plasma membranes of adjacent cells appear to fuse together in a series of one or more contacts (Fig. 31-2). Early models of tight junctions proposed a fusion between the lipid bilayers of the two membranes to account for the barrier to ion diffusion, but freeze-fracture images revealed that the strands consist of integral membrane proteins. The contacts correspond to continuous strands of intramembranous particles that form a branching network in the plane of the lipid bilayer.

Transmembrane proteins forming the strands observed by freeze-fracture were difficult to identify until investigators found a monoclonal antibody that bound to the cytoplasmic side of the plasma membrane at tight junctions. Using this antibody, they isolated an integral membrane protein and named it **occludin.** The amino acid sequence of occludin suggested four transmembrane strands and two hydrophobic extracellular loops that are extremely rich in tyrosine and glycine residues (Fig. 31-3). The same group then discovered that mice lacking the single occludin gene survive with normal tight junctions, revealing the existence of other tight junction proteins. It is now believed that a family of more than 20 proteins, called **claudins,** constitutes the main structural proteins of tight junction strands. Claudins have four transmembrane sequences, but they are not related in sequence to occludin. Close

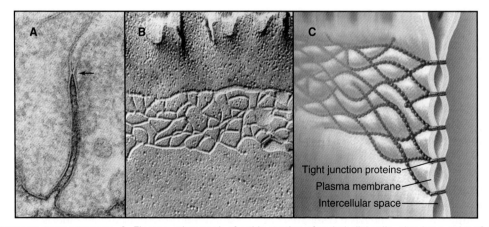

Figure 31-2 **EPITHELIAL TIGHT JUNCTIONS. A,** Electron micrograph of a thin section of endothelial cells, showing a point of contact between the plasma membranes at a tight junction *(arrow).* **B,** Electron micrograph of a replica of a freeze-fractured cell. This method exposes proteins within the lipid bilayer and reveals strands aligned along the points of contact between the plasma membranes. **C,** Interpretive drawing, showing the strands at points of contact as rows of transmembrane proteins. (A, Courtesy of George Palade, University of California, San Diego. B, Courtesy of Don W. Fawcett, Harvard Medical School, Boston, Massachusetts.)

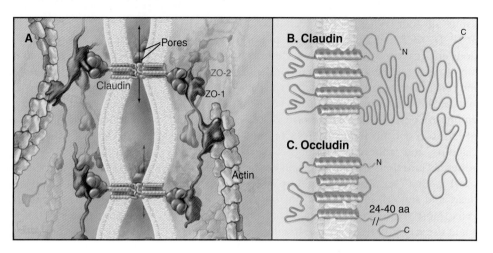

Figure 31-3 TIGHT JUNCTION PROTEINS: OCCLUDIN AND CLAUDIN. **A,** Preliminary model of tight junction structure with claudin linking the two membranes together and peripheral protein ZO-1 linking the cytoplasmic tail of claudin to actin filaments. **B–C,** Transmembrane topology of claudin and occludin.

association of claudins limits diffusion in the extracellular space between cells as well as diffusion of lipids and proteins in the plane of the membrane.

The extracellular domains of claudins form rows of pores along the tight junction contacts. Each claudin has a unique selectivity for cations or anions, and the selection of claudins expressed in various epithelia creates their distinct selectivities. The pores of all claudins probably restrict diffusion of solutes larger than about 1 nm in diameter. Larger solutes may cross the barrier by traversing transient breaks in the strands of claudins.

The cytoplasmic tails of claudins interact with numerous proteins with roles as scaffolds and in actin binding, signaling, and cell polarity. **ZO-1, ZO-2,** and **ZO-3,** peripheral membrane adapter proteins containing PDZ protein-interaction domains (see Fig. 25-11), interact with the long C-terminal cytoplasmic tail of occludin and JAM (junctional adhesion molecule). These ZO-adapters link the transmembrane proteins to cytoplasmic proteins including actin filaments, cingulin, and a small GTPase. ZO-2 and cingulin are specific for tight junctions, whereas ZO-1 also associates with cadherins in adherens junctions and connexins in gap junctions.

Tight junctions are the barrier that segregates different pumps, carriers, receptors, and lipids in the apical and basolateral domains of the plasma membrane. These domains allow polarized cells to create different extracellular environments in the basal and apical compartments. For example, intestinal epithelial cells take up nutrients from the lumen of the intestine and transport them into the extracellular space beneath the cells (see Fig. 11-2). Tight junctions and epithelial polarity are required for many physiological functions (see Figs. 11-3 and 11-4). Separating the apical and basal compartments also regulates some types of signaling. For instance, airway epithelial cells release the growth factor heregulin from the apical surface, but it activates cell growth only by activating the receptor tyrosine kinase erbB2 (see

Fig. 25-4) on the basolateral surface when the epithelium is damaged or the tight junctions compromised.

Circumferential tight junctions account for the electrical resistance across sheets of epithelial cells. The quality of the seal, reflected in the electrical resistance, varies by several orders of magnitude depending on the cell type and is matched to the physiological function of the epithelium. Permeability in the two directions across the junction is identical. The number and continuity of claudin/occludin strands as well as the specific claudin proteins that are expressed determine the tightness of the barrier to diffusion of ions in the extracellular space. Most tight junctions are more permeable to cations than to anions and generally restrict the diffusion of all solutes larger than about 1 nm in diameter. Along with variations in ion and solute permeability, the ability for water to flow through tight junctions also appears to differ among epithelia. Extremely tight barriers with many strands and distinct claudin forms are found where epithelia must maintain high ion gradients, such as in the distal tubules of the kidney, where urine is concentrated. Leaky tight junctions with fewer strands and different claudins are found where ion gradients across epithelia are small but a barrier is required for large solutes, proteins, and leukocytes (e.g., in most blood vessels).

The transepithelial barrier that is established by tight junctions is regulated by extracellular stimuli (e.g., hormones such as vasopressin and aldosterone and cytokines such as tumor necrosis factor; see Chapter 27), their downstream second messengers (e.g., Ca^{2+} and cyclic adenosine monophosphate [cAMP]; see Chapter 26), and effectors (e.g., protein kinases A and C; see Chapter 25). The mechanisms are not yet well understood, but posttranslational modifications of tight junctions might modulate their assembly. Another possibility is that tension on associated actin filaments might physically open passages through tight junctions. The metabolic state of the cell also influences tight junctions;

depletion of ATP causes tight junctions to leak without destroying the barrier between the apical and basolateral domains of the plasma membrane. Cells migrating across epithelia, such as white blood cells moving from the blood to the connective tissue, open tight junctions locally without disrupting the tight seal across the epithelium (see Fig. 30-13). Migratory cells induce a localized increase in cytoplasmic Ca^{2+} in the epithelial cells that is required for opening the tight junctions.

Several bacterial toxins affect the tight junction barrier. The ZO-toxin of *Vibrio cholerae* induces diarrhea by loosening tight junctions, independent of the classic cholera toxin, which induces secretion. *Helicobacter pylori* injects a protein toxin into the cells lining the stomach. This toxin disrupts tight junctions, breaking the barrier that protects the underlying tissues and predisposing to ulcers. Mutation of individual human claudin genes can result in highly selective defects in epithelial barriers, such as reduced ability of the kidney to reabsorb potassium (claudin-16) or deafness due to loss of ion gradients in the inner ear (claudin-14).

Gap Junctions

For many years, the dominance of the cell theory in biology, which suggested that isolation of cells was a general principle, discouraged curiosity about the possibility of direct intercellular communication. Early electrophysiological experiments on nerves and skeletal muscles reinforced the widespread belief that cells were autonomous. By chance, the cells that were used in these experiments *were* electrically isolated and communicated exclusively by secreting chemical messengers that bound to receptors on target cells (see Figs 11-8 and 11-9). However, nerve and skeletal muscle cells were found to be exceptions to the general principle, which emerged only later, that cells in animal tissues communicate with each other by gap junctions. The generality of gap junctional communication means that sharing cytoplasmic components is common in animal cell biology. Cells in plant tissues also communicate with each other, but they use direct cytoplasmic connections, called **plasmodesmata,** rather than gap junctions (Box 31-1 and Fig. 31-4).

In 1959, electrophysiological experiments on synapses between giant axons and the motor neurons that drive the flipper muscles of crayfish provided the first convincing evidence for direct electrical communication between cells. These **electrical synapses** transmit action potentials (see Fig. 11-6) directly from one cell to the next without the delay required for secretion and reception of a chemical transmitter. This, in turn, allows exceptionally fast responses to escape predators. Heart muscle cells were found to be connected by similar electrical junctions.

Plants lack gap junctions, but many cells in plant tissues maintain cytoplasmic continuity with their neighbors through plasmodesmata, membrane-lined channels across the cell wall (Fig. 31-4). A strand of modified endoplasmic reticulum fills most of the pore. Specialized proteins on the cytoplasmic surfaces of the surrounding plasma membrane and central endoplasmic reticulum are thought to line the pore, although few molecular components of plasmodesmata have been identified. Most plasmodesmata form by incomplete cytokinesis, but secondary plasmodesmata can form independently.

Molecules smaller than about 1 kD diffuse freely through plasmodesmata, but larger molecules, even whole viral genomes, can pass selectively through these channels. Constitutive diffusion of small molecules allows exchange of metabolites between cells. Regulated passage of larger molecules, including double-stranded RNAs and proteins such as transcription factors, allows developmental signals to move between cells and tissues.

Permeability varies among tissues and with physiological states and developmental stages. For example, all cells in embryos are connected, whereas cells in some adult tissues are isolated. Actin filaments contribute to regulation of the pore size, but the signals controlling permeability are not known. Specialized viral proteins are required for viruses or their nucleic acids to move between cells.

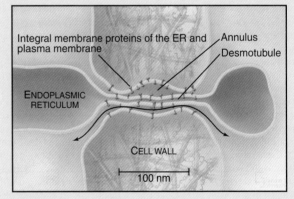

Figure 31-4 A PLASMODESMA CONNECTING TWO PLANT CELLS.

Over the next decade, three approaches revealed coupling between many nonexcitable cells. Using microelectrodes, physiologists established that plasma membrane depolarization of one cell was transmitted with little resistance to adjacent epithelial cells (Fig. 31-5), although the amplitude of the response declined with distance. Similarly, it was discovered that fluorescent molecules, radioactive tracers, and essential nutrients pass from the cytoplasm of one cell to the cytoplasm of

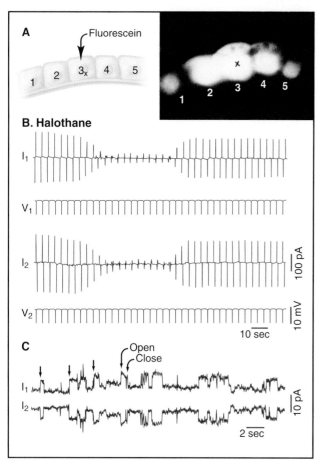

Figure 31-5 GAP JUNCTION PHYSIOLOGY. **A,** Drawing and fluorescence micrograph, showing the movement of a tracer dye between epithelial cells from the salivary gland of *Chironomus*. Cell 3 was injected with fluorescein (molecular weight: 330), which spread to adjacent cells via gap junctions. **B–C,** Electrical recordings from pairs of cells coupled by gap junctions. **B,** Two cells (1 and 2) were voltage-clamped (see the text that describes Fig. 11-6) and subjected alternately to small depolarizing voltage changes (V_1, V_2). Being electrically coupled, they responded with opposite currents (I_1, I_2). The anesthetic halothane closes most of the channels, reducing the current in response to depolarization. **C,** When the cells are held at a constant depolarizing voltage in the presence of halothane, current records reveal the opening and closing of individual gap junction channels as opposite step changes in current. (A, From Lowenstein W: Physiol Rev 61:829, 1991. B, From Eghbali B, Kessler JA, Spray DC: Expression of gap junction channels in communication-incompetent cells. Proc Natl Acad Sci 87:1328–1331, 1990. C, Courtesy of Mark Ellisman, University of California, San Diego; reprinted with permission from Gaietta G, Deernick TJ, Adams SR, et al: Multicolor and electron microscopic imaging of connexin trafficking. Science 296:503–507, 2002. Copyright 2002 AAAS.)

neighboring cells. Electron microscopists associated low-resistance communication between cells with the presence of plasma membrane specializations that they called gap junctions owing to the regular 2-nm separation of the adjacent cell membranes (Fig. 31-6). Light microscopy with antibody probes is used to survey tissues for junctions, while fluorescent fusion proteins are the best approach to study gap junction assembly and dynamics.

Gap junctions are plaques that contain large *intercellular* channels that connect the cytoplasms of a pair of cells. These plaques exclude other transmembrane proteins and contain a few to thousands of channels. Half channels in each membrane are called **connexons.** They consist of six protein subunits, named **connexins,** which are proteins with four transmembrane α-helices (Fig. 31-7). Connexons assemble in vesicles along the secretory pathway. New connexons add around the periphery of gap junction plaques and old connexons are removed from the middle of plaques (Fig. 31-6C).

A hexagonal ring of connexins forms a central aqueous channel across the lipid bilayer. In the narrow intracellular gap, each connexon pairs with a connexon from the adjacent cell, forming a tight extracellular seal that precludes leakage of ions out of either cell. The use of six subunits creates a larger pore than tetrameric voltage-gated ion channels (see Fig. 10-7) or pentameric ligand-gated ion channels (see Fig. 10-12). The cylindrical transmembrane pore is 10 nm long with a diameter of 1.2 nm. This pore passes hydrophilic molecules up to about 1 kD in size, including ions (to establish electrochemical continuity between the cells), second messengers (to establish a common network of information), small peptides, and metabolites (to allow sharing of resources). Recent evidence shows that connexon hemichannels (the ring of six connexins in one plasma membrane) can open rarely for the nonspecific passage of ions and solutes as large as ATP.

Vertebrates have genes for a family of about 20 connexins isoforms ranging in size from 26 to 60 kD. These isoforms make channels that differ somewhat in terms of their permeability and charge selectivity. The transmembrane helices and extracellular loops are more conserved than are the variable N- and C-terminal cytoplasmic sequences. Connexins are named by molecular weight; for instance, connexin-43 (Cx-43) is the name for the 43-kD isoform.

Remarkably, gap junctions were invented twice during evolution. Connexins are found exclusively in chordates. The earliest metazoan branches (see Fig. 2-9) have a gene for proteins called innexins, for invertebrate connexins. Innexins have four transmembrane domains and form functional gap junctions but lack any sequence similarity to connexins. Vertebrates have a few innexin genes, expressed in the central nervous system.

In cells that express more than one connexin, the hexameric connexons may consist of one or more than one type of subunit. Most connexons pair with identical connexons on the partner cell to form homotypic gap junctional channels, but nonidentical pairs can form heterotypic channels with novel properties. Homotypic channels pass molecules equally well in both directions, but heterotypic channels can be asymmetrical. These hybrid channels may pass fluorescent tracers more readily in one direction than the other or react more sensitively to the transjunctional potential of one polar-

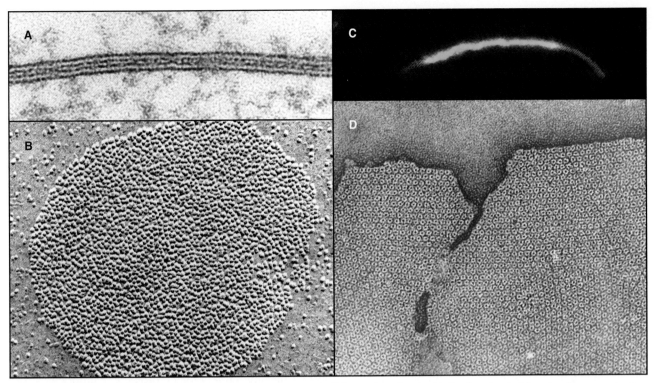

Figure 31-6 LIGHT AND ELECTRON MICROGRAPHS OF GAP JUNCTIONS. **A,** Thin section of embedded cells, showing the closely apposed membranes of adjacent cells separated by a gap of 2 nm. **B,** Replica of a freeze-fractured cell, showing an irregular array of particles exposed in the plane of the lipid bilayer. **C,** Fluorescence micrograph of a gap junction plaque between cultured HeLa cells expressing connexin-43 with a tetracysteine peptide tag. The cells were first exposed to a *green* fluorescent dye that binds tightly to the tetracysteine tag and then, after four hours of growth without the *green* dye, the same cells were incubated with a second *red* fluorescent dye that binds to the tetracysteine tag on newly synthesized connexin-43. The older central part of this plaque is *green.* The newer peripheral regions of the plaque are *red.* **D,** Negative staining of an isolated gap junction reveals the intercellular connexon channels packed together in a regular, two-dimensional array. Each connexon has a central channel filled with stain. (A–B and D, Courtesy of Don W. Fawcett, Harvard Medical School, Boston, Massachusetts; from the work of N. B. Gilula, Scripps Research Institute, La Jolla, California. C, Courtesy of Mark Ellisman, University of California, San Diego; and from Gaietta G, Deernick TJ, Adams SR, et al: Multicolor and electron microscopic imaging of connexin trafficking. Science 296:503–507, 2002.)

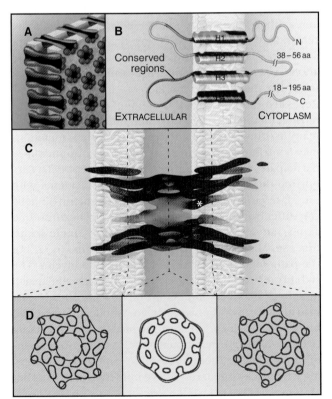

Figure 31-7 MOLECULAR STRUCTURE OF THE GAP JUNCTION CONNEXON. **A,** Drawing of gap junction connexons forming channels between the cytoplasms of adjacent cells. **B,** Transmembrane topology of connexins. Judging from the X-ray diffraction pattern and reconstructions from electron micrographs, the polypeptide chain crosses the lipid bilayer four times as α-helices. A linear array of conserved polar residues on one face of helix 3 suggests that it lines the channel. Conserved residues *(maroon)* form the transmembrane and extracellular loops required for channel assembly. Cytoplasmic loops between helix 2 and 3 and the C-terminal tails vary in length among connexin isoforms. Removal of the C-terminal tail from connexin-43 alters its gating properties. **C,** Three-dimensional reconstruction of a gap junction channel at 7.5-Å resolution by electron crystallography. The specimen was a two-dimensional crystal composed of a mutant connexin α₁-Cx-263T lacking most of the C-terminal tail, which would project into the cytoplasm. This cutaway side view shows the interior of the channel and transmembrane densities formed by α-helices. The *yellow asterisk* marks the narrowest part of the channel. **D,** Cross-sectional views at three levels. The *pink* contours are cross sections of the 24 α-helices. Secondary structures forming the tightly sealed channel across the extracellular gap are not resolved *(middle panel).* (C–D, Courtesy of Mark Yeager, Scripps Research Institute, La Jolla, California. Reference: Unger VM, Kumar NM, Gilula NB, Yeager M: Three-dimensional structure of a recombinant gap junctional membrane channel. Science 283:1176–1180, 1999.)

ity than the other. This might explain the asymmetrical coupling that is sometimes observed between both excitable and nonexcitable cells, such as neuronal gap junctions, which pass action potentials in one direction but not the other.

Biophysicists have studied the properties of single connexon channels by patch-clamping pairs of cells with few channels, a state that can be achieved conveniently by expressing connexins in cells lacking them, or by measuring electrical properties of purified connexons incorporated into lipid bilayers (see Fig. 10-16A). Like other channels, connexons flip back and forth between two states: open and closed (Fig. 31-5). The structural basis for this difference in conductance is not yet established. The conductance of the open state depends on the connexin isoform and varies from about 30 pS to 300 pS. Given the permeability of gap junctions to relatively large solutes, it is surprising that their conductance is in the same range as narrower ligand- and voltage-gated ion channels. Both the greater length and the arrangement of charged residues lining the channel may contribute to the unexpectedly low conductance of connexons.

Gap junctional communication is conditional, depending on both the number of channels and the fraction that are open or closed. The fraction of open channels is usually less than 1.0; it is about 0.2 in heart and as low as 0.01 in one nerve cell that was tested. Many factors regulate the reversible opening and closing of connexon channels, including the transjunctional voltage, cytoplasmic H^+ and Ca^{2+} concentrations, and protein kinases. Oleamide, a fatty acid amide produced by the brain, blocks gap junctional communication and induces sleep in animals. Organic alcohols (heptanol and octanol) and general anesthetics (halothane) can also close gap junction channels reversibly (see Fig. 31-5), but these agents are not specific for gap junctions. The transjunctional potential (i.e., the potential difference between the coupled cells) gates most connexons, regardless of the plasma membrane potentials of these cells. Like other voltage-gated channels, individual transitions are fast, but the response to potential changes, on the scale of seconds, is very slow in comparison with other channels (see Fig. 10-7). High concentrations of cytoplasmic Ca^{2+} (100 to 500 μM) and cytoplasmic acidification also close connexons. These effects of membrane potential, H^+, and Ca^{2+} allow cells to terminate communication with neighboring cells that are damaged (depolarizing the plasma membrane and admitting high concentrations of Ca^{2+}) or metabolically compromised (allowing Ca^{2+} to leak out of intracellular stores and acidifying the cytoplasm).

Second messengers generated by signaling pathways control gap junction activity in two ways. For example, on a time scale of hours, cAMP also promotes the assembly of gap junctions. On a time scale of seconds, cAMP

activates protein kinase A, which phosphorylates the C-terminal tail of some connexins, increasing or decreasing the fraction of open channels (depending on the connexin isoform and the cell type). In the retina of the eye, the neurotransmitter dopamine) (see Fig. 11-7) regulates the size of a network of electrically coupled neurons. Dopamine activates a seven-helix receptor on these "horizontal cells," stimulating the production of cAMP (see Fig. 26-1). This second messenger activates protein kinase A to phosphorylate connexons, reducing their open probability and the size of the neuronal network.

Cells in most metazoans communicate by gap junctions. Coupled cells in vertebrates include epithelial cells of the skin, endocrine glands, exocrine glands, gastrointestinal tract, and renal-urinary tract as well as smooth muscle, cardiac muscle, bone, some neurons, and glial cells. Epithelial cells can coordinate their activities with their neighbors, as in synchronizing the beats of cilia (see Fig. 38-14C). Fragments of viral proteins can spread from infected cells to neighboring cells, which then become targets for cytotoxic T lymphocytes (see Fig. 28-9). Gap junctions allow osteocytes buried deep in bone to maintain a cellular supply line to acquire nutrients from distant blood vessels (see Fig. 32-4). Passage of action potentials between cardiac and smooth muscle cells sets off waves of contraction (see Fig. 39-18). Electrical synapses between neurons can transmit action potentials at very high frequencies (>1000 per second). In some parts of the brain, gap junctions also coordinate action potentials in groups of neurons. Even white blood cells may form transient gap junctions with endothelial cells.

Mutations in connexin genes cause human disease and pathology in mice (Table 31-2). The defects are remarkably specific, considering that most connexins are expressed in several tissues. This might reflect situations in which other connexins cannot compensate or in which the absolute number of channels is crucial. Recessive mutations in the connexin-26 gene are the most common causes of inherited human **deafness.** As many as 1 in 30 people are carriers, and their mutations may contribute to hearing loss late in life. Connexin-26 participates in the transport of K^+ in the epithelia supporting the sensory hair cells in the ear. Patients with one of a variety of mutations in the connexin-32 gene can suffer from degeneration of the myelin sheath around axons, an X-linked variant of **Charcot-Marie-Tooth disease.** Many human tissues express connexin-32, but the pathological processes are confined to myelin. The stability of myelin might depend on intracellular gap junctions between layers of the myelin sheath that provide a pathway between the metabolically active cell body and the deep layers of the sheath near the axon. (Defects in myelin membrane proteins cause other forms of Charcot-Marie-Tooth disease.) In contrast to humans, mice that lack connexin-32 have mild myelin defects but

Table 31-2

PHENOTYPES OF HUMANS AND MICE WITH MUTATIONS IN GAP JUNCTION SUBUNITS

Connexin	Species	Phenotype
Cx-26β2	Human	Dominant and recessive mutations with deafness; skin disease
	Mouse	Embryonic lethal defect due to defective glucose transport across the placenta
Cx-30β6	Human	Recessive deafness; skin disease
Cx-31β3	Human	Recessive deafness; skin disease
Cx-32β1	Human	X-linked point mutations, defective myelin, peripheral nerve degeneration; deafness
	Mouse	Defective liver glucose metabolism, liver tumors, mild nerve defect
Cx-37α4	Mouse	Female infertility, defect in communication of granulosa cells with oocyte
Cx-40α5	Mouse	Partial block of impulse conduction in heart
Cx-43α1	Human	Deafness
	Mouse	Embryonic lethal heart defects (heterozygote mild heart conduction defect)
Cx-46α3	Mouse	Cataracts in lens of the eye
Cx-50α8	Mouse	Cataracts in lens of the eye, small eyes
	Human	Cataracts in lens of the eye

Note: Mutations are homozygous loss of function mutations unless noted otherwise. The nomenclature used here combines the Cx- "molecular mass in kDa" and molecular phylogeny αβ-number systems.

more serious defects in liver function (metabolic defects and a high incidence of tumors). Mice with null mutations in connexin-43, the main connexin of gap junctions in heart and other tissues, die shortly after birth. Their hearts beat, but a malformation of the heart is fatal. Other organs are only mildly abnormal.

Adherens Junctions

Adherens junctions and desmosomes are two types of adhesive junctions using homophilic (like to like) interactions of cadherins (see Fig. 30-6) to bind epithelial cells to their neighbors. Cytoplasmic actin filaments reinforce adherens junctions (Fig. 31-8A), whereas cytoplasmic intermediate filaments anchor desmosomes (Fig. 31-8B).

Homophilic interactions between densely clustered **E-cadherins** bind adjacent cells together at adherens junctions. β-Catenin and a related protein called plakoglobin bind the cytoplasmic domains of E-cadherin (see Fig. 7-9F). β-Catenin not only regulates gene expression when it enters the nucleus as part of the Wnt signaling pathway (see Fig. 30-8) but also interacts with several cytoskeletal and signaling proteins associated with adherens junctions. α-Catenin has been a candidate to connect cadherins to actin filaments, since it can bind both β-catenin and actin filaments. However, these two interactions appear to be mutually exclusive, so the link between cadherins and actin is still under investigation.

Adherens junctions are the first connections that are established between developing sheets of epithelial cells. Contact begins when cadherins on the tips of filopodia engage partner cadherins of the same type on another cell. The contact spreads laterally as more cadherins are recruited along with associated actin filaments, as is illustrated by dorsal closure of the ectoderm by *Drosophila* embryos (see Fig. 38-5). These pioneering adherens junctions eventually allow like cells to associate in epithelial sheets (see Fig. 30-7) and to influence the maturation of the epithelium. Adherens junctions are a prerequisite for the tight junctions that allow epithelial cells to establish polarity with different proteins and lipids in the apical and basal plasma membranes. The shape of the cells depends on Rho family GTPases and protein kinases associated with the adherens junction, which regulate the assembly and contraction of the associated actin cytoskeleton. The junctions and polarity of the cells determine the orientation of the mitotic spindle and the plane of division. This allows for asymmetrical division of stem cells, such as those at the base of stratified epithelia (see Figs. 35-6 and 41-15). In mature columnar epithelia, a belt-like adherens junction, called the **zonula adherens,** encircles the cells near their apical surface (see Fig. 31-1D) and maintains the physical integrity of the epithelium.

Desmosomes

Desmosomes (*desmos* = "bound", *soma* = "body") provide strong adhesions between epithelial and muscle cells. In epithelia, these junctions are small, disk-shaped, "spot welds" between adjacent cells. Desmosomes in the heart are more complicated because they are mixed with adherens junctions (see Fig. 39-18). Cellular adhesion at desmosomes is mediated by two families of

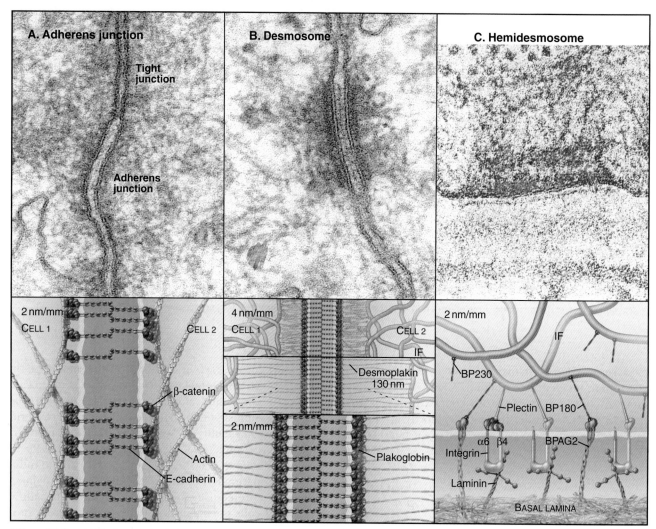

Figure 31-8 COMPARISON OF ADHERENS JUNCTION, DESMOSOME, AND HEMIDESMOSOME. **Top,** Electron micrographs of thin sections. **Bottom,** Molecular models. **A,** Adherens junction. Electron micrograph from the intestinal epithelium. E-cadherins link two cells together. β- and α-catenin link the cytoplasmic domain of E-cadherin to actin filaments. **B,** Desmosome. Two types of cadherins—desmoglein and desmocollin—link adjacent cells together. The central dense stratum seen in the micrograph presumably corresponds to the interaction sites of the cadherins, although accessory proteins may participate. Desmoplakin and other accessory proteins link the cadherins and associated plakoglobin (related to catenin) to keratin intermediate filaments. Desmoplakin molecules are shown extended to their full length in the *middle drawing,* whereas in desmosomes, they must be kinked or folded (as shown in the *upper drawing*), since the thickness of the desmoplakin layer is half that expected from extended molecules. **C,** Hemidesmosome. Integrin $\alpha_6\beta_4$ and type XVII collagen (also called BPAG2) attach to the basal lamina. Plectin and BPAG1 link the membrane proteins to keratin intermediate filaments. (A–B, Micrographs courtesy of Hilda Pasolli and Elaine Fuchs, Rockefeller University, New York; from Perez-Moreno M, Jamora C, Fuchs E: Sticky business: Orchestrating cellular signals at adherens junctions. Cell 112:535–548, 2003. C, Micrograph courtesy of Jonathan Jones, Northwestern University, Chicago, Illinois.)

desmosomal cadherins, named **desmogleins** and **desmocollins** (see Fig. 30-5 and Table 30-2). These cadherins link the plasma membranes of adjacent cells and connect to cytoplasmic intermediate filaments via adapter proteins. The most distal of five extracellular CAD domains interact head to head with CAD1 domains from the partner cells and laterally with other cadherins in a dense tangle midway between the two plasma membranes (see Fig. 30-6).

Plakoglobin (also called γ-catenin, since it is similar to β-catenin) binds to the ICS domains of desmogleins

and desmocollins, forming a link to **desmoplakin,** plakophilin, and intermediate filaments. Desmoplakin and accessory proteins link desmosomal cadherins to intermediate filaments. Desmoplakin I and II, dimeric proteins related to plectin (see Fig. 35-7), consist of a coiled-coil rod with globular domains at each end. N-terminal globular domains bind plakoglobin and desmosomal cadherins, whereas domains called "plakin repeats" at the C-terminus bind directly to the N-terminal, nonhelical domains of **epidermal keratins.** Mutations in this part of epidermal keratins can cause blistering skin diseases by compromising the integrity of desmosomes (see Fig. 35-6).

Although all desmosomes share a common plan, their molecular compositions vary in particular tissues. Mammals have four genes for desmogleins and three genes for desmocollins. Desmocollin mRNAs are also alternatively spliced (see Fig. 16-6). Desmoglein-2 and desmocollin-2 are found in most desmosomes. Expression of the other isoforms is more restricted. For example, in epidermis, desmoglein-1 and desmocollin-1 are found only in the upper layers, whereas desmoglein-3 is in the basal layers. This explains the pathology in autoimmune blistering diseases. Patients with **pemphigus foliaceus** make antibodies that react with desmoglein-1 and disrupt desmosomes in the upper layers of the epidermis, whereas patients with **pemphigus vulgaris** produce autoantibodies to desmoglein-3 that have the same effect on the basal layers. Antibodies are directly responsible; transfusion of human autoantibodies into a mouse reproduces the disease. Other organs are spared, owing to the restricted expression of these two isoforms. Mutations in these desmoglein genes in mice compromise desmosomes and cause skin blisters similar to pemphigus.

The development of animal tissues depends on desmosomes and their constituent proteins. Loss-of-function mutations can lead to mechanical failures; mutations in the plakoglobin gene can be lethal in mice and humans during embryogenesis, owing to disruption of the heart. Similarly, mutations in the desmoplakin gene cause skin and cardiac defects. Less direct evidence suggests that desmosomes might also transduce signals, perhaps deploying plakoglobin in a manner similar to that of β-catenin (see Fig. 30-8).

Adhesion to the Extracellular Matrix: Hemidesmosomes and Focal Contacts

Adhesion to the extracellular matrix is fundamentally different from intercellular adhesion because integrins, rather than homophilic interactions of cadherins, provide the transmembrane link between the cytoskeleton and ligands in the extracellular matrix (see Fig. 30-9). At focal contacts and related assemblies, transmembrane integrins link cytoplasmic actin filaments to the extracellular matrix (see Fig. 30-11).

Hemidesmosomes are another type of integrin-based adhesive junction that links cytoplasmic intermediate filaments to the basal lamina. The morphologic resemblance of hemidesmosomes to half of a conventional desmosome belies the fact that they are fundamentally different at the molecular level (Fig. 31-8). Like desmosomes, hemidesmosomes have a dense plaque on the cytoplasmic surface of the plasma membrane that anchors loops of intermediate filaments. The similarity ends there.

Two transmembrane proteins—$\alpha_6\beta_4$ **integrin** and **type XVII collagen**—concentrate in hemidesmosomes; both are essential for assembly and stability. Outside the cell, $\alpha_6\beta_4$ integrin binds **laminin-5** in the basal lamina. Type XVII collagen is a trimeric transmembrane protein. The extracellular collagen triple helix is thought to form anchoring filaments between the membrane and the basal lamina. In a blistering skin disease called **bullous pemphigoid,** autoantibodies attack type XVII collagen, so the protein is also called bullous pemphigoid antigen-2, or BPAG2. This clinical observation and genetic deletions have established that both $\alpha_6\beta_4$ integrin and type XVII collagen are required for stable hemidesmosomes.

In the cytoplasm, plectin links the long tail of β_4 integrin to keratin intermediate filaments. The dense cytoplasmic plaque also contains BPAG1 (bullous pemphigoid antigen-1), a relative of plectin and desmoplakin, which might help to bind intermediate filaments. Human mutations in plectin cause skin blisters associated with late-onset muscular dystrophy. A mouse null mutation of BPAG1 causes skin blisters, as well as defects in motor neurons.

ACKNOWLEDGMENTS

Thanks go to James Anderson and Dan Goodenough for their suggestions on revisions to this chapter.

SELECTED READINGS

Cilia ML, Jackson D: Plasmodesmata form and function. Curr Opin Cell Biol 16: 500–506, 2004.

Coulombe PA: A new fold on an old story: Attachment of intermediate filaments to desmosomes. Nat Struct Biol 9:560–562, 2002.

Dejana E: Endothelial cell-cell junctions. Nat Rev Mol Cell Biol 5:261–270, 2004.

Fleishman SJ, Unger VM, Yeager M, Ben-Tal N: A C-alpha model of the transmembrane alpha-helices of gap junction intercellular channels. Mol Cell 15:879–888, 2004.

Garrod DR, Merritt AJ, Nie Z: Desmosomal cadherins. Curr Opin Cell Biol 14:537–545, 2002.

Getsios S, Nuen AC, Green KJ: Working out the strength and flexibility of desmosomes. Nat Rev Mol Cell Biol 5:271–281, 2004.

Gonzalez-Mariscal L, Betanzoa A, Nava P, Jaramillo BE: Tight junction proteins. Prog Biophys Mol Biol 81:1–44, 2003.

Harris AL: Emerging issues in connexin channels: Biophysics fills the gap. Quart Rev Biophys 34:325–472, 2001.

Heinlein M, Epel BL: Macromolecular transport and signaling through plasmodesmata. Int Rev Cytol 235:93–164, 2004.

Jones JE, Hopkinson SB, Goldfinger LE: Structure and assembly of hemidesmosomes. BioEssays 20:488–494, 1998.

Knust E, Bossinger O: Composition and formation of intercellular junctions in epithelial cells. Science 298:1955–1959, 2002.

Payne AS, Hanakawa Y, Amagai M, Stanley JR: Desmosomes and disease: Pemphigus and bullous impetigo. Curr Opin Cell Biol 16:536–543, 2004.

Perez-Moreno M, Jamora C, Fuchs E: Sticky business: Orchestrating cellular signals at adherens junctions. Cell 112:535–548, 2003.

Powell AM, Sakuma-Oyama Y, Oyama N, Black MM: Collagen XVII/BP180: A collagenous transmembrane protein component of the dermoepidermal anchoring complex. Clin Exp Derm 30:682–687, 2005.

Stout C, Goodenough DA, Paul DL: Connexins: Functions without junctions. Curr Opin Cell Biol 16:507–512, 2004.

Tsukita A, Furuse M: Claudin-based barrier in simple and stratified cellular sheets. Curr Opin Cell Biol 14:531–536, 2002.

Van Itallie CM, Anderson JM: The molecular physiology of tight junction pores. Physiology 19:331–338, 2004.

Wei C-J, Xu X, Lo CW: Connexins and cell signaling in development and disease. Annu Rev Cell Dev Biol 20:811–838, 2004.

Yap AS, Brieher WM, Gumbiner BM: Molecular analysis of cadherin-based adherens junctions. Annu Rev Cell Dev Biol 13:119–146, 1998.

CHAPTER 32

Connective Tissues

Animals use different proportions of matrix macromolecules to construct connective tissues with a range of mechanical properties to support their organs. Bone is a stiff, hard solid; blood vessel walls are flexible and elastic; and the vitreous body of the eye is a watery gel. Plant cell walls are conceptually similar to the animal extracellular matrix but are composed of completely different molecules. This chapter begins with a discussion of simple connective tissues but concentrates on cartilage, bone, development of the skeleton, and the mechanisms that repair wounds, finishing with a discussion of the plant cell wall.

Loose Connective Tissue

Loose connective tissue consists of a sparse extracellular matrix of **hyaluronan** and **proteoglycans** supported by a few **collagen fibrils** and **elastic fibrils.** In addition to fibroblasts, the cell population is heterogeneous, including both indigenous and emigrant connective tissue cells (see Fig. 28-3). The loose connective tissue underlying the epithelium in the gastrointestinal tract is a good example of this heterogeneity (Fig. 32-1A), with lymphocytes, plasma cells, macrophages, eosinophils, neutrophils, and mast cells, as well as fibroblasts and occasional fat cells (see Chapter 28 for details on these cells). This variety of defensive cells is appropriate for a location near the lumen of the intestine, which contains microorganisms and potentially toxic materials from the outside world. Loose connective tissue is also found in and around other organs. The optically transparent vitreous body of the eye is an extremely simple loose connective tissue in which fibroblasts produce a highly hydrated gel of hyaluronan and proteoglycans, supported by a loose network of type II collagen. Few defensive cells are required, as the interior of the eye is sterile.

Dense Connective Tissue

Collagen fibers, with or without elastic fibers, predominate over cells in dense connective tissue (Fig. 32-1B). Fibroblasts are present to manufacture extracellular matrix but are relatively sparse. Other connective tissue cells are even rarer, as these tissues are not usually exposed to microorganisms. Collagen fibers can be arranged precisely, as in tendons or cornea (see Fig. 29-3), or less so, as in the wall of the intestine or the skin. Tendons consist nearly exclusively of type I collagen fibers, all aligned along the length of the tendon to provide the tensile strength that is required to transmit forces

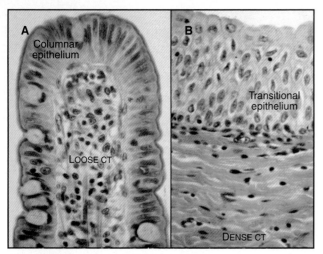

Figure 32-1   CONNECTIVE TISSUES. **A,** Loose connective tissue (CT) underlying the columnar epithelium of the small intestine. Light micrograph of a section stained with Masson trichrome stain. **B,** Dense connective tissue (CT) underlying transitional epithelium in the wall of the ureter. Light micrograph of a section stained with hematoxylin-eosin. (Courtesy of D. W. Fawcett, Harvard Medical School, Boston, Massachusetts.)

from muscle to bone. The cornea that forms the transparent front surface of the eye is also well organized into orthogonal layers of collagen fibrils.

Dense connective tissues can also be elastic. For example, the walls of arteries (see Fig. 29-8) and the dermal layer of skin consist of both collagen and elastic

fibers. Energy from each heartbeat stretches the elastic fibers in the walls of arteries. Recoil of these elastic fibers propels blood between heartbeats.

About 1 of 5000 humans inherits a mutation in a gene for fibrillar collagens type III or type IV, which causes a range of connective tissue defects called **Ehlers-Danlos syndrome.** Most affected individuals have thin skin and lax joints. Severe mutations lead to rupture of arteries, bowel, or uterus, often with fatal consequences. Ehlers-Danlos syndrome illustrates the importance of these collagens with regard to the integrity of the affected tissues. Inheritance is dominant, as these collagens consist of trimers of three identical subunits. Given one mutant gene, only one in eight ($\frac{1}{2} \times \frac{1}{2} \times \frac{1}{2}$) procollagen molecules is normal.

Cartilage

Cartilage (Fig. 32-2) is tough, resilient connective tissue that is well suited for a variety of mechanical roles. It covers the articular surfaces of joints and supports large airways, such as the trachea, and skeletal appendages, such as the nose and ears. Cartilage also forms the entire skeleton of sharks and the embryonic precursors of many bones in higher vertebrates. The mechanical properties of cartilage are attributable to abundant extracellular matrix consisting of fine collagen fibrils and high concentrations of glycosaminoglycans and proteoglycans (Fig. 32-3).

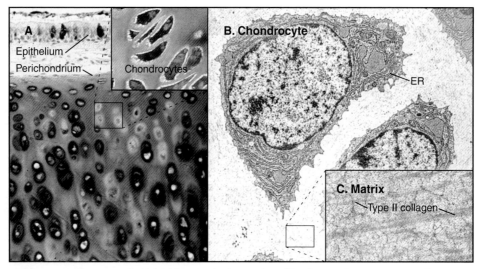

Figure 32-2   CARTILAGE AND CHONDROCYTES. **A,** Light micrograph of a section of hyaline cartilage in the wall of the respiratory tree stained with periodic acid–Schiff stain and alcian *blue*. The cartilage capsule of dense connective tissue (perichondrium) and the columnar epithelium lining the respiratory passage are at the top. **Inset,** Light micrograph of hyaline cartilage stained with toluidine *blue*. The proteoglycans in the matrix stain *pink*. The rough endoplasmic reticulum stains *blue*. Shrinkage during fixation and embedding creates the artifactual cavity or lacuna around each cell. **B,** Electron micrograph of a thin section of hyaline cartilage showing chondrocytes embedded in dense extracellular matrix. **C,** Electron micrograph of cartilage matrix at high magnification. This specimen was rapidly frozen and prepared by freeze-substitution to avoid collapse of the proteoglycans during dehydration and embedding. ER, endoplasmic reticulum. (A, Courtesy of D. W. Fawcett and E. D. Hay, Harvard Medical School, Boston, Massachusetts. B, Courtesy of E. D. Hay, Harvard Medical School, Boston, Massachusetts. C, Courtesy of E. B. Hunziker, M. Müller Institute, University of Bern, Switzerland.)

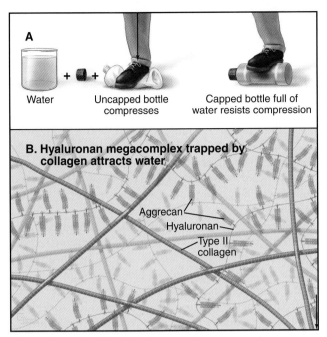

A

Water   Uncapped bottle   Capped bottle full of
         compresses   water resists compression

**B. Hyaluronan megacomplex trapped by
collagen attracts water**

Aggrecan
Hyaluronan
Type II
collagen

Figure 32-3 MACROMOLECULAR STRUCTURE AND MECHANICAL PROPERTIES OF HYALINE CARTILAGE MATRIX. **A,** Hydrostatic model of the mechanical properties of cartilage. Water trapped in the extracellular matrix resists compression. Neither water alone (in beaker) nor a pliable container (uncapped plastic bottle) resists compression. However, if water fills a capped bottle, it resists compression. **B,** In the cartilage matrix, flexible strands of type II collagen trap proteoglycans, which attract large amounts of water. Trapped water resists compression because its "container," the network of collagen fibrils, does not stretch.

Chondrocytes synthesize and secrete macromolecules for the cartilage matrix, which eventually surrounds them completely. Chondrocytes replenish the matrix as the macromolecules turn over slowly, but their ability to remodel and repair the matrix is limited. No blood vessels penetrate cartilage, owing to production of several inhibitors of endothelial cell growth by chondrocytes. Thus, all nutrients must diffuse into cartilage from the nearest blood vessel in the **perichondrium,** a dense capsule of fibrous connective tissue that covers the surface of cartilage. This capsule contains mesenchymal stem cells (see Box 41-1) that are capable of differentiating into chondrocytes.

A meshwork of **type II collagen fibrils,** accounting for about 25% of the dry mass, fills the extracellular matrix. These slender collagen fibrils are hard to see even in electron micrographs but are extremely stable, with lifetimes that are estimated to be many years. Fibrils tend to line up parallel to surfaces but otherwise are arranged randomly. Minor collagens type IX and type XI bind to the surface of type II fibrils. Type IX might be a cross-linker, and type XI might limit fibril size. Expression of type X collagen is restricted to cartilage that is undergoing conversion to bone. The matrix

contains several minor adhesive proteins, and other proteins inhibit invasion of blood vessels.

Glycosaminoglycans, including hyaluronan, constitute the second major class of matrix macromolecules. Molecules of the proteoglycan **aggrecan** attach to a hyaluronan backbone like the bristles of a test tube brush, forming so-called **megacomplexes** (see Fig. 29-14). Aggrecan also binds type II collagen. Highly charged glycosaminoglycans fill the extracellular space and attract water, the most abundant component of the matrix.

A hydrostatic mechanism allows cartilage to resist deformation (Fig. 32-3). Collagen fibrils provide tensile strength (i.e., resistance to stretching) but do not resist compression or bending. Glycosaminoglycans strongly attract water, resulting in an internal swelling pressure that pushes outward against collagen fibrils aligned parallel to the surface of the cartilage. The force of internal hydrostatic swelling pressure is balanced by the force produced by tension on the collagen fibrils. Remarkably, this internally stressed material can resist strong external forces such as those on the articular surfaces of joints. A macroscopic analog is a thin-walled plastic bottle filled with water. One can stand on the bottle provided that it is sealed, whereas neither the empty bottle nor the water could separately support any weight.

Specialized Forms of Cartilage

Hyaline cartilage, described earlier, is most common. It provides mechanical support for the respiratory tree, nose, articular surfaces, and developing bones. Elastic cartilage has abundant elastic fibers in addition to collagen, making the matrix much more elastic than hyaline cartilage. Elastic cartilage supports structures subjected to frequent deformation, including the larynx, epiglottis, and external ear. Fibrocartilage has features of both dense connective tissue (an abundance of thick collagen fibers) and cartilage (a prominent glycosaminoglycan matrix). It is tough and deformable, appropriate for its role in intervertebral disks and insertions of tendons.

Differentiation and Growth of Cartilage

Cartilage grows by expansion of the extracellular matrix either from within or on the surface. For surface growth, mesenchymal cells in the perichondrium differentiate into chondrocytes that synthesize and secrete matrix materials. For internal growth, chondrocytes trapped in the matrix divide and manufacture additional matrix, which is sufficiently deformable to allow for internal expansion.

Many growth factors cooperate to influence the differentiation of precursor cells into chondrocytes, the proliferation of chondrocytes, and the production of cartilage matrix molecules. These include Indian hedgehog (Ihh), members of transforming growth factor-β family (TGF-β and bone morphogenetic factors), fibroblast growth factors (FGFs), parathyroid hormone–related protein (PTHrP), and insulin-like growth factors (IGF-I and IGF-II). Chondrocytes produce some of these growth factors (TGF-β, FGFs, and IGFs). During development, adjacent tissues can induce cartilage formation by secreting TGF-β and FGF. SOX9 is the key transcription factor mediating expression of cartilage-specific genes.

Diseases Involving Cartilage

Cartilage fails in common human diseases, including arthritis and ruptured intervertebral disks. Mutations in the genes for cartilage proteins and growth factors cause human disease (Appendix 32-1). Chondrocytes fail to proliferate in the absence of PTHrP or certain receptors for FGF, causing severe deformities of the skeleton. More than 25 different mutations of the human gene for type II collagen cause disorders of cartilage, ranging in severity from death in utero to dwarfism or osteoarthritis. Mutations in genes for minor cartilage collagens cause a variety of symptoms, including degenerative joint disease. A premature stop codon in chicken aggrecan causes lethal skeletal malformations.

Bone

For most vertebrates, bones provide mechanical support and serve as a storage site for calcium. The great strength and light weight of bones are attributable both to the mechanical properties of the extracellular matrix and to efficient overall design, including tubular form and lamination (Fig. 32-4). A superficial layer of compact bone surrounds a medullary cavity that is filled with marrow, fat, or both and is supported by struts of bone arranged precisely along lines of mechanical stress. External surfaces of bones are covered either by dense connective tissue, called **periosteum,** or by cartilage at joint surfaces. A monolayer of bone-forming cells called osteoblasts line the internal surfaces. Blood vessels supply the medullary cavity and penetrate compact bone through a network of channels. Although bone is durable and strong, continuous remodeling makes bone much more dynamic than it appears.

Extracellular Matrix of Bone

Bone is a composite material consisting of collagen fibrils (providing tensile strength) embedded in a matrix of calcium phosphate crystals (providing rigidity) (Fig. 32-4E). Macroscopic analogs of the bone matrix are concrete reinforced by steel rods and fiberglass consisting of a brittle plastic reinforced by glass fibers. Each of these composites is stronger than its separate components. Simple extraction experiments illustrate the contributions of the two components. After removal of calcium phosphate with a calcium chelator, bone is so rubbery that it bends easily. After destruction of collagen by heating, bone is hard but brittle.

Fibrils of type I collagen, the dominant organic component of the matrix (Table 32-1), are arranged in sheets or a meshwork. Covalent cross-links between the collagen molecules in fibrils make them inextensible. The matrix contains more than 100 minor proteins, including growth factors and adhesive glycoproteins, but few proteoglycans.

Calcium-phosphate crystals, similar to **hydroxyapatite** $[Ca_{10}(PO_4)_6(OH)_2]$, make up about two thirds of the dry weight of bone. These crystals begin growing within collagen fibrils and in holes between the ends of the staggered collagen molecules, eventually filling the spaces between the collagen molecules within the fibrils. The mechanisms that control nucleation of hydroxyapatite and the orientation of the crystals are still under investigation.

Bone Cells

Bone is an active tissue that is maintained by a balance of cellular activities. Osteoblasts and osteocytes produce extracellular matrix and establish conditions for its calcification. Osteoclasts resorb bone, as is required for growth and remodeling. An imbalance of these opposing cellular activities causes human diseases. Osteoblasts arise from the same mesenchymal stem cells that give rise to fibroblasts and chondrocytes (see Fig. 28-3). Osteoclasts form by fusion of blood monocytes.

A monolayer of **osteoblasts** on the surface of growing bone tissue uses a well-developed secretory pathway to synthesize and secrete organic components of the matrix (Fig. 32-5). Unmineralized bone matrix consists largely of type I collagen but includes factors that promote crystallization of calcium phosphate on the surface of these fibrils. Osteoblasts also control the differentiation, but not the activity, of osteoclasts (see Fig. 32-6).

Once an osteoblast has enclosed itself within bone matrix, it is called an **osteocyte.** Osteocytes are connected to each other by long, slender filopodia that run through narrow channels in the matrix (see Fig. 32-4D–E). Gap junctions between the processes of osteocytes provide a continuous network of intercellular communication that stretches from cells adjacent to blood vessels to the most deeply embedded osteocyte. Osteocytes can lay down or resorb matrix in their immediate vicinity.

Osteoblasts differentiate from mesenchymal cells under the control of growth factors, including Indian hedgehog, bone morphogenetic proteins (BMPs; see

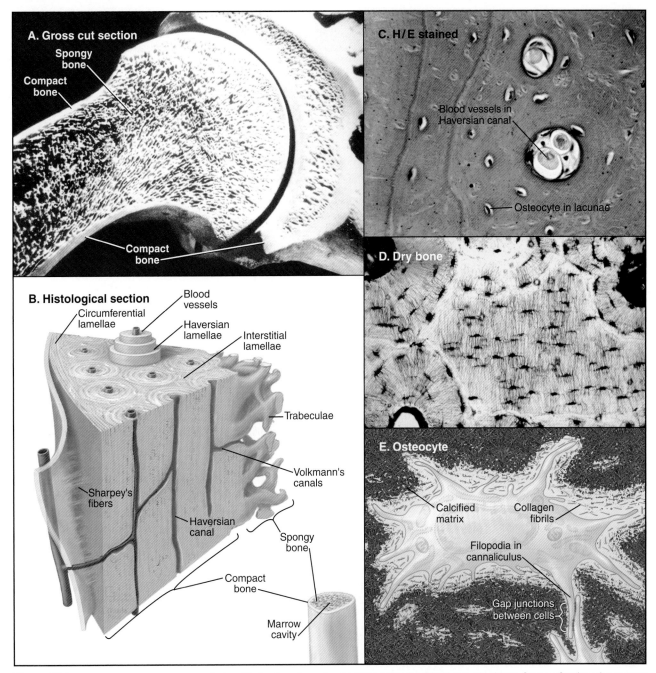

Figure 32-4 ORGANIZATION OF LONG BONES. **A,** Longitudinal section of a shoulder joint of a dried bone specimen. Struts of trabecular spongy bone reinforce compact bone in the cortex. **B,** A wedge of long bone. Circumferential lamellae form the outer layer just beneath the periosteum *(blue)* covering the surface. Osteons (Haversian systems) consist of concentric lamellae of calcified matrix and osteocytes arranged around a channel containing one or two capillaries or venules. Interstitial lamellae are fragments of osteons that remain after remodeling (Fig. 32-10). Radial vascular channels connect longitudinal vascular channels to the medullary cavity or periosteum. **C,** Light micrograph of a cross section stained with hematoxylin-eosin showing circumferential lamellae on the *left* and two Haversian canals. **D,** Light micrograph of a cross section of dried bone showing a central interstitial lamella surrounded by three osteons. Narrow canaliculi connect the lacunae housing osteocytes. **E,** An osteocyte surrounded by calcified matrix and extending filopodia into canaliculi. (Micrographs courtesy of D. W. Fawcett, Harvard Medical School, Boston, Massachusetts.)

Fig. 24-8), and Wnts (see Fig. 30-8). Humans with loss-of-function mutations in a Wnt coreceptor have few osteoblasts and low bone density, while loss-of-function mutations in a BMP competitor have the opposite effect. Inside osteoblasts, **Runx2/Cbfa1** is the master tran-

scription factor controlling the expression of genes that are required to make bone matrix. Mouse embryos lacking Runx2/Cbfa1 have no osteoblasts or osteoclasts. They make a cartilage skeleton that never transforms to bone. Humans and mice with just one active Runx2/

Table 32-1

BONE PROTEINS

Name	Content	Functions
Bone morphogenic proteins	Minor	TGF-β homologs; cartilage stimulation and bone development and repair
Collagen type I	90%	Forms fibrils in the bone matrix
Osteocalcin	1%–2%	Network of aspartic acid and γ-carboxylated glutamic acid side chains bind hydroxyapatite; promotes calcification; attracts osteoclasts and osteoblasts
Osteonectin	2%	Synthesized in developing and regenerating bone; binds collagen and hydroxyapatite; may nucleate hydroxyapatite crystallization in bone matrix
Osteopontin	Minor	RGD sequence; binds osteoclast integrins to bone surface
Proteoglycans	Minor	Decorin, biglycan, osteoadherin; may bind TGF-β
Sialoproteins	2%	RGD sequence; binds osteoclast integrins to bone surface

Cbfa1 gene lack collarbones and experience a delay in the fusion of joints between skull bones. This syndrome is the most common human skeletal defect. Runx2/Cbfa1 is part of a network of transcription factors with positive and negative influences on osteoblast differentiation and function.

Circulating hormones influence the activity of osteoblasts and osteocytes. In response to the calcium concentration in blood, parathyroid glands secrete **parathyroid hormone,** which stimulates osteocytes to mobilize calcium from the surrounding matrix. This feedback loop maintains a constant concentration of calcium in the blood.

Osteoclasts are multinucleated giant cells specialized for bone resorption (Fig. 32-6). They attach like a

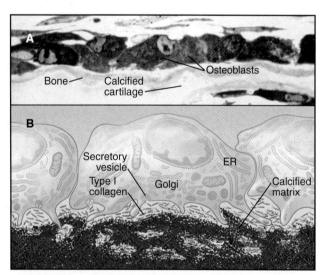

Figure 32-5 **OSTEOBLASTS. A,** Light micrograph of a section of forming bone stained with toluidine *blue.* Osteoblasts with abundant, *blue-stained,* rough endoplasmic reticulum lay down bone matrix *(light green)* on the surface of calcified cartilage *(light pink).* **B,** Drawing of osteoblasts. ER, endoplasmic reticulum. (A, Courtesy of R. Dintzis and from the work of D. Walker, Johns Hopkins Medical School, Baltimore, Maryland.)

suction cup to the surface of bone. Interactions of a plasma membrane integrin ($\alpha_v\beta_3$) with bone matrix proteins (osteopontin and sialoprotein) help to create a leak-proof compartment on the bone surface. Osteoclasts amplify the plasma membrane lining this closed space, forming a "ruffled border" composed of microvilli enriched with a **V-type H⁺** transporting adenosine triphosphatase (ATPase, see Fig. 8-5) and chloride channels (see Fig. 10-13). The combined activities of the H⁺ pump and chloride channels allow the cell to secrete hydrochloric acid into the sealed extracellular compartment on the bone surface. This closed space acts like an extracellular lysosome: Acid dissolves calcium phosphate crystals, and secreted proteolytic enzymes, including **cathepsin K,** digest collagen and other organic components. Degradation products are taken up by endocytosis and transported across the cell in vesicles for secretion on the free surface. Amino acids are reused, but collagen cross-linking groups are not, so they are excreted in the urine, where their concentration is a measure of bone turnover.

Bone marrow supporting cells, osteoblasts, and activated T lymphocytes produce two proteins, which stimulate blood monocytes to fuse and differentiate into multinucleated osteoclasts (Fig. 32-6). These key factors are **macrophage colony–stimulating factor (M-CSF)** and **RANKL** (RANK ligand, also called osteoprotegerin ligand [OPGL] or TRANCE). Both factors are produced locally in bone marrow as transmembrane proteins with the growth factor domain on the cell surface. These proteins control differentiation through binding to their receptors by either direct cell-to-cell contact or release of the active domain by proteolytic cleavage. First, M-CSF activates a cytokine receptor (see Fig. 24-6) on macrophages. The resulting stimulation of a JAK-STAT pathway (see Fig. 27-9) turns on expression of genes required for the monocyte to differentiate into a pre-osteoclast. An important change is the expression of a receptor called RANK (receptor for activation of NF-κB, a member of the TNF receptor family; see Fig. 24-10).

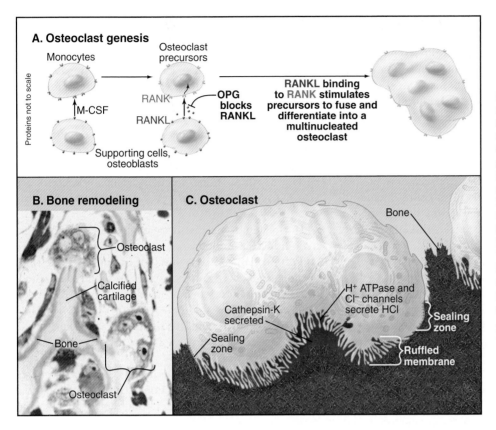

A. Osteoclast genesis

Proteins not to scale

Monocytes

Osteoclast precursors

M-CSF

RANK

RANKL

OPG blocks RANKL

Supporting cells, osteoblasts

RANKL binding to RANK stimulates precursors to fuse and differentiate into a multinucleated osteoclast

B. Bone remodeling

Osteoclast

Calcified cartilage

Bone

Osteoclast

C. Osteoclast

Bone

Cathepsin-K secreted

Sealing zone

H⁺ ATPase and Cl⁻ channels secrete HCl

Sealing zone

Ruffled membrane

Figure 32-6 OSTEOCLASTS. **A,** Formation of a multinucleated osteoclast by fusion of monocytes stimulated by RANKL, M-CSF, and other factors. **B,** Light micrograph of a section of forming bone stained with toluidine *blue* showing two osteoclasts degrading bone and calcified cartilage. **C,** An osteoclast attached to the bone matrix by a sealing zone, forming a resorption cavity *(pink)*. The cell pumps H⁺ and secretes lysosomal enzymes into this cavity to resorb the surface of the matrix. (B, Courtesy of R. Dintzis and from the work of D. Walker, Johns Hopkins Medical School, Baltimore, Maryland.)

Once this receptor is expressed, RANKL can activate preosteoclasts through the transcription factor NF-κB (see Fig. 15-22C) to express the proteins that are required for cell fusion and further differentiation into an osteoclast. Mice that lack RANKL form no osteoclasts, so bone resorption fails.

Other growth factors, including TNF itself, contribute to this process by acting directly on osteoclasts, but many stimulators of osteoclast differentiation (e.g., parathyroid hormone, vitamin D, leptin) act indirectly by stimulating supporting cells to make RANKL. For example, **leptin,** a satiety hormone secreted by fat cells, acts on neurons of the hypothalamus in the brain that regulate not only appetite but also bone metabolism indirectly via the sympathetic nervous system. Norepinephrine released by sympathetic nerves activates osteoblasts to secrete RANKL. This explains why animals and people that lack leptin or its receptor not only are obese but also have dense bones. Osteoclast growth factors RANKL, TNF, and interleukin-1 mediate excess bone resorption at sites of chronic inflammation in rheumatoid arthritis and gum diseases.

Differentiation of osteoclasts is subject to negative regulation by a soluble **decoy receptor** for RANKL called OPG (osteoprotegerin), which binds RANKL and blocks activation of RANK. Estrogens inhibit osteoclast differentiation by stimulating osteoblasts to produce OPG, so circulating OPG declines in parallel with estro-

gen levels after menopause. The resulting increase in osteoclasts contributes to bone loss in older women.

Formation and Growth of the Skeleton

Both genetic and environmental information direct formation of the skeleton. Genetic information predominates in the master plan and initial development of skeletal tissues, as the size and shape of bones are characteristic for each species. Subsequently, environmental information is important in remodeling of the skeleton in response to use. Mutations in genes for structural and informational molecules have provided valuable clues about the genetic blueprint for the skeleton, but the understanding of these complex regulatory pathways is far from complete (Appendix 32-1).

Genetic information is read out on at least two levels. First, master genetic regulators—including transcription factors encoded by **HOX (homeobox)** and **PAX (paired box)** genes—specify the developmental fate of each embryonic segment. Homeoboxes are DNA sequences that encode a family of 60-residue protein domains that bind DNA (see Fig. 15-17). The human genome contains 39 HOX genes arrayed in four linear arrays, similar to those in other animals, including flies and nematodes. HOX genes were discovered in flies as a result of mutations that cause "homeotic conversion," whereby the fate of one segment is converted into another, sometimes with bizarre results, such as the substitution of a leg for an antenna. The same thing happens in vertebrates: Mouse embryos express Hoxd-4 in the second cervical (neck) vertebra and more posterior segments. Mutation of Hoxd-4 results in a failure of the second cervical vertebra to form normally. Instead, it takes on some of the features of the first cervical vertebra. Mutations in other HOX genes cause congenital malformations in humans. HOX transcription factors control the expression of downstream genes, including growth factors, but the pathways from HOX genes to determinants of three-dimensional architecture are incompletely understood.

Second, systematically circulating and locally secreted growth factors control the proliferation and differentiation of the cells of cartilage and bone. Mutations in these factors and their receptors also cause surprisingly specific human skeletal malformations. Circulating **growth hormone** produced by the pituitary gland is a major determinant of skeletal size. Individuals who are deficient in growth hormone are short in stature. Locally produced growth factors, including bone morphogenetic proteins (BMPs) and fibroblast growth factors (FGFs) and their receptors, control the development and growth of cartilage and bone during embryogenesis, in addition to stimulating repair after fractures. FGF receptors are tyrosine kinases. BMPs are related in structure and mechanism to TGF-β and are expressed in tissues other than bone and cartilage (see Fig. 24-8). BMPs are part of a system of positive and negative factors that regulates formation of cartilage, bone, and joints. For example, a BMP called GDF-5 specifies the position of joints, but joints form only if noggin protein, an inhibitor of other BMPs, is present.

Embryonic Bone Formation

Bone always forms by replacement of preexisting connective tissue. During embryonic development, flat bones, such as the skull and shoulder blades, form from **neural crest cell** precursors in loose connective tissue (Fig. 32-7). Somehow, one-dimensional information in the genome is read out as the three-dimensional pattern of a skull. Growth factors, vitamins (e.g., retinoic acid), and local matrix molecules, such as glycosaminoglycans all influence the differentiation of these cells into osteoblasts at specific locations in connective tissue. Osteoblasts lay down struts of bone matrix in the loose connective tissue. As new bone is laid down on the surface of these bone spicules, some osteoblasts are trapped and become osteocytes. A similar process heals fractures.

During embryonic and postnatal development, genetic information precisely controls changes in the size and proportions of flat bones. For example, for the skull to increase in size both externally and internally, osteoclasts on the outer surface lay down new bone at the same rate at which osteoclasts resorb old bone inside (Fig. 32-9). These cellular activities are carefully coordinated to change the proportions of the skull as the individual matures.

Long bones, such as the humerus, begin as cartilage models that are replaced by bone (Fig. 32-8). The initial steps are only vaguely understood at the cellular and molecular levels. Multiple, genetically programmed factors induce clusters of mesenchymal cells at specific locations to differentiate into chondrocytes that secrete type II collagen and glycosaminoglycans. This produces a miniature cartilaginous version of the adult bone.

Bone replaces this cartilage precursor in a series of steps that are coordinated locally by production of growth factors. Perichondrial cells and proliferating chondrocytes secrete parathyroid hormone-related protein (PTHrP), which promotes chondrocyte division and growth. In supporting roles, BMPs promote and FGFs inhibit chondrocytes growth and differentiation. More mature chondrocytes produce Indian hedgehog, which directs the terminal differentiation of neighboring chondrocytes. These **hypertrophic chondrocytes** cause the bone to grow longer as they grow in size,

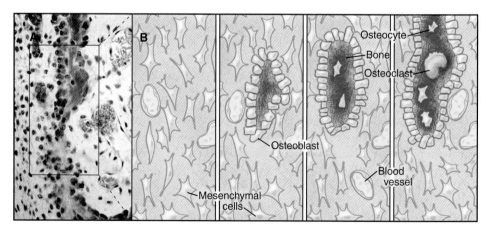

Figure 32-7 BONE FORMATION BY INTRAMEMBRANOUS OSSIFICATION. **A,** Light micrograph of a section of forming bone stained with hematoxylin-eosin. Calcified bone matrix is *maroon*. **B,** Interpretive drawings. Connective tissue mesenchymal cells differentiate into osteoblasts, which lay down bone matrix *(blue)*. Osteoblasts become trapped as the matrix grows. (A, Courtesy of D. W. Fawcett, Harvard Medical School, Boston, Massachusetts.)

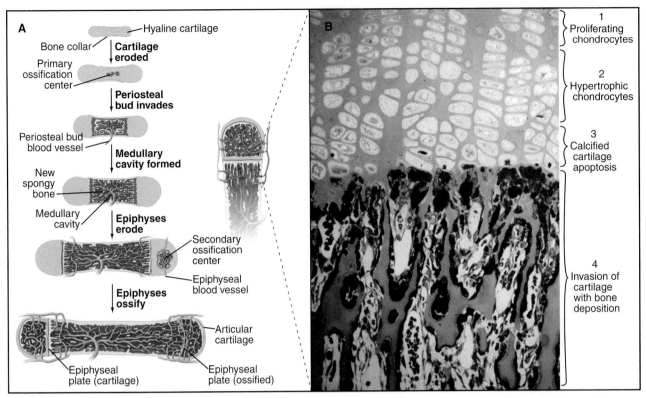

Figure 32-8 FORMATION OF A LONG BONE BY REPLACEMENT OF CARTILAGE. **A,** The shaft grows in diameter as osteoblasts lay down bone *(tan)* on the outer surface of the primary collar of bone and osteoclasts remove bone from the inner surface to form and maintain the marrow cavity. The bone grows in length by interstitial expansion of the cartilage in the epiphyseal plate and its replacement by bone. **B,** Light micrograph of a section of an epiphyseal plate stained with toluidine *blue.* Cartilage growth, differentiation, and replacement by bone occur in several zones. Proliferation of chondrocytes and their production of matrix *(pink)* containing type II collagen are solely responsible for the longitudinal growth of the bone *(1).* Hypertrophic chondrocytes enlarge and make type X collagen, as well as matrix metalloproteinases that resorb some of the surrounding matrix *(2).* Chondrocytes die by apoptosis (see Chapter 46), and the matrix calcifies *(3).* Blood vessels and osteoblasts move into spaces vacated by chondrocytes and lay down bone *(blue)* on the surface of calcified cartilage *(4).* (Micrograph courtesy of R. Dintzis and from the work of D. Walker, Johns Hopkins Medical School, Baltimore, Maryland.)

secrete type X collagen, and use matrix metalloproteinases to resorb some of their surrounding matrix. They direct the calcification of the cartilage matrix before undergoing apoptosis. Osteoblasts lay down bone matrix on the surface of the calcified cartilage. Cartilage is avascular, owing to expression of inhibitors of blood vessel growth, but hypertrophic cartilage ceases to inhibit endothelial cell growth. This allows FGF-2, TGF-β, and vascular endothelium growth factor to attract capillaries as part of the transformation of cartilage to bone.

For a long bone to maintain its shape as it grows in size, deposition and removal of bone tissue must be highly selective. For the shaft to grow in diameter, new bone is laid down on the outer surface by osteoblasts at the same time as old bone is removed inside by osteoclasts (Fig. 32-9). Bones grow longer as a result of interstitial growth of cartilage in the **epiphyseal plate** and its continual replacement by bone. Growth of long bones stops at puberty, when high concentrations of estrogen and testosterone stop proliferation of

epiphyseal chondrocytes so that bone replaces this cartilage. This closure of the epiphyses occurs over several years in a predictable order, so one can judge the maturity of a child by examining epiphyses by radiographic studies. Genetic variations in this process of maturation give rise to differences in stature. Metabolic and endocrine disorders can also affect the timing of epiphyseal closure.

Bone Remodeling

Bone is amazingly dynamic and is remodeled continuously in response to stresses. Bone cells and matrix turn over every few years. Reorganization of bone requires two carefully coordinated steps: breakdown of preexisting bone by osteoclasts and replacement with new bone by osteoblasts. More than 100 years ago, Wolff realized that the strength of a bone depends on use. For example, bones of the racquet arm of tennis players are more robust than the bones of their other arm. Thus, mechanical forces on the bones must generate modulatory

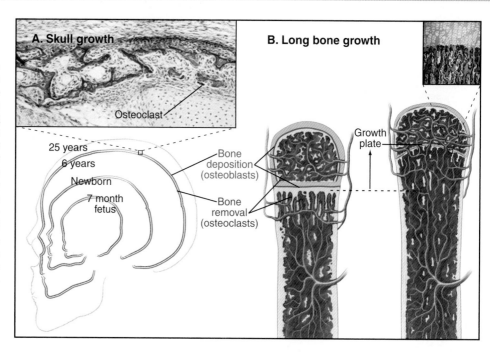

Figure 32-9 BONE GROWTH. A, Light micrograph of a section of skull stained with Mallory's trichrome stain and an interpretive drawing. The skull expands during fetal development and growth to adulthood as osteoblasts lay down new bone on the outer surface *(blue)* and osteoclasts resorb bone *(pink)* on the inner surface. **B,** Long bones grow entirely by expansion of cartilage in the epiphyseal plate and its replacement by bone *(tan),* followed by resorption *(pink).* (A, Courtesy of D. W. Fawcett, Harvard Medical School, Boston, Massachusetts.)

signals that control remodeling, but the molecular mechanisms are still uncertain.

Formation of the cylindrical units of long bones called **osteons** is a good example of well-coordinated remodeling. The process involves two steps (Fig. 32-10). First, osteoclasts resorb preexisting bone to form long, cylindrical, resorption channels in the same way that a plumber's snake (such as the Roto-Rooter) clears debris from drain pipes. The second step is slower, as osteoblasts take weeks to fill in these channels by depositing concentric layers of lamellar bone against the walls. They lay down matrix at a rate of about 1 μm of thickness per day until bone completely surrounds the blood vessels trapped in the middle of the newly formed osteon. Because resorption channels cut randomly through the bone, fragments of older osteons are left behind during the remodeling of mature bone. These fragments are called **interstitial lamellae.** Resorption may release growth and differentiation factors from the mineralized matrix that provide a local stimulus for the next round of bone formation by new osteoblasts.

Bone Diseases

Osteoporosis, a thinning of bones, is common in elderly people as a result of an imbalance of bone resorption over renewal. In the United States, osteoporosis results in 1.5 million painful fractures, costing $16 billion annually. Almost 50% of women suffer from such a fracture at some time in their lives. Osteoporosis also occurs at reduced gravitational forces during space flight. The pathogenesis is not understood, but both behavioral (e.g., inactivity, poor nutrition, smoking) and multiple genetic factors have modest effects. One genetic factor among many might be naturally occurring variants of the nuclear receptor for vitamin D. This receptor is a transcription factor that is required for vitamin D to stimulate intestinal calcium uptake and calcification of bone. Variations in the genes for type I collagen or bone growth factors may also contribute. To date, treatments (e.g., vitamin D, estrogen, calcium, strontium, bisphosphonates) are only partially effective. Injection of either OPG or antibodies to RANKL strongly inhibits bone resorption, but long-term clinical confirmation of efficacy in osteoporosis is not yet available.

Osteopetrosis is failure of bone resorption, leading to an imbalance of renewal over resorption. This rare disease of osteoclasts is fatal in humans, owing to bone marrow failure. Recessive mutations in the genes for the proton-ATPase pump (60%) and chloride channel (~15%) account for most human cases. Naturally occurring or engineered mutations in the genes for essentially any protein required for osteoclast differentiation or function cause osteopetrosis in mice. The disease can be cured in humans and mice by transplantation of bone marrow stem cells to replace defective osteoclast precursors, an early example of stem cell therapy.

Osteogenesis imperfecta is the name of a variety of congenital fragile bone syndromes. Severely affected fetuses die in utero from multiple broken bones. Mildly affected individuals are born but suffer multiple fractures resulting in skeletal deformities. All of the patients have mutations in the gene for type I collagen. Some are deletions or insertions, which may be mild. Most patients with severe disease have point mutations leading to replacement of a glycine by a larger amino acid. This

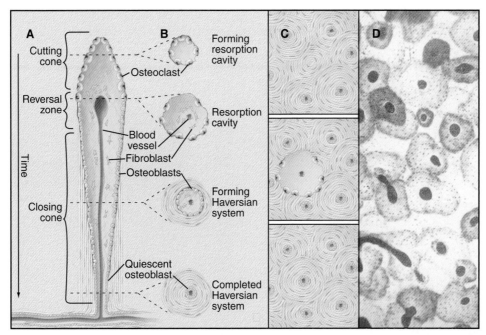

Figure 32-10 BONE REMODELING. **A–B,** Longitudinal and cross sections of a time line illustrating the formation of an osteon. Osteoclasts cut a cylindrical channel through bone. Osteoblasts follow, laying down bone on the surface of the channel until the matrix surrounds the central blood vessel of the newly formed osteon. **C,** Steps in the formation of a new osteon. Parts of older osteons are left behind as interstitial lamellae. **D,** Microradiograph of a cross section of a long bone, illustrating the range of ages of the structures. A section of bone is placed on X-ray film, exposed to X-rays, developed, and examined by light microscopy. Older parts of the bone, such as the interstitial lamellae, are more heavily calcified and therefore absorb more of the X-rays, appearing lighter. Newly formed osteons appear the darkest, as they are the least calcified. Vascular spaces are empty and fully exposed by the X-rays. (A, Redrawn from Parfitt AM: The action of parathyroid hormone on bone. Metabolism 25:809–844, 1976. D, Courtesy of D. W. Fawcett, Harvard Medical School, Boston, Massachusetts.)

prevents the zipper-like folding of the collagen triple helix (see Fig. 29-1), even if only one chain is defective per molecule. This poisons assembly and accounts for the dominant phenotype. No one knows why these mutations in type I collagen do not affect other tissues, such as skin, which are rich in type I collagen.

Repair of Wounds and Fractures

Healing of minor skin wounds is a familiar occurrence that illustrates the mechanisms that control the assembly of connective tissue. Repair of connective tissue in the dermis underlying the epithelium proceeds in three stages: formation of a blood clot, assembly of provisional connective tissue, and remodeling of the connective tissue (Fig. 32-11).

Tissue damage ruptures blood vessels, releasing blood that clots to stem the hemorrhage and fill the damaged area. The clot forms when injury activates the blood plasma proteolytic enzyme **thrombin,** which cleaves the plasma protein **fibrinogen** to form **fibrin.** Fibrin polymerizes and is cross-linked to itself and to **plasma fibronectin.** This provisional extracellular matrix of fibrin and fibronectin provides physical integ-

rity for the clot and an environment for wound repair. Platelets that are activated during clotting secrete matrix molecules (thrombospondin, fibrinogen, fibronectin, and von Willebrand's factor) and growth factors (platelet-derived growth factor [PDGF], TGF-β, and TGF-α) that initiate the cellular events required to complete wound repair.

Chemotactic factors attract phagocytes from the blood into the wound. These factors include PDGF, chemokines, peptides cleaved from fibrinogen by thrombin, and peptides from any contaminating bacteria. Neutrophils arrive first from the nearby blood vessels, having attached to activated endothelial cells (see Fig. 30-13) and migrated into the connective tissue and clot. They ingest any bacteria. Second, monocytes (using a similar mechanism) migrate into the clot and clear foreign material and any dead neutrophils. The environment in a wound promotes transformation of monocytes into macrophages, which synthesize and secrete cytokines and growth factors that mediate the cellular events that complete the repair process. In this way, platelets, monocytes, and fibroblasts form a relay, passing information from one cell to the next.

During the next phase of repair, macrophages, fibroblasts, and capillary endothelial cells migrate into the

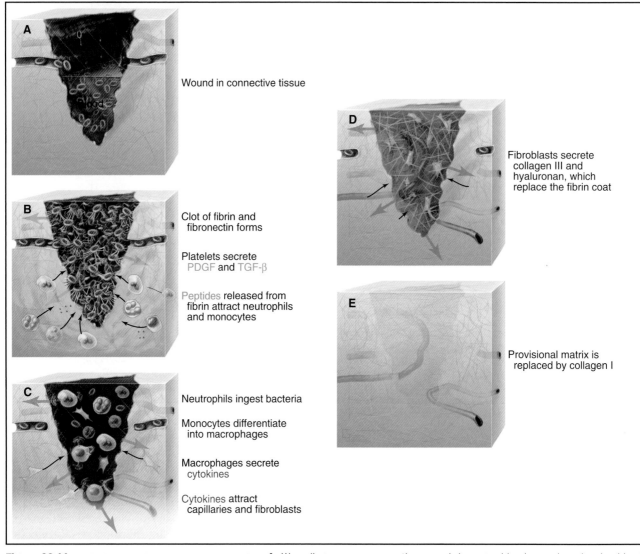

A, Wound in connective tissue

B, Clot of fibrin and fibronectin forms

Platelets secrete PDGF and TGF-β

Peptides released from fibrin attract neutrophils and monocytes

C, Neutrophils ingest bacteria

Monocytes differentiate into macrophages

Macrophages secrete cytokines

Cytokines attract capillaries and fibroblasts

D, Fibroblasts secrete collagen III and hyaluronan, which replace the fibrin coat

E, Provisional matrix is replaced by collagen I

Figure 32-11 REPAIR OF A WOUND IN CONNECTIVE TISSUE. **A,** Wounding removes some tissue and damages blood vessels, releasing blood into the defect. **B,** Blood forms a clot of fibrin and fibronectin, releasing fibrin peptides, and platelets secrete PDGF and TGF-β, all of which attract neutrophils and monocytes. **C,** Neutrophils ingest any bacteria. Monocytes clean up debris and differentiate into macrophages, which secrete cytokines, attracting fibroblasts and blood vessels. **D,** Fibroblasts secrete type III collagen and hyaluronan, which, in turn, replace the fibrin clot. **E,** Fibroblasts remodel the provisional connective tissue with type I collagen, and blood vessels grow back into the new tissue.

fibrin clot and reestablish the connective tissue. Endothelial cells form capillary loops that allow blood to flow and to provide oxygen. Initially, the endothelial cells are attracted by growth factors released by platelets, but macrophages and dissolution of fibrin provide a more sustained supply of chemoattractants and growth factors. Integrin receptors for fibronectin allow fibroblasts to migrate into the clot. They secrete more fibronectin as they move. Within the clot, PDGF and TGF-β from macrophages stimulate fibroblasts to secrete type III collagen, hyaluronan, SPARC (secreted protein acidic and rich in cysteine), and tenascin. Initially, this loose connective tissue is disorganized and weak. Hyaluronan predominates transiently, but after about five days,

it is gradually replaced by proteoglycans and type I collagen.

Two events complete the repair of the matrix. First, fibroblasts differentiate into (smooth muscle–like) **myofibroblasts,** which contract the collagen matrix, closing the edges of the wound. This step is particularly important for large wounds. Second, fibroblasts remodel the provisional connective tissue to restore its original architecture with nearly normal physical strength. This requires resorption of provisional collagen fibrils by metalloproteinases (see Fig. 29-20) and assembly of more robust type I collagen fibrils.

While fibroblasts repair the connective tissue, the epithelium bordering the wound spreads by cell division and migration to cover the defect. This process of migration is initiated within hours of wounding. Both the loss of contacts with neighboring cells at the edge of the wound and the release of growth factors in the wound are thought to transform the static epithelial cells into migrating cells. Keratin filaments that predominate in the cytoskeleton of the skin epithelial cells are replaced with actin filaments. Hemidesmosomes that anchor the skin epithelial cells to the basal lamina are lost, and the cells migrate over the surface of the underlying matrix, which consists initially of fibrin and fibronectin and later of collagen. As they go, epithelial cells lay down a new basal lamina. Depending on the size of the defect, proliferation of epithelial cells might be required to complete coverage of the surface. When it is covered, the cells begin to differentiate into stratified epithelium.

Many parallels exist between repair of a fractured bone and repair of a skin wound. Blood escapes from damaged blood vessels and clots at the fracture site. PDGF that has been released by platelets stimulates mesenchymal cells to proliferate in the surrounding tissue. These cells migrate into the clot along with blood vessels and macrophages. Stimulated by growth factors released initially by platelets and in a more sustained fashion by macrophages, mesenchymal cells differentiate into chondrocytes and osteoblasts that recapitulate the development of new bone to fill in the defect. Although the bone that is initially produced to join the fractured ends is poorly organized, fractures are mechanically stable within about six weeks. The fibrin clot is converted directly into bone if the broken bone is immobilized. A cartilage intermediate may form first if the fracture is allowed to move. Over a period of months, remodeling reestablishes the normal pattern of the bone. With time, remodeling can even straighten out bones that are mildly bent at fracture sites.

In all of these examples, wound healing is coordinated by a variety of growth factors and cytokines and is supported by the environment provided by the extracellular matrix. For example, PDGF from platelets stimulates the proliferation of fibroblasts and attracts them to the fibrin clot at the site of a wound. TGF-β inhibits fibroblast proliferation but stimulates fibroblasts to make matrix molecules. The actions of cytokines and growth factors depend on the local environment in the matrix. In a fibrin clot, TGF-β binds to its receptor on cells rather than the matrix. In the normal connective tissue matrix, TGF-β binds to proteoglycans in preference to its cell surface receptors, and its effects are not felt. In a fibrin/fibronectin clot, cellular fibronectin receptors bind the matrix, stimulating production of matrix metalloproteinases that are appropriate for remodeling the matrix. In normal connective tissue with less fibronectin, cells produce less metalloproteinase.

The mechanisms that mediate physiological wound repair can also contribute to disease. For example, PDGF that is released from activated platelets in clots at the sites of wounds initiates the cellular events that are required for repair. On the other hand, when the endothelium lining of large arteries is damaged, platelets are activated by binding to the exposed basal lamina. This stimulates them to release PDGF, which promotes proliferation of fibroblasts and smooth muscle cells in the artery wall, an early step in the development of arteriosclerosis.

Plant Cell Wall

The cell walls of land plants are composite materials consisting of cellulose, other polysaccharides, and glycoproteins (Fig. 32-12). Wood and cotton are two familiar examples of cell wall material that is left behind after plant cells have died. Like the extracellular matrix of animals, plant cell walls not only provide mechanical support but also may influence development. Two types of forces act on cell walls. Internally, the vacuole of the plant cell applies turgor pressure. Cell walls also resist a variety of external mechanical forces that tend to deform the cell.

The main constituent of cell walls is **cellulose,** the most abundant biopolymer on earth. It is a long, unbranched polymer of glucose (see Fig. 3-25). Several dozen cellulose polymers associate laterally into 5- to 7-nm bundles called **microfibrils** (Fig. 32-12B). Two types of branched polysaccharides—**hemicellulose** and **pectin**—associate with cellulose in microfibrils.

A complex of plasma membrane enzymes termed **cellulose synthases** synthesize cellulose. *Arabidopsis* has genes for about 30 different cellulose synthases. Genetic evidence suggests that active enzymes consist of two different synthase polypeptides. These transmembrane enzymes form a rosette of six particles that are visible by electron microscopy. Glucose polymers are initiated with a lipid anchor and then elongated by the rosettes, which extrude 36 cellulose polymers across the plasma membrane. Outside the cell, these polymers self-assemble into linear crystals called microfibrils. Hydrogen bonds constrain the glucose units to face in alternate directions in planar ribbons (see Fig. 3-25A). These ribbons self-assemble laterally into planar crystalline sheets, which stack vertically into paracrystalline bundles that are held together by C-H•••O hydrogen bonds. Cellulose microfibrils in the cell wall are usually organized like barrel hoops perpendicular to the axis of cellular growth to allow for expansion. Cytoplasmic microtubules tend to have the same orientation. Cellulose synthesis moves the rosettes of cellulose synthase in the plane of the plasma membrane along paths defined by the cytoplasmic microtubules.

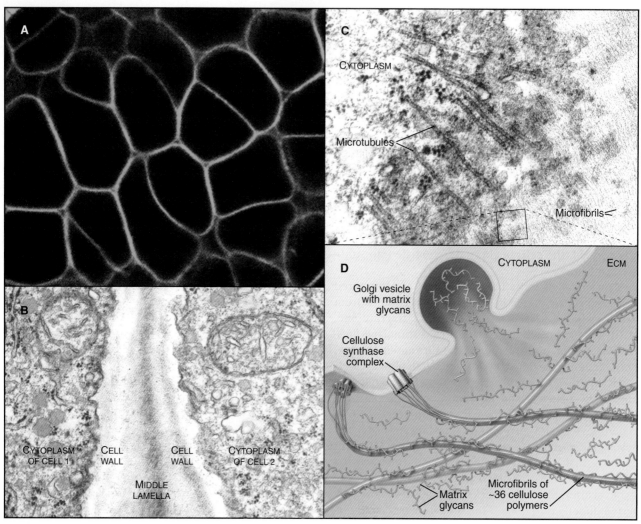

Figure 32-12   PLANT CELL WALL. **A,** Confocal fluorescence micrograph of an Arabidopsis leaf with cell walls stained by the periodic acid Schiff's reaction using Acriflavin as the Schiff's reagent. **B–C,** Electron micrographs of thin sections of cell walls in the root-like append-ages of the parasitic weed dodder. **B,** Two cells are separated by an electron-translucent cell wall consisting of cellulose, xylogycan, and pectins. The darker area between the two cell walls is the middle lamella, which contains a high concentration of pectins. **C,** At high mag-nification, an oblique section through the plasma membrane and cell wall shows cellulose microfibrils aligned roughly parallel to cortical microtubules inside the plasma membrane. **D,** Biosynthesis of the cell wall. ECM, extracellular matrix. (A, Courtesy of Steven E. Ruzin, Uni-versity of California, Berkeley. B–C, Courtesy of K. C. Vaughn, U.S. Department of Agriculture, Stoneville, Maryland. D, Redrawn from Cos-grove DJ: Loosening of plant cell walls by expansins. Nature 407:321–326, 2000.)

Glycosyltransferases in the Golgi apparatus synthe-size hemicellulose and pectin, which are transported in vesicles to the surface for secretion. Hemicellulose is a branched polysaccharide that coats microfibrils. Pectin is an acidic polysaccharide that forms a gel between microfibrils. Primary cell walls, laid down at the time of cellular growth and expansion, mature with the addi-tion of glycoproteins and organic molecules, such as **lignins** (polymers of phenylpropanoid alcohols and acids), which contribute to the integrity of the "second-ary" cell wall. Covalent and noncovalent bonds are thought to link cellulose and these other matrix mole-cules. The great strength and flexibility of tree branches

illustrate the remarkable mechanical properties of mature cell walls.

Cellulose microfibrils are flexible and have a tensile strength greater than that of steel, so they do not stretch. For a plant tissue to expand, microfibrils must rear-range. Slippage and rearrangement of microfibrils are facilitated by **expansins,** a recently recognized class of matrix proteins unique to plants. Genetic defects in expansins inhibit the growth of plant tissues and the ripening of some fruits, such as tomatoes. Cell wall expansion apparently does not involve cleavage of sugar polymers, so it is speculated that expansins break non-covalent links between the polymers transiently, allowing turgor pressure to expand the volume of the cell. Expansins in grass pollen are one allergen responsible for hay fever.

Little is known about the molecular basis of plant cells adhering to their cell walls. By virtue of their physical connection with their product, cellulose synthases offer one means of attachment. Other plasma membrane proteins, including a family of serine/threonine kinases and some proteins with glycosylphosphatidylinositol anchors, may contribute to adhesion by binding cell walls. Integrins are conspicuously missing from plant cells.

ACKNOWLEDGMENT

Thanks go to Roland Baron for his suggestions on revisions to this chapter.

SELECTED READINGS

Boyle WJ, Simonent WS, Lacey DL: Osteoclast differentiation and activation. Nature 423:337-342, 2003.

Cosgrove DJ: Assembly and enlargement of the primary cell wall in plants. Annu Rev Cell Dev Biol 13:171-201, 1997.

Cosgrove DJ: Loosening of plant cell walls by expansins. Nature 407:321-326, 2000.

Goldstein AL, Hannappel E, Kleinmann HK: Thymosin β4: Actin sequestering protein moonlights to repair injured tissues. Trends Mol Med 11:421-429, 2005.

Harada S, Rodan GA: Control of osteoblast function and regulation of bone mass. Nature 423:349-355, 2003.

Kohorn BD: Plasma membrane-cell wall contacts. Plant Physiol 124:31-38, 2000.

Kronenberg HM: Developmental regulation of the growth plate. Nature 423:332-336, 2003.

Mariani FV, Martin GR: Deciphering skeletal patterning: Clues from the limb. Nature 423:319-325, 2003.

Marx SJ: Hyperparathyroid and hypoparathyroid disorders. N Engl J Med 343:1863-1875, 2000.

Olsen BR, Reginato AM, Wang W: Bone development. Annu Rev Cell Dev Biol 16:191-220, 2000.

Ortega N, Behonick DJ, Werb Z: Matrix remodeling during endochondral ossification. Trends Cell Biol 14:86-93, 2004.

Pyeritz RE: Ehlers-Danlos syndrome. N Engl J Med 342:730-732, 2000.

Raisz LG: Pathogenesis of osteoporosis: Concepts, conflicts and prospects. J Clin Invest 115:3318-3325, 2005.

Reid JG: Cementing the wall: Cell wall polysaccharide synthesizing enzymes. Curr Opin Plant Biol 3:512-516, 2000.

Somerville C: Cellulose synthesis in higher plants. Annu Rev Cell Dev Biol 22:53-78, 2006.

Teitelbaum SL: Bone resorption by osteoclasts. Science 289:1504-1508, 2000.

Tolar J, Teitelbaum SL, Orchard PJ: Osteopetrosis. 351:2839-2849, 2004.

Wasteneys GO, Galway ME: Remodelling the cytoskeleton for growth and form: An overview with some new views. Ann Rev Plant Biol 54:691-722, 2003.

Watanabe H, Yamada Y, Kimata K: Roles of aggrecan, a large chondroitin sulfate proteoglycan, in cartilage structure and function. J Biochem 124:687-693, 1998.

Zlezer E, Olsen BR: The genetic basis of skeletal disease. Nature 423:343-348, 2003.

APPENDIX **32-1**

Examples of Genetic Defects of Cartilage and Bone

Protein	Species	Mutation	Phenotype
Transcription Factors			
c-fos	Mouse	Null	Osteopetrosis; no osteoclasts
hoxa-2	Mouse	Null	Deletion of the second branchial arch; duplication of first branchial arch
hoxd-13	Mouse	Null	Deletion fourth sacral derivatives; duplication third sacral derivatives
msx-1	Mouse	Null	Cleft palate
msx-2	Mouse	Null	Craniosynostosis (fusion of skull bones)
Runx2/Cbfa-1	Human	+/−	Dominant skeletal defects (cleidocranial dysplasia)
	Mouse	Null	No osteoblasts or bone
SOX9	Human	Point mutations	Dominant cartilage & skeletal defects (compamelic dysplasia)
Growth Factors			
BMP-4	Human	Overexpression	Fibrodysplasia progressiva; ectopic bone formation
BMP-5	Mouse	Null	Defective ears and sternum (*Shortear mutation*)
CSF-1	Mouse	Null	Osteopetrosis; reduced osteoclasts (*op mutation*)
GDF-5 (TGF-β family)	Mouse	Null	Reduced size of long bones; no joints (*Brachypodism mutation*)
Growth hormone	Human	Null	Reduced size of bones
OPG (osteoprotegerin)	Human	Null	Recessive juvenile Paget's disease with excess bone remodeling
PTHrP	Human	Null	Reduced chondrocyte growth; epiphyseal plates fused at birth
RANKL	Mouse	Null	Osteopetrosis; no osteoclasts
Signal Transduction Components			
c-Src	Mouse	Null	Osteopetrosis; osteoclasts fail to attach to or degrade bone
FGF receptor 1	Human	Point mutation	Pfeiffer's syndrome; cranial synostosis; long bone defects
FGF receptor 2	Human	Point mutation	Jackson-Weiss syndrome; cranial synostosis; long bone defects
FGF receptor 2	Human	Point mutation	Crouzon's disease; cranial synostosis
FGF receptor 3	Human	Point mutation	Gain of function mutation; achondroplasia; short, wide bones
Collagen and Other Structural Components of Cartilage and Bone			
Aggrecan	Mouse	Missense	Recessive cartilage deficiency; dwarfism; cleft palate
Cathepsin-K	Mouse	Deletion	Osteopetrosis
CLC7	Human	Point mutations	Osteopetrosis
COL1	Human	Missense, deletions	Dominant osteogenesis imperfecta; fragile bones
COL2	Human	Nonsense	Dominant Stickler's syndrome; chondrodysplasia, eye defects
	Human	Point mutations	Dominant chondrodysplasia and osteoarthritis of variable severity
COL9A2	Human	Splicing mutation	Defective cartilage with degeneration of knee joint
COL10A1	Human	Point mutations	Dominant Schmid's metaphyseal chondrodysplasia with short bones
COL11A2	Human	Exon skipping	Dominant Stickler's syndrome; chondrodysplasia, eye defects
	Human	Point mutation	Recessive severe chondrodysplasia; deafness; cleft palate
Lysyl hydroxylase	Human	Point mutation	Bruck's disease; fragile bones
Perlecan	Mouse	Deletion	Recessive defects in cartilage and bone formation
Proton ATPase	Human	Point mutations	Osteopetrosis
Sulfate transporter	Human	DTDST gene	Recessive cartilage defects; short limbs; joint deformation

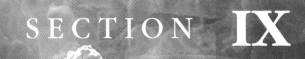

Cytoskeleton and Cellular Motility

SECTION IX OVERVIEW

The seven chapters in this section of the book cover the cytoskeleton and cellular motility. These topics are intimately related, because two of the protein polymers constituting the cytoskeleton, the internal scaffolding of the cell, are also tracks for motor proteins that power many cellular movements. Assembly and disassembly of the cytoskeletal polymers also produce some types of cell movements.

Most organisms depend on motility to sustain life itself. Without a motile sperm, the egg would not be fertilized. Without cellular motility, a fertilized egg would not progress past the single-cell stage. Without active changes in cell shape and cellular migrations, complex embryos would not form. Without cellular motility, white blood cells would neither accumulate at sites of inflammation nor ingest invading microorganisms. Without active and rapid movements of organelles in axons and large plant cells, the peripheral parts of these cells would not be nourished. Without muscle contractions, we would be paralyzed and unable to move. Even a yeast, prevented from locomotion by its rigid cell wall, depends on internal movements for cell division and endocytosis. Many prokaryotes use rotary flagella for locomotion. Therefore, an understanding of the basis of cellular motility is central to our understanding of the functioning of all cells and organisms.

This section of the book starts with Chapters 33 to 35, which introduce the three cytoskeletal polymers, and Chapter 36, which explains the mechanisms of motor proteins. Three concluding chapters show how

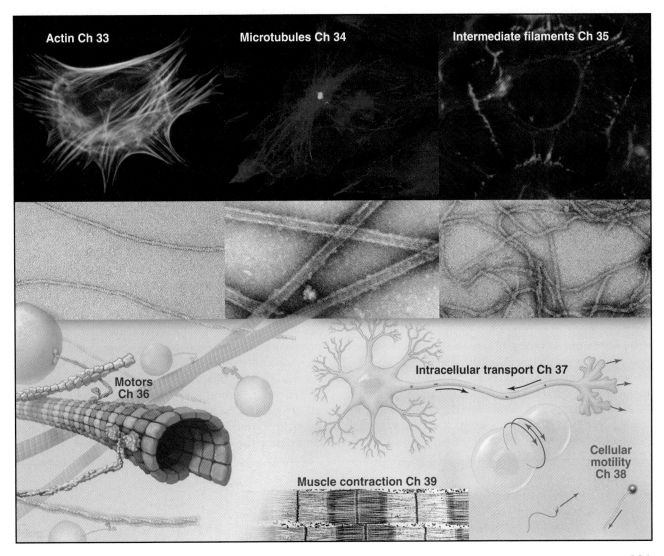

Actin Ch 33

Microtubules Ch 34

Intermediate filaments Ch 35

Motors Ch 36

Intracellular transport Ch 37

Cellular motility Ch 38

Muscle contraction Ch 39

cells use cytoskeletal polymers and motors to produce a vast variety of movements: intracellular movements (Chapter 37); cell shape changes, cellular locomotion, and swimming (Chapter 38); and muscle contraction (Chapter 39). Mitosis and cytokinesis appear in the discussion of the cell cycle (see Chapter 44).

Actin filaments (Chapter 33) and **microtubules** (Chapter 34) have much in common, including their evolutionary origins in prokaryotes. Both assemble spontaneously into polymers that are used as tracks by molecular motors. The protein subunits of both polymers bind a nucleoside triphosphate: ATP in the case of actin and GTP for tubulin. Hydrolysis of these bound nucleotides after polymerization destabilizes the polymer, much more so in the case of microtubules than in the case of actin filaments. Both polymers can turn over rapidly in cells or remain as stable components. Cells use many proteins to regulate the assembly of these polymers: Some proteins bind to the cytoplasmic pools of the subunit proteins; others initiate the assembly; some stabilize the polymers, others sever or depolymerize; still others link the polymers together or to other cellular constituents.

Actin filaments and microtubules cooperate with a third polymer called **intermediate filaments** (Chapter 35) to form the **cytoskeleton,** which resists deformation and transmits mechanical forces. Microtubules are rigid, hollow reinforcing rods that sustain both compression and tension. These mechanical properties make microtubules useful for supporting asymmetrical cellular processes and for bidirectional traffic generated by the motor proteins kinesin and dynein. Actin filaments are more flexible, so they must be cross-linked into bundles to bear compression forces or support asymmetrical processes. High tensile strength allows actin filaments to bear forces produced by myosins. Intermediate filaments are flexible cables that have considerable tensile strength but little capacity to resist compression. Both intermediate filaments and actin filaments reinforce whole tissues by anchoring cadherins, transmembrane proteins that are used for cell to cell adhesion (see Chapter 30). Intermediate filaments prevent excessive stretching of cells in multicellular animals by external forces. If intermediate filaments are defective, tissues are mechanically fragile.

Most movements of eukaryotic cells depend on actin filaments and microtubules. Assembly and disassembly of actin filaments and microtubules produce force for several types of cellular movements (Chapter 37). Actin polymerization drives extension of pseudopods at the leading edge of motile cells. Hydrolysis of ATP bound to actin regulates recycling of subunits rather than being used directly to produce force. Growth of microtubules supports the extension of some asymmetrical cellular processes, including nerve cell processes.

Many other cellular movements result from the physical movement of protein motors (Chapter 36) along actin filaments and microtubules in cytoplasm. Different motors move along these two polymers: **Myosins** move on actin filaments, and **dyneins** and **kinesins** move along microtubules. These motors use energy released from the hydrolysis of adenosine triphosphate to take nanometer steps along their protein polymer tracks. These small steps apply force and move cargo attached to the motor. The cargo includes membrane-bound organelles, macromolecular complexes, and cytoskeletal polymers. Microtubule motors power most organelle movements in animal cells (Chapter 37), chromosomal movements during mitosis (see Chapter 44), and beating of cilia and flagella (Chapter 38). The actin-myosin system is responsible for cytokinesis (see Chapter 44), some organelle movements (especially in plants and fungi [Chapter 37]), and muscle contraction (Chapter 39).

Several motility systems do not depend on actin filaments or microtubules (Chapter 38). Nematode sperm use the reversible assembly of another protein to make pseudopods for their movements. Calcium-sensitive contractile fibers cause rapid contractions of some protozoa. A proton or sodium ion gradient across the plasma membrane powers the rotary motor that turns bacterial flagella. Although not usually considered to be molecular motors, nucleic acid polymerases and helicases use ATP hydrolysis to move along polymers of DNA or RNA.

The ability of actin filaments and microtubules to resist mechanical deformation and to transmit forces from motors allows the cytoskeletal-motility system to determine cell shape and hence the structure of both tissues and whole organisms. Furthermore, the dynamic nature of cytoskeletal polymers allows cells to change shape rapidly, in a time frame of seconds. At each cell division, a band of actin filaments and myosin pinches the daughter cells apart. Active extension of cellular processes and active changes in shape produce asymmetrical cell shapes. Movements of chromosomes during mitosis and organelles in cytoplasm determine the cellular distribution of these components that are otherwise too large to move by diffusion. Together with the extracellular matrix, the shapes of individual cells define the shapes of tissues and organs.

CHAPTER 33

Actin and Actin-Binding Proteins

Actin filaments form a cytoskeletal and motility system in all eukaryotes (Fig. 33-1). Cross-linked actin filaments resist deformation, transmit forces, and restrict diffusion of organelles. A network of cortical actin filaments excludes organelles (Fig. 33-2C), reinforces the plasma membrane, and restricts the lateral motion of some integral membrane proteins. The **cortex** varies in thickness from a monolayer of actin filaments in red blood cells (see Fig. 7-10) to more than 1 μm in amoeboid cells (Fig. 33-2C). Like fingers in a glove, bundles of actin filaments support slender protrusions of plasma membrane called **microvilli** or **filopodia** (Fig. 33-2B). Microvilli expand the cell surface for transport of nutrients and participate in sensory processes, including hearing. The actin cytoskeleton complements and interacts physically with cytoskeletal structures composed of microtubules (see Chapter 34) and intermediate filaments (see Chapter 35).

Actin contributes to cell movements in two ways. First, polymerization and depolymerization of the network of actin filaments just inside the plasma membrane contribute to the extension of pseudopods, cell locomotion (Fig. 33-2D–E), and phagocytosis (see Fig. 22-3). Second, actin filaments are tracks for movements of the myosin family of motor proteins (see Fig. 36-7). Actin filaments and myosin filaments form the highly ordered, stable contractile apparatus of muscles (Fig. 33-3B; also see Fig. 39-3), as well as the transient **contractile ring** that pinches the two daughter cells apart at the end of mitosis (Fig. 33-3A; also see Fig. 44-23). Myosins also power movements of membranes and other cargo along actin filaments, complementing organelle movements by other motors along microtubules (see Fig. 37-1). Actin, myosin, and accessory proteins form intracellular bundles called **stress fibers** (Fig. 33-1B) that apply tension between adhesive junctions on the plasma membrane (see Fig. 30-11), where cells attach to each other or to the extracellular matrix. Stress fibers are prominent in tissue culture cells grown on glass or plastic and in endothelial cells lining major arteries.

Actin and myosin are thought to be among the five most abundant eukaryotic proteins on the earth. Actin is often the most abundant protein in a cell, composing up to 15% of total protein, and the many types of actin-binding proteins may account for another 10% of cellular protein. In muscle, actin and myosin constitute more than 60% of the total protein. Given this abundance, it is curious that actin was discovered in muscle only in the 1940s and in nonmuscle cells in the late 1960s. Since the 1970s, scientists have discovered new actin-binding proteins every year, but the inventory is probably still incomplete. Genetic defects in components of the actin cytoskeletal and

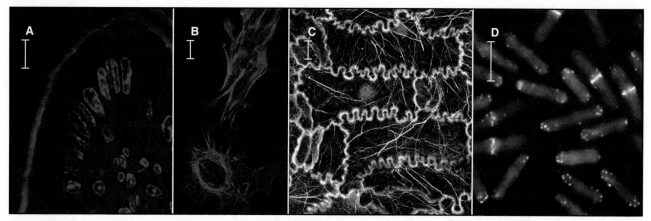

Figure 33-1 FLUORESCENCE MICROGRAPHS ILLUSTRATING THE DISTRIBUTION OF ACTIN FILAMENTS IN CELLS. **A,** Intestinal epithelial cells stained *red* with rhodamine-labeled phalloidin, a cyclic peptide that binds tightly to actin filaments. Actin filaments are concentrated in microvilli bordering the intestinal lumen. Nuclei are stained *blue* with DAPI. **B,** Cultured vascular smooth muscle cells. Actin filaments, stained *red* with a fluorescent antibody, are concentrated in stress fibers and in the cortex around the edges of these cells. **C,** Maize epidermis stained with rhodamine-labeled phalloidin. Actin filaments are concentrated in the cortex and in cytoplasmic bundles in these plant cells. **D,** Fission yeast *Schizosaccharomyces pombe,* stained with rhodamine-labeled phalloidin. Actin filaments are found in patches at the tips of growing cells and in the cleavage furrow of dividing cells. Scale bars are 10 μm. (A, Courtesy of C. Rahner, Yale University, New Haven, Connecticut. B, Courtesy of I. Herman, Tufts Medical School, Boston, Massachusetts. C, Courtesy of M. Frank, University of California, San Diego. D, Courtesy of W.-L. Lee, Salk Institute, La Jolla, California.)

motility system cause many human diseases, including muscular dystrophy (see Table 39-2), hereditary fragility of red blood cells (i.e., hemolytic anemias, see Fig. 7-10), and hereditary heart diseases called cardiomyopathies (see Table 39-4).

Actin Molecule

Actin is folded into two domains that are stabilized by an adenine nucleotide lying in between (Fig. 33-4). The polypeptide of 375 residues crosses twice between the two domains, with the N- and C-termini located near each other. The two domains are folded similarly, suggesting that the actin gene arose by duplication of an ancestral gene. Remarkably, the adenine nucleotide binding site, fold, and overall shape of actin closely resemble those of two other proteins with very different functions: the glycolytic enzyme hexokinase (see Fig. 3-12) and the heat shock protein Hsc70. All three proteins might have evolved originally in prokaryotes from the same primordial nucleotide-binding protein.

Actin binds adenosine triphosphate (ATP) or adenosine diphosphate (ADP) and a divalent cation, Mg^{2+} in cells, with nanomolar affinity. The affinity of actin for ATP is higher than that for ADP, so given the higher concentration of ATP in cells, unpolymerized actin is saturated with ATP. The bound nucleotide exchanges relatively slowly with nucleotide in the medium (Fig. 33-11). Actin monomer–binding proteins can inhibit or accelerate nucleotide exchange. Bound nucleotide stabilizes the molecule but is not required for polymeriza-

tion in vitro. ATP-actin and ADP-actin polymerize at different rates.

Posttranslational modifications of actins include acetylation of the N-terminus and (in most cases) methylation of histidine-68. In some insect flight muscles, the small protein ubiquitin (see Fig. 23-7) is attached covalently to about one in six actin molecules, yielding a 55-kD polypeptide that is incorporated with unmodified actin into filaments. Some invertebrate actins are phosphorylated on tyrosine-211. The functional significance of these modifications is still being investigated.

Actin genes originated in prokaryotes, where they are required for rod-shaped bacteria to maintain their asymmetric shapes. Other bacterial actins help to segregate DNA plasmids to the two daughters during cell division. Eukaryotic actin genes are highly conserved, but through divergent evolution, they encode subtly different proteins, some with novel functions. Most organisms have multiple actin genes, and all known actin isoform diversity arises from multiple genes rather than from alternative splicing of mRNAs. Humans have six actin genes; *Dictyostelium* has more than ten; but budding yeast has only one. Muscle actin genes diverged from cytoplasmic actins in primitive chordates (see Fig. 2-9). To fulfill special developmental functions, plant actin genes diverged among themselves more than animal actin genes.

The biochemical similarities of **actin isoforms** are more impressive than their differences (Fig. 33-5). The sequences of pairs of actins are generally more than 90% identical, even between highly divergent species. Humans express β and γ isoforms in nonmuscle cells

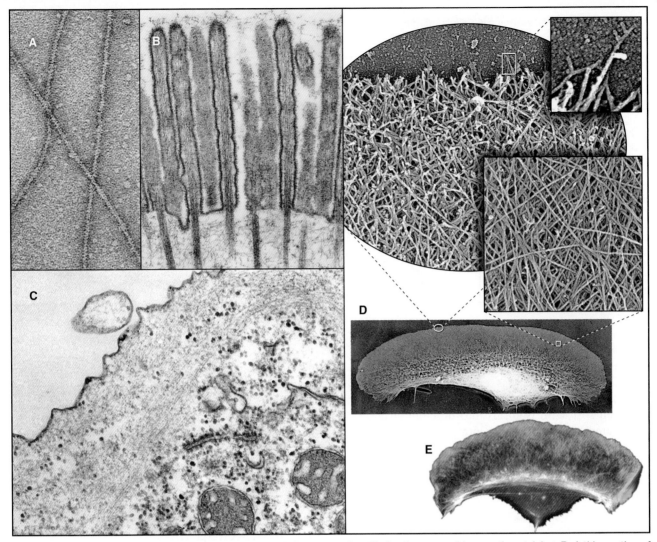

Figure 33-2 ELECTRON MICROGRAPHS OF ACTIN FILAMENTS. **A,** Filaments of purified actin prepared by negative staining. **B,** A thin section of an intestinal epithelial cell illustrating finger-like microvilli with tightly packed bundles of actin filaments linked to the surrounding plasma membrane by myosin-I. The barbed ends of these filaments (see Fig. 33-9) are located at the tips of the microvilli. **C,** A thin section of Acanthamoeba showing the actin filament meshwork in the cortex beneath the plasma membrane. **D–E, Cultured fish scale keratocytes, fixed while actively migrating toward the *top* of the figure. D,** Electron micrograph of a whole mount of a cell illustrating the meshwork of branched filaments near the leading edge and longer, unbranched filaments deeper in the cytoplasm. Most filaments are oriented with their barbed ends forward. **E,** Fluorescence micrograph with phalloidin staining actin filaments *(blue)* and antibodies staining myosin II *(red)*. (A, Courtesy of U. Aebi, University of Basel, Switzerland. B, Courtesy of L. Tilney, University of Pennsylvania, Philadelphia, and M. Mooseker, Yale University, New Haven, Connecticut. D–E, Courtesy of T. Svitkina and G. Borisy, University of Wisconsin, Madison.)

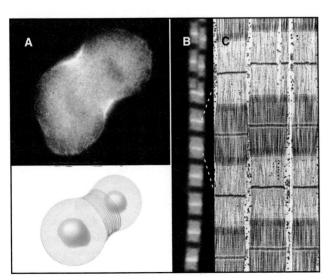

Figure 33-3 MICROGRAPHS OF CONTRACTILE BUNDLES OF ACTIN FILAMENTS. **A,** Fluorescence micrograph of a dividing normal rat kidney cell stained with fluorescein-phalloidin. Actin filaments are concentrated in the contractile ring in the constricting cleavage furrow. The drawing illustrates the filaments in the contractile ring. **B,** Fluorescence micrograph of a myofibril isolated from skeletal muscle and stained with fluorescein-phalloidin for actin filaments *(green)* and rhodamine-antibody to α-actinin for Z disks *(yellow)*. **C,** Electron micrograph of a thin section of skeletal muscle. (A, Micrograph courtesy of Y.-L. Wang, University of Massachusetts, Worcester. B, Courtesy of V. Fowler, Scripps Research Institute, La Jolla, California. C, Courtesy of H. E. Huxley, Brandeis University, Waltham, Massachusetts.)

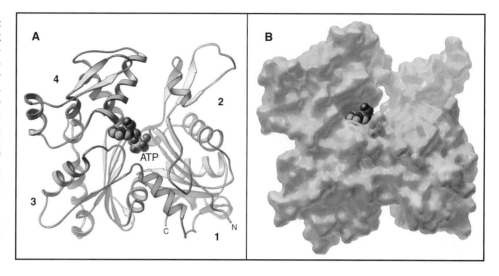

Figure 33-4 ATOMIC STRUCTURE OF ACTIN. **A,** Ribbon model showing the polypeptide fold and the location of Mg-ATP, shown as space-filling. Numbers indicate the four subdomains. **B,** Surface rendering. ATP is almost completely buried in the cleft between the two lobes of the protein, where it makes extensive contacts with the protein. The barbed end of the molecule (Fig. 33-9) is at the *bottom* in this orientation. (PDB file: 1ATN. Reference: Kabsch W, Mannherz HG, Suck D, et al: Atomic structure of the actin-DNase I complex. Nature 347:37–44, 1990.)

and four different α and β isoforms in various muscle cells. Many nonmuscle cells express both the β and γ isoforms, but red blood cells use only β-actin.

In every case that was examined, actin isoforms copolymerize in the test tube, so it is remarkable that cells can sort actin isoforms into different structures. For example, β-actin is concentrated near the plasma membrane of cultured cells, whereas γ-actin is concentrated in stress fibers (Fig. 33-6). In muscle, α-actin forms the thin filaments of the contractile apparatus, whereas γ-actin localizes around mitochondria. Even

the full array of known actin-binding proteins cannot yet explain how cells prevent copolymerization of the isoforms or concentrate isoforms at different locations.

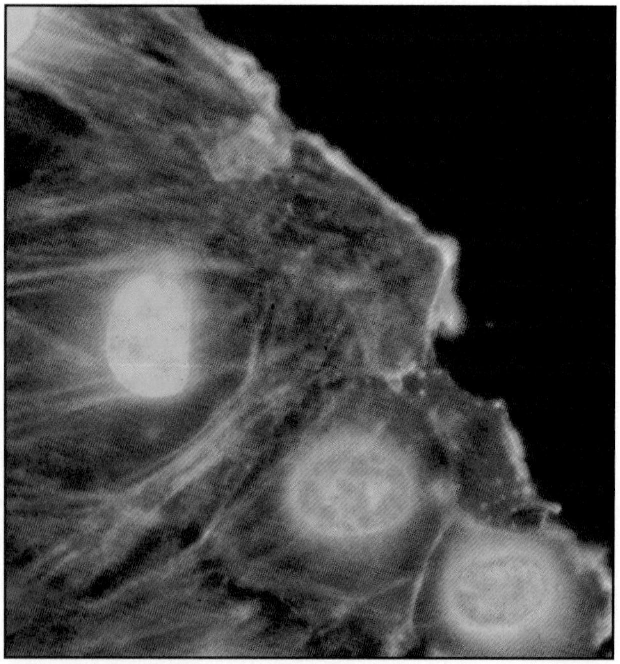

Actin-Related Proteins

After believing for 20 years that actins are one of the most evolutionarily conserved protein families, scientists discovered several families of highly divergent **actin-related proteins (Arps)** in the 1990s (Fig. 33-6). Genes for Arps diverged from actin genes after the earliest branches in the eukaryotic tree and are now found in eukaryotic species ranging from amoebas to humans. Arps share with actin the fold of the polypeptide chain and residues forming the nucleotide-binding site, but fewer than 60% of the residues are identical to actin. Divergent surface residues allow Arps to participate in molecular interactions different from actin. Arp1 forms a short filament as part of the dynactin complex that promotes cargo movement by the microtubule motor dynein (see Fig. 37-2). Arp2 and Arp3 are two of seven subunits in a protein complex that nucleates branched actin filaments in the cell cortex (Fig. 33-13). Eight additional types of Arps are widespread in eukaryotes. Several participate in complexes that regulate chromatin structure.

Actin Polymerization

Actin filaments are polarized, owing to the uniform orientation of the asymmetrical subunits along the polymer (Fig. 33-7). One end is called the barbed end, the other is called the pointed end. This nomenclature arises from the asymmetrical arrowhead pattern created when myosin bind along the length of actin filaments (Fig. 33-8). The helical arrangement of subunits in actin

Figure 33-5 SORTING OF ACTIN ISOFORMS IN CELLS. Fluorescence micrograph of cultured cells doubly stained with fluorescent antibodies specific for β-actin concentrated at the leading edge *(orange)* and γ-actin concentrated in stress fibers *(green)*. Nuclei are stained *blue* with DAPI. (Courtesy of I. Herman, Tufts Medical School, Boston, Massachusetts.)

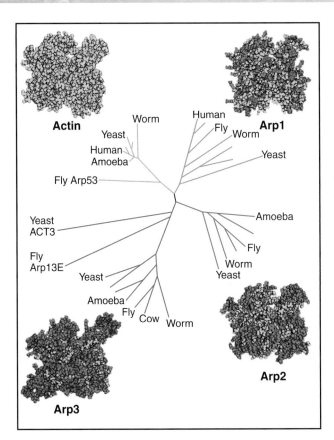

Figure 33-6 COMPARISON OF ACTIN AND ACTIN-RELATED PROTEINS. Space-filling models are based on the atomic structure of actin and the sequences of the Arps. *Yellow* residues are identical to actin, *green* residues are conservative substitutions, *blue* residues are nonconservative substitutions, and *red* residues are insertions. All of these proteins have similar internal architectures, including identical contacts with ATP, but their surfaces differ considerably. The phylogenetic tree, based on sequence comparisons, shows that the genes for actins and for all of the Arps had a common ancestor. (From the work of J. Kelleher, Johns Hopkins Medical School, Baltimore, Maryland; illustration redrawn from Mullins D, Kelleher J, Pollard TD: Actin' like actin. Trends Cell Biol 6:208–212, 1996.)

filaments was originally revealed in the 1960s by electron microscopy and X-ray fiber diffraction of whole muscle and actin gels. These low-resolution data are used to orient the atomic structure of the actin monomer in current models.

Actin self-assembles into filaments by means of a series of bimolecular reactions (Fig. 33-9; see also Fig. 5-6). Actin is isolated from cells as a monomer at low salt concentrations. Physiological concentrations of monovalent and divalent cations bind to low-affinity

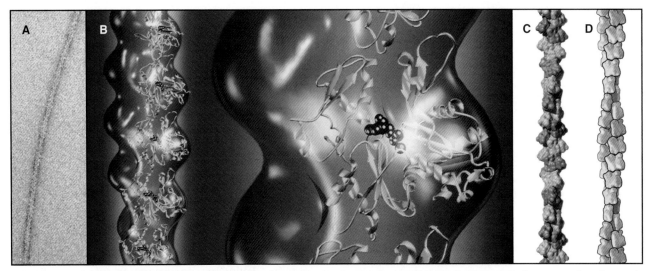

Figure 33-7 STRUCTURE OF THE ACTIN FILAMENT. **A,** Electron micrograph of a negatively stained actin filament. **B,** Reconstruction of an actin filament by image processing of electron micrographs *(blue)* with ribbon models of the subunits *(gold)* along one strand of the double helix. One subunit is enlarged to the *right.* The pointed end of the subunits with the nucleotide cleft is at the *top,* and the faster-growing barbed end is at the *bottom.* This orientation of the actin molecule in the filament uniquely accounts for the X-ray fiber diffraction pattern of oriented filaments and agrees with electron microscopy with probes on specific actin residues and with chemical cross-linking between residues of adjacent subunits. **C,** Surface rendering of the molecular model. Subunits in the two long-pitch helices are shown as *yellow-orange* and *blue-green* (see Fig. 5-5 for nomenclature). The short pitch helix, including every subunit, follows a *yellow-green-orange-blue* pattern. **D,** Scale drawing used throughout this text. (A–B, Courtesy of U. Aebi, University of Basel, Switzerland. C, Courtesy of R. Milligan, Scripps Research Institute, La Jolla, California.)

sites on actin and promote polymerization. In vitro, actin trimers appear to be the nucleus that initiates polymer growth in the sense that the reactions that are required to form trimers are very unfavorable in comparison with reactions for elongation of polymers larger than trimers. To initiate new filaments, cells use regulatory proteins to overcome these unfavorable nucleation reactions.

Actin filaments grow and shrink by the addition and loss of subunits at the two ends of the polymer. The reactions at the two ends have different rate constants (Fig. 33-8). Association of subunits is rapid at both ends. Subunit association is a diffusion-limited reaction (see Chapter 4) at the rapidly growing barbed end and somewhat slower at the other end. Subunit dissociation is relatively slow at both ends, between 0.3 and 8 subunits per second. The rates of these reactions depend on the nucleotide bound to the monomer associating with or dissociating from a filament.

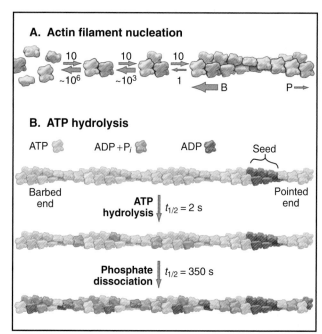

Figure 33-9 ACTIN FILAMENT NUCLEATION, GROWTH, AND NUCLEOTIDE HYDROLYSIS. **A,** Nucleation. Formation of dimers and trimers is very unfavorable, owing to rapid dissociation of subunits. Actin trimers are called nuclei because they initiate the highly favorable elongation reactions. This mechanism is based on kinetic modeling of experimental data. Estimated rate constants have units of $\mu M^{-1} s^{-1}$ for association reactions and s^{-1} for dissociation reactions. **B,** ATP hydrolysis by a polymer of ATP-actin (yellow subunits) is random and irreversible at a rate of $0.3 s^{-1}$, yielding subunits with bound ADP and inorganic phosphate (orange). Phosphate dissociates slowly at a rate of $0.002 s^{-1}$, converting half of the newly polymerized subunits to ADP-actin (pink) in 6 minutes. ADP bound to polymerized subunits does not exchange with nucleotide in the medium. Phosphate binding is reversible, but the affinity is low, so most subunits bind only ADP. (Reference: Pollard TD, Blanchoin L, Mullins RD: Biophysics of actin filament dynamics in nonmuscle cells. Annu Rev Biophys Biomol Struct 29:545–576, 2000.)

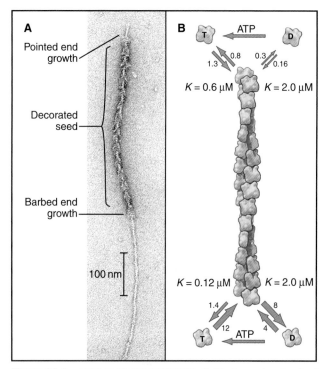

Figure 33-8 ACTIN FILAMENT ELONGATION. **A,** Electron micrograph of growth from an actin filament seed decorated with myosin heads to reveal the polarity. Growth is faster at the barbed end than at the pointed end. **B,** Rate constants for association (units: $\mu M^{-1} s^{-1}$) and dissociation (units: s^{-1}) for Mg-ATP-actin (T) and Mg-ADP-actin (D) were determined by measuring the rate of elongation at the two ends as a function of monomer concentration. Ratios of the rate constants yield critical concentrations (K, units: μM) for the various reactions. The critical concentrations at the two ends are the same for ADP-actin but differ for ATP-actin. (A, Courtesy of M. Runge, Johns Hopkins Medical School, Baltimore, Maryland. B, Reference: Pollard TD: Rate constants for the reactions of ATP- and ADP-actin with the ends of actin filaments. J Cell Biol 103:2747–2754, 1986.)

In the presence of ATP, purified actin assembles almost completely, leaving as monomers the **critical concentration** of about 0.1 μM ATP-actin. The critical concentration is the monomer concentration giving equal rates of association and dissociation, $1.4 s^{-1}$ at the barbed end (see Figure 5-6). The critical concentration for ADP-actin is about 20 times higher than for ATP-actin.

Hydrolysis of bound ATP and dissociation of the γ-phosphate during assembly modifies the behavior of actin filaments, including their affinity for regulatory proteins. Following incorporation of an ATP-actin subunit into a filament, bound ATP is hydrolyzed irreversibly to ADP and phosphate with a half time of 2 s (Fig. 33-9). These ADP-Pi subunits behave much like ATP subunits. Phosphate dissociates slowly and reversibly over several minutes. This yields filaments with a core of subunits with tightly bound ADP. At the

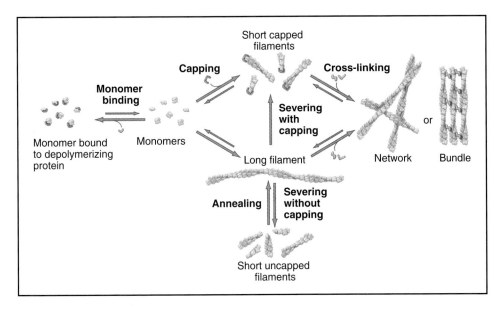

Figure 33-10 FAMILIES OF ACTIN-BINDING PROTEINS. Monomer-binding proteins generally favor either ATP-actin (profilin and thymosin-β_4) or ADP-actin (ADF/cofilins). Capping proteins bind to either the barbed end (capping protein, gelsolin) or the pointed end (tropomodulin, Arp2/3 complex) of filaments. Some severing proteins also cap (gelsolin, fragmin), whereas others do not (ADF/cofilins). Cross-linking proteins can form networks or bundles.

millimolar concentrations of phosphate in cytoplasm, phosphate rebinds to some ADP-actin subunits.

The critical concentrations for ATP-actin differ at the two ends of the filament. This results from differences in the probability of nucleotide hydrolysis and phosphate release at the two ends, which is more likely to expose ADP-subunits at the pointed end. At steady state in the presence of ATP, the actin monomer concentration falls between the critical concentrations at the two ends. Though the polymer and monomer concentrations remain constant, net addition of subunits at the barbed end and net loss of subunits at the pointed end result in the slow migration of subunits through the polymer from the barbed end to the pointed end. This process is called *treadmilling*. Neither end exhibits rapid fluctuations in length like those of microtubules (see Fig. 34-7).

In many cell types, the barbed ends of the filaments are associated with the plasma membrane (Fig. 33-2). Actin filaments in muscle are also anchored at their barbed ends (Fig. 33-3C; also see Fig. 39-3). This makes mechanical sense, as actin filaments sustain tension better than compression and because (with one interesting exception) all known myosins pull filaments in a direction away from the barbed end. The plasma membrane is a prominent actin filament–anchoring site, allowing force that is produced in the cytoplasmic actin network to change the shape of the membrane and to be transmitted to the substrate on which the cell sits or to adjacent cells (see Fig. 38-5).

Actin-Binding Proteins

In contrast to the slow treadmilling of filaments of purified actin, actin filaments in live cells can polymerize and depolymerize rapidly under the control of more than 60 families of actin-binding proteins (Fig. 33-10 and Appendix 33-1). Broadly, these proteins fall into families that bind monomers, sever filaments, cap filament ends, nucleate filaments, cross-link filaments, stabilize filaments, or move along filaments. Like actin, actin-binding proteins are ancient. Many families arose in early eukaryotes and are found in protozoa, yeast, plants, and vertebrates.

No actin-binding protein functions in isolation. Typically, two or more proteins collaborate to control each aspect of actin dynamics. This section introduces examples of each class of actin-binding protein. Following sections explain how ensembles of these proteins work together to regulate actin filament dynamics in cells.

Actin Monomer–Binding Proteins

Proteins that bind actin monomers cooperate with capping proteins to maintain a pool of unpolymerized actin in cells and regulate the nucleotide bound to actin.

Profilins are abundant proteins, found in all branches of the eukaryotic tree. Cells require three different profilin activities for viability: binding actin monomers, catalyzing the exchange of nucleotides bound to actin (Fig. 33-11) and binding to polyproline sequences on other protein such as formins (Fig. 33-12). Profilins also bind acidic membrane lipids (polyphosphoinositides). The nucleotide bound to actin monomers determines the affinity for profilin: highest for nucleotide-free actin monomers, followed by ATP-actin and ADP-actin. Profilins bind to the barbed end of actin monomers, thereby sterically blocking nucleation and pointed end elongation but not association of the profilin-actin complex with the barbed end of filaments. Profilin dissociates

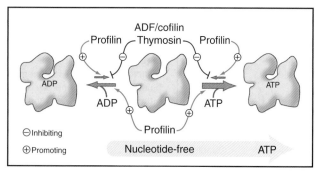

Figure 33-11 REGULATION OF ACTIN NUCLEOTIDE EXCHANGE BY ACTIN-BINDING PROTEINS. The rate-limiting step is dissociation of the bound nucleotide, which requires opening the nucleotide cleft. ADF/cofilins and β-thymosins inhibit dissociation of both ATP and ADP. Profilin competes with both inhibitors for binding actin monomers and increases the rates of both nucleotide dissociation and binding. The ability of profilin to promote nucleotide exchange, the higher affinity of actin for ATP than for ADP, and the higher concentration of ATP than ADP in cytoplasm drive the reactions to the right, accounting for why essentially all unpolymerized actin in cells has bound ATP.

rapidly after the profilin-actin complex binds to a barbed end.

Found only in vertebrates, **β-thymosins** are peptides of 43 residues that bind ATP-actin monomers with higher affinity than ADP-actin monomers. They inhibit both actin polymerization and nucleotide exchange. Thymosin-β4 is the most abundant actin-binding protein in some animal cells, where it sequesters most of the unpolymerized actin.

Members of the **ADF/cofilin** family are essential for the viability of many eukaryotes. They bind ADP-actin monomers with higher affinity than ATP-actin and inhibit nucleotide exchange but not polymerization. Their major roles are to bind and destabilize ADP-actin filaments (Figs. 33-15 and 33-19) and to nucleate filaments.

Actin Filament Nucleation Factors

Spontaneous nucleation of new filaments from actin monomers is intrinsically unfavorable and further inhibited by profilin, so cells use nucleation factors to specify when and where new filaments form. The best characterized are formins, Arp2/3 complex, and spire. Each has a different evolutionary origin, mechanism of action, and physiological function.

Formins initiate unbranched actin filaments that are incorporated into the contractile ring and bundles of actin filaments such as cables in yeast (see Fig. 37-11) and stress fibers in animal cells (Fig. 33-1B). Each of the three formins in fission yeast assembles actin filaments for a specific function: the cytokinetic contractile ring, interphase actin cables, or mating structures. Thus, the 15 different mammalian formins are also likely to have specific functions. These proteins have in common a formin homology-2 (FH2) domain (Fig. 33-12). Pairs of FH2 domains form a doughnut-shaped ring that fits around the barbed end of an actin filament. Interactions with two actin monomers nucleate a filament that grows by adding subunits to the barbed end. An FH2 domain can track faithfully on the growing end as it adds thousands of new subunits. When associated with a membrane in a cell or a microscope slide in an experiment,

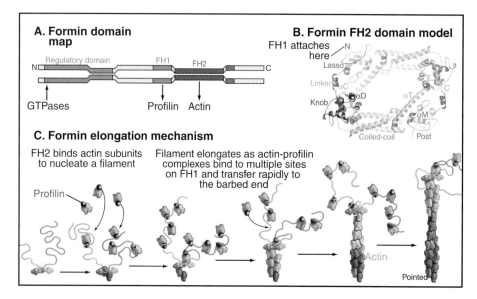

Figure 33-12 NUCLEATION OF ACTIN FILAMENTS BY FORMINS. **A,** Domain structure of a generic formin similar to mouse mDia1. Rho-family GTPases activate formins by disrupting intramolecular associations that autoinhibit the FH2 domains. **B,** Ribbon diagram of the structure of the homodimer of FH2 domains of budding yeast Bni1p. The linker segments must be extended for the dimer to fit around an actin filament. **C,** Proposed pathway of actin filament nucleation and elongation in association with formin FH1 and FH2 domains. Elongation is favored by concentrating and orienting profilin-actin near the barbed end by binding to multiple polyproline sequences in FH1. (B, PDB file: 1UX5. C, Reference: Kovar D, Harris ES, Mahaffy R, et al: Control of the assembly of ATP- and ADP-actin by formins and profilin. Cell 724:423–435, 2006.)

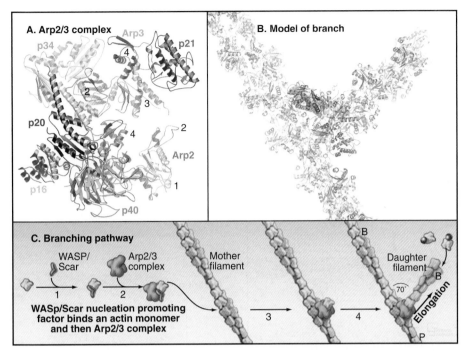

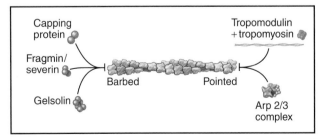

Figure 33-13 Nucleation of branched actin filaments by Arp2/3 complex. **A,** Ribbon diagram of the crystal structure of Arp2/3 complex. The seven subunits are color coded and labeled. Numbers label the subdomains of Arp2 and Arp3. **B,** Model of branch based on a 3D reconstruction from electron micrographs. **C,** Steps in branch formation (also refer back to panel **A**): A WASp/Scar nucleation promoting factor binds an actin monomer *(1)*. This binary complex binds Arp2/3 complex, bringing together the actin subunit with Arp2 and Arp3 *(2)*. The ternary complex binds to the side of an actin filament, completing the activation process *(3)*. A new daughter filament grows at its barbed end from the side of the older mother filament *(4)*. B is the barbed end. P is the pointed end. (A, PDB file: 1K8K. References: Robinson R, Turbedsky K, Kaiser DA, et al: Crystal structure of Arp2/3 complex. Science 294:1679–1684, 2001. B, Based on the work of I. Rouiller, N. Volkmann, and D. Hanein, Burnham Institute, La Jolla, California. C, Marchand J-B, Kaiser DA, Pollard TD, Higgs HN: Interaction of WASp/Scar proteins with actin and vertebrate Arp2/3 complex. Nat Cell Biol 3:76–82, 2001.)

a formin molecule can extrude a growing actin filament for many minutes. Profilin enhances elongation by targeting profilin-actin complexes to multiple polyproline sequences in the FH1 domain adjacent to FH2. Some well-studied formins are autoinhibited by interactions between parts of the polypeptide flanking the FH1FH2 domains. Rho family GTPases regulate foramins by overcoming this autoinhibition.

Arp2/3 complex consists of two actin-related proteins (Arp2 and Arp3) tightly bound to five novel proteins (Fig. 33-13). Arp2/3 complex binds to the side of actin filaments and forms branches by nucleating filaments that grow at their free barbed ends. The complex caps the pointed end of the new filament and attaches it to the side of the older filament. Growth of the free barbed ends of these branches produces the force that pushes the plasma membrane forward at the leading edge of motile cells (Fig. 33-2D).

Spire was discovered in *Drosophila* as a gene required for the development of eggs and embryos and later found in other metazoans but not fungi or protozoa. Spire proteins have multiple domains (corresponding to the V domains in Fig. 33-17A) that bind actin monomers and stabilize oligomers on the pathway to nucleation of unbranched filaments. The biological functions of these proteins are being investigated.

Actin Filament–Capping Proteins

Capping proteins bind to either the barbed or pointed end of actin filaments, where they block subunit addition and dissociation (Fig. 33-14). Some capping proteins also stimulate the formation of new filaments and/or sever actin filaments (Fig. 33-15).

Gelsolins consist of six domains with similar folds but different sequences and functions. They bind tightly to the sides and barbed ends of actin filaments, blocking both the dissociation and association of actin subunits. Gelsolin also binds actin dimers, forming a nucleus that

Figure 33-14 ACTIN FILAMENT–CAPPING PROTEINS. Interactions of capping proteins with the ends of actin filaments. Most of these proteins bind with high affinity to a filament end. Tropomodulin requires tropomyosin for high-affinity binding.

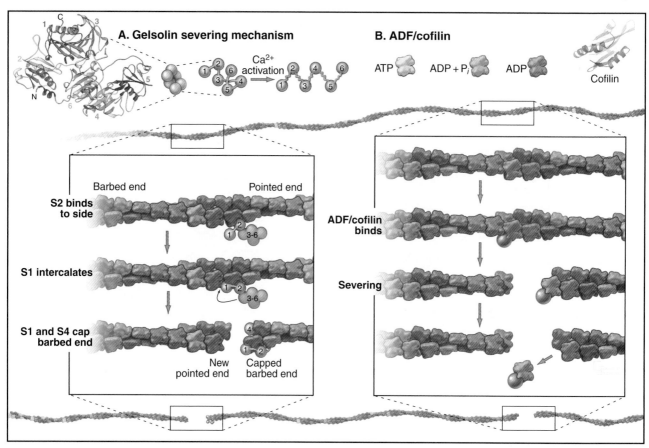

Figure 33-15 **ACTIN FILAMENT–SEVERING MECHANISMS. A,** Severing by gelsolin. Ribbon model of the atomic structure of gelsolin, showing the six homologous domains labeled 1 to 6. When activated by Ca^{2+}, gelsolin domains 2 to 6 bind to the side of an actin filament, increasing the likelihood that domain 1 will insert between actin subunits and disrupt the filament. The products are two filaments: one with a new pointed end and another with a new barbed end tightly capped by gelsolin. **B,** Severing by ADF/cofilins. ADF/cofilins bind to sites on ADP-actin filaments with a rare but naturally occurring tighter helical twist. Binding destabilizes and severs the filament. The products are two uncapped ends that are available for subunit association and dissociation. (A, PDB file: 1DON. Reference: Robinson R, Mejillano M, Le VP, et al: Domain movement in gelsolin: A calcium-activated switch. Science 286:1939–1942, 1999. B, References: McGough A, Pope B, Chin W, Weeds AG: Cofilin changes the twist of F-actin. J Cell Biol 138:771–781, 1997; Blanchoin L, Pollard TD: Mechanism of interaction of *Acanthamoeba* actophorin (ADF/cofilin) with actin filaments. J Biol Chem 274:15538–15546, 1999.)

grows at the pointed end. Phosphatidyl 4,5-bisphosphate (PIP$_2$) competes with actin for binding gelsolin. Three-domain capping proteins, such as **fragmin** and **severin,** are similar in structure and function to the first three domains of gelsolin. Genes for these capping proteins, found widely across the phylogenetic tree, are likely to have duplicated during evolution to give rise to gelsolin genes.

Heterodimeric capping proteins consist of two subunits of approximately 30 kD. They cap barbed ends with high affinity, independent of Ca^{2+}, and promote nucleation of new pointed ends by stabilizing small actin oligomers. As with gelsolins, PIP$_2$ inhibits capping by these proteins. Heterodimeric capping proteins are found in most eukaryotic cells. In striated muscle, they cap the barbed end of actin filaments in the Z disk (see Fig. 39-5).

Tropomodulin caps the pointed end of stable actin filaments in muscle, red blood cells, and other cells of higher organisms. High-affinity binding to pointed ends

requires tropomyosin, an α-helical protein that binds along the length of actin filaments (see Fig. 39-4).

Actin Filament–Severing Proteins

Three classes of proteins just introduced—gelsolin, fragmin/severin, and ADF/cofilin—also sever actin filaments into short fragments (Fig. 33-15). Domain 2 of gelsolin binds to the side of an actin filament, positioning domain 1 to bind between subunits and disrupt the filament. This requires micromolar concentrations of Ca^{2+}. One gelsolin isoform is found inside cells; another is secreted into blood plasma, where it may sever actin filaments released from damaged cells. Fragmin and severin from slime molds (but not their vertebrate homologs) have similar Ca^{2+}-dependent severing activity. Independent of Ca^{2+}, ADF/cofilins bind ADP-actin subunits in filaments and promote severing and depolymerization.

Proteins That Bind the Side of Actin Filaments

Tropomyosin, nebulin, and **caldesmon** are extended proteins that bind along the sides of actin filaments. Tropomyosin increases the tensile strength of actin filaments; in striated muscles, it is also an essential component of the Ca^{2+}-sensitive regulatory machinery that controls the interaction of myosin and actin (see Fig. 39-4). Nebulin may determine the length of the actin filaments in skeletal muscle (see Chapter 39). Caldesmon, together with tropomyosin and Ca^{2+}-calmodulin, regulates interaction of actin and myosin in smooth muscle (see Fig. 39-21) and nonmuscle cells. Phosphorylation of caldesmon by cell cycle kinases and may play a role in the reorganization of actin filaments during mitosis.

Actin Filament Cross-Linking Proteins

Possession of two actin-binding sites enables cross-linking proteins (Fig. 33-16) to bridge filaments and to stabilize higher-order assemblies of actin filaments. Some have a greater tendency to cross-link filaments in regular bundles, like those in microvilli (Fig. 33-2A), but depending on protein concentrations and filament lengths, most of these proteins can promote the formation of both random networks and regular bundles of filaments.

Many of these proteins share a homologous actin binding domain associated with other domains that form dimers. α-**Actinin** is found in the cortical actin network, at intervals along stress fibers, on the cytoplas-

mic side of cell adhesion plaques (see Fig. 30-11), and in the Z-disk of striated muscles (see Fig. 39-5). Fimbrin and villin (a relative of gelsolin with an extra actin-binding site) stabilize the regular actin filament bundles in microvilli. Filamin cross-links filaments in the cortex of many cells and also anchors these filaments to an integrin, a plasma membrane receptor for adhesive glycoproteins (see Fig. 30-11). Actin filament cross-linking proteins of the plasma membrane skeleton, such as spectrin (see Fig. 7-10) and dystrophin (see Fig. 39-9) are anchored to integral membrane proteins. Relatively little is known about how cells regulate cross-linking proteins, although Ca^{2+} inhibits binding of some α-actinins to actin.

Adapter Proteins

Eukaryotic cells use multidomain proteins as adapters between signaling pathways and actin assembly (Fig. 33-17). The multidomain protein **WASp** is defective in the inherited immunodeficiency and bleeding disorder called Wiskott-Aldrich syndrome. The C-terminal domains of WASp (and related proteins N-WASp and Scar/WAVE) activate the Arp2/3 complex to nucleate new actin filaments on the side of existing filaments (Fig. 33-13). Intramolecular interactions autoinhibit WASp. Rho-family GTPases (guanosine triphosphatase), membrane polyphosphoinositides, and polyproline-binding proteins with SH3 domains cooperate to overcome the autoinhibition by binding to parts of WASp involved with the intramolecular interactions. Rac activates Scar by interacting with a complex of regulatory

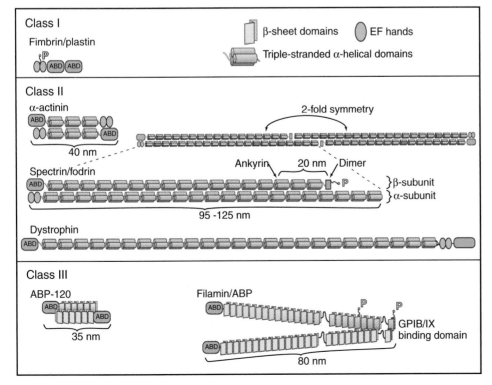

Figure 33-16 Actin filament cross-linking proteins sharing homologous actin-binding domains *(red)*. Cross-linking requires two actin-binding sites, which can be part of one polypeptide (fimbrin) or on different subunits of dimeric proteins (α-actinin, filamin). Dystrophin has a second actin-binding site in the middle of the tail. (Redrawn from Matsudaira P: Modular organization of actin cross-linking proteins. Trends Biochem Sci 16:87–92, 1991.)

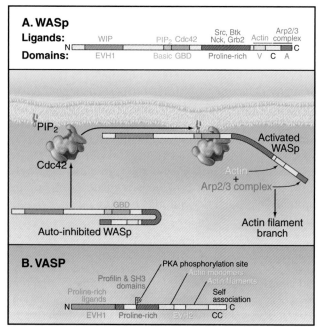

A. WASp

Ligands: WIP   PIP₂ Cdc42   Src, Btk   Actin   Arp2/3
                              Nck, Grb2   complex
N   C
Domains: EVH1   Basic GBD   Proline-rich   V C A

PIP₂
Cdc42
Auto-inhibited WASp
GBD
Activated WASp
Actin + Arp2/3 complex
Actin filament branch

B. VASP

PKA phosphorylation site
Profilin & SH3 domains
Actin monomers
Actin filaments
Proline-rich ligands
Self association
N   C
EVH1   Proline-rich   EVH2   CC

Figure 33-17 ADAPTER PROTEINS. A, WASp (Wiskott-Aldrich syndrome protein). Domains called V (for verprolin homology), C (for connecting), and A (for acidic) activate Arp2/3 complex. VC binds an actin monomer, and CA binds Arp2/3 complex. C also binds intramolecularly to the GBD (GTPase-binding domain), autoinhibiting VCA. Membrane-bound Rho-family GTPases and polyphosphoinositides compete C from GBD, releasing VCA to interact with actin and Arp2/3 complex. SH3 domain proteins such as Nck also activate WASp by binding the proline-rich domain. The N-terminal EVH1 (Ena-VASP homology) domain binds WIP (WASp interacting protein), the mammalian homolog of yeast verprolin. **B,** VASP (vasodilator-stimulated phosphoprotein). The EVH1 domain (see Fig. 25-11B) binds polyproline ligands, including vinculin and zyxin in focal contacts; the proline-rich domain binds profilin, profilin-actin complexes, and proteins with certain SH3 domains; the EVH2 domain binds both actin monomers and filaments; and the C-terminal coiled-coil (CC) mediates the formation of VASP tetramers.

proteins. An unrelated protein called **VASP** (vasodilator-stimulated phosphoprotein) also has EVH1 and proline-rich domains as well as an actin-binding domain. These domains allow VASP and related proteins to bind proline-rich ligands in focal adhesions and on the surface of the bacterium *Listeria,* profilin-actin complexes, and actin filaments. These interactions stimulate actin polymerization in filopodia and "comet tails" assembled by *Listeria* (see Fig. 37-12).

Functional Redundancy of Actin-Binding Proteins

The diversity and the apparent redundancy of actin-binding proteins are striking. Why should most organisms retain genes for 60 different actin-binding proteins if they have such a limited repertoire of functions: monomer binding, nucleation, capping, severing, cross-linking, stabilizing, and motility? Null mutations show that some proteins are essential for normal physiology.

These include myosin-II, Arp2/3 complex, profilin, and cofilin in yeast. On the other hand, organisms can survive genetic deletion of some actin-binding proteins, suggesting that parts of the system are redundant. For example, in a laboratory environment, *Dictyostelium* tolerates the loss of cross-linking proteins (α-actinin or ABP-120), severin, or one of two profilin genes with only minor defects in behavior and growth. Humans who lack dystrophin develop and grow normally for a few years but later succumb to muscle wasting (see Table 39-2). Mice without their single gelsolin gene reproduce normally, with only mild defects in platelets and other cells.

The data suggest that each actin-binding protein has a distinct function, conferring a small selective advantage. Multiple proteins sharing overlapping functions make the actin system relatively fail-safe so that it is difficult to detect the phenotypic consequences of the loss of particular proteins in mutant animals. Alternatively, these proteins may have other unknown functions distinct from actin binding.

Actin Dynamics in Live Cells

Cellular actin filaments vary widely in stability. In muscle, the ends of actin filaments exchange subunits over hours. Four proteins stabilize these filaments (see Fig. 39-6). Tropomyosin and nebulin run along the length of the filament, CapZ binds to the barbed end, and tropomodulin binds to the pointed end. These proteins inhibit breakage of the filaments and allow limited exchange of actin subunits at the barbed ends. On the other hand, amoebae and white blood cells protrude and remodel actin-rich pseudopods on a time scale of seconds. Several methods are available to document actin filament dynamics in cells.

Although light microscopes lack the resolution to observe individual actin filaments crowded together in cytoplasm, assemblies of actin filaments can be imaged directly in favorable cases by DIC or phase contrast microscopy. For example, the parallel arrays of actin filaments in muscle are observed to be very stable, whereas networks of actin filaments in nerve growth cones constantly assemble and move away from the leading edge (Fig. 33-18).

A second approach is to observe the effects of drugs that bind actin such as **cytochalasin** or **latrunculin** (Box 33-1). Neither disassembles actin filaments directly, but they both interfere with assembly from monomers, so their effects reveal if filaments are turning over naturally. Muscle actin filaments are relatively resistant to these drugs, but they disrupt the cortical actin filament network in other cells in seconds (Fig. 33-18). When the drug is removed, the cortical actin network reforms rapidly from the leading edge. This response indicates that many cellular filaments turn over rapidly.

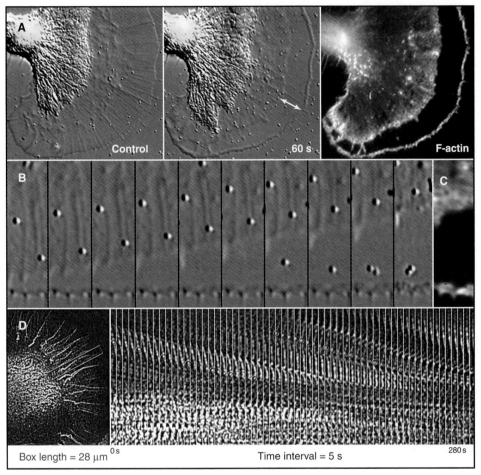

Figure 33-18 ACTIN FILAMENT DYNAMICS AT THE LEADING EDGE OF A GIANT GROWTH CONE OF A NEURON ISOLATED FROM THE MOLLUSK *APLYSIA*. A network of actin filaments forms continuously at the leading edge of the growth cone, moves inward by retrograde flow, and disassembles near the central organelle-rich zone. **A–C, Effect of the drug cytochalasin D on the growth cone. A,** DIC micrograph before application of the drug, showing the broad lamellum at the leading edge *(left)*. DIC *(middle)* and fluorescence *(right)* micrographs of this growth cone 60 s after the application of the drug, which disrupts the network of actin filaments at the leading edge. The *arrows* mark the zone cleared of actin filaments, stained with rhodamine phalloidin in the *right panel*. A narrow rim of filaments survives at the leading edge. **B,** Time series of differential interference contrast micrographs at 6-s intervals, showing that cytochalasin blocks the formation of new filaments at the leading edge, but retrograde flow of existing filaments (toward the cell body) continues, separating the network from the leading edge. Small beads on the surface move at the same rate. **C,** This growth cone fixed after 60 s and stained with rhodamine-phalloidin. The fluorescence micrograph shows that few filaments survive at the leading edge. If cytochalasin is removed from a live cell, the actin filament network recovers, beginning near the leading edge. **D,** Fluorescence micrographs of a growth cone injected with rhodamine-phalloidin to mark actin filaments. **Left,** Bundles of actin filaments arranged radially in the lamellum. **Right,** A time series of one actin filament bundle showing the steady retrograde flow of irregularities in the actin filament network at a rate of about 3 to 6 μm/min (equivalent to filaments growing by 19 to 38 subunits per second) from the leading edge *(top)* to the organelle-rich central zone *(bottom)*. (Courtesy of Paul Forscher, Yale University, New Haven, Connecticut; based on Forscher P, Smith SJ: Actions of cytochalasins in a neuronal growth cone. J Cell Biol 107:1505–1516, 1988, by copyright permission of The Rockefeller University Press.)

Actin can also be observed in live cells if labeled with a fluorescent probe. Purified actin can be labeled with a fluorescent dye and microinjected into live cells, where it is incorporated into the actin-containing structures. Expression of actin tagged with green fluorescent protein is even more convenient for following actin in live cells, although caution is required because the bulky green fluorescent protein can interfere with interactions with formins and perhaps other molecules. In muscle, fluorescent actin slowly incorporates, through exchange, at the pointed ends of the filaments. In non-muscle cells, fluorescent actin is quickly incorporated into all of the filaments. If low levels of fluorescent actin are used, random incorporation into filaments can result in fluorescent "speckles" that can be used to follow the movements and turnover of these subunits (Fig. 33-18D). Figure 38-9 illustrates how bleaching or activating fluorescent actin in a live cell can reveal where filaments assemble and disassemble at the leading edge of motile cells. The associated text explains the biochemical mechanism.

Biochemical and genetic experiments identified the same minimal set of proteins that are essential for maintaining the pool of unpolymerized actin, initiating

Tools to Study Actin Filaments: Natural Products Can Stabilize or Destabilize Actin Filaments

Destabilizers Cytochalasins, complex organic compounds synthesized by fungi, inhibit actin assembly in two ways. High-affinity binding to the barbed end of actin filaments inhibits subunit association and dissociation. Low-affinity binding to actin monomers promotes their dimerization and the hydrolysis of ATP bound to one subunit. In this way, cytochalasins catalyze the conversion of ATP-actin to ADP-actin. Cytochalasin (meaning "cell relaxing") is so named because it causes regression of the cleavage furrow during cytokinesis and disrupts many structures containing actin filaments in cells. Cytochalasins are used to test for the participation of actin filaments in cellular processes, but observations must be interpreted cautiously, given the complicated mechanism of action. Sponges synthesize toxins that destabilize actin filaments in cells by sequestering actin monomers (latrunculin A and B) or severing actin filaments (swinholide A).

Stabilizers Phallotoxins (such as phalloidin) are cyclic peptides that are synthesized by poisonous mushrooms. They bind and stabilize actin filaments by reducing the rate of subunit dissociation to near zero at both ends of the polymer. When introduced into cells by microinjection, phallotoxins inhibit processes that depend on actin filament turnover, including amoeboid movement. They are toxic to humans because they interfere with bile secretion. Fluorescent derivatives of phallotoxins are widely used to localize actin filaments in cells and tissues (Fig. 33-1), as well as to quantify polymerized actin in cells and cell extracts. A sponge toxin, jasplakinolide, has effects similar to phallotoxins.

C2 toxin produced by *Clostridium botulinum* is an enzyme that catalyzes the ADP-ribosylation of cytoplasmic actins on arginine-177. *Clostridium perfringens* iota toxin does the same to muscle actin. ADP-ribosylated actin polymerizes poorly and caps the barbed end of actin filaments. The ability of these protein toxins to penetrate live cells, cap actin filaments, and alter actin polymerization accounts for their disruption of the actin cytoskeleton in cells and may contribute to their toxicity.

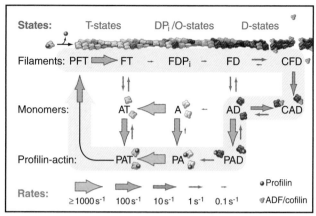

Figure 33-19 ACTIN POLYMERIZATION CYCLE SHOWING REACTION RATES ADJUSTED FOR PHYSIOLOGICAL CONCENTRATIONS *(ARROWS)*. Note the main pathway followed by an actin molecule as it recycles between the monomer pool and filaments *(shading)*. A pool of ATP-actin bound to profilin elongates actin filaments with free barbed ends. Profilin rapidly dissociates, and filamentous actin hydrolyzes ATP and dissociates phosphate. ADF/cofilins promote phosphate dissociation and sever ADP-actin filaments. ADP subunits dissociate from filaments. Profilin competes with ADF/cofilin for actin monomers and promotes the exchange of ADP for ATP. Thymosin-β_4, when present, sequesters a pool of unpolymerizable ATP-actin. Profilin transfers actin from this thymosin-actin pool to actin filaments. A, actin monomer; C, ADF/cofilin; D, ADP bound to actin; F, filamentous actin; P, profilin; Pi, phosphate bound to actin; T, ATP bound to actin.

The Pool of Unpolymerized Actin

Cells can respond rapidly to stimuli such as chemoattractants by assembling actin filaments where needed, because they have a large pool of unpolymerized actin to grow the new filaments. Roughly half of the actin in the cytoplasm of resting cells is unpolymerized, corresponding to 50 to 100 μM monomers, 500 to 1000 times higher than the critical concentration.

Two complementary mechanisms maintain the pool of unpolymerized actin: monomer binding to profilin and capping of actin filament ends. In vertebrate cells another protein, thymosin-$\beta4$, augments the effects of profilin. Thymosin-$\beta4$ buffers the free monomer concentration by sequestering actin monomers. Rapid exchange allows monomers to move between profilin and thymosin-$\beta4$. The concentrations of profilin and thymosin-$\beta4$ exceed the concentration of unpolymerized actin, and these proteins bind tightly enough to reduce the free monomer concentration to the micromolar level. Actin monomers bound to profilin or thymosin-$\beta4$ do not nucleate new filaments. However, for profilin to maintain a monomer pool, the barbed ends of most filaments must be capped, since rapid addition of actin-profilin complexes to free barbed ends would quickly deplete the pool of unpolymerized actin. Cells contain enough heterodimeric capping protein, gelsolin, or both to cap the barbed ends of most filaments. Together, monomer

and terminating new filaments, and controlling disassembly (Fig. 33-19). For example, biochemical reconstitution of actin filament assembly and recycling in the comet tail of the intracellular bacterium *Listeria* (see Fig. 37-12) requires (in addition to a regulatory protein on the surface of the bacterium) only actin, Arp2/3 complex, ADF/cofilin, profilin, and a capping protein.

binding and capping allow cells to maintain a large pool of actin subunits ready to elongate any barbed ends created by uncapping, severing, or nucleation.

Initiation and Termination of Actin Filaments

A variety of external agonists and internal signals stimulate the conversion of actin from the unpolymerized pool into actin filaments. Examples include the ability of chemoattractants to direct pseudopod formation in slime molds (see Fig. 38-12) and white blood cells (see Fig. 30-13), and the influence of the mitotic spindle on the assembly of the cytokinetic contractile ring (see Fig. 44-22). Polymerization depends on creation of barbed ends, which grow rapidly at rates estimated to be 50 to 500 subunits per second, depending on the concentration of actin-profilin.

Three mechanisms are thought to create free barbed ends: uncapping, severing, and de novo formation of new barbed ends. In many cases, new barbed ends appear to form de novo. At the leading edge of motile cells, small Rho-family GTPases associated with the plasma membrane and polyphosphoinositides activate WASp/Scar proteins, which stimulate Arp2/3 complex to nucleate branches with free barbed ends on the side of older filaments (Figs. 33-2D and 33-13). Formins nucleate filaments for the cleavage furrow and appear to either initiate or sustain the growth of actin filaments in filopodia (see Fig. 38-2A). When thrombin activates platelets (see Fig. 30-14), plasma membrane polyphosphoinositides uncap barbed ends by dissociating gelsolin. Transient increases in the cytoplasmic Ca^{2+} concentration may also induce gelsolin to sever actin filaments, creating capped barbed ends. Dephosphorylation activates ADF/cofilin proteins, which can sever and nucleate filaments, creating free barbed ends.

The duration of growth depends on the nucleation mechanism and the local environment. At the leading edge, new branches nucleated by Arp2/3 complex grow rapidly but transiently, as the concentration of free capping protein is high enough to terminate growth by capping barbed ends in a few seconds. On the other hand, barbed ends growing in association with a formin are protected from capping and grow persistently, as is observed at the tips of filopodia and the barbed ends of actin cables located in the buds of yeast cells.

Actin Filament Turnover and Subunit Recycling

Actin filaments are long lived if protected by tropomyosin and capping, as in muscle and stress fibers, but many actin filaments, such as those at the leading edge of motile cells, turn over quickly. A possible mechanism involves the hydrolysis of ATP and dissociation of the γ-phosphate, reactions that provide a timer to mark older filaments for depolymerization by regulatory proteins (Fig. 33-19). After phosphate dissociates, ADF/cofilin proteins bind ADP-actin subunits in filaments and sever these older filaments. After ADP-actin dissociates from filaments (the details are not yet clear), profilin replaces ADF/cofilin and stimulates the exchange of ADP for ATP. This process recycles actin back to the pool of ATP-actin monomers interacting with profilin. In cells with a high concentration of thymosin-β4, much of the ATP-actin is stored bound to thymosin. Profilin shuttles ATP-actin from this thymosin-β4 buffer to growing filaments. Tropomyosin stabilizes a subset of old filaments by protecting them against ADF/cofilins.

How Do Cells Organize Actin Assemblies?

Cells organize actin filaments in a variety of structures, including cortical networks, microvilli or filopodia, and contractile bundles (Figs. 33-1 to 33-3). Although each cell in a population is unique, all cells of a particular type achieve a similar pattern of organization. How are these patterns specified? Although not yet understood in detail, the mechanisms appear to depend on expression of an appropriate mixture of actin-binding proteins, a prerequisite for self-assembly of particular structures. For example, actin forms bundles similar to microvilli and filopodia when polymerized in the presence of fimbrin and villin, the two major cross-linking proteins found in microvilli. Overexpression of villin in cells induces extension of existing filopodia and formation of new filopodia. Thus, the pool of villin and fimbrin and other components sets the number of microvilli.

The **Rho-family GTPases Cdc42, Rac, and Rho** regulate the assembly of many actin filament structures (Fig. 33-20). A complex of proteins including Cdc42 in the bud of yeast cells anchors formins, which mediate the continuous assembly of a cable of actin filaments. The formins anchor the growing barbed ends as the pointed ends extend into the mother cell. These cables are tracks for myosin-V to move cargo into the bud. In motile cells, signals downstream of chemotactic receptors activate Cdc42 and Rac (see Fig. 38-8), which activate WASp/Scar proteins. They in turn stimulate Arp2/3 complex to generate the branched filament network that pushes the membrane forward. *Listeria* use a surface protein, ActA, to activate Arp2/3 complex, which generates a "comet tail" of actin filaments to push the bacterium through the cytoplasm (see Fig. 37-12). Proteins that mediate endocytosis activate homologs of WASp and other proteins to assemble actin patches in budding yeast (see Fig. 37-11) and fission yeast (Fig. 33-1D).

Physical forces also help to organize actin filaments. Bundles of actin filaments in stress fibers (Fig. 33-1) and

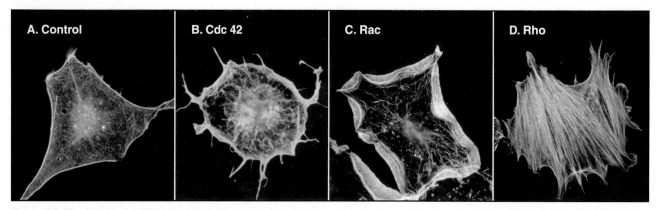

Figure 33-20   Rho-family GTPases promote the assembly of actin-based structures. Fluorescence micrographs of Swiss 3T3 fibroblasts stained with rhodamine-phalloidin to reveal actin filaments. **A,** Resting cells. **B,** Cells microinjected with activated Cdc42 form many filopodia. **C,** Cells microinjected with activated Rac have a thick cortical network of actin filaments around the periphery. **D,** Stress fibers anchored at their ends by focal contacts are abundant in cells microinjected with an activated form of Rho. (Courtesy of Alan Hall, University of London, England.)

the contractile ring during cytokinesis (Fig. 33-3; also see Fig. 44-23) appear to be aligned, at least in part, by tension generated by myosin motors. Activated Rho is required for cytokinesis and also stimulates formation of stress fibers (Fig. 33-20) by activating **myosin II.** Rho stimulates two kinases that phosphorylate the regulatory light chain and inhibit a phosphatase that reverses the phosphorylation of the light chain (see Fig. 39-21). The success of forces in organizing actin filaments depends on anchoring of the filaments to the plasma membrane—focal contacts in the case of stress fibers (see Fig. 30-11) and the equatorial plasma membrane for the contractile ring (see Fig. 44-23). Cross-linking proteins, such as α-actinin, help to maintain the integrity of these bundles under mechanical stress.

Mechanical Properties of Cytoplasm

Actin filaments provide the molecular basis for many of the mechanical properties of cytoplasm, a complicated, viscoelastic material. *Viscoelastic* means that cytoplasm can both resist flow, like a viscous liquid (e.g., molasses),

and store mechanical energy when stretched or compressed, like a spring.

The physical properties of actin filaments depend on their lengths and their interactions. At physiological concentrations, purified actin filaments are viscoelastic. At high concentrations, actin filaments also align spontaneously into large parallel arrays called liquid crystals. Cross-linking networks of actin filaments increases both their viscosity and stiffness. Severing actin filaments decreases their viscoelasticity. On the other hand, shorter filaments have an increased tendency to form bundles in the presence of cross-linking proteins, so severing can actually promote the formation of rigid actin filament bundles.

Many cross-linking proteins, including α-actinin, have a low affinity for actin filaments with a K_d in the micromolar range. At steady state in vitro, bonds between these cross-linking proteins and actin filaments break and reform on a second or subsecond time scale. Consequently, gels of actin filaments and α-actinin are much more rigid when deformed rapidly than slowly (Fig. 33-21), because cross-links resisting the displacement of the filaments can rearrange if given sufficient

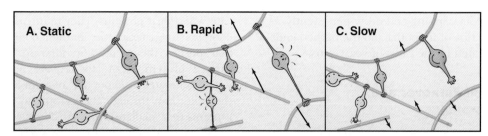

Figure 33-21   **DYNAMIC CROSS-LINKING OF ACTIN FILAMENTS.** Rapid binding and dissociation of cross-linking proteins allow networks of actin filaments to resist rapid deformations but to change shape passively when force is applied for a prolonged time. **A,** Cross-linked network in a static region. **B,** Cross-linking proteins resist deformation if force is applied rapidly. **C,** Cross-linking proteins provide little resistance to deformation if force is applied slowly, since the cross-links rearrange faster than the filaments are displaced. (Redrawn from Pollard TD, Satterwhite L, Cisek L, et al: Actin and myosin biochemistry in relation to cytokinesis. Ann N Y Acad Sci 582:120–130, 1990.)

time. Dynamic cross-links between filaments allow actin networks to remodel passively as cells move. Cells also remodel the actin cytoskeleton actively by nucleating, severing or depolymerizing filaments.

ACKNOWLEDGMENTS

Thanks go to Charmaine Chan and Aditya Paul for their suggestions on revisions to this chapter.

SELECTED READINGS

Amos LA, van den Ent F, Löwe J: Structural/functional homology between the bacterial and eukaryotic cytoskeletons. Curr Opin Cell Biol 16:24-31, 2004.

Bamburg JR, Wiggan OP: ADF/cofilin and actin dynamics in disease. Trends Cell Biol 12:598-605, 2002.

Blessing CA, Ugrinova GT, Goodson HV: Actin and ARPs: Action in the nucleus. Trends Cell Biol 14:435-442, 2004.

Janmey PA, Weitz DA: Dealing with mechanics: Mechanisms of force transduction in cells. Trends Biochem Sci 29:364-370, 2004.

Krause M, Dent EW, Bear JE, et al: Ena/VASP proteins: Regulators of the actin cytoskeleton and cell migration. Annu Rev Cell Dev Biol 19:541-564, 2003.

Kreis T, Vale R (eds): Guidebook to the Cytoskeletal and Motor Proteins, 2nd ed. New York, Oxford University Press, 1999.

Kwiatkowski AV, Gertler FB, Loureiro JJ: Function and regulation of Ena/VASP proteins. Trends Cell Biol 13:386-392, 2003.

Löwe J, van den Ent F, Amos LA: Molecules of the bacterial cytoskeleton. Annu Rev Biophys Biomolec Struct 33:177-198, 2004.

Pollard TD, Blanchoin L, Mullins RD: Biophysics of actin filament dynamics in nonmuscle cells. Annu Rev Biophys Biomol Struct 29:545-576, 2000.

Quinlan M, Heuser JE, Kerkhoff E, Mullins RD: Drosophila spire is an actin filament nucleation factor. Nature 433:382-388, 2005.

Stossel TP, Condeelis J, Cooley L, et al: Filamins as integrators of cell mechanics and signalling. Nat Rev Mol Cell Biol 2:138-145, 2001.

Wallar BJ, Alberts AS: The formins: Active scaffolds that remodel the cytoskeleton. Trends Cell Biol 13:435-445, 2003.

Wear MA, Cooper JA: Capping protein: New insights into mechanism and regulation. Trends Biochem Sci 29:418-428, 2004.

Weaver AM, Young ME, Lee W-L, Cooper JA: Integration of signals to the Arp2/3 complex. Curr Opin Cell Biol 15:23-30, 2003.

Welch MD, Mullins RD: Cellular control of actin nucleation. Annu Rev Cell Dev Biol 18:247-288, 2002.

Winder SJ: Structural insights into actin-binding, branching and bundling proteins. Curr Opin Cell Biol 15:14-22, 2003.

Zigmond SH: Formin-induced nucleation of actin filaments. Curr Opin Cell Biol 16:99-105, 2004.

APPENDIX 33-1

Classification of Actin-Binding Proteins

Protein (Homologs and Synonyms)	Distribution	Subunits (N × kD)	K_d Actin Binding	Other Ligands	Diseases and Mutations
Monomer Binding					
Actobindin	Pr	1 × 9.8	3.3 µM dimers	—	—
β Thymosins	An	1 × 5	0.7 µM monomer	—	—
DNase I	An	1 × 29	0.1 nM monomer and pointed end	Calcium, DNA	—
Profilin	Eu	1 × 13-15	0.1 µM monomer	PIP₂, VASP, Polyproline	Yst, Dros, mouse
Vitamin D–binding protein (Gc globulin)	An	1 × 58	1 nM monomer	Vitamin D, C5A complement	—
Small Severing					
ADF/cofilin (actophorin, depactin, destrin)	Eu	1 × 15-19	0.1 µM ADP monomer, 0.5 µM ADP filament	PIP₂	Yst, Dros., *C. elegans*
Capping					
Arp2/3 complex	Eu	1 × 49, 1 × 44, 1 × 40, 1 × 35, 1 × 21, 1 × 20, 1 × 16	10 nM pointed end 0.5 µM filament side	Profilin Scar, WASp, cortactin	Yst

An, animals; Dd, Dictyostelium discoideum; Dros, Drosophila melanogaster; Eu, all eukaryotes; Fu, fungi; Hs, Homo sapiens; MAP-2, microtubule-associated protein 2; NMDA, N-methyl-d-aspartate; Pl, plants; Pr, protozoa; TM, tropomyosin; TNC, troponin C; TNI, troponin I; TNT, troponin T; tRNA, transfer RNA; Yst, yeast.

Continued

Protein (Homologs and Synonyms)	Distribution	Subunits (N × kD)	K_d Actin Binding	Other Ligands	Diseases and Mutations
Capping protein (CapZ)	Eu	1×32–$36(\alpha) +$ 1×28–$32(\beta)$	<1 nM barbed end	Dynactin complex, PIP_2	Yst, Dros, Dd
Fragmin (severin, gCAP39)	Pr, An	1×40	1 nM barbed end	—	Dd
Gelsolin (scinderin)	Pr, An	1×80 or 83	50 nM barbed end, μM dimers, sides	Calcium, PIP_2	Dros, mouse, Hs Finnish amyloidosis
Tensin	An	1×96	Barbed end	P-tyrosine	
Tropomodulin	An	1×40	Pointed end, 1 nM with TM, 0.4 μM without TM	Tropomyosin (TM)	Dros
Villin (Cap 100)	Pr, An	1×93	7 μM filament, 0.3 μM filament for head domain	Calcium, PIP_2	—
Filament Side Binding					
Abp1p	Fu, An	1×67		—	Yst
Adducin	An	$1 \times 100 +$ 1×105	0.3 μM filament	Spectrin	—
Caldesmon	An	1×90 or 1×61	1 μM filament with tropomyosin	Calmodulin, tropomyosin, myosin	—
Calponin	An	1×34	0.2 μM filament with tropomyosin	Calmodulin, tropomyosin	
Coronin	Pr, Fu, An	1×51	5–40 nM filament	—	Dd, yst
Drebrin	An	1×95	0.1 μM filament	—	—
Nebulin		1×750	Filament		Hs Nemaline myopathy
Nuclear actin-binding protein	Pr	2×34	0.25 μM filament	DNA	—
Tropomyosin	Pr, Fu, An	2×28–32	Filament, cooperative	Self, troponin, caldesmon, calponin	Yst, Dros, Hs cardiomyopathy
Troponin	An	1×18, TNC 1×21, TNI 1×31, TNT	Filament	Tropomyosin, calcium	TNT in Hs cardiomyopathy
Cross Linking					
ABP-120	Pr	2×92	<1 μM filament	—	Dd
α-Actinin (actinogelin)	Pr, Fu, An	2×100	1-5 μM filament	Vinculin, zyxin, integrin, PIP_2, NMDA receptor, selectin	Dd, Dros, Hs muscular dystrophy
Anillin	An, Fu	1×132	Filament	—	Dros, Yst
Cortexillin	Pr	2×51	0.2 μM filament	—	Dd
Dematin (Band 4.9)	An	3×43–45	Filament	RBC membrane	—
eEF1A (ABP-50)	Eu	1×50	0.1-10 μM filament	GTP, ribosome, aminoacyl-tRNA, tubulin	Yst
Espin	An	1×95 or 29	0.1-0.2 μM filaments	—	Hs deafness
Fascin	An	1×56	Filament	β-catenin	Dros
Filamin (ABP-280)	An	2×240–280	0.5 μM filament	$GP1B^h1X$	—
Fimbrin (plastin)	Eu	1×68	Filament	Ca^{2+}	Yst
Scruin	An	1×102	Filament	Calmodulin	—

Protein (Homologs and Synonyms)	Distribution	Subunits (N × kD)	K$_d$ Actin Binding	Other Ligands	Diseases and Mutations
Small cross-linking proteins (gelactins)	Pr	1 × 34	Filament	Ca^{2+}	Dd
Transgelin	Fu, An	1 × 23	Filament	—	—
Membrane Associated					
Actolinkin	An	1 × 20	Filament	Membranes	—
Annexin-II (calpactin I, Lipocortin II)	An, Pl	2 × 38 + 2 × 10	0.2 μM filament	Calcium, acidic, phospholipids	—
Dystrophin/ utrophin	An	1 × 427/1 × 395	Filament, head 44 μM, tail 0.5 μM	β-dystroglycan	Hs muscular dystrophies
Ezrin/moesin/ radixin	An	1 × 68 + oligomers	Filament	Self	—
Hisactophilin	Pr	1 × 13.5	Filament, 0.2 μM monomer	Membranes	Dd
Ponticulin	Pr, An	1 × 17	0.3 μM filament	Membranes	Dd
Protein 4.1	An	1 × 80	Filament	Spectrin, band 3, glycophorin	Hs hereditary elliptocytosis
Spectrin (fodrin, calspectin)	Pr, An	2 × 280 (α) + 2 × 246 (β)	1–25 μM filament	Ca^{2+}, self, ankyrin, calmodulin, band 4.1, adducin	Hs hereditary spherocytosis
Talin	Pr, An	1 × 272	Filament, 0.25 μM monomer	Vinculin, integrins, p125FAK	—
Microtubule Binding					
MAP-2	An	1 × 210	Filament sides	Microtubules, PKA, intermediate filaments	—
Tau	An	1 × 43–86	Filament sides	Microtubules	Alzheimer's disease
Intermediate Filament Binding					
BPAG1	An	? × 280 or ? × 230	0.2 μM filaments	Intermediate filaments	Mouse dystonia musculorum
Motors					
Myosins I–XII	Eu	Various	1–100 μM with ATP, 4nM without ATP	Various (self, membranes)	Hs cardiomyopathy, deafness, retinitis

CHAPTER 34

Microtubules and Centrosomes

Microtubules are stiff, cylindrical polymers of α- and β-**tubulin** (Fig. 34-1) that provide support for a variety of cellular components and tracks for movements powered by motor proteins called kinesins and dyneins. Microtubules are 25 nm in diameter and can grow longer than 20 μm in cells and 3 mm in vitro. The head-to-tail arrangement of dimers of α- and β-tubulin in the wall of microtubules give the polymer a molecular polarity. The **"plus" (β-tubulin) end** grows faster than the **"minus" end.**

A great simplifying principle is that microtubules have a radial organization in many types of cells (Fig. 34-2A). Typically, the plus end is peripheral, and the minus end is anchored in a **microtubule-organizing center.** One exception to this radial organization is found in dendrites of nerve cells, where about 40% of the microtubules are oriented with the minus end away from the cell body.

In most animal cells, the organizing center for cytoplasmic microtubules is the **centrosome.** Centrosomes consist of centrioles and a surrounding matrix containing the active component in microtubule nucleation—a complex of proteins including the specialized tubulin isoform **γ-tubulin.** The microtubule-organizing center is more diffuse in columnar epithelial cells, where microtubules originate from a broad zone containing γ-tubulin near the apex of the cell (Fig. 34-2B). In plant cells, γ-tubulin and microtubules are found throughout the cortex rather than in a discrete array, although they form a bipolar **mitotic spindle** during cell division (Fig. 34-2C). Microtubules in fungi grow from a **spindle pole body,** an organizing center containing γ-tubulin that is associated with the nuclear envelope (Fig. 34-2D). Animals and protozoa with cilia and flagella use **basal bodies** (Fig. 34-3B) to nucleate the assembly of microtubules for their motile structure, called an axoneme.

Microtubules vary considerably in stability. Those that form the **axonemes** in eukaryotic cilia and flagella are stable for days to weeks. Cytoplasmic microtubules turn over much more rapidly, within minutes in the case of the interphase array of microtubules and within tens of seconds for mitotic spindle microtubules. These dynamic microtubules randomly undergo rapid depolymerization and then regrow over a period of seconds to minutes. This **"dynamic instability"** helps to remodel the network of microtubules in cytoplasm and contributes to some forms of motility, including the assembly of the mitotic spindle and movements of chromosomes during mitosis (see Fig. 44-7).

Because the same tubulin dimers can form dynamic single microtubules in cytoplasm and stable doublet microtubules in axonemes, it is believed that accessory

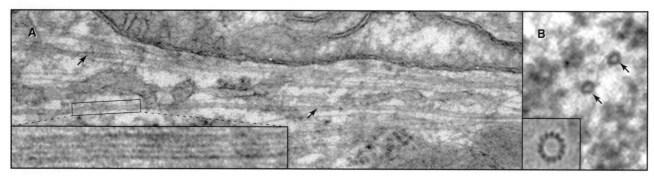

Figure 34-1 MICROTUBULES *(ARROWS)* VISUALIZED IN ELECTRON MICROGRAPHS OF THIN SECTIONS OF A CULTURED MAMMALIAN CELL. **A,** Longitudinal section. **B,** Cross section. **Insets,** Electron micrographs of microtubules in frozen hydrated rat hepatoma cells. (Main panels, Courtesy of R. Goldman, Northwestern University, Evanston, Illinois. Insets, Courtesy of Cédric Bouchet-Marquis and Jacques Dubochet, University of Lausanne, Switzerland.)

proteins specify both the stability and diverse structures assembled from tubulin. The various families of **microtubule-associated proteins (MAPs)** bind tubulin dimers, stabilize polymers, associate with microtubule ends, or sever cytoplasmic microtubules. In the axonemes of cilia and flagella, more than 100 accessory proteins organize and stabilize the regular array of nine outer doublet microtubules and two central single microtubules (see Fig. 38-16).

Microtubule motor proteins (see Figs. 36-13 and 36-14) power movements ranging from the slow movements of chromosomes on the mitotic spindle (see Fig. 44-14) to the rapid beating of cilia and flagella (see Fig. 38-14). Different motors move toward the plus and minus ends of microtubules. The main minus-end-directed motor, dynein, drives the beating of cilia and flagella. Dynein and the kinesin family of plus-end motors move membrane-bound organelles, RNA particles, viruses, and other cargo along microtubules (see Fig. 37-7). These active movements determine, to a great extent, the distribution of cellular organelles and the shape of cells.

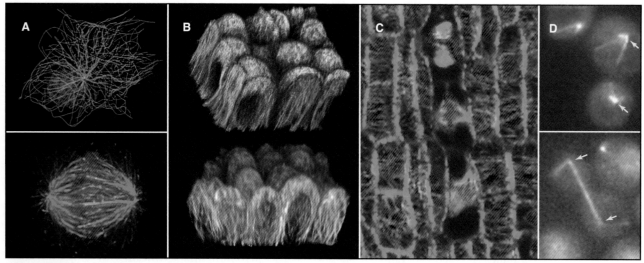

Figure 34-2 ARRANGEMENTS OF MICROTUBULES IN VARIOUS CELLS. **A–C,** Fluorescence micrographs of microtubules stained with antibodies to tubulin. **A,** Vertebrate tissue culture cells. *Green* microtubules radiate from the *red* centrosome near the *blue* nucleus of an interphase cell *(upper panel)*. A HeLa cell in mitosis with *green* microtubules radiating from the two poles toward the *blue* chromosomes and *red* centromeres (stained with anticentromere antibody) *(lower panel)*. **B,** Columnar epithelial cells in tissue culture. Three-dimensional reconstructions show microtubules oriented along the long axis of the cell. **C,** Plant cells. Maize epidermal cells with *green* microtubules in the cortex and in the mitotic spindles of three dividing cells near the middle of the field. Nuclei are stained *orange*. **D, Live budding yeast.** Two interphase cells with microtubules radiating from the spindle pole bodies *(arrows)* associated with the nuclear envelope; these microtubules are marked with dynein fused to *green* fluorescent protein *(upper panel)*. A cell late in mitosis with a bundle of microtubules extending from one spindle pole body to the other inside the nucleus; these microtubules are marked with tubulin fused to *green* fluorescent protein *(lower panel)*. (A, Upper panel, Courtesy of A. Khodjakov, Wadsworth Center, Albany, New York; lower panel, Courtesy of D. W. Cleveland, University of California, San Diego. B, Courtesy of R. Bacallao, University of Indiana Medical School, Indianapolis. C, Courtesy of L. Smith, University of California, San Diego. D, Courtesy of P. Maddox, University of North Carolina, Chapel Hill.)

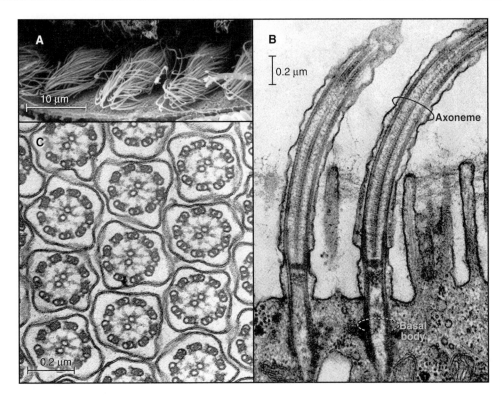

Figure 34-3 CILIA ON MUSSEL GILL EPITHELIAL CELLS. **A,** A scanning electron micrograph reveals how the bending movements of the thread-like cilia are coordinated in waves. **B–C,** Transmission electron micrographs of cilia. **B,** Longitudinal section showing basal bodies and proximal parts of two cilia. **C,** Cross section of many cilia showing the nine outer doublets and the central pair of microtubules. (Courtesy of P. Satir, Albert Einstein College of Medicine, Bronx, New York. Reference: Satir P: How cilia move. Sci Am 231:44–52, 1974.)

Tubulin Structure

The tubulin molecule is a heterodimer of α and β subunits that share a common fold and 40% identical residues (Fig. 34-4). Dimers of α- and β-tubulin are stable and rarely dissociate at the 10- to 20-μM concentrations of tubulin found in cells. γ-Tubulins have the same fold.

Each tubulin subunit binds a guanine nucleotide, either guanosine triphosphate (GTP) or guanosine diphosphate (GDP). The fold and the GTP-binding site of tubulin do not resemble those of other GTP-binding proteins (see Fig. 25-7). GTP on α-tubulin is buried in the dimer, so it does not exchange with solution GTP; hence, it is called the nonexchangeable N-site. GTP on β-tubulin is exposed in the dimer and exchanges slowly ($K_d = 50$ nM), so this is known as the exchangeable site, or E-site. When incorporated into a microtubule, contacts with the adjacent α subunit bury the GTP on the β subunit and promote its hydrolysis. Neither bound guanine nucleotide can exchange when tubulin is buried in the wall of a microtubule. As is explained later in this chapter, the nature of the nucleotide on the β subunit profoundly affects microtubule assembly.

Most Archaea and Bacteria have a protein called **FtsZ** with the same fold as tubulin. The two proteins are most likely to have had a common ancestor, but their sequences have diverged considerably. FtsZ also forms polymers and is required for cytokinesis of prokaryotes (see Fig. 44-21). One group of Bacteria lost their FtsZ

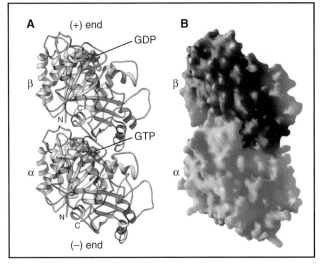

Figure 34-4 STRUCTURE OF THE α-TUBULIN/β-TUBULIN DIMER. **A,** Ribbon diagrams with space-filling GTP on α-tubulin and GDP on β-tubulin. **B,** Surface rendering. This historic structure was the first high-resolution structure of a nonmembrane protein to be determined by electron crystallography, using sheets of tubulin protofilaments as the specimen. Each subunit consists of about 450 residues arranged in two domains. Each domain is a β-sheet flanked by α-helices. The nucleotides bind in pockets similar to the binding site for nicotinamide-adenine dinucleotide (NAD) on the enzyme glyceraldehyde-3-phosphate dehydrogenase. (PDB file: 1TUB. Reference: Nogales E, Downing K: Structure of the α/β tubulin dimer by electron crystallography. Nature 391:199–203, 1998.)

but have acquired genes for both α- and β-tubulin, most likely by lateral transfer from an eukaryote.

Tubulins are modified in a number of different ways in cells. Over time, stable microtubules accumulate two modifications—acetylation of lysine-40 and removal of the C-terminal tyrosine of α-tubulin—but neither modification is responsible for the stability. The enzyme carboxypeptidase B removes the tyrosine, leaving a glutamic acid exposed. Another enzyme, tyrosine-tubulin ligase, can replace the tyrosine. Other microtubules are modified by the addition of a polymer of up to six glutamic acid residues to the γ-carboxyl groups of glutamic acid residues of both α-tubulin and β-tubulin. Addition of one or more glycines to the γ-carboxyl of other glutamate residues stabilizes the central pair of microtubules in axonemes (see Fig. 38-16).

Tubulin Diversity

Tubulins are remarkably conserved across the phylogenetic tree; more than 75% of the residues of animal α- or β-tubulins are identical to their plant homologs. On the other hand, species differ considerably in their variety of tubulin isoforms. Vertebrates have six to eight genes each encoding variants of α- and β-tubulin, whereas budding yeast have but two α-tubulin genes and one β-tubulin gene. Unicellular ciliates such as *Tetrahymena* assemble a greater variety of microtubule-based structures than humans have in their various tissues, but they do this using only one α- and one β-tubulin polypeptide. Most vertebrate cells express several tubulin isoforms, but exceptional cases, such as bird red blood cells, express a single α-tubulin and β-tubulin. It is impressive that the sequences of orthologous tubulins vary little, if at all, between different vertebrate species, whereas the paralogous β-tubulin isoforms in one organism differ by about 10% in primary structure. The sequences of γ-tubulins are also conserved between species.

Two views rationalize the significance of multiple α- and β-tubulin isoforms. On one hand, isoforms have different assembly properties and affinities for microtubule-associated proteins (MAPs) that may confer some advantage to the organism. This is illustrated by the failure of paralogous tubulin genes to substitute for each other in flies. Alternatively, the proteins themselves may be largely interchangeable (and all isoforms appear to copolymerize), but different genes may be required to ensure precise control of biosynthesis in particular cells at appropriate times during development. For example, the two α-tubulin proteins of the filamentous fungus *Aspergillus* can substitute for each other, but two genes are required to control the expression of tubulin at specific times in the life cycle.

Four tubulin isoforms called δ-, ε-, ζ-, and η-tubulin are found in protozoa, algae, and vertebrates but are conspicuously missing from fungi and most plants. All of these isoforms are required for the structure or function of centrioles or basal bodies. Their absence accounts for the lack of centrioles in plants and fungi.

Structure of Microtubules

Microtubules are cylinders constructed of longitudinally oriented **protofilaments** with a 4-nm longitudinal repeat arising from the tubulin subunits (Fig. 34-5). Most cytoplasmic microtubules have 13 protofilaments, but microtubules in some cells have 11, 15, or 16 protofilaments. Microtubules assembled in vitro can have 11 to 15 protofilaments, but 13 is the favored number. For years, microtubules were thought to be true helices, but

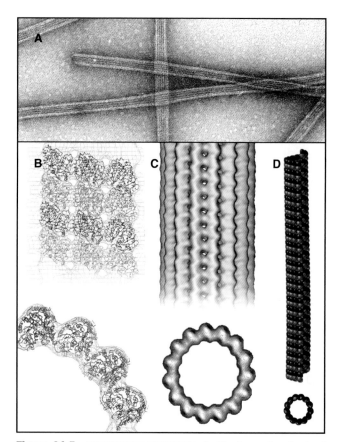

Figure 34-5   MICROTUBULE STRUCTURE. A, Electron micrograph of negatively stained microtubules. **B–C,** Longitudinal and cross sections of a reconstruction of a 13-protofilament microtubule made by image processing of electron micrographs. **B,** Atomic model made by fitting the tubulin dimer model into the reconstruction of the microtubule. **C,** Surface rendering of the reconstruction. **D,** Drawing of the microtubule used throughout this book. It shows the longitudinal seam between two protofilaments, which breaks the helical repeat of tubulin dimers. (A, Courtesy of D. B. Murphy, Johns Hopkins Medical School, Baltimore, Maryland. B–C, Courtesy of R. Milligan, Scripps Research Institute, La Jolla, California. Note that a higher resolution is now available: Li H, DeRosier D, Nicholson WV et al: Microtubule structure at 8 Å resolution. Structure 10:1317–1328, 2002.)

microtubules with 13 protofilaments have a longitudinal seam or discontinuity between two of the protofilaments, breaking up perfect helical packing of the subunits (Fig. 34-5D). The other protofilaments are aligned identically with respect to their neighbors.

Microtubules are polar because all of the dimers have the same orientation. β-tubulin is oriented toward the plus end; α-tubulin is oriented toward the minus end. This polarity results in different rates of growth at the two ends. The plus end grows faster than the minus end. For the purpose of marking polarity in electron micrographs, microtubules in extracted cells can be decorated with either exogenous dynein or with excess tubulin, which can form curved "hooks" under nonphysiological conditions. These hooks provided the primary evidence that the minus ends are usually associated with microtubule-organizing centers.

As might be expected from their cylindrical structure, microtubules are much stiffer than are either actin filaments or intermediate filaments. If enlarged 1 million–fold to a diameter of 25 mm, microtubules would have mechanical properties similar to those of a plastic pipe: quite stiff locally but flexible over distances of several meters (micrometers in the cell). On the same scale, actin filaments would be like 8-mm plastic rods, and intermediate filaments would be akin to 10-mm braided plastic ropes. Thus, microtubules are resistant to compression and support asymmetrical structures much more effectively than the other cytoskeletal polymers. Interactions of microtubules with both actin filaments and intermediate filaments reinforce the cytoskeleton.

The stiffness, length, and polarity of microtubules make them valuable both for cytoskeletal support and as tracks for microtubule-based motors. Because they resist compression, microtubules are called on more frequently than actin filaments or intermediate filaments to support asymmetrical cellular structures, including axonemes, the mitotic spindle, and elaborate surface processes of some protozoa (see Fig. 38-4). Plants provide a spectacular example of the influence of microtubules on morphology: Point mutations in tubulin influence whether climbing plants wrap in a left-handed or right-handed helix around their supports.

Microtubule Assembly from GTP Tubulin

Microtubules assemble from pure GTP-tubulin subunits much like actin filaments do using subunits with bound ATP (see Figs. 5-6 and 33-8). Superficially, the assembly of microtubules is a simple bimolecular reaction of tubulin dimers with the ends of the polymer. Association and dissociation of tubulin occurs only at the ends, not from the walls of microtubules. Growth is faster at

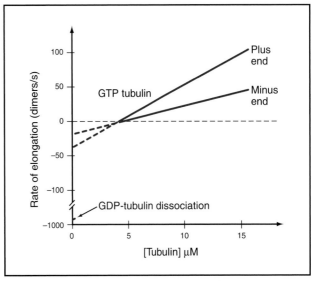

Figure 34-6 ELONGATION OF PURE TUBULIN MICROTUBULES. The rate of elongation at plus and minus ends depends on the concentration of GTP-tubulin dimers. Slopes give association rate constants, x-intercepts give the critical concentrations, and the y-intercepts (after linear extrapolation [*dashed lines*] from positive growth rates to the y-axis) give the dissociation rate constants for GTP tubulin. The dissociation rate of GDP tubulin is shown as a single point at 733 s^{-1} on the y-axis. (Data from Walker RA, O'Brien ET, Pryer NK, et al: Dynamic instability of individual microtubules. J Cell Biol 107:1437–1448, 1988.)

the plus end than at the minus end (Fig. 34-6), and assembly of GTP-tubulin is much more favorable than that of GDP-tubulin. The rate of elongation is proportional to the concentration of GTP-tubulin dimers above the **critical concentration** at each end. The rate constants measured from the slopes and intercepts in elongation experiments (Table 34-1) are similar to those for actin (see Fig. 33-8), although this similarity might be misleading, as the number of sites growing at the end of a microtubule is unknown and is most likely to be greater than one as on actin filaments.

Drugs (Box 34-1) and environmental conditions can depolymerize microtubules. Pioneering light microscopic observations of live cells established that mitotic spindle fibers (later shown to be microtubules) are sensitive to both cold and high hydrostatic pressure. This makes it possible to purify microtubules and tightly associated proteins by cycles of depolymerization in the cold and repolymerization at higher temperatures. Dissociated microtubule components in ice-cold cellular extracts polymerize when rewarmed to body temperature. Pelleting in a centrifuge separates microtubules and any associated proteins from soluble components. Resuspension in cold buffer with GTP depolymerizes the microtubules. The cycle is repeated until the desired degree of purity is achieved. Adaptations of tubulins or accessory proteins allow cold-water organisms to assemble microtubules at temperatures near freezing.

Table 34-1

RATE CONSTANTS FOR THE ASSEMBLY OF MICROTUBULES IN VITRO AND IN CELLS

Reaction	Plus End	Minus End
In Vitro Elongation of Purified Tubulin		
Association of GTP tubulin	$9\ \mu M^{-1}\ s^{-1}$	$4\ \mu M^{-1}\ s^{-1}$
Dissociation of GTP tubulin	$44\ s^{-1}$	$23\ s^{-1}$
Association of GDP tubulin	Unknown	Unknown
Dissociation of GDP tubulin	$733\ s^{-1}$	$915\ s^{-1}$
Steady-State Dynamic Instability		
Frequency of catastrophe in vitro at 7 μM tubulin	$0.0045\ s^{-1}$	$0.003\ s^{-1}$
Frequency of rescue in vitro at 7 μM tubulin	$0.02\ s^{-1}$	$0.06\ s^{-1}$
Microtubule Dynamic Instability in Live Cells		
Frequency of catastrophe in vivo (interphase)	$0.014\ s^{-1}$	
Frequency of catastrophe in vivo (mitosis)	$0.017\ s^{-1}$	
Frequency of rescue in vivo (interphase)	$0.046\ s^{-1}$	
Frequency of rescue in vivo (mitosis)	0	

Data from Walker RA, O'Brien ET, Pryer NK, et al: Dynamic instability of individual microtubules. J Cell Biol 107:1437–1448, 1988.

Microtubule-Organizing Centers

Spontaneous nucleation of microtubules from tubulin dimers is so unfavorable that it is probably irrelevant to living cells. In vitro, this slow nucleation of pure tubulin accounts for a substantial lag of minutes during the formation of microtubules. Presumably, tubulin dimers form oligomers that assemble into small sheets of protofilaments and eventually close to form a cylinder, but the details are still under investigation.

Instead of spontaneous nucleation, virtually all cellular microtubules arise from **microtubule-organizing centers.** Microtubules in cilia and flagella grow directly from basal bodies (see Fig. 38-17), but other microtubules originate in the pericentrosomal material surrounding centrioles in the centrosome (Figs. 34-2A and 34-18), from fungal spindle pole bodies (Fig. 34-19) or nuclear envelopes and less-organized material in the cortex of some epithelial cells (Fig. 34-2B) and plant cells (Fig. 34-2C). As is described in the section on centrosomes later in this chapter, these organizing centers use assemblies of γ-tubulin to initiate microtubules.

Steady-State Dynamics of Microtubules in Vitro

If the GTP-tubulin reactions were all that contributed to assembly, microtubules would grow until the concentration of free tubulin dimers decreased to the critical concentration, after which polymers would be relatively stable, since the critical concentrations are similar at the two ends. Under these conditions, assembly at one end would be balanced by disassembly at the other. However, this is not what happens at steady state in either test tubes or cells. In vitro, the overall microtubule polymer and monomer concentrations are stable over time, but the microtubule number declines as some microtubules disappear, and the survivors grow longer. Direct observation by light microscopy (Fig.

BOX 34-1
Pharmacologic Tools for Studying Tubulin and Microtubules

Tubulin binds several therapeutically active plant alkaloids and synthetic chemicals, including two of the most successful drugs used to treat cancer. *Vinblastine* (from periwinkle) interferes with microtubule dynamics by binding between tubulin dimers at the ends of microtubules. *Taxol* (from the bark of the Western yew) binds β-tubulin and stabilizes microtubules. At substoichiometric concentrations, vinblastine and taxol are effective in cancer chemotherapy because they interfere with the dynamic instability of mitotic spindle microtubules and block cell division. *Colchicine* (from the autumn crocus) and *nocodazole* (a synthetic chemical) inhibit microtubule assembly by binding dissociated tubulin dimers. Colchicine binds dimers between the two subunits, stabilizing a bent conformation that cannot fit into the microtubule lattice. Colchicine is used empirically to treat gout, a painful condition that results from the accumulation of uric acid crystals in joints and other tissues, but no one knows precisely how it works or why it is not more toxic.

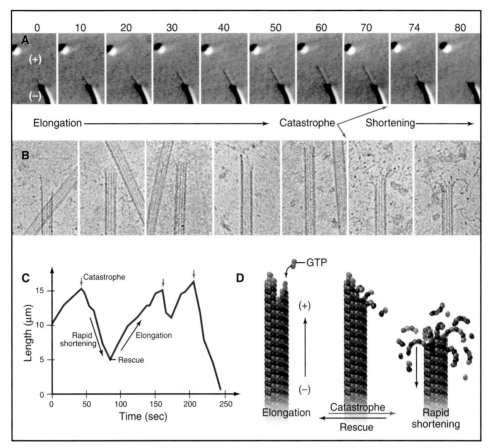

Figure 34-7 DYNAMIC INSTABILITY OF MICROTUBULES IN VITRO. **A,** Time series of differential interference contrast light micrographs of a microtubule growing from the broken end of an axoneme in the presence of 11 μM GTP tubulin. At 70 s, a catastrophe occurs, and the microtubule shortens rapidly. **B,** Electron micrographs of frozen samples. Growing microtubules have flat or oblique ends interpreted as sheets of polymerized tubulin that have not yet closed up into a tube. Rapidly shortening microtubules have protofilaments and sheets peeling from the end. **C,** Time course of the fluctuations in the length of a microtubule from an experiment similar to **A. D,** Model for the transitions during steady-state dynamic instability of microtubules in vitro. GTP tubulin is *blue-green;* GDP tubulin is *red-orange.* (A, Reproduced from Walker RA, O'Brien ET, Pryer NK, et al: Dynamic instability of individual microtubules. J Cell Biol 107:1437–1448, 1988, by copyright permission of The Rockefeller University Press. B, Reproduced from Mandelkow E-M, Mandelkow E, Milligan RA: Microtubule dynamics and microtubule caps: A time-resolved cryo-electron microscopy study. J Cell Biol 114:977–991, 1991, by copyright permission of The Rockefeller University Press. C, Reference: Erickson HP, O'Brien E: Microtubule dynamic instability and GTP hydrolysis. Annu Rev Biophys 21:145–166, 1992.)

34-7A) shows that this behavior is attributable to random, rapid fluctuations in the length of microtubules. Amazingly, growing and shrinking microtubules coexist at steady state; some shrinking microtubules disappear while others grow. This behavior is called **dynamic instability.**

At steady state, individual microtubules grow slowly until they undergo a random transition to a phase of rapid shortening. This transition is called a **catastrophe.** As they shorten, tubulin is lost from the end at a rate of nearly 1000 dimers per second, so the polymer shrinks more than 0.5 μm per second. Electron micrographs of rapidly shortening microtubules show curved segments of protofilaments peeling out from the end (Fig. 34-7B). Dimers dissociate from these curved protofilaments and sheets before or after they break free from an end. Rapid shortening can be terminated by another stochastic event called a **rescue,** after which

the microtubule grows again at a steady rate. Rescue is more likely at the minus end than at the plus end (Table 34-1). Occasionally, a microtubule disappears completely during a shortening phase if its length reaches zero before a rescue event occurs.

Hydrolysis of GTP bound to the (exchangeable) E-site on β-tubulin drives dynamic instability. Dimeric tubulin hydrolyzes E-site GTP very slowly, but when it is incorporated into a microtubule, interactions with the adjacent α subunit stimulate hydrolysis 250-fold ($k = 0.3$ s^{-1}, corresponding to a half time of 2 s). The γ-phosphate then dissociates ($k = 0.02$ s^{-1}, corresponding to a half time of 35 s). In contrast, GTP bound to the α subunit is not hydrolyzed because the β subunit does not provide the residues required to complete the active site. Thus, "GDP-tubulin" has GDP on the β subunit and GTP on the α subunit. Microtubules composed of GDP-tubulin are extremely unstable in comparison to microtubules assembled from dimers with slowly hydrolyzed GTP analogs bound to the β subunit.

Because the active site for GTP hydrolysis is formed by both the α and β subunits, incorporation of each new dimer on the plus end of a microtubule stimulates hydrolysis of the GTP on the adjacent β subunit already incorporated into the polymer. At the minus end, the same mechanism presumably stimulates hydrolysis of GTP bound to the incoming subunit. This creates microtubules with an unstable core capped at both ends with less dynamic GTP tubulin. GTP caps are maintained by exchange of GTP-tubulin dimers at the ends and by direct exchange of GTP onto the β tubulin subunits exposed at the plus end. The size of the GTP cap is expected to be small and is difficult to measure, as few subunits are involved compared with the large number of GDP subunits in the core of a microtubule (1600 per μm).

Loss of the GTP cap has been suggested to cause a catastrophe. No one knows how many terminal subunits must have GDP before a catastrophe occurs, but the available data and quantitative models based on reasonable assumptions (including a single layer of GTP subunits forming the cap) predict many features of dynamic instability. If the GTP cap is lost, the end shortens rapidly, because of the large dissociation rate constant of GDP tubulin. The energy derived from GTP hydrolysis is released during disintegration of the end of the microtubule, so hydrolysis can be viewed as a step that prepares the polymer for rapid depolymerization. The lattice of GDP-tubulin is also slightly different from that of GTP-tubulin, and this also promotes disassembly. Thus, the strategy of assembling microtubules from GTP-tubulin and converting after assembly to GDP-tubulin creates a polymer that is poised for explosive disassembly. Michael Caplow of the University of North Carolina provides this apt description: "A catastrophe of an elongating microtubule is like removing the cork from a shaken bottle of champagne." The tendency of GDP-tubulin protofilaments to curve into inside-out rings might contribute to their peeling rapidly off the ends of microtubules. The proteins discussed later can regulate this behavior. Some proteins promote catastrophes, while others stabilize microtubules.

The GTP-cap hypothesis is an attractive explanation for catastrophes and is most likely to be valid in many respects. As is expected, the frequency of catastrophes is inversely proportional to the concentration of GTP-tubulin dimers, declining to near zero at high concentrations. However, GDP ends do not inevitably shorten. If a microtubule is physically cut in the middle (presumably exposing two GDP ends), the plus end usually shortens as expected, but the newly exposed minus end continues to grow. If simply exposing GDP tubulin initiated a catastrophe, both ends would shorten. However, both ends do rapidly shorten within several seconds

after dilution of the tubulin pool, indicating that long-term stability of both ends depends on GTP-tubulin association.

If rapid dissociation of GDP tubulin drives shortening, it is logical to assume that recapping with GTP tubulin might rescue shortening microtubules. This hypothesis is also most likely to be true in some ways, but the actual mechanism is complicated. For example, the frequency of rescue depends only weakly on the concentration of GTP tubulin.

In the test tube most microtubules grow at steady state at the expense of other microtubules suffering catastrophes. The catastrophes liberate GDP-tubulin subunits that exchange their bound GDP for GTP. This regenerates a pool of GTP-tubulin dimers at a concentration above the critical concentration to support elongation of the surviving microtubules.

Microtubule Dynamics in Cells

Microtubule dynamics in cells (Fig. 34-8A) are remarkably similar to those in simple buffers in vitro (Table 34-1). The centrosome nucleates and stabilizes the minus ends of most microtubules. At any moment in time, the plus ends of these microtubules are growing, as revealed by the presence of tip-binding proteins (Fig. 34-14). Despite catastrophes about once each minute ($k = 0.01\ \mathrm{s}^{-1}$), during which they shorten rapidly (0.28 μm s^{-1}), interphase microtubules generally are long, both because the chance of rescue is high ($k = 0.05\ \mathrm{s}^{-1}$) and because steady growth during the elongation phase (at a rate of 0.11 μm s^{-1}) restores their length before the next catastrophe. As a result of dynamic instability, the

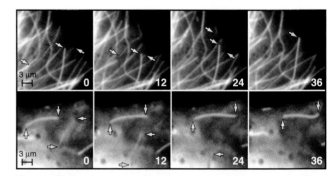

Figure 34-8 DYNAMIC INSTABILITY OF MICROTUBULES IN VIVO. Time series of fluorescence micrographs of a cultured vertebrate cell microinjected with rhodamine-labeled tubulin. **Upper row,** The plus ends of microtubules anchored at the centrosome grow and shrink randomly in the same cell (arrows). **Lower row,** Free microtubules treadmill, growing at their plus end at about the same rate as shortening proceeds at their minus end. Marking a spot on such microtubules shows that this is treadmilling rather than transport of a stable microtubule through cytoplasm. (Courtesy of G. Borisy, University of Wisconsin, Madison.)

bulk of interphase microtubules have a half-life of about 10 minutes.

Dynamic instability allows the plus ends of microtubules to explore the entire cytoplasm as they search for targets such as kinetochores on chromosomes during mitosis (Fig. 34-2A) and to deliver tip-binding proteins, including signaling proteins, to the cell cortex. Fluctuations in microtubule length can do mechanical work such as moving cargo away from the center of the cell (see Fig. 37-6), positioning the nucleus in the center of fission cells as in yeast, or locating the mitotic spindle off center in cells that divide asymmetrically. Reciprocally, the local environment can influence the behavior of the microtubules as they explore the cytoplasm. For example, signaling pathways in the cortex involving Rho-family GTPases and kinases can stabilize microtubules locally and polarize the microtubule array.

Microtubules can also treadmill in the cytoplasm, growing at one end and shrinking at the other. This behavior is common in plants in which dynamic stability at the plus end is biased toward net growth and minus ends depolymerize steadily. Treadmilling is seen in animal cells when an occasional microtubule detaches from the centrosome (Fig. 34-8B).

Regulation by Microtubule-Associated Proteins

The properties of pure tubulin cannot explain all microtubule behavior in cells, which use microtubule-associated proteins (MAPs) to regulate initiation, elongation, shortening, catastrophes, and rescues (Appendix 34-1 and Fig. 34-9). MAPs stabilize some microtubules, such as those in ciliary axonemes. Tubulin purified from axonemes forms microtubules that are just as labile as cytoplasmic microtubules, but microtubules in axonemes with their associated MAPs are stable for days, even under conditions that would depolymerize cytoplasmic microtubules. Modulation of the activity of MAPs allows cells to change the dynamics of microtu-

bules, as when dynamic instability becomes more pronounced when the cell enters mitosis (Fig. 34-2A). Developmentally programmed gene expression establishes the mix of MAPs in each cell type.

MAPs were discovered when they copurified from vertebrate brains along with microtubules during cycles of microtubule assembly and disassembly. Copurification selects a subset of MAPs that bind tightly to microtubules, but it misses important proteins that bind weakly. Functional assays yielded additional MAPs. For example, a light microscopic assay for microtubule fragmentation led to the discovery of the severing protein katanin. Genetic screens have also uncovered proteins that regulate microtubules, such as specialized kinesins and several of the plus-end-binding proteins.

Cells appear to regulate the activity of most MAPs, varying their activity across the cell cycle and locally in the cytoplasm. The following section discusses selected examples of regulation, as this subject is too complex to cover completely.

Microtubule-Stabilizing MAPs

At least a dozen distinct MAPs stabilize microtubules (Appendix 34-1). Most bind along the length of microtubules, but some interact only at or near ends. Some are expressed widely, but others are restricted to specialized cells. Members of the **tau** family, including **MAP2** and **MAP4,** differ in size and pattern of expression but share many common features (Fig. 34-10). These MAPs are abundant in brain, the historical tissue of choice for isolation of microtubules.

- They share similar tubulin-binding motifs consisting of 18 residues arrayed in three or four imperfect tandem repeats separated by flexible linkers of 13 variable residues. Each repeat binds independently to a tubulin subunit along the length of a single protofilament.
- N-terminal domains of tau family members project from the surface of microtubules (Fig. 34-11). The long side arm of MAP2 excludes structures, includ-

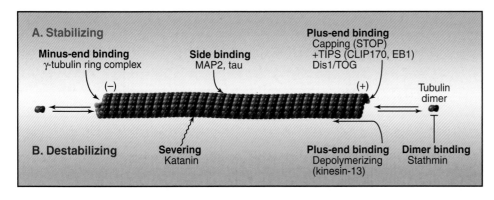

Figure 34-9 FAMILIES OF MICRO-TUBULE-BINDING PROTEINS. **A,** Proteins that stabilize microtubules. **B,** Proteins that destabilize microtubules. These MAPs can bind to the end or the side of the polymer or to tubulin dimers.

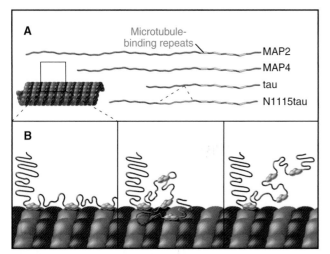

Figure 34-10   Tau, MAP2, and MAP4. **A,** Comparison of the domain organization, showing the homologous tubulin-binding motifs. **B,** The tubulin-binding motifs bind to either α- or β-tubulin and are thought to exchange rapidly among tubulin subunits along a protofilament. (Redrawn from Butner KA, Kirschner M: Tau protein binds to microtubules through a flexible array of distributed weak sites. J Cell Biol 115:717–730, 1991.)

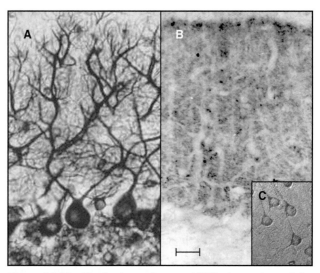

Figure 34-12   Distributions of tau and MAP2 in sections of the cerebellum from rat brain labeled with antibodies and subjected to a histochemical method producing a dark stain. **A,** MAP2 is concentrated in the cell bodies and dendrites of Purkinje cells. **B,** Tau is concentrated in the axons of granule cells, which appear here as *small dark dots*. **C,** Tau staining in the cell body and neurites of a pyramidal cell from another part of the brain. Scale bar is 20 μm. (Courtesy of L. Binder, Northwestern University Medical School, Evanston, Illinois.)

ing other microtubules (see Fig. 35-9), accounting for the wider spacing of microtubules in dendrites compared with axons, where the smaller tau predominates. Neither tau nor MAP2 cross-links microtubules, but MAP2 links microtubules to actin filaments.

- Tau family MAPs stabilize microtubules. For example, in the presence of tau, microtubules grow three times faster, shorten more slowly, and have catastrophes only 2% as frequently as pure tubulin microtubules. The rapid equilibrium of individual tubulin-binding repeats with the micro-

tubule surface might allow tau to dampen microtubule dynamics without stopping tubulin association and dissociation altogether.

- Phosphorylation of the microtubule-binding motifs of these MAPs inhibits microtubule binding and destabilizes microtubules.

Tau, named for tubulin-associated protein, is the major MAP in the axons of neurons in vertebrate brains (Fig. 34-12B). It is also present in some neuronal cell

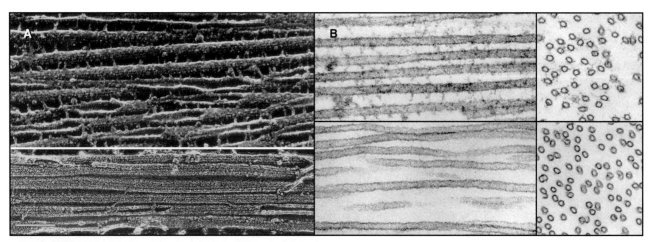

Figure 34-11   Electron micrographs of tau and MAP2 bound to microtubules. **A,** Frozen, deep-etched, and shadowed specimens of microtubules with tau *(upper panel)* and pure tubulin microtubules *(lower panel)*. **B,** Thin sections of microtubules with MAP2 showing 40- to 100-nm projections *(upper panels)* and bare pure tubulin microtubules *(lower panels)*. (A, Courtesy of N. Hirokawa, Tokyo University, Japan. Reference: Hirokawa N, Shiomura Y, Okabe S: Tau proteins: The molecular structure and mode of binding on microtubules. J Cell Biol 107:1449–1459, 1988. B, Courtesy of D. B. Murphy, Johns Hopkins Medical School, Baltimore, Maryland.)

bodies and glial cells. Alternate splicing produces seven tau isoforms from a single tau gene. Most of these isoforms have molecular weights of 40 to 50 kD, but a higher-molecular-weight tau is found in peripheral nerves. As is expected from its ability to stabilize microtubules in vitro, reduction in the tau concentration in cultured nerve cells by depletion of the mRNA reduces the numbers of microtubules. Nevertheless, mice survive the loss of their single tau gene with only minor alterations of their neurons. Compensation by other MAPs is postulated to account for the differences in the acute and chronic loss of tau.

In **Alzheimer's disease,** the most common dementia of older persons, as well as other neurodegenerative diseases and strokes, tau forms intracellular **paired helical filaments** (Fig. 34-13) that aggregate in "neurofibrillary tangles." These tangles are a hallmark of Alzheimer's disease, and their number judged by light microscopy correlates with the severity of the dementia. Dozens of different tau mutations are responsible for rare cases of inherited dementia, but for individuals with normal tau, excess phosphorylation can cause tau to dissociate from microtubules and leads to its fragmentation by proteolysis. Over time, short, phosphorylated

tau fragments assemble into highly insoluble paired helical filaments and tangles. It is not known which molecular species along this pathway cause neuronal degeneration. Inhibition of the several kinases that initiate the conversion of tau into tangles is a possible therapeutic strategy.

MAP2 is concentrated in dendrites of neurons (Fig. 34-12A). The mechanism giving preferential distribution of MAP2 in dendrites and tau in axons of the same cell is still largely a mystery. MAP4 shares many features with MAP2 but is expressed by glial cells in the nervous system and by many other cells and tissues. High-molecular-weight **MAP1A** and **1B** are related proteins that are distinct from the tau family, but they also form rod-shaped projections on the surface of microtubules in neurons. As in the case of tau, mice with null mutations of MAP1B are viable with minimal defects.

A variety of other proteins stabilize microtubules in distinct ways. Vertebrates have a protein called STOP that binds microtubules, making them resistant to depolymerization by cold, dilution, or drugs. Bird red blood cells express syncolin, which stabilizes the marginal band of microtubules. Tektins are fibrous proteins that stabilize microtubules in axonemes (see Fig. 38-16) and centrioles.

Microtubule-Destabilizing MAPs

Cells destabilize microtubules in three different ways. First, the small protein **stathmin** destabilizes microtubules by sequestering tubulin dimers. The protein has a long α-helix that binds laterally to a pair of tubulin dimers, blocking their polymerization. This sequestration of dimers may promote catastrophes. Thus, overexpression of stathmin in cell lines reduces tubulin available for polymerization. Phosphorylation of the tubulin-interacting sites regulates the activity of stathmin. Inhibition of stathmin by mitotic kinases promotes assembly of the mitotic spindle. Many malignant cells express unusually high levels of stathmin (hence its synonym Op18, for oncoprotein 18).

Second, two classes of microtubule motor proteins, **kinesin-13** and kinesin-8, promote microtubule disassembly by forming rings around the microtubules. These kinesins were discovered independently in several systems, leading to a variety of historic names. Most kinesins have a motor domain at one end of the polypeptide and use ATP hydrolysis to move cargo along the sides of microtubules (see Fig. 36-13). Kinesin-13 is not a typical motor. The ATPase domain in the middle of the polypeptide binds with high affinity to curved protofilaments that peel off the ends of microtubules. Energy from ATP hydrolysis is used to promote catastrophes and disassembly. Different isoforms of kinesin-13 are concentrated at the two ends of microtubules in the mitotic spindle—with minus ends at the poles and plus

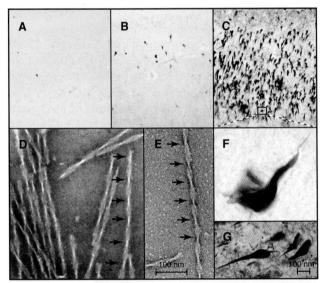

Figure 34-13 NEUROFIBRILLARY TANGLES OF PAIRED HELICAL FILAMENTS IN THE BRAINS OF PATIENTS WITH ALZHEIMER'S DISEASE. **A–C,** Light micrographs of sections of the hippocampus of human brains stained with silver for neurofibrillary tangles. **A,** Stage I with few tangles. **B,** Stage III with moderate numbers of tangles. **C,** Stage V, advanced Alzheimer's disease, showing abundant tangles. **D,** Electron micrograph of paired helical filaments isolated from Alzheimer's neurofibrillary tangles and prepared by negative staining. **E,** Electron micrograph of a negatively stained, paired, helical filament reassembled in vitro from recombinant tau protein. **F–G,** High-powered micrographs of neurofibrillary tangles from the brain of an Alzheimer's patient stained *brown* with an antibody to tau. (A–C and G, Courtesy of E. and H. Braak, University of Frankfurt, Germany. D–E, Courtesy of E.-M. Mandelkow, Max Planck Institute, Hamburg, Germany. F, Courtesy of L. Binder, Northwestern University Medical School, Evanston, Illinois.)

ends at kinetochores—where they regulate the lengths of the two ends (see Chapter 44).

Third, **katanin**, an AAA ATPase (see Box 36-1), uses ATP hydrolysis as the energy source to sever microtubules into short fragments. It disrupts the noncovalent bonds between the subunits in the microtubule wall. Tubulin dimers dissociate from the cut ends and return to the cytoplasmic pool for reassembly. Activation of severing at the onset of mitosis might contribute to remodeling the interphase microtubule network.

MAPs Associated with Growing Microtubule Plus Ends

Given the dynamic way that microtubules probe the cytoplasm, the plus-end is an ideal location for proteins that regulate microtubule dynamics and connect microtubules to membranes. Indeed, several proteins concentrate at the plus ends of growing microtubules (Fig. 34-14). These plus-end tracking proteins (+TIPs) are widely distributed in eukaryotes. End-binding protein 1 (EB1 in vertebrates) is also found in plants and Giardia. **CLIP-170** is found in vertebrates as well as budding and fission yeasts. Dynamic microtubules carry CLIP-170/Tip1p and an associated protein, Tea1p, to the ends of *S. pombe* cells (see Fig. 6-3D), where Tea1p directs the polar growth of the cell. EB1 and CLIP-170 interact with each other and a complex of other proteins. Both stabilize plus ends by reducing the frequency of catastrophes. +TIPS are involved in membrane transport along microtubules (see Fig. 37-6), but the details are still being investigated.

Three different mechanisms contribute to the association of +TIPs with plus ends. Experiments in budding and fission yeast provide evidence that some +TIPs are carried to plus ends by kinesin motors or relocated onto

newly incorporated GTP subunits. Animal CLIP-170 and EB1 do not actually move along microtubules but are concentrated on plus ends because of a higher affinity for tubulin dimers than microtubules. Tubulin dimers carry CLIP-170 piggyback onto plus ends, where it dissociates quickly and recycles back to the cytoplasm. Consequently, such +TIPs are not found on the plus ends of shortening microtubules (Fig. 34-14).

The **Dis1/TOG** family of proteins (called XMAP215 in frogs) also associate with microtubule plus ends in animals, plants, and fungi. They appear to regulate microtubule assembly and dynamics and are required for the organization of mitotic spindle poles in animals and the cortical array of microtubules in plants. Mixtures of tubulin, XMAP215, and a depolymerizing kinesin-13 recapitulate microtubule dynamic instability in test tubes very similar to that seen in extracts from mitotic cells. Members of the Dis1/TOG family might also stabilize the plus ends of stable cytoplasmic microtubules by reducing the frequency of catastrophes. Human colonic-hepatic tumor overexpressed gene (ch-TOG) was so named because it is particularly abundant in tumor cells. The binding partner that targets ch-TOG to spindle poles is also implicated in human cancer. However, the role, if any, of these proteins in promoting cancer is not yet known.

Several other proteins that function at or near the plus ends of microtubules are not classical +TIPS. These include the chromosomal passenger protein INCENP (see Fig. 44-10), which targets the aurora-B kinase to the central spindle and regulates its kinase activity toward spindle components. An emerging family of MAPs that includes human CLASP appears to be required to regulate the dynamic behavior of microtubule plus ends near the cell cortex in interphase and at kinetochores during mitosis.

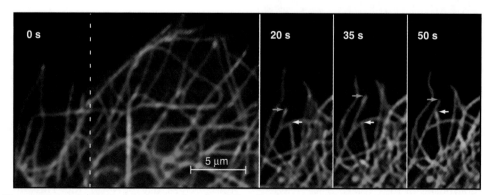

Figure 34-14 Time series of fluorescence micrographs of a CHO cell expressing the microtubule tip-binding protein CLIP-170 tagged with GFP *(red)* and microinjected with Cy3-tubulin to mark microtubules *(green)*. CLIP-170 concentrates at the plus ends of growing microtubules but dissociates from shrinking microtubules. (Courtesy of Yulia Komarova, Northwestern University, Evanston, Illinois. Modified from Komarova Y, Vorobjev IA, Borisy GG: Life cycle of microtubules: Persistent growth in the cell interior, asymmetric transition frequencies and effects of the cell boundary. J Cell Sci 115:3527–3539, 2002.)

Linker Proteins

Protein connectors link microtubules to many other cellular structures. For example, MAP2 links to actin filaments, and plectin links to intermediate filaments. Gephyrin binds microtubules and is required for clustering glycine receptors (see Fig. 10-12) in the plasma membrane of neurons.

The Centrosome

The **centrosome** is the dominant microtubule-organizing center in most animal somatic cells. It is the only major organelle in the cytoplasm that (1) is not bounded by a membrane and (2) is duplicated in a semi-conservative manner. Remarkably, the complete reproduction of a centrosome takes more than one full cell cycle. Current interest in centrosomes stems from their role as the microtubule-organizing center during interphase and mitosis, as well as their roles in cell cycle progression, cytokinesis, cell polarity, and organization of primary cilia. A variety of evidence has also linked centrosomal abnormalities to cancer.

When Flemming and Van Beneden discovered the centrosome in 1875, it was thought to be one of the three main cell components, together with the nucleus and the cell body. In fact, it was correctly regarded as a key organelle that regulates mitosis and was called the "dynamic centre" of the cell by Boveri, who coined the term *centrosome*. The large centrosomes of certain eggs appeared to contain one or two central granules, which Boveri called **"centrioles"** (Fig. 34-15). Centrioles are the "architects of centrosomes," spatially organizing the organelle, but some cells possess bona fide centrosomes that lack centrioles.

Most metazoan cells have a centrosome containing a centriole. Multinucleated animal cells such as megakaryocytes (see Fig. 28-7) and osteoclasts (see Fig. 32-6) have multiple centrosomes. On the other hand, vertebrate muscle cells and mature oocytes lack centrosomes, as do the cells of lower plants such as ferns, which have basal bodies only in male gametes. Since diverging from animals about a billion years ago, most plants and fungi lost their centrioles but retain other structures that serve as microtubule-organizing centers.

Organization of the Centrosome

In most cells, the centrosome is organized around two cylindrical centrioles about 0.5 μm long by about 0.2 μm in diameter and composed of nine microtubule triplets (Fig. 34-16). Centrioles and basal bodies, located at the base of cilia and flagella (see Fig. 38-17), are equivalent structures. Both were present in ancient eukaryotes, since they are found in organisms that branched earliest

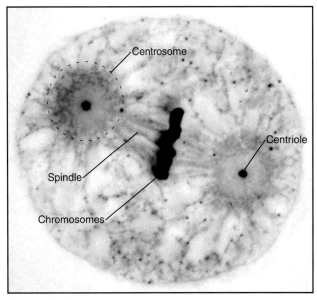

Figure 34-15 METAPHASE SPINDLE IN AN EGG OF *PARASCARIS EQUORUM*. In this micrograph taken by Joe Gall from a classic slide prepared by Boveri in the early 20th century, the centrosomes are particularly prominent, and the centrioles are clearly visible within them. (Micrograph courtesy of Joseph Gall, Carnegie Institution, Baltimore, Maryland.)

from the eukaryotic lineage (see Fig. 2-4). In most vertebrate tissues, centrioles retain the capacity to grow a nonmotile **primary cilium,** which serves as a sensory organelle (see Fig. 38-21). Similarly, flagella grow from both poles of the meiotic spindle of dividing spermatocytes of species such as the silk moth *Bombyx mori.*

Centrioles organize specific proteins into a surrounding matrix, called the **pericentriolar material (PCM).** This matrix links pairs of centrioles together and contains γ-tubulin ring complexes, which nucleate microtubules. The pericentriolar material and its direct surroundings form the **centrosphere,** which contains proteins that interact with the Golgi apparatus and has a composition that varies during the course of the cell cycle.

Cells that are about to enter mitosis have three types of centrioles that differ in age, structures, and activities. Two distinct **mother centrioles,** M^{old} and M^{new}, are each linked to one of two identical **daughter centrioles.** M^{old} was assembled at least two cell cycles previously. M^{new} was assembled in the previous cell cycle, and the daughter centrioles were assembled during the S phase (DNA synthesis phase) of the present cell cycle. M^{old} is characterized by the presence of distal and subdistal appendages (Fig. 34-16C), which function in microtubule anchoring. Although the pericentriolar material that surrounds both mother and daughter centrioles nucleates microtubules, the microtubules are predominantly anchored near M^{old}. Consequently, M^{old}

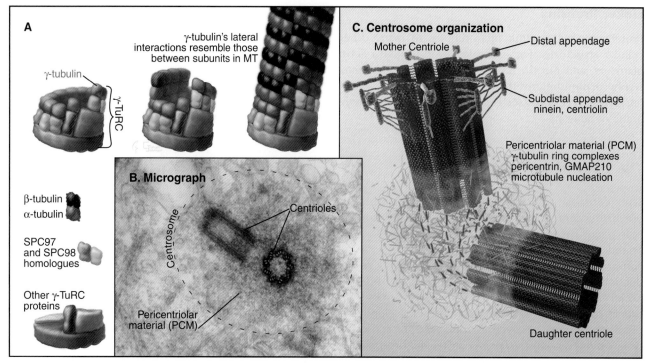

Figure 34-16 **STRUCTURE OF CENTRIOLES. A,** Gamma tubulin ring complex, γTuRC. Low-resolution model of the subunit composition and a proposal for how the complex initiates a microtubule, which is capped on its minus end and grows on its free plus end. Crystals of γ-tubulin have the molecules arranged with lateral interactions similar to those shown in this model. Here, γ-tubulin's GTP-binding site is oriented toward the plus end, where it interacts with α-tubulin at the minus ends of the protofilaments. **B,** Paired centrioles surrounded by pericentriolar material at telophase in a PtK1 (rat kangaroo) cell. **C,** Diagram of the structure of the centrioles. Locations of a number of proteins referred to in the text are indicated. (A, Redrawn from Job D, Valiron O, Oakley B: Microtubule nucleation. Curr Opin Cell Biol 15:111–117, 2003. B, Micrograph courtesy of Conly Rieder, Wadsworth Center, Albany, New York.)

acts as the cell center, surrounded by a radial array of microtubules (Fig. 34-2A) with their minus ends at the centrosome and plus ends at the periphery. In some G_0 cells (cells that are no longer actively proliferating—see Chapter 41), the daughter centriole is motile. Centrosomes usually associate tightly with the nucleus, allowing the microtubule network to anchor it to the cell cortex during cell migration. This is important for nuclear positioning and migration in fungi, as well as during brain development in vertebrates.

Centrosomes and their associated microtubules contribute to the shape of specialized cells. The array of polarized microtubules radiating from the centrosome in leukocytes and fibroblasts accounts for the fact that membrane bound organelles have a specific distribution within the cell. Membranes associated with minus-end-directed motors such as cytoplasmic dynein accumulate near the centrosome. The most prominent example is the Golgi apparatus. After disruption of centrosomes by RNA interference or by laser microsurgery, cytoplasmic microtubules emanating from the centrosome disappear, but other cytoplasmic microtubules persist (Fig. 34-17). In many differentiated cells, microtubules initially nucleated at centrosomes subsequently detach and

become anchored elsewhere in the cytoplasm, for example at the apical membrane in epithelial cells (Fig. 34-2B). In neurons, microtubules detach from the centrosome and are transported along axons and dendrites (see Fig. 37-5).

A Few Key Proteins of the Centrosome

The most prominent protein components of centrioles are α-, β-, δ-, and ε-tubulin (Fig. 34-16). Centriolar microtubules are more stable than most cytoplasmic microtubules, exchanging only about 10% of their tubulin per cell cycle. Like other stable microtubules, the α- and β-tubulins of centrioles are highly modified by polyglutamylation. Microinjection of cells with antibodies to glutamylated tubulin causes centrioles and centrosomes to disassemble.

Centrioles also contain multiple isoforms of centrin (see Fig. 38-6), EF-hand, Ca^{2+} binding proteins similar to calmodulin (see Fig. 3-12). Centrins are essential for the biogenesis of centrioles and spindle pole body biogenesis in yeasts. In *Chlamydomonas,* centrins form links between the centrioles and the nucleus. Despite their association with centrioles, most centrins are

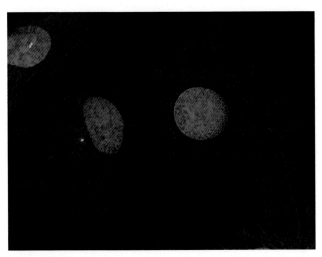

Figure 34-17 Destruction of the centrosome with a laser does not block cytoplasmic microtubule assembly, but the assembled microtubules are disorganized. Centrioles, *green;* nuclei, *blue;* microtubules, *red.*

cytoplasmic; and in the cytoplasm, their functions are unknown.

Additional proteins make up other functionally important centriolar structures (Appendix 34-2). The subdistal appendages of the mother centriole contain ninein, centriolin, and presumably a number of other proteins. Ninein is thought to play some role in anchoring the minus ends of microtubules to the centrosome. Centriolin appears to both anchor cell cycle control proteins to the centrosome and regulate microtubule stability.

The pericentriolar material contains many more proteins; up to 110 were identified in one proteomic study. The best characterized are components of the γ-tubulin ring complex (usually abbreviated γTuRC), which is primarily responsible for nucleating microtubules with 13 protofilaments in higher eukaryotes. This complex of 10 to 13 γ-tubulin molecules and 8 associated polypeptides resembles a dislocated ring or lock washer. It is now

thought that the γTuRC acts as a seed from which α/β tubulin dimers polymerize in a polar manner (Fig. 34-16A). Consistent with this, the complex appears to cap the minus ends of microtubules that it initiates. Many microtubules initiated by γ-tubulin ring complexes subsequently detach, possibly as a result of being severed by katanin (Fig. 34-9). The pericentriolar material surrounding the mother centriole is then thought to recapture the slow-growing minus ends of these microtubules.

The other pericentriolar material proteins assemble a matrix around the centrioles. About 75% of these proteins are predicted to contain α-helical coiled-coils. Well-studied proteins include pericentrin/kendrin, C-NAP1 (see later), and GMAP210, among many others. Pericentrin/kendrin is a large coiled-coil protein that was identified using autoantisera from scleroderma patients (see Fig. 13-22). It binds calmodulin plus several regulatory enzymes, including protein kinases and phosphatases. Pericentrin can also bind dynein and the γ-tubulin ring complex, presumably contributing to the transport and organization of centrosomal components. Another coiled-coil protein, GMAP210 appears to be involved in, among other things, clustering of the Golgi apparatus around the centrosome.

Centrosome Duplication

The cycle of semiconservative centrosome duplication and division is closely linked to the cell cycle (Fig. 34-18; see Chapter 40 for an introduction to the cell cycle). Centrosome replication begins during S phase, when the nuclear DNA is also replicated. This connection plus the semiconservative mode of duplication initially suggested that centrioles, like mitochondria and chloroplasts, might have their own genomes. However, genetic experiments in the green alga *Chlamydomonas* showed that nuclear genes regulate centriolar behavior, and careful morphologic analysis showed that centrioles lack their own DNA. Centriole duplication requires two

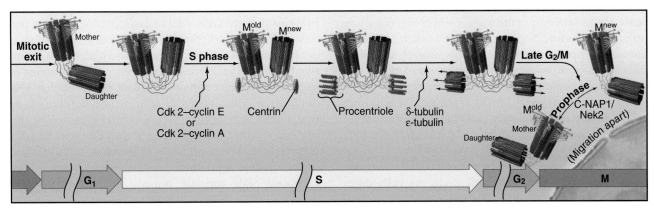

Figure 34-18 The pathway of centriole duplication is linked to the cell cycle.

cyclin dependent kinases (Cdk2–cyclin E and/or Cdk2–cyclin A; the latter is more important in mammalian cells). However, the critical phosphorylated target proteins are unknown.

The mother and daughter centrioles lose their strict orthogonal orientation during the exit from mitosis but remain linked at their proximal ends, possibly by protein fibers of the centrosomal matrix (Fig. 34-18). In G_1 phase, the daughter moves slightly away from its mother. In S phase, each centriole initiates the formation of a new daughter, thus converting the previous daughter into a new mother centriole, M^{new}. Newly formed daughter centrioles are oriented at right angles to what is known as the proximal end of the mother centrioles. Centriole formation is thought to begin with a disk-like structure containing centrin, which nucleates the assembly of a ring of nine single microtubules, the procentriole. The ring is converted into an array of nine triplets in a process that requires δ- and ε-tubulin. In organisms such as *Drosophila* and *Caenorhabditis elegans,* that lack these specialized tubulin isoforms, centrosomes are built of doublet and singlet microtubules. The daughter centrioles gradually lengthen during the remainder of the cell cycle, reaching their mature length just before mitosis. Then M^{new} acquires distal and subdistal appendages and becomes morphologically and biochemically equivalent to M^{old}. The two replicated centrosome pairs separate during prophase of mitosis and in many cells then migrate apart over the surface of the nuclear envelope to set up the two poles of the mitotic spindle.

The cohesion of the centriole pair is controlled by a trimeric complex of a coiled-coil protein, C-NAP1, plus the protein kinase Nek2 and the protein phosphatase PP1. These two enzymes regulate each other. The complex is concentrated at the proximal end of both centrioles. Phosphorylation of C-NAP1 by Nek2 is thought to trigger centriole separation.

Daughter centrioles usually arise next to a preexisting mother centriole, but is the mother centriole required? New centrioles do not appear in normal vertebrate cells after their centrioles are destroyed experimentally. However, this might be because normal cells sense the absence of centrosomes and block cell cycle progression before S phase when daughter centrioles normally form. Cancer cells lack this control, so even if they lack a centrosome, they progress into S phase and can form multiple new centrioles from scratch at the time centrioles would normally replicate. Thus mother centrioles are not absolutely essential to form daughter centrioles. Similarly, epithelial cells with multiple cilia make multiple basal bodies de novo.

The capacity of centrosomes to nucleate microtubules fluctuates during the cell cycle. As cells enter mitosis, the microtubule-nucleating activity of centrosomes increases dramatically. This "maturation" is asso-

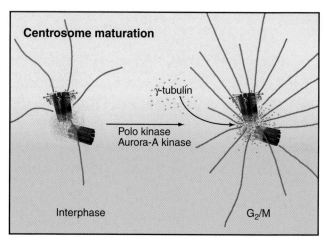

Figure 34-19 Centrosome maturation as cells enter mitosis involves the recruitment of γ-tubulin ring complexes and is triggered by the Polo-like and Aurora-A kinases.

ciated with accumulation of γ-tubulin, apparently driven by the action of the Polo and Aurora-A kinases (Fig. 34-19).

Centrosomes and astral microtubules also contribute to both the initiation of cytokinesis (by helping to specify the position of the contractile ring; see Fig. 44-22) and the completion of cytokinesis. As the cleavage furrow forms during late anaphase, mother and daughter centrioles detach from each other. In some cells, the mother centriole moves transiently into the intercellular bridge between the two daughter cells just before they separate. These movements of the mother centriole might somehow influence the cleavage of the bridge.

The "Centrosome" of Yeasts

For many fungi, including budding and fission yeasts, the role of the centrosome is played by the **spindle pole body** (SPB), a plaque-like structure embedded in the nuclear envelope (Fig. 34-20). Like centrosomes, SPBs organize the microtubule cytoskeleton, particularly during mitosis. Centrin and γ-tubulin are two of the 45 proteins that are known to be associated with SPBs, but few of the other proteins have been found in vertebrate centrosomes. A small tetrameric complex containing two γ-tubulins and two distinct but related proteins is sufficient for yeast SPBs to nucleate microtubules. SPB duplication is analogous to centrosome duplication in that a new SPB forms adjacent to and attached to the original SPB during the S phase of the cell cycle. As with centrosomes, SPB duplication is therefore tightly linked to cell cycle progression.

Fungal SPBs regulate mitosis and cytokinesis. In fission yeast, a GTPase and a series of three kinases associate transiently with SPBs before triggering con-

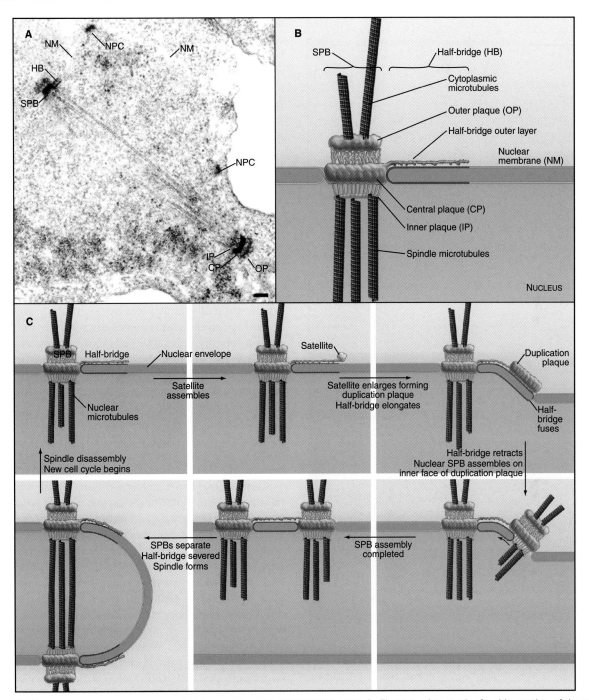

Figure 34-20 STRUCTURE AND DUPLICATION OF THE BUDDING YEAST SPINDLE POLE BODY. **A,** Electron micrograph of a thin section of the mitotic spindle of *Saccharomyces cerevisiae,* with both poles ending in an SPB. **B,** Diagram of the parts of the SPB. **C,** Pathway of duplication of the budding yeast SPB. (A, Micrograph courtesy of John Kilmartin. Reference: Adams IR, Kilmartin JV: Spindle pole body duplication: A model for centrosome duplication? Trends Cell Biol 10:329–335, 2000. B–C, Redrawn from the Adams and Kilmartin review.)

striction of the contractile ring and formation of septa (see Fig. 44-24). The corresponding GTPase in budding yeast, Tem1p, is anchored to the SPB by a protein that resembles a portion of mammalian centriolin. The guanine nucleotide exchange factor that activates Tem1p is concentrated in the bud, far from either SPB, until the elongating mitotic spindle relocates an SPB to the bud during anaphase. Only then can the guanine nucleotide

exchange factor activate the GTPase and trigger a signaling cascade that ultimately drives the cell out of mitosis.

Centrosomes and Cancer

The rediscovery that centrosome abnormalities are common in cancer cells has contributed to the

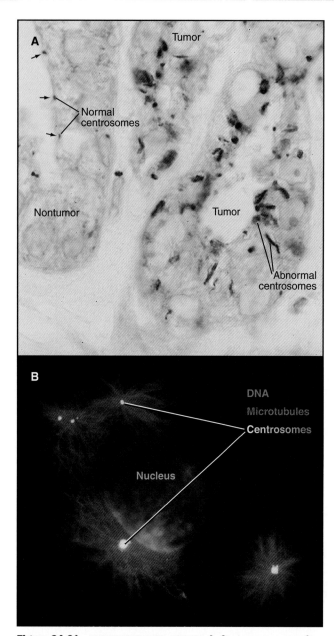

Figure 34-21 **CENTROSOMES AND CANCER. A,** Centrosomes are often abnormal in human tumors. Prostate tissue labeled by antibodies coupled to an enzyme (peroxidase) that produces a *brown* stain shows single uniform centrosomes in normal tissue *(left, arrows)* and abnormal centrosomes in tumor cells *(right)*. Abnormal centrosomes are greater in number, elongated, and much larger than those in normal cells. Centrosome defects lead to spindle abnormalities, mistakes in the segregation of chromosomes, and abnormal numbers of chromosomes, a hallmark of tumors. **B,** Tumor cells have abnormal centrosomes. Fluorescence micrograph of a single prostate tumor cell: DNA is stained *blue* with DAPI, microtubules are stained *red* with a fluorescent antibody, and pericentrin in the centrosomes is stained *green* (showing as *yellow* where it overlaps *red*) with a second fluorescent antibody. Cells were treated with nocodazole to depolymerize microtubules and were then released briefly to allow microtubule regrowth before processing. Tumor cells have abnormal numbers of centrosomes, which are heterogeneous in size, but they remain competent to nucleate microtubules. Normal cells typically have a single centrosome with a single focus of microtubules (not shown). (A–B, Courtesy of S. Doxsey, G. Pihan, and A. Purohit, University of Massachusetts, Worcester.)

resurgence of interest in centrosomes. Centrosomal defects in malignant cells include enlarged size (5 to 10 times larger than normal), abnormal shape, and increased number (Fig. 34-21). In one study, 217 out of 227 high-grade tumors had centrosomal abnormalities. Overexpression of the Aurora-A protein kinase can cause centrosomal abnormalities. The Aurora-A genetic locus is amplified in certain cancers. Furthermore, the kinase can function as an oncogene when overexpressed in tissue culture cells, causing the cells to lose their normal growth regulation and to form tumors when the cells are injected into mice.

A link between centrosomes and cell cycle progression was discovered when researchers studied the results of surgically removing the centrosome. Cells that lack centrosomes complete the cell cycle, enter mitosis, and assemble apparently normal bipolar mitotic spindles (presumably by a pathway that involves the organization of spindle poles by microtubule motor proteins that bundle and remodel microtubule networks). After a lengthy delay, the cells exit mitosis, and about 40% manage to complete cytokinesis. The surprise is that after completing mitosis, these cells never rereplicate their DNA or enter a subsequent mitotic cycle. Thus, the centrosome appears to be required to pass the G_1 restriction point and to enter S phase (see Fig. 41-7). Chapter 41 explains how defects in this key control point in the cell cycle are common in many types of cancer.

Centrosomal abnormalities in cancer arise when cells fail to complete cytokinesis, giving rise to progeny that have twice the normal content of DNA, number of chromosomes, and number of centrosomes. It has been suggested that normal cells have a checkpoint that is dependent on the p53 tumor suppressor protein (see Fig. 41-13) that arrests the cycle of cells that fail to complete cytokinesis. Cell lines from mice that lack p53 often have multiple centrosomes. Cancer cells with multiple centrosomes are prone to error when they attempt to segregate their chromosomes during subsequent divisions. The loss or gain of chromosomes can contribute to uncontrolled cell proliferation if the balance between growth-promoting oncogenes and growth-regulating tumor suppressor genes is upset.

ACKNOWLEDGMENTS

Thanks go to Michael Caplow, Steve Doxsey, Holly Goodson, and Alexey Khodjakov for their suggestions on revisions to this chapter.

SELECTED READINGS

Akhmanova A, Hoogenraad CC: Microtubule plus-end-tracking proteins: Mechanisms and functions. Curr Opin Cell Biol 17:47–54, 2005.

Beisson J, Wright M: Basal body/centriole assembly and continuity. Curr Opin Cell Biol 15:96-104, 2003.

Bornens M: Centrosome composition and microtubule anchoring mechanisms. Curr Opin Cell Biol 14:25-34, 2002.

Cassimeris L: The oncoprotein 18/stathmin family of microtubule destabilizers. Curr Opin Cell Biol 14:18-24, 2002.

Dogterom M, Kerssenmakers JWJ, Romet-Lemonne G, Janson ME: Force generation by dynamic microtubules. Curr Opin Cell Biol 17:67-74, 2005.

Doxsey S: Re-evaluating centrosome function. Nat Rev Mol Cell Biol 2:688-698, 2001.

Doxsey S, McCollum D, Theurkauf W: Centrosomes in cellular regulation. Annu Rev Cell Dev Biol 21:411-434, 2005.

Drewes G: MARKing tau for tangles and toxicity. Trends Biochem Sci 29:548-555, 2004.

Dutcher SK: Long-lost relatives appear: Identification of new members of the tubulin superfamily. Curr Opin Microbiol 6:634-640, 2003.

Gundersen GG, Gomes ER, Wen Y: Cortical control of microtubule stability and polarization Curr Opin Cell Biol 16:106-112, 2004.

Job D, Valiron O, Oakley B: Microtubule nucleation. Curr Opin Cell Biol 15:111-117, 2003.

Kreis T, Vale R (eds): Guidebook to the Cytoskeletal and Motor Proteins, 2nd ed. New York, Oxford University Press, 1999.

Lange BM: Integration of the centrosome in cell cycle control, stress response and signal transduction pathways. Curr Opin Cell Biol 14:35-43, 2002.

Marshall WF: Centrioles take center stage. Curr Biol 11:R487-R496, 2001.

Moritz M, Agard DA: Gamma-tubulin complexes and microtubule nucleation. Curr Opin Struct Biol 11:174-181, 2001.

Nigg EA: Centrosome aberrations: Cause or consequence of cancer progression? Nat Rev Cancer 2:815-825, 2002.

Nogales E: Structural insights into microtubule function. Annu Rev Biophys Biomol Struct 30:397-420 , 2001.

Ohkura H, Garcia MA, Toda T: Dis1/TOG universal microtubule adaptors: One MAP for all? J Cell Sci 114:3805-3812, 2001.

Westerman S, Weber K: Post-translational modifications regulate microtubule function. Nature Rev Molec Cell Biol 4:938-947, 2003.

Wordeman L: Microtubule depolymerizing kinesins. Curr Opin Cell Biol 17:81-88, 2005.

APPENDIX 34-1

Some Microtubule-Associated Proteins

Name (Synonyms)	Distribution	Composition	Properties	Functions
Destabilizers				
Stathmin/Op18 (prosolin, metablastin)	Vertebrate cells	1×18 kD	Binds tubulin dimers	Enhances dynamic instability; null mice viable without defects
MCAK/ kinesin 13	Vertebrate	2×82 kD	Kinesin-related but not a motor	Promotes microtubule disassembly at kinetochores
Severing				
Katanin	Metazoans, plants	1×84 kD 1×60 kD	MT-stimulated ATPase; ATP-dependent MT severing	
Stabilizers				
E-MAP 115	Vertebrate epithelial cells	$? \times 84$ kD	Phosphorylation inhibits MT binding	May stabilize MTs
MAP1A	Axons of vertebrate neurons, glia, and other cells	1×277 kD 1×30 kD 1×28 kD 1×16 kD	150-nm rod	Promotes MT assembly
MAP1B (MAP5)	Vertebrate neurons and other cells	1×243 kD 1×30 kD 1×28 kD 1×16 kD	200-nm rod; expressed during brain development	Promotes MT assembly; null mutation well tolerated by mice
MAP2	Dendrites of vertebrate neurons	One gene, 4 isoforms: MAP2a 1×200 kD MAP2b 1×200 kD MAP2c 1×42 kD	200-nm rod; three or four 18-residue MT-binding repeats	Promotes MT assembly; binds regulatory subunit of PKA; binds actin

Continued

Name (Synonyms)	Distribution	Composition	Properties	Functions
MAP 4 (MAP3, MAPU)	Vertebrate brain glia, many other cell types	1 × 135 kD	Three or four 18-residue MT-binding repeats; phosphorylation inhibits MT binding	Promotes MT assembly and stability
STOP	Vertebrate cells	100 kD	Inhibited by either calcium/calmodulin or phosphorylation	Stabilizes MT against cold depolymerization
Syncolin	Chicken red blood cells	? × 280 kD	Relative of MAP2	Stabilizes marginal band MTs in red blood cells
Tau	Vertebrates; axon of neurons and other; cells big tau in peripheral nerves	One gene, six isoforms 1 × 40-50 kD; big tau 1 × 80 kD	Three or four 18-residue MT-binding repeats; paired helical filaments in Alzheimer's disease	Promotes MT assembly and stability; mice tolerate null mutation
Tektin	Metazoan axonemes and cytoplasmic MTs	2 × 47-53 kD	Coiled-coil proteins	Stabilizes MTs in axonemes and centrioles
XMAP230	Various *Xenopus* cell types	1 × 230 kD	Phosphorylated by mitotic kinases with lowered MT affinity	Stabilizes MTs against catastrophes
Linkers				
Gephyrin	Vertebrate neurons	? × 93 kD		Anchors glycine receptors to MTs
Other				
Mapmodulin	Vertebrate cells	1 × 28 kD	Binds MT-binding repeats of tau, MAPs	Promotes dynein-driven organelle movements on MTs
+TIPs (Plus End Binding Proteins)				
CLIP-170	Eukaryotes	170 kD	Phosphorylation inhibits MT binding	Binds endosomes to plus ends of MT
CLASP (Mast/Orbit)	Eukaryotes	? × 165 kD	Binds MT plus ends, CLIP-170, and EB1	Regulates MT dynamics in the cell cortex and at kinetochores
APC	Vertebrates, insects	1 × 300 kD	Binds EB1 and β-catenin	Regulates β-catenin; acts as tumor suppressor; loss of causes predisposition to colon cancer
EB1 (Bim1p, Mal3p)	Eukaryotes	? × 30 kD	Binds MT plus ends and APC	Promotes MT assembly
XMAP215 (other Dis1/TOG family members)	Eukaryotes	215 kD		Regulates MT dynamics and spindle pole
LIS1	Eukaryotes	2 × 50 kD	Interacts with dynein, dynactin, CLIP-170	May regulate catastrophe rate; loss of leads to type 1 lissencephaly, a brain development defect
KMN network	Eukaryotes	Many subunits	Includes KNL-1, Mis12 complex, NCD80 complex	Forms MT binding sites at kinetochores
Motors				
Kinesins	Eukaryotes	Multiple isoforms (see Chapter 36)	MT-stimulated ATPase plus-end motors	Organelle transport; mitotic spindle function
Cytoplasmic Dynein (MAP1C)	Eukaryotes	2 × 410 kD 3 × 74 kD 4 × 55-59 kD ? × 8-21 kD	MT-stimulated ATPase; plus-end motors MT-stimulated ATPase; minus-end motor; binds dynactin complex	Organelle transport; mitotic spindle function

MT, microtubule; PKA, protein kinase A.

APPENDIX 34-2

Some Centrosomal Proteins

Name	Distribution	Composition (Subunit Size)	Properties	Functions
γ-Tubulin Ring Complex	Eukaryotes	10–13 × 50 kD (δ tubulin) + eight other proteins	Polymeric lockwasher-like rings in pericentriolar material and yeast spindle pole bodies	Binds minus end of microtubules and nucleates their assembly
Pericentrin (Kendrin)	Animals Plants	~350 kD	Human autoantigen. Coiled-coil protein in pericentriolar matrix	Required for spindle formation. Binds calmodulin, dynein, γ-tubulin ring complex, kinases, and phosphatases
GMAP 210		~210 kD		Clustering Golgi at centrosome
C-NAP1		~220 kD	Located at proximal end of centrioles	Involved in regulating cohesion of centriole pairs, regulated by the protein kinase Nek2
Ninein		~240 kD	Coiled-coil protein in subdistal appendages	Microtubule anchoring
Centriolin		~240 kD	Coiled-coil protein in subdistal appendages	May function in cell cycle control, may regulate microtubule stability
AKAP-450	Animals	453 kD	Coiled-coil protein similar to pericentrin located in centrosomal matrix	Anchoring factor for components of cell signaling machinery including cAMP-dependent protein kinase, protein kinase C, several phosphatases and Ran
NuMA	Vertebrates	236 kD	Coiled-coil protein; nucleus in interphase; centrosome in mitosis	Interacts with dynein to focus microtubules at spindle poles
PCM-1	Vertebrates	230 kD	In centriolar satellites	Required for centrin, pericentrin and ninein localization to centrosomes and for microtubule anchoring
TACC	Animals	~125 kD	Gene amplified in human breast cancer	Targets Dis1/ch-TOG family proteins to centrosomes
SAS-6	Animals	?	Coiled-coil protein	Binds SAS-5. Required for daughter centriole formation
SAS-4	*C. elegans*	92 kDa	Coiled-coil protein	Controls centrosome size
Centrosomin	*Drosophila*	115 kD	Coiled-coil protein in centrosomes	Required for spindle formation and recruitment of CP60 and CP190 to poles
CP60	*Drosophila*	48-kD oligomers	Nucleus in interphase; centrosome in mitosis	Binds microtubules; copurifies with CP190
CP190	*Drosophila*	120 kDa	Nucleus in interphase; centrosome in mitosis	Binds microtubules; copurifies with CP60

CHAPTER 35

Intermediate Filaments

I ntermediate filaments (Fig. 35-1) are strong but flexible polymers that provide mechanical support for cells ranging from bacteria to human tissues. These filaments were named *intermediate* because their diameter of about 10 nm is intermediate between the diameters of the thick and thin filaments in striated muscles (see Figs. 39-3 and 39-8). Cytoplasmic intermediate filaments tend to cluster into wavy bundles that vary in compactness, forming a branching network between the plasma membrane and the nucleus. Desmosomes anchor intermediate filaments to the plasma membrane (see Fig. 31-7) and transmit mechanical forces between adjacent cells. Hemidesmosomes connect intermediate filaments across the plasma membrane to the extracellular matrix.

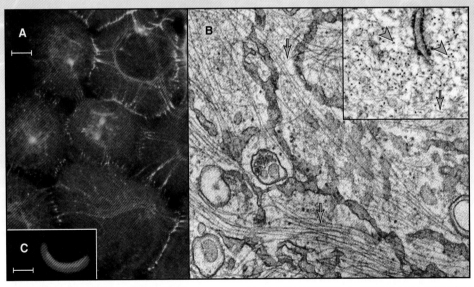

Figure 35-1 LIGHT AND ELECTRON MICROGRAPHS OF INTERMEDIATE FILAMENTS. **A,** Fluorescence light micrograph of cultured epithelial cells stained with antibodies to keratin intermediate filaments *(orange)*. Desmosomes are stained *green*. The network of keratin filaments stabilizes the cell against physical forces and reinforces desmosomal attachments between cells. Scale bar is ~10 μm. **B,** Electron micrograph of a thin section of a cultured baby hamster kidney cell showing longitudinal *(arrows)* and cross sections *(arrowheads)* of vimentin intermediate filaments. **C,** Fluorescence micrograph of crescentin intermediate filaments labeled with a *red* fluorescent dye in the bacterium *Caulobacter crescentus*. Scale bar is 2 μm. (A, Courtesy of E. Smith and E. Fuchs, University of Chicago, Illinois. B, Courtesy of R. Goldman, Northwestern University, Chicago, Illinois. C, Courtesy of M. Cabeen and C. Jacobs-Wagner, Yale University, New Haven, Connecticut.)

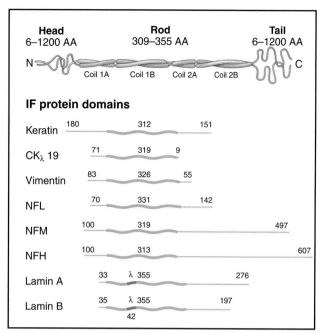

Figure 35-2 Intermediate filament (IF) proteins have head and tail domains of variable lengths flanking a central rod domain. Rod domains consist of a coiled-coil of about 310 residues and are 46.5 nm long. Lamins have an additional 42 residues in the rod (λ). The residues that are most important for assembly are at the beginning and end of the rod. End domains differ in sequence and size from 6 to 1200 residues.

The continuum of intermediate filaments and junctions prevents excessive stretching of the cells and gives tissues such as epithelia their mechanical integrity. Hair, which is built from cross-linked intermediate filaments, nicely illustrates their flexibility and high tensile strength. Molecular defects in cytoplasmic intermediate filaments or junctions associated with intermediate filaments result in rupture of skin cells and blistering diseases. Defects in lamins cause a bewildering array of diseases (see Fig. 14-9).

The nearly 70 human genes for intermediate filament proteins are expressed selectively in various cell types. All intermediate filament proteins possess an α-helical coiled-coil domain that forms the core of the filaments, while the flanking N- and C-terminal domains vary considerably in size (Fig. 35-2). These variable domains give each type of intermediate filament distinctive features but made it difficult to appreciate the general features of intermediate filament structure and function until the sequences of the proteins were determined in the 1980s.

Structure of Intermediate Filament Subunits

Each intermediate filament protein isoform has a unique amino acid sequence, but all have a rod-like domain between head and tail domains of variable length at the

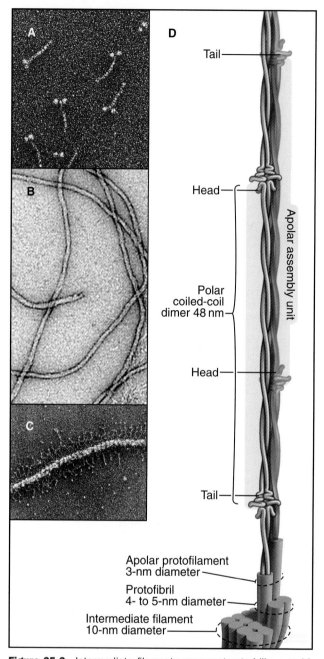

Figure 35-3 Intermediate filaments are constructed like a multistrand rope. **A–C,** Electron micrographs. **A,** Metal-shadowed lamin molecules consisting of two polypeptides joined by a long coiled-coil with globular tail domains at the C-terminus. **B,** Negatively stained keratin filaments. **C,** Rotary shadowed intermediate filament showing lateral projections. **D,** A model for intermediate filament structure. Antiparallel molecular dimers (referred to as tetramers because they have four polypeptides) are the building blocks. They polymerize in a staggered fashion to make apolar protofilaments. Two protofilaments associate laterally to make a protofibril. Four protofibrils associate to form the 10-nm intermediate filament. This model is consistent with X-ray fiber diffraction patterns, chemical cross-linking, and other data, but details of the subunit packing remain to be determined. (A–C, Courtesy of U. Aebi, University of Basel, Switzerland. D, Based on Steinert P, Marekov LN, Parry DA: Conservation of the structure of keratin intermediate filaments. Biochemistry 32:10046–10056, 1993.)

two ends. The rod is a parallel coiled-coil of two α-helices, usually about 47 nm long (Fig. 35-3A). Analysis of sequences, spectroscopic data, and X-ray fiber diffraction from materials composed of intermediate filaments, like wool, established this coiled-coil structure of the rod. Like other coiled-coils (see Fig. 3-10), **rod domains** of intermediate filament proteins have a heptad repeat of amino acids, the first and fourth residues providing a continuous row of hydrophobic interactions along the interface of the two helices. Zones of positive and negative charge alternate along the rod. When staggered appropriately, these zones provide complementary electrostatic bonds for assembly of filaments. About 20 highly conserved residues at each end of the rod are essential for filament elongation through head-to-tail interactions between dimeric molecules. Assembly studies with mutant proteins suggest that these parts of the rod contribute to lateral associations within filaments. Amino acid sequences indicate three interruptions in the coiled-coil (Fig. 35-2).

Less is known about the structures and functions of the nonhelical N- and C-terminal domains. They can influence assembly and in some cases project from the filament surface (Fig. 35-3C) to interact with other cellular components.

Intermediate filament protein molecules are commonly referred to as *dimers,* as they consist of two polypeptide chains. Some intermediate filament molecules are homodimers; others are heterodimers. **Lamins** and class III intermediate filament molecules are parallel dimers of identical polypeptides (Fig. 35-3A), whereas **keratins** are obligate heterodimers of one acidic (class I) and one basic (class II) keratin polypeptide. Many intermediate filament molecules form stable, partially overlapping, antiparallel molecular dimers (referred to as *tetramers;* Fig. 35-3D) that are believed to be intermediates in polymer assembly.

The evolution of genes for intermediate filament proteins remains a mystery. These genes are found in both Bacteria and the higher branches of the animal lineage, but their presence has not been verified in eukaryotes that branched before animals. Given this large gap in the history of these genes, the bacterial and animal genes might have evolved separately, a rare example of convergent evolution, or the genes might have moved between these domains of life by lateral transfer.

In Bacteria, the intermediate filaments are required for the asymmetrical shape of *Caulobacter crescentus* (Fig. 35-1C). Genes for animal intermediate filament proteins arose in early metazoan cells, encoding nuclear lamins (see Fig. 14-7). Most metazoans including chordates, mollusks, insects, and nematodes (see Fig. 2-9) retain genes for lamins. An invertebrate organism in the lineage leading to chordates duplicated a lamin gene, which was subsequently modified by deletion of the nuclear localization sequence and the CAAX box (a C-terminal prenylation site, see Fig. 7-9) giving rise to cytoplasmic intermediate filaments. (Cytoplasmic intermediate filaments of mollusks and nematodes retain more features of lamins, so they seem to have evolved separately.) After deletion of the codons for 42 residues of the coiled-coil in early chordates, further gene duplication and divergence produced the four families of genes for cytoplasmic intermediate filaments of vertebrates (Table 35-1).

These gene families have further diverged, so today sequence similarities are greater between species for each family of intermediate filament protein than for the different families of intermediate proteins within one species. For example, human desmin is much more similar to frog desmin than it is to human keratin. This suggests that unique functional requirements of each class of intermediate filament protein have conferred strong selective pressure on their genes.

Polymer Structure

Intermediate filaments are about 10 nm in diameter with wavy profiles in electron micrographs of thin sections of cells (Fig. 35-1B) or after negative staining isolated filaments (Fig. 35-3B). In some cases, the N- or C-terminal domains project from the surface (Fig. 35-3C). The most carefully studied intermediate filaments are built from four-chain, antiparallel molecular dimers that associate end to end in protofibrils like the strands of a rope (Fig. 35-3D). A cross section has up to 16 coiled-coils, but their internal arrangement is not known. Since tetramers lack polarity, intermediate filaments are considered to be apolar (i.e., both ends of the filament are equivalent; Fig. 35-3D). This is a striking difference from actin filaments (see Fig. 33-8) and microtubules (see Fig. 34-5), which depend on their polarity for many functions, including the unidirectional motion of motor proteins.

Assembly and Dynamics of Intermediate Filaments

Dissociated intermediate filament subunits spontaneously polymerize within a few minutes under physiological conditions in vitro. Assembly is highly favored, judging from the low critical concentration. Subunits add to both the ends and sides of polymers, in contrast to actin filaments and microtubules, which grow only at their ends. The nucleation mechanism that initiates polymerization and the elongation reactions are still being investigated. Rod domains of some intermediate filaments can assemble in vitro and in vivo without one of the end domains. In other cases, end domains modulate assembly.

Table 35-1

CLASSIFICATION OF INTERMEDIATE FILAMENT PROTEINS BASED ON ROD DOMAIN SEQUENCES

Class	Type	Genes	Molecule	Distribution	Diseases
I	Acidic keratin	>15	40–65 kD, obligate heterodimer with class II	Epithelial cells	Blistering skin, corneal dystrophy, brittle hair and nails
II	Basic keratin	>15	51–68 kD, obligate heterodimer with class I	Epithelial cells	Similar to class I
III	Desmin	1	53 kD, homopolymers	Muscle cells	Cardiac and skeletal myopathies
	GFAP	1	50 kD, homopolymers	Glial cells	Alexander disease; mouse null viable
	Peripherin	1	57 kD	Peripheral > CNS neurons	
	Synemin	1	190 kD, interacts with other class III IFs	Muscle cells	
	Vimentin	1	54 kD, homopolymers and heteropolymers	Mesenchymal cells	Mouse null viable
IV	Neurofilament				
	NFL	1	Obligate heteropolymers with NFM, NFH	Neurons	Mouse null viable; neuropathies
	NFM	1	Obligate heteropolymers with NFL, NFH	Neurons	
	NFH	1	Obligate heteropolymers with NFL, NFM	Neurons	Mutations a risk factor in amyotrophic lateral sclerosis
	α-Internexin	1	55 kD, homopolymers	Embryonic neurons	
V	Lamins	4	7 Isoforms, 62–72 kD, homodimers	Animal, plant nuclei	Cardiomyopathy, lipodystrophy, one form of Emery-Dreifuss muscular dystrophy, two forms of progeria plus many others
VI	Nestin	1	230 kD, homopolymers	Embryonic neurons, muscle, other cells	

IF, intermediate filament; NFH, neurofilament heavy; NFL, neurofilament light; NFM, neurofilament medium.
Reference: Omary MB, Coulombe PA, McLean WHI: Intermediate filament proteins and their associated diseases. New Engl J Med 351:2087–2100, 2004.

Intermediate filaments are among the most chemically stable cellular components, resisting solubilization by extremes of temperature as well as high concentrations of salt and detergents (Fig. 35-4). Nevertheless, intermediate filaments in some cells exchange their subunits within minutes to hours during interphase. For example, if **vimentin** is labeled with a fluorescent dye and injected into live cells, fluorescent vimentin incorporates into cytoplasmic filaments (Fig. 35-5). After a spot of fluorescent filaments is photobleached with a laser, the fluorescence recovers over a period of several minutes, indicating that subunits along the length of the filaments exchange with a pool of unpolymerized molecules. (Fig. 38-9 shows a similar experiment with actin.) Observations on cells expressing vimentin fused to GFP confirm these properties. Vimentin and lamin filaments, but not all intermediate filaments, disassemble reversibly during mitosis in response to phosphorylation by mitotic kinases in some cells (Fig. 35-4C; also see Fig. 44-6). Other intermediate filaments appear to be very stable, including keratin filaments in epithelial cells.

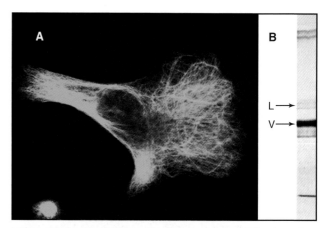

Figure 35-4 Intermediate filaments resist solubilization when cells are extracted. **A,** A fluorescence micrograph shows the network of vimentin filaments remaining after extraction of a CHO cell with the detergent Triton X-100, DNase, and a high concentration of salt to remove lipids, DNA, and soluble proteins. **B,** Gel electrophoresis reveals that lamins (L) and vimentin (V) are among the few proteins remaining in the detergent-resistant cytoskeletal fraction. (Courtesy of R. Goldman, Northwestern University, Chicago, Illinois.)

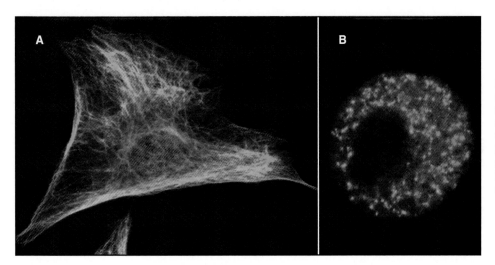

Figure 35-5 FLUORESCENCE MI-CROGRAPHS OF INTERMEDIATE FILA-MENTS. **A,** A cultured fibroblast stained with antibodies to vimen-tin filaments *(green)* and microtu-bules *(red)*. **B,** Vimentin filaments dispersed in mitosis. (Courtesy of R. Goldman, Northwestern Univer-sity, Chicago, Illinois.)

Although no known motors move on intermediate filaments, motor proteins move the filaments along microtubules. A spectacular example is found in nerve cells (see Fig. 37-5C).

Posttranslational Modifications

Many types of intermediate filaments are phosphory-lated, and these phosphates tend to turn over rapidly. Phosphorylation can dramatically affect polymer assem-bly and dynamics. The story is complex and incom-pletely understood, as each class of intermediate filament has multiple phosphorylation sites, and many protein kinases can phosphorylate these sites. The impact of phosphorylation depends critically on the particular residue modified.

In several cases, phosphorylation destabilizes the fila-ments and blocks assembly. The best examples are phos-phorylation of lamins and vimentin by Cdkl : cyclin B kinase during mitosis. The enzyme phosphorylates serine residues near the ends of the rod domain. This destabilizes the filaments and contributes to the break-down of the nuclear lamina (see Figs. 16-7 and 44-6) and depolymerization of cytoplasmic vimentin filaments (Fig. 35-5B). Keratins are also phosphorylated during mitosis but not directly by Cdkl : cyclin B kinase. During mitosis, the organization of keratins changes subtly without complete disassembly as in other intermediate filaments. The role of phosphorylation of intermediate filaments during interphase is less clear, but it might influence the structure of the cytoskeleton in response to various signals.

Neurofilaments, abundant intermediate filaments in nerve axons and dendrites (Fig. 35-9), are an excep-tion to the rule that phosphorylation destabilizes inter-mediate filaments. The most stable neurofilaments are heavily phosphorylated in the large C-terminal end domain (Fig. 35-2), whereas the pool of unpolymerized molecules is not phosphorylated. The end domain con-taining the phosphorylation sites is not essential for assembly, so phosphorylation might influence other functions of these intermediate filaments.

Keratin intermediate filaments in hair are chemically cross-linked to each other and associated with matrix proteins by disulfide bonds and amide bonds between lysines and acidic residues, creating a tough composite material built on the same principles as fiberglass. Beau-ticians take advantage of these cross-links to modify the shape of hairs during "permanents." They first reduce disulfide bonds and then re-form them after molding the hair into a new shape.

Expression of Intermediate Filaments in Specialized Cells

With rare exceptions, animal and plant cells express nuclear lamins, whereas the repertoire of cytoplasmic intermediate filaments varies greatly in different cell types (Table 35-1). It is assumed that each isoform has unique properties appropriate for cells that use them. Most cells express predominantly one class of cytoplas-mic intermediate filament. For example, epithelial cells express keratin and muscle cells express desmin. A few cells, such as the basal myoepithelial cells of the mammary gland, express two types of intermediate fila-ment subunits that sort into separate filaments with different distributions in the cytoplasm. Similarly, micro-injection or expression of foreign intermediate filament subunits usually (but not invariably) results in correct sorting to the homologous class of filaments.

In tissues such as skin and brain, cells express a suc-cession of intermediate filament isoforms as they mature and differentiate. Human epidermis and its appendages (hair and glands) express 12 different keratin isoforms

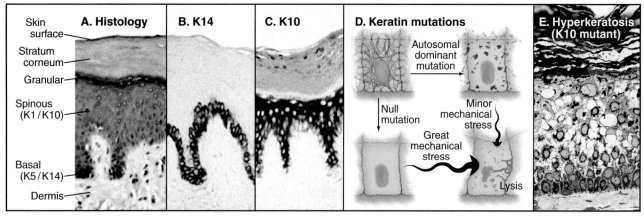

Figure 35-6 EXPRESSION OF KERATIN AND EFFECTS OF KERATIN MUTATIONS ON THE STRATIFIED SQUAMOUS EPITHELIUM OF SKIN. **A,** Light micrograph of a section of mouse skin stained with hematoxylin-eosin. **B,** Localization of keratin 14 in a section of skin using antibodies and a histochemical procedure that leaves a *brown* deposit. Proliferating cells in the basal layer express keratin 5 and keratin 14. **C,** Localization of keratin 10 to differentiating cells in intermediate layers of the epithelium. These cells eventually lose their nuclei and form the surface layers of cornified cells. **D,** Drawings illustrating the effects of keratin mutations on the structure of the epithelium. Dominant negative keratin mutations affect the assembly of keratin filaments wherever they are expressed. Human patients with epidermolysis bullosa have point mutations in keratin 5 or keratin 14 that disrupt the filaments in the basal cells, causing mechanical fragility and cellular rupture with mild trauma, resulting in blisters. Mutations in keratin 1 or keratin 10 cause cell rupture in the middle layers where they are expressed. Null mutations in keratin genes disrupt the epithelium to a lesser extent than dominant negative point mutations. **E,** Light micrograph of a histologic section of skin illustrating how a mutation in keratin 10 disrupts cells in the spinous layer and causes hyperkeratosis (excess scaling of surface layers). (A–C and E, Courtesy of P. Coulombe, Johns Hopkins University, Baltimore, Maryland. D, Based on a drawing with permission from Fuchs E, Cleveland DW: A structural scaffolding of intermediate filaments in health and disease. Science 279:514–519, 1998. Copyright 1998 AAAS.)

as they differentiate. Dividing cells at the base of the epidermis express mainly keratins 5 and 14, whereas terminally differentiating cells express keratins 1 and 10 (Fig. 35-6). The switch in keratin expression is associated with a marked increase in filament bundling, a feature that might contribute to the resistance of the surface layers of the skin to chemical dissociation. In the nervous system, supporting glial cells use a class III intermediate filament, whereas embryonic neurons first express α-internexin and later express the three different neurofilament isoforms (Table 35-1). Although the smallest neurofilament isoform (NFL) can assemble on its own in vitro, NFL plus one of the larger isoforms (NFM or NFH) is required to form intermediate filaments in neurons.

Tumors often express the intermediate filament protein that is characteristic of the differentiated cells from which the tumor arose. This is helpful to pathologists in diagnosing poorly differentiated cancers. For example, tumors of muscle cells express desmin rather than keratin, like epithelial cells, or vimentin, like mesenchymal cells.

Proteins Associated with Intermediate Filaments

A number of proteins bind intermediate filaments and link them to membranes and other cytoskeletal polymers (Table 35-2). Integral membrane proteins anchor nuclear lamins to the nuclear membrane. Filaggrin helps to aggregate keratin filaments in the upper layers of skin.

Plakins are the largest family of proteins that interact with intermediate filaments. These giant proteins typically have binding sites for other cytoskeletal polymers and certain adhesive junctions, so they can link the various elements of the cytoskeleton to each other and membranes. Like several other plakins, **plectin** has globular domains on both ends of a 200-nm coiled-coil. Binding sites in the globular domains allow plectin to serve as an all-purpose cytoskeletal glue, cross-linking intermediate filaments to each other, to actin filaments and microtubules (Fig. 35-7), and to β4 integrins in hemidesmosomes (see Fig. 31-7). Recessive mutations in human plectin cause a rare form of muscular dystrophy associated with skin blisters. **BPAG1e** also links intermediate filaments to another transmembrane protein in hemidesmosomes and can bind actin filaments. Mice that lack BPAG1 have skin blisters secondary to compromised hemidesmosomes, as well as disorganized neuronal intermediate filaments that result in the death of sensory neurons. **Desmoplakin** links keratin to desmosomes (see Fig. 31-7).

Functions of Intermediate Filaments in Cells

Intermediate filaments function primarily as flexible but inextensible intracellular tendons that prevent

Table 35-2

PROTEINS ASSOCIATED WITH INTERMEDIATE FILAMENTS

Name	Molecule	Distribution	Partners	Diseases
Plakins				
BPAG-1	Multiple splice isoforms (a, b, e, n) with ABDs and plakin domains ± spectrin and plakin repeats	a: Hemidesmosomes b: Muscle, cartilage e: Epithelial hemidesmosomes n: Neurons	IFs, MTs, actin	Autoimmune bullous pemphigoid
Desmoplakin	Two splice isoforms with plakin and coiled-coil domains and plakin repeats	Desmosomes	IFs; cadherin and other desmosome proteins	Autoimmune pemphigus; genetic striate palmoplantar keratoderma
Plectin	Multiple splice isoforms; ABD, plakin domain and plakin repeats	Most tissues except neurons	IFs, actin, MTs, spectrin, $\beta 4$ integrin	Autoimmune pemphigus; genetic epidermolysis bullosa with muscular dystrophy
Epidermal				
Filaggrin	Ten 37-kD filaggrins cut by proteolysis from profilaggrin	Cornified epithelia	Aggregates keratin	?
Lamin Associated				
LAP1	57–70 kD isoforms	Integral nuclear membrane proteins	Binds laminin to nuclear envelope	
LAP2	50 kD	Integral nuclear membrane protein	Binds laminin to nuclear envelope	
LBR	73 kD	Integral nuclear membrane protein	Binds laminin to nuclear envelope	Pelger-Huët anomaly; Greenberg skeletal dysplasia
Emerin	34 kD	? Peripheral protein of the inner nuclear membrane	? Nucleates and binds actin filaments to the nuclear envelope	Emery-Dreifuss muscular dystrophy

ABD, actin binding domain; IFs, intermediate filaments; MTs, microtubules.

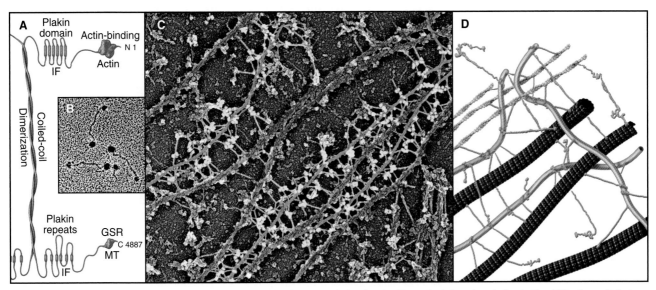

Figure 35-7   **PLECTIN STRUCTURE AND ACTIVITIES. A,** Domain structure of plectin: the N-terminal domain, similar to the ABD of α-actinin (see Fig. 33-16), binds actin and intermediate filaments; the 200-nm long coiled-coil forms dimers; six C-terminal plakin repeats include a second binding site for intermediate filaments; the C-terminal GSR domain binds microtubules (MT). **B,** Electron micrograph of plectin molecules. **C,** Electron micrograph of an extracted fibroblast cell reacted with gold-labeled antibodies to plectin. Gold particles *(yellow)* identify plectin molecules *(blue)* as linkers between intermediate filaments *(orange)* and microtubules *(red)*. The specimen was prepared by rotary shadowing. The molecules are pseudocolored for clarity. **D,** Drawing of plectin *(blue)* connecting cytoskeletal polymers to each other. (B, Courtesy of G. Wiche, University of Vienna, Austria. C, Courtesy of G. Borisy, University of Wisconsin, Madison.)

excessive stretching of cells that are subjected to external or internal physical forces. This function is facilitated by interactions with microtubules, actin filaments, and membranes. For example, if a relaxed smooth muscle is stretched, the intracellular network of desmin filaments between cytoplasmic dense bodies and the plasma membrane (see Fig. 39-20) reorganizes from a polygonal three-dimensional network into a continuous strap that runs the length of the cell (Fig. 35-8). Up to the point at which this network is taut, the cell offers little resistance to stretching. Once the network is taut, the cell strongly resists further stretching. Actin filaments anchored to dense bodies apply contractile force to the network of intermediate filaments.

Although the geometry is different in striated muscles, the concept is remarkably similar to smooth muscle. Desmin filaments surround the Z disks in addition to forming a looser, longitudinal basket around the myofibrils (see Fig. 39-8). The ends of both skeletal and cardiac muscle cells must be anchored to transmit their contractile forces. This is accomplished by intercellular junctions that combine features of desmosomes or hemidesmosomes (anchoring intermediate filaments) and adherens junctions (anchoring actin filaments).

Keratin intermediate filaments are the major proteins in skin, where they form a dense network connected to numerous desmosomes and hemidesmosomes (Figs. 35-1 and 35-6). These junctions anchor a physically continuous network of intermediate filaments,

imparting mechanical stability to the epithelium. If either the junctions or keratin filaments fail, cells pull apart or rupture, and the skin blisters. Mutations that compromise intermediate filament assembly or their anchoring junctions illustrate the importance of this network. Point mutations near the ends of the keratin rod cause especially severe forms of skin diseases (such as **epidermolysis bullosa** simplex) characterized by blistering and sensitivity to mechanical stress. Similar mutations engineered in transgenic mice reproduce the human disease. Which epithelial cells are affected depends on the expression pattern of the defective keratin. For example, a mutation in the rod domain of keratin 14 or keratin 5 leads to disruption of the basal cells in the epidermis where these keratins are expressed. Similarly, mutations in keratin 10 or keratin 1 cause cellular rupture at higher levels in the epidermis where these keratins are found. Mutations in keratin 12 or keratin 3 cause sores on the cornea of the eye where they are expressed.

A mutant keratin can cause disease in heterozygotes with one normal keratin gene. This is called a **dominant negative mutation.** Defective subunits assemble imperfectly with normal keratin subunits and compromise the physical integrity and strength of the filaments. The affected cells can grow, divide, and even form desmosomes with neighboring cells, but they tear apart physically when subjected to the shearing forces that affect the skin during normal life activities. Young children are severely affected, but some patients improve with age. They learn to avoid physical trauma to their skin and may also adapt biochemically in some way.

In contrast to these dominant negative keratin mutations, complete loss of an intermediate filament protein can be less severe (Fig. 35-6D). Mice and humans that lack keratin 14 suffer from milder blistering than do patients with dominant negative point mutations. Mice without functional keratin 8 or keratin 18 genes may die during embryonic development, but some survive with only modest defects in their colon and liver. Remarkably, mice also survive deletion of both copies of the genes for class III intermediate filaments. Mice that lack desmin are viable but with mildly disorganized muscle architecture that is aggravated by vigorous exercise. Humans who are heterozygous for desmin mutations can suffer severely from generalized muscle failure, including signs of heart disease.

Neurofilaments have a second function that is equal in importance to their mechanical properties. Once a nerve cell forms synapses (see Figs. 11-8 and 11-9), it produces neurofilaments to fill the axon and expand its diameter (Fig. 35-9). This enhances electrical communication in the nervous system because the velocity of action potentials (see Fig. 11-6) depends on the diameter of axons.

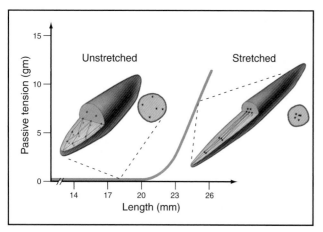

Figure 35-8 Smooth muscle cell intermediate filaments form an inextensible intracellular tendon that resists excessive stretching. The graph shows that a relaxed smooth muscle resists stretching very little up to a length of 21 mm. Resistance increases dramatically with further stretching. At short lengths, the three-dimensional network of intermediate filaments and dense bodies is open, offering little resistance to stretching. At the inflection point of the resistance curve, the filaments are extended linearly from one end of the cell to the other and so resist further stretching. (Based on Cooke P, Fay R: Correlation between fiber length, ultrastructure, and the length tension relationship of mammalian smooth muscle. J Cell Biol 52:105–116, 1972.)

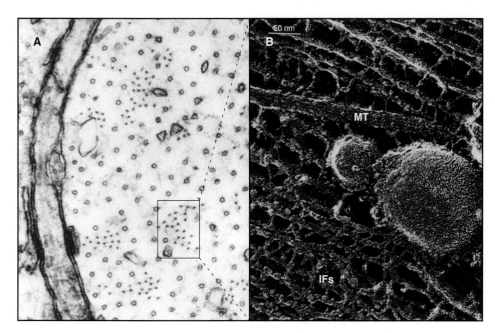

Figure 35-9 ELECTRON MICRO-GRAPHS OF INTERMEDIATE FILAMENTS (CALLED NEUROFILAMENTS) IN AXONS OF NERVE CELLS. **A,** A thin cross section shows clusters of intermediate filaments and microtubules. **B,** A longitudinal freeze-fracture preparation shows a microtubule (MT [red]) with associated vesicles and many intermediate filaments (IF [orange]). (A, Courtesy of P. Eagle, Kings College, London, England. B, Courtesy of N. Hirokawa, University of Tokyo, Japan.)

Lamins were originally thought to be a simple support network for the nuclear envelope, but they have other important functions. For example, perturbation of lamin assembly by expressing toxic fragments of lamins in cells can interfere with DNA replication. This may reflect a role for the lamina in organizing the chromosomal architecture in the interphase nucleus. Mutations in the lamin A/C gene cause diverse human diseases, including premature aging (see Fig. 14-9), the Emery-Dreifuss form of muscular dystrophy as well as disorders of fat tissue and nerves. These high tissue-specific deficiencies are remarkable given the expression of lamins A and C in all tissues.

SELECTED READINGS

Braun S, Panatel K, Muller P, et al: Cytokeratin-positive cells in the bone marrow and survival of patients with stage I, II or III breast cancer. N Engl J Med 342:525-533, 2000.

Erber A, Riemer D, Bovenschulte M, Weber K: Molecular phylogeny of metazoan intermediate filament proteins. J Mol Evol 47:751-762, 1998.

Fuchs E, Cleveland DW: A structural scaffolding of intermediate filaments in health and disease. Science 279:514-519, 1998.

Helfand BT, Chang L, Goldman RD: The dynamic and motile properties of intermediate filaments. Annu Rev Cell Dev Biol 19:445-467, 2003.

Herrmann H, Aebi U: Intermediate filaments: Molecular structure, assembly mechanism, and integration into functionally distinct intracellular scaffolds. Annu Rev Biochem 73:749-789, 2004.

Hutchison CJ: Lamins, building blocks or regulators of gene expression? Nat Rev Mol Cell Biol 3:848-858, 2002.

Leung CL, Green KJ, Liem RKH: Plakins: A family of versatile cytolinker proteins. Trends Cell Biol 12:37-45, 2002.

Moller-Jensen J, Löwe J: Increasing complexity of the bacterial cytoskeleton. Curr Opin Cell Biol 17:75-81, 2005.

Omary MB, Coulombe PA, McLean WHI: Intermediate filament proteins and their associated diseases. New Engl J Med 351:2087-2100, 2004.

Wiche G: Role of plectin in cytoskeleton organization and dynamics. J Cell Sci 111:2477-2486, 1998.

Worman HJ, Courvalin J-C: The nuclear lamina and inherited disease. Trends Cell Biol 12:591-598, 2002.

CHAPTER 36

Motor Proteins

Molecular motors use ATP hydrolysis to power movements of subcellular components, such as organelles and chromosomes, along the two polarized cytoskeletal fibers: actin filaments and microtubules. No motors are known to move on the apolar intermediate filaments. Motor proteins also produce force locally within the network of cytoskeletal polymers, which transmits these forces to determine the shape of each cell and, ultimately, the architecture of tissues and whole organisms. Chapters 37 to 39 and 44 illustrate how motors move cells and their parts.

Just three families of motor proteins—**myosin, kinesin,** and **dynein**—power most eukaryotic cellular movements (Fig. 36-1 and Table 36-1). During evolution myosin, kinesin, and Ras family GTPases appear to have shared a common ancestor (Fig. 36-1), whereas dynein is a member of the **AAA ATPase** family (Box 36-1). Although the ancestral genes appeared in prokaryotes, and prokaryotes have homologs of both actin and tubulin, none of these motor proteins has been found in prokaryotes. Over time, gene duplication and divergence in eukaryotes gave rise to multiple genes for myosin, dynein, and kinesin, each encoding proteins with specialized functions. Even the slimmed down genome of budding yeast includes genes for five myosins, six kinesins, and one dynein. Table 36-1 lists other protein machines that produce molecular movements during protein and nucleic acid synthesis, proton pumping, and bacterial motility.

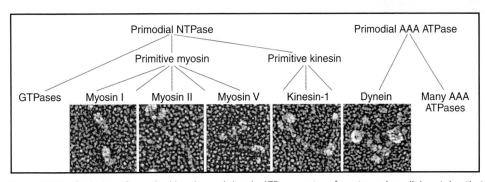

Figure 36-1 Evolution of myosin, kinesin, and dynein ATPase motors from two primordial proteins that bound and hydrolyzed nucleoside triphosphates. The electron micrographs illustrate a selection of contemporary motor molecules prepared by rotary shadowing. (Images courtesy of J. Heuser, Washington University, St. Louis, Missouri.)

Table 36-1

EXAMPLES OF MECHANOCHEMICAL ATPASES AND OTHER SYSTEMS

Families	Track	Direction	Cargo	Energy
ATPases				
Myosins				
Muscle myosin	Actin	Barbed end	Myosin filament	ATP
Myosin II	Actin	Barbed end	Myosin, actin	ATP
Myosin I	Actin	Barbed end	Membranes	ATP
Myosin V	Actin	Barbed end	Organelles	ATP
Myosin VI	Actin	Pointed end	Endocytic vesicles	ATP
Dyneins				
Axonemal	Microtubule	Minus end	Microtubules	ATP
Cytoplasmic	Microtubule	Minus end	Membranes, chromosomes	ATP
Kinesins				
Conventional	Microtubule	Plus end	Membranes, intermediate filaments	ATP
Ncd	Microtubule	Minus end	? Microtubules	ATP
Other Mechanochemical Systems				
Polymerases				
Ribosome	mRNA	5′ to 3′	None	GTP
DNA polymerase	DNA	5′ to 3′	None	ATP
RNA polymerase	DNA	5′ to 3′	None	ATP
Conformational System				
Spasmin/centrin	None	None	Cell, basal body	Ca^{2+}
Polymerizing Systems				
Actin filaments	None	Barbed end	Membranes	ATP
Microtubules	None	Plus end	Chromosomes	GTP
Worm sperm MSP	None	Not polar	Cytoskeleton	
Rotary Motors				
Bacterial flagella	None	Bidirectional	Cell	H^+ or Na^+ gradient
F-type ATPase	None	Bidirectional	None	H^+ or ATP
V-type ATPase pump	None		None	ATP

mRNA, messenger RNA; MSP, major sperm protein.

Motor proteins have two parts: a **motor domain** that utilizes adenosine triphosphate (ATP) hydrolysis to produce movements and a **tail** that allows the motors to self-associate or to bind particular cargo. Within the three families, the tails are more diverse than the motor domains, allowing for specialized functions of each motor isoform.

All motor proteins are enzymes that convert chemical energy stored in ATP into molecular motion to produce force upon an associated cytoskeletal polymer (Fig. 36-2). If the *motor* is anchored, the polymer may move. If the *polymer* is anchored, the motor and any attached cargo may move. If *both* are anchored, the force stretches elastic elements in the molecules transiently, but nothing moves, and the energy is lost as heat. Cells use all of these options (see Chapters 37 to 39).

Biochemists originally discovered and purified these motors by means of enzyme activity or in vitro motility assays (Fig. 36-11). With the prototype enzymes identified, investigators found further examples and variant isoforms of each motor by purification of the proteins, molecular cloning of DNAs, genomewide DNA sequencing, or genetic screening.

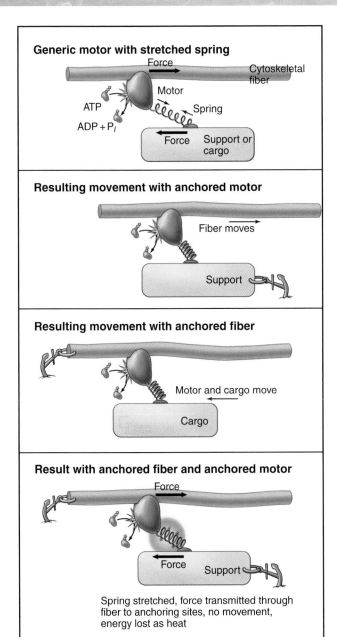

Figure 36-2 General features of ATPase motors. Motors bind stably to a support or cargo and transiently to a cytoskeletal fiber (actin filament or microtubule). Energy liberated by ATP hydrolysis produces force to stretch an elastic element somewhere in the physical connection between the cargo and the cytoskeletal fiber. The resulting motion depends on whether the force in the spring exceeds the resistance of the fiber or the cargo.

Myosins

Myosins are the only motors that are known to use actin filaments as tracks. As is discussed in the section entitled "The Myosin Superfamily," the members of this diverse family arose from a common ancestor and share a common motor unit called a **myosin "head"** that produces force on actin filaments (Fig. 36-3). Myosins have one or two heads attached to various types of tails that are adapted for diverse purposes, including polymerization into filaments, binding membranes, and interacting with various cargos.

Myosin heads consist of two parts. A catalytic domain at the N-terminus of the myosin **heavy chain** binds and hydrolyzes ATP and interacts with actin filaments. Light chain domains consist of an α-helical extension of the heavy chain from the catalytic domain associated with one to seven **light chains.** Calmodulin (see Fig. 3-12) serves as a light chain for some cytoplasmic myosins, but many light chains are specialized relatives of calmodulin.

Myosin Mechanochemistry

Studies of skeletal muscle myosin established general principles that apply, with some interesting variations, to energy transduction by all myosins. This founding member of the myosin family is responsible for the forceful contraction of skeletal muscle. Like other types of myosin-II, it has two heads on a long tail formed from an α-helical coiled-coil. These tails polymerize into bipolar filaments (see Figs. 5-7 and 39-6).

The head of muscle myosin was originally isolated as a proteolytic fragment called subfragment-1 (Fig. 36-3). The N-terminal 710 residues of the heavy chain form the globular **catalytic domain.** The nucleotide binding site in the core of the catalytic domain is formed by a β-sheet flanked by α-helices with a topology similar to Ras GTPases (see Fig. 4-6) despite little sequence similarity.

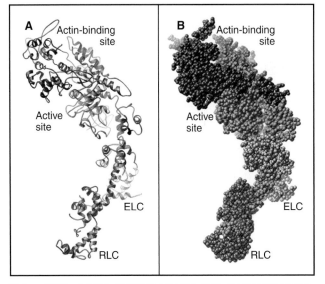

Figure 36-3 ATOMIC STRUCTURE OF THE HEAD OF MUSCLE MYOSIN. **A,** Ribbon drawing of the polypeptide backbones. **B,** Space-filling model. Heavy chain residues 4–204 *(green);* heavy chain residues 216–626 *(red);* heavy chain residues 647–843 *(purple):* essential light chain (ELC *[yellow]*); regulatory light chain (RLC *[orange]*). The myosin light chains consist of two globular domains connected by an α-helix, like calmodulin and troponin C. (PDB file: 2MYS.)

The γ-phosphate of ATP inserts deeply into the nucleotide-binding site with the adenine exposed on the surface. Actin binds more than 4 nm away from the nucleotide on the other side of the head. The **light-chain domain** has an essential light chain and a regulatory light chain wrapped around and stabilizing a long α-helix formed by the heavy chain (Fig. 36-3). The interaction of light chains with the heavy chain α-helix is similar to calmodulin binding its target proteins (see Fig. 3-12).

Myosin heads bind tightly and rigidly to actin filaments in the absence of ATP. This is called a **rigor** complex because it forms in muscle during rigor mortis when ATP is depleted after death. Myosin heads bound along an actin filament form a polarized structure, resembling a series of arrowheads when viewed from the side (Fig. 36-4). The heads bind at an angle and wrap around the filament. Their orientation defines the barbed and pointed ends of the actin filament (see Fig. 33-8). All known myosins except myosin-VI move toward the barbed end of the filament.

The atomic structures of the myosin head and actin filament fit nicely into the three-dimensional structure of the decorated filament determined by electron microscopy, providing a reasonable model of the complex at near atomic resolution (Fig. 36-4). The model shows each head in contact with two adjacent actins but does not reveal important details, including atomic contacts, between the proteins. This model is the structural starting point for understanding the mechanics of force production.

Actomyosin ATPase Cycle

Myosin uses energy from ATP hydrolysis to move actin filaments, so an appreciation of the mechanism requires an understanding of the steps in the biochemical reaction. Figure 36-5A looks intimidating, but working through it one step at a time reveals its logic and simplicity. Note that the mechanism consists of two parallel lines of chemical intermediates. This series of reactions explains why myosin alone turns over ATP remarkably slowly, at a rate of only about 0.02 s^{-1}. First, consider the bottom line, which shows how myosin hydrolyzes ATP in the absence of actin:

Step 1. At physiological concentrations of ATP, myosin binds ATP in less than 1 ms, so this is not the rate-limiting step. Binding is accompanied by a conformational change in the myosin that can be detected by a change in the fluorescence of the protein itself.

Step 2. The enzyme catalyzes the hydrolysis of ATP. This reaction is moderately fast (>100 s^{-1}) and readily reversible. The equilibrium constant for hydrolysis on the enzyme is near 1, so each ATP is hydrolyzed to adenosine diphosphate (ADP) and inorganic phosphate and is resynthesized several times before the products eventually dissociate from the enzyme. ATP splitting provides energy for a second conformational change, reflected in a further increase in the fluorescence of the myosin. It is presumed that this conformational change completes the "cocking" of the myosin in a structure prepared to undergo the molecular rearrangements that subsequently produce movement.

Step 3. Inorganic phosphate (P) slowly dissociates from the active site (at a rate of about 0.02 s^{-1}), perhaps by escaping through a narrow "back door" on the far side of the enzyme. This is the

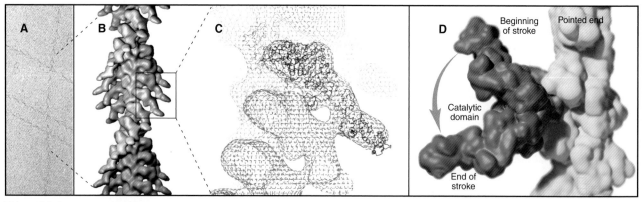

Figure 36-4   ACTIN FILAMENTS DECORATED WITH MYOSIN HEADS. **A,** Electron micrograph of frozen-hydrated actin filaments fully occupied with myosin heads. **B,** Three-dimensional reconstruction from electron micrographs of an actin filament saturated with myosin heads. **C,** Superimposition of atomic models of the actin filament and one myosin head on the reconstruction of the decorated filament (*blue* cage-like surface). **D,** Space-filling atomic model of an actin filament with one attached muscle myosin head showing the light-chain domain in two positions: (1) the end of the power stroke as observed in the absence of ATP (*blue*), and (2) the postulated beginning of the power stroke (*pink*) deduced from X-ray structures of isolated heads and spectroscopic studies. The catalytic domain (*red*) is fixed in one position on actin (*yellow*). (Courtesy of R. Milligan, Scripps Research Institute, La Jolla, California.)

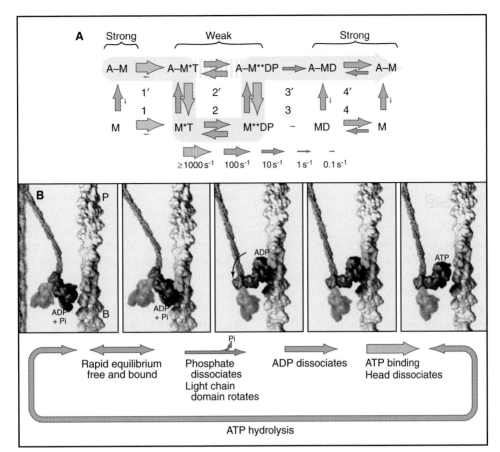

Figure 36-5 Myosin ATPase mechanisms. **A,** A diagram of the actomyosin ATPase cycle of striated muscle myosin-II showing the actin filament (A), myosin head (M), ATP (T), ADP (D), and inorganic phosphate (P). Transient-state kinetics revealed the major chemical intermediates and the rate constants for their transitions. *Arrows* are proportional to the rates of the reactions, with second-order reactions adjusted for physiological concentrations of reactants. *One* or *two asterisks* indicate conformational changes in the myosin head induced by ATP binding and hydrolysis. Myosin without nucleotide (M) and myosin with ADP (MD) bind much more tightly to actin filaments than do AMT and AMDP. The weakly bound AMT and AMDP intermediates are in a rapid equilibrium with free MT and MDP. The beige highlight shows the main pathway through the reaction. **B,** The postulated force-producing structural changes in the orientation of the light-chain domain (*purple* and *blue*) coupled to the myosin ATPase cycle. (B, Based on sketches and data from R. Vale, University of California, San Francisco, and R. Milligan, Scripps Research Institute, La Jolla, California.)

rate-limiting step of the reaction pathway. The loss of phosphate is coupled to conformational changes that return the myosin toward its "uncocked" basal state. The phosphate dissociation step has the largest negative free energy change, so it is presumed that energy derived from ATP binding and hydrolysis and stored in conformational changes in the myosin head is used to do work or dissipated as heat at this point in the reaction pathway.

Step 4. Once phosphate dissociates, ADP leaves rapidly from the "front door."

To summarize, in the absence of actin filaments, ATP binds rapidly to myosin and is rapidly but reversibly split, and the products slowly dissociate from the active site. The overall cycle of the enzyme is limited by a slow conformational change coupled to product dissociation,

not binding or hydrolysis. Energy derived from ATP binding and hydrolysis is used for a conformational change in the myosin head that is dissipated when phosphate dissociates.

Now focus on the upper line in Figure 36-5A, where myosin is associated with an actin filament. The chemical intermediates are the same, but some of the key rate constants differ for the actin-bound and free enzymes. Steps 1 and 2 are similar to those of free myosin, but step 3—the dissociation of phosphate—is much faster when a head is bound to an actin filament. As a result, myosin bound to actin traverses the ATPase cycle about 200 times faster than myosin free in solution, and ATP hydrolysis becomes the rate-limiting step. This effect of actin is referred to as "actin activation of the myosin ATPase." A practical advantage of this mechanism is that the ATPase cycle is essentially turned off unless a head interacts with an actin filament.

Finally, consider the vertical arrows representing transitions between bound and free states of each myosin chemical intermediate. All myosin intermediates bind rapidly to actin filaments, but the dissociation rate constants vary over a wide range depending on the nucleotide that is bound to the active site of the myosin. Myosin with no nucleotide or with bound ADP alone dissociates very slowly and therefore binds tightly to actin filaments. Myosin with bound ATP or ADP+P_i dissociates rapidly from actin, so these states bind actin weakly.

These rapid binding and dissociation reactions allow myosin intermediates (MT and MDP) to hop on and off actin filaments on a millisecond time scale, a key feature of muscle contraction (see Chapter 39). As a result of this rapid equilibrium, a single pathway cannot be drawn through the reaction mechanism of ATP, myosin, and actin. One cycle of ATP hydrolysis takes about 50 ms. Starting with AM, ATP binds very rapidly and sets up a rapid, four-way equilibrium including AMT, MT, AMDP, and MDP—the major intermediates during steady-state ATP turnover. Because the products of ATP hydrolysis dissociate much more rapidly from AMDP than from MDP, the favored pathway out of this four-way equilibrium is through AMDP to AMD and back to AM. Because the fraction of myosin heads bound to actin in the AMDP state depends on the actin concentration, the overall ATPase rate depends on the actin concentration. At the high actin concentrations in cells, a significant fraction of myosin heads are associated with actin (about 10% in contracting muscle), but each molecule continues to exchange on and off actin filaments.

Transduction of Chemical Energy into Molecular Motion

Myosin heads produce force during the transition from the AMDP state to the AMD and AM states. Production of force at this step makes sense for two reasons: First, the large free-energy difference between AMDP and AMD provides energy to produce force; second, the force-producing AMD and AM intermediates bind tightly to actin, so any force between the motor and the actin track is not dissipated. However, for many myosins, including skeletal muscle myosin, these force-producing states occupy a small fraction of the whole ATPase cycle. The fraction of the time in force producing states is called the **duty cycle.** ADP dissociates rapidly from AMD, and ATP binds rapidly to AM, dissociating myosin from the actin filament and initiating another ATPase cycle.

Establishing the structural basis for the conversion of free energy into force has been the most challenging question in this field of research for 50 years. A combination of mechanical measurements, static atomic struc-

tures of myosin heads with various bound nucleotides, and spectroscopic observations of contracting muscle have revealed the most likely mechanism: a dramatic conformational change in the myosin head associated with phosphate dissociation (Fig. 36-5B).

One approach has been to measure the size of the mechanical step produced by a myosin during one cycle of ATP hydrolysis. Elegant mechanical experiments on live muscles first suggested that each cycle of ATP hydrolysis moves an actin filament about 5 to 10 nm relative to myosin. Now light microscopy makes it possible to observe myosin moving single actin filaments. An array of myosin heads attached to a microscope slide can utilize ATP hydrolysis to push actin filaments over the surface (Fig. 36-6A–C). More complicated assays with single myosin molecules show that each cycle of ATP hydrolysis can move an actin filament up to 5 to 15 nm and develops a force of about 3 to 7 pN (Fig. 36-6D). At low ATP concentrations, the interval between the force-producing step and the binding of the next ATP is relatively long, so single steps can be observed.

Further insights emerged from biophysical studies of muscle and purified proteins using X-ray diffraction, electron microscopy, electron spin resonance spectroscopy, and fluorescence spectroscopy. These experiments showed that the light-chain domain pivots around a fulcrum just within the catalytic domain, which is stationary relative to the actin filament. For example, spectroscopic probes on light chains reveal a change in orientation when muscle is activated to contract, whereas the same probes on the catalytic domain do not rotate. Crystal structures of myosin heads with various bound nucleotides and nucleotide analogs show that the light-chain domain can pivot up to 90° (Fig. 36-4D). The light-chain domain is bent more acutely in the AMT and AMDP intermediates and pivots to a more extended orientation, when phosphate dissociates. ADP dissociation extends this rotation of some classes of myosin. Consistent with this concept of rotation of the light-chain domain, the rate of actin filament gliding in an in vitro assay is proportional to the length of the light-chain domain. The observed range of orientations of the light-chain domain relative to the catalytic domain can account for the observed step size of 10 nm for muscle myosin. This conformational change on phosphate release depends on rearrangements in the polypeptide chain around the γ-phosphate of ATP, similar to the changes in the Ras family of GTPases (see Fig. 4-6), but many mechanistic details remain to be resolved.

Rotation of the light-chain domain is believed to produce movement indirectly in the sense that force-producing intermediates stretch elastic elements in the system. This mechanism is represented by a spring in Figure 36-2. The elastic elements in the myosin-actin complex are most likely to be mainly in the myosin head, with small contributions from the actin and

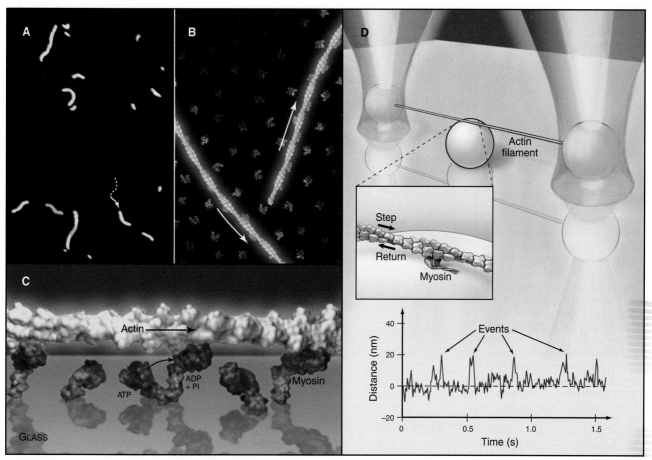

Figure 36-6 IN VITRO MOTILITY ASSAYS WITH PURIFIED MUSCLE MYOSIN AND ACTIN FILAMENTS. **A–C, Actin filament gliding assays. A,** Filaments are labeled with rhodamine-phalloidin to render them visible by light microscopy. ATP hydrolysis by myosin moves actin filaments over the surface with the pointed end leading as the myosins walk toward the barbed end of the filaments. **B–C,** Drawings of actin filaments moving over myosin heads immobilized on a glass coverslip. **D, Measurement of the muscle myosin step size.** An actin filament is attached between two plastic beads, which are suspended by laser optical traps. The optical traps move the filament near a myosin molecule on the surface of another bead attached to the microscope slide, allowing a myosin head to attach to the actin filament. When supplied with ATP, a single myosin head can move the actin filament a short distance corresponding to the step size. The graph shows the time course of displacements of the actin filament and attached beads. Brownian motion limits the precision of the measurement of the size of these steps to a range of 5 to 15 nm. The duration of the step depends on the ATP concentration, because ATP dissociates the force-producing AM state, allowing the force of the optical traps to return the beads and the actin filament to their original position. (A, Courtesy of A. Bresnick, Albert Einstein College of Medicine, New York. D, Reference: Finer JT, Simmons RM, Spudich JA: Single myosin molecule mechanics: Piconewton forces and nanometer steps. Nature 368:113–119, 1994.)

myosin filaments. Movement of the light-chain domain tensions the spring transiently in the AMD and AM states. Dissociation of ADP and rebinding of ATP to the AM intermediate reverts the system to the rapid equilibrium of weakly bound intermediates, including dissociated heads. Any force left in the spring is lost as soon as the head dissociates from the actin filament.

The actual motion depends on the mechanical resistance in the system (Fig. 36-2). If both myosin and actin are fixed, elastic elements are stretched for the life of the force-producing states (AMD and AM), and the energy is lost as heat when the head dissociates. This happens when one tries to lift an immovable object. If the resistance is less than the force in the stretched elastic elements, the actin filament moves relative to

myosin, as in muscle contraction. The distance moved in each step depends on the resistance, as the spring stops shortening when the forces are balanced.

The Myosin Superfamily

All 18 classes of myosin arose from a common genetic ancestor in an early Eukaryote more than a billion years ago (Fig. 36-7). Gene duplication and divergence produced myosins specialized for particular biological functions owing to variations of the mechanochemical ATPase cycle and acquisition of diverse tails to interact with cargo. Extreme examples include myosin-V, which takes giant processive steps; myosin-VI, the only myosin that is capable of moving toward the pointed end of an

Figure 36-7 MYOSIN FAMILY. A, Phylogenetic relationships based on sequences of motor domains. Note the very early branching of 15 myosin classes denoted by roman numerals and of many isoforms within these classes (e.g., cytoplasmic versus striated muscle myosin-II). Thus, much of myosin diversity is very ancient. Genes for myosins in related species (for clarity, illustrated here only by mouse and chicken myosin-V) branched only recently. Many of the specific names are based on gene names and are not enumerated here. **B,** Drawing of myosin heavy chain domains and molecular models of myosin isoforms showing catalytic domains (rose); IQ motifs, light-chain-binding sites (rose bars); basic domains with affinity for membrane lipids (violet); SH3 domains (dark green); coiled-coil (orange); kinase domain (light blue); and pleckstrin homology domain (blue). (Redrawn with permission from Mermall V, Post P, Mooseker MS: Unconventional myosins in cell movement, membrane traffic and signal transduction. Science 279:527–533, 1998. Copyright 1998 AAAS. See also Myosin Home Page, available at http://www.mrc-lmb.cam.ac.uk/myosin/myosin.html.)

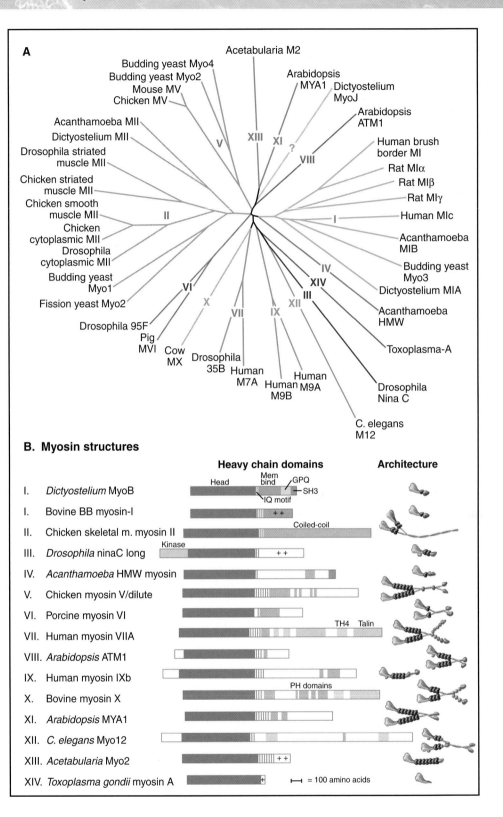

actin filament; and plant myosins, which move at very high speeds (see Fig. 37-9). Within a myosin class, the tails are similar to each other, but between classes, tails are diverse in terms of their ability to polymerize and interact with other cellular components including membranes and ribonucleoprotein particles.

No organism has genes for all 18 classes of myosin. Humans have 40 myosin genes from 12 classes. Yeast have five myosin genes, including types I, II, and V, which are widely dispersed among eukaryotes. Plants have lost the genes for these ancient myosins and are the only organisms with the highly diverged relatives of myosin-V, called myosin-VIII and myosin-XI. Gene duplications gave rise to multiple isoforms within most classes of myosin. For instance, vertebrate smooth muscle myosin genes arose from duplication of a gene for a cytoplasmic myosin-II.

Establishing the biological functions of the various classes of myosin has been challenging. Biochemical characterization of cargo and localization in cells provide some clues, but genetic or biochemical knockouts often have mild effects, probably owing to overlapping functions of the myosins and the capacity of some cells to adapt to their loss, at least under laboratory conditions.

Myosin-I was the first "unconventional myosin" discovered—unconventional in the sense that it differed from the type II myosin originally isolated from skeletal muscle. These myosins have one head and short tails with various types of domains, including a basic domain with affinity for acidic phospholipids. Those with an SH-3 domain (see Fig. 25-11) can bind proline-rich sequences in other proteins. Those with an actin filament–binding domain separate from the motor domain can cross-link actin filaments. Some types of myosin-I have ATPase cycles similar to skeletal muscle myosin, but others differ considerably. With duty cycles less than 10%, multiple myosin heads must work together to move membranes. Mutations show that myosin-I participates in endocytosis, as expected from its concentration at sites of phagocytosis and macropinocytosis. In microvilli of intestinal epithelial cells, myosin-I links actin filaments laterally to the plasma membrane (see Fig. 33-2B). Heavy chain phosphorylation activates myosin-I from lower eukaryotes, whereas calcium binding to calmodulin light chains regulates myosin-I from the intestinal brush border.

The **myosin-II** class includes various muscle myosins and cytoplasmic myosins that also have two heads and long coiled-coil tails. Assembly of tails into bipolar filaments (see Figs. 5-7 and 6-4) allows myosin-II to pull together oppositely polarized actin filaments during muscle contraction (see Chapter 39) and cytokinesis (see Fig. 44-23). As in smooth muscle (see Fig. 39-21), phosphorylation of the regulatory light chain activates myosin-II in animal nonmuscle cells. In addition, phosphorylation of the heavy chain regulates the polymerization of some myosin-IIs. Lower eukaryotes use both light-chain phosphorylation to activate myosin-II and heavy-chain phosphorylation to inhibit myosin-II.

Myosin-V participates in the movement of pigment granules and other cellular components (see Fig. 37-11). Myosin-V takes long, processive steps along an actin filament by virtue of the fact that it has a long light-chain domain and each of its two heads spends most of each ATPase cycle attached to the filament (Fig. 36-8). This is accomplished by very slow ADP dissociation from the AMD intermediate. This rate-limiting step allows plenty of time for the other head to take a long step, binding to an actin subunit 36 nm along the barbed end. Mechanical strain after the step may modestly increase the rate of ADP dissociation from the trailing head. This cooperation between the heads initiates ATP binding and the next ATPase cycle, as the motor walks deliberating along the filament. These features of myosin-V provide strong support for the light-chain domain serving as the lever arm for movements of the whole myosin family.

In animal cells, **myosin-VI** moves some types of endocytic vesicles from the plasma membrane into the cytoplasm and contributes to the organization of the Golgi apparatus. Myosin-VI is the only myosin that is known to move toward the pointed end of actin filaments. The force-producing AMD and AM states occupy a large fraction of the ATPase cycle, owing to slow ADP dissociation from AMD state and slow ATP binding to AM. Several mysteries remain. Measurements on dimeric myosin-VI suggest that the motor takes huge steps of about 30 nm along an actin filament. A flexible connector between the head and tail might allow large steps in spite of a small light-chain domain that binds a single calmodulin. Agreement has not been reached on whether there are one or two heads; in fact, formation of dimers might be a form of regulation.

Myosin mutations can cause disease. Loss-of-function mutations in the genes for myosins-IIA, -IIIA, -VI, -VIIA, and -XV cause deafness and vestibular dysfunction in mice and humans. Similarly, fly photoreceptor cells degenerate without myosin-III.

Microtubule Motors

The kinesin and dynein families of molecular motors are responsible for movements of vesicles, membrane-bound organelles, chromosomes, and other cargo along microtubules in cells (see Fig. 37-1). Dynein also powers bending motions of eukaryotic flagella and cilia (see Fig. 38-14). Dyneins move themselves and any cargo toward the minus end of microtubules. Most kinesins move in the opposite direction, toward the plus end, but some kinesin family members are minus-end-directed motors (Table 36-2). Like myosins, microtubule motors have heads with ATPase activity and tails that serve as adapters for interacting with cargo.

Kinesins

Kinesins use ATP hydrolysis to move along microtubule tracks. Some can move processively along a microtubule, using cooperation between two heads to maintain physical contact with the microtubule. Processive movement allows single kinesin molecules to move

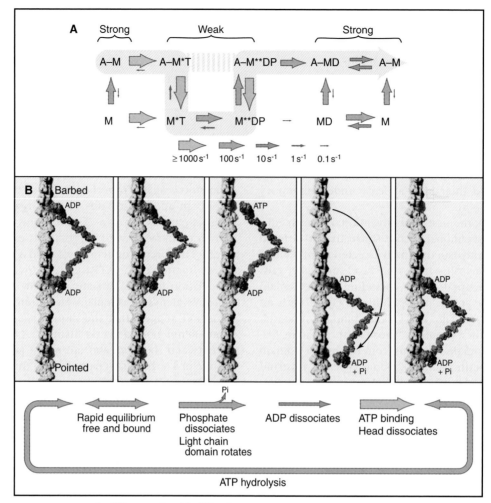

Figure 36-8   MYOSIN-V MECHANISM. **A,** ATPase cycle with ADP release as the rate-limiting step rather than phosphate dissociation as for muscle myosin (Fig. 36-5A). **B,** Relationship of mechanical steps to the ATPase cycle. Shown are actin filament (A), myosin head (M), ATP (T), ADP (D), and inorganic phosphate (P). (Reference: De La Cruz EM, Ostap EM: Relating biochemistry and function in the myosin super-family. Curr Opin Cell Biol 16:61–67, 2004.)

Table 36-2				
KINESIN SUPERFAMILY: CLASSIFICATION AND EXAMPLES OF KINESIN-FAMILY MOTOR PROTEINS				
Class	**Examples**	**Subunits (kD)**	**Velocity ($\mu m\ s^{-1}$)**	**Functions**
N-terminal Motor				
Kinesin-1	Human KHC	$2 \times 110, 2 \times 70$	+0.9	Organelle movement
Kinesin-2	Urchin KRP85/95	$1 \times 79, 1 \times 84, 1 \times 115$	+0.4	Organelle movement
Kinesin-3	Mouse KIF1B	1×130	+0.7	Mitochondria movement
Kinesin-4	*Xenopus* Kp11	2×139	+0.2	Chromosome movement
Kinesin-5	Fly KLP61F	4×121	+0.04	Pole separation, mitosis
Kinesin-7	Human CENP-E	2×340	+0.1	Kinetochore-microtubule binding
Internal Motor				
Kinesin-13	MCAK	2×83	—	Microtubule disassembly
C-terminal Motor				
Kinesin-14	Fly ncd	2×78	−0.2	Mitotic/meiotic spindle

Adapted from Vale RD, Fletterick RJ: The design plan of kinesin motors. Annu Rev Cell Dev Biol 13:745-777, 1997. More data on kinesins are available at the Kinesin Home Page, http://www.proweb.org/kinesin.

cargo, such as an organelle, toward the plus end of a microtubule.

Classic kinesin or kinesin-1 has two heads at the N-terminus of an α-helical coiled-coil tail, much like myosin-II, except both the heads and coiled-coil are smaller (Fig. 36-9). The tail of kinesin-1 is called the stalk. Each head, consisting of about 340 residues, is a motor unit that binds microtubules and catalyzes ATP hydrolysis. With some variation in amino acid sequence, this motor unit is common to the whole kinesin family. In kinesin-1, light chains are associated with the C-terminal bifurcation of the tail. Other members of the kinesin family have the motor domain (Fig. 36-13) attached to a variety of tails that are believed to interact with cargo. Most kinesin motor domains are located at the N-terminus of the polypeptide chain, but a few are at the C-terminus or even in the middle.

Because the **kinesin head** is less than half the size of a myosin head and because the proteins lack appreciable sequence homology, determination of the atomic structure of kinesin-1 (Fig. 36-9) revealed a major surprise: The small kinesin head is folded like the core of the catalytic domain of myosin! In fact, this core consisting of a central, mixed β-sheet flanked by helices is similar to the considerably smaller Ras family GTPases

(see Fig. 4-6). This provided strong evidence that all three families of nucleoside triphosphatases evolved from a common ancestor. ATP binds to a site on kinesin that is homologous to the GTP-binding site of Ras, but the enzyme mechanisms differ in important ways. The microtubule-binding site is some distance from the ATP-binding site, as seen by fitting the atomic model of the head into three-dimensional reconstructions of kinesin-1 bound to microtubules (Fig. 36-10).

Kinesin Mechanochemistry

In vitro motility assays (Fig. 36-11) revealed that a two-headed kinesin-1 can move along a single (or two parallel) microtubule protofilaments for long distances at 0.8 μm/s. Kinesin-1 moves in discrete steps of 8 nm, the spacing of successive tubulin dimers in a microtubule, so the motor takes a step every 10 ms when moving at full speed. This large step of 8 nm is remarkable for the small (<10 nm) kinesin heads linked together at the neck region. Processive movement depends on the ability of kinesin to remain associated with the microtubule as it moves.

Single kinesin-1 heads, produced experimentally by expression of truncated complementary DNAs (cDNAs), traverse a microtubule-stimulated ATPase cycle much

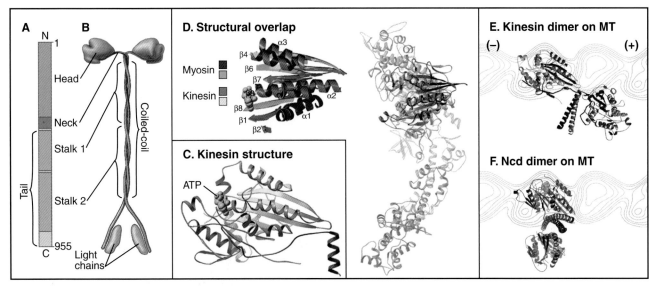

Figure 36-9 STRUCTURE OF KINESINS. **A,** Domain architecture of the polypeptide sequence of the heavy chain of kinesin-1. **B,** Sketch of kinesin-1 showing two heads and the coiled-coil tail with light chains bound at the distal end. **C,** Ribbon diagram of the polypeptide backbone of the kinesin head showing ATP as a space-filling model *(green)*, the neck-linker residues *(red)*, and the proximal part of the coiled-coil stalk. **D,** Superimposition of the core of the kinesin-1 head on the catalytic domain of myosin showing the structural homology of the proteins. The detailed ribbon diagram shows only the homologous elements of secondary structure. The overview *(right)* shows kinesin-1 *(blue)* superimposed on the structure of the whole head of skeletal muscle myosin *(pink)*. **E,** Ribbon model of dimeric kinesin-1 superimposed on a microtubule (MT) protofilament with the leading head toward the plus end of the microtubule *(right)*. **F,** Ribbon model of dimeric Ncd *Drosophila* kinesin-14 superimposed on a microtubule protofilament. The N-terminus of Ncd attaches to the coiled-coil stalk in approximately the same position as the C-terminus of kinesin-1. The two heads are positioned asymmetrically on the stalk, with the leading head toward the minus end of the microtubule *(left)*. (C, PDB file: 3KIN. Reference: Sack S, Muller J, Marx A, et al: X-ray structure of motor and neck domains from rat brain kinesin. Biochemistry 36:16155–16165, 1997. F, PDB file: 1N6M. Reference: Yun M, Bronner CE, Park CG, et al: Rotation of the stalk/neck and one head in a new crystal structure of the kinesin motor protein, Ncd. EMBO J 22:5382–5389, 2003. E, PDB file: 3KIN. *Note:* Superimposed ribbon diagrams courtesy of R. Vale, University of California, San Francisco.)

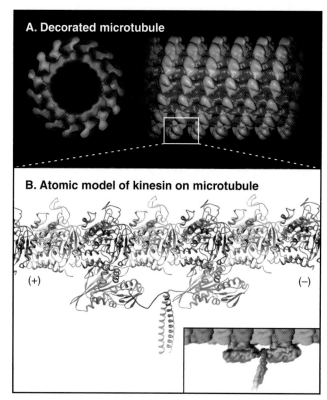

Figure 36-10 INTERACTION OF KINESIN-1 WITH MICROTUBULES. **A,** Three-dimensional reconstruction from electron micrographs of kinesin-1 heads *(blue)* bound to a microtubule *(brown)*. The primary interaction is with β-tubulin *(red* in panel **B**). **B,** Atomic model of dimeric kinesin-1 bound to the surface of a microtubule with the neck-linker peptide unfolded on the leading head *(brown,* toward the plus end) and the neck-linker peptide folded on the trailing head *(green).* (A, Courtesy of R. Milligan, Scripps Research Institute, La Jolla, California. B, Courtesy of R. Vale, University of California, San Francisco.)

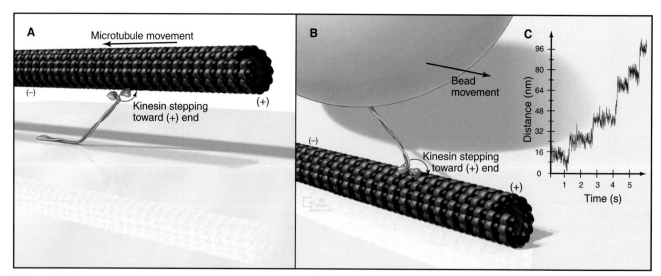

Figure 36-11 IN VITRO MOTILITY ASSAYS FOR MICROTUBULE MOTORS. **A,** Gliding assay. Kinesin or dynein that is attached to a microscope slide uses ATP hydrolysis to move microtubules over the surface. A single kinesin-1 molecule can move a microtubule in this assay. Microtubules can be imaged by video-enhanced differential interference contrast microscopy (see Fig. 34-7). **B,** Bead assay. Kinesin or dynein that is attached to a plastic bead uses ATP hydrolysis to move the bead along a microtubule attached to the microscopic slide. **C,** Experimental measurement of the kinesin-1 step size using the bead assay. The bead is held in a laser optical trap so that 8-nm steps can be recorded, as a single, two-headed kinesin-1 moves a bead processively along a microtubule, as in **B**. The position of the bead is recorded with nanometer precision by interferometry. (Reference: Svoboda K, Schmidt CF, Schnapp BJ, Block SM: Direct observation of kinesin stepping by optical trapping interferometry. Nature 365:721–727, 1993.)

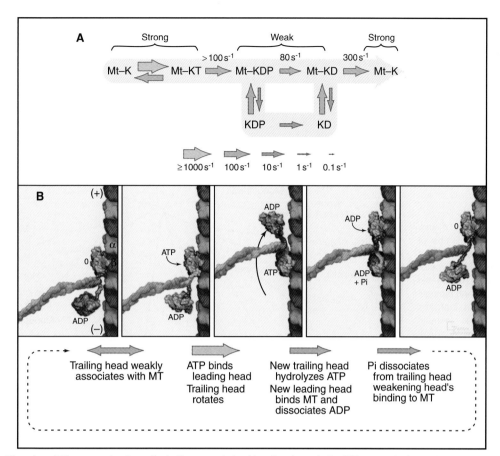

Figure 36-12 Kinesin-1 ATPase mechanism. **A,** A diagram of the kinesin-microtubule ATPase cycle for a single kinesin-1 head showing the kinesin (K), microtubule (Mt), ATP (T), ADP (D), and inorganic phosphate (P). *Arrows* are proportional to the rates of the reactions, with second-order reactions adjusted for physiological concentrations of reactants. Depending on the length of the polypeptide chain, some but not all single-headed kinesin-1 preparations remain associated with a microtubule for multiple rounds of ATP hydrolysis. The *beige* highlight shows two pathways through the reaction, one along the top line without dissociation, and the other with dissociation from the microtubule. **B,** Postulated structural changes in double-headed kinesin-1 coupled to the ATPase cycle resulting in hand-over-hand, processive stepping along of a microtubule. ATP binding to the empty head, bound to the microtubule, causes folding of its neck-linker *(green),* thereby thrusting the detached head with its unfolded *(pink)* neck-linker forward. The new leading head binds the microtubule and dissociates its ADP, whereas the trailing head hydrolyzes ATP and dissociates phosphate, returning the heads to the original condition, but with the heads advanced 8 nm and in the opposite chemical states. (B, Based on sketches and data from R. Vale, University of California, San Francisco, and R. Milligan, Scripps Research Institute, La Jolla, California.)

like myosin (Fig. 36-12A). Like myosin, kinesin-1 binds and hydrolyzes ATP rapidly followed by slower release of phosphate and ADP. Some kinesin head preparations dissociate from the microtubule during each cycle of ATP hydrolysis, but others (differing in the length of the polypeptide) appear to remain bound to the microtubule (presumably a single tubulin dimer) through multiple cycles of ATP hydrolysis.

Kinesin-1 with two heads moves processively along a microtubule, remaining attached through more than a hundred cycles of ATP hydrolysis (Fig. 36-12B). The presence of a second head introduces a key feature: The two heads strongly influence each other, leading to reciprocal affinities of the heads for nucleotide (either ATP or ADP) and microtubules. One head binds nucleotide strongly and microtubules weakly; the other does the opposite. Hence, one head tends to bind the tubule and

to dissociate its bound nucleotide rapidly. For example, if kinesin-1 with ADP bound to both heads is mixed with microtubules, only one of the two heads binds the microtubule and dissociates its ADP. Given an excess of ATP over ADP in cells, ATP will bind to this open site on the head associated with the microtubule, starting a processive cycle of stepping, each step coupled to one ATP turnover. ATP binding drives the conformational change or switch that propels the rearward head forward to bind the next tubulin subunit toward the plus end of the microtubule. ATP hydrolysis on the rearward head leads to tight binding of the forward head, whose active site is now empty. Phosphate release from the rearward head weakens its affinity for the microtubule, resulting in detachment of the rearward head.

Cooperation between the two heads ensures that at least one head is bound to the microtubule at every

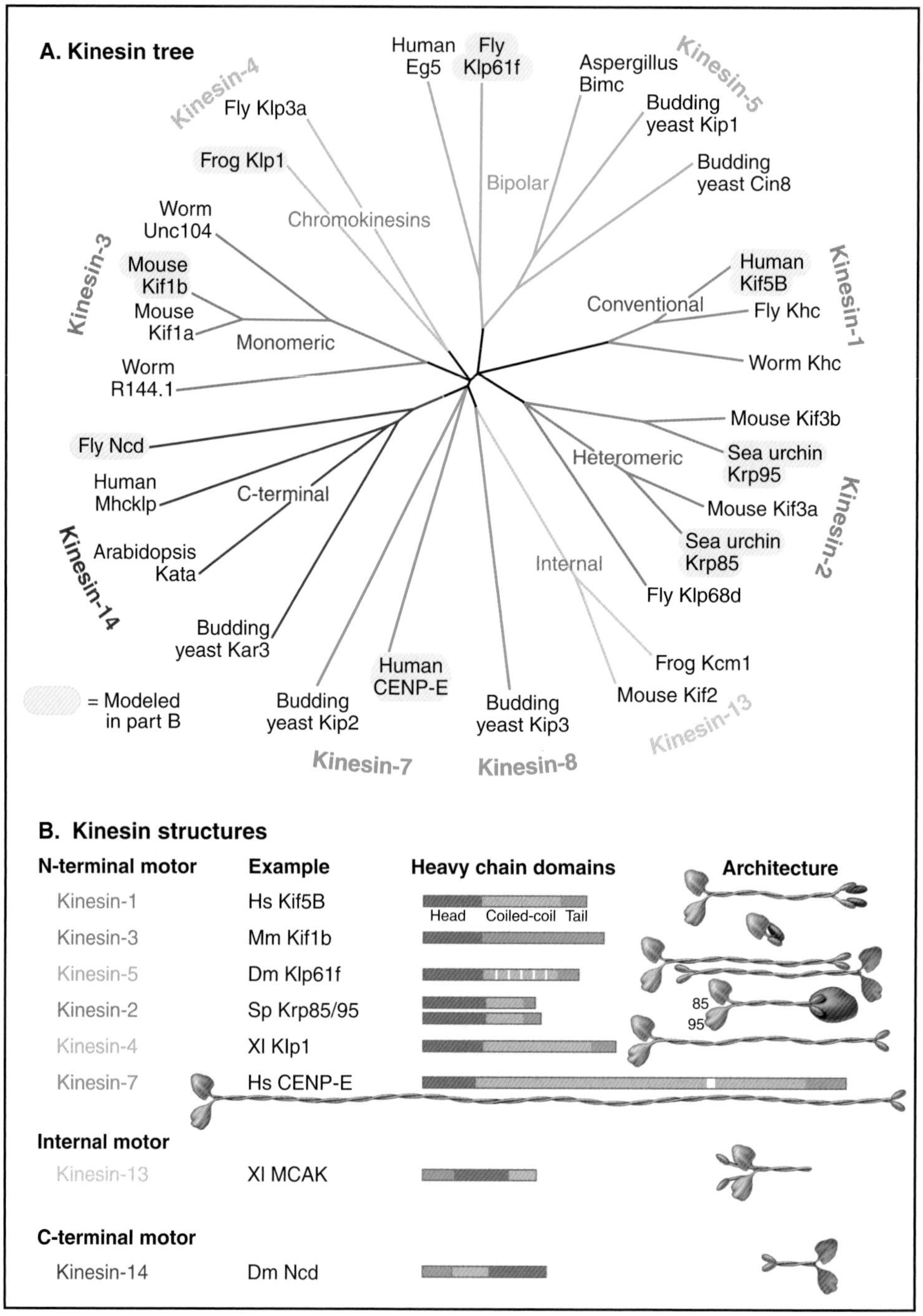

Figure 36-13 KINESIN FAMILY. **A,** Phylogenetic relationships of a selection of kinesins based on the sequences of the motor domains. **B,** Drawing of kinesin heavy chain domains and molecular models of kinesin isoforms showing the catalytic domain *(red),* coiled-coil stalk *(orange),* and tails *(blue).* (Based on data of R. Case and R. Vale, University of California, San Francisco. References: Lawrence CJ, Dawe RK, Christie KR, et al: Standardized kinesin nomenclature. J Cell Biol 167:19–22, 2004; Dagenbach EM, Endow S: A new kinesin tree. J Cell Sci 117:3–7, 2004; see also the Kinesin Home Page at http://www.proweb.org/kinesin.)

point in the ATPase cycle (Fig. 36-12B). The reciprocal affinities for nucleotide and microtubules allows the two heads to alternate between microtubule binding and dissociation. During this interchange, the trailing ADP head steps past the bound ATP head and binds to the tubulin dimer 8 nm beyond the ATP head. A simple mechanism might have the trailing head always step around the same side of the leading head, resulting in a 360° rotation every two steps. However, microtubules moved by kinesin-1 attached to a slide do not rotate. This result together with several types of experiments

with single kinesin-1 heads labeled with fluorescent dyes showed that kinesin walks asymmetrically, alternating steps on the right and left sides of the microtubule like a person walking on a beam.

The mechanism of stepping is postulated to be the folding and unfolding of a segment of the kinesin-1 heavy chain linking the motor domain to the coiled-coil neck/stalk. When ATP is bound to the motor domain, this "neck-linker" peptide is postulated to associate tightly with the motor domain, as in the X-ray structure of dimeric kinesin (Fig. 36-9). When no nucleotide or

ADP is bound to the motor domain, the neck-linker peptide is thought to be flexible and only loosely bound to the motor domain.

The Kinesin Superfamily

Early in evolution, gene duplication and recombination produced at least 14 families of kinesins having motor domains associated with a variety of coiled-coil stalks and tails (Fig. 36-13 and Table 36-2). Classification systems based on the sequences of motor domains turn out to group kinesins that also have similar coiled-coil stalks and tails, and functions. Most kinesins are dimeric, with two polypeptides joined in a coiled-coil. Most are homodimers, but the kinesin-2 class consists of two different polypeptides with motor domains plus another large subunit. Most kinesins move along microtubules toward their plus ends, but C-terminal kinesin-14 motors, such as Ncd, move toward the minus end, and internal motor kinesins-13 might not move at all but function to destabilize microtubules (see Fig. 34-9). Whether located at the N- or C-terminus, the motor domains are similar in structure; peptide sequences that link the head to the neck/stalk determine the direction of movement on microtubules.

Kinesins transport a variety of cargo, including chromosomes and organelles, along microtubules. A variety of evidence implicates kinesin-1 in the movement of membrane vesicles toward the plus end of microtubules in nerve axons and other cells (see Fig. 37-1). **Chromokinesins** or kinesin-4 motors have DNA-binding sites that allow them to bind to the surface of mitotic chromosomes and carry them toward the metaphase plate (see Fig. 44-7). Kinesin-7 or **CENP-E** is concentrated at kinetochores. **Bipolar kinesin-5 motors** form an antiparallel tetramer of two dimeric kinesins that can interact with a pair of oppositely polarized microtubules and push apart the poles of the mitotic spindle (see Fig. 44-7).

Most kinesins appear to be constitutively active, so there is most likely still much to learn about their regulation. One regulatory mechanism involves the tail of kinesin-1 folding over and inhibiting the heads. This shuts off the motor when no cargo is bound to the tail, thereby conserving ATP.

Some kinesins, such as the *Drosophila* kinesin-14, Ncd, move backward, toward the minus rather than the plus end of microtubules. This difference is not explained by the structural architecture of the motor domain, as Ncd is nearly identical to plus-end kinesin-1 (Fig. 36-9). The Ncd ATPase mechanism is similar to kinesin-1, although there is less cooperation between the heads and no processivity. The most obvious difference is that the Ncd motor domain is attached to the coiled-coil stalk by its N-terminus, rather than C-terminus, as in kinesin-1. However, this does not explain backward movement, because transplantation of kinesin-1 heads to the C-terminus of a coiled-coil stalk or Ncd heads to the N-terminus of a coiled-coil stalk does not necessarily reverse their motor activity. Experiments with more complicated chimeric proteins suggest that the neck-linker peptide and the proximal part of the Ncd coiled-coil stalk determine the direction of movement. Interactions of the heads with the neck/stalk are important in directing the motor toward the microtubule minus end.

Dyneins

Dynein microtubule-based motors are AAA ATPases (Box 36-1), so they have a different evolutionary origin than myosins and kinesins. Unique in the AAA family,

---

BOX 36-1
AAA ATPases

The common ancestor of life on the earth had a gene for a versatile ATP-binding domain. Through gene duplication and divergence this progenitor gave rise to the AAA family of ATPases in all branches of the phylogenic tree. Given the remarkable variety of functions of the contemporary proteins, the name "ATPases Associated with Diverse Activities" is apt. The family now includes regulatory subunits of proteasomes (see Fig. 23-5); proteases from prokaryotes, chloroplasts, and mitochondria; Hsp100 protein folding chaperones; dynein microtubule motors (Fig. 36-14); the microtubule severing protein katanin (see Fig. 34-9); activators of origins of replication (including ORC1, 4, and 5 and Mcm-7 [see Fig. 42-7]); clamp loader proteins for DNA polymerase processivity factors (see Fig. 42-11); two proteins required for peroxisome bio-

genesis (see Appendix 18-1); and proteins involved in vesicular traffic such as NSF (the N-ethylmaleimide-sensitive factor [see Fig. 21-12]).

AAA domains have a common fold with a catalytic site that binds and hydrolyzes ATP. A "Walker A" motif of conserved residues interacts with the β- and γ-phosphates of ATP, and "Walker B" motif residues participate in ATP hydrolysis. Many AAA ATPases form ring-shaped hexamers of identical subunits or up to six different AAA subunits although the dynein heavy chain has six AAA domains. Often, an arginine residue from the adjacent subunit in the hexamer inserts into the active site and facilitates conformational changes in response to ATP binding and release of the γ-phosphate.

dyneins consist of six ATPase domains concatenated in a giant heavy chain of nearly 500 kD (Fig. 36-14). The globular head is formed from the six AAA domains, each predicted to be folded like the known crystal structures of other AAA ATPases, and a seventh domain of unknown structure. The N-terminal half of the heavy chain forms a tail that interacts with accessory polypeptides (called light and intermediate chains) and cargo molecules. The segment of dynein heavy chain between the fourth and fifth AAA domains forms a coiled-coil stalk. The globular end of the stalk binds to a site on microtubules similar to the kinesin binding site.

Dynein Mechanochemistry

AAA domain 1 binds and hydrolyzes ATP during force-producing interactions with microtubules. Full motor function requires ADP or ATP binding to domains 2 to 4, but ATP hydrolysis by these domains is not coupled

directly to motility. The dynein ATPase cycle of AAA domain 1 resembles the actomyosin ATPase mechanism in broad outline but differs in important details, particularly the rate-limiting reactions (Fig. 36-15). Remarkably, ATP binding to AAA domain 1 dissociates the stalk from microtubules that are more than 20 nm distant. The dynein-ADP-P_i intermediate also binds weakly to microtubules. After rapid dissociation of inorganic phosphate, the dynein-ADP complex rebinds to the microtubule. Binding to a microtubule stimulates the rate of ADP dissociation from dynein about 10-fold, from about 3 s^{-1} to about 33 s^{-1}, by accelerating a rate-limiting conformational change. Consequently, microtubules stimulate the dynein ATPase to levels required for the rapid beating of cilia at up to 100 cycles per second. Free dynein turns over ATP relatively rapidly (3 s^{-1}). However, in cilia and flagella, control mechanisms keep dynein turned off except during beating, as ATP hydrolysis is tightly coupled to the production of motion (see Fig. 38-14).

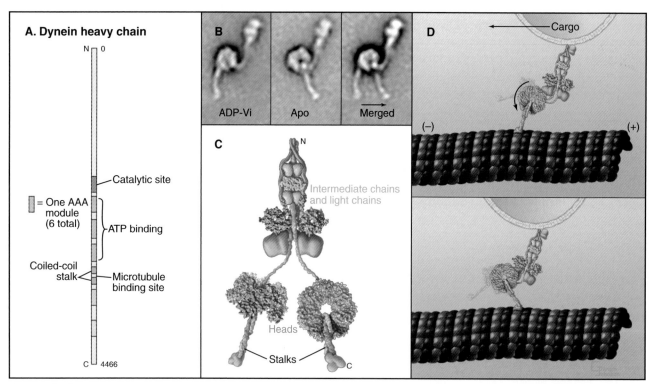

Figure 36-14 DYNEIN STRUCTURE. A, Domain organization of a dynein heavy chain showing the location of six AAA modules and two sequences that form an antiparallel coiled-coil stalk with an ATP-sensitive microtubule-binding site in the connecting loop. The first AAA module forms the catalytic site. Modules 2, 3, and 4 bind ATP, but hydrolysis is not coupled to movement. Modules 5 and 6 do not bind ATP. **B,** Ensemble averages of electron micrographs of single dynein molecules show the shaft *(top)*, head *(middle)*, and stalk *(bottom)*. The relationship of the head to the shaft differs with no nucleotide (Apo) or ADP and the phosphate analog vanadate bound to the head. This conformational change might contribute to producing motion. **C,** Model for cytoplasmic dynein based on electron micrographs of the whole molecule, crystal structures of some light chains, and a homology model of the heads based on crystal structures of other AAA ATPases. **D,** Drawing of cytoplasmic dynein with two heads interacting with a microtubule and cargo. Light and intermediate chains bind cargo and 10-nm stalks link the globular heads to the microtubule. (B, Reprinted by permission from Macmillan Publishers Ltd. from Burgess SA, Walker ML, Sakakibara H, et al: Dynein structure and power stroke. Nature 421:715–718, 2003. Copyright 2003. C, Modified from a drawing by Graham Johnson for Vale RD: The molecular motor toolbox for intracellular transport. Cell 112:467–480, 2003. Copyright 2003, with permission from Elsevier.)

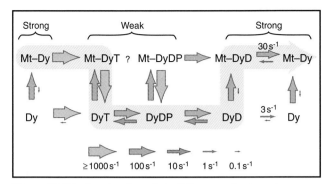

Figure 36-15 Dynein-microtubule ATPase mechanism. *Arrows* are proportional to the rates of the reactions, with second-order reactions adjusted for physiological concentrations of reactants. The *beige* highlight shows the main pathway through the reaction. D, ADP; Dy, dynein; Mt, microtubule; P, inorganic phosphate; T, ATP.

If dynein is immobilized on a surface in an in vitro motility assay, the plus end of a microtubule moving on the bound motors will lead as the dynein "walks" toward the minus end of the microtubule.

Crystal structures of the various chemical intermediates will be required to learn how the ATPase cycle drives the motion of dynein toward the minus end of microtubules. An attractive hypothesis that is consistent with electron micrographs of isolated dynein (Fig. 36-14B) is that the microtubule-binding stalk is used as a lever arm to amplify conformational changes in the globular domain during the ATPase cycle. However, it is not understood how ATP binding to the active site dissociates a distant binding site from the microtubule or how phosphate release moves the stalk, particularly since the whole molecule appears to be quite flexible. The size of the mechanical step associated with each ATP hydrolysis in most often 8 nm, but cytoplasmic dynein can take larger steps when the load is low.

The Dynein Superfamily

Animals have multiple genes for dynein heavy chains, multiple splice isoforms of intermediate chains, and multiple isoforms of light chains. The full extent of dynein diversity is not yet known, owing to the technical challenge of working with such large genes and proteins. However, this genetic diversity provides the potential to construct a variety of different dyneins with specialized functions. Cytoplasmic dynein has two heavy chains, while axonemal dyneins consist of one to three heavy chains and the corresponding number of heads. Each isoform has particular light chains and intermediate chains.

Tissues express these dynein isoforms differentially and target them to specific cellular locations. In axonemes of cilia and flagella, at least seven different dynein isoforms bind to unique sites on the outer doublets (see Fig. 38-16). Cytoplasmic dynein isoforms associate with organelles for transport along microtubules toward the cell body in nerve axons and with ER vesicles for transport to the Golgi apparatus located at the cell center. A null mutation in the gene for a mouse cytoplasmic dynein heavy chain leaves the Golgi apparatus dispersed throughout the cytoplasm and is lethal during embryogenesis. During mitosis, dyneins in the cell cortex and bound to kinetochores of chromosomes apply forces to microtubules of the mitotic spindle (see Fig. 44-7). A temperature-sensitive mutation in *Caenorhabditis elegans* dynein heavy chain results in defects in mitosis at the restrictive temperature.

Calcium and a cyclic adenosine monophosphate (cAMP)–dependent protein kinase (see Fig. 25-3D) regulate dynein in cilia and flagella, but little is known about the regulation of cytoplasmic dynein.

ACKNOWLEDGMENTS

Thanks go to Chip Asbury, Enrique De La Cruz, Sharyn Endow, Susan Gilbert, Martin Latterich, and Mike Ostap for their suggestions on revisions to this chapter.

SELECTED READINGS

Asbury CL: Kinesin: World's tiniest biped. Curr Opin Cell Biol 17:89–97, 2005.

Berg JS, Powell BC, Cheney RE: A millennial myosin census. Mol Biol Cell 12:780–794, 2001.

Burgess SA, Knight PJ: Is the dynein motor a winch? Curr Opin Struct Biol 14:138–146, 2004.

Buss F, Spudich G, Kendrick-Jones J: Myosin VI: Cellular functions and motor properties. Annu Rev Cell Dev Biol 20:649–676, 2004.

De La Cruz EM, Ostap EM: Relating biochemistry and function in the myosin superfamily. Curr Opin Cell Biol 16:61–67, 2004.

Erzberger JP, Berger JM: Evolutionary relationships and structural mechanisms of AAA+ proteins. Annu Rev Biophys Biomol Struct 35:93–114, 2006.

Geeves MA, Holmes KC: Structural mechanism of muscle contraction. Annu Rev Biochem 68:687–728, 1999.

Hackney DD: The kinetic cycles of myosin, kinesin and dynein. Annu Rev Physiol 58:731–750, 1996.

Hirokawa N, Takemura R: Biochemical and molecular characterization of diseases linked to motor proteins. Trends Biochem Sci 28:558–565, 2003.

Kull FJ, Endow SA: A new structural state of myosin. Trends Biochem Sci 29:103–106, 2004.

Mandelkow E, Johnson KA: The structural and mechanochemical cycle of kinesin. Trends Biochem Sci 23:429–433, 1998.

Miki H, Okada Y, Hirokawa N: Analysis of the kinesin superfamily: Insights into structure and function. Trends Cell Biol 15:467–476, 2005.

Oiwa K, Sakakibara H: Recent progress in dynein structure and mechanism. Curr Opin Cell Biol 17:98–103, 2005.

Spudich JA, Motors take tension in stride. Cell 126:242–244, 2006.

Tyska MJ, Mooseker MS: Myosin-V motility: These levers were made for walking. Trends Cell Biol 13:447–451, 2003.

Vale RD: The molecular motor toolbox for intracellular transport. Cell 112:467–480, 2003.

CHAPTER 37

Intracellular Motility

V irtually every component inside living cells moves to some extent, but the magnitude and velocity of these movements vary by orders of magnitude depending on the cell (Table 37-1 and Fig. 37-1). At one extreme, the bulk cytoplasm of algae and giant amoebas streams tens of micrometers per second. At the other extreme, small molecules and macromolecules diffuse through cytoplasm essentially unnoticed. The network of cytoskeletal polymers has a pore size of less than 50 nm, so particles that are larger than the pores must be transported actively. For example, messenger RNA (mRNA) moves from its site of synthesis in the nucleus through nuclear pores into the cytoplasm and then may be carried actively to specific parts of the cell. The nucleus rotates back and forth in most cells. Lysosomes, mitochondria, secretory vesicles, and endosomes all move around actively in cytoplasm, frequently between the centrosome and the cell periphery. Intracellular pathogenic bacteria and viruses subvert the host cell's actin system to propel themselves randomly through the cytoplasm. Virus particles move along microtubules.

Table 37-1

VELOCITIES OF INTRACELLULAR MOVEMENTS

System	Velocity ($\mu m\,s^{-1}$)	Mechanism
Microtubule Motors		
Anterograde fast axonal transport, squid	1	Individual kinesin motors
Retrograde fast axonal transport, squid	2	Individual dynein motors
Chromosome movement in anaphase of mitosis	0.003–0.2	Motors plus depolymerization
Endoplasmic reticulum sliding, Newt cell	0.1	Individual kinesin motors
Slow axonal transport, rat nerves	0.002–0.1 net 1 (intermittent)	Motors on microtubules
Microtubule Polymerization		
Endoplasmic reticulum tip elongation, Newt cell	0.1	Microtubule polymerization
Actin-Myosin Motors		
Cytoplasmic streaming, *Nitella*	60	Myosin motors on tracks
Cytoplasmic streaming, *Physarum*	500	Actin-myosin contraction
Actin Polymerization		
Actin-propelled comet, *Listeria*	0.5	Actin polymerization

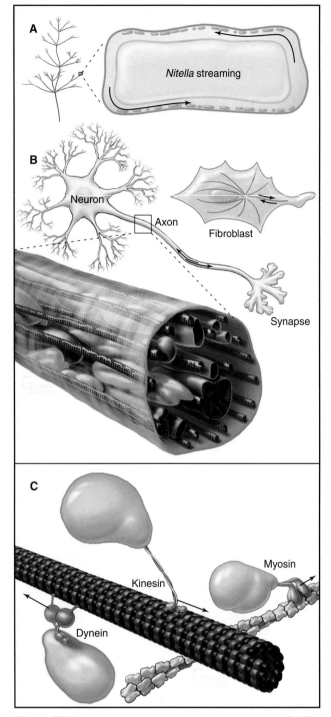

Figure 37-1 MECHANISMS OF INTRACELLULAR MOVEMENT. **A,** The green alga *Nitella* moves cytoplasmic organelles along bundles of actin filaments *(yellow)* located in the cell cortex. **B,** Fibroblasts and neurons move organelles bidirectionally along microtubules *(red)*. **C,** Microtubule-based and actin filament–based motors.

forms of myosin, kinesin, and dynein are dedicated to particular movements. In most cases, transport involves single organelles, but vigorous organelle transport can even result in bulk movement of the cytoplasm. Alternatively, cytoplasmic contractions generated by myosin and actin filaments can produce cytoplasmic streaming, like squeezing toothpaste from a tube. Polymerization and depolymerization of microtubules and actin filaments also produce special types of intracellular movements.

Motor-driven movements on microtubules in animal cells generally receive the most attention, but this chapter takes a broad view across biology, highlighting all of the mechanisms for intracellular transport. Chapters on membrane traffic (see Chapters 20 to 22) and mitosis (see Chapter 44) cover more examples of intracellular movements.

Strategies to Identify Tracks and Motors

Historically, experiments with drugs that depolymerize or stabilize actin filaments or microtubules (see Boxes 33-1 and 34-1) provided the first clues about the cytoskeletal polymers that support various biological movements. Identifying the participating motors, if any, has been much more challenging, given a minimum five myosin genes, six kinesin genes, and one dynein gene in budding yeast and about ten times more motor protein genes in humans. A limited number of pharmacologic agents (Box 37-1) can implicate some motors, but the most definitive approach is to alter motor activity or abundance genetically or by RNAi-mediated depletion. Some motors are essential, so deletion mutations are lethal. Conditional mutations have allowed many definitive tests for the functions of these motors in yeast and, in a few cases, in more complex organisms. Other motors are not essential in the sense that cells have alternative strategies that can compensate if the protein is missing or inactive; nevertheless, the protein may have an important function. For example, dynein contributes to mitosis, but *Drosophila* tissue culture cells that are depleted of dynein can complete mitosis, though only after a long delay during which other motors take over.

Rapid Movements along Microtubules

Organelles in most cells are capable of moving at relatively high velocities, on the order of 1 μm s^{-1} (Table 37-1) along linear microtubule tracks. Thus, the organi-

Two ancient mechanisms (Fig. 37-1) account for most intracellular movements in eukaryotes. Transport along microtubules by kinesin or dynein predominates in animal cells. Transport along actin filaments by myosin is more important in plants and fungi. Specialized iso-

Few selective pharmacologic agents were available to inhibit motor proteins until recently, when academic and biotech labs discovered small organic molecules that inhibit particular motors. A small compound named monasterol inhibits kinesin-5, resulting in monopolar mitotic spindles that fail to segregate the chromosomes. Higher-affinity inhibitors of kinesin-5 are being tested for cancer therapy. A chemical called blebbistatin inhibits cytoplasmic and skeletal muscle myosin-II (but not smooth muscle myosin-II) and blocks cytokinesis. Vanadate and ultraviolet light can inactivate dynein. Vanadate binds to the γ-phosphate site of dynein-ADP, but it binds similarly to other ATPases, so it is not specific. However, ultraviolet light has a novel effect on the dynein-ADP-vanadate complex: It cleaves and inactivates the dynein heavy chain.

zation of microtubules determines the patterns of these movements (Fig. 37-1; also see Fig. 34-2). Such movements are typically intermittent.

Microtubule-based motor proteins, kinesins and dyneins, power organelle movement along microtubules. Kinesins move organelles toward microtubule plus ends, which are located near the periphery of cells with microtubules radiating from centrosomes. Dyneins are responsible for organelle movements toward the minus ends of microtubules, located at the cell center. Intraflagellar transport of proteins in cilia and flagella (see Fig. 38-20) shares many features with the movements of organelles. Movements of organelles along microtubules have been reconstituted with purified dynein and kinesin. Final proof of the responsible motors usually depends on genetic tests.

An assembly of proteins called the **dynactin complex** regulates the ability of dynein to transport membranes along microtubules (Fig. 37-2). This complex consists of a short filament of the actin-related protein Arp1 and seven other subunits, including heterodimeric capping protein. The 150-kD subunit (p150^{glued}) binds to an intermediate chain of dynein. The Arp-1 filament interacts with spectrin associated with the membrane. Mutations in *Drosophila* p150^{glued} cause developmental defects in the eye and brain. Some patients with inherited forms of motor neuron degeneration also have mutations of p150^{glued}.

Several different proteins link kinesins to transported membranes. Each link is intriguing for reasons independent of intracellular motility. For example, the transmembrane amyloid precursor protein not only binds directly to kinesin-1 light chain but in Alzheimer's disease also is cleaved to produce amyloid-β peptide—a toxic peptide that is implicated in neuronal death.

Another transmembrane protein, JIP-3, binds MAP kinase cascade kinases in addition to kinesin-1 light chains. Mutations in the gene for *Drosophila* JIP-3 disrupt axonal transport and clog axons with clumps of vesicles. Adapter proteins link kinesin-1 light chains to transmembrane receptor proteins or AMPA glutamate receptors. A PH-domain on kinesin-3 targets the protein to membrane polyphosphoinositides and promotes the formation of dimers, which makes the motor processive. These examples illustrate that many mechanisms exist to link specific kinesin motors to a wide variety of transported vesicles and that much interesting biology will emerge from further characterization.

Fast Axonal Transport

Analysis of microtubule-based movements is particularly favorable in axons of nerve cells because axons are long (up to 1 m) but narrow, the microtubules have a uniform polarity, and organelles move at steady rates in both directions. Furthermore, nerve cells contain high concentrations of microtubules and microtubule motors; indeed, cytoplasmic tubulin, cytoplasmic dynein, and kinesin were all originally isolated from brain.

High-contrast light microscopy of living axons reveals that most membrane-bound organelles move either toward (anterograde) or away from (retrograde) the end of the axon (Fig. 37-3) with some pauses and even occasional changes of direction. **Retrograde movements** (2.5 μm s^{-1} or 22 cm/day) are faster than **anterograde movements** (0.5 μm s^{-1} or 4 cm/day). At these rates, a round trip from a cell body in the spinal cord of a human

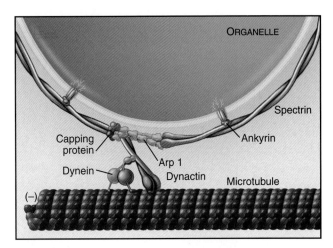

Figure 37-2 **ATTACHMENT OF CYTOPLASMIC DYNEIN TO MEMBRANES BY THE DYNACTIN COMPLEX.** Dynein moves toward the minus end of a microtubule. It is linked to a vesicle by the dynactin complex associated with spectrin on the membrane surface. The dynactin complex consists of a short filament of Arp1 (capped on its barbed end by the capping protein), p50 dynamitin, and by p150^{glued}, which binds both Arp1 and microtubules. (Redrawn from Holleran E, Karki S, Holzbaur EL, et al: The role of the dynactin complex in intracellular motility. Int Rev Cytol 182:69–109, 1998.)

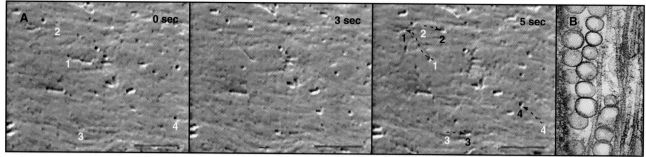

Figure 37-3 FAST TRANSPORT IN CYTOPLASM ISOLATED FROM SQUID GIANT AXONS. **A,** Three frames from a series of video-enhanced differential interference contrast micrographs show movement of organelles in both the anterograde *(right)* and retrograde *(left)* directions. Four large organelles are marked with numbers and colored *green* at zero time, *blue* at 3 seconds, and *red* at 5 seconds. Movement *(arrows in right panel)* is from the *white* to the *black number*. The original video record shows hundreds of smaller organelles moving steadily in either an anterograde or a retrograde direction at 1 to 2 μm/second. **B,** Electron micrograph of a thin section showing vesicles associated with microtubules in axoplasm. (A, Courtesy of S. Brady, University of Texas Southwestern Medical School, Dallas. B, Courtesy of R. H. Miller, Case Western Reserve Medical School, Cleveland, Ohio.)

to the foot and back takes only three weeks. This might seem slow, but if a 0.1-μm vesicle were the size of a small car, it would be moving anterograde at 50 miles per hour and retrograde at 250 miles per hour. In the axons of vertebrate neurons, mitochondria and autophagic vesicles move back and forth in both directions. Their net movement toward the nerve terminal or cell body depends on physiological conditions.

Biochemical reconstitution showed that the plus-end motors of the kinesin family are responsible for anterograde movements toward the nerve terminal and the minus-end motor dynein is responsible for movement in the retrograde direction. Proofs of function are more

complicated in animals, owing to multiple plus-end motors with partially overlapping functions. Nevertheless, kinesin mutations in flies result in paralysis of the back half of larvae, because transport fails in the longest axons. Mutations in three different kinesin genes also cause human nerve degeneration. Point mutations resulting in amino acid substitutions in the mouse dynein heavy chain cause apparently mild defects in retrograde axonal transport in motor neurons, but the affected neurons die with pathology similar to that of human motor neuron diseases.

Classic nerve ligation experiments revealed the cargo carried in each direction by fast transport (Fig. 37-4).

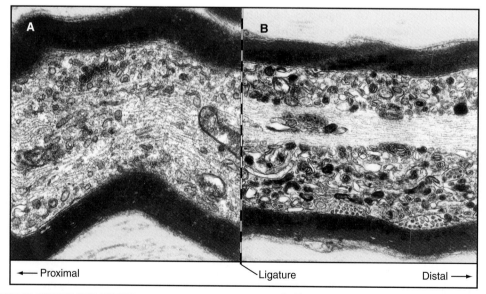

Figure 37-4 ELECTRON MICROGRAPHS SHOWING THE RESULT OF NERVE LIGATION. **A,** The cytoplasm proximal to the ligation demonstrates the accumulation of vesicles and mitochondria, which were being transported toward the nerve terminal to the right. **B,** The cytoplasm distal to the ligation shows the accumulation of lysosomes, multivesicular bodies, and mitochondria, which were being transported toward the cell body to the left. (B, Reproduced from Hirokawa N, Sato-Yoshitake R, Yoshida T, Kawashima T: Brain dynein (MAP1C) localizes on both anterogradely and retrogradely transported membranous organelles in vivo. J Cell Biol 111:1027–1037, 1990, by copyright permission of The Rockefeller University Press.)

When mechanical constriction blocks transport, different organelles pile up on either side. Small, round, and tubular vesicles, including components of synaptic vesicles (see Fig. 11-8), accumulate on the side near the cell body. Fast anterograde transport carries these cargoes from the cell body toward the end of the axon, where they enter the cycle of synaptic vesicle turnover. Endosomes and multivesicular bodies moving by fast retrograde transport pile up on the distal side of the constriction. Retrograde transport can also move signals from nerve terminals to the cell body. For example, when nerve growth factor activates the TrkA receptor tyrosine kinase (see Fig. 24-4) at nerve terminals, the activated receptor is taken up by endocytosis and transported in endosomes to the perinuclear region, where the MAP kinase pathway regulates cell growth. Some viruses also move by retrograde transport.

Dynein piles up on both sides of nerve ligatures. It is associated with vesicles moving in the anterograde direction (toward microtubule plus ends). At nerve terminals, an unknown mechanism activates dynein and reverses the direction of transport. Vesicles that move on microtubules can transfer to and move along actin filaments, using myosin to power local movements at the nerve terminus and in the cortex of the axon.

Many questions remain regarding the control of microtubule motors during fast transport, including how kinesins remain active and dynein remains inactive during the long trip to the nerve terminal, how cytoplasmic dynein on retrograde cargo is activated locally at the nerve terminal and kept active during movement to the cell body, how the bidirectional movements of mitochondria are biased by the physiological state of the cell to achieve net transport, and how defects in fast transport may contribute to neurodegenerative diseases.

Slow Transport of Cytoskeletal Polymers and Associated Proteins in Axons

Many neuronal proteins move slowly from their site of synthesis in the cell body toward the ends of axons and dendrites. This transport is essential, as most protein synthesis occurs in the cell body, whereas more than 99% of cell volume can be in axons and dendrites. If nerve cells were smaller or less asymmetrical, we might not even notice such slow movements. These movements along axons can be followed by labeling the proteins with radioactive amino acids during their synthesis in the cell body (Fig. 37-5A). Proteins that are moved by slow axonal transport are classified into two groups based on their velocities. Tubulin, intermediate filament proteins, and spectrin, which compose the "slow component–a," move exceedingly slowly, about 0.1 to 1.0 mm per day (or 1 to 10 nm s^{-1}). In a human, these molecules take more than 3 months to travel from their site of synthesis in the spinal cord to the foot. "Slow component–b" moves about 10 times faster and includes 10 times more protein than slow component–a. It is a heterogeneous mixture of proteins, including clathrin, glycolytic enzymes, and actin.

Defining the mechanism of slow transport was challenging because various experimental approaches yielded apparently conflicting results. Radioactive labeling established the existence of slow movements and showed that the moving proteins become spread out and diluted as they move away from the cell body (Fig. 37-5A). Photobleaching of fluorescent tubulin and actin in axons of cultured neurons demonstrated that the bulk of these cytoskeletal polymers are stationary (Fig. 37-5B), whereas fluorescent tubulin, photoactivated inside an axon of a cultured *Xenopus* neuron, moves as a block at a rate that is characteristic of slow transport.

This puzzle was resolved by imaging single fluorescent intermediate filaments in axons of live nerve cells. These filaments are stationary most of the time (up to 99%), but occasionally, they move rapidly (0.2 to 2 μm s^{-1}) for up to 20 μm. Most but not all of these movements are away from the cell body, accounting for the net anterograde movement. These rapid but intermittent movements depend on microtubules and are presumably driven by motor proteins. The movements of whole microtubules are similar to those of intermediate filaments. Thus, fast but intermittent transport appears to be slow in assays for bulk transport.

Other Microtubule-Dependent Movements

Other cells use the same molecular mechanisms as neurons to move organelles in the cytoplasm. Secretory vesicles use plus-end motors to move from the Golgi apparatus to the plasma membrane. Endosomes use dynein to move from the plasma membrane toward the cell center. Herpes virus and rabies virus also use dynein for long-distance transport on microtubules from the terminals of sensory nerves to the cell body, where viral DNA enters the nucleus for replication.

The distribution of the endoplasmic reticulum depends on intact microtubules. Strands of the endoplasmic reticulum align with microtubules in cultured cells (Fig. 37-6). This codistribution is achieved in two ways: (1) Motors transport strands of endoplasmic reticulum bidirectionally on microtubules, and (2) other strands of the endoplasmic reticulum attach to the plus end of microtubules and ride the microtubule tip as it grows and shrinks during dynamic instability. This is the best example of movement of an organelle driven by microtubule assembly. The concentration of the

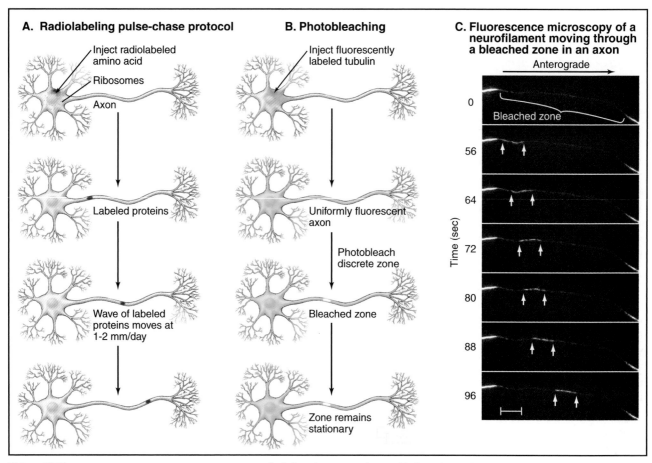

Figure 37-5 EXPERIMENTS ON SLOW AXONAL TRANSPORT. **A,** Pulse-chase experiment. Radioactive amino acids are injected into the spinal cord or eye of an experimental animal. In the nerve cell body, radioactive tracer is incorporated into proteins, which are transported along the axon. Some proteins are incorporated into stationary structures and are left along the way. **B,** Photobleaching experiment. A cultured nerve cell is injected with tubulin labeled with a fluorescent dye. Tubulin fills the cytoplasm and axon as it grows out. A section of the axon is then bleached with a strong pulse of light. This bleached zone is stationary over a period of minutes. **C,** Fluorescence micrographs of the axon of a cultured rat neuron showing rapid transport of a neurofilament labeled with subunits fused to GFP. Note the photobleached region *(bracket)* and the ends of the moving neurofilament *(arrows)*. The neurofilament moves rapidly into the bleached region, but the bleached region does not move because most of the neurofilaments are stationary. Scale bar is 5 μm. (A–B, Redrawn from Cleveland DW, Hoffman PN: Slow axonal transport models come full circle. Cell 67:453–456, 1991. C, From Wang L, Brown A: Rapid intermittent movement of axonal neurofilaments observed by fluorescence photobleaching. Mol Biol Cell 12:3257–3267, 2001. Reprinted from *Molecular Biology of the Cell* [12:3257–3267, 2001] with the permission of The American Society for Cell Biology.)

Golgi apparatus near the centrosome depends on microtubules, because dynein motors transport Golgi vesicles toward the minus ends of the microtubules. Mitochondria move bidirectionally on microtubules in animal cells but depend on actin filaments in yeast. These examples illustrate how not only the dynamics of the organelles but also the overall organization of a cell depend on the activity of microtubule motors. Thus, cellular architecture is determined actively, not passively.

The cellular distribution of nucleoprotein complexes in the cell also depends on active movements. The most obvious example is the movement of chromosomes during mitosis, which depends on microtubule assembly and microtubule motors (see Fig. 44-7). Another example is the asymmetric localization in fly oocytes of certain mRNAs that help to establish the polarity of the

embryos. Specific RNA sequences promote the assembly of protein-containing particles that move at steady rates on microtubules over long distances in the cell (Fig. 37-7). Kinesins and dynein are believed to power these movements, but most of the details remain to be determined. Dynein also anchors localized RNAs in oocytes.

Intracellular Movements Driven by Microtubule Polymerization

Microtubule polymerization and depolymerization have long been known to play a central role in the assembly of the mitotic apparatus and the movement of chromosomes (see Fig. 44-7), as well as the establish-

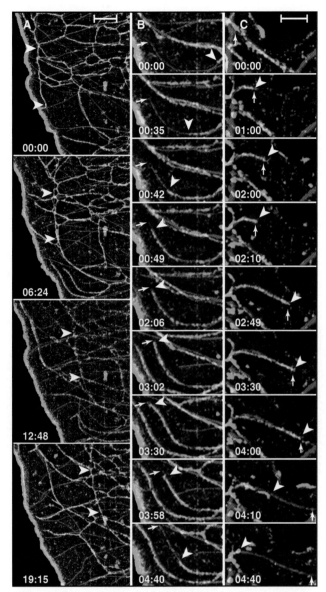

Figure 37-6 **TWO MODES OF MICROTUBULE-DEPENDENT MOVEMENT OF THE ENDOPLASMIC RETICULUM IN A NEWT EPITHELIAL CELL.** The cell was microinjected with rhodamine-labeled tubulin, which incorporates into microtubules, and a lipophilic fluorescent dye (DiOC₆), which labels endoplasmic reticulum (ER). Time series are indicated in minutes and seconds. Scale bar for all panels is 5 μM. **A,** This column of fluorescence micrographs illustrates the dynamics of microtubules *(red)* and ER *(green),* over a period of 19 minutes. Note the strand of ER moving away from the leading edge *(arrowheads).* **B,** Time course of the movement of a strand of ER toward the end of a microtubule, followed by retraction. This type of movement is thought to be driven by a kinesin motor attached to the tip of the elongating membrane *(arrowhead).* **C,** Time course of the movement of a strand of ER attached to the tip of a growing microtubule *(arrowhead),* followed by retraction of the membrane along the microtubule. (Courtesy of C. Waterman-Storer and E. D. Salmon, University of North Carolina, Chapel Hill. Reference: Waterman-Storer C, Salmon ED: Endoplasmic reticulum membrane tubules. Curr Biol 8:798–806, 1998.)

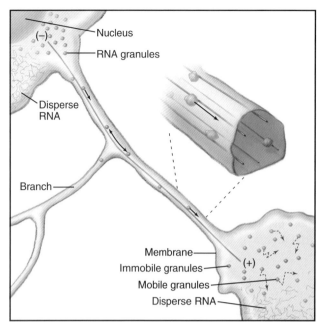

Figure 37-7 Transport of mRNA for myelin basic protein in a cultured oligodendrocyte, a glial cell isolated from brain. mRNA synthesized in the cell body (or, in this case, labeled with a fluorescent dye and microinjected into the cell body) is packaged with proteins in a ribonucleoprotein particle, transported from the cell center along microtubules at a steady rate of 0.2 μm s⁻¹, and released at the periphery, where it moves randomly at 1 μm/s. (Redrawn from Ainger K, Avossa D, Morgan F, et al: Transport and localization of exogenous myelin basic protein mRNA microinjected into oligodendrocytes. J Cell Biol 123:431–441, 1993, by copyright permission of The Rockefeller University Press.)

ment of cellular asymmetry (see Fig. 34-2). Polymerizing microtubules can exert substantial forces, but the force will buckle microtubules longer than about 10 μm. Consequently, microtubule pushing mechanisms work best over short distances, such as for positioning the nucleus in fission yeast cells and the mitotic spindle in budding yeast cells.

Remarkably, the depolymerizing end of a microtubule can also pull on attached cargo. An in vitro proof-of-principle experiment (Fig. 37-8) showed that

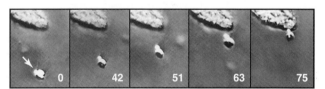

Figure 37-8 **TRANSPORT OF AN ISOLATED CHROMOSOME ON A SHORTENING MICROTUBULE IN VITRO.** A microtubule was grown from brain tubulin nucleated by a basal body in the extracted carcass of a ciliate, *Tetrahymena.* A chromosome *(arrow)* was added as a test cargo and captured by the end of the microtubule. When the concentration of tubulin was reduced, the microtubule shortened, carrying along the chromosome attached to its tip. This transport occurs in the absence of ATP or GTP. (Courtesy of J. R. McIntosh, University of Colorado, Boulder.)

chromosomes can ride along on the end of a depolymerizing microtubule, even in the absence of ATP or GTP. Presumably, multiple weak bonds between the chromosome and the side of the microtubule near its end rearrange rapidly enough to maintain attachment, even as tubulin subunits dissociate from the end. In budding yeast, the link between the chromosome and the end of the microtubule is a ring-shaped complex of ten proteins. This ring may slide along the microtubule as protofilaments peel away from the end as it shortens.

Endoplasmic reticulum provides the best example of an intracellular organelle that harnesses microtubule growth for movement as an alternative to motor-driven movements along microtubules (Fig. 37-6). A "tip attachment complex," yet to be characterized, maintains a connection between the endoplasmic reticulum and the end of a microtubule as its length varies secondary to cycles of polymerization and depolymerization.

Bulk Movement of Cytoplasm Driven by Actin and Myosin

Bulk streaming of cytoplasm is most spectacular in plant cells (Fig. 37-1A). Although confined within rigid walls, plant cell cytoplasm streams vigorously at very high velocities (up to 60 μm s^{-1}). At this rate, cytoplasm moves 5 m/day. Such **cytoplasmic streaming** is best understood in the giant cells of the green alga *Nitella*. Streaming occurs continuously in a thin layer of cyto-

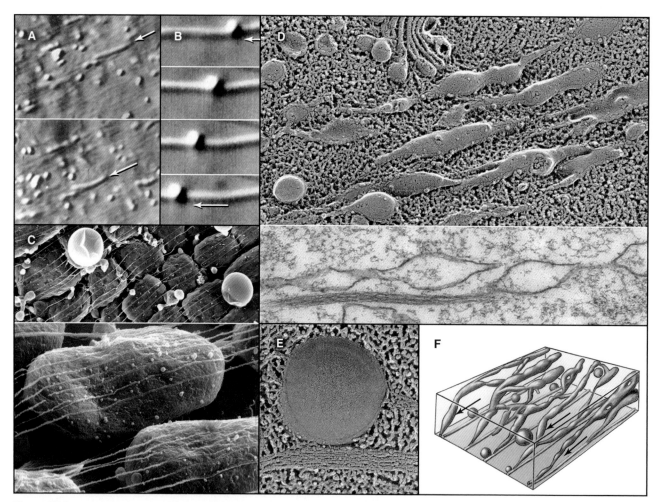

Figure 37-9   CYTOPLASMIC STREAMING IN THE GREEN ALGA *NITELLA*. **A,** A pair of differential interference contrast (DIC) light micrographs showing the movement of organelles in cytoplasm. Note the strand of endoplasmic reticulum (ER *[arrow]*). **B,** Time series of DIC light micrographs showing movement of a vesicle isolated from *Nitella* along a bundle of actin filaments isolated from *Nitella*. **C,** Scanning electron micrographs of the cortex isolated from *Nitella* showing the bundles of actin filaments associated with chloroplasts. **D,** Transmission electron micrographs of a freeze-fracture preparation *(upper)* and thin section *(lower)* showing ER associated with actin filament bundles. **E,** Freeze-fracture preparation of a vesicle associated with an actin filament bundle. **F,** Movement of ER along actin filament bundles dragging along bulk cytoplasm. (Courtesy of B. Kachar, National Institutes of Health. Reference: Kachar B, Reese T: The mechanism of cytoplasmic streaming in characean algal cells. J Cell Biol 106:1545–1552, 1988.)

plasm between the large central vacuole and chloroplasts immobilized in the cortex. On each side of the cell, a zone of stationary cytoplasm separates streams moving in opposite directions. The physiological function of this streaming is not clearly understood.

Bulk streaming in *Nitella* is brought about by movement of endoplasmic reticulum along tracks consisting of bundles of polarized actin filaments associated with chloroplasts (Fig. 37-9C). All of the actin filaments in these bundles have the same polarity, and cytoplasm streams toward their barbed ends. In *Nitella* extracts, membrane vesicles move along actin filament bundles at the same high velocities that are characteristic of the cytoplasmic streaming. An extraordinary type XI myosin pulls endoplasmic reticulum along cortical actin tracks, dragging along other cytoplasmic components, including organelles and soluble molecules. This myosin moves nearly 10 times faster than the fastest muscle contraction, apparently by taking large steps and by the cooperation of several motors working rapidly on the same membrane.

A completely different actomyosin mechanism produces equally spectacular cytoplasmic streaming in the acellular slime mold *Physarum*. In these giant, multinucleated cells, cytoplasm flows back and forth rhythmically at high velocities through tubular channels (Fig. 37-10). Cycles of contraction and relaxation of cortical actin filament networks push the relatively fluid endoplasm back and forth in a manner akin to squeezing a toothpaste tube. Myosin-II is thought to generate the cortical contraction, as it is present in high concentration in this cell and can contract actin filament gels in vitro. (This, incidentally, was the first nonmuscle myosin to be purified in the late 1960s.) The cortical contractions that are so prominent in *Physarum* are also used by giant amoebas for cell locomotion (see Fig. 38-1), cytokinesis (see Fig. 44-23), and movements of some embryonic tissues (see Fig. 38-5).

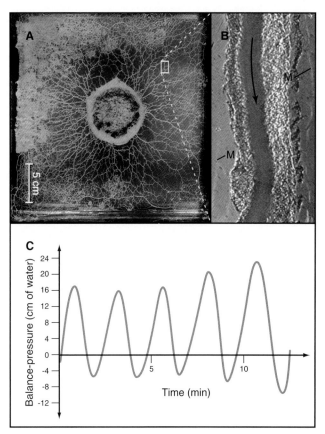

Figure 37-10 CYTOPLASMIC STREAMING IN THE ACELLULAR SLIME MOLD *PHYSARUM POLYCEPHALUM*. **A,** Photograph of *Physarum*, a giant multinucleated single cell growing in a baking dish. **B,** Blur photomicrograph made with polarization optics by taking a time exposure showing the bulk streaming of the endoplasm in a cytoplasmic strand *(long arrow)*. Mucus is designated by "M." **C,** Time course of pressure changes produced by shuttle streaming of cytoplasm through a strand. (B, From Nakajima H: The mechanochemical system behind streaming in *Physarum*. In Allen RD, Kamiya N (eds): Primitive Motile Systems in Cell Biology. New York, Academic Press, 1964, pp 111–123. C, Reference: Kamiya N: The mechanism of cytoplasmic movement in a myxomycete plasmodium. Symp Soc Exp Biol 22:199–214, 1968.)

Actin-Based Movements of Organelles in Other Cells

Like *Nitella*, budding yeasts transport vesicles along bundles of actin filaments from the mother to the bud (Fig. 37-11), although the movements of these solitary vesicles do not produce cytoplasmic streaming. Myosin-V is the motor, so vesicles fail to move from mother to bud in null mutants of myosin-V genes. A myosin-V also transports certain mRNAs along actin filament cables from the mother to the bud, where they determine cell fate.

Animal cells generally use extended microtubules for long-distance movements and shorter actin filaments for local transport. For example, fish skin cells can change color by using dynein to aggregate and kinesin to dis-

perse pigment granules called melanophores along radial microtubule tracks. Myosin-V contributes by moving dispersed melanophores laterally between microtubules. Similarly, mutations causing light coat color in mice revealed that myosin-V is required for some aspects of the transport of pigment granules called melanosomes within and between cells in the skin. A protein called melanophilin links the tail of myosin-V to a small GTPase on melanosomes.

Cytoplasmic Movements Driven by Actin Polymerization

Some intracellular pathogenic bacteria, including *Listeria* and *Shigella*, use actin polymerization to move

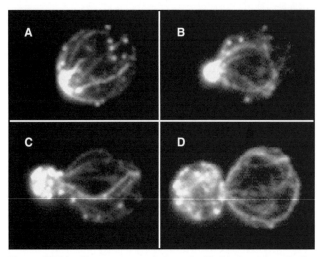

Figure 37-11 Fluorescence micrographs **(A–D)** showing actin fila- ment bundles and patches at various stages in the cell cycle of the budding yeast *Saccharomyces cerevisiae*. Myosin-V uses these actin filament bundles to deliver vesicles (including the vacuole), certain mRNAs, and at least one enzyme (chitin synthase) from the mother to the bud. (Courtesy of J. A. Cooper, Washington University, St. Louis, Missouri.)

through the cytoplasm of their animal cell hosts at about 0.5 μm s^{-1} (Fig. 37-12A). These bacteria hijack the machinery that is used to move the leading edge of motile cells to polymerize a comet tail of actin filaments that pushes the bacterium forward. One end of the

bacterium has a concentration of proteins that directly *(Listeria)* or indirectly *(Shigella)* activate Arp2/3 complex to polymerize a network of branched actin fila- ments (see Fig. 33-13). Growth of this network pushes the bacterial cell forward. The comet tail of cross-linked actin filaments is stationary and depolymerizes distally at the same rate at which it grows next to the bacterium, so it remains a constant length. Under some conditions, cellular endosomes can induce actin filament comets and move similar to *Listeria* rather than using microtu- bules. It is not yet known how widely this phenomenon is used for intracellular motility.

Vaccinia viruses attached to the outer surface of animal cells also use transmembrane proteins to usurp the cytoplasmic actin assembly system to drive their movements at one stage in its life cycle (Fig. 37-12B). Placement of a plastic bead coated with adhesion pro- teins on the plasma membrane of some animal cells can induce similar propulsive actin comet tails in the cytoplasm.

Fungal and animal cells use Arp2/3 complex to assemble small comets of actin filaments associated with endocytic vesicles. Mutations show that endocy- tosis in yeast depends on actin assembly, but questions remain about the contribution of actin to the various steps in endocytosis (vesicle invagination, fission of the vesicle from the plasma membrane and movement of the vesicle from the plasma membrane), which is still being investigated.

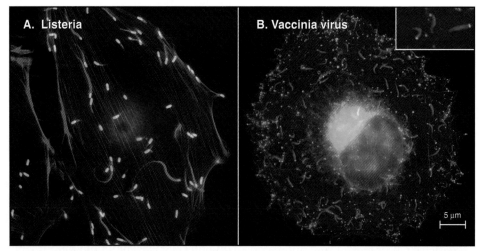

Figure 37-12 Fluorescence micrographs of actin filament comet tails in animal epithelial cells infected with the bacterium *Listeria mono- cytogenes* **(A)** or Vaccinia virus **(B)**. Both pathogens are stained *green* with fluorescent antibodies. They use host cell proteins to assemble a cross-linked network of actin filaments shaped like a comet tail. Actin filaments are stained *red* with rhodamine-phalloidin. **A,** The comet tail pushes *Listeria* in a PtK cell through the cytoplasm and into projections of the plasma membrane at the edge of the cell. **B,** When the replicated Vaccinia viruses in this HeLa cell reach the cell surface 8 hours after infection, they activate Arp2/3 complex to assemble a cytoplasmic comet tail of actin filaments that are thought to enhance the spread of the virus from cell to cell. Actin-based motility of Vaccinia virus depends on tyrosine phosphorylation of a viral transmembrane protein A36R that remains inserted in the plasma membrane. (A, Courtesy of K. Skoble, D. Portnoy, and M. Welch, University of California, Berkeley. B, Courtesy of T. P. Newsome and M. Way, Cancer Research UK, London, England. Reference: Frischknecht F, Moreau V, Rottger S, et al: Actin-based motility of Vaccinia virus mimics receptor tyrosine kinase signaling. Nature 401:926–929, 1999.)

ACKNOWLEDGMENT

Thanks go to Larry Goldstein for his suggestions on revisions to this chapter.

SELECTED READINGS

Chou YH, Helfand BT, Goldman RD: New horizons in cytoskeletal dynamics: Transport of intermediate filaments along microtubule tracks. Curr Opin Cell Biol 13:106-109, 2001.

Cossart P, Pizarro-Cerdá J, Lecuit M: Invasion of mammalian cells by *Listeria monocytogenes:* Functional mimicry to subvert cellular functions. Trends Cell Biol 13:23-31, 2003.

Engqvist-Goldstein AEY, Drubin DG: Actin assembly and endocytosis: From yeast to mammals. Annu Rev Cell Dev Biol 19:287-332, 2003.

Frank DJ, Noguchi T, Miller KG: Myosin VI: A structural role in actin organization important for protein and organelle localization and trafficking. Curr Opin Cell Biol 16:189-194, 2004.

Guzik BW, Goldstein LSB: Microtubule-dependent transport in neurons: Steps towards an understanding of regulation, function and dysfunction. Curr Opin Cell Biol 16:443-450, 2004.

Hathaway NA, King RW: Dissecting cell biology with chemical scalpels. Curr Opin Cell Biol 17:12-19, 2005.

Kamal A, Goldstein LSB: Principles of cargo attachment to cytoplasmic motor proteins. Curr Opin Cell Biol 14:63-68, 2002.

Kashina A, Rodionov V: Intracellular organelle transport: Few motors, many signals. Trends Cell Biol 15:396-398, 2005.

Lopez de Heredia M, Jansen R-P: mRNA localization and the cytoskeleton. Curr Opin Cell Biol 16:80-85, 2004.

Mandelkow E, Mandelkow E-M: Kinesin motors and disease. Trends Cell Biol 12:585-591, 2002.

Mermall V, Post PL, Mooseker MS: Unconventional myosins in cell movement, membrane traffic and signal transduction. Science 279:527-533, 1998.

Pruyne D, Legesse-Miller A, Gao L, et al: Mechanisms of polarized growth and organelle segregation in yeast. Annu Rev Cell Dev Biol 20:559-591, 2004.

Schroer TA: Dynactin. Annu Rev Cell Dev Biol 20:759-779, 2004.

Shah JV, Cleveland DW: Slow axonal transport: Fast motors in the slow lane. Curr Opin Cell Biol 14:58-62, 2004.

Shimmen T, Yokota E: Cytoplasmic streaming in plants. Curr Opin Cell Biol 16:68-72, 2004.

Stokin GB, Goldstein LSB: Axonal trnasport and Alzheimer's disease. Annu Rev Biochem 75:607-627, 2006.

38

Cellular Motility

Cells move at rates that range over four orders of magnitude (Fig. 38-1 and Table 38-1). At one extreme, ciliates, bacteria, and sperm swim rapidly through water, and giant amoebas crawl rapidly over solid substrates. At the other extreme, fungal, algal, and plant cells with rigid cell walls are immobile. However, even some plant cells move, such as pollen, which extends tubular pseudopods. Most cells, including white blood cells, nerve growth cones, and fibroblasts move at intermediate rates.

Cells produce forces for motility in many different ways, most commonly using the same four mechanisms that produce intracellular movements (see Chapter 37): contraction of actin-myosin networks, movement of motors on microtubules, reversible assembly of actin filaments, or reversible assembly of microtubules. These mechanisms often complement each other, even where movement depends mainly on one system. For example, microtubules contribute to actin-based pseudopod extension by helping to specify the polarity of the cell. The chapter compares these standard mechanisms with a few novel mechanisms: contraction of calcium-sensitive fibers of ciliates, reversible assembly of novel cytoskeletal polymers of nematode sperm, and rotation of bacterial flagellar motors.

Most cells possess the proteins that are required for cellular motility, so the striking variation in their rates of movement arises from differences in the abundance and organization of this machinery. For example, both nonmotile yeasts and contractile muscle cells contain actin, myosin-II, heterodimeric capping protein, α-actinin, and tropomyosin. Yeasts use these proteins for cytokinesis (see Fig. 44-24), while muscle assembles high concentrations of similar proteins into sarcomeres (see Figs. 39-2 and 39-3) for powerful, fast contractions.

Cell Shape Changes Produced by Extension of Surface Processes

Simple alteration of cellular shape can be brought about by assembly of new cytoskeletal polymers or by rearrangement of preexisting assemblies of actin filaments or microtubules. One example that is dependent on assembly of actin filaments is the extension of cell surface projections called filopodia (Fig. 38-2).

Studies of echinoderm sperm revealed that actin polymerization drives the formation of filopodia. Fertilization is accomplished when the sperm extend a long filopodium to penetrate the protective jelly surrounding the egg (Fig. 38-3A). Actin subunits for this **acrosomal process** are stored with profilin (see Figs. 1-4 and 33-19) in a concentrated packet near the nucleus. Contact with an egg stimulates actin filaments to

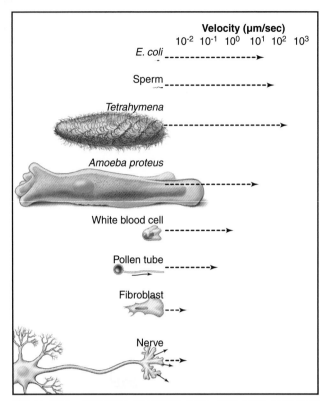

Figure 38-1 VELOCITIES OF MOVING CELLS SPAN MORE THAN FOUR ORDERS OF MAGNITUDE. Scale drawings of cells with a range of velocities.

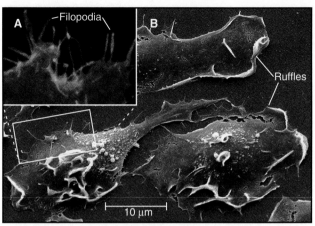

Figure 38-2 **A,** Fluorescence micrograph of the edge of a mouse NIH 3T3 cell expressing formin mDia2 and activated Rif, an Rho-family GTPase that activates mDia2. mDia2 concentrated at the tips of filopodia is stained *red* with fluorescent antibodies. **B,** Scanning electron micrograph of mouse macrophages spreading on a glass slide, illustrating the flat peripheral lamellum, wave-like "ruffles" on the upper surface, and finger-like filopodia. (A, Courtesy of S. Pellegrin and H. Mellor, University of Bristol, England; and from Pellegrin S, Mellor H: The Rho family GTPase Rif induces filopodia through mDia2. Curr Biol 15:129–133, 2005. B, Courtesy of V. Chitu and E. R. Stanley, Albert Einstein College of Medicine, Bronx, New York; and from Chitu V, Pixley FJ, Macaluso F, et al: The PCH family member MAYP/PSTPIP2 directly regulates F-actin bundling and enhances filopodia formation and motility in macrophages. Mol Biol Cell 16:2947–2969, 2005.)

polymerize, starting from a dense structure near the nucleus. Addition of subunits to the distal (barbed) end of growing filaments drives the elongation of the process and the surrounding membrane at a rate of 5 to 10 μm s^{-1} (an astounding maximum of 3700 subunits per second). Actin subunits diffuse rapidly enough from their storage site to drive this rapid elongation, which pushes the plasma membrane forward.

Filopodia on macrophages, nerve growth cones (Fig. 38-7), fibroblasts, and epithelial cells grow much more slowly and depend on formins at their tips (Fig. 38-2) to guide barbed-end assembly. Microvilli of the brush border of epithelial cells (see Fig. 33-2) are short, stable filopodia. The bundles of actin filaments supporting microvilli are cross-linked to each other (by fimbrin and villin) and to the plasma membrane by myosin-I.

Table 38-1

VELOCITIES OF CELLULAR MOVEMENTS

System	Unitary Velocity (μm s^{-1})	Summed Velocity (μm s^{-1})	Motile Mechanism
Striated muscle contraction (biceps)	5–10	4–8×10^5	Actin-myosin ATPase
Filopodium extension, *Thyone* sperm	10	10	Actin polymerization
Pseudopod extension, fibroblast	0.02	0.02	Actin polymerization
Pseudopod extension, human neutrophil	0.1	0.1	Actin polymerization
Pseudopod extension, *Amoeba proteus*	?	10	?Actin-myosin ATPase
Pseudopod extension, nematode sperm	1	1	Assembly of major sperm protein
Retraction of axopodium, heliozoan	>100	>100	Disassembly of microtubules
Spasmoneme contraction, *Vorticella*	?	23,000	Calcium-induced conformational change
Swimming, *E. coli*		25	Flagellum powered by rotary motor
Swimming, sea urchin sperm		15	Microtubule-dynein ATPase

Note: Unitary velocity refers to a single molecular unit. Summed velocity is the overall motion of the cell.

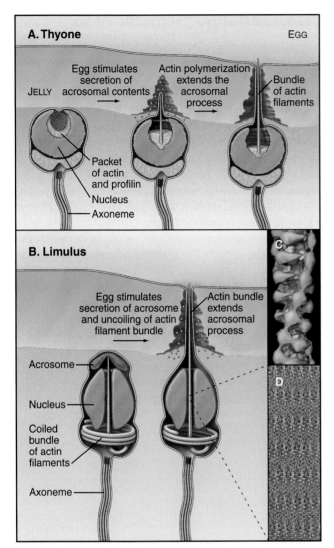

A. Thyone
EGG

Egg stimulates secretion of acrosomal contents
JELLY

Actin polymerization extends the acrosomal process

Bundle of actin filaments

Packet of actin and profilin
Nucleus
Axoneme

B. Limulus

C

Egg stimulates secretion of acrosome and uncoiling of actin filament bundle

Actin bundle extends acrosomal process

Acrosome

D

Nucleus

Coiled bundle of actin filaments

Axoneme

Figure 38-3 SPERM ACROSOMAL PROCESSES. **A,** Actin polymerization drives the growth of the acrosomal process in the sperm of the sea slug, *Thyone*. The acrosome *(red)* is a membrane-bound secretory vesicle, which fuses with the plasma membrane and releases its hydrolytic enzymes prior to growth of the acrosomal process. When the acrosomal process reaches the egg, the plasma membranes of the two cells fuse. **B,** Uncoiling of a bundle of actin filaments extends the acrosomal process of the sperm of the horseshoe crab, *Limulus*. **C–D,** Electron micrograph of the actin filament bundle from the acrosomal process of *Limulus* and a three-dimensional reconstruction of one filament *(yellow)* decorated with cross-linking proteins *(green)*. (A–B, Drawings based on the work of L. Tilney, University of Pennsylvania, Philadelphia. C–D, Courtesy of W. Chiu, Baylor College of Medicine, Houston, Texas.)

Synthesis of these accessory proteins during embryonic development triggers assembly of microvilli. Similarly, cells with few microvilli can be induced to make more simply by increasing the level of villin.

Sperm of the horseshoe crab, *Limulus*, use a novel acrosomal process to fertilize an egg (Fig. 38-3B). They preassemble a coiled bundle of actin filaments cross-linked by a protein called scruin. This bundle is a tightly

coiled spring. An encounter with an egg stimulates rearrangement of the cross-links, causing the actin bundle to unwind. Uncoiling drives the bundle through a channel in the nucleus followed by extension of a process surrounded by plasma membrane that literally screws its way through the egg jelly to fuse with the egg plasma membrane.

A group of ciliates called heliozoans, named for their similarity to a cartoon of the sun, are unique in using microtubules instead of actin filaments to extend, support, and retract long, thin processes bounded by the plasma membrane (Fig. 38-4). Microtubules in these **axopodia** are cross-linked into a precise geometrical array that accounts for the rigidity of these long processes. After mechanical stimulation by prey organisms, axopodia collapse in a few seconds, dragging the prey toward the cell body for phagocytosis. The collapse is caused by rapid depolymerization of the microtubules. Ca^{2+} influx appears to trigger depolymerization of

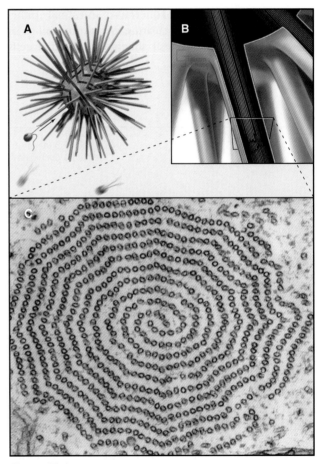

Figure 38-4 DYNAMIC CELL SURFACE PROJECTIONS SUPPORTED BY MICROTUBULES. **A–B,** Drawings of the radiolarian *Echinospherium* (a protozoan) showing projections called axopodia, which capture prey and draw them toward the cell body. **C,** Electron micrograph of a thin section across an axopodium, showing the double spiral array of microtubules. (Courtesy of L. Tilney, University of Pennsylvania, Philadelphia.)

the microtubules, but the details of the mechanism are not known.

Cell Shape Changes Produced by Contraction

Contraction by Actin and Myosin

Cells can change shape by localized or oriented cytoplasmic contractions. Muscle contraction (see Chapter 39) and cytokinesis (see Chapter 44) are the best examples, but contractions remodel many embryonic tissues. Localized contractions at the base or apex of cells in a planar epithelium cause evaginations or invaginations that form the neural tube and glands that bud from the gastrointestinal tract and respiratory tract (Fig. 38-5). Closure of the epidermis over a *Drosophila* embryo also requires contraction of a circumferential ring of cells. Tension generated by myosin-II and actin filaments deforms each cell and, collectively, the whole epithelium. Similarly, contraction of a ring of actin filaments associated with the zonula adherens of intestinal epithelial cells is one factor regulating the permeability of the tight junctions that seal sheets of epithelial cells (see Fig. 31-2).

Calcium-Sensitive Contractile Fibers

The ciliate *Vorticella* avoids predators by contracting a stalk that anchors them to leaves or other supports (Fig. 38-6A). The contractile fibril, called a **spasmoneme,** contracts faster than any muscle. Ca^{2+} released from tubular membranes associated with the spasmoneme triggers contractions, when it binds to a calmodulin-like protein, spasmin, that forms 3-nm filaments in the spasmoneme. Ca^{2+} binding changes the conformation of spasmin and results in rapid shortening, because many spasmin subunits are assembled in series. The spasmoneme relaxes when Ca^{2+} dissociates. Energy for contraction is supplied indirectly by ATP hydrolysis. ATP-driven pumps create a Ca^{2+} gradient between the lumen of the membrane system and cytoplasm. Movement of Ca^{2+} down this gradient drives contraction.

Proteins similar to spasmin are found not only in other ciliates but also in algae, fungi, and animals, where they are called **centrin** or **caltractin.** These calmodulin-like proteins form fibrils that anchor centrosomes and the basal bodies of cilia and flagella. Mutations that inactivate caltractin in algae or yeast compromise the duplication and separation of the microtubule organizers (centrosomes or spindle pole bodies; see Figs. 34-16 and 34-19) used for mitosis.

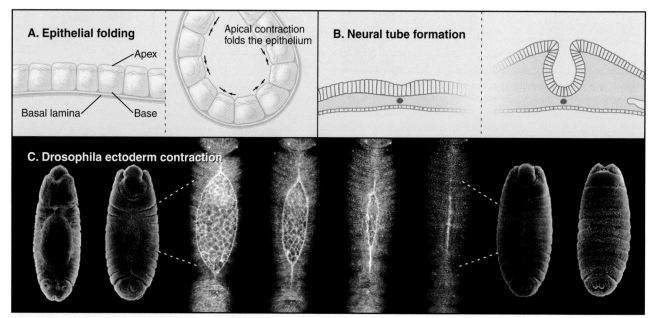

Figure 38-5 ACTOMYOSIN CONTRACTIONS MOLD THE SHAPE OF EPITHELIA DURING EMBRYONIC DEVELOPMENT. **A,** Folding of a planar epithelium into a tube. **B,** Formation of the neural tube by contraction of the apical pole of columnar epithelial cells and cell shape change and invagination of the epithelium. **C,** Contraction around the margin of the ectoderm pulls this epithelium over the surface of a *Drosophila* embryo. The scanning electron micrographs (SEMs [*left* and *right*]) show the steps in the dorsal closure of the epithelium. The time series of fluorescence micrographs (*center*) show live embryos expressing an actin-binding fragment of the protein moesin, which has been fused to green fluorescent protein. (C, SEMs courtesy of Thom Kaufman, Indiana University, Bloomington [see his movie "Fly Morph-o-genesis" at http://www.sdbonline.org/archive/dbcinema/kaufman/kaufman.html]; light micrographs courtesy of D. Kiehart, Duke University, Durham, North Carolina. Reference: Kiehart DP, Galbraith CG, Edwards KA, et al: Multiple forces contribute to cell sheet morphogenesis for dorsal closure in *Drosophila*. J Cell Biol 149:471–490, 2000.)

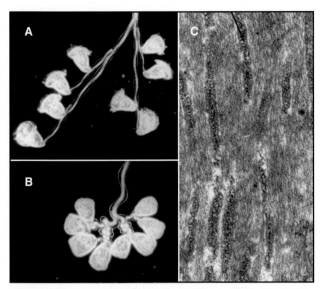

Figure 38-6 CALCIUM-SENSITIVE CONTRACTILE FIBERS. **A–B,** Light micrographs of a group of vorticellid protozoa suspended from the bottom of a leaf, taken before **(A)** and after **(B)** contraction of their spasmonemes. **C,** Electron micrograph of a thin section of contractile fibers and tubular membranes that store and release calcium. (Courtesy of W. B. Amos, MRC Laboratory of Molecular Biology, Cambridge, England.)

Locomotion by Pseudopod Extension

The ability to crawl over solid substrates or through extracellular matrix is essential for many cells. Perhaps the most spectacular example is the slowly moving **growth cone** of a nerve axon (Fig. 38-7A). Although moving less than 50 nm s^{-1}, growth cones navigate precisely over distances ranging from micrometers to meters to establish all of the connections in the human nervous system, which consists of billions of neurons and about 1 million miles of cellular processes. Some epithelial cells (Fig. 38-7B) and white blood cells move much faster, about 0.5 μms^{-1}. These movements enable epithelial cells to cover wounds and allow leukocytes to move from the blood circulation to sites of inflammation (see Fig. 30-13) and to engulf microorganisms by phagocytosis (see Fig. 22-3). During vertebrate embryogenesis, neural crest cells also migrate long distances before differentiating into pigment cells and sympathetic neurons. Fibroblasts lay down collagen fibrils as they move through the extracellular matrix (see Fig. 29-4).

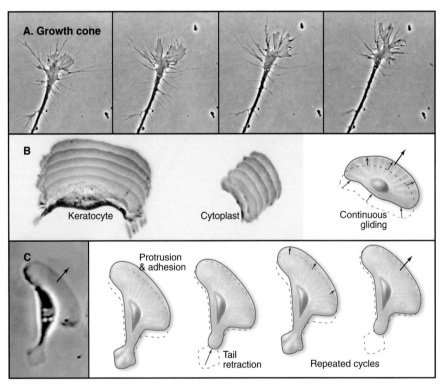

Figure 38-7 MOTILITY BY PSEUDOPOD EXTENSION. **A,** Phase-contrast micrographs of a cultured nerve cell's growth cone at one-minute intervals. The growth cone extends filopodia and fills in the space between with an actin-filled lamella. **B,** Gliding movements of a fish epidermal keratocyte and a keratocyte cytoplast, a cell fragment consisting of the leading edge with most of the cell body including the nucleus removed. Differential interference contrast micrographs at 15-second intervals were superimposed. Drawing shows the pattern of movement. **C,** Phase-contrast micrograph of a keratocyte on glass. This cell moved toward the upper right using cycles of expansion of the broad leading lamella and retraction of the trailing edge from the surface as shown by the drawings. (A, Courtesy of D. Bray, University of Cambridge, England. B, Courtesy of T. Svitkina and G. G. Borisy, Northwestern University, Evanston, Illinois; From Pollard TD, Borisy GG: Cellular motility driven by assembly and disassembly of actin filaments. Cell 112:453–465, 2003. C, Courtesy of J. Lee, University of Connecticut, Storrs.)

This type of locomotion requires coordination of three different events. The cell must extend its leading edge, adhere to the underlying substrate, and (if the whole cell is to move) retract any attachments of its tail to the substrate. Most cells use assembly of actin filaments to extend pseudopods, but nematode sperm accomplish the same thing with a completely different protein (Fig. 38-11).

Pseudopod Extension

Pseudopods that lead the way in cell migration are filled with a dense, branched network of actin filaments with their fast-growing barbed ends generally facing the plasma membrane (Fig. 38-8). Only the leading lamellum is required for locomotion, since it moves normally after amputation from the rest of the cell (Fig. 38-7B). Generally, the leading lamellum is very flat, on the order of 0.25 µm thick, but some cells extend the lamellum

up from the substrate into a wave-like fold of membrane called a ruffle (Fig. 38-2). Microtubules help cells to maintain the polarized shape that is required for persistent directional locomotion, but they are not required for pseudopod extension. A role for actin polymerization in pseudopod extension was originally indicated by the ability of the drug cytochalasin to inhibit the process (see Fig. 33-18).

Microscopic observations of cells injected with fluorescent actin molecules show that filaments assemble continuously near the **leading edge** of pseudopods (Fig. 38-9). Purified actin can be labeled with a fluorescent dye and microinjected into live cells, where it incorporates into actin-containing structures, including the cortical network, pseudopods, stress fibers, and surface microspikes. If the dye bound to actin is bleached locally with a strong pulse of light inside a stationary cell (Fig. 38-9A), the bleached spot moves away from the edge of the cell. The spot recovers as bleached actin is replaced with fluo-

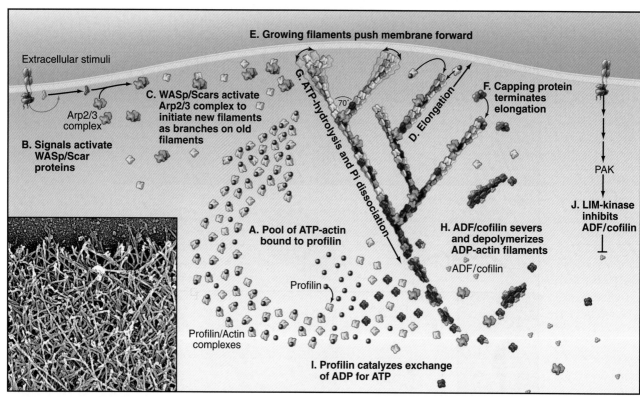

Figure 38-8   A MODEL FOR ACTIN FILAMENT ASSEMBLY AND DISASSEMBLY AT THE LEADING EDGE. The reactions are separated in space for clarity but actually occur together along the leading edge. **A,** Cells contain a large pool of unpolymerized actin bound to profilin. **B,** Stimulation of cell surface receptors produces activated Rho-family guanosine triphosphatases (GTPases) and other signals that activate WASp/Scar proteins. **C,** These proteins, in turn, activate nucleation of new actin filaments by Arp2/3 complex on the side of existing filaments. **D,** The new filaments grow at their barbed ends until they are capped (see **F**). **E,** Growing filaments push the plasma membrane forward. **F,** Capping protein terminates elongation. **G,** Polymerized ATP-actin (*yellow*) hydrolyzes the bound ATP to ADP and inorganic phosphate (P$_i$) (*orange*), followed by slow dissociation of phosphate yielding ADP-actin (*red*). **H,** ADF/cofilins bind and sever ADP-actin filaments and promote disassembly of ADP-actin. **I,** Profilin promotes the exchange of ADP for ATP, restoring the pool of unpolymerized ATP-actin bound to profilin. **J,** Some of the same stimuli that initiate polymerization can also stabilize filaments when LIM-kinase phosphorylates ADF/cofilins, inhibiting their depolymerizing activity. **Inset,** Electron micrograph of the branched network of actin filaments at the leading edge. PAK, p21-activated kinase. (Redrawn from Pollard TD, Blanchoin L, Mullins RD: Biophysics of actin filament dynamics in nonmuscle cells. Annu Rev Biophys Biomol Struct 29:545–576, 2000, with permission from the *Annual Review of Biophysics and Biomolecular Structure*, Volume 29, © 2000 by Annual Reviews, www.annualreviews.org. Inset, Courtesy of T. Svitkina and G. Borisy, Northwestern University, Evanston, Illinois.)

rescent actin through a combination of diffusion and active movement of filaments, assembly of new filaments, or subunit flux through filaments. To assess the contribution of each process, a cell can be injected with actin carrying a "caged" dye. The caged dye is not fluorescent until a blocking group is removed locally by photolysis with a pulse of light (Fig. 38-9B). Fluorescent actin monomers diffuse away quickly, so any fluorescent filaments can be observed. In rapidly moving cells, marked filaments remain relatively stationary with respect to the substrate as the front of the cell advances, confirming that new filaments are assembled at the leading edge. The fluorescence of the marked filaments declines over a period of minutes, as fluorescent subunits are released from filaments and diffuse away. In a third approach, a low concentration of fluorescent actin is injected such that it incorporates irregularly into filaments, producing spots of fluorescence that can be tracked over time (see Fig. 33-18). Analysis of these fluorescent speckles confirms that filaments assemble at the leading edge and turn over rapidly deeper in the cytoplasm.

The molecular mechanism that assembles actin filaments at the leading edge (Fig. 38-8) shares many features with the formation of actin filament comet tails by intracellular bacteria (see Fig. 37-12) and by actin patches in yeast (Figs. 6-3 and 37-11). Chemotactic stimuli (Fig. 38-12) or intrinsic signals transduced by Rho-family GTPases, membrane polyphosphoinositides, and proteins with SH3 domains activate **WASp/Scar proteins,** which promote the formation of actin filament branches by **Arp2/3 complex** (see Fig. 33-13). The pool of unpolymerized actin maintained by profilin (and thymosin-

β4, where it is present) drives the elongation of actin filament branches at 50 to 500 subunits per second. The growing filaments are generally oriented toward the leading edge and push against the inside of the plasma membrane with forces in the piconewton range. Heterodimeric **capping protein** terminates elongation of the branches before they grow longer than 1 μm. Longer filaments are less effective at pushing, since they buckle under piconewton forces.

Actin filament cross-linking proteins stabilize pseudopods. Human melanoma cells that lack **filamin** form unstable pseudopods all around their peripheries and locomote abnormally (Fig. 38-10). These tumor cells recover their normal behavior when provided with filamin. Similarly, *Dictyostelium* cells that lack a homolog of filamin form fewer pseudopods.

The recycling of actin and accessory proteins is essential for multiple rounds of assembly as the cell moves forward. Severing proteins such as **ADF/cofilins** are thought to promote the disassembly of aged ADP-actin filaments located away from the leading edge, although the details are not established. One mystery is how the branched network is rapidly converted into long, unbranched filaments a short distance behind the leading edge (see Fig. 33-2D–E). The side-binding protein tropomyosin protects these longer filaments from ADF/cofilins.

Adhesion: Influence of the Substrate

Pseudopods must establish contacts with the substrate for a cell to move forward. Cells tend to move up gradi-

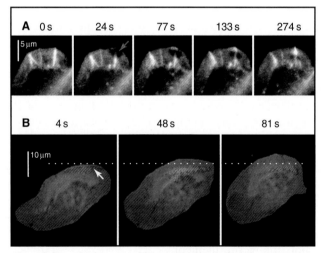

Figure 38-9 DOCUMENTATION OF ACTIN FILAMENT DYNAMICS AT THE LEADING EDGE WITH FLUORESCENT ACTINS. **A,** Fluorescence photobleaching experiment with a stationary cell. Fluorescent actin is injected into a cultured epithelial cell and allowed to incorporate into filaments. A laser pulse bleaches some of the fluorescent actin, leaving a dark spot *(arrow)* that reveals movement of the filaments toward the cell center. **B,** Caged fluorescent actin experiment with a motile cell. Fluorescent dye bound to actin is masked with a chemical group preventing fluorescence. After incorporation into actin filaments of a fish keratocyte (see Fig. 33-2E), dyes in one area of the cell are uncaged with a light pulse *(arrow)*, and red fluorescence is followed with time. Fluorescent actin filaments are stationary with respect to the substrate as the cell moves forward (upward). The fluorescent spot of marked filaments fades with time, owing to depolymerization and dispersal of the fluorescent subunits. (A, Reproduced from Wang Y-L: Exchange of actin subunits at the leading edge of living fibroblasts: Possible role of treadmilling. J Cell Biol 101:597–602, 1985, by copyright permission of The Rockefeller University Press. B, From Theriot JA, Mitchison TJ: Actin microfilament dynamics in locomoting cells. Nature 352:126–131, 1991.)

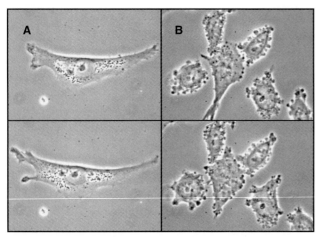

Figure 38-10 CONTRIBUTION OF THE ACTIN FILAMENT CROSS-LINKING PROTEIN FILAMIN TO THE STABILITY OF THE LEADING EDGE OF HUMAN MELANOMA CELLS. Pairs of phase-contrast light micrographs, taken at different times, of living cells grown in serum-containing medium on a plastic surface. **A,** Melanoma cells expressing filamin have normal leading lamella. **B,** Melanoma cells lacking filamin form spherical blebs around their margins and migrate very little. (Courtesy of C. Cunningham and T. P. Stossel, Harvard Medical School, Boston, Massachusetts. Reference: Cunningham C, Gorlin JB, Kwiatkowski DJ, et al: Actin-binding protein requirement for cortical stability and efficient locomotion. Science 255:325–327, 1992.)

ents of adhesiveness but stop if adhesion is too strong, so adhesion with movement requires a compromise. Adhesion must be strong enough for the internal forces to propel the cell forward but not so strong that it prevents movement. Rapidly reversible binding of integrins and other adhesion proteins to extracellular matrix molecules, such as fibronectin, allows adhesion without immobilization. Rapidly moving white blood cells attach weakly and transiently, whereas slowly moving fibroblasts form longer-lasting focal contacts (see Fig. 30-11). Both the chemical nature and the physical nature of the substrate influence adhesion and movement. Cultured cells move up gradients of fibronectin coated on glass. Similarly, neural crest cells migrate preferentially through regions of embryonic connective tissue marked by adhesive proteins.

The growing actin network at the leading edge will either push the membrane forward or slip backward depending on how well it is connected to the substrate across the plasma membrane. In highly motile cells such as epithelial cells from fish scales (Fig. 38-7B) transmembrane adhesion proteins anchor the actin filament network to the substrate, so the polymerization results in forward motion. In stationary cells (Fig. 38-9A), actin polymerizes at the edge of the cell but the entire network moves en masse away from the membrane, a phenomenon called *retrograde flow*. Fibroblasts are an intermediate state, in which actin polymerization produces some forward movement in addition to considerable retrograde flow. Another variation of this theme is seen

in nerve growth cones (Fig. 38-7A), which extend short filopodia and then fill the spaces in between with a lamellum filled with new actin filaments.

Tail Retraction and Other Roles for Myosin in Motility

Growth cones draw out a long process from a stationary cell body, but most cells must break adhesions at their trailing edge to advance. Adherent, slowly moving cells such as fibroblasts exert significant tension on the underlying substrate, when myosin pulls on the actin filaments associated with focal contacts. When tension overcomes the attachments, the rear of the cell shortens elastically and then contracts further (Fig. 38-7C). Myosin also contributes to the retrograde flow of actin filaments in the zone between the leading edge and the cell body. Super-fast giant amoebas (Fig. 38-1) appear to use myosin to generate contractions in the cortex or the front of the pseudopod to drive the bulk streaming of cytoplasm into advancing pseudopods.

An Actin Substitute in Nematode Sperm

Nematode sperm use amoeboid movements to find an egg rather than swimming with flagella like other sperm (Fig. 38-11). The behavior of these sperm is so similar to a small amoeba cell that anyone would have guessed that it is based on the assembly of actin filaments. However, actin is a minor protein in nematode sperm. Instead, sperm pseudopods are filled with 10-nm filaments assembled from a 14-kD protein called **major sperm protein.** Proteins in the cytoplasm and associated with the plasma membrane guide the assembly of the filaments, which function remarkably like actin, despite the fact that they have no bound nucleotide and no known associated motor protein. Light microscopy of migrating cells shows that 10-nm filaments assemble at the leading edge of the pseudopod and remain stationary with respect to the substrate as the expanding pseudopod advances. Filament bundles depolymerize at the interface between the pseudopod and the spherical cell body. A pH gradient is thought to influence assembly at the front and disassembly at the rear of the pseudopod. This highly efficient motility system is still unknown in other parts of the phylogenetic tree.

Chemotaxis of Motile Cells

Extracellular chemical clues direct locomotion by influencing the formation and persistence of pseudopods. Movement toward a positive signal is called *chemotaxis.* The best-characterized example is the attraction of *Dictyostelium* to cAMP (Fig. 38-12), the extracellular chemical that these amoebas use to communicate as they form colonies before making spores. Remarkably, these

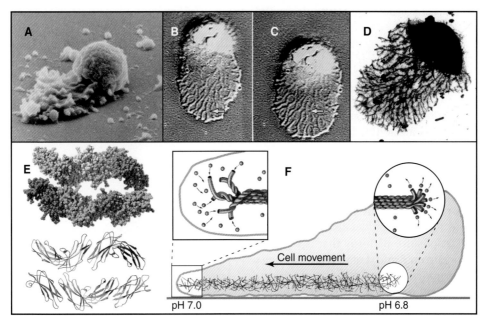

Figure 38-11 MOTILITY OF NEMATODE SPERM. **A,** Scanning electron micrograph of an amoeboid sperm showing the anterior pseudopod and trailing cell body. **B–C,** Time series of differential interference contrast light micrographs showing movement of a live sperm by assembly of a network of fibers at the leading edge. *Arrows* mark the same point in the network, which is stationary with respect to the substrate. **D,** Transmission electron micrograph of an extracted sperm showing the fibers. **E,** Atomic model of a short segment of the sperm filaments consisting of a polymer of major sperm protein (MSP). **F,** Cycle of MSP assembly at the leading edge and disassembly at the cell body. (Courtesy of T. Roberts, Florida State University, Tallahassee, and M. Stewart, MRC Laboratory of Molecular Biology, Cambridge, England.)

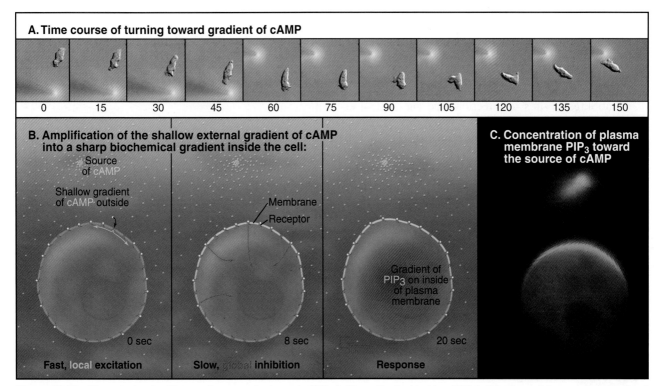

Figure 38-12 Chemotaxis of a *Dictyostelium* amoeba toward cAMP. **A,** Live cell attracted to cAMP *(gold)* released from a micropipette. A time series of differential interference micrographs shows the rapid formation of a new pseudopod and reorientation of the direction of movement when the position of the micropipette is moved at the 60-second time point. **B,** Cells have a uniform distribution of cAMP receptors *(yellow and red dots)* over their surface. A shallow gradient of cAMP activates these seven-helix receptors *(red)*, which activate a trimeric G-protein and phosphatidylinositol-3 kinase, an enzyme that rapidly converts PIP_2 to PIP_3. On a slower time scale, the active G-protein activates PTEN, a PIP_3 phosphatase, throughout the cell. The combination of these two signals creates a steep gradient of PIP_3 across the cell. **C,** Fluorescence micrograph of a cell exposed to a point source of cAMP *(yellow)*. A GFP-PH domain fusion protein inside the cell binds to PIP_3 *(green)* on the inside of the plasma membrane, revealing the steep gradient of PIP_3. (A, Courtesy of Susan Lee and Richard Firtel, University of California, San Diego. B, Redrawn from a sketch by Pablo Iglesias, Johns Hopkins University, Baltimore, Maryland. C, Courtesy of Pablo Iglesias, Johns Hopkins University, Baltimore, Maryland. Reference: Janetopoulos C, Ma L, Devreotes PN, Iglesias PA: Chemoattractant-induced phosphatidylinositol 3,4,5 trisphosphate accumulation is spatially amplified and adapts, independent of the actin cytoskeleton. Proc Natl Acad Sci U S A 101:8951–8956, 2004.)

cells can sense a gradient of cAMP corresponding to a concentration difference of less than 2% along their length. This small difference is amplified into strong internal signals that control motility. Binding of cAMP to seven-helix receptors in the plasma membrane activates trimeric G-proteins inside the cell (see Fig. 25-9). The G-proteins activate pathways that regulate the activity of enzymes that control the concentration of the lipid second messenger phosphatidylinositol 3,4,5 trisphosphate, PIP_3, in the plasma membrane: phosphatidylinositol 3-kinase (PI3K) synthesizes and PTEN phosphatase degrades PIP_3. (See Fig. 26-7 for details on polyphosphoinositides.) A fast positive pathway that is sensitive to local receptor occupancy and a slower global negative signal that is proportional to total receptor occupancy produce a gradient of PI3K activity inside the cell that is steeper than the external gradient of cAMP. These pathways have the opposite effect on PTEN, concentrating it on the plasma membrane away from the source of cAMP. This complementary regulation of the kinase and phosphatase creates an internal gradient of PIP_3 three to seven times steeper than the external gradient of cAMP. Transduction of this internal gradient of PIP_3 into motility requires Rho-family GTPases and formation of new actin filaments. Local polymerization and cross-linking of these actin filaments expand the cortex facing the source of cAMP into a new pseudopod and move the cell toward the cAMP.

Leukocytes are attracted to chemokines and bacterial metabolites at sites of infection (see Fig. 30-13), especially small peptides from the N-termini of bacterial proteins, such as **N-formyl-methionine-leucine-phenylalanine** (referred to as FMLP in the scientific literature). Activation of seven-helix receptors and trimeric G-proteins amplifies shallow external gradients of FMLP into steeper internal gradients of PIP_3 and other signals that control pseudopod formation.

Negative signals also influence pseudopod persistence and the direction of motility. A classic example is the negative effect of contact with another cell. Loss of **contact inhibition** of motility by tumor cells contributes to their tendency to migrate among other cells and spread throughout the body.

Growth Cone Guidance: A Model for Regulation of Motility

Growth cones of embryonic nerve cells use a combination of positive and negative cues to navigate with high reliability to precisely the right location to create a synapse (Fig. 38-13). This combinatorial strategy is much more complex than the simple chemoattraction of *Dictyostelium* to cAMP, as expected for the more complicated task of connecting billions of neurons to each other and to targets, such as specific muscle

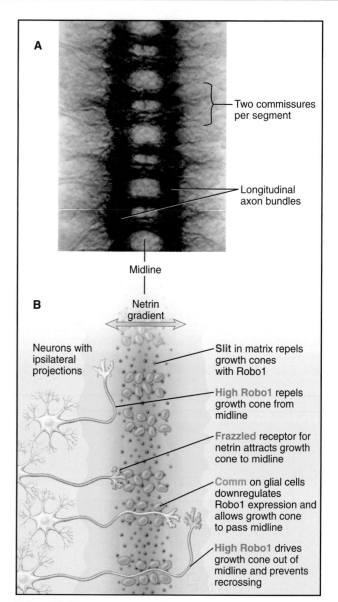

Figure 38-13 *DROSOPHILA* GROWTH CONE GUIDANCE. **A,** Light micrograph of a filleted embryo showing the nerve cord stained *brown* with an axon marker. The axons of about 90% of neurons cross the midline a single time in a transverse nerve bundle called a commissure before running longitudinally in fascicles on each side of the midline. **B,** Drawing showing the ligands and receptors that guide growth cones across the midline and prevent their return to the ipsilateral (original) side. Frazzled receptors for netrin attract the growth cone to the midline where Comm downregulates the activity of Robo1, a repulsive receptor for Slit, allowing axons to cross the midline. (A, Courtesy of John Thomas, Salk Institute, La Jolla, California.)

cells. Cues for growth cone guidance come from soluble factors and cell surface molecules, each requiring a specific receptor on the growth cone. As in other systems, extracellular matrix molecules provide a substrate for growth cone movements. Precisely positioned expression of cue molecules and their receptors guides growth cones along a staggering number of different pathways. The following are some well-characterized examples.

Chemoattractants

Localized cells in the nervous system, such as those in the floor plate of the developing spinal cord, secrete soluble chemoattractant proteins such as **netrin.** Gradients of netrin provide long-range guidance for growth cones of cells that possess netrin receptors (members of the DCC family, including Frazzled) to migrate toward a netrin source. Growth cones without these receptors are insensitive to this cue.

Chemorepellents

A variety of transmembrane and secreted proteins repel growth cones that express appropriate receptors. Netrin is a bifunctional soluble cue, since it also repels growth cones that express other receptors.

Matrix Repellents

Slit, a large extracellular matrix protein, repels growth cones with Slit receptors, which are immunoglobulin cell adhesion molecules (Ig-CAMs) called Robo1, Robo2, and Robo3. Mutations in the genes for these receptors cause growth cones to ignore Slit.

Cell Adhesion Proteins

Ig-CAM cell surface adhesion proteins (see Fig. 30-3), such as **fasciculin II,** prompt growing axons to bundle together in bundles called fascicles by homophilic interactions. Growth cones can be attracted out of these bundles to particular targets, such as muscle cells, that secrete chemoattractants or proteins that antagonize fasciculin II adhesion.

Navigation of growth cones in *Drosophila* embryos illustrates these multiple guidance cues (Fig. 38-13). The original insights came largely from studying the effects of mutations in genes for the various receptors and their ligands. Growth cones of neurons on one side of the nerve cord migrate across the midline to the opposite side and then navigate faithfully to their targets. Netrins secreted by cells at the midline attract growth cones expressing the netrin receptor. However, midline cells also secrete high levels of the matrix protein Slit, which repels growth cones. Growth cones cross the midline by downregulating the slit receptor. Once growth cones complete their journey across the midline, they upregulate the slit receptor, so they never cross back to the side of origin. Local cues alert particular growth cones of motor neurons to branch off of fascicles to innervate individual muscle cells. Path finding by

capillaries uses some of the same guidance mechanisms to grow blood vessels.

Locomotion by Cilia and Flagella

Microtubule-containing axonemes that produce the beating of cilia and flagella are not only exceedingly complex but also remarkably ancient. Diplomonads that branched early in the eukaryotic radiation (see Fig. 2-4) have flagella that share the essential features of human cilia and flagella. This highly efficient organelle for rapid swimming developed well over a billion years ago and is retained essentially unchanged in many parts of the eukaryotic phylogenetic tree. Most protists, algae, and animals have axonemes, but most fungi, ferns, and plants have lost the genes for axonemes.

Cilia and flagella are distinguished from each other by their beating patterns (Fig. 38-14), but are nearly identical in structure. In fact, the flagella of the green alga *Chlamydomonas* can alternate between propagating waves typical of flagella and the oar-like rowing motion of cilia. Subtle differences in the mechanism that converts the dynein-powered sliding of the axonemal microtubules into movements determine which beating pattern is produced.

Both cilia and flagella can propel cells as they cycle rapidly, beating up to 100 times per second. Propaga-

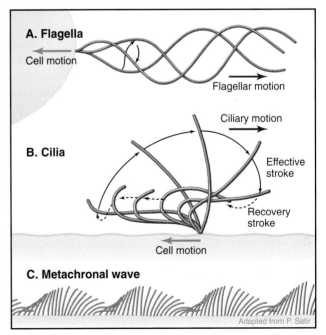

Figure 38-14 BEATING PATTERNS OF CILIA AND FLAGELLA. **A,** Waves of a sperm flagellum. **B,** Ciliary power and recovery strokes. **C,** Coordinated beating of cilia on the surface of an epithelium. (Adapted from a drawing by P. Satir, Albert Einstein College of Medicine, Bronx, New York.)

tion of bends along the length of individual flagella pushes the cell forward. Coordinated beating of many cilia can move large cells (Fig. 38-15). Reversal of the direction of the power stroke allows a cell to swim forward or backward. Alternatively, if the cell is immobilized, like epithelial cells lining an animal respiratory tract, coordinated beating of cilia propels fluid and particles over their apical surface. Ctenophores fuse the membranes of many cilia together to make macrocilia that propel the organism in a manner similar to that of fins.

Although nature has produced some fascinating variations, most cilia and flagella consist of **axonemes** composed of a 9 + 2 arrangement of microtubules surrounded by the plasma membrane (Figs. 38-16 and 38-17). The 9 **outer doublets** consist of one complete A-microtubule of the usual 13 protofilaments, with an incomplete B-microtubule composed of 10 protofilaments attached to its side. Tektin, a filamentous protein in the wall of the A-microtubule, might help to attach the B-microtubule. Like most microtubular structures, the distal end of axonemal microtubules is the plus end. The **central pair** are typical 13-protofilament microtubules.

More than 200 accessory proteins reinforce the 9 + 2 microtubules (Fig. 38-16A), making axonemes stiff but elastic. Genetic analysis established the locations of many of these polypeptides, such as the 17 proteins that make up the radial spokes between the central sheath and the outer doublets. Circumferential links join outer doublets to each other. Central pair microtubules are connected by a bridge and decorated by elaborate projections.

A family of axonemal **dyneins** bound to outer doublets generates force for movement. Each dynein consists of a large heavy chain with globular AAA ATPase domain and a flexible stem anchored to an A-tubule by light and inter-

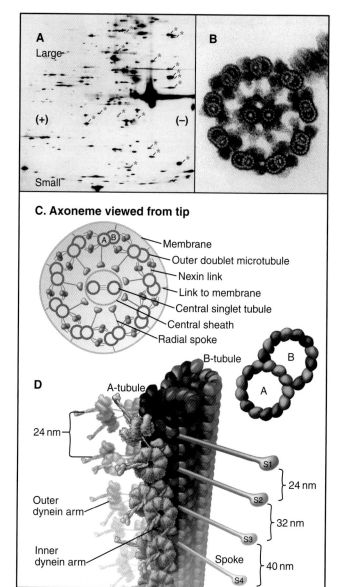

C. Axoneme viewed from tip

Membrane
Outer doublet microtubule
Nexin link
Link to membrane
Central singlet tubule
Central sheath
Radial spoke

B-tubule
A-tubule
24 nm
Outer dynein arm
Inner dynein arm
Spoke
S1
S2
S3
S4
24 nm
32 nm
40 nm

Figure 38-16 COMPOSITION AND STRUCTURE OF THE AXONEME. **A,** Two-dimensional gel electrophoresis separating more than 100 polypeptides of the axoneme of *Chlamydomonas*. Marked polypeptides *(blue asterisks)* are components of radial spokes. **B,** Electron micrograph of a thin cross section of a ciliary axoneme stained with tannic acid. **C,** Cross section of a cilium. **D,** A short section of an outer doublet showing inner and outer dynein arms and radial spokes. In this example, the outer arm dyneins have two heads. In some species, they have three heads. The dimensions indicate the longitudinal spacing between dynein arms and radial spokes. (A, Courtesy of B. Huang, Scripps Research Institute, La Jolla, California. B, Courtesy of R. Linck, University of Minnesota, Minneapolis. D, Redrawn from Amos LA, Amos WB: Molecules of the Cytoskeleton. New York, Guilford Press, 1991.)

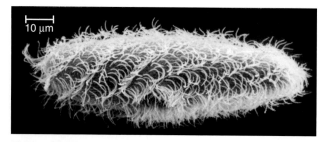

Figure 38-15 SCANNING ELECTRON MICROGRAPH OF COORDINATED BEATING OF CILIA OF *PARAMECIUM*. Waves of effective strokes pass regularly over the cell surface from one end to the other to keep the cell moving steadily forward. (Courtesy of T. Hamasaki, Albert Einstein College of Medicine, Bronx, New York. From Lieberman SJ, Hamasaki T, Satir P: Ultrastructure and motion analysis of permeabilized Paramecium. Cell Motil Cytoskel 9:73–84, 1988. Copyright © 1988 John Wiley & Sons, Inc. Reprinted with permission of Wiley-Liss Inc., a subsidiary of John Wiley & Sons, Inc.)

mediate chains. A thin stalk projecting from the catalytic domain exerts force on the adjacent B-tubule during part of the ATPase cycle (see Figs. 36-14 and 36-15). The outer row of dynein arms in *Chlamydomonas* axonemes are all the same three-headed molecules (Fig. 38-16D).

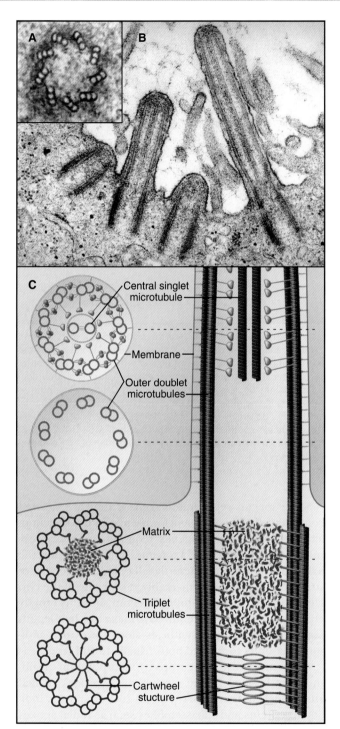

Figure 38-17 BASAL BODIES. **A,** Electron micrograph of a thin cross section of a basal body. **B,** Electron micrograph of thin longitudinal section of basal bodies and proximal axonemes of cilia. **C,** Drawings of a longitudinal section and cross sections of the flagella of *Chlamydomonas*. (A–B, Courtesy of D. W. Fawcett, Harvard Medical School, Boston, Massachusetts. C, Redrawn from Amos LA, Amos WB: Molecules of the Cytoskeleton. New York, Guilford Press, 1991; originally from Cavalier-Smith T: Basal body and flagellar development. J Cell Sci 16:529–556, 1974.)

Labels in figure: Central singlet microtubule; Membrane; Outer doublet microtubules; Matrix; Triplet microtubules; Cartwheel stucture

Seven different inner-arm dyneins are arranged in an orderly pattern that repeats every 96 nm along the A-tubule of each outer doublet.

Dynein-powered sliding of outer doublets relative to each other bends axonemes. Sliding was first inferred from electron micrographs of the distal tips of microtubules in bent cilia. Later, sliding was observed directly by loosening connections between outer doublets with proteolytic enzymes and then adding ATP to allow dynein to push the microtubules past each other (Fig. 38-18B). Sliding can be followed precisely in axonemes stripped of their membrane by marking outer doublets with small gold beads (Fig. 38-18A). As outer doublets slide past each other, the relative positions of the beads change. Dynein attached to one doublet "walks" toward the base of the adjacent microtubule, pushing its neighbor toward the tip of the axoneme.

Biochemical extraction or genetic deletion of specific dynein isoforms alters the frequency and wave form of axonemal bending. Inner dynein arms are required for flagellar beating, and deletion of even a single type of inner-arm dynein can alter the wave form. Outer dynein arms are not essential but influence the beat frequency and add power to the inner arms. Humans with **Kartagener's syndrome** lack visible dynein arms and have immotile sperm and cilia. As a result, affected males are infertile, and both men and women have serious respiratory infections, owing to poor clearance of bacteria and other foreign matter from the lungs.

The mechanism of beating is intrinsic to the axoneme, as sperm tail axonemes swim normally when provided with ATP, even without the plasma membrane or soluble cytoplasmic components (Fig. 38-18A). Experiments with these demembranated sperm models revealed that the dynein adenosine triphosphatase (ATPase) activity is tightly coupled to movement. The beat frequency is proportional to ATPase activity, regardless of whether the frequency is limited by increasing the viscosity of the medium or the enzyme activity is limited by decreasing the ATP concentration.

The bending that produces the sinusoidal waves of flagella or the power and recovery strokes of cilia results from local variation in the rate of sliding of the outer doublet microtubules and along the length of an axoneme. Coordination of these events is not well understood, but at least two factors are involved. Mutations show that the central pair and radial spokes help to coordinate the activity of the dyneins around the circumference of the axoneme as it bends. Mechanical constraints are also required to convert microtubule sliding into coordinated bending. Destruction of the links between outer doublets frees them to slide past each other rather than bending the axoneme.

A **basal body,** a modified centriole similar to those in the centrosome of animal cells, anchors each axoneme

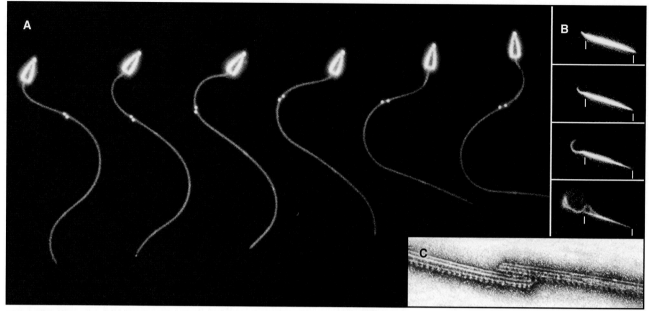

Figure 38-18 SLIDING MOVEMENTS OF OUTER DOUBLETS OF AXONEMES. **A–B,** Time series of dark-field light micrographs. **A,** Sea urchin sperm extracted with the detergent Triton X-100 and reactivated with ATP. Gold microbeads attached to two different outer doublets allow the visualization of their displacement as the tail bends. **B,** Fragment of a sea urchin flagellar axoneme treated with trypsin. The addition of ATP results in outer doublets sliding past each other out of the ends of the axonemal fragment. **C,** Electron micrograph of two outer doublets that have slid past each other in an experiment similar to that in panel **B.** (A, Courtesy of Charles Brokaw, California Institute of Technology, Pasadena. Reproduced from Brokaw CJ: Microtubule sliding in swimming sperm flagella. J Cell Biol 114:1201–1215, 1991, by copyright permission of The Rockefeller University Press. B, Courtesy of Ian Gibbons, University of California, Berkeley. Reference: Summers KE, Gibbons I: ATP-induced sliding of tubules in trypsin-treated flagella of sea-urchin sperm. Proc Natl Acad Sci U S A 68:3092–3096, 1971. C, Courtesy of P. Satir, Albert Einstein College of Medicine, Bronx, New York. Reference: Sale WS, Satir P: Direction of active sliding of microtubules in Tetrahymena cilia. Proc Natl Acad Sci U S A 74:2045–2049, 1977.)

in the cortex of the cell (Fig. 38-17; see also 34-3B). Note that the nine outer doublets of the axoneme grow directly from an extension of the nine outer triplet microtubules of the basal body rather than from amorphous pericentriolar material that initiates interphase microtubules (see Fig. 34-16). In sperm, one centriole serves as the basal body. In some protozoa, basal bodies are used as centrioles during mitosis. In ciliated cells, basal bodies replicate simultaneously from amorphous filamentous material to provide a basal body for each of the numerous axonemes.

Although axonemes function autonomously, they are regulated by signal transduction pathways. Phototaxis of *Chlamydomonas* is a particularly clear example of how fluctuations in intracellular Ca^{2+} can modify flagellar activity. The release of Ca^{2+} affects the two flagella of the organism differentially and allows a cell to steer toward or away from light (Fig. 38-19). Ciliates also have mechanosensitive channels that depolarize the plasma membrane when the organism collides with something. Depolarization opens voltage-sensitive plasma membrane Ca^{2+} channels, admitting Ca^{2+} into the cell. This reverses the direction of ciliary beat. Both calcium and cAMP-dependent phosphorylation of outer-arm dynein can change the beat frequency (all the way to zero) or alter the wave form.

Some species regenerate flagella if they are severed from the cell (Fig. 38-20A–B). Absence of the flagellum activates expression of genes required to supply subunits for regrowth of the axoneme. In about 1 hour, the cell regrows a replacement flagella, and the genes are turned off. Even more remarkably, if only one of the two flagella is lost, the remaining flagellum shortens rapidly to provide components required to make two half-length flagella. Then protein synthesis slowly provides additional subunits to restore both flagella to full length.

Axonemes grow at their tips by incorporation of subunits synthesized in the cytoplasm. A process called **intraflagellar transport** (Fig. 38-20C–D) carries individual proteins and subassemblies such as radial spokes to the growing tip. Kinesin-2 motors move the packets of proteins toward the tip of the axoneme along the outer doublets just beneath the plasma membrane. Cytoplasmic dynein 1b transports particles back toward the cell body. Transmembrane proteins of the plasma membrane also move bidirectionally along microtubules of the underlying axoneme, presumably powered by motor proteins. Intraflagellar transport is remarkably similar to fast axonal transport (see Fig. 37-1) but on a smaller scale. In neither case is it known how transport is reversed for the return trip from the tips of the microtubules.

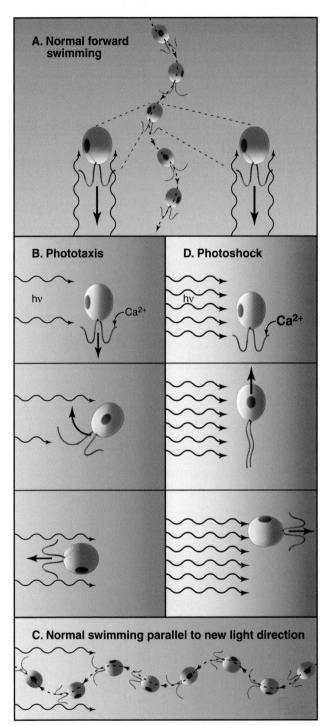

Figure 38-19 *CHLAMYDOMONAS PHOTOTAXIS.* **A,** Normal swimming toward the light using a cilia-like rowing motion of the flagella. Absorption of light by a sensory rhodopsin (related to sensory rhodopsins in Archaea) in the eyespot keeps the cell oriented. **B,** Moderate-intensity light from the side causes Ca^{2+} to enter the cytoplasm from outside the cell. The two flagella react differently, causing the cell to turn toward the light. **C,** Once the cell is reoriented, the flagella beat equally, and the cell swims toward the light. **D,** High-intensity light releases a high concentration of Ca^{2+} and causes transient wave-like motion of the flagella. This backward swimming allows the cell to reorient and to swim away from the light.

Primary Cilia

With the exception of blood cells, most differentiated cells in metazoan tissues produce a single **primary cilium** by growth of an axoneme from their older centriole (Fig. 38-21). The axonemes lack the central pair, and most lack dynein, so they are immotile. Many primary cilia are sensory organelles with special receptors in the plasma membrane. Nematode olfactory neurons have their odorant receptors concentrated in the membranes of primary cilia. Rod and cone photoreceptors in the eye are modified cilia with a basal body and a vestigial axoneme (see Fig. 27-2). Primary cilia on the epithelial cells of kidney tubules act as flow sensors, admitting Ca^{2+} into the cell through mechanosensitive channels in the plasma membrane when bent. Deficiencies in either intraflagellar transport or these ion channels result in polycystic kidney disease, a relatively common cause of kidney failure.

Primary cilia in the "ventral node" of vertebrate embryos are required for the asymmetric location of some internal organs, such as the heart and liver, on one side of the body. These nodal cilia lack the central pair but do have dynein arms on their nine outer doublet microtubules. Asymmetrical beating of the nodal cilia propels the extracellular fluid carrying certain growth factors toward the left side of the embryo. Humans with Kartagener's syndrome and mice that are missing a single dynein heavy chain have an equal chance of having their internal organs, such as heart and liver, on either the normal side or the opposite side, a condition called **situs inversus.**

Specialized Microtubular Organelles

Some protozoa use dynein to generate beating movements of large arrays of cytoplasmic microtubules called **axostyles** (Fig. 38-22). The mechanism seems to be similar to an axoneme, although the organization clearly differs. Cross-linking structures hold together sheets of singlet microtubules, which slide past each other as a result of the action of dynein motors on adjacent sheets. Coordinated beats of the axostyle distort the whole organism, allowing it to wiggle about.

Bacterial Flagella

Bacteria use a reversible, high-speed, rotary motor driven by H^+ or Na^+ gradients to power their flagella (Figs. 38-23 and 38-24). Bacterial flagella differ in every respect from eukaryotic cilia and flagella. The bacterial flagellum is an extracellular protein wire (see Fig. 5-9), not a cytoskeletal structure like an axoneme inside the plasma membrane. Bacteria with multiple flagella are more common than those with single flagella.

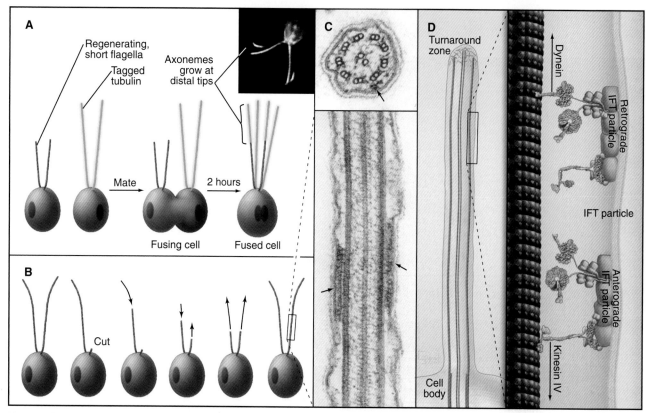

Figure 38-20 FLAGELLAR GROWTH AND INTRAFLAGELLAR TRANSPORT. **A,** Incorporation of protein subunits at the tip of growing *Chlamydomonas* flagella is revealed by an experiment involving the fusion of two cells, one expressing tubulin with an epitope tag that reacts with a specific antibody and the other regenerating its flagella. As is shown in the fluorescence micrograph, tagged tubulin is incorporated only at the distal tips of the growing flagella. Cells with paralyzed flagella made this experiment more convenient. **B,** Time course of regeneration of *Chlamydomonas* flagella following amputation of one flagellum. The surviving flagellum shortens transiently before both grow out together. **C,** Electron micrographs of thin sections of *Chlamydomonas* flagella showing intraflagellar transport particles. **D,** Model for intraflagellar transport. (A, Courtesy of K. Johnson, Haverford College, Haverford, Pennsylvania. Inset, Reproduced from Johnson KA, Rosenbaum JL: Polarity of flagellar assembly in Chlamydomonas. J Cell Biol 119:1605–1611, 1992, by copyright permission of The Rockefeller University Press. B, Based on the work of J. Rosenbaum, Yale University, New Haven, Connecticut. C, Courtesy of Joel Rosenbaum, Yale University, New Haven, Connecticut.)

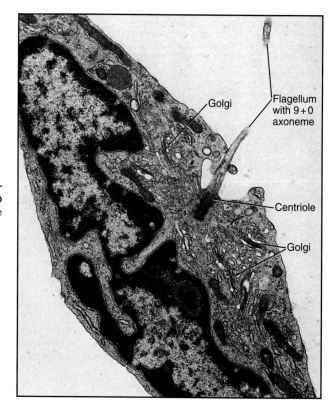

Figure 38-21 ELECTRON MICROGRAPH OF A THIN SECTION OF A MESEN-CHYMAL CELL WITH A PRIMARY CILIUM ASSEMBLED FROM ONE OF THE TWO CENTRIOLES, WHICH SERVES AS THE BASAL BODY. (From Fawcett DW: The Cell. Philadelphia, WB Saunders, 1981.)

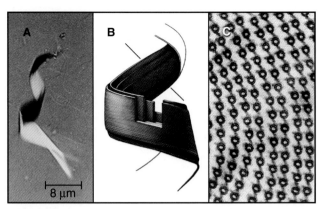

Figure 38-22 MOTILE AXOSTYLE OF *SACCINOBACULUS*, A PROTOZOAN PARASITE OF TERMITES. The twisting motions of this intracellular assembly of microtubules cause the whole parasite to twist and turn in the gut of termites. **A,** Polarization light micrograph of an isolated axostyle. **B,** Drawing of part of the axostyle showing the arrangement of sheets of cross-linked microtubules. **C,** Transmission electron micrograph of a cross section of the axostyle showing microtubules cross-linked into sheets with dynein arms between the sheets. (Courtesy of R. Linck, University of Minnesota, Minneapolis. Reproduced from Woodrum D, Linck R: Structural basis of motility in the microtubular axostyle. J Cell Biol 87:404–414, 1980, by copyright permission of The Rockefeller University Press.)

A motor, embedded in the plasma membrane, turns the bacterial flagellum either clockwise or counterclockwise (viewed from the tip of the flagellum) like the propeller of a motor boat. When multiple flagella are present, counterclockwise rotation forms a bundle. Four flagella propel *Escherichia coli* 30 μm s⁻¹, a velocity of 15 cell lengths per second, equivalent to 400 miles per hour if the bacterium were the size of an automobile. When one or more flagella reverse their direction and

rotate clockwise, the bundle flies apart, and the cell tumbles in one place. Figures 27-12 and 27-13 explain how chemotactic stimuli control the probability of clockwise rotation, favoring steady runs toward nutrients and allowing for more frequent tumbles to change direction to avoid harm.

Assays for rotation of single flagella provide insights about the mechanism of flagellar motion (Fig. 38-23). When a flagellum is attached to a glass slide by means of antibodies to the flagellar filament, the bacterium rotates, providing decisive evidence for rotation of flagella. Similarly, beads attached to short flagella are observed to rotate. The rotational speed depends on the resistance. The motor of a single immobilized flagellum can rotate a whole *E. coli* 10 to 50 times per second, whereas in some species, unloaded motors rotate up to 1600 times per second (100,000 rpm)!

The rotary engine driving the flagellar filament is constructed from two parts: a rotating, cylindrical **basal body** on the end of the filament and a surrounding ring of stationary proteins embedded in the plasma membrane and anchored to the peptidoglycan layer (Fig. 38-24). Genetic screens for motility mutants identified all of the protein components of the motor, and their functions were defined by analysis of the behavior of these mutants. Most of these proteins are present in isolated basal bodies. Two proteins essential for rotation—MotA and MotB—are found in the cell membrane surrounding the basal body. MotA has four hydrophobic segments that are believed to be transmembrane helices. MotB has transmembrane segment in addition to a periplasmic domain anchored to the peptidoglycan layer (Fig. 38-24). Flagella are immotile in cells that lack either one of these proteins. If the missing protein is replaced

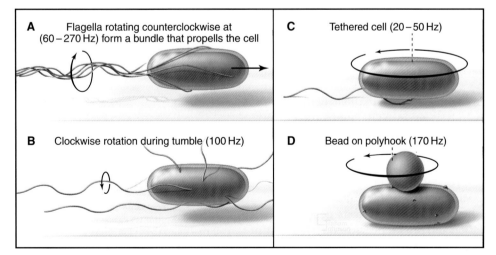

Figure 38-23 DIFFERENT MANIFESTATIONS OF THE ROTATION OF FLAGELLA. **A,** If the flagella rotate counterclockwise, they form a bundle that propels the cell forward. **B,** If one or more flagella rotate clockwise, the bundle falls apart and the cell tumbles in one place. **C,** If a flagellum is tethered to a surface, the bacterium rotates. **D,** If the flagellar filament is replaced by an elongated hook region with an attached bead, the bead rotates. (Redrawn from Schuster SD, Khan S: The bacterial flagellar motor. Annu Rev Biophys Biomol Struct 23:509–539, 1994, with permission from the *Annual Review of Biophysics and Biomolecular Structure*, Volume 23, © 1994 by Annual Reviews, www.annualreviews.org.)

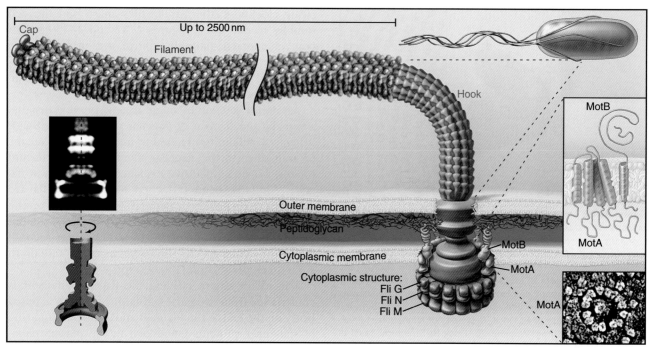

Figure 38-24 BACTERIAL ROTARY MOTOR. **Left,** Averaged electron micrographs of isolated flagellar basal bodies and a three-dimensional reconstruction of this large structure, estimated to have a molecular mass of 4400 kD. **Middle,** Molecular model of the rotary motor in place in the bacterial membrane. **Lower right,** Electron micrograph of a freeze-fractured bacterium illustrating the ring of intramembranous particles thought to correspond to MotA and MotB. (Left, Courtesy of D. DeRosier, Brandeis University, Waltham, Massachusetts. Reference: Thomas DR, Morgan DG, DeRosier DJ: Rotational symmetry of the C ring. Proc Natl Acad Sci U S A 96:10134–10139, 1999. Middle, Redrawn from Schuster SD, Khan S: The bacterial flagellar motor. Annu Rev Biophys Biomol Struct 23:509–539, 1994, with permission from the *Annual Review of Biophysics and Biomolecular Structure*, Volume 23, © 1994 by Annual Reviews, www.annualreviews.org. Lower right, Courtesy of S. Khan, Albert Einstein College of Medicine, Bronx, New York.)

by initiating its biosynthesis, the paralyzed flagellum begins to turn, increasing its speed of rotation in a stepwise fashion, as independent, torque-producing units are added one after another. At the same time, the ring of 10 to 12 transmembrane proteins reappears surrounding the basal body, so these particles are believed to be the motors.

The energy to turn the motor comes from protons (or, in some bacteria, Na^+) that move down an electrochemical gradient from outside the bacterium through the motor to the cytoplasm. Transfer of one proton across the membrane provides approximately the same energy as the hydrolysis of an ATP. Pumps driven by light, oxidation, or ATP hydrolysis (see Table 8-1) generate the **proton gradient.** Flagellar rotation stops when bacteria are starved, and it resumes when nutrients are supplied to allow reestablishment of the membrane proton gradient. MotA is the prime candidate for the proton channel, because mutations in its gene inhibit both flagellar rotation and proton permeability. Roughly 1000 protons cross the membrane for each rotation, corresponding to two protons for each tiny rotational step. Proton transfer is tightly coupled to rotation of the basal body, and the efficiency is near 100%. Detailed understanding of the mechanism awaits determination of atomic structures of the proteins.

ACKNOWLEDGMENTS

Thanks go to Pablo Iglesias, Aditya Paul, and Elke Stein for their suggestions on revisions to this chapter.

SELECTED READINGS

Beisson J, Wright M: Basal body/centriole assembly and continuity. Curr Opin Cell Biol 15:96–104, 2003.

Berg HC: The rotary motor of bacterial flagella. Annu Rev Biochem 72:19–54, 2003.

Bray D: Cell Movements, 2nd ed. New York, Garland Publishing, 2000.

Carmeliet P, Tessier-Lavigne M: Common mechanisms of nerve and blood vessel wiring. Nature 436:193–2000, 2005.

Condeelis J, Singer RH, Segall JE: The great escape: When cancer cells hijack the genes for chemotaxis and motility. Annu Rev Cell Dev Biol 21:695–718, 2005.

Huber AB, Kolodkin AL, Ginty DD, Cloutier JF: Signaling at the growth cone, ligand-receptor complexes and the control of axon growth and guidance. Annu Rev Neurosci 26:509–563, 2003.

Jaffe AB, Hall A: Rho GTPases: Biochemistry and biology. Annu Rev Cell Dev Biol 21:247–269, 2005.

Kamiya R: Functional diversity of axonemal dyneins as studied in Chlamydomonas mutants. Int Rev Cytol 219:115–155, 2002.

Levin M: Left-right asymmetry in embryonic development: A comprehensive review. Mech Dev 122:3–25, 2005.

Manahan CL, Iglesias PA, Long Y, Devreotes PN: Chemoattractant signaling in Dictyostelium discoideum. Annu Rev Cell Dev Biol 20:223–253, 2004.

Moriyama Y, Okamoto H, Asai H: Rubber-like elasticity and volume changes in the isolated spasmoneme of giant Zoothamnium sp. under Ca^{2+}-induced contraction. Biophys J 76:993-1000, 1999.

Parent CA: Making all the right moves: Chemotaxis in neutrophils and Dictyostelium. Curr Opin Cell Biol 16:4-13, 2004.

Pazour GJ, Rosenbaum JL: Intraflagellar transport and cilia-dependent diseases. Trends Cell Biol 12:551-555, 2002.

Pazour GJ, Witman GB: The vertebrate primary sensory cilium is a sensory organelle. Curr Opin Cell Biol 15:105-110, 2003.

Pollard TD, Borisy GG: Cellular motility driven by assembly and disassembly of actin filaments. Cell 112:453-465, 2003.

Praetorius HA, Spring KR: A physiological view of the primary cilium. Annu Rev Physiol 67:515-529, 2003.

Rafelski SM, Theriot JA: Crawling toward a unified model of cell motility: Spatial and temporal regulation of actin dynamics. Annu Rev Biochem 73:209-239, 2004.

Ridge KD: Algal rhodopsins: Phototaxis receptors found at last. Curr Biol 12:R588-R590, 2002.

Ridley AJ, Schwartz MA, Burridge K, et al: Cell migration: Integrating signals from front to back. Science 302:1704-1709, 2003.

Roberts TM, Stewart M: Actin' like actin. The dynamics of the nematode major sperm protein (msp) cytoskeleton indicate a push-pull mechanism for amoeboid cell motility. J Cell Biol 149:7-12, 2000.

Scholey JM: Intraflagellar transport. Annu Rev Cell Dev Biol 19:423-443, 2003.

Weaver AM, Young ME, Lee W-L, Cooper JA: Integration of signals to the Arp2/3 complex. Curr Opin Cell Biol 15:23-30, 2003.

Witman G: Chlamydomonas phototaxis. Trends Cell Biol 3:403-408, 1993.

CHAPTER 39

Muscles

Vertebrates have three types of specialized contractile cells—smooth muscle, skeletal muscle, and cardiac muscle—that use actin and myosin to generate powerful, unidirectional movements (Fig. 39-1). These muscles have much in common but differ in their activation mechanisms, arrangement of contractile filaments, and energy supplies. This provides three options for physiological responses. The nervous system controls the timing, force, and speed of skeletal muscle contraction over a wide range. Cardiac muscle generates its own rhythmic, fatigue-free contractions that spread through the heart in a highly reproducible fashion. Neurotransmitters, acting like hormones, regulate the force and frequency of heartbeats over a narrow range. Nerves, hormones, and intrinsic signals control the activity of smooth muscles, which contract slowly but maintain tension very efficiently.

This chapter explains the molecular and cellular basis for the distinctive physiological properties of the three types of muscle. These specialized muscle cells adapt and exaggerate the same molecular strategies that other cells use to produce contractions, to adhere to each other and the extracellular matrix, and to control their activity.

Skeletal Muscle

Skeletal muscle cells are optimized for rapid, forceful contractions. Accordingly, they have a massive concentration of highly ordered contractile units composed of actin, myosin, and associated proteins (Fig. 39-2). Actin and myosin filaments are organized into **sarcomeres,** aligned contractile units that give the cells a striped appearance in the microscope. For this reason, they are called striated muscles. Myosin uses ATP hydrolysis to power contraction, which results from myosin-powered sliding of actin-based thin filaments past myosin-containing thick filaments. Speed is achieved by linking many sarcomeres in series. Force is determined by the number of sarcomeres contracting in parallel.

Although skeletal muscle *cells* have only two states—inactive (relaxed) or active (contracting)—skeletal *muscles* produce a wide range of contractions, varying from slow and delicate to rapid and forceful. These **graded contractions** are achieved by varying the *number* of muscle cells activated by voluntary or reflex signals from the nervous system (Fig. 39-14). Nerve impulses stimulate a transient rise in cytoplasmic calcium that activates the contractile proteins.

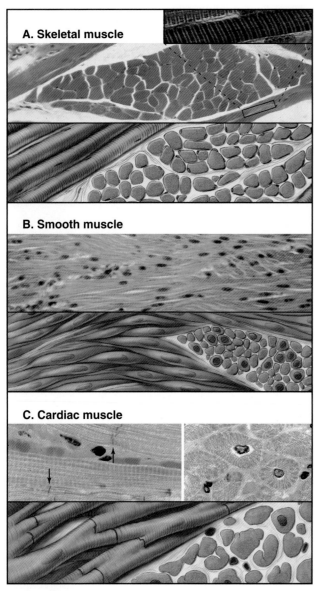

Figure 39-1 LIGHT MICROGRAPHS AND INTERPRETIVE DRAWINGS OF HISTOLOGIC SECTIONS OF SKELETAL, CARDIAC, AND SMOOTH MUSCLES. **A,** Skeletal muscle cells are shaped like cylinders and may be up to 50 cm long. Multiple nuclei are located near the plasma membrane. Striations are seen in the inset, a longitudinal section at high magnification. **B,** Smooth muscle cells are spindle-shaped with homogeneous cytoplasm and single nuclei. **C,** Cardiac muscle cells are striated and have one or two nuclei. Adhesive junctions called intercalated disks (*bright pink vertical bars* in the longitudinal section, *top left arrows*) bind these short cells together end to end.

Organization of the Skeletal Muscle Contractile Apparatus

Skeletal muscle cells (also called muscle fibers in the physiological literature) are among the largest cells of vertebrates. During development, mesenchymal stem cells give rise to progenitor cells with single nuclei called myoblasts. A family of master transcription factors, including MyoD and myogenin, coordinates the expression of specialized muscle proteins. As they differentiate, numbers of myoblasts fuse and elongate to form muscle cells with multiple nuclei and lengths of millimeters to tens of centimeters. The number of muscle cells is determined genetically and is relatively stable throughout life even as the size of the cells varies with the level of exercise and nutrition. Mature muscles harbor small numbers of stem cells (called satellite cells [see Fig. 41-15]) with a limited capacity to differentiate and repair damage.

A basal lamina (see Fig. 29-18C) surrounds and supports each muscle cell. At the ends of each cell, actin thin filaments are anchored to the plasma membrane at myotendinous junctions, which are similar to focal contacts (see Fig. 30-11). Integrins spanning the membrane link actin filaments to the basal lamina and to collagen fibrils of tendons. These physical connections transmit contractile force to the skeleton.

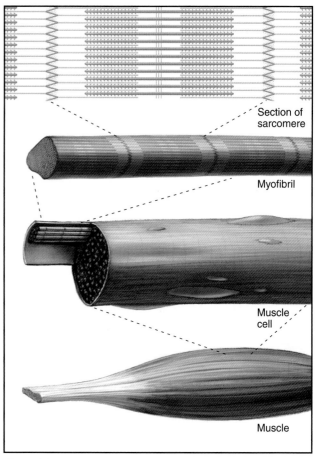

Section of sarcomere

Myofibril

Muscle cell

Muscle

Figure 39-2 CONTRACTILE APPARATUS OF STRIATED MUSCLES. The contractile unit is the sarcomere, an interdigitating array of thick and thin filaments. Sarcomeres are arranged end to end into long, rod-shaped myofibrils that run the length of the cell. Mitochondria and smooth endoplasmic reticulum separate myofibrils, which can readily be isolated for functional and biochemical studies.

Organization of the Actomyosin Apparatus

Interdigitation of thick, bipolar, myosin filaments and thin actin filaments in the sarcomeres of living muscle cells is so precise (Fig. 39-3) that it yields an X-ray diffraction pattern (Fig. 39-13) revealing the spacing of the filaments and the helical repeats of their subunits to a resolution of about 3 nm. **Z disks** at both ends of the sarcomere anchor the barbed ends of the actin fila-

ments, so their pointed ends are near the center of the sarcomere. Myosin heads project from the surface of **thick filaments,** whereas their tails are anchored in the filament backbone. Thick and **thin filaments** overlap, with the myosin heads only a few nanometers away from adjacent actin filaments. The alignment and interdigitation of the filaments facilitate the sliding interactions required to produce contraction.

An important, simplifying architectural feature is that sarcomeres are symmetrical about their middles (Fig. 39-3). Consequently, the polarity of myosin relative to the actin filaments is the same in both halves of the sarcomere, allowing the same force-generating mechanism to work at both ends of the bipolar myosin filaments. Sarcomeres are organized end to end into long, cylindrical assemblies called **myofibrils** (Fig. 39-2) that retain their contractility even after isolation from muscle.

Thin Filaments

Thin filaments consist of actin and the tightly bound regulatory proteins **troponin** and **tropomyosin** (Fig. 39-4). When the concentration of Ca^{2+} is low in cytoplasm, troponin and tropomyosin inhibit the actin-activated ATPase of myosin. Tropomyosin, a 40-nm long coiled-coil of two α-helical polypeptides (see Fig. 3-10), binds laterally to seven contiguous actin subunits as well as head to tail to neighboring tropomyosins, forming a continuous strand along the whole thin filament. Troponin (TN) consists of three different subunits called TNC, TNI, and TNT (Table 39-1). TNT anchors troponin to tropomyosin. Like calmodulin (see Fig. 3-12 and Chapter 26), TNC is a dumbbell-shaped protein with four EF-hand motifs to bind divalent cations. In resting muscle the C-terminal globular domain of TNC binds two Mg^{2+} ions and an N-terminal α-helix of TNI, while the two low-affinity sites in the N-terminal globular domain of TNC are empty. Ca^{2+} binding to the low-affinity sites during muscle activation exposes a new binding site for TNI. The resulting conformational change in TNI allows tropomyosin to expose myosin-binding sites on the actin filament.

A protein meshwork in the Z disk anchors the barbed end of each thin filament (Fig. 39-5). Some cross-links between actin filaments consist of α-actinin, a short rod with actin-binding sites on each end (see Fig. 33-16). At least a half dozen structural proteins stabilize the Z disk through interactions with α-actinin, actin, and titin in the Z disk.

Proteins cap both ends of thin filaments. **Cap-Z,** the muscle isoform of capping protein (see Fig. 33-14), binds the barbed ends of thin filaments with high affinity, limiting actin subunit addition or loss. **Tropomodulin** associates with both tropomyosin and actin to cap and stabilize the pointed end of thin filaments (Fig. 39-4B).

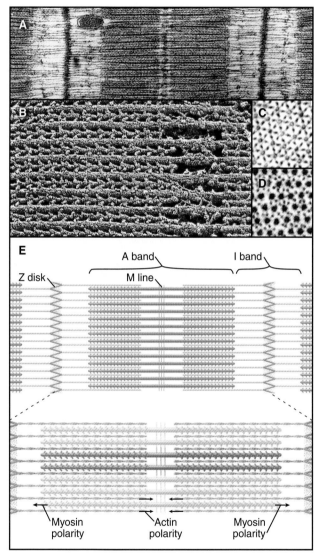

Figure 39-3 ELECTRON MICROGRAPHS AND DRAWINGS OF SARCOMERES. **A,** Longitudinal thin section showing the array of thin filaments anchored to Z disks and overlapping bipolar thick filaments cross-linked in the middle at the M line. **B,** Longitudinal freeze-fractured, etched, and shadowed sarcomere showing myosin cross-bridges attached to thin filaments near the bare zone in the center *(right)* of a sarcomere. **C–D,** Cross-sections of insect flight muscle and vertebrate skeletal muscle showing the double hexagonal arrays of thick and thin filaments. **E,** Drawings indicating the polarity of the thick and thin filaments. (A and C, Courtesy of H. E. Huxley, Brandeis University, Waltham, Massachusetts. B and D, Courtesy of J. Heuser, Washington University, St. Louis, Missouri.)

Figure 39-4 **THIN FILAMENT STRUCTURE. A,** Three-dimensional reconstruction from electron micrographs of a thin filament from vertebrate skeletal muscle showing actin and the position of tropomyosin in relaxed muscle. **B,** Drawing of a model of a thin filament from active muscle. Each tropomyosin is associated with seven actin subunits. The structure and binding sites of troponin and tropomodulin have been inferred from biochemical experiments. **C,** Ribbon diagrams of the atomic structures of troponin C, free and bound to a troponin I peptide. Two divalent cation-binding EF-hands are found at each end, separated by a long α-helix. In cells, two high-affinity sites at the C-terminal end are permanently occupied with Mg^{2+}. Two low-affinity sites at the other end are unoccupied in relaxed muscle but bind Ca^{2+} when muscle is activated. (A, Courtesy of W. Lehman, Boston University, Massachusetts. C, PDB files: 1AX2 and 1TROP.)

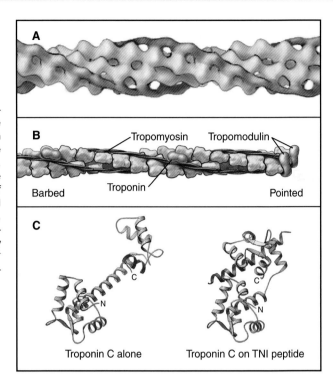

Table 39-1

SARCOMERE PROTEINS OF VERTEBRATE STRIATED MUSCLES

Name	Size (kD)	Domains	Functions
Thick Filament			
Myosin	2 × 200	Heavy chain	Motor, backbone of thick filament
	2 × 20	Light chain	
	2 × 18 or 25	Light chain	
C protein	128	Ig, FNIII	Stabilizes thick filament
M Line			
MM-creatine phosphokinase	2 × 43		Glycolytic enzyme
M protein	165	IgC2, FNIII	M-line structure
Myomesin (skelemin)	185	IgC2, FN III	Link M-disk to desmin
Thin Filament			
Actin	43		Backbone of thin filaments
Tropomyosin	2 × 35	Coiled-coil	Blocks myosin binding to actin filament
Troponin C	18	4 × EF-hand	Calcium-binding component of troponin
Troponin I	21		Inhibitory component of troponin
Troponin T	31		Tropomyosin-binding component of troponin
Tropomodulin	43		Binds tropomyosin at pointed end of actin filament
Nebulin	500–900	>200 × 35 residues	Binds thin filament
Z Disk			
α-Actinin	2 × 100	Actin binding	Cross-links thin filaments in the Z disk
CapZ	31 + 32		Blocks barbed end of thin filaments
Elastic Filaments			
Titin	3700	FNIII, IgC2, MLCK	Elastic connection from Z disk to M line

FN, fibronectin; Ig, immunoglobulin; MLCK, myosin light-chain kinase.

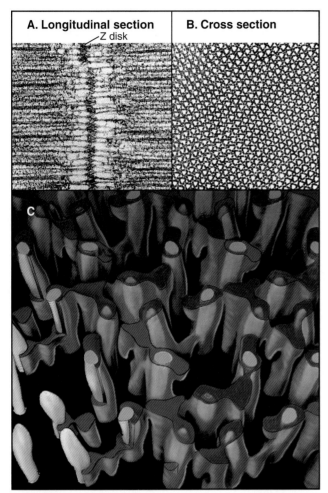

A. Longitudinal section	B. Cross section

Figure 39-5 Z DISK STRUCTURE. **A–B,** Electron micrographs of thin sections perpendicular to and in the plane of the Z disk. **C,** Three-dimensional reconstruction, based on electron micrographs of the Z disk, showing the network of protein cross-links that anchor the barbed ends of the *yellow* actin filaments. (Courtesy of J. Deatherage, National Institutes of Health, Bethesda, Maryland; modified from Cheng NQ, Deatherage JF: Three dimensional reconstruction of the Z disk of sectioned bee flight muscle. J Cell Biol 108:1761–1774, 1989, by copyright permission of The Rockefeller University Press.)

Tropomyosin and a gigantic filamentous protein, **nebulin,** stabilize thin filaments laterally. Nebulin consists of about 185 imperfect repeats of 35 amino acids that interact with each actin subunit, tropomyosin, and troponin along the length of thin filaments. Interactions with tropomodulin and Z disk proteins anchor nebulin at the two ends of the thin filament. Acting as a ruler and a cap, nebulin and tropomodulin help to set the length of thin filaments.

Thick Filaments

The self-assembly of myosin II (see Fig. 5-7) establishes the bipolar architecture of striated muscle thick filaments (Fig. 39-6). Some features of thick filaments are

invariant, such as a backbone consisting of myosin tails, a surface array of myosin heads, the 14.3-nm stagger between rows of heads, and a central bare zone formed by antiparallel packing of tails. Filaments may vary in length, diameter, and organization of the helical array of heads in various species. Invertebrate thick filaments have a core of paramyosin, a second coiled-coil protein, which is not found in vertebrates.

Several accessory proteins stabilize thick filaments (Table 39-1). Thick filaments in most striated muscles are girdled at intervals by semicircular bands of a protein

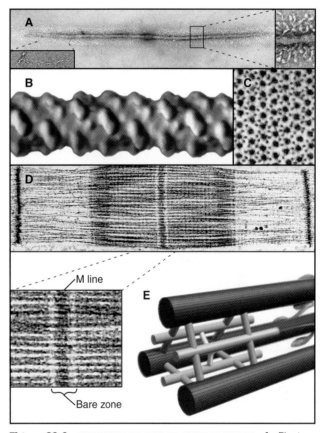

Figure 39-6 STRUCTURE OF BIPOLAR THICK FILAMENTS. **A,** Electron micrograph of a thick filament isolated directly from skeletal muscle and prepared by negative staining. A myosin molecule is shown at the same magnification at the *lower left*. The myosin tails form the backbone of the thick filament and allow the two myosin heads to swing out from the side (see the enlarged *inset* on the *right*). **B,** Reconstruction from electron micrographs of part of a rabbit skeletal muscle thick filament. The surface bumps are myosin heads. **C,** Cross section of vertebrate skeletal muscle showing the double hexagonal arrays of thick and thin filaments. **D,** Electron micrograph of a highly stretched sarcomere with the M line in the middle. **E,** Drawing of protein links between thick filaments in the M line. (A, Courtesy of John Trinick, University of Bristol, England. Reference: Knight P, Trinick J: Structure of the myosin projections on native thick filaments from vertebrate skeletal muscle. J Mol Biol 177:461–482, 1984. B, Courtesy of M. Stewart, MRC Laboratory of Molecular Biology, Cambridge, England. C, Courtesy of J. Heuser, Washington University, St. Louis, Missouri. D, Courtesy of H. E. Huxley, Brandeis University, Waltham, Massachusetts.)

that is, coincidentally, called *C-protein*. C-protein consists of fibronectin III and immunoglobulin domains. The "**M line**" in the center of the sarcomere is a three-dimensional array of protein cross-links that maintains the precise registration of thick filaments. At least three structural proteins and the enzyme MM-creatine phosphokinase (which transfers phosphate from creatine-phosphate to ADP) are located in the M line.

Titin Filaments

A third array of protein filaments lies parallel to the thin and thick filaments, connecting the Z disk to the thick filaments and the M line (Fig. 39-7). Hard to preserve for electron microscopy, these diaphanous filaments were neglected for years. Each filament is a single polypeptide named **titin** (after mythological giants), so named because of its remarkable size: more than 30,000 amino acids folded into a linear array of 300 immunoglobulin and fibronectin II domains measuring more than 1.2 µm long. Titin is thought to be the largest protein encoded by the human genome.

Titin molecules are elastic, and this accounts for the passive resistance to stretching of relaxed muscle. Their connections to the Z disk and thick filaments provide elastic continuity from one sarcomere to the next and keep the thick filaments centered in the sarcomere during contraction. If titin molecules are broken experimentally, thick filaments slide out of register toward one Z disk during contraction. Two features provide the elasticity during short (~0.3 µm per titin), physiological stretches: The irregular chain of immunoglobulin domains in the I band straightens out, and a segment of the polypeptide rich in proline, glutamic acid, valine, and lysine (the PEVK domain) stretches. Stretching decreases entropy and provides the energy for elastic recoil. (See Fig. 29-12 for another example of an entropic spring in biology.) Extreme stretching unfolds Ig domains one by one.

Intermediate Filaments

Desmin intermediate filaments (see Chapter 35) help to align the sarcomeres laterally (Fig. 39-8) by linking each Z disk to its neighbors and to specialized attachment sites on the plasma membrane. Myofibrils near the cell surface are attached to the plasma membrane at specializations called costameres. In addition to desmin, costameres contain several cytoskeletal proteins (vinculin, talin, spectrin, and ankyrin) found in focal contacts

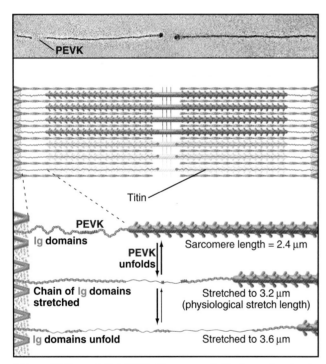

Figure 39-7 TITIN FILAMENTS. Upper panel, Electron micrographs of single, isolated titin molecules prepared by heavy metal shadowing. Titin molecules are long enough to extend from the Z disk to the M line. **Middle panel,** Drawing of a sarcomere, to the same scale as the electron micrograph, with the thick filaments removed from the bottom half to illustrate how titin molecules anchor thick filaments to the Z disk and extend to the M line. **Lower panel,** Drawing illustrating a model for the elasticity of titin. Modest stretches within the physiological range reversibly extend the chain of Ig domains in the I-band and the PEVK domain. Extreme extension can unfold immunoglobulin domains. (Modified from Reif M, Gautel M, Oesterhelt F, et al: Reversible unfolding of individual titin immunoglobulin domains by AFM. Science 276:1090–1092, 1997. Reference: Leake MC, Wilson D, Gautel M, Simmons RM: The elasticity of single titin molecules using a two-bead optical tweezers assay. Biophys J 87:1112–1135, 2004.)

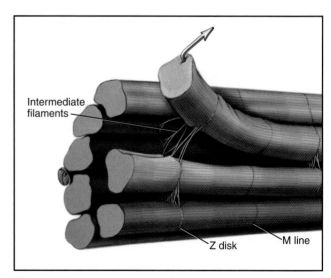

Figure 39-8 DESMIN INTERMEDIATE FILAMENTS IN SKELETAL MUSCLE. Desmin filaments connect Z disks laterally to each other and to the plasma membrane at specializations called costameres. (Redrawn from Lazarides E: Intermediate filaments as mechanical integrators of cellular space. Nature 283:249–256, 1980.)

and adherens junctions of nonmuscle cells (see Figs. 30-11 and 31-7). Desmin mutations in humans cause disorganization of myofibrils, resulting in generalized muscle failure.

Organization of the Muscle Membrane System

Structural Proteins of the Plasma Membrane: Defects in Muscular Dystrophies

In addition to providing a permeability barrier, the plasma membrane of the muscle cell must maintain its integrity while being subjected to years of forceful contractions. Accordingly, the membrane is stabilized by a transmembrane complex of proteins, the **dystroglycan-sarcoglycan complex,** that links the internal membrane skeleton to the basal lamina outside (Fig. 39-9 and Table 39-2). Occasional breaches of the membrane are inevitable, so muscle cells also depend

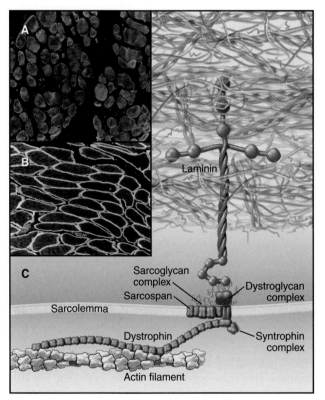

Figure 39-9 DYSTROPHIN AND ASSOCIATED PROTEINS STABILIZE THE PLASMA MEMBRANE OF SKELETAL MUSCLE. **A–B,** Fluorescent antibody staining of cross sections of human skeletal muscle showing the localization of dystrophin at the plasma membrane of a normal individual **(B)** and its absence in an individual with Duchenne's muscular dystrophy **(A). C,** Model of the transmembrane complex of proteins that links dystrophin and actin filaments in cytoplasm to laminin in the basal lamina outside the cell. (A–B, Courtesy of L. Kunkel, Harvard Medical School, Boston, Massachusetts. C, Based on a drawing by K. Amann and J. Ervasti, University of Wisconsin, Madison.)

on a repair process that reseals holes. If membrane damage exceeds the repair capacity, muscle cells degenerate locally (segmental necrosis) or globally. Cell death beyond the ability of muscle stem cells to repair the tissue results in **muscular dystrophy.** The age of onset and clinical features of inherited muscular dystrophies depend on the molecular defect. Patients with severe defects develop progressive muscle weakness as children. Ultimately, failure of respiratory muscles is fatal.

Mutations in more than 40 human genes have been linked to muscular dystrophies (Table 39-2), so it is possible that the malfunction or lack of any molecule in the system that maintains the integrity of the plasma membrane will cause disease. Disease-causing mutations occur in genes for the proteins of the dystroglycan-sarcoglycan complex, extracellular matrix proteins, Golgi apparatus enzymes that process these structural proteins, and the membrane repair machinery. Some of these mutations also affect the nervous system. Mutations are usually autosomal-recessive and are not uncommon. About one in several thousand humans develops some form of muscular dystrophy, because they inherit mutations in both copies of one of the sensitive genes. The mechanism of disease in muscular dystrophies is similar to that in hereditary spherocytosis, in which deficiencies of the membrane skeleton make red blood cells susceptible to mechanical damage (see Fig. 6-10).

The proteins that stabilize muscle membranes escaped detection until the late 1980s, when x-linked mutations in the **dystrophin** gene were discovered to cause Duchenne's muscular dystrophy, the most common human form of the disease. Dystrophin is an enormous member of the α-actinin superfamily of actin-binding proteins (see Fig. 33-16). The dystroglycan-sarcoglycan complex was found when it copurified with dystrophin after solubilizing the membrane with detergents. Loss of any protein of the dystrophin-dystroglycan-sarcoglycan complex typically leads to secondary loss of the other proteins from muscles.

Studies of mutations in muscular dystrophy patients led to the identification of most of the other genes in this system. α2 laminin is the extracellular ligand for dystroglycan in the basal lamina. Glycosylation of the transmembrane complex by Golgi apparatus glycosyltransferases is required for their mechanical functions. Proteins in cytoplasmic vesicles are used to repair damaged plasma membranes. The mechanical activity of muscle cells might make them more sensitive than other cells to deficiencies in proteins that support the nuclear envelope (lamin A/C and emerin).

Dystroglycans and a dystrophin homolog, utrophin, participate in clustering acetylcholine receptors at the neuromuscular junction, the chemical synapse between motor neurons and skeletal muscle (see Fig. 11-8). When, during development, a motor neuron arrives at the surface of its target muscle cell, the neuron secretes an

Table 39-2

PROTEINS REQUIRED TO STABILIZE AND REPAIR MUSCLE PLASMA MEMBRANES

Protein	Partners/Functions	Expression	Inheritance, Diseases Associated with Mutations
Membrane Skeleton			
Dystrophin	β-Dystroglycan, actin	Muscle, brain	XR, DMD, BMD, mdx mouse
Utrophin	β-Dystroglycan, actin	Muscle, other tissues	
α-Syntrophins	Dystrophin	Muscle > other tissues	None detected in humans
β-Syntrophins	Dystrophin, utrophin	Muscle > other tissues	None detected in humans
Transmembrane Proteins			
Caveolin-3	Cholesterol	Muscle	AD, LGMD
α-Dystroglycan	Laminin, agrin	Many tissues	Embryonic lethal
β-Dystroglycan	Dystrophin, utrophin	Many tissues	Embryonic lethal
α-Sarcoglycan	Sacroglycans, biglycan	Muscle	AR, LGMD, cardiomyopathy
β-Sarcoglycan	Sarcoglycans	Muscle	AR, LGMD
γ-Sarcoglycan	Sarcoglycans, biglycan	Muscle	AR, LGMD
Integrin α7	Laminin	Many tissues	AR, CMD
Extracellular Matrix			
Collagen VI α1, α2, α3	Biglycan	Muscle, other tissues	AD, Bethlem myopathy, Ulrich syndrome
α2-Laminin	α-Dystroglycan	Muscle, other tissues	AR, CMD, dy/dy mouse
Agrin	α-Dystroglycan, AChR	Muscle	
Sarcomeric Proteins			
Titin	Myosin, Z-disk	Muscle	AR, LGMD, tibial MD
Myotilin	α-actinin, Z-disk	Muscle	AR, LGMD
Golgi Enzymes That Process Membrane and ECM Proteins			
Fukutin	Glycosyltransferase	Many tissues	AR, Fukuyama CMD
LARGE	Glycosyltransferase	Many tissues	AR, CMD
POMGnT1	Glycosyltransferase	Many tissues	AR, Muscle eye brain disease
POMTi	O-mannosyltransferase	Many tissues	AR, Walker-Warburg syndrome
Membrane Repair Machinery			
Dysferlin		Muscle	AR, LGMD, Miyoshi myopathy
Nuclear Envelope Proteins			
Emerin	Lamins, actin	All cells	XR, Emery-Dreifuss MD
Lamin AC	Nuclear envelope	All cells	AD/AR, LGMD, Emery-Dreifuss MD

AD, autosomal dominant; AR, autosomal recessive; BMD, Becker's muscular dystrophy; CMD, childhood muscular dystrophy; DMD, Duchenne muscular dystrophy; LGMD, limb-girdle muscular dystrophy; XR, X-linked recessive.

adhesive protein called agrin, which is incorporated into the basal lamina, immediately adjacent to the nerve terminal. Dystroglycan binds agrin and positions associated acetylcholine receptors at the site where they receive acetylcholine secreted by the nerve in response to an action potential.

Interaction of Plasma Membrane Invaginations with the Smooth Endoplasmic Reticulum

The plasma membrane of skeletal muscle cells, like the plasma membrane of nerve cells, is excitable (see Fig. 11-6) and invaginates deeply to form so-called **T tubules** that run across the entire cell (Fig. 39-10). Depending on the species and type of striated muscle (skeletal versus cardiac), T tubules may be located either at the level of the Z disks or at the thick filament ends. Inside the muscle cell, T tubules interact extensively with the smooth endoplasmic reticulum (SER) that surrounds each myofibril. Historically, this SER has been called **sarcoplasmic reticulum.** Terminal cisternae of SER are closely associated with the passing T tubules by foot processes that can be visualized by electron microscopy. Together, T tubules and

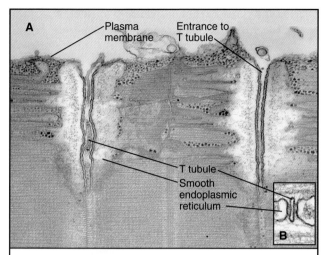

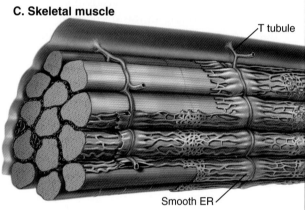

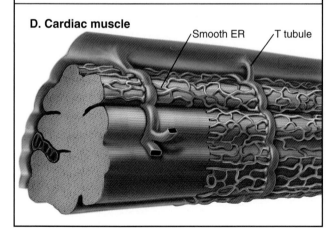

Figure 39-10 PLASMA MEMBRANE SPECIALIZATIONS OF STRIATED MUSCLES. **A–B,** Electron micrographs of thin sections of fish skeletal muscle showing invaginations called T tubules, which cross the whole muscle cell and associate closely with smooth endoplasmic reticulum (ER). The complex of a T tubule with smooth ER on both sides is called a triad. Foot processes, consisting of voltage-sensitive calcium channels in a T tubule paired with calcium release channels in the ER, connect the T tubule to the smooth ER. (Fig. 39-15 provides molecular details.) **C–D,** Drawings of the three-dimensional arrangement of T tubules and smooth ER relative to the sarcomeres in skeletal and cardiac muscle. (A–B, Courtesy of C. Franzini-Armstrong and K. Porter, University of Pennsylvania, Philadelphia.)

SER constitute a signal-transducing apparatus that converts depolarizations of the plasma membrane into a spike of cytoplasmic Ca^{2+} that triggers contraction (Fig. 39-15).

Molecular Basis of Skeletal Muscle Contraction

The Sliding Filament Mechanism

The key to understanding muscle contraction was the discovery that thick and thin filaments maintain constant lengths and slide past each other as sarcomeres (and the muscle) shorten (Fig. 39-11). About the same time, it was appreciated that cross-bridges (now recognized to be myosin heads) can connect actin and myosin filaments and that tension produced during contraction is proportional to the overlap of actin and myosin filaments (Fig. 39-12). Supported by biochemical and ultrastructural evidence for actin-myosin interaction, these pioneering observations led to the theory that cross-bridges between the thick and thin filaments produce force for contraction. Fifty years of research on cross-bridges have yielded a detailed picture of the chemistry and molecular mechanics underlying the force-producing reactions. A review of the steps of the actomyosin-ATPase cycle (see Fig. 36-5) is helpful in understanding the contraction mechanism. Three different physiological states reveal information about cross-bridge mechanisms.

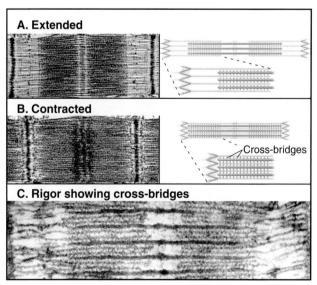

Figure 39-11 SLIDING FILAMENTS. Electron micrographs and interpretive drawings of longitudinal sections of a sarcomere from a relaxed muscle **(A)** and a contracted skeletal muscle **(B).** The lengths of the thin and thick filaments are constant as the sarcomere shortens, demonstrating that the filaments slide past each other during contraction. **C,** Cross-bridges between thick and thin filaments from a muscle in rigor. (Micrographs courtesy of H. E. Huxley, Brandeis University, Waltham, Massachusetts.)

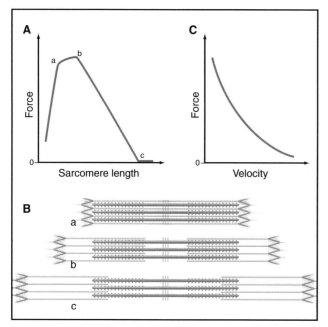

Figure 39-12 PHYSIOLOGICAL PROPERTIES OF SKELETAL MUSCLE. **A,** Dependence of maximum tension on the length of the sarcomeres. **B,** Interpretive drawings. Each relates to a point on graph **A. C,** Relationship of force and velocity during muscle contraction. (A, Reference: Gordon AM, Huxley AF, Julian F: The variation in isometric tension with sarcomere length in vertebrate muscle fibres. J Physiol 171:28P–30P, 1964. C, From Ruch TC, Patton HD (eds): Physiology and Biophysics, 19th ed. Philadelphia, WB Saunders, 1965.)

Relaxed. One extreme is relaxed muscle. When the concentration of cytoplasmic Ca^{2+} is low, tropomyosin and troponin inhibit the interaction of myosin heads with actin filaments, so few myosin heads are bound. Lacking long-lived physical connections between the filaments, muscle offers little resistance to passive stretching. X-ray diffraction (Fig. 39-13) shows that the myosin heads (with bound ATP or ADP and phosphate) are closely associated with the backbone of thick filaments and arranged in a helical array determined by the thick filament structure (Fig. 39-6B).

Rigor. The other extreme occurs after death. Depletion of ATP allows all myosin heads to bind tightly to actin filaments (Figs. 39-3B and 39–11C). By X-ray diffraction, the myosin heads bound to actin filaments contribute to the strength of the reflections from the actin filament helix. The strong physical connections between the filaments prevent stretching, making the muscle stiff (hence the term *rigor mortis*). This extreme condition is informative because it illustrates what happens structurally and mechanically when all of the cross-bridges engage actin filaments.

Contracting. The most interesting, but most complicated, state is *actively contracting* muscle. Myosin heads "walk" along actin filaments toward their

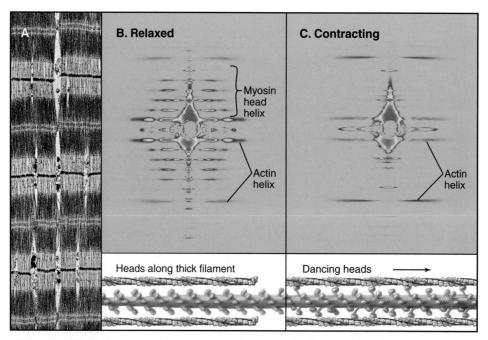

Figure 39-13 CROSS-BRIDGE DYNAMICS REVEALED BY X-RAY DIFFRACTION PATTERNS OF WHOLE MUSCLE. **A,** Electron micrograph showing the orientation of the muscle in the X-ray beam. **B–C,** Fiber diffraction patterns from relaxed and contracting skeletal muscles with interpretive drawings of cross-bridges in each state. Reflections from myosin heads arranged on the thick filament helix are strong in relaxed muscle. Reflections from the actin helix are stronger than the thick filament helix in contraction. The myosin and actin reflections are each labeled in only one of four equivalent quadrants. During contraction, a few myosin heads attach transiently to actin, increasing the strength of the actin helix reflections, but most are disordered. (Micrograph and X-ray patterns courtesy of H. E. Huxley, Brandeis University, Waltham, Massachusetts.)

barbed ends, pulling Z disks toward the center of the sarcomere. Thousands of sarcomeres shorten in series, causing the whole muscle to shorten. ATP is consumed, and force is produced. The thick filament helical pattern is very weak by X-ray diffraction (Fig. 39-13). Actin reflections are stronger than relaxed muscle but not as strong as rigor. Disordered myosin heads must lie between the thick and thin filaments as each one dances asynchronously on and off of actin filaments.

Most myosin heads in contracting muscle have bound ATP or ADP-P_i and oscillate rapidly among the four "weakly bound" states illustrated in Figure 36-5. During some of the transient interactions of myosin-ADP-P_i with actin, phosphate dissociates from myosin, and the light-chain domain rapidly reorients (see Figs. 36-4 and 36-5). This stretches elastic elements in the myosin heads and both thick and thin filaments. Energy in these elastic elements can be used over a period of milliseconds to displace the actin filament relative to the cross-bridge and contract the muscle. When ADP dissociates from the actin-myosin-ADP intermediate, ATP rapidly binds to the actin-myosin complex, dissociating the cross-bridge and starting a new ATPase cycle.

Relationship of Cross-Bridge Behavior to the Mechanical Properties of Muscle

Under normal conditions, each sarcomere shortens less than 1 μm. However, the whole muscle shortens macroscopically because it has thousands of sarcomeres in series. For example, a human biceps muscle 20 cm long has about 80,000 sarcomeres in series from end to end. When each contracts 0.25 μm, the muscle shortens 2 cm. Because the system maintains a constant volume, each sarcomere and the whole muscle increase in diameter as they shorten. Although the individual filaments slide past each other relatively slowly (about 5 μm s^{-1}), muscles contract rapidly because the motion of each sarcomere in the series is added together. In our example, without resistance, the biceps contracts 2 cm in 100 to 200 ms.

The behavior of cross-bridges explains why the velocity of muscle contractions of an active muscle depends on the external load (Fig. 39-12). Contraction velocity is maximal when opposed by no load. Without a load, the molecular motion stored in elastic elements of each cross-bridge is largely converted into movement of actin filaments relative to myosin filaments. Under these conditions, the filaments in muscle slide past each other at a rate of about 5 μm s^{-1}, the same speed that is observed for free actin filaments moving over myosin heads in vitro (see Fig. 36-6). For this rapid sliding to occur,

myosin heads that do not produce force must not impede movement. If bound tightly to actin, they would interfere mechanically with rapid sliding. This is avoided by the rapid equilibrium of the myosin intermediates between being bound to actin and being free. Myosin heads with bound ATP or ADP-P_i do not produce force when they bind transiently to a given actin subunit. Nor do these brief encounters retard sliding driven by force-producing cross-bridges.

Muscle produces maximum force when the contraction rate is zero (Fig. 39-12). The conformational change in the myosin head stretches elastic elements in the cross-bridge, but the force cannot overcome the resistance from the load on the muscle. Consequently, the filaments do not slide, and energy stored in each stretched elastic element is lost as heat when the cross-bridge dissociates at the end of the ATPase cycle. The maximum force depends on the numbers of sarcomeres in parallel, that is, the cross-sectional area of the muscle. Thus, muscles respond to strengthening exercises by growing in diameter.

Regulation of Skeletal Muscle Contraction

Control of Skeletal Muscle by Motor Neurons

Neural stimuli that activate skeletal muscles arise in two ways (Fig. 39-14). In organisms with well-developed

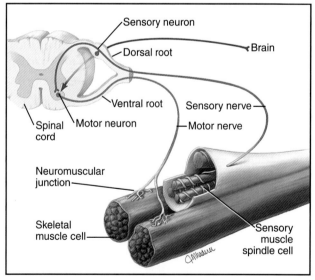

Figure 39-14 INNERVATION OF SKELETAL MUSCLE. Motor neurons in the spinal cord stimulate one or (usually) more skeletal muscle cells. Two neural pathways control motor neurons. Some stimuli come from neurons in higher centers of the brain. This pathway provides voluntary control over muscle contraction. Other stimuli come through local reflex circuits from sensory detectors, including muscle spindle cells. These signals help to coordinate muscle contraction in response to changing forces on the muscle.

central nervous systems, most neural signals that activate skeletal muscles result from conscious decisions, providing voluntary control over skeletal muscles. Other signals result from reflex responses to stimulation of sensory nerves. Specialized muscle cells innervated with both motor and sensory nerves function as stretch receptors, relaying information about length and tension back to the spinal cord, where reflexes coordinate the motor neuron output. Neural inputs from both sources converge on **motor neurons** located in the brain stem and spinal cord of vertebrates. Axons of these motor neurons branch in the muscle to contact one or more muscle cells. A motor neuron together with its target muscle cells forms a **motor unit.** In the most precisely controlled muscles, such as the extraocular muscles, some motor neurons innervate single muscle cells.

The contractile activity of a muscle is graded in terms of the speed and force of the contraction, so individual muscles can produce both delicate and powerful movements. Nerve stimulation determines the contractile force in two ways: (1) The number of active motor units determines how many muscle cells produce force, and (2) the rate of stimulation adjusts the force produced by active cells. Every time a muscle cell is stimulated, all of the sarcomeres are activated, but the force that they produce increases as the rate of stimulation increases, up to a maximum of about 200 stimuli per second. The shortening velocity of an active muscle depends simply on force produced and the resistance (Fig. 39-12C). If a large force or high velocity of contraction is required, many motor units are called into action and stimulated repetitively. To sustain contraction, motor nerves fire repeatedly. By varying the number of active cells in a muscle and the rate of stimulation, the nervous system sets the force required for a particular movement.

Synaptic Transmission at Neuromuscular Junctions

The terminal branch of each motor neuron axon forms a synapse called the **motor end plate** or **neuromuscular junction** on the muscle surface (see Fig. 11-8). These nerve endings are filled with synaptic vesicles containing the neurotransmitter **acetylcholine.** Arrival of an action potential at the nerve terminal stimulates fusion of synaptic vesicles with the nerve plasma membrane, releasing acetylcholine into the cleft between nerve and muscle. In less than a millisecond, acetylcholine diffuses across the extracellular space and binds to acetylcholine receptors concentrated in the adjacent muscle plasma membrane. Acetylcholine binding opens the receptor cation channel, initiating a new action potential that spreads over the muscle cell plasma membrane and down into the T tubules.

Coupling Action Potentials to Contraction

An action potential in a T tubule triggers the release of Ca^{2+} from SER into the cytoplasm (Fig. 39-15). Ca^{2+} binding to troponin allows myosin to interact with the thin filament, initiating contraction. This signal transduction process is called excitation-contraction coupling. Ca^{2+} release in skeletal muscle is the best-characterized example of a general regulatory mechanism used by many cells (see Chapter 26).

Three transmembrane proteins located in the T tubule and the terminal cisternae of the SER cooperate to generate the transient Ca^{2+} signal (Fig. 39-16). The operation of this system is described after its components are introduced:

1. A voltage-sensitive calcium channel (see Chapter 10) senses action potentials in the T tubule. These channels are called **dihydropyridine (DHP) receptors,** owing to their affinity for this class of drugs. The actual Ca^{2+} channel of dihydropyridine receptors is not essential for skeletal muscle, as is shown by the fact that external Ca^{2+} is not required for contraction in the short term.

2. Ca^{2+} release channels (see Fig. 26-13), concentrated in the terminal cisternae of SER, release Ca^{2+} into the cytoplasm. A drug called ryanodine binds these channels and inhibits Ca^{2+} release. Every second **ryanodine receptor** is connected to a cytoplasmic loop of a DHP receptor, forming bridges called *feet* between the T tubule and the endoplasmic reticulum (Fig. 39-10B).

3. The P-type **calcium-ATPase** (see Fig. 8-7) actively pumps Ca^{2+} from cytoplasm into the endoplasmic reticulum against a concentration gradient greater than 10^4. Several low-affinity, high-capacity Ca^{2+}-binding proteins buffer the millimolar concentration of Ca^{2+} inside the SER. For example, numerous carboxyl groups on the surface of calsequestrin bind Ca^{2+} with a millimolar K_d. This rapidly reversible reaction increases the Ca^{2+} storage capacity of endoplasmic reticulum without sacrificing the speed of Ca^{2+} release. Accessory subunits anchor calsequestrin to the Ca^{2+} release channel, ensuring a local supply of Ca^{2+} for release into cytoplasm when muscle is activated.

An action potential in a T tubule results in a transient rise in cytoplasmic Ca^{2+}, from $0.1\,\mu M$ to about $2\,\mu M$ (Fig. 39-16), in the following way. The action potential causes a short-lived conformational change in the DHP receptors that is transmitted directly to associated ryanodine receptor Ca^{2+} release channels. Many Ca^{2+} channels open transiently, allowing Ca^{2+} to diffuse down the steep concentration gradient from the SER lumen to cytoplasm. Physical connections between ryanodine

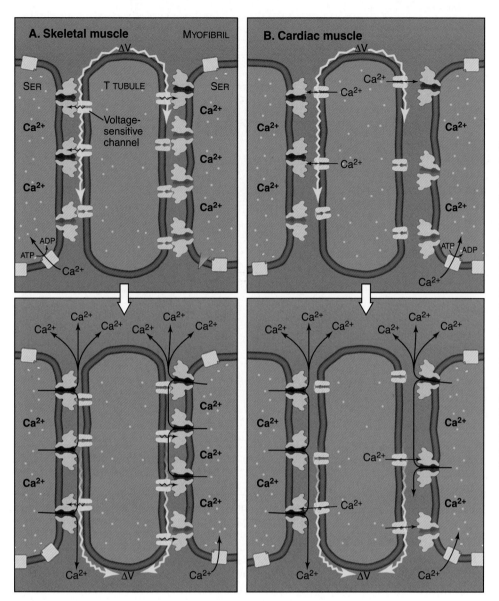

Figure 39-15 MECHANISM OF CALCIUM RELEASE IN SKELETAL AND CARDIAC MUSCLES. Both muscles use voltage-sensitive calcium channels in the T tubule membrane and calcium release channels in the smooth endoplasmic reticulum (SER). **A,** Direct coupling in skeletal muscle. An action potential in the T tubule (ΔV) activates the voltage sensor (turning from *gray* to *blue*). This direct contact opens the calcium release channel (turning from *gray* to *pink*). Cytoplasmic Ca^{2+} levels rise only briefly because calcium-ATPase pumps Ca^{2+} back into the lumen of the SER. **B,** Calcium-induced Ca^{2+} release in cardiac muscle. An action potential opens the voltage-sensitive Ca^{2+} channel in the T tubule, releasing Ca^{2+} into the cytoplasm. This Ca^{2+} opens the calcium release channel in the SER.

Figure 39-16 Ca^{2+} triggers contraction of skeletal muscle. In these experiments, the Ca^{2+}-sensitive protein aequorin was injected into live muscle cells to provide a signal for the cytoplasmic Ca^{2+} concentration. **A,** Single stimulus. Cytoplasmic Ca^{2+} concentration increases transiently, followed by a short contraction. This brief contraction persists after cytoplasmic Ca^{2+} decreases to the resting level. **B,** Multiple stimuli. Each stimulus releases a new pulse of Ca^{2+}, prolonging the contraction in so-called tetanus. (Reference: Ridgway EB, Ashley CC: Calcium transients in single muscle fibers. Biochem Biophys Res Comm 29:229–234, 1967.)

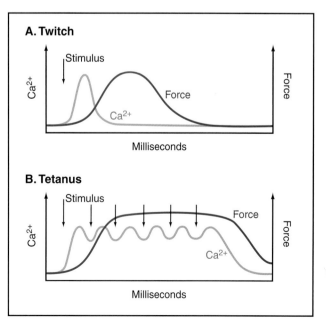

receptors may spread their activation laterally, ensuring synchronous activation of a patch of channels. The structural changes in these channels that release Ca^{2+} are not yet understood.

After a single action potential, the rise in the cytoplasmic Ca^{2+} level lasts but a few milliseconds for three reasons. First, Ca^{2+} release channels close quickly. Second, cytoplasmic Ca^{2+} binds to troponin C and other proteins. Third, Ca^{2+} pumps efficiently transport cytoplasmic Ca^{2+} back into the lumen of the smooth endoplasmic reticulum, even before the muscle develops maximum force. Ca^{2+} pumps are continuously active, keeping the cytoplasmic Ca^{2+} concentration low. Repeated action potentials are required to prolong the rise in cytoplasmic Ca^{2+} (Fig. 39-16B).

Transduction of the Calcium Spike into Contraction

Troponin-tropomyosin on thin filaments cooperates with myosin to turn on contraction in response to a Ca^{2+} spike. At rest, two Ca^{2+}-binding sites of troponin C are largely unoccupied (owing to their low affinity for Ca^{2+} and the low Ca^{2+} concentration), and the troponin-tropomyosin complex partially blocks the binding site for myosin heads on actin (Fig. 39-17). This prevents most of the weak-binding myosin intermediates with ATP or ADP-P_i in the active site from binding the thin filament. When released into cytoplasm, Ca^{2+} binds troponin C, causing a conformational change that creates a binding site for a helical region of TNI. This interaction attracts the C-terminus of TNI away from actin and tropomyosin, allowing a small shift in the position of tropomyosin on the thin filament. This shift increases the probability that myosin-ADP-P_i heads will bind to the thin filament, dissociating their bound P_i and producing force. The initial binding of the first force-producing heads shifts the long tropomyosin molecule a bit farther away from the myosin-binding sites, allowing adjacent actins to interact freely with other myosin heads. The end-to-end association of tropomyosins facilitates this cooperative switch by exposing the myosin-binding sites on more distant actin subunits in the thin filament.

Thus, the combined influence of Ca^{2+} and myosin makes the thin filament receptive to myosin binding. Activation is cooperative because both Ca^{2+}-binding sites on troponin C must be occupied, because the effects of Ca^{2+} binding and myosin binding are transmitted to neighboring tropomyosins through their end-to-end attachments, and because every myosin that binds accentuates the response. This cooperativity makes the on-off switch respond very sharply to a relatively small, 10- to 20-fold change in the cytoplasmic Ca^{2+} concentration. The efficiency of this switch is underscored by the fact that the energy consumption of a muscle cell

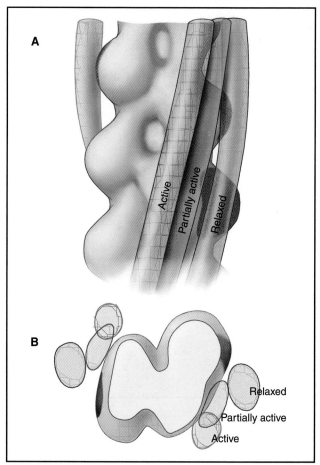

Figure 39-17 THIN FILAMENT ACTIVATION MECHANISM. Reconstructions from electron micrographs showing a short segment of thin filament **(A)** and a cross section of a thin filament **(B)**. Ca^{2+} binding to troponin C partially activates the filament by moving tropomyosin away from its lateral position in relaxed muscle, where it overlaps the myosin-binding site on actin *(red)*. Myosin binding to the partially activated filament moves tropomyosin further out of the way into the active position. (Redrawn from data of W. Lehman, Boston University, Massachusetts.)

increases more than 1000-fold when it is activated. Activation of slow skeletal muscle (Table 39-3) and cardiac muscle is less cooperative, as their troponin C has only one Ca^{2+}-binding site.

Note the delay between the Ca^{2+} spike and the onset of tension (Fig. 39-16). The Ca^{2+}-sensitive switch is sharp but slow owing to the slow response of thin filaments to Ca^{2+} binding. Note also that muscle continues to produce force well after the cytoplasmic Ca^{2+} concentration returns to resting levels. Ca^{2+} binds troponin C rapidly (milliseconds) but dissociates slowly (tens of milliseconds). Thus, the Ca^{2+} spike saturates troponin C, and the muscle remains active even after free Ca^{2+} has returned to the endoplasmic reticulum lumen. Force declines slowly as Ca^{2+} dissociates from troponin C and returns to the smooth endoplasmic reticulum without raising the cytoplasmic Ca^{2+} concentration.

Table 39-3

MUSCLE CELL TYPES

Physiological Type	Myosin Type	Mitochondria	Fatigue
Fast, white	Fast	Few	Rapid
Intermediate	Fast	Medium	Medium
Fast, red	Fast	Many	Slow
Slow, red	Slow	Many	Slow

A single action potential produces a short contractile "twitch" (Fig. 39-16). Maximum contractile force is produced by a series of closely spaced action potentials, leading to a sustained rise in cytoplasmic Ca^{2+} and prolonged activation of actomyosin. The extended contraction is called tetanus.

Regulation by Myosin Light Chains

The participation of skeletal muscle myosin light chains in the regulation of contraction varies among species. The skeletal muscles of mollusks are one extreme; myosin light chains bind Ca^{2+} and provide the main on/off switch for contraction. When the Ca^{2+} concentration is low in resting muscle, no Ca^{2+} binds to light chains, and the actin-myosin ATPase is off. Ca^{2+} that is released during activation binds to the light chains, turning on the ATPase and contraction. At the other extreme, the light chains of vertebrate skeletal muscle myosin do not bind Ca^{2+} and do not participate in activation. However, *phosphorylation* of vertebrate skeletal muscle light chains modulates contractile activity by increasing force production at suboptimal Ca^{2+} concentrations. Horseshoe crab skeletal muscle uses a dual system: Ca^{2+} binding to troponin-tropomyosin on thin filaments and Ca^{2+}-regulated phosphorylation of myosin light chains both stimulate contraction.

Specialized Skeletal Muscle Cells

All skeletal muscle cells are built on the same principles, but vertebrates actually have several different types of skeletal muscle cells, each with distinct contractile protein isoforms and metabolic enzymes. The myosin and actin isoforms are coded by different genes, whereas alternative splicing of one primary transcript (see Fig. 16-6) creates more than 50 isoforms of troponin T. Mutations in the genes for myosin, actin, tropomyosin, troponin-T, and nebulin can each cause defects in human skeletal muscles.

Physiological properties, such as the speed of contraction and the rate of fatigue, provide criteria for classifying muscle cells (Table 39-3). The isoforms of myosin (and probably the other contractile proteins) determine the speed of contraction, whereas the content of mito-

chondria and myoglobin determines the endurance and overall color of the muscle. White muscle cells depend largely on glycolysis to supply ATP, accounting for their rapid fatigue compared with red muscle cells, which are specialized for oxidative metabolism with abundant mitochondria and myoglobin.

Some muscles consist of only fast-twitch white muscle cells or slow-twitch red muscle cells, but most muscles are a mixture of two or more cell types. For example, in chickens, the leg muscles that are responsible for supporting the body, walking, and maintaining balance over long periods of time are rich in red muscle cells. On the other hand, the chicken breast muscles, used for energetic flapping of the wings for short periods, are mainly white muscle cells.

Remarkably, the pattern of *nerve stimulation* determines the muscle cell type by controlling which genes are expressed (and presumably, how the troponin T messenger RNA is processed). This was demonstrated by transplanting motor nerves between fast and slow muscles. Over a period of weeks, slow isoforms replace fast isoforms and vice versa. Even more surprising, the same result is achieved by stimulating muscles electrically with fast or slow patterns of impulses. Chronic low-level stimulation biases gene expression toward the proteins that are found in slow muscle cells. Calcium and calmodulin provide one prominent link between activity and gene expression. The concentration of active calmodulin tracks with the pattern of stimulation, because Ca^{2+} is released in the cytoplasm each time a muscle contracts. Among other things, calcium-calmodulin activates protein phosphatase PP2b (calcineurin; see Fig. 25-6), which dephosphorylates transcription factors (see Fig. 15-21). These activated transcription factors move into the nucleus and cooperate with other transcription factors including a nuclear receptor to turn on expression of proteins found in slow muscles, including contractile proteins and enzymes for oxidative metabolism.

The proportions of slow and fast muscle cells are determined genetically, so world-class sprinters (with a high proportion of fast, white fibers) and marathoners (with a high proportion of slow, red fibers) are born with advantages for their specialties. Training can lead to hypertrophy of specific muscle cell types and improved performance. Endurance training also leads to an increased proportion of slow cells. Without training, muscle strength declines with age as a constant number of cells each decreases in size.

Cardiac Muscle

To maintain the circulation of blood, heart muscle is specialized for repetitive (~100,000 times per day), fatigue-free contractions driven at regular intervals by action potentials from specialized pace-making cells. Gap junctions allow these action potentials to spread from one muscle cell to the next. The arrangement of the contractile apparatus into sarcomeres is similar to that in skeletal muscle.

The Contractile Apparatus of Cardiac Muscle

Cardiac muscle cells have sarcomeres with thick and thin filaments like skeletal muscle (Fig. 39-18), but they have more mitochondria, larger T tubules, less smooth endoplasmic reticulum, and a smaller version of nebulin called nebulette. The atrium has one major myosin isoform. Two ventricular myosin isoforms (one shared with slow skeletal muscle) differ in ATPase activity and speed of contraction. Humans almost exclusively express only one of these isoforms. In rats, thyroid hormone regulates expression of these isoforms. Both are expressed normally, but one predominates in hypothyroidism, and the other predominates in hyperthyroidism. Heart expresses different isoforms of TNI and TNT than does skeletal muscle. If damaged in a heart attack, cardiac cells release TNI and TNT into the blood. Measurement of cardiac TNI and TNT in blood is now the most sensitive chemical test for heart attacks.

Short, modestly branched, cardiac muscle cells have centrally located nuclei and squared-off ends (Fig. 39-1) where neighboring cells attach to each other at specialized adhesive junctions called **intercalated disks** (Fig. 39-18). These junctions have properties of both adherens junctions (links to actin filaments) and desmosomes (links to intermediate filaments). Ca^{2+}-dependent cadherins form the physical connections between adjacent cells (see Fig. 30-5).

Pacemaker Cells

Modified cardiac muscle cells in the right atrium (**sinoatrial node**) spontaneously depolarize their plasma membrane at regular intervals to initiate each heartbeat (Fig 39-19; see also Fig. 11-11). Special nonselective cation channels allow Na^+ to leak into these cells and K^+ to leak out, depolarizing the plasma membrane and triggering an action potential. The action potential spreads from cell to cell through gap junctions (see Fig. 31-6), activating all cells in the atrium within a few hundred milliseconds. After a brief delay in the **atrioventricular node,** the action potential and contraction spread through the ventricle.

As in skeletal muscle, plasma membrane action potentials stimulate cardiac muscle cells to contract by releasing Ca^{2+} to activate troponin-tropomyosin. However, the Ca^{2+} release mechanism differs in important details from skeletal muscle. In particular, extracellular Ca^{2+} is required for heart but not skeletal muscle. Action potentials open voltage-sensitive calcium channels (dihydropyridine receptors) in T tubules, releasing Ca^{2+} locally. This small burst of Ca^{2+} opens nearby ryanodine receptors in the smooth endoplasmic reticulum, releasing a flood of Ca^{2+} to trigger contraction. This excitation-contraction coupling can be defective when heart muscle cells grow larger in response to abnormal demands, such as high blood pressure. The defect may be explained by growth separating T tubules from smooth endoplasmic reticulum, either physically or functionally, thereby decreasing the probability that Ca^{2+} entering through dihydropyridine receptors will trigger Ca^{2+} release from the endoplasmic reticulum.

Motor nerves do not stimulate cardiac muscle directly, but the heart is rich in autonomic nerves from the sympathetic and parasympathetic nervous systems.

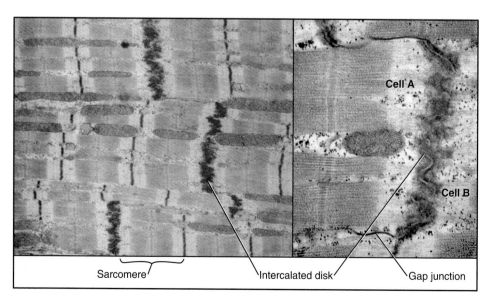

Figure 39-18 ELECTRON MICROGRAPHS OF A LONGITUDINAL SECTION OF TWO CARDIAC MUSCLE CELLS. Sarcomeres are similar to skeletal muscle. Intercalated disks anchor neighboring cells together, and gap junctions couple the cells electrically. (Courtesy of D. W. Fawcett, Harvard Medical School, Boston, Massachusetts.)

Cell A

Cell B

Sarcomere   Intercalated disk   Gap junction

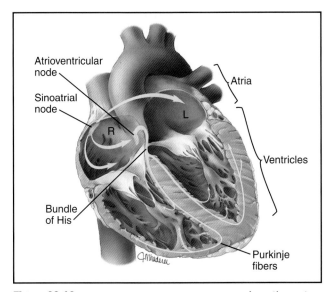

Figure 39-19 ACTIVATION OF CARDIAC CONTRACTION. An action potential (*yellow arrows*) starts at the sinoatrial node and travels through atrial muscle cells to the atrioventricular node. After a short delay at the atrioventricular node, the action potential spreads through the interventricular septum in modified cardiac muscle cells, called Purkinje's fibers, and then through muscle cells to the whole ventricle. The action potential follows the same path each time, giving rise to electrical signals that can be detected on the body surface by electrocardiogram (EKG). Damage during myocardial infarctions changes the EKG pattern and may cause arrhythmias.

These nerves secrete acetylcholine and norepinephrine, which act as hormones to modulate the rate and force of contraction (see Fig. 11-12). Norepinephrine acting through the β-adrenergic receptor and cAMP, activates PKA (see Fig. 27-3), which phosphorylates TNI. This increases the rate of cross-bridge cycling and the strength of contraction.

Molecular Basis of Inherited Heart Diseases

Because the heart is so vital to survival, relatively minor molecular defects command attention in humans. About 1 of 500 individuals carries a mutation in a gene that compromises cardiac function (Table 39-4). For example, many different point mutations in the myosin heavy chain can compromise its function. Affected individuals are typically heterozygous for these mutations, and the mutant myosin interferes with the function of the normal myosin (i.e., they are dominant negative mutations). Over a period of years, the heart attempts to compensate for the contractility defect through hypertrophy, but the thickened heart wall compromises cardiac relaxation and filling of the chambers with blood. More serious, heart hypertrophy eventually causes defects in activation and abnormal rhythms that

Table 39-4

GENETIC DEFECTS IN CARDIAC AND SKELETAL MUSCLE DISEASE

Gene/Protein	Normal Function	Disease Manifestations
Contractile Proteins		
Actin	Thin filament	Dilated cardiomyopathy, heart failure, myopathy
Titin	Passive elasticity	Dilated cardiomyopathy, heart failure, muscular dystrophy
Nebulin	Thin filament	Myopathy
Dystrophin	Membrane stabilization	Dilated cardiomyopathy, heart failure, Duchenne muscular dystrophy
β-Myosin heavy chain	Thick-filament motor	Hypertrophic cardiomyopathy, arrhythmias, myopathy
Myosin essential light chain	Myosin motor	Hypertrophic cardiomyopathy, arrhythmias
Myosin regulatory light chain	Myosin motor	Hypertrophic cardiomyopathy, arrhythmias
Myosin C protein	Thick-filament structure	Hypertrophic cardiomyopathy, arrhythmias
Troponin T	Calcium regulation	Hypertrophic cardiomyopathy, arrhythmias, myopathy
Troponin I	Calcium regulation	Hypertrophic cardiomyopathy, arrhythmias, myopathy
Tropomyosin	Calcium regulation	Hypertrophic cardiomyopathy, arrhythmias, myopathy
Electrophysiology		
HERG	Potassium channel	Long QT syndrome, arrhythmias
KVLQT1	Potassium channel	Long QT syndrome, arrhythmias
minK	Potassium channel	Long QT syndrome, arrhythmias
SCN5A	Sodium channel	Long QT syndrome, arrhythmias
Ankyrin	Membrane scaffold	Long-QT syndrome, arrhythmias
Other Functions		
NKX2-5	Transcription factor	Congenital atrioseptal defects
TBX5	Transcription factor	Multiple congenital defects between heart chambers

can be fatal. The rate of progress of these so-called **hypertrophic cardiomyopathies** depends on not only the particular mutation but also other factors that vary from person to person. Individuals with defects in C protein develop hypertrophy in their fifties and can live normal life spans. By contrast, those with defects in troponin T can be affected as teenagers and die of arrhythmias in their twenties. These severe mutations of cardiac contractile proteins account for about half of the deaths of apparently healthy young athletes. Myosin mutations are intermediate in severity. Mutations in actin and dystrophin cause a disease of an opposite sort. Individual cells hypertrophy, but many die and are replaced by connective tissue, leading to thinning of the wall of the heart and defective contractility.

Smooth Muscle

The Contractile Apparatus

Smooth muscle cells are specialized for slow, powerful, efficient contractions under the control of a variety of involuntary mechanisms. Smooth muscle cells are generally confined to internal organs, such as blood vessels (where they regulate blood pressure), the gastrointestinal tract (where they move food through the intestines), and the respiratory system (where their excessive contraction contributes to asthma and other allergic reactions). The cytoplasm of spindle-shaped smooth muscle cells (Fig. 39-1) appears homogeneous by light microscopy because the contractile proteins are not organized in regular arrays like sarcomeres of skeletal and cardiac muscle. A basal lamina and variable amounts of collagen and elastic fibers surround each cell.

In terms of organization and biochemistry, smooth muscle cells (Fig. 39-20) resemble nonmuscle cells more than they do skeletal or cardiac muscle. For example, the gene for smooth muscle myosin arose relatively recently from a cytoplasmic myosin II gene (see Fig. 36-7). These myosins also share the same regulatory light chain. Long myosin thick filaments are interspersed among the thin filaments but not in a regular way like striated muscles. Thin filaments are composed of actin and tropomyosin, along with two regulatory proteins, caldesmon and calponin, rather than troponin. Thin filaments are arranged obliquely in the cell, some with their barbed ends attached to dense plaques on the plasma membrane, others to **dense bodies** in the cytoplasm. Like Z disks in striated muscles, dense bodies anchor desmin intermediate filaments, forming a continuous, inextensible, internal "tendon" running from end to end into the cell, preventing excess stretching (see Fig. 35-8).

Smooth muscle cells contract like a concertina (Fig. 39-21) because tension generated by myosin and actin is applied to discrete spots on the plasma membrane. This compression can be seen in light micrographs as irregular cells with "corkscrew" nuclei. Given that smooth muscle cells have less myosin than striated muscle cells do, it is remarkable that they develop the same force. This is explained by two factors. First, the force-generating unit, the myosin filament, is larger in smooth muscle than in skeletal muscle. Deploying a given amount of myosin in large, thick filaments in a long sarcomere produces more force than does the same myosin in smaller filaments arranged in a series of short sarcomeres. Second, individual smooth muscle myosin molecules produce a larger force than skeletal muscle myosin, at least in vitro assays.

Regulation of Smooth Muscle Contraction

Stimuli that trigger smooth muscle contraction vary widely, but they all seem to act through seven-helix receptors coupled to trimeric G-proteins. Hormones stimulate contraction of the uterus, whereas motor nerves stimulate intrinsic eye muscles that close the pupil. Gap junctions couple some groups of smooth muscle cells, so their activation is propagated and coordinated within the tissue.

Depending on the muscle, Ca^{2+} for contraction enters the cytoplasm through either voltage-dependent calcium channels in the plasma membrane or IP_3 (inositol, 1,4,5-triphosphate)–induced Ca^{2+} release from smooth endoplasmic reticulum (Fig. 39-21). Drugs that block plasma membrane calcium channels can distinguish these two pathways experimentally. In intestines, parasympathetic nerves release acetylcholine to stimulate seven-helix muscarinic receptors (see Figs. 11-7 and 11-12). Associated trimeric G-proteins activate cation channels that depolarize the plasma membrane and allow Ca^{2+} to enter through voltage-sensitive calcium channels. Gap junctions couple gut smooth muscle cells, allowing excitation to spread from cell to cell. Calcium channel blockers strongly inhibit activation of gut smooth muscle. At the other end of the spectrum, vascular smooth muscle depends on IP_3 to release Ca^{2+} from intracellular stores rather than from outside the cell.

Following stimulation, intracellular Ca^{2+} increases rapidly but transiently, declining to a value above resting level as the receptors desensitize (see Fig. 24-3). Ca^{2+} pumps in both smooth endoplasmic reticulum and plasma membrane clear the cytoplasm of Ca^{2+} so that Ca^{2+} levels decrease to resting levels and the muscle relaxes when the activating stimulus is removed. Relaxing agents, acting through cyclic guanosine monophosphate (cGMP) or cAMP (see Fig. 26-1), promote clearance of cytoplasmic Ca^{2+}. Epinephrine relaxes smooth muscles of the respiratory system by another method. Stimulation of β-adrenergic receptors activates

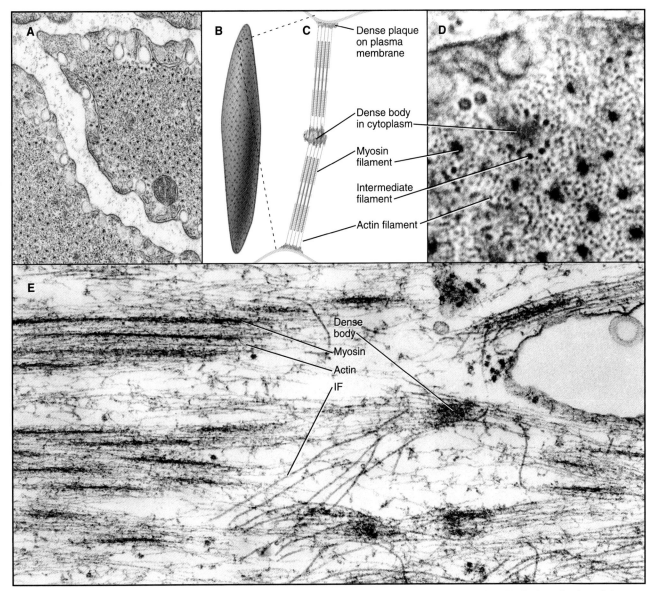

Figure 39-20 **CONTRACTILE APPARATUS OF SMOOTH MUSCLE. A,** Electron micrograph of a thin cross section. **B–C,** Organization of the contractile units, which stretch across the cell between plasma membrane attachment plaques. Contractile units consist of myosin filaments connecting thin filaments attached to a dense body or plasma membrane plaque. **D,** High-power electron micrograph showing a dense body and cross sections of three types of filaments. **E,** Electron micrograph of a longitudinal section of an extracted vascular smooth muscle cell illustrating associations of actin filaments and intermediate filaments (IF) with dense bodies, and myosin filaments interacting with actin filaments. (A, D, and E, Courtesy of A. V. Somlyo and A. P. Somlyo, University of Virginia, Charlottesville. References: Somlyo AP, Devine CE, Somlyo AV, Rice RV: Filament organization in vertebrate smooth muscle. Philos Trans R Soc Lond [Biol] 265:223–229, 1973; Bond M, Somlyo AV: Dense bodies and actin polarity in vertebrate smooth muscle. J Cell Biol 95:403–413, 1982.)

potassium channels that hyperpolarize the plasma membrane and reduce Ca^{2+} entry. This approach is widely used to treat asthma.

After a considerable delay (>200 ms) following the Ca^{2+} spike, contractile force develops slowly. The delay is attributable to the time required for a sequence of three biochemical reactions: Ca^{2+} binding to calmodulin, calcium-calmodulin activation of **myosin light-chain kinase** (see Fig. 25-4), and phosphorylation of myosin regulatory light chains, turning on the myosin-actin ATPase cycle (Fig. 39-21). Unphosphorylated myosin-II from smooth muscle and vertebrate nonmuscle cells is inactive.

Phosphorylation of myosin light chains is required to initiate but not maintain contraction, so slowly cycling, unphosphorylated myosins maintain peak force with

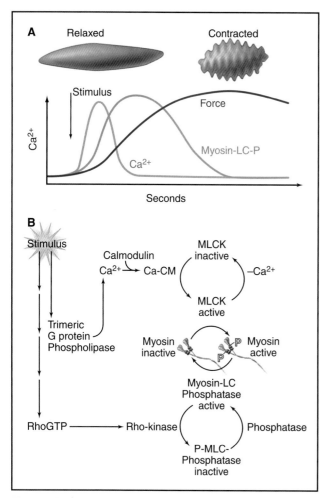

Figure 39-21 ACTIVATION OF SMOOTH MUSCLE CONTRACTION. **A,** The spindle-shaped smooth muscle cell becomes pleated as it contracts, owing to the attachment of the actin filaments at intervals along the plasma membrane. The graph shows the time course of activation, consisting of release of Ca^{2+} into the cytoplasm, phosphorylation of myosin regulatory light chains, and then the slow development of force. Myosin light-chain phosphorylation (LC-P) is required to initiate, but not to prolong, the contraction of smooth muscle. **B,** Biochemical pathways controlling phosphorylation of myosin regulatory light chains. Receptor stimulation leads to production of IP_3 by phospholipase C and release of Ca^{2+} into cytoplasm. Ca^{2+} binds calmodulin (CM), which activates myosin light-chain kinase (MLCK) by binding the kinase's autoinhibitory peptide and displacing it from the active site. Active MLCK phosphorylates activating sites on the regulatory light chain. Light-chain phosphatase reverses phosphorylation of myosin. Activation of the small GTPase Rho with GTP stimulates Rho-kinase, which phosphorylates and inactivates light-chain phosphatase. This makes the system more sensitive to any level of Ca^{2+}, as light-chain phosphorylation is prolonged. P-MLC-, phosphorylated myosin light chain. (A, Redrawn from the work of K. Kamm and J. Stull, University of Texas Southwestern Medical School, Dallas.)

little expenditure of energy. Regulation of unphosphorylated cross-bridges is not well understood, but they appear to be activated cooperatively by a small population of phosphorylated myosin heads. Caldesmon, a calcium-calmodulin-binding protein associated with

tropomyosin on actin filaments, may contribute to activation and/or allow myosin heads to cycle very slowly even in the presence of ATP.

The sensitivity of light-chain phosphorylation to Ca^{2+} depends on a parallel signaling pathway that partially inhibits myosin phosphatase, thus increasing the number of phosphorylated myosin cross-bridges and force at any given Ca^{2+} concentration (Fig. 39-21). Receptors coupled to trimeric G-proteins activate the small GTPase RhoA, which stimulates a protein kinase that inhibits myosin light-chain phosphatase. Malfunction of this Ca^{2+}-sensitizing mechanism may contribute to some forms of high blood pressure, since in hypertensive animals, drugs that inhibit Rho-activated kinase relax smooth muscle and lower blood pressure.

SELECTED READINGS

Agarkova I, Perriard J-C: The M-band: An elastic web that crosslinks thick filaments in the center of the sarcomere. Trends Cell Biol 15:477–485, 2005.

Bansal D, Campbell KP: Dysferlin and the plasma membrane repair in muscular dystrophy. Trends Cell Biol 14:206–213, 2004.

Bassel-Duby R, Olson EN: Role of calcineurin in striated muscle: Development, adaptation and disease. Biochem Biophys Res Comm 311:1133–1141, 2003.

Bolton TB, Prestwich SA, Zholos AV, Gordienko DV: Excitation-contraction coupling in gastrointestinal and other smooth muscles. Annu Rev Physiol 61:85–115, 1999.

Clark KA, McElhinny AS, Beckerle MC, Gregorio CC: Striated muscle cytoarchitecture: An intricate web of form and function. Annu Rev Cell Dev Biol 18: 637–706, 2002.

Dalkilic I, Kunkel, LM: Muscular dystrophies, genes to pathogenesis. Curr Opin Gen Dev 13:231–238, 2003.

Davies KE, Nowak KJ: Molecular mechanisms of muscular dystrophies: Old and new players. Nature Rev Mol Cell Biol 7:762–773, 2006.

Fatkin D, Graham RM: Molecular mechanisms of inherited cardiomyopathies. Physiol Rev 82:945–980, 2002.

Fischer RS, Fowler VM: Tropomodulin: Life at the slow end. Trends Cell Biol 13:593–601, 2003.

Franzini-Armstrong C, Protasi F, Ramesh V: Comparative ultrastructure of Ca^{2+} release units in skeletal and cardiac muscle. Ann N Y Acad Sci 853:20–30, 1998.

Geeves MA, Holmes KC: Structural mechanism of muscle contraction. Annu Rev Biochem 68:687–728, 1999.

Goody RS: The missing link in the muscle cross-bridge cycle. Nat Struct Biol 10:773–775, 2003.

Gordon AM, Homsher E, Regnier M: Regulation of contraction in striated muscle. Physiol Rev 80:853–924, 2000.

Horowits R: Nebulin regulation of actin filament lengths: New angles. Trends Cell Biol 15:121–124, 2005.

Kiriazis H, Kranias EG: Genetically engineered models with alterations in cardiac membrane calcium-handling proteins. Annu Rev Physiol 62:321–351, 2000.

McElhinny AS, Kazmierski ST, Labeit S, Gregorio CC: Nebulin, the nebulous, multifunctional giant of striated muscle. Trends Cardiovasc Med 13:195–201, 2003.

Olson EN, Williams RS: Remodeling muscles with calcineurin. Bioessays 22:510–519, 2000.

Pownall ME, Gustafsson MK, Emerson CP Jr: Myogenic regulatory factors and the specification of muscle progenitors in vertebrate embryos. Annu Rev Cell Dev Biol 18:747-783, 2002.

Severs NJ: The cardiac muscle cell. Bioessays 22:188-199, 2000.

Somlyo AP, Somlyo AV: Signal transduction by G-proteins, Rho-kinase and protein phosphatase to smooth muscle and non-muscle myosin-II. J Physiol (Lond) 522:177-185, 2000.

Squire JM, Morris EP: A new look at thin filament regulation in vertebrate striated muscle. FASEB J 12:761-771, 1998.

Takeda S, Yamashita A, Maeda K, Maeda Y: Structure of the core domain of human cardiac troponin in the Ca^{2+}-saturated form. Nature 424:35-41, 2003.

Tskhovrebova L, Trinick J: Titin: Properties and family relationships. Nat Rev Mol Cell Biol 4:679-689, 2003.

Wehrens XH, Lehnart SE, Marks AR: Intracellular calcium release and cardiac disease. Annu Rev Physiol 67:69-98, 2005.

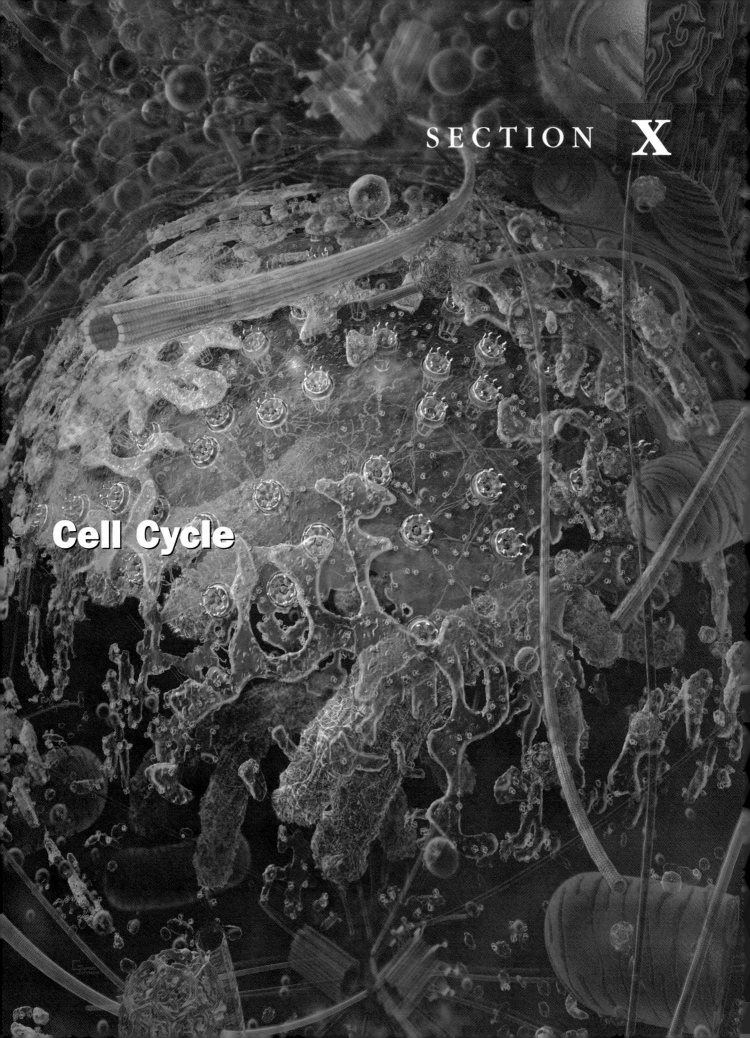

Cell Cycle

SECTION X OVERVIEW

This last section of the book pulls together principles from previous chapters to explain some of the rules that govern the lifestyles of cells. Cells exhibit a remarkable diversity in their patterns of growth, proliferation, and death. For example, some human cells (neurons) are born around the time of birth and live until the person dies—over 100 years in some cases. The fate of other cells is to live for only a day or two (e.g., cells in the gut lining). Many differentiated cells form by elaborate pathways that employ a carefully choreographed series of cues from within the cell and from its neighbors. Other cells, such as many in the immune system, are spawned in excess, followed by random selection of the few with correctly rearranged genes or with productive connections to partner cells. The unlucky majority of their siblings whose differentiation did not go so well then commit suicide.

Very different strategies maintain populations of cells. Really long-lived cells divide seldom, if at all. In contrast, the cells that are involved in producing the gut lining

grow and divide at top speed. Most human cells differentiate to carry out specific functions and then no longer proliferate. How do cells decide whether to proliferate, to stop proliferating and differentiate, or to die? This section answers these and other questions.

Chapter 40 begins the section with an introduction to the language of the cell cycle. The cell cycle is driven by changing states of the cytoplasm created by shifting balances of protein phosphorylation and degradation machinery. For the cell cycle, the key kinases are **cyclin-dependent kinases** (Cdks), which require an associated **cyclin** subunit for activity. Cdks are also regulated by phosphorylation and by additional protein cofactors that bind and inactivate them. Cdks are usually stable, but cyclin levels fluctuate, owing to targeted destruction at particular points in the cell cycle. In fact, targeted proteolytic destruction by the proteasome is a key aspect of cell-cycle control. Each cell-cycle phase is characterized by the activity of one or more E3 ubiquitin ligases. Each of these targets particular proteins for

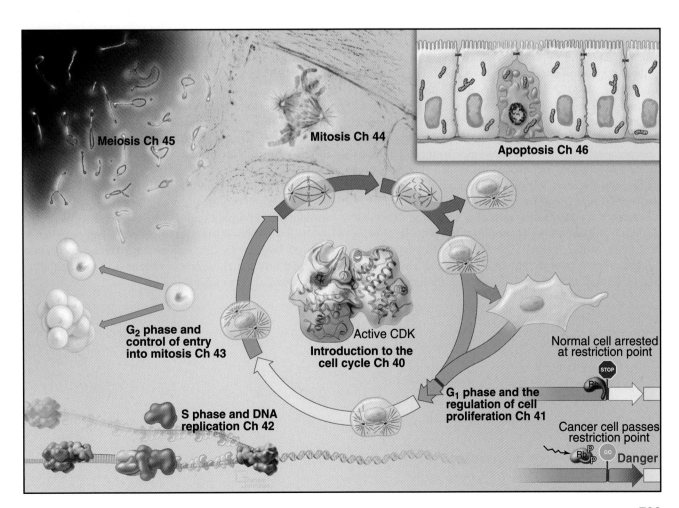

Meiosis Ch 45

Mitosis Ch 44

Apoptosis Ch 46

G₂ phase and control of entry into mitosis Ch 43

Active CDK
Introduction to the cell cycle Ch 40

Normal cell arrested at restriction point

STOP

Rb

G₁ phase and the regulation of cell proliferation Ch 41

S phase and DNA replication Ch 42

Cancer cell passes restriction point

Rb

GO

Danger

destruction by decorating them with chains of ubiquitin, a protein that was introduced in Chapter 23.

The chapters that follow explain how the cell-cycle machinery controls each step in the proliferation and differentiation of cells. Chapter 41 begins with newly born cells in the **G₁ phase** of the cell cycle. These cells need to decide whether to commit themselves to a round of proliferation or to withdraw from the proliferation rat race and enter a quiescent or differentiated state called **G₀.** Cells that are considering proliferation must first pass two inspections. The first is the **restriction point,** a biochemical control circuit that determines whether internal and external conditions are suitable for proliferation. Malfunctions of this restriction point lead to one of the most terrifying perturbations of the cell cycle: cancer. The second quality control (the G₁ phase **checkpoint**) verifies that the chromosomes are intact before allowing the cell to replicate its DNA. The chapter includes a large section on **stem cells** and concludes by considering the role of one of the most famous cell-cycle proteins, **p53,** in cell-cycle control.

Cells that decide to proliferate must replicate their DNA in a timely and accurate manner. Chapter 42 explains the mechanism of DNA replication during the **S phase,** including the selection of sites on DNA to initiate replication, the enzymes that copy the DNA, the regulation of replication by the cell-cycle machinery, the organization of replicating chromosomes within the nucleus, and the cell-cycle checkpoints that help the cells to cope with various problems that they encounter along the way. Chapter 43 discusses the **G₂ phase,** during which cells conduct a final "cockpit check" before embarking on the great adventure of division. Another key cell-cycle checkpoint looks for damaged or unreplicated DNA and restrains cells from entering into mitosis before it is repaired. This is also the last point in the cell cycle at which the genome is scanned for damage so that it can be repaired before division.

Chapter 44 describes **mitosis,** certainly the most dramatic and complex program in the cell cycle. Mitosis has been studied since the 1800s, but very recent advances have considerably advanced our understanding of how it is accomplished at the molecular level.

Division requires wholesale reorganization of cellular structures, including condensation of the chromosomes and the assembly of the mitotic spindle. In many cells, the nuclear envelope breaks down. Once the chromosomes are all attached to the microtubules of the mitotic spindle (yet another important checkpoint here), they are separated equally and form two daughter nuclei. Finally, **cytokinesis** separates the two daughter cells.

Chapter 45 takes a step to the side to consider **meiosis,** a specialized form of division that is irrelevant for most cells but absolutely critical for the continuation of many species. Meiosis is the program that is used to produce gametes that form the basis of sexual reproduction. In this division, DNA recombination is key to segregation of the chromosomes. A number of arcane terms are used to describe the specialized structures and processes involved. Meiosis provides another example of how recent research has greatly advanced the understanding of a process that has been studied for over 100 years. For example, the chapter explains how problems with meiosis can lead to genetic diseases and how studies of chromosome segregation in yeast led to an understanding of why birth defects become more prevalent as human mothers age.

Chapter 46 closes the book with a discussion of what happens when cells commit suicide by **apoptosis.** This is not, strictly speaking, a cell-cycle event but instead represents an alternative pathway with its own machinery and signaling systems. Apoptosis sometimes results when it all "runs off the rails" and cells receive insults from which they cannot recover. But cell death is not always bad, since apoptosis is an essential part of development of metazoan organisms as well as the homeostasis of their organs and tissues. Malfunctions of apoptotic pathways can lead to particularly nasty types of cancer.

The concepts that are discussed in this section of the book build on the ideas in earlier sections. Cells are wonderfully complex systems whose behavior is driven by the laws of chemistry and physics. A major challenge for cell biology in the future is to devise molecular explanations for the complex behaviors exhibited in this closing section of our book.

CHAPTER 40

Introduction to the Cell Cycle

T he **cell cycle,** is the series of events that leads to the duplication and division of a cell. Research on the molecular events of cell-cycle control revealed that variations of similar mechanisms operate the cell cycles of all eukaryotes from yeasts to humans. Furthermore, the components that regulate cell growth and division also play key roles in the cessation of cell division that accompanies cell differentiation. Control of the cell cycle is of major importance to human health because cancer, which is usually caused by perturbations of cell-cycle regulation, affects 46% of males and 38% of females in the United States.

Although animal cells have a wide variety of specialized cell cycles, the cells in the stratified epithelium that forms skin illustrate the most common lifestyles (Fig. 40-1). The basal layer of the epithelium is composed of **stem cells** that divide only occasionally. (See Box 41-1.) They can activate the cell cycle on demand and then return to a nondividing state. When specific signals induce stem cells to proliferate, one daughter cell usually remains a stem cell and the other enters a pool of rapidly dividing cells. These dividing cells populate the upper layers of the epithelium, stop dividing, and gradually differentiate into the specialized cells that cover the surface.

Similarly, the nervous system contains a few stem cells and a few dividing cells, but most neurons, once differentiated, can live for more than 100 years without dividing again. Like stem cells, fibroblasts of the connective tissue (see Fig. 28-2) are typically nondividing, but they can be stimulated to enter the cell cycle following wounding or other stimuli (see Fig. 32-11).

Principles of Cell-Cycle Regulation

The goal of the cell cycle in most cases is to produce two daughter cells that are accurate copies of the parent (Fig. 40-2). The cell cycle integrates a continuous **growth cycle** (the increase in cell mass) with a discontinuous **division** or **chromosome cycle** (the replication and partitioning of the genome into two daughter cells). The chromosome cycle is driven by a sequence of enzymatic cascades that produce a sequence of discrete biochemical "states" of the cytoplasm. Each state arises by destruction or inactivation of key enzymatic activities characteristic of the preceding state and expression or activation of a new cohort of activities. Later sections of this chapter explain these mechanisms.

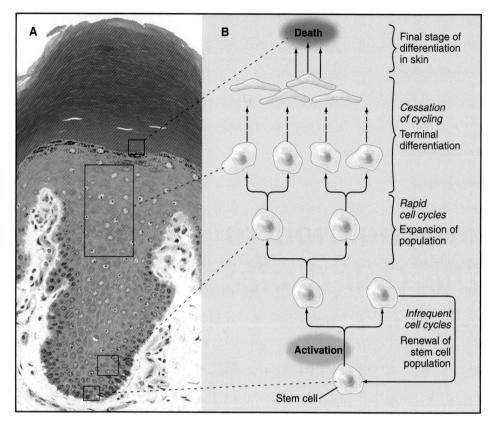

Figure 40-1 A, Light micrograph of a section of skin, a stratified squamous epithelium, stained with hematoxylin and eosin. **B,** Diagram showing the different types of cell cycles at the various levels of this epithelium.

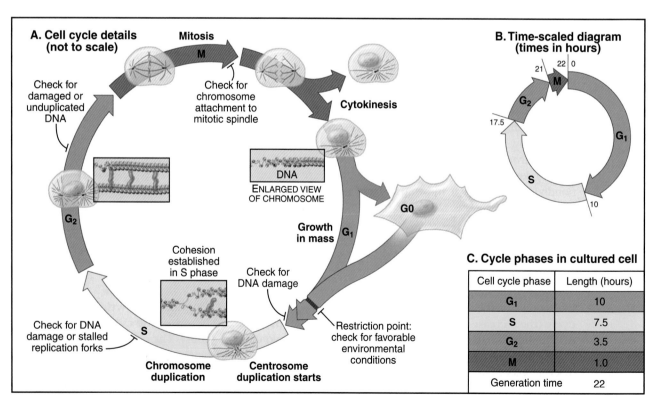

Figure 40-2 INTRODUCTION TO THE CELL-CYCLE PHASES. A, Diagrams of cellular morphology and chromosome structure across the cell cycle. **B,** Time scale of cell-cycle phases. **C,** Length of cell-cycle phases in cultured cells.

Phases of the Cell Cycle

In thinking about the cell cycle, it is convenient to divide the process into a series of phases. Recognition of cell-cycle phases began in 1882, when Flemming named the process of nuclear division **mitosis** (from the Greek *mito,* or "thread") after the appearance of the condensed chromosomes. It initially appeared that cells were active only during mitosis, so the rest of the cell cycle was called **interphase** (or resting stage) (Box 40-1).

Once DNA was recognized as the agent of heredity in the 1940s, it was deduced that DNA must be duplicated at some time during interphase so that daughter cells can each receive a full complement of genetic material. A key experiment identified the relationship between the timing of DNA synthesis and the mitotic cycle (Fig. 40-3) and defined the four cell-cycle phases as they are known today (Fig. 40-2).

Each cell is born at the completion of the **M phase,** which includes **mitosis,** the partitioning of the chromosomes and other cellular components, and **cytokinesis,** the division of the cytoplasm. The chromosomal DNA is replicated during **S phase** (synthetic phase). The remaining two phases are gaps between mitosis and the S phase. The **G$_1$ phase** (first gap phase) is the interval between mitosis and DNA replication. The **G$_2$ phase** (second gap phase) is the interval between the completion of DNA replication and mitosis. All cycling cells have an M phase and an S phase; however, some early embryos have minimal G$_1$ and G$_2$ phases. The following sections describe the stages of the cell cycle in order, starting just after the birth of the cell.

G$_1$ Phase

The G$_1$ phase is typically the longest and most variable cell-cycle phase. When cells are "born" at cytokinesis, they are half the size they were before mitosis, and during G$_1$, they grow back toward an optimal size. During this time, many genes involved in cell-cycle progression are switched off so that the cell cannot initiate a new round of proliferation. This repressive system is termed the **restriction point.** If the supply of nutrients is poor or if cells receive an antiproliferative stimulus such as a signal to embark on terminal differentiation, they delay their progress through the cell cycle in G$_1$ or exit the cycle to enter G$_0$ (see the next section). However, if appropriate positive stimuli are received, cells overcome the restriction point block and trigger a program of gene expression that commits them to a new cycle of DNA replication and cell division. Faulty restriction point control may result in cell proliferation under inappropriate conditions. Cancer cells often have defects in restriction point control and continue to attempt to divide even in the absence of appropriate environmental signals.

G$_0$ and Growth Control

Most cells of multicellular organisms differentiate to carry out specialized functions and no longer divide. Such cells are considered to be in the **G$_0$ phase.** G$_0$ cells are not dormant; indeed, they are often actively engaged in protein synthesis and secretion, and they may be highly motile. The G$_0$ phase is not necessarily permanent. In some cases, G$_0$ cells may be recruited to reenter the cell cycle in response to a variety of stimuli. This process must be highly regulated, as the uncontrolled proliferation of cells in a multicellular organism can lead to cancer.

S Phase

Chromosomes of higher eukaryotes are so large that replication of the DNA must be initiated at many different sites, termed **origins of replication.** In budding yeast, the approximately 400 origins are spaced an average of 30,000 base pairs apart. An average human chromosome contains about 150×10^6 base pairs of DNA, about 10 times the size of the entire budding yeast genome, so many more origins are required. Each region

---

BOX 40-1
Selected Key Terms

M phase: Cell division, comprising *mitosis,* when a fully grown cell segregates the replicated chromosomes to opposite ends of a molecular scaffold, termed the spindle, and *cytokinesis,* when the cell cleaves between the separated chromosomes to produce two daughter cells. In general, each daughter cell receives a complement of genetic material and organelles identical to that of the parent cell.

Interphase: The portion of the cell cycle when cells grow and replicate their DNA. Interphase has three sections. The *G$_1$ (first gap) phase* is the interval between mitosis and the onset of DNA replication. The *S (synthetic) phase* is the time when DNA is replicated. The *G$_2$ (second gap) phase* is the interval between the termination of DNA replication and the onset of mitosis. In multicellular organisms, many differentiated cells no longer actively divide. These nondividing cells (which may physiologically be extremely active) are in the *G$_0$ phase,* a branch of the G$_1$ phase.

Checkpoints: Biochemical circuits that regulate cell-cycle transitions in response to the physiological condition of the cell and the state of its environment. Checkpoints detect the presence or absence of external signals telling the cell to proliferate, damage to the DNA, and problems that arise during DNA replication and chromosome segregation.

of the chromosome that is replicated from a single origin is referred to as a **replicon.**

Proliferating diploid cells must replicate their DNA once and only once each cell cycle. Each origin of replication is prepared for replication by the formation of a prereplication complex (a process that is referred to as *licensing*) during G_1. As each origin "fires" during S phase, the prereplication complex is dismantled and cannot be reassembled until the next G_1 phase. This ensures that each origin fires only once per cell cycle. The cyclic nature of origin licensing is driven at least in part by fluctuations in the activity of cyclin-dependent kinases (discussed later).

During replication, the duplicated DNA molecules, called **sister chromatids,** become linked to each other by a protein complex called cohesin (see Fig. 13-19). This pairing of sister chromatids is important for their symmetrical segregation later in mitosis (see Fig. 44-16).

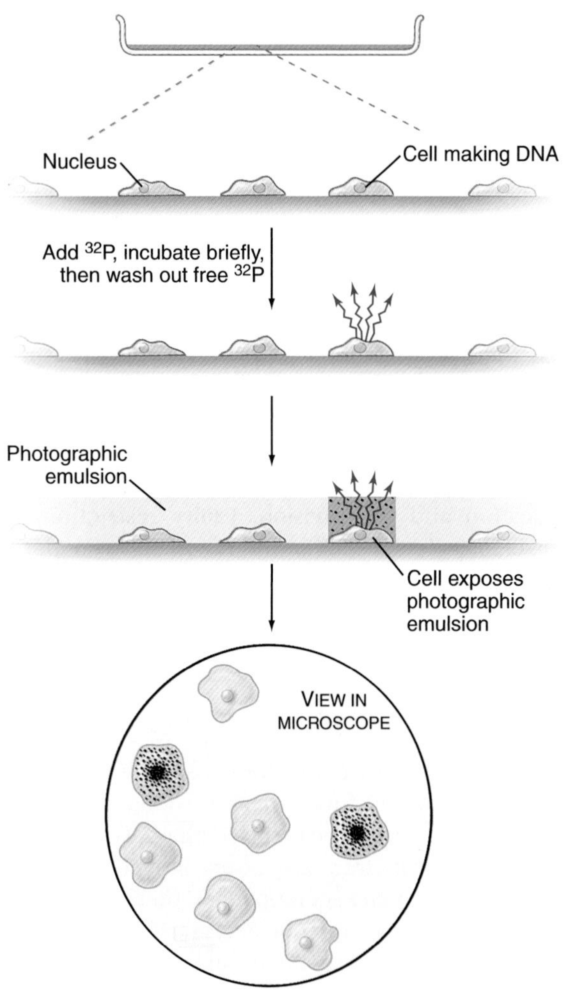

G_2 Phase

In most cells of metazoans, G_2 is a relatively brief period during which key enzymatic activities that will trigger the entry into mitosis gradually accumulate and are converted to active forms. When their activities reach a critical threshold level, the cell enters mitosis. In parallel, the chromatin and cytoskeleton are prepared for the dramatic structural changes that will occur during mitosis. If unreplicated or damaged DNA is detected during G_2, a mechanism called a checkpoint delays entry of the cell into mitosis.

M Phase

During M phase (**mitosis** and the subsequent **cytokinesis**), chromosomes and cytoplasm are partitioned into two daughter cells. Mitosis is normally divided into five discrete phases.

Prophase is defined by the onset of chromosome condensation inside the intact nucleus and is actually the final part of G_2 phase. In the cytoplasm, a dramatic change in the dynamic properties of the microtubules decreases their half-lives from ~10 minutes to ~30 seconds. The duplicated centrosomes (centrioles and associated pericentriolar material in animal cells) separate and form the two poles of the **mitotic spindle.**

Prometaphase begins when the nuclear envelope breaks down (in higher eukaryotes) and chromosomes begin to attach randomly to microtubules emanating from the two poles of the forming mitotic spindle. Chromosomes may also nucleate some spindle microtubules.

Figure 40-3 To determine whether cells synthesize DNA during a defined portion of the cell cycle or constantly throughout the entire cycle (as is the case in bacteria, for example), Howard and Pelc fed a radioactive component of DNA (^{32}P) to onion root tip cells, spread the cells in a thin layer on a microscope slide, washed away the ^{32}P that had not become incorporated into DNA, and overlayered the slide with photographic emulsion. After incubation in the dark, the emulsion was developed like film and examined with a light microscope. The nuclei of cells that were engaged in active DNA replication during the period of exposure to ^{32}P incorporated the radioactive label into DNA and exposed the photographic emulsion above them. Two possible outcomes were predicted. If cells synthesized DNA constantly during interphase, then all cells would incorporate the radioactive label. Conversely, if each cell synthesized DNA only during a discrete portion of the cell cycle, then only those cells that were engaged in active replication during the period of exposure to ^{32}P would expose the photographic emulsion. When the slides were examined, 20% of the interphase cell nuclei were labeled, proving that cells synthesize DNA only during a discrete portion of interphase. Mitotic cells were unlabeled. Assuming that the cells traverse the cycle at a more or less constant rate, it was possible to calculate the length of the synthetic phase. Overall, the time between successive divisions—the generation time—was about 30 hours in the root tip cells. If about 20% of the cells were labeled, then about 20% of the 30-hour generation time must be spent in DNA synthesis. Thus, 0.2 × 30, or 6 hours, was spent in replication. (Drawing based on the work of Pelc HA Sr: Synthesis of DNA in normal and irradiated cells and its relation to chromosome breakage. Heredity Suppl 6:261–273, 1953.)

Once both kinetochores on a pair of sister chromatids are attached to opposite spindle poles, the chromosome slowly moves to a point midway between the poles. When all chromosomes are properly attached, the cell is said to be in **metaphase.**

The exit from mitosis begins at **anaphase** with the abrupt separation of the two **sister chromatids** from one another. The metaphase-anaphase transition is triggered by the proteolytic degradation of molecules that regulate sister chromatid cohesion. During anaphase, the separated sister chromatids move to the two spindle poles **(anaphase A),** which themselves move apart **(anaphase B).** As the chromatids approach the spindle poles, the nuclear envelope reforms on the surface of the chromatin. At this point, the cell is said to be in **telophase.**

Finally, during telophase, a **contractile ring** of actin and myosin assembles as a circumferential belt in the cortex midway between spindle poles and constricts the equator of the cell. The separation of the two daughter cells from one another is called **cytokinesis.**

Checkpoints

The cell cycle is highly regulated, and **checkpoints** control transitions between cell-cycle stages. Checkpoints are biochemical circuits that detect external or internal problems and send inhibitory signals to the cell-cycle system. There are four major types of checkpoints. The **restriction point** in the G_1 phase is sensitive to the physiological state of the cell and to its interactions with the surrounding extracellular matrix. Cells that do not receive appropriate growth stimuli from their environment do not progress past this point in the G_1 phase and may commit suicide by apoptosis (see Chapter 46).

DNA damage checkpoints operate in G_1, S, and G_2 phases of the cell cycle. In general, these checkpoints block cell-cycle progression, but they can also trigger cell death by apoptosis. The **DNA replication checkpoint** detects the presence of unreplicated or stalled DNA replication forks. This checkpoint shares some components with the DNA damage checkpoints but has the additional feature that it specifically stabilizes stalled replication forks so that they can be repaired. During mitosis, the **spindle assembly checkpoint** (also called the **metaphase checkpoint)** delays the onset of chromosome segregation until all chromosomes have attached properly to the mitotic spindle.

The checkpoints in G_1, S, and G_2 use common strategies to regulate cell-cycle progression (Fig. 40-4). DNA damage is detected by *sensors.* These activate *transducers,* which are often protein kinases but may also be transcriptional activators. The transducers act on *effectors,* which ultimately block cell-cycle progression and may also fulfill other functions. Two key protein kinases, ataxia-telangiectasia mutated (ATM) and ataxia-

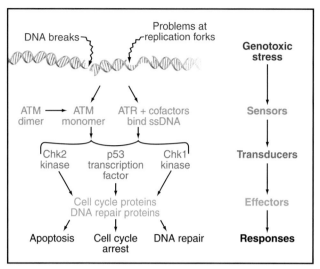

Figure 40-4 Elements of the DNA damage checkpoint system.

telangiectasia and Rad9 related (ATR), lie at the head of the pathway and may act as sensors of DNA damage. They activate two transducer kinases Chk1 and Chk2 and also stabilize a transcription factor called p53 that induces the expression of a cohort of genes involved in halting cell-cycle progression as well as genes that trigger cell death by apoptosis. Chapters 41 and 43 discuss these proteins in detail. In general, DNA damage checkpoints block cell-cycle progression by inhibiting the cyclin-dependent kinases by a variety of mechanisms.

The Biochemical Basis of Cell-Cycle Transitions

Transitions between cell-cycle phases are triggered by a network of protein kinases and phosphatases that is linked to the discontinuous events of the chromosome cycle by the periodic accumulation, modification, and destruction of several key components. This section provides a general introduction to the most important components of this network.

Cyclin-Dependent Kinases

Genetic analysis of the cell cycle in the fission yeast *Schizosaccharomyces pombe* identified a gene called cell division cycle-2+ $(cdc2^+)$ that is essential for cell-cycle progression during both the $G_1 \rightarrow S$ and $G_2 \rightarrow M$ transitions (Box 40-2). The product of this gene, a protein kinase of 34,000 D originally called p34^{cdc2}, is the prototype for a family of protein kinases that is crucial for cell-cycle progression in all eukaryotes. This mechanism of cell-cycle control is so well conserved that a human homolog of p34^{cdc2} can replace the yeast protein, restoring a normal cell cycle to a *cdc2* mutant yeast. Boxes 40-3 and 40-4 present a number of the key experiments and

BOX 40-2
Use of Genetics to Study the Cell Cycle

Studies of the distantly related budding and fission yeasts *Saccharomyces cerevisiae* and *Schizosaccharomyces pombe* (see Fig. 2-9) have been extremely important for understanding the cell cycle for several reasons. First, the proteins that control the cell cycle are remarkably conserved between yeasts and mammals. Second, both yeast genomes are sequenced and annotated, simplifying characterization of novel gene products. Third, genetic analysis is facilitated, as both yeasts grow as haploids, and both efficiently incorporate cloned DNA into their chromosomes by homologous recombination.

These two yeasts evolved very different strategies for cell division. Budding yeasts divide by assembling a single bud on the surface of the cell every cell cycle. Fission yeasts divide by fission across the center of an elongated cell. A useful feature of using yeast to study the cell cycle is that the stage of the cell cycle is revealed by the cellular morphology in the light microscope. For budding yeast, unbudded cells are in G_1, cells with buds smaller than the mother cell are in S phase, and cells whose buds are similar in size to the mother cell are in G_2 or M. For fission yeast, cell length provides a yardstick for estimating cell-cycle position.

The cell cycles of both yeasts differ from those of animal cells. In budding yeast, much of the 90-minute cell cycle is spent in G_1. Thus, the system controlling the $G_1 \rightarrow S$ transition is particularly amenable to study. In contrast, a fission yeast spends most of its two-hour cell cycle in G_2. S phase follows separation of sister chromatids and occurs prior to cytokinesis. Thus, the control of the $G_2 \rightarrow M$ transition is readily studied in fission yeast. During mitosis, the nuclear envelopes of both yeasts remains intact, so chromosomes segregate on a spindle inside the nucleus.

Genetic studies revealed that the yeast cell cycle is a *dependent pathway* whereby events in the cycle occur normally only after earlier processes are completed. The cell cycle can be modeled as a line of dominoes, each domino corresponding to the action of a gene product that is essential for cell-cycle progression (Fig. 40-5) and the *n*th domino falling only when knocked down by the (*n* − 1)th domino. According to the model, mutations in genes that are essential for cell-cycle progression cause an entire culture of yeast to accumulate at a single point in the cell cycle (the point at which the defective gene product *first becomes essential*). This is referred to as the **arrest point.** Figure 40-5 shows this by including a "mutant" domino that does not fall over when struck by the upstream domino. Mutants that meet this criterion are called **cell division cycle mutants** or **CDC mutants.** (Cdc is used in fission yeast.) Genetic screens for CDC mutants have identified many important genes involved in cell-cycle control.

Because CDC genes are essential for cell-cycle progression, it is impossible to propagate strains of yeast carrying CDC mutants unless the mutants have a **conditional lethal** phenotype. The most commonly used conditional lethal mutations are **temperature sensitive (ts).** Many yeast temperature-sensitive mutants are viable at 23°C (the **permissive temperature**) but cease dividing at 36°C (the

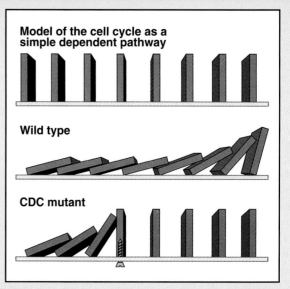

Figure 40-5 THE CELL CYCLE MAY BE MODELED AS A SIMPLE DEPENDENT PATHWAY. A CDC mutation can block further progression along the pathway, typically at a characteristic point in the cell cycle.

restrictive temperature). Temperature-sensitive proteins often have an altered amino acid sequence, but occasionally, the lack of a gene product altogether can cause a *ts* phenotype.

Fission yeasts with CDC mutants affecting the entry into mitosis have distinctive morphologies. Cells that are mutant in Wee1 (a kinase that keeps Cdk1 inactive prior to mitosis) enter mitosis prematurely and are shorter than normal (Fig. 40-6B). In contrast, cells lacking Cdc25 (a phosphatase that counteracts Wee1 and activates Cdk1) are unable to undergo mitosis but continue their growth cycle, therefore becoming greatly elongated (Fig. 40-6C). This simple morphologic assay allowed straightforward classification of yeast CDC genes into those that stimulate progression through mitosis and those that retard entry into mitosis.

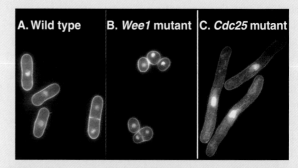

Figure 40-6 FLUORESCENCE MICROGRAPHS OF FISSION YEAST CELLS ILLUSTRATING PHENOTYPES OF CELL CYCLE MUTATIONS. Cell walls and nuclei are stained. **A,** Wild-type cells. **B,** Mutant *wee1* that accelerates entry into mitosis at the restrictive temperature. **C,** Mutant *cdc25* that delays entry into mitosis at the restrictive temperature. (Courtesy of H. Ohkura, Wellcome Trust Institute for Cell Biology, University of Edinburgh, Scotland.)

Studies of the Cell Cycle in Vitro

Amphibian oocytes and eggs are storehouses of most components needed for cell-cycle progression. Oocytes are arrested in G_2 until a surge of the hormone progesterone causes them to "mature" into eggs, which are then naturally arrested in metaphase of the second meiotic division (see Chapter 45). After fertilization, the embryo of the South African clawed frog *(Xenopus laevis)* undergoes a rapid burst of cell divisions. An initial cell cycle that is 90 minutes long is followed by a rapid succession of 11 cleavages spaced only 30 minutes apart to produce an embryo of 4096 cells (Fig. 40-7).

Thirty minutes per cycle is insufficient to transcribe and translate all of the genes needed to make the daughter cells that are produced at each division. The frog solves this problem by making oocytes extremely large (~500,000 times the volume of a typical somatic cell) and storing within them vast stockpiles of the structural components needed to make cells. As a result, only DNA and a very few proteins need be synthesized during early embryonic divisions. In addition to structural components, many factors that regulate normal cell-cycle progression are also stockpiled in oocytes. These features make *Xenopus* oocytes an excellent source of material for cell-cycle analyses.

Remarkably, it is possible to make cell-free extracts from *Xenopus* eggs that progress through the cell cycle in vitro (Fig. 40-8). Nuclei from G_1 cells, when added to

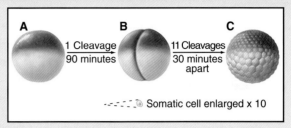

Figure 40-7 **SUMMARY DIAGRAM OF THE EARLY DEVELOPMENT OF** ***XENOPUS*** **SHOWING HOW CLEAVAGES SUBDIVIDE THE EGG. A,** Fertilized egg. **B,** Two-cell stage. **C,** Multicellular embryo. Compare size of somatic cell and egg.

these extracts, efficiently replicate their DNA and proceed through the cell cycle into mitosis, complete with chromosome condensation, nuclear envelope breakdown, chromosome alignment on a spindle, and anaphase segregation of sister chromatids without any additions to the tube. Because these events occur in a cell-free milieu, they are readily accessible to biochemical manipulation. For example, antibodies and other proteins can be added to the extracts, and their effect on the cell cycle can readily be determined. Thus, the *Xenopus* extract system offers one of the best tools for testing the role of various proteins in the cell cycle in higher eukaryotes.

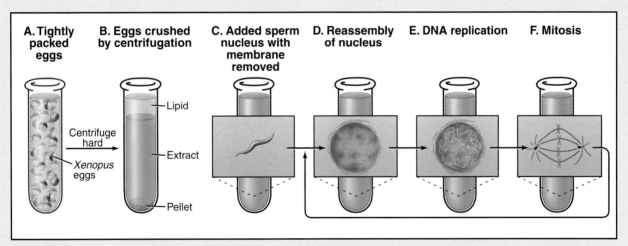

Figure 40-8 A–B, The procedure for making an extract from *Xenopus* eggs that is competent to carry out cell-cycle oscillations in vitro. **C–F,** The sequence of cell-cycle events that occur in a cycling *Xenopus* extract. These cycles consist of alternating S and M phases. G_1 and G_2 phases are minimal (as they are during early development of the frog).

BOX 40-4
Discovery of Factors Essential for Cell-Cycle Progression

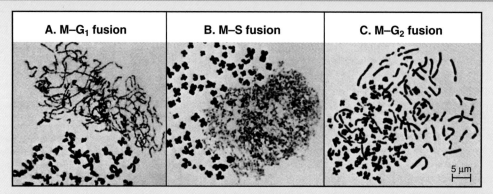

A. M–G₁ fusion   **B. M–S fusion**   **C. M–G₂ fusion**

5 µm

Figure 40-9   FUSION OF MITOTIC AND INTERPHASE CELLS CAUSES THE INTERPHASE CELLS TO ENTER MITOSIS PREMATURELY, NO MATTER WHERE THEY ARE IN THE CELL CYCLE. The resulting prematurely condensed chromosomes are single threads if the interphase cell was in G_1 phase **(A)**, or double threads if the cell was in G_2 phase **(C)**, and a complex mixture of both interspersed with uncondensed regions if the cell was in S phase **(B)**. (From Hanks SK, Gollin SM, Rao PN, et al: Cell cycle-specific changes in the ultrastructural organization of prematurely condensed chromosomes. Chromosoma 88:333–342, 1983.)

The best early evidence for the existence of positive inducers of cell-cycle transitions in mammals was obtained in cell fusion experiments. When cultured cells in S phase were fused with cells in G_1, the G_1 nuclei initiated DNA replication shortly thereafter. In contrast, if S phase cells were fused with G_2 cells, the G_2 nuclei did not rereplicate their DNA until after passing through mitosis. The most dramatic results were obtained when mitotic cells were fused with interphase cells. This caused the interphase cells to enter into mitosis abruptly (as judged by nuclear envelope breakdown and chromosome condensation). The phenomenon was termed **premature chromosome condensation (PCC).** The mitotic inducer could work in any cell-cycle phase (Fig. 40-9). If mitotic cells were fused with cells in G_1 phase, interphase chromosomes condensed into long, single filaments. If the interphase cell was in G_2 phase, the duplicated chromosomes appeared as double filaments. If the interphase cell was in the S phase, the partially replicated chromosomes condensed into a

complex pattern of single and double condensed regions separated by regions of decondensed chromatin corresponding to sites where DNA was actively replicating at the time of fusion.

Working independently, developmental biologists who were interested in the control of cell division during early development in frogs also discovered an activity that could cause interphase cells to enter the M phase. They used a micropipette to extract a tiny bit of cytoplasm from a mature egg that was arrested in metaphase of meiosis II and inject it into oocytes (which are in G_2 phase). The oocytes rapidly entered M phase, with concomitant chromosome condensation and nuclear envelope disassembly (Fig. 40-10). This stimulation to enter M phase is called *maturation,* and the unknown factor present in the egg cytoplasm that induced oocyte maturation was termed **MPF,** or **maturation-promoting factor** (now often referred to as **M phase**-promoting factor). It was realized early on that MPF might be related to the inducer of mitosis

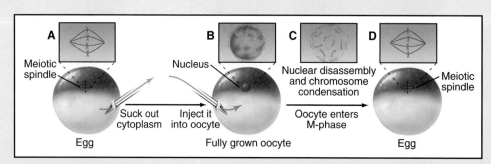

A Meiotic spindle   **B** Nucleus   **C** Nuclear disassembly and chromosome condensation   **D** Meiotic spindle

Suck out cytoplasm   Inject it into oocyte   Oocyte enters M-phase

Egg   Fully grown oocyte   Egg

Figure 40-10   DIAGRAM OF THE EXPERIMENTAL PROTOCOL THAT IDENTIFIED MATURATION PROMOTING FACTOR. **A,** The *box* shows the meiotic spindle in a *Xenopus* egg arrested in metaphase II of meiosis. **B,** The *box* shows the interphase nucleus in a mature oocyte. Following injection of MPF, the nucleus disassembles **(C),** and the cell assembles a meiotic spindle **(D).** Disassembly of the oocyte nucleus and entry into M phase is called maturation, and the factor triggering this event was named maturation promoting factor (MPF).

Discovery of Factors Essential for Cell-Cycle Progression—cont'd

detected in the PCC experiments. In fact, extracts from mitotic tissue culture cells could induce meiotic maturation when injected into oocytes. Similar extracts from cells in other phases of the cell cycle did not cause the G_2/M phase transition in oocytes.

Other cell biologists studying protein synthesis in starfish and sea urchin embryos noticed a curious protein that seemed to accumulate across the cell cycle but was then destroyed during mitosis. They were well aware of the work on MPF, and immediately suspected that their protein, which they called cyclin, might be somehow involved in MPF activity (Fig. 40-11).

In a third line of investigation, geneticists working on yeasts realized that the cell cycle could be dissected through the isolation of cell division cycle (CDC) mutants (Box 40-2). The analysis of the cell cycle with these mutants

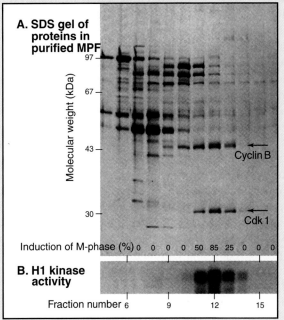

Figure 40-12 PURIFICATION OF MPF. **A,** SDS polyacrylamide gel electrophoresis of fractions from the final column used in purification. The numbers at the bottom show the percentage of oocytes that entered M phase when a portion of each column fraction was injected (the classical MPF assay). The roughly 32-kD band is Cdk1 ($p34^{cdc2}$). The roughly 45-kD band is cyclin B. **B,** Assay of the ability of the column fractions to phosphorylate histone HI. This is now the standard assay for active Cdk enzymes. (Redrawn from Lohka M, Hayes MK, Maller JL: Purification of maturation-promoting factor, an intracellular regulator of early mitotic events. Proc Natl Acad Sci U S A 85:3009–3013, 1988.)

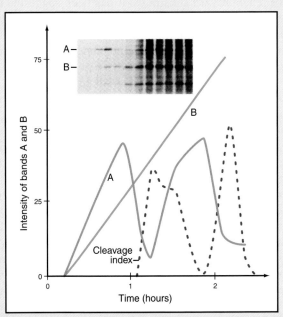

Figure 40-11 THE ORIGINAL IDENTIFICATION OF A CYCLIN. Newly synthesized proteins (labeled with ^{35}S-methionine) in fertilized sea urchin eggs were separated by SDS polyacrylamide gel electrophoresis. It was noted that the protein labeled A (which was named cyclin) first accumulated, was greatly reduced at the metaphase/anaphase transition, and then began to accumulate again. Protein B, which is not involved in cell-cycle regulation, accumulated progressively over this time. "Cleavage index" refers to the percentage of dividing cells observed in the microscope at varying times after fertilization. (From Evans T, Rosenthal ET, Youngblom J, et al: Cyclin: A protein specified by maternal mRNA in sea urchin eggs that is destroyed at each cleavage division. Cell 33:389–396, 1983.)

dominated cell-cycle research to such an extent that many human genes that are important in cell-cycle control bear the CDC name if they are related to well-characterized yeast genes. The best-known genes to emerge from this analysis were *Cdc2* (Cdk1) and *Cdc25,* both of which were determined genetically to encode proteins that actively promote the G_2/M transition. Other genes, such as *Wee1,* were found to encode activities that act as antagonists that inhibit the G_2/M transition.

When active MPF was eventually purified from *Xenopus* eggs (Fig. 40-12), the purified fractions turned out to consist primarily of two polypeptide chains of 45,000 D and 32,000 D. The 32,000-D component of MPF is the *Xenopus* equivalent of the fission yeast Cdc2 (now known as Cdk1) gene product. The 45,000-D component of MPF is a *Xenopus* B-type cyclin.

experimental systems that led to the identification of the molecules that drive the cell cycle.

Humans have more than 10 distinct protein kinases related to p34[cdc2], although only a few are involved in cell-cycle control. To be active, these enzymes must each associate with a regulatory subunit called a cyclin. Thus, they have been termed **cyclin-dependent kinases (Cdks).** p34[cdc2], now termed Cdk1, seems to function primarily in the regulation of the $G_2 \rightarrow M$ transition in animal cells. A second family member, Cdk2, is involved in regulation of the $G_1 \rightarrow S$ and $G_2 \rightarrow M$ transitions, whereas two other family members—Cdk4 and Cdk6—are involved in passage of the restriction point (Appendix 40-1). Cdk7 is important for activation of other Cdks, and also appears to participate in RNA transcription and repair of damaged DNA. Other Cdks participate in diverse processes ranging from transcriptional regulation to neuronal differentiation and may play as-yet-undiscovered roles in cell-cycle regulation. Surprisingly, fibroblasts from mice that lack Cdk2, Cdk4, or Cdk6 are viable; other Cdks must be able to drive the cell cycle if necessary. The mice themselves suffer difficulties because the genes are needed for the differentiation of particular cell types.

Cyclins

The defining feature of Cdks is that they require binding of **cyclins** for catalytic activity. Cyclins are a diverse group of proteins ranging in size between 35 kD and 130 kD, all with a similar core structure based on two symmetrical domains of five α-helices (Fig. 40-13). One of these domains, the cyclin box, is highly conserved and is the defining structural feature of these proteins. Cyclins were discovered in rapidly dividing invertebrate embryos as proteins that accumulate gradually during interphase and are abruptly destroyed during mitosis (Fig. 40-11). This process of cyclic accumulation and destruction is the derivation of their name. Subsequently, at least 16 different cyclins have been identified in humans, although only a handful are involved in cell-cycle control. Of those that are, some function during G_1 phase, others during G_2 phase, and still others during M phase.

Positive Regulation of Cyclin-Dependent Kinase Structure and Function

The activity of Cdks is regulated with extraordinary care. Like other eukaryotic protein kinases (see Fig. 25-3), Cdks have a bilobed structure with the active site in a deep cleft between a small N-terminal and larger C-terminal domain. However, newly synthesized monomeric Cdks differ from other kinases in that they appear to be incompletely folded: a flexible loop (T loop) blocks the mouth of the catalytic pocket. In addition, misorientation of a short α-helix causes a glutamic acid required for adenosine triphosphate (ATP) hydrolysis to point away from the catalytic cleft. As a result, ATP bound by the monomeric kinase is distorted and cannot transfer its α-phosphate to protein substrates (Fig. 40-13A).

At least four different mechanisms regulate Cdk activity (Fig. 40-14). On one hand, cyclin binding and phosphorylation of the T loop stimulate enzyme activity. On the other, phosphorylation of residues adjacent to the ATP-binding site and binding of inhibitory proteins inhibit Cdks.

Cyclin binding profoundly changes Cdk structure, causing the retraction of the T loop back from the mouth of the catalytic pocket (Fig. 40-13B). In addition, the secondary structure of the N-terminal domain is altered, reorienting the short helix by 90 degrees so that the critical glutamate can interact with the ATP phosphates. This causes the bound ATP to assume a conformation suitable for reaction with substrates. It has been suggested that cyclin binding also causes two residues—threonine[14] and tyrosine[15] in the roof of the ATP-binding pocket—to reorient so that they become accessible to protein kinases that regulate Cdk1 activity (see later section).

Despite these changes, the Cdk-cyclin complex has only partial catalytic activity. Complete activation of most Cdks requires the action of a kinase called Cdk-activating kinase (CAK), which phosphorylates threonine[160] in the T loop of Cdk2-cyclin A (this threonine gives the loop its name). In vertebrates, CAK is composed of Cdk7-cyclin H. Phosphorylated threonine[160] fits into a charged pocket on the surface of the enzyme, flattening the T loop back even farther from the mouth of the catalytic pocket (Figs. 40-13C and 40-14A). This stimulates the catalytic activity up to 300-fold, in part because the flattened T loop forms part of the substrate-binding surface. In addition, threonine[160] phosphorylation stabilizes the association of Cdk2 with cyclin A.

In addition to their cyclin partner, Cdk1 and Cdk2 bind an additional small Cdc kinase subunit (Cks) protein to their C-terminal domain, away from the active site. Bound Cks influences substrate recognition and increases the efficiency of substrate phosphorylation by the Cdk-cyclin-Cks kinase. In addition, Cks proteins play an important role in promoting the destruction of cyclin B and the Cdk inhibitor p27[Kip1].

Negative Regulation of Cyclin-Dependent Kinase Structure and Function

At least two mechanisms slow or stop the cell cycle by inactivating Cdks (Fig. 40-14). During G_2 phase, the protein kinases Myt1 and Wee1 hold Cdk1 in check by phosphorylating threonine[14] and tyrosine[15] in the roof

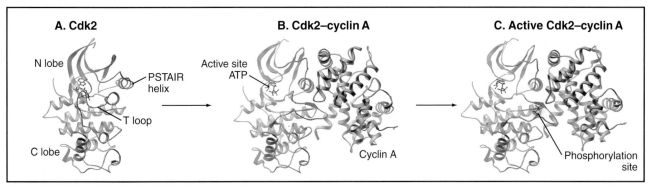

A. Cdk2

N lobe

PSTAIR helix

T loop

C lobe

B. Cdk2–cyclin A

Active site
ATP

Cyclin A

C. Active Cdk2–cyclin A

Phosphorylation site

Figure 40-13   ATOMIC STRUCTURES OF CYCLIN-DEPENDENT KINASES. **A,** Cdk2. The PSTAIR helix, found in most Cdks, is named after a sequence of six amino acids (one letter code). (PDB file: 1DM2.) **B,** Cdk2–cyclin A (kinase at basal activity level). (PDB file: 1FIN.) **C,** Cdk2–cyclin (kinase fully active following phosphorylation of threonine[160]). (PDB file: 1JST.)

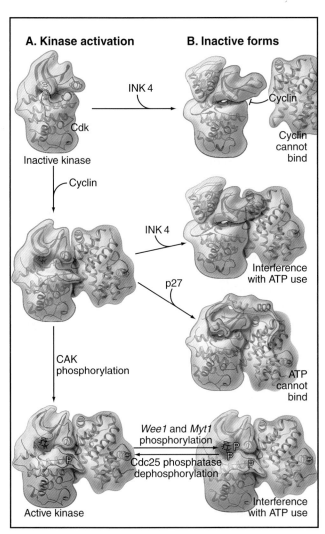

A. Kinase activation   **B. Inactive forms**

INK 4

Cyclin

Cdk

Inactive kinase

Cyclin cannot bind

Cyclin

INK 4

p27

Interference with ATP use

CAK phosphorylation

ATP cannot bind

Wee1 and *Myt1* phosphorylation

Cdc25 phosphatase dephosphorylation

Active kinase

Interference with ATP use

Figure 40-14   POSITIVE AND NEGATIVE REGULATION OF CYCLIN-DEPENDENT KINASES. **A,** Pathway of activation by cyclin binding and phosphorylation. **B,** Pathways of inactivation by inhibitor binding and phosphorylation. (PDB files: Cdk2-INK4 is 1BI7; Cdk2-INK4-cyclin A is a composite of 1FIN and 1BI7; Cdk2-p27-cyclin A is 1JSU.)

of the ATP-binding site. These phosphates interfere with ATP binding and hydrolysis. Because threonine[14] and tyrosine[15] are accessible to the regulatory kinases only following cyclin binding, this phosphorylation of Cdks depends, at least in part, on the availability of cyclins.

Three Cdc25 phosphatases (see Fig. 25-5) reverse these inhibitory phosphorylations. Cdc25A is involved in the regulation of both the $G_1 \rightarrow S$ and $G_2 \rightarrow M$ transitions and is essential for life of the cell. Ccd25B is dispensable for mitosis, but it is essential for the production of gametes in meiosis. Cdc25C is a target of the G_2 DNA damage checkpoint that prevents cells from undergoing mitosis with damaged DNA (see Fig. 43-12), but cells can survive without it.

A second strategy for inactivating Cdks involves the binding of small inhibitory subunits of the cyclin-dependent kinase inhibitor (CKI) and inhibitor of Cdk4 (INK4) families (for their names, see Appendix 40-1). CKI molecules inactivate Cdk-cyclin A complexes most efficiently. The CKI p27[Kip1] inactivates Cdk2–cyclin A complexes in two ways (Fig. 40-15A). One part of p27[Kip1] associates with the cyclin subunit, while another invades the N-terminal domain of the Cdk, profoundly disrupting its structure and competing with ATP for binding to the active site.

Members of the INK4 family preferentially inactivate Cdk4 and Cdk6. They do this in two ways (Fig. 40-15B). First, interaction with monomeric Cdk opposite the catalytic cleft distorts the orientation of the N- and C-terminal lobes so that cyclin D does not bind. INK4 family inhibitors also inhibit preformed Cdk4/6–cyclin D complexes by binding the Cdk and distorting the ATP-binding site so that the kinase uses ATP much less efficiently.

Cdk inhibitors are important for growth regulation during the G_1 and G_0 phases of the cell cycle (see Chapter 41). They also play a critical role in the cell-cycle arrest

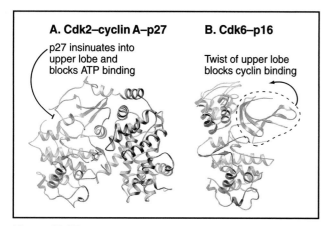

A. Cdk2–cyclin A–p27

p27 insinuates into upper lobe and blocks ATP binding

B. Cdk6–p16

Twist of upper lobe blocks cyclin binding

Figure 40-15 ATOMIC STRUCTURES OF CYCLIN-DEPENDENT KINASES WITH BOUND INHIBITORS. **A,** Cdk2–cyclin A with bound p27^{Kip1}. **B,** Crystal structures of Cdk4 with bound inhibitor p16^{Ink4a}.

that occurs in response to DNA damage and to anti-proliferative signals.

Role of Protein Destruction in Cell-Cycle Control

Mitosis is a state of the cytoplasm dominated by high levels of active Cdk1-cyclin B-Cks. Phosphorylation of key components by this kinase leads to dramatic reorganization of the cell and, ultimately, to separation of sister chromatids on the mitotic spindle. Once chromatids are separated, the cell must return to a state with low levels of Cdk activity so that nuclear envelope reassembly, spindle disassembly, and cytokinesis can occur. Thus, exit from mitosis requires Cdk inactivation. This occurs through the action of the ubiquitin-directed proteolytic machinery that targets, among other key proteins, A- and B-type cyclins and a protein called securin, which

regulates the onset of sister chromatid separation at anaphase. Destruction of cyclins inactivates the Cdk1 and Cdk2 kinases, allowing various phosphatases to reverse the action of Cdks and bring mitosis to a close.

Ubiquitin-mediated destruction of cyclins involves the action of a series of enzymes (see Fig. 23-8). First, an E1 enzyme (**ubiquitin-activating enzyme**) activates the small protein **ubiquitin** by forming a thioester bond between the C-terminus of ubiquitin and a cysteine on the enzyme. Activated ubiquitin is then transferred to another thioester bond on an E2 enzyme (**ubiquitin-conjugating enzyme**). E2 may either transfer ubiquitin directly to the ε-amino group of a lysine of a target protein or combine with a third component (an E3 or ubiquitin-protein ligase) to do so. E3s are particularly important for imparting substrate specificity. Finally, the same enzymes build a chain of ubiquitins by successive conjugations of the C-terminus of a new ubiquitin to a lysine side chain of the previous ubiquitin.

The resulting polyubiquitinated proteins are usually targets for destruction by the cylindrical 26S **proteasome** (see Fig. 23-5), although depending on the way the ubiquitins are linked together, they may alternatively serve as signaling intermediates. The proteasome is a large multienzyme complex that functions like a cytoplasmic garbage disposal, grinding target proteins down to short peptides and spitting out intact ubiquitin monomers for reuse in further rounds of protein degradation. Its role was originally thought to be the removal of damaged proteins from the cytoplasm; however, it is now recognized as a central factor in cell-cycle control.

The key factor regulating proteolysis of cyclins is a large (20S) complex with E3 activity consisting of 12 to 13 subunits called the **anaphase-promoting complex/cyclosome (APC/C)** (Fig. 40-16). The APC/C is inactive during the S and G_2 phases of the cell cycle. Binding of protein "specificity factors" such as Cdc20

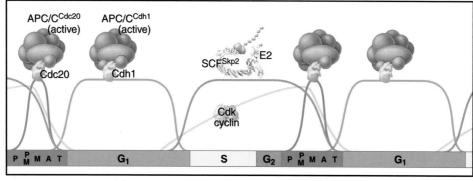

Figure 40-16 THE ROLES OF THE TWO FORMS OF ANAPHASE-PROMOTING COMPLEX/CYCLOSOME IN CELL-CYCLE CONTROL. At the metaphase-anaphase transition, the APC/C with associated Cdc20 triggers the onset of anaphase by signaling the degradation of securin and cyclin B. During mitosis Cdh1 phosphorylated by Cdk1–cyclin B is unable to bind APC/C, so APC/C^{Cdh1} activity is low. As Cdk1–cyclin B activity declines in anaphase, Cdh1 binds APC/C and APC/C^{Cdh1} drives the exit from mitosis into G_1. APC/C^{Cdh1} remains active throughout G_1 until phosphorylation by Cdk2–cyclin A again causes Cdh1 to dissociate from APC/C. After the onset of S phase, SCF (shown here adding a ubiquitin chain to a docked substrate) directs the degradation of cell cycle substrates such as p27^{Kip1}, following their phosphorylation by protein kinases.

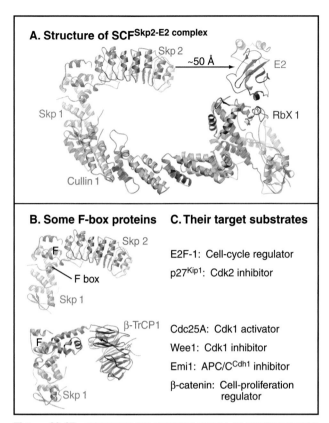

A. Structure of SCF^{Skp2-E2} complex

Skp 2
~50 Å
E2
Skp 1
RbX 1
Cullin 1

B. Some F-box proteins

Skp 2
F
F box
Skp 1

β-TrCP1
F
Skp 1

C. Their target substrates

E2F-1: Cell-cycle regulator

p27^{Kip1}: Cdk2 inhibitor

Cdc25A: Cdk1 activator

Wee1: Cdk1 inhibitor

Emi1: APC/C^{Cdh1} inhibitor

β-catenin: Cell-proliferation regulator

Figure 40-17 STRUCTURE AND FUNCTION OF SCF, AN E3 THAT TARGETS PROTEINS FOR CELL-CYCLE-REGULATED DESTRUCTION, USUALLY AFTER THEY HAVE BEEN PHOSPHORYLATED BY CYCLIN-DEPENDENT KINASES (AND OTHER KINASES). **A,** Structure of SCF^{Skp2}. **Left,** SCF recognizes target proteins through its F-box subunit (Skp2 in this case). **Right,** Ubiquitin is then transferred from an E2 enzyme. The whole is assembled on a rigid bow-like scaffold composed of the cullin subunit. Structures of F-box proteins Skp2 and β-Trcp **(B)** and a list of several of their known target proteins **(C)**.

and phosphorylation by Cdk1-cyclin B-Cks1 activate the APC/C in early mitosis. APC/C^{Cdc20} is responsible for triggering the metaphase-anaphase transition.

Later in mitosis, the APC/C binds a second specificity factor, Cdh1. Cdk phosphorylation blocks Cdh1 binding to APC/C, so APC/C^{Cdh1} forms only after cyclin levels (and therefore Cdk activity) start to fall late in mitosis. Further repression of Cdk activity and destruction of Cdc20 by APC/C^{Cdh1} are critical both for mitotic exit and during G₁ phase in preparing chromatin for the initiation of DNA replication (see Chapter 42). As cells pass from G₁ into S phase, a newly synthesized protein, Emi1, binds to APC/C^{Cdh1} and inactivates it. This allows the accumulation of cyclins during S and G₂. Remarkably, APC/C^{Cdh1} also has a role in nondividing neurons, where it is involved with regulating the activity of synapses.

A different E3 activity functions after the G₁ → S transition and throughout the remainder of interphase to regulate the levels of Cdk activity that ultimately results in mitotic entry. This activity is called SCF after

three of its four key subunits: Skp1, Cullin, and F-box (Fig. 40-17). SCF is a molecular toolbox built on a bow-shaped scaffold formed by the cullin subunit. The fourth subunit, Rbx1, binds near the C-terminus of cullin and uses a protein motif called a RING finger to dock to an E2 enzyme. Skp1 binds to the other end of cullin, where it provides a docking site for the F-box protein that actually recognizes and binds the substrate. (The F-box got its name because it was first discovered in cyclin F.) Humans have 78 F-box proteins (*Caenorhabditis elegans* has 350), and this gives SCF an enormous versatility. We discuss two of these: Skp2, which targets the Cdk inhibitor p27, and β-Trcp, which targets Cdc25A, Wee1, and Emi1. SCF is fundamentally different from the APC/C because many F-box proteins bind substrates only after they have been phosphorylated, often by Cdks.

Figure 40-18 shows the activities of two of the major SCF complexes: SCF^{Skp2}, which helps to drive the G₁ → S transition, and SCF^{β-Trcp}, which functions throughout the cycle, sometimes as an inhibitor and sometimes as a stimulator of cell-cycle progression.

Changing States of the Cytoplasm during the Cell Cycle

The cell cycle is characterized by five discrete physiological states of the cytoplasm, including two phases of mitosis (Fig. 40-18). Transitions between these states are driven by changing levels of Cdk activity, which are sometimes counteracted and sometimes reinforced by targeted proteolysis.

1. Early mitosis. Starting in prophase, mitotic Cdks (Cdk1 and Cdk2, in combination with cyclins A and B) are highly active. At prometaphase, the APC/C^{Cdc20} degrades cyclin A, but the spindle checkpoint inhibits destruction of other substrates. When the last chromosome has attached correctly to both spindle poles, the checkpoint block is released, and APC/C^{Cdc20} starts to gradually degrade cyclin B and securin, an inhibitor of a key protease called separase. This degradation continues throughout metaphase.

2. Anaphase and mitotic exit. When securin levels fall below a critical threshold, separase is activated and cleaves a key substrate in the cohesin complex (see Fig. 13-19). This triggers sister chromatid separation. Cyclin destruction continues throughout anaphase and telophase, and falling Cdk1 activity allows the formation of APC/C^{Cdh1}, which destroys Cdc20 and completes destruction of the B-type cyclins. SCF^{β-Trcp} destruction of Emi1 allows APC/C^{Cdh1} to be active when it forms.

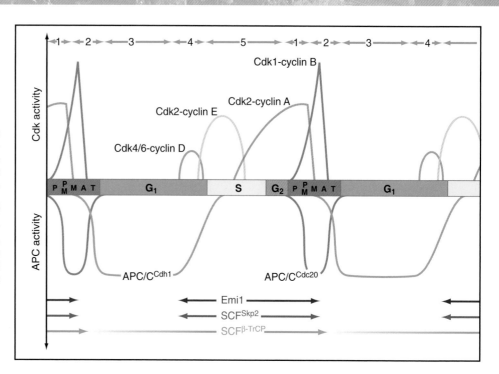

Figure 40-18 DIAGRAM SHOWING THE CHANGING PATTERNS OF CYCLIN-DEPENDENT KINASE, ANAPHASE-PROMOTING COMPLEX, AND SCF ACTIVATION IN THE VARIOUS CELL-CYCLE STATES. Between G_2 and G_1 are shown the various stages of mitosis: P, prophase; PM, pro-metaphase; M, metaphase; A, anaphase; T, telophase. The states of the cytoplasm discussed in the text are shown as *green arrows* across the top.

3. G_1 phase. APC/C^{Cdh1} and Cdk inhibitors of the CKI and Ink4 family cooperate to inhibit Cdk activity. Low Cdk activity is required for cytokinesis, spindle disassembly, chromosome decondensation, nuclear envelope reassembly, reactivation of transcription, reassembly of the Golgi apparatus, and assembly of prereplication complexes on the chromosomes.

4. G_1–S phase transition. Growth signals from the environment stimulate the cell to synthesize D-type cyclins. If the levels pass a critical threshold, a pulse of Cdk4/6 and Cdk2 activity triggers passage of the restriction point, leading to synthesis of proteins required for DNA replication and cell-cycle progression. Cdk phosphorylation targets the CKI peptides for destruction by SCF allowing Cdk2 to become activated. In addition, APC/C^{Cdh1} is inactivated by newly synthesized Emi1. Rising levels of Cdk2-cyclin A ultimately trigger the onset of DNA replication.

5. S–G_2 phase. Cdk activity remains high throughout the remainder of the cell cycle, and SCF continues to degrade selected proteins targeted by the Cdks. In addition, SCF$^{\beta-Trcp}$ destruction of Cdc25A keeps Cdk1 inactive, preventing a premature entry into mitosis. The APC/C remains switched off, allowing accumulation of mitotic cyclins. It is not known what ultimately triggers entry into mitosis, but a switch in the specificity of SCF$^{\beta-Trcp}$, which now spares Cdc25A and instead degrades the Cdk-inhibitory kinase Wee1, may be an important factor.

Although this sounds complicated, the underlying principles are actually quite straightforward. The following chapters discuss the cell-cycle transitions in greater detail and show how checkpoints modulate the process in response to a changing environment.

ACKNOWLEDGMENTS

Thanks go to David Morgan, Jan-Michael Peters, Jonathon Pines, and Claude Prigent for their suggestions on revisions to this chapter.

SELECTED READINGS

Hartwell LH, Weinert TA: Checkpoints: Controls that ensure the order of cell cycle events. Science 246:629–634, 1989.

Kastan M, Bartek J: Cell-cycle checkpoints and cancer. Nature 432:316–323, 2004.

Morgan DO: Cyclin-dependent kinases: Engines, clocks and microprocessors. Annu Rev Cell Biol 13:261–291, 1997.

Murray AW: Recycling the cell cycle: Cyclins revisited. Cell 116:221–234, 2004.

Nasmyth K: A prize for proliferation. Cell 107:689–701, 2001.

Nigg EA: Cell division: Mitotic kinases as regulators of cell division and its checkpoints. Nat Rev Mol Cell Biol 2:21–32, 2001.

Nurse P: A long twentieth century of the cell cycle and beyond. Cell 100:71–78, 2000.

Peters JM: The anaphase-promoting complex: Proteolysis in mitosis and beyond. Mol Cell 9:931–943, 2002.

Pines J: Four-dimensional control of the cell cycle. Nat Cell Biol 1: E73–E79, 1999.

Russell P: Checkpoints on the road to mitosis. Trends Biochem Sci 23:399–402, 1998.

Sherr CJ: Cancer cell cycles. Science 274:1672–1677, 1996.

APPENDIX 40-1

Inventory of the Enzymes of the Cell Cycle Engine

Cyclin-Dependent Kinases and Their Cyclin Partners

Kinase	Cyclin (+ Other) Partner	Function
Cdk1 (p34^{cdc2})	A B_1, B_2 (Xenopus has 5 B-type cyclins) Cdk1–cyclin B binds Cks1.	Mammals: triggers $G_2 \to M$ transition. Yeasts: triggers $G_1 \to S$ and $G_2 \to M$ transitions. Cyclin A is synthesized in S and destroyed starting at prometaphase. Cyclins B are synthesized in S/G_2 and destroyed following the completion of chromosome attachment to the spindle.
Cdk2	A, E	Triggers $G_1 \to S$ transition. Can be replaced by other Cdks in mouse.
Cdk3	?	Poorly understood. May trigger $G_1 \to S$ transition.
Cdk4, Cdk6	D_1–D_3	Phosphorylation of the retinoblastoma susceptibility protein (pRb) in G_1. Triggers passage of the restriction point and cyclin E synthesis. Extracellular growth factors control synthesis of D cyclins. Can be replaced by other Cdks in mouse.
Cdk5	p35 (G)	Neuronal differentiation
Cdk7 (CAK)	H; also binds assembly factor MAT1.	Cdk activation by phosphorylation of the T loop. Also in TFIIH, important for regulation of RNA polymerase II transcription and DNA repair.
Cdk8	C	Regulation of RNA polymerase II transcription.
Cdk9	T	Regulation of RNA polymerase II transcription.

Cyclin Inhibitors

Inhibitor	Cdk Substrates	Function
CKI: p21$^{Cip1/Waf1}$	most Cdk-cyclin complexes	Induced by p53 tumor suppresser. Cell cycle arrest after DNA damage. Binds PCNA (see Chapter 42) and inhibits DNA synthesis. Promotes cell cycle arrest in senescence and terminal differentiation. At low levels, may help to assemble active Cdk-cyclin complexes.
CKI: p27^{Kip1}	most Cdk-cyclin complexes	Cell cycle arrest in response to growth suppressers like TGF-β and in contact inhibition and differentiation.
CKI: p57^{Kip2}	most Cdk-cyclin complexes	Important in development of the palate.
INK4: p15^{Ink4b}	Cdk4, Cdk6	Cell cycle arrest in response to TGF-β. Also altered in many cancers.
INK4: p16^{Ink4a}	Cdk4, Cdk6	Cooperates with the retinoblastoma susceptibility protein (pRb) in growth regulation. Cell cycle arrest in senescence. Altered in a high percentage of human cancers. This gene overlaps the gene for p19^{ARF}, an important regulator of the p53 tumor suppresser protein.
INK4: p18^{Ink4c}	Cdk4, Cdk6	Cell cycle arrest in response to growth suppressers.
INK4: p19^{Ink4d}	Cdk4, Cdk6	Cell cycle arrest in response to growth suppressers.

Other Components

Enzyme	Substrates	Functions
Wee1 kinase	Cdk1 Y^{15}	Nuclear kinase. Inhibits Cdk1-cyclinB in G_2.
Myt1 kinase	Cdk1 T^{14} + Y^{15}	Cytoplasmic kinase. Inhibits Cdk1-cyclin B in G_2.
Cdc25A phosphatase	Cdk1 T^{14}, Y^{15}	Promotes $G_1 \to S$ transition and $G_2 \to M$ transition. Essential for life of the cell.
Cdc25B phosphatase	Cdk1 T^{14}, Y^{15}	Promotes $G_2 \to M$ transition. Essential in meiosis.
Cdc25C phosphatase	Cdk1 T^{14}, Y^{15}	Promotes $G_2 \to M$ transition. Dephosphorylates Cdk1 complexed to cyclins A, B at T^{14} and Y^{15}. Not essential for life.
APC/C^{CDC20}	Cyclin B, many others	E3 ubiquitin ligase active during M. Requires high Cdk activity to function. Destruction of cyclins and other substrates essential for exit from mitosis. Contains 12-13 subunits + the CDC20 activator/specificity factor.

Continued

Enzyme	Substrates	Functions
APC/C^{Cdh1}	Cyclins A, B, many others	E3 ubiquitin ligase active during G$_1$. Requires low Cdk activity to function. Keeps Cdk activity low in G$_1$ through cyclin proteolysis. Contains 12–13 subunits + the Cdh1 activator/specificity factor.
SCF	Cyclin E, many others	Class of E3 ubiquitin ligases containing Skp1 + cullin + Rbx1 + an F-box protein. C. elegans has over 60 F-box proteins, acting as specificity factors for substrates phosphorylated at specific sites, including cyclin E and Cdk inhibitors.

CHAPTER 41

G_1 Phase and Regulation of Cell Proliferation

During the G_1 phase of the cell cycle, each cell makes a key decision: whether to continue through another cycle and divide or to remain in a nondividing state either temporarily or permanently. During development of metazoans, this is the time when cells exit the cell cycle as the first step toward forming differentiated tissues. In adults, strict regulation of the timing and location of cell proliferation is critical to avoid cancer.

Cells enter G_1 phase at the end of a proliferation cycle, after completing mitosis. To make an unbiased decision whether to proliferate or differentiate, the cell must erase the bias toward proliferation that was carried over from the preceding cell cycle. This is accomplished by inactivating cyclin-dependent kinases (Cdks [see Chapter 40]) through proteolytic destruction of cyclin subunits and synthesis of inhibitory proteins. The absence of Cdk activity turns on a regulatory network that represses the transcription of many genes that promote cell-cycle progression. While this repressive network is active, the cell cannot proceed through the cell cycle. The repression can be switched off if the cell is continuously stimulated by growth-promoting signals from the surrounding medium, extracellular matrix, and other cells (see Chapters 27 and 30). These stimuli can trigger another round of DNA replication and mitosis, but first, the cell must pass a major decision point in G_1 called the **restriction point** (Fig. 41-1). Factors that promote the growth of cell mass are referred to herein as **growth factors,** and factors that promote cell-cycle proliferation are referred to herein as **mitogens.**

In metazoans, many cells cease cycling in the G_1 phase, either temporarily or permanently, exiting the cell cycle into a state known as G_0 (Fig. 41-1). This frequently accompanies their acquisition of specialized, differentiated characteristics. Occasionally, it is desirable in tissues for cells in G_0 to reenter the cell cycle to replace cells lost through death. These cells reenter the cycle in G_1 phase. During the G_1 phase, cells also screen continuously for damage to their DNA. If damage is detected, the cell either stops cycling or undergoes apoptosis (see Chapter 46).

This chapter describes how cells regulate their progress through the G_1 phase, exit into the G_0 phase, and return to the cycle. It also considers some of the points at which defects in growth control lead to cancer.

The G_0 Phase and Growth Control

Most cells in multicellular organisms are differentiated (adapted to carry out specialized functions) and no longer divide. They typically form specialized tissues, each of

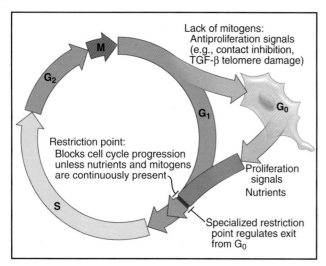

Figure 41-1 THE CELL CYCLE, SHOWING MAJOR LANDMARKS IN THE G_1 PHASE.

which has a distinctive structural organization that is important for function. Unscheduled cell division can severely disrupt the organization of such tissues (Fig. 41-2). Accordingly, tissues strictly regulate both the location and the frequency of cell division. These divisions normally occur at a low rate, producing new cells in numbers just sufficient to replace those that die. Under special circumstances, however, such as in response to

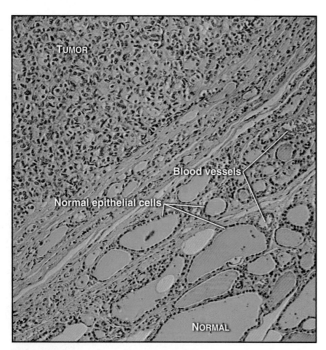

Figure 41-2 DISRUPTION OF NORMAL TISSUE ARCHITECTURE BY CANCER CELLS PROLIFERATING WITHOUT PROPER CELL-CYCLE REGULATION. **Lower right,** Normal thyroid tissue. **Upper left,** A thyroid tumor with loss of the normal gland structure. (Courtesy of Clara Sambade, IPATIMUP, Porto, Portugal.)

wounding (see Fig. 32-11), the rate of cell division increases dramatically. This highlights an important constraint on cell-cycle control in multicellular organisms: *To make organized tissues, cells must exit from the cell cycle, but some cells must also retain the ability to reenter the active cell cycle when needed to repair injuries or replace worn-out cells.*

Cells that stop cycling to differentiate normally do so in the G_1 phase. Such cells are said to have left the cycle and entered a nonproliferating state called **G_0** (Fig. 41-1). G_0 may last hours or days or even for the life of the organism, as it does for most neurons. It is important to note that *nondividing cells are not dormant:* G_0 cells continue to expend energy for many ongoing processes. Because of turnover, all cells must continuously synthesize housekeeping proteins. They must also expend energy to maintain intracellular pH and ionic composition and to power intracellular motility. In addition, many specialized G_0 cells consume large amounts of energy to synthesize and secrete protein products and generate action potentials. Energy metabolism is particularly dramatic in muscle cells that are responsible for all body movements. Thus, most G_0 cells should be regarded as active cells that just happen no longer to be engaged in cell division.

How do cells stop cycling and enter the G_0 phase? First, cells may receive external signals that stimulate withdrawal from the cell cycle. This often initiates differentiation of tissues. Second, cells may find themselves in an environment with insufficient mitogens to drive proliferation. Such conditions trigger many cell types to undergo suicide by apoptosis (see Chapter 46), but other cells enter a nondividing state. Third, at least in cell culture, cells that have divided more than a critical number of times or that have received certain types of unfavorable input from their environment undergo **senescence,** entering a viable but nondividing state. Senescence is a terminal G_0 state from which cells normally cannot exit. One particularly interesting signal that can lead to senescence is stress caused by a critical shortening of the telomere regions of the chromosomes. In fact, overexpression of telomerase (see Fig. 12-15) can, when combined with suitable mitogenic stimuli, prevent cells from undergoing senescence in tissue culture.

Transforming growth factor–β (TGF-β) is an example of an external signal that arrests progress through the cycle and regulates differentiation and tissue morphogenesis (Fig. 41-3). TGF-β acts through a receptor serine/threonine kinase that activates the Smad transcription factors (see Fig. 27-10) and increases the expression of the Ink4 class Cdk inhibitor, p15^{Ink4b}, by up to 30-fold (see Appendix 40-1). Like other Ink4 family members, p15^{Ink4B} specifically inactivates Cdk4–cyclin D and Cdk6-cyclin D complexes. p15^{Ink4B} binding also displaces CKI class inhibitors from the Cdk4–cyclin D complexes, per-

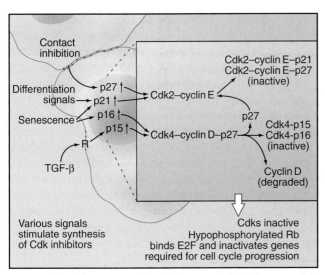

Figure 41-3 Mechanisms by which external stimuli act on Cdk inhibitors to cause cells to enter the nondividing G₀ state from the G₁ phase of the cell cycle.

mitting them to transfer to Cdk2–cyclin E complexes in the nucleus and further inhibit cell-cycle progression.

In addition to its role in stopping cell-cycle progression in response to TGF-β, the CKI inhibitor p27^{Kip1} helps to arrest the cell cycle when normal cells become crowded by neighboring cells (contact inhibition; see Fig. 30-8) or when the environment lacks mitogens. Genetic analysis in mice indicates that p27^{Kip1} regulates cell-cycle progression during development. Indeed, mice that lack p27^{Kip1} are 30% larger than their normal littermates by several weeks of age. This increase in size occurs at least partly because cells in many organs undergo extra rounds of division.

An analogous mechanism appears to arrest the cell cycle during the differentiation of muscle cells. The transcription factor MyoD is a master regulator of muscle differentiation. MyoD activates transcription of the CKI inhibitor p21^{Cip1}, which helps to arrest proliferation and start muscle differentiation (Fig. 41-3). p21^{Cip1} stops cell-cycle progression in at least two ways. First, by binding Cdk-cyclin complexes, it blocks them from promoting cell-cycle progression. Second, p21^{Cip1} binds to the DNA replication factor proliferating cell nuclear antigen (PCNA [see Chapter 42]) in a way that blocks chromosomal replication but not repair of DNA damage.

Several of these mechanisms, including increased expression of both p16^{Ink4a} and p21^{Cip1}, are responsible for permanent cell-cycle arrest of aged cells (senescence). Furthermore, formation of heterochromatin permanently inactivates some genes required for proliferation. This is accomplished when inhibitory proteins of the Rb and E2F families (see later) bind to promoters and recruit histone methyltransferases (see Fig. 13-9).

Once cells exit the cycle, multiple redundant pathways block reentry by reinforcing the primary inhibition of Cdk activity. In addition, a specialized histone variant H1° replaces histone H1 in G₀ cells, resulting in more condensed chromatin, which represses transcription and replication generally. However, not all gene expression is suppressed in differentiated cells, many of which synthesize large amounts of specific proteins (e.g., digestive enzymes secreted by the pancreas).

Exit from the G₀ Phase

Cells in the G₀ phase may reenter the growth cycle in response to specific stimulation, often induced by injury or normal cell turnover. Cultured fibroblasts are favored for studies of this process, as they readily enter the G₀ phase when deprived of serum (i.e., mitogens and growth factors) and rapidly reenter the cell cycle when serum is restored. The pattern of gene expression induced by serum in culture reproduces that found in wounded tissues. When a living tissue is wounded (see Fig. 32-11), fibroblasts are exposed to serum. In response, they divide and colonize the wound, where they lay down new extracellular matrix to repair the damage.

Serum stimulates three waves of gene expression in cultured fibroblasts in G₀ (Fig. 41-4). The first wave includes more than 100 **"immediate early"** genes, including transcription factors of the Jun, fos, myc, and zinc finger families (see Chapter 15) that activate numerous downstream genes required for cell growth and division. Other immediate early genes encode tissue remodeling factors, cytokines (growth factors), extracellular matrix components (fibronectin), plasma membrane receptors (integrins), and cytoskeletal proteins (actin, tropomyosin, vimentin), as well as activities involved in angiogenesis (blood vessel formation),

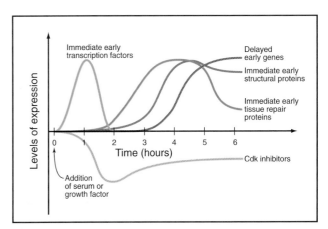

Figure 41-4 PATTERNS OF EXPRESSION OF IMMEDIATE AND DELAYED EARLY GENES DURING THE RETURN OF GROWTH-ARRESTED FIBROBLASTS FROM G₀ TO ACTIVE PROLIFERATION AND THE CELL CYCLE.

inflammation, and coagulation. These proteins facilitate the movement of fibroblasts into wounds and initiate the repair of tissue damage.

Expression of a second wave of **"delayed early"** genes precedes the onset of the S phase. Genes activated after the onset of the S phase are referred to as **"late"** genes. Both delayed early gene transcription and late gene transcription require synthesis of proteins, including the transcription factors that are encoded by immediate early genes. Delayed early genes encode a variety of proteins that are required for cell growth and proliferation, including cyclin D and several other proteins that regulate cellular proliferation.

These waves of transcription in response to mitogens enable the G_0 cells to pass through a "gate" and reenter the active cell cycle. This gate is a specialized form of the restriction point, a critical aspect of G_1 control that regulates the proliferation of all normal cells.

The Restriction Point: A Critical G_1 Decision Point

All eukaryotes have a mechanism that operates during the G_1 phase to ensure that cells proliferate only when the environment is supportive and the chromosomes are undamaged. Whether cells also monitor their size is controversial. Healthy yeast cells do not embark on a round of DNA replication and division until they reach an appropriate minimum size (actually, they probably measure their ribosome content and ongoing rate of protein synthesis). This is important because after cell division, the daughter cell (bud) is smaller than the mother. The daughter cell needs more time to grow before it divides, if the population is to maintain a constant cell size.

The influence of cell size on the division cycle was first demonstrated in an elegant microsurgery experiment (Fig. 41-5). Two *Amoeba proteus* cells were grown under identical conditions in parallel cultures. Each day, a portion of the cytoplasm was amputated from one amoeba, and the other was left untouched as a control. Under those circumstances, the cell that suffered the amputations did not divide for 20 days. During this time, the control amoeba divided 11 times. When the amputations were stopped, the amoeba that had been operated on divided within 38 hours. The interpretation of this experiment was that the repeated amputations prevented the experimental amoeba from ever attaining a size sufficient to undergo division. Evidence suggests that some types of human cells have a similar size control while others do not.

An essential aspect of growth control during the G_1 phase involves monitoring the external environment for nutrient availability and for signals to proliferate (**mitogenic** signals) coming from other cells and from the extracellular matrix. In a classic experiment, when three populations of cells proliferating in culture were starved by deprivation of amino acids, serum, or phosphate, they stopped cycling in G_1. When the missing ingredients were restored, all three populations of treated cells resumed the cell cycle and entered the S phase at about the same time. This was surprising because amino acids are needed to make protein, serum provides growth factors and mitogens, and phosphate is needed for synthesis of DNA phospholipids (needed to make membranes). This experiment was interpreted as evidence that all three types of starvation caused cells to arrest at an equivalent point in the G_1 phase, termed the **restriction point.** The restriction point is defined as the point after which the cell cycle will proceed even if mitogenic factors are withdrawn (Fig. 41-6). This

Figure 41-5 A MICROSURGERY EXPERIMENT DEMONSTRATES THAT AMOEBAE WILL NOT DIVIDE IF THEY ARE KEPT FROM ATTAINING A SUFFICIENT SIZE. **A,** Control cell continues to divide. **B,** Experimental cell does not divide. (Reference: Prescott DM: Relation between cell growth and cell division. II: The effect of cell size on cell growth rate and generation time in Amoeba proteus. Exp Cell Res 11:86–98, 1956.)

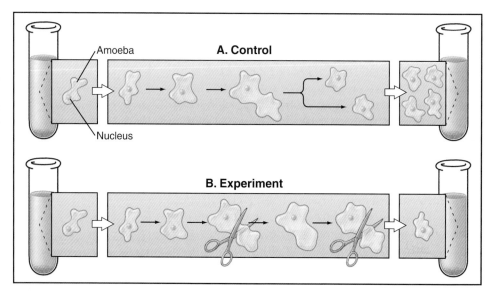

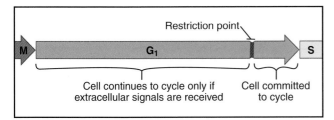

Figure 41-6 AT THE RESTRICTION POINT, CELLS ASSESS EXTERNAL AND INTERNAL STIMULI AND DECIDE WHETHER TO COMMIT TO A FURTHER ROUND OF DNA REPLICATION AND DIVISION.

supremely important aspect of cell-cycle control prevents cells from dividing at inappropriate times and in inappropriate places. Defects in restriction point control are among the most common causes of cancer.

Genetic analysis of budding yeast also revealed a point in the G₁ phase after which cells appear to be committed to completion of the cycle. Cells that are starved for nutrients arrest at, or just prior to, this point, termed **START.** The mammalian restriction point resembles yeast START in a number of aspects, but they are not exactly equivalent, owing to differences between animal and yeast cell cycles.

Regulation of Cell Proliferation by the Restriction Point

The restriction point is a molecular "gate" that regulates the expression of genes required for cell-cycle progression. The gate is based on proteins that are related to the retinoblastoma susceptibility protein (**pRb**) and a family of essential transcription factors known as **E2F.** Mammals have three Rb-related proteins (pRb, p107, and p130) and ten E2F family members, which together constitute a complex multifunctional network with particular pairs doing specific jobs. This account refers to the families generically as Rb and E2F. An alternative way around the restriction point gate depends on a potent transcriptional regulator called Myc to be discussed separately later.

Rb regulates the ability of E2F to activate genes required for cell-cycle progression. E2F forms a heterodimer with one of two DP family members and associates with the promoter region of its target cell-cycle genes (Fig. 41-7A). Rb binding blocks the ability of E2F to activate transcription. In addition, Rb recruits histone deacetylases, enzymes that remove acetyl groups from the amino-terminal tails of histones (see Fig. 13-9). This causes compaction of chromatin structure and represses genes required for cell-cycle progression.

Phosphorylation of Rb by Cdks causes it to dissociate from E2F, allowing E2F/DP to activate, rather than repress, transcription of the target genes. Cells that can

phosphorylate Rb pass the restriction point and complete a cell cycle, whereas cells that cannot phosphorylate Rb remain arrested in the G₁ or G₀ phase. The E2F/DP heterodimer remains bound to its target promoter regions after phosphorylated Rb dissociates from E2F. If activated as a result of DNA damage, E2F can also act as a potent inducer of cell death by apoptosis (see Chapter 46).

E2F/DP that is free of Rb is a potent transcription factor, promoting expression of genes that stimulate both reentry of G₀ cells back into the cycle and their

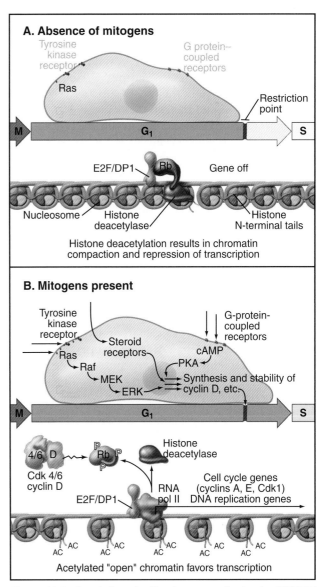

Figure 41-7 Regulation of cell-cycle progression by the E2F/DP/Rb complex. **A,** The E2F/DP/Rb complex recruits histone deacetylases (see Chapter 13) and represses specific genes that are required for cell-cycle progression. This blocks cell-cycle progression at the restriction point. **B,** Phosphorylation of Rb by Cdks alleviates this block and permits passage of the restriction point. cAMP, cyclic adenosine monophosphate; MEK, mitogen-activated protein kinase kinase; PKA, protein kinase A.

subsequent passage through the cell cycle. These target genes encode proteins that are required for DNA synthesis (DNA polymerase α_1, accessory factors, and enzymes that synthesize nucleotide precursors; see Chapter 42), proteins that promote cell-cycle progression (cyclins E and A, Cdk1 and Cdc25), and proteins that regulate cell-cycle progression (pRb, p107, Emi1).

Passage through the restriction point therefore hinges on Cdk activation (Fig. 41-7B; see also Chapter 40 and Appendix 40-1), which leads to Rb phosphorylation and activation of E2F/DP dimers on the promoters of essential cell-cycle genes. The normal pathway of Rb phosphorylation is started by Cdk4–cyclin D and Cdk6–cyclin D (referred to hereafter as Cdk4/6–cyclin D) and is carried forward by Cdk2–cyclin E and Cdk2–cyclin A. Cdk activity in early G_1 is regulated by adjusting the relative levels of the three D-type cyclins and the CKI class Cdk2 inhibitors p27^{Kip1} and p21^{Cip1}. Regulation of cyclin D levels provides the crucial link between extracellular mitogens and the cell cycle.

Nonproliferating cells control cyclin levels in G_1 cells in two ways. First, cyclin D mRNA levels are so low that little protein is made. Second, the little cyclin D that is made is kept in the cytoplasm, where it is phosphorylated by glycogen synthase kinase-β (GSK [see Fig. 30-8]) and degraded by SCF (see Fig. 40-17). E2F controls the expression of the genes for cyclins E and A, so these cyclins are present at only low levels, while E2F/Rb/DP acts as an inhibitor. Furthermore, levels of the CKI class Cdk2 inhibitor p27^{Kip1} are high in prerestriction point G_1 cells. Thus, any Cdk2–cyclin E or Cdk2–cyclin A that happens to be present is inactive (see Figs. 40-14 and 40-15).

How do cells convert signals from mitogens and the extracellular matrix into a decision to open the restriction point gate? Stimulation of receptor tyrosine kinases (see Chapters 25 and 27) or integrins (see Chapter 30) initiates a signal transduction pathway starting with Ras activation of Raf and leading to activation of the mitogen-activated protein (MAP) kinase/extracellular signal–regulated kinase (ERK) cascade (see Fig. 27-6). The output of this cascade stimulates transcription of D-type cyclins (Figs. 41-7 and 41-8) and also inactivates GSK. This allows cyclin D to accumulate in nuclei.

In addition to promoting the accumulation of cyclin D, mitogens stimulate transcription of the CKI class Cdk2 inhibitor p21^{Cip1}. This protein and p27^{Kip1} actually promote the *activation* of Cdk4/6–cyclin D complexes in two ways. First, they enhance assembly of complexes of cyclin D with Cdk4 and Cdk6. Second, they promote the nuclear import of Cdk4/6–cyclin D, thereby leading to activation of Cdks by Cdk-activating kinase (a nuclear enzyme; see Chapter 40), as well as an increase in the stability of cyclin D. All of this depends on the continuous presence of mitogenic signals; if these cease, then cyclin D stability rapidly declines again.

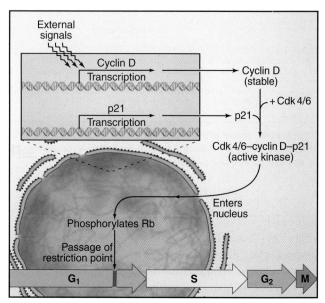

Figure 41-8 How growth factors regulate Cdk4/6 activity: the role of D-type cyclins and p21.

The response to mitogens breaks the blockade on cell-cycle progression imposed by Rb in a positive feedback loop as follows. Cdk4/6–cyclin D-p21^{Cip1}/p27^{Kip1} complexes begin to phosphorylate Rb. This releases some E2F and permits the initial expression of genes that encode cyclin E, cyclin A, and CDC25A. Cdk4/6–cyclin D also acts as a "sponge," soaking up p21^{Cip1} and p27^{Kip1} and liberating active Cdk2–cyclin E enzyme. The restriction point probably is passed here.

Cdk2–cyclin E is responsible for a second wave of Rb phosphorylation on many sites, leading to the wholesale liberation of E2F and a surge in transcription of genes that promote cell-cycle progression. These factors are needed for DNA replication and trigger the onset of the S phase and progression through the cell cycle. As the cell cycle proceeds, Rb phosphorylation is maintained first by Cdk2–cyclin A and then later by Cdk1–cyclin B until the exit from mitosis. Rb is dephosphorylated at the mitosis-G_1 transition. This enables it once again to bind E2F and close the restriction point gate to progression through the next G_1.

The transcriptional regulator **Myc,** drives an alternative pathway for G_1 exit, which is also stabilized by mitogenic signals. When associated with one partner, myc activates the transcription of cyclins E and D2. When associated with a different partner, myc downregulates the transcription of Cdk inhibitors of both the CKI and INK class. Both effects promote cell-cycle progression and can, under some conditions, promote passage of the restriction point. This partly explains why Myc can act as an **oncogene**—a protein that helps to transform normal cells into cancer cells (explained further later).

The Restriction Point and Cancer

Cancer is a complex class of diseases in which genetic changes within clones of cells lead to production of cell populations whose uncontrolled growth can disrupt tissue function and can ultimately kill the individual. Two in five Americans will be affected by cancer during their lifetimes. This sounds very high, but considering the number of cell cycles that are required to produce a human composed of about 10^{14} cells, the disease is actually remarkably rare on a per cell basis. Why is this so? One reason is that multiple genetic alterations are required to transform a normal cell into a cancer cell. This is because the cell cycle is highly regulated, and activities that tend to drive cellular proliferation are held in check by a web of negative feedback pathways. As a result, some cancer-causing mutations are actually deleterious in normal cells. In fact, most cells with disturbed growth control pathways are eliminated by backup mechanisms that cause them to commit suicide by apoptosis (see Chapter 46).

Almost all types of cancer are caused by a disregulation of cell proliferation in the G₁ phase. This is readily seen in the laboratory when cells are grown on plastic tissue culture dishes. Most normal cells proliferate until they cover the surface completely, forming a monolayer. When the monolayer is confluent (i.e., when cells are touched by other cells on all sides), signaling initiated by cadherin proteins (see Fig. 30-8) causes cells to arrest their cell-cycle progression in G₁. This is called **contact inhibition** of growth (see Chapter 30, in the section titled "Cadherin Family of Adhesion Receptors"). Cancer cells lack this control, so they keep proliferating and piling up on top of one another as long as nutrient and mitogen supplies last (Fig. 41-9). Cells that lose this aspect of growth regulation are said to be **transformed.**

Malfunction of the restriction point is an extremely common contributor to transformation. In fact, one or more components of the p16/cyclin D/Cdk-4/Rb system are mutated in most human cancers. In addition, several cancer-causing viruses, such as simian virus 40 (SV40), papillomaviruses, and adenovirus, make proteins that facilitate the G₁ → S transition by binding Rb and liberating E2F.

Cancer cells have abnormalities in the activities of two classes of genes. **Oncogenes** are genes whose inappropriate *activation* can cause oncogenic (cancerous) transformation of cells. The protein products of most oncogenes are regulators of cellular growth and proliferation, typically, components of signal transduction pathways that are controlled by feedback mechanisms. **Tumor suppressors** are genes whose *inactivation* can lead to cancerous transformation. Their protein products typically inhibit products of oncogenes or negatively regulate cell proliferation. Several genes that are involved in restriction point control can act as oncogenes, and at least two can act as tumor suppressors.

More than 100 oncogenes have been identified thus far. Most normally function in signal transduction pathways that lie downstream of signals that stimulate cell-cycle progression. Their inappropriate activation can mimic the effects of persistent mitogenic stimulation, thereby uncoupling cells from normal environmental controls and leading to uncontrolled proliferation and cancer. For example, Ras proteins are key components of signaling pathways that lead to activation of the MAP/ERK kinase cascade and accumulation of cyclin D (Fig. 41-7). They are mutated in about 15% of human cancers. Inappropriate activation of Ras tricks the cell into thinking that it is receiving mitogenic signals, leading it to express cyclin D, phosphorylate Rb, and proliferate. Luckily, in normal cells, this usually activates a checkpoint mechanism and leads to rapid cell-cycle arrest. Other proteins that are involved in restriction point control can also act as oncogenes if hyperactivated. These include E2F1, cyclin D (overexpressed in 50% of breast cancers), and Cdk4. In each case, activation of the protein causes inappropriate transcription of genes promoting cell-cycle progression, bypassing the restriction point, and leading to uncontrolled cell cycles and cancerous transformation (Fig. 41-10).

Rb is one of the best-characterized tumor suppressor genes. As was discussed earlier, a primary function of Rb is to block cell-cycle progression until mitogenic stimulation results in its inactivation. It is therefore not surprising that loss of Rb can lead to inappropriate cell-cycle progression and cancer. Rare individuals who inherit one defective Rb gene usually develop retinoblastomas as children and osteosarcomas as adults. The cancer arises when the "good" allele is inactivated in a proliferating cell (this is called a somatic mutation). Such cancers are rare and occur only later in life in

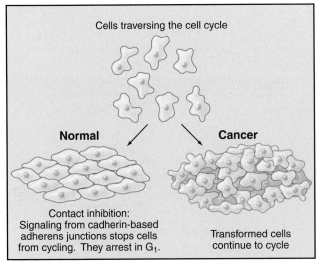

Cells traversing the cell cycle

Normal   **Cancer**

Contact inhibition: Signaling from cadherin-based adherens junctions stops cells from cycling. They arrest in G₁.

Transformed cells continue to cycle

Figure 41-9   LOSS OF GROWTH CONTROL IN TRANSFORMED CELLS.

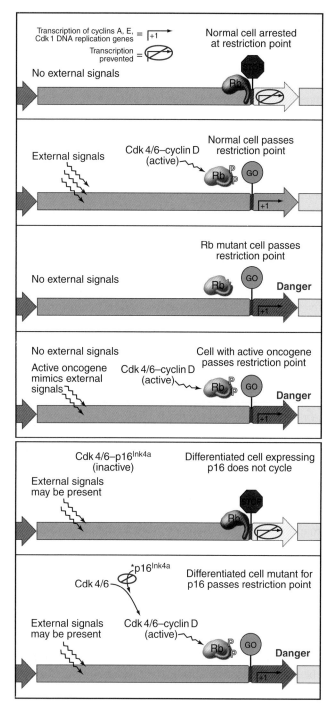

Figure 41-10   How activated oncogenes or mutations in the Rb or p16 tumor suppressor proteins can lead to abnormal passage of the restriction point and cancer.

individuals who inherit two good Rb genes, as two independent somatic mutations (two "hits") are required in the same proliferating cell. Homozygous loss of pRb is lethal during embryogenesis. This is partly because under some circumstances, the unleashed E2F can act as a potent inducer of apoptotic cell death (see Chapter 46).

$P16^{Ink4a}$ is another important tumor suppressor that is involved in G_1 growth control. Normally, it suppresses Cdk4/6 activity in nondividing cells (see next section; also see Chapter 40), thereby reinforcing the ability of Rb to maintain the growth arrest of G_1 cells (Fig. 41-10). Mutations in the $p16^{Ink4a}$ gene are very commonly seen in cancer, but this is partly because this gene is fascinatingly complex (see Fig. 41-14). Mutations in other INK4 Cdk inhibitors and the CKI $p27^{Kip1}$ are also found in cancer, though less frequently.

Proteolysis and G_1 Cell Cycle Progression

Just as controlled destruction of proteins is key to the transition of cells from mitosis to the G_1 phase (see Chapter 40), proteolysis also fulfills a number of key roles during progression through G_1 into the S phase (Fig. 41-11). For example, when Cdk2-cyclin E is activated following synthesis of cyclin D, it phosphorylates its $p27^{Kip1}$ inhibitor. This allows $p27^{Kip1}$ to be recognized by a specific class of ubiquitin ligase (E3) called SCF^{Skp2} (see Figs. 40-16 and 40-17). The resulting destruction of $p27^{Kip1}$ helps to produce a burst of Cdk2-cyclin E activation in a feedback loop that allows for rapid amplification of Cdk activity and contributes to initiation of the S phase. Later in the S phase, phosphorylation of the DP subunit of E2F causes its dissociation from DNA, recognition by SCF, and destruction. This is essential to complete the S phase. SCF also targets cyclins D1 and E for destruction, the former when mitogens are limiting and the latter during progression through the S phase.

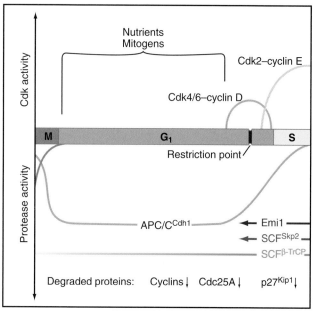

Figure 41-11   PROTEOLYTIC ACTIVITIES IN G_1.

Integrity of Cellular DNA Monitored by a G₁ Checkpoint

The S phase is a point of no return in the history of any dividing cell. Because of the semiconservative mechanism of DNA replication, whereby existing DNA strands serve as templates for the newly synthesized strands, any DNA defect that passes unnoticed through the S phase becomes perpetuated as a mutation that is transmitted to all future progeny of the cell. Furthermore, any single-stranded nick in DNA becomes a full-fledged chromosome break if present during replication. To avoid these problems, cells have a quality control mechanism to ensure that chromosomal DNA is undamaged prior to replication in the S phase.

This quality control mechanism involves a **checkpoint** that operates throughout the G₁ phase (Fig. 41-12). Checkpoints are biochemical circuits superimposed on the normal cell cycle. When activated, checkpoints block progression through the cycle, either temporarily or, in some cases, permanently. In certain cases, checkpoint activation leads to cell death by apoptosis. Checkpoints are activated by sensor proteins that detect problems—typically, DNA damage in the case of the G₁ checkpoint. Sensor proteins activate protein kinases that modify target proteins, which then block cell-cycle progression (see Fig. 40-4).

DNA damage checkpoints have fast and slow components: The former is analogous to applying the brakes in a car; the latter is analogous to removing the wheels and putting it up on blocks. Both components depend on the protein kinases, ATM and ATR (see Fig. 40-4). ATM and ATR are related to the lipid kinase phosphatidylinositol 3-kinase (see Chapters 25 and 27), but their only known substrates are proteins (see Chapter 40). People who lack ATM have the disease ataxia-telangiectasia, which is characterized by immunodeficiency, photosensitivity, cerebellar degeneration, and an elevated incidence of leukemias and lymphomas. ATR is essential for life.

When ATR is activated, primarily by DNA damage that disrupts ongoing DNA replication, it phosphorylates and activates a downstream kinase called Chk1, one of whose targets is the essential phosphatase CDC25A (Fig. 41-12). This phosphorylation signals CDC25A for destruction. Since CDC25A is required to remove inhibitory phosphate groups from inactive Cdks, its destruction applies a rapid brake to cell-cycle progression.

ATM is activated selectively by DNA double-strand breaks. ATM activation results directly and indirectly in the stabilization and activation of a critical tumor suppresser, **p53.**

p53 is a transcription factor whose role in the G₁ DNA damage checkpoint is to activate a set of target genes, including the Cdk inhibitor p21^Cip1. The result is a stable block to cell-cycle progression (putting the car up on blocks). However, p53 is also thought to induce G₁ arrest by mechanisms that do not require p21^Cip1.

p53 is mutated or deleted in about half of all human cancers. Families that carry a mutated p53 allele have Li-Fraumeni syndrome, a condition that is associated with an elevated risk of cancers. Mice that lack p53 are viable but lack the G₁ DNA damage checkpoint and develop cancers while young. This reveals an important fact about checkpoints. In many cases, checkpoint components are not essential for life as long as nothing untoward occurs. Checkpoints exist primarily as backup mechanisms to deal with problems that arise during cell-cycle progression. However, the elevated cancer rates in Li-Fraumeni syndrome patients indicate that although p53 is not essential for the passage of every cell cycle, it is essential for genetic stability and for maintaining a proper balance among cell proliferation, differentiation, and death during the lifetime of a mammal.

p53 is very powerful medicine for the cell cycle. If present in excessive amounts, it is extremely toxic. For this reason, p53 is regulated by a partner protein called

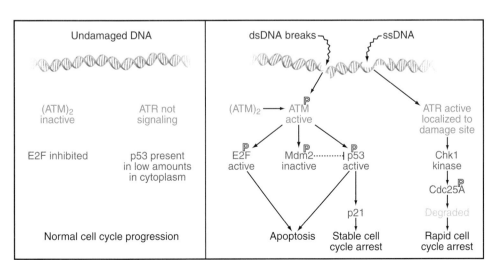

Figure 41-12 THE G₁ CHECKPOINT.

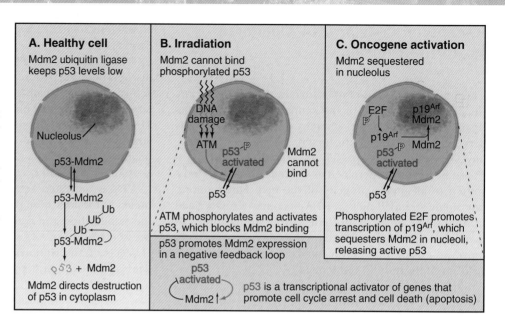

Figure 41-13 p53 regulation and the DNA damage checkpoint in G_1. **A,** Healthy cell. **B,** After irradiation, Mdm2 can no longer bind p53, which accumulates in active form in the nucleus. **C,** After oncogene activation, Mdm2 is sequestered in the nucleolus, and active p53 accumulates in the nucleus. Activated p53 can induce either cell-cycle arrest or cell death.

Mdm2 (mouse double minute 2; the human ortholog of this is Hdm2), a ubiquitin ligase (E3) whose job is to keep p53 levels low when the cell cycle is running normally (Fig. 41-13A). Loss of the Mdm2 gene in mice is lethal unless the p53 gene is also lost. Mdm2 protein shuttles in and out of the nucleus (see Chapter 14). p53 also has a nuclear export signal, and when these two proteins associate in the cytoplasm, Mdm2 promotes the rapid degradation of p53 by the ubiquitin/proteasome system (see Chapter 23). Because p53 directly stimulates expression of Mdm2, a negative feedback loop keeps levels of p53 low.

Both p53 and Mdm2 are phosphorylated following DNA damage (Fig. 41-13B). These phosphorylations prevent Mdm2 from binding, so p53 is stabilized, and its concentration in the nucleus increases dramatically. The phosphorylations also make p53 a more potent transcriptional activator. The result is a burst of transcription of p53-regulated genes.

A different mechanism is used to defend the cell against cancer caused by inappropriate activation of oncogenes that disrupt normal cell-cycle controls. Dysregulated cell-cycle progression allows E2F to stimulate expression of the tumor suppressor protein $p19^{Arf}$, which binds and sequesters Mdm2 (but not p53) in the nucleolus (Fig. 41-13C). This allows p53 to accumulate in the nucleus, where it activates a pathway promoting apoptotic cell death by stimulating transcription of a number of genes involved in cell killing, including *Bax,* BH3-domain proteins, CD95 (*Fas/Apo1*), and *Apaf-1* (Fig. 41-13, also discussed in Chapter 46). Thus, aberrantly proliferating cells are removed, and the body is protected.

The $p19^{Arf}$ gene (in humans, the protein is smaller and so is called $p14^{Arf}$) is quite unusual, as it is encoded in a common gene with $p16^{Ink4a}$ (Fig. 41-14). In fact, the genes not only overlap but also share a common exon. Nevertheless, the two proteins have no common amino acid sequences because the shared exons are read in different frames in the mature messenger RNAs (mRNAs) for the two proteins. Thus, the $p16^{Ink4a}/p14^{Arf}$ locus encodes two vital protective factors with different jobs. It is not surprising that mutations in this key locus are found in between 25% and 70% of human cancers.

Moving into and out of G_0: Stem Cells

Some cells are professionals at moving back and forth between G_0 and more active cell cycles. Without doubt, the champions at this are **stem cells,** one of whose roles is to replace worn-out parts of tissues as differentiated cells age or die as a result of various misadventures. Box 41-1 provides a brief introduction to the very topical world of stem cells.

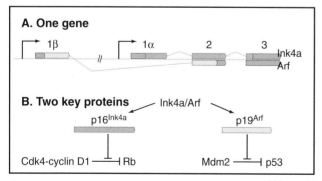

Figure 41-14 Dual control of G_1 progression by the $p16^{Ink4a}/p19^{Arf}$ gene. This gene encodes two completely different proteins that are key to avoiding cancer. **A,** The intron/exon structure of the $p16^{Ink4A}/p19^{Arf}$ gene. **B,** $p16^{Ink4A}$ and $p19^{Arf}$ negatively regulate the restriction point via Rb and the DNA damage checkpoint via p53, respectively.

The defining feature of **stem cells** is their capacity to produce, through asymmetrical cell division, both a self-renewing stem cell and a second cell with the capacity to differentiate into more specialized cells. Stem cells play a key role in the development of multicellular organisms in addition to providing cells for the renewal and regeneration of adult tissues.

Each multicellular organism begins as a single cell with a genome encoding the information required to produce an adult. The first embryonic cell divisions produce a small group of **embryonic stem cells** that go on to form the embryo. The other cells that are produced at this stage are specialized to support the embryo. Embryonic stem cells are termed **pluripotent** because their progeny can form all of the specialized cells of the adult. This requires many rounds of division followed by differentiation to produce cells as diverse as skeletal muscle and red blood cells.

Most adult tissues set aside a few **tissue stem cells** that have the capacity to renew themselves and to produce daughter cells that differentiate into a limited range of specialized cells (see Figs. 28-1, 28-5, and 40-1). Adult stem cells have diverse patterns of cell-cycle regulation. Some of these tissue stem cells cycle continuously throughout life. For example, epithelial stem cells give rise to mature cells that continuously replace the skin and the lining of the gastrointestinal tract. Hematopoietic stem cells in bone marrow give rise to several different types of short-lived blood cells. Plant meristematic stem cells produce cells for roots and shoots. In other organs such as liver and skeletal muscle, tissue stem cells are held in reserve unless the tissue is damaged, when they produce daughter cells to repair the damage. Stem cells are present but largely inactive in organs such as the nervous system, which have limited capacity for renewal and regeneration. The potential for regeneration from stem cells has stimulated research to find ways of using embryonic or tissue stem cells to repair damaged or diseased organs in human patients. Stem cells have also been useful for production of transgenic animals for scientific research (e.g., knockout mice) or for production of therapeutically important proteins.

Discovery and Defining Features of Stem Cells

Pioneering work on blood cell development (see Fig. 28-5) established the existence of stem cells and defined many of the concepts that apply to all types of stem cells. The key experiment was to inject bone marrow cells from a normal mouse into a mouse that had been irradiated to kill all of the cells that produce blood cells. Transplantation of bone marrow cells rescued these irradiated mice from death from anemia, bleeding, and infections. The transplanted bone marrow contained precursor cells that formed colonies of proliferating cells that regenerated the full range of blood cells. The blood-forming colonies in the spleen, each of which formed from a single stem cell, con-

tained either one or, infrequently, several types of differentiating blood cells.

This experimental system first revealed the existence of several different types of hematopoietic stem cells in bone marrow with the dual capacity to renew themselves and to give rise to differentiated cells (see Fig. 28-5). Very rare **pluripotent hematopoietic stem cells** can give rise to all types of blood cells, including themselves. Other **committed stem cells** with a more restricted capacity for self-renewal can give rise to specific subsets of blood cells, such as red blood cells, platelets, granulocytes, or lymphocytes. Antibodies for surface markers can now be used to distinguish and purify the various types of hematopoietic stem cells from mice and humans. Once separated from the far more numerous mature and differentiating cells in bone marrow, stem cells can be used for transplantation into patients with bone marrow defects.

Most pluripotent hematopoietic stem cells are in the G$_0$ phase of the cell cycle. A low level of metabolic activity is thought to contribute to their longevity, which can potentially exceed the life span of the individual. When stimulated by demand for more blood cells, growth factors drive pluripotent stem cells into a cell cycle that culminates in an asymmetrical division. One daughter cell is another pluripotent stem cell. The second daughter cell enters the proliferating pool of blood cell precursors as a committed stem cell. Committed stem cells and their progeny proliferate massively and differentiate into mature blood cells. An adult human produces more than one million blood cells every second.

Cytokines and other growth factors regulate proliferation and differentiation at every stage of blood cell production. The later stages are best understood. For example, the cytokine erythropoietin acts through a kinase-coupled receptor to activate a cytoplasmic transcription factor that stimulates the proliferation and differentiation of the red blood cell lineage. Other cytokines guide the differentiation of granulocytes and monocytes. Hematopoietic stem cells respond to the same families of growth factors that control other aspects of development, including Wnts (see Fig. 30-8), Notch (see Chapter 24), fibroblast growth factor (see Fig. 24-4), and insulin-like growth factor (see Fig. 24-4). However, too little is yet known about these regulatory mechanisms to grow hematopoietic stem cells in the laboratory.

Properties of Adult Stem Cells

Years of detailed analysis in the laboratory and clinic established hematopoietic stem cells as a model for stem cells in other tissues. General features include the capacity for self-renewal and the production of daughters that proliferate and differentiate. This dichotomy is achieved by asymmetrical cell divisions guided by the same types of internal cues that control unequal divisions of cells in early embryos (Fig. 41-15). Symmetrical divisions (to give two daughter stem cells) can also expand the numbers of stem cells

Continued

BOX 41-1
Stem Cells—cont'd

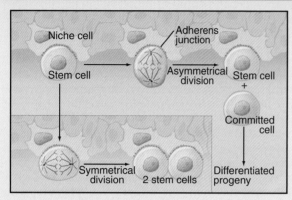

Figure 41-15 TWO PATTERNS OF STEM CELL DIVISION. Asymmetrical divisions create two daughter cells: a stem cell that remains associated with its niche cell to maintain the pool of stem cells and one that is committed to multiply and produce differentiated progeny. Symmetrical divisions produce two stem cells to expand the pool of stem cells.

during growth to maturity and during regeneration of damaged tissues.

Stem cells depend on local environmental cues to maintain their status as stem cells. These special environments, called **stem cell niches,** are created by tissue cells and the extracellular matrix. Niche cells anchor stem cells with adherens junctions and provide cell surface and secreted proteins that activate the signaling pathways that regulate the cell cycle of the stem cell. Some of these factors stimulate division; others inhibit differentiation. The niches that are occupied by germ cells and neural stem cells from invertebrates are particularly well characterized. During asymmetrical divisions of germ stem cells, the renewed stem cell stays behind in the niche, while the daughter that is destined to differentiate into an egg, sperm, or neuron

is released. In bone marrow, osteoblasts (see Fig. 32-5) and endothelial cells (see Fig. 30-13) provide niches for hematopoietic stem cells.

Epidermal Stem Cells

Skin is an example of a continuously renewing organ with a considerable capacity for regeneration (see Fig. 40-1). Multipotential and committed stem cells contribute to both renewal and regeneration. Committed stem cells reside in the basal layer of the epidermis. Asymmetrical cell divisions oriented at right angles to the basal lamina produce two daughter cells. The daughter on the basal lamina carries on as the stem cell. The apical daughter cell divides multiple times and differentiates into a column of cells, forming the superficial layers of the epidermis (see Fig. 35-6). Multipotential stem cells associated with hair follicles give rise to all of the cells of the hair follicle and also serve as a reserve for the committed epidermal stem cells in the event of injury (Fig. 41-16). Like other adult stem cells, the stem cells of the skin are relatively quiescent, are responsive to growth and differentiation factors, and are influenced by their local environments.

Skeletal Muscle Stem Cells

Small numbers of stem cells reside in a niche between the basal lamina and the giant multinucleated muscle cells. If the muscle is damaged, these quiescent "satellite cells" multiply and produce cells that regenerate the tissue. Positive signals for proliferation and differentiation come through receptor tyrosine kinases and the MAP kinase pathway (see Fig. 27-6) and other pathways. Restraining signals are provided by myostatin, a member of the TGF-β family (see Fig. 27-10). Inactivation of the myostatin pathway results in massive enlargement of muscles in mice and humans. Muscles are capable of regenerating multiple times, so the stem cell population renews itself

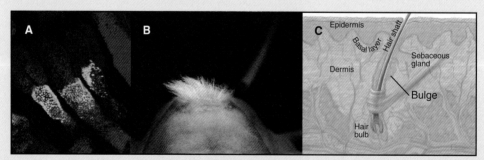

Figure 41-16 STEM CELLS FROM SKIN. Multipotent stem cells of the skin reside in the hair follicle bulge (*green* cells in **A**, diagram in **C**). They move up and repair the epidermis during wound healing, and they move down and generate new hair growth during the hair cycle. **B,** Depicts a *Nude* mouse grafted with the cultured cell progeny of a single "bulge" stem cell and displaying a large tuft of hair, all derived from a single stem cell. (A and C, From Fuchs E, Tumbar T, Guasch G: Socializing with the neighbors: Stem cells and their niche. Cell 116:769–778, 2004. [A is from Fig. 3A, p. 773, and C is redrawn from Fig. 3C, p. 773]. B, From Blanpain C, Lowry WE, Geoghegan A, et al: Self-renewal, multipotency, and the existence of two cell populations within an epithelial stem cell niche. Cell 118, 635–648, 2004 [B is from Fig. 4A, p. 641]. Images were the gift of Elaine Fuchs and her collaborators: Valentina Greco [A] and Cedric Blanpain and William Lowry [B].)

BOX 41-1
Stem Cells—cont'd

during regeneration or is augmented by stem cells that migrate through the blood from bone marrow or other tissues.

Neural Stem Cells

The brain is the prime example of an organ with little capacity for regeneration. Nevertheless, certain parts of the adult brain near the ventricles contain stem cells that give rise to a few progeny that develop into functioning neurons throughout life.

Cancer Stem Cells

Stem cells may play a role in cancer, acting as a source for proliferating cells that make up the bulk of the tumor. If this concept is true, it helps to explain why it is relatively easy to reduce the size of tumors by targeting dividing cells but difficult to eliminate residual tumor stem cells, which may divide less frequently.

Meristematic Stem Cells

The growth of plants depends on carefully orchestrated proliferation and differentiation of cells that are derived from stem cells called meristems. Through asymmetrical divisions, these relatively inactive cells give rise to daughters that proliferate at the tips of shoots and roots. These proliferating cells differentiate into specialized tissues such as flowers, while the stem cells maintain a pool of slowly replicating cells in a special niche.

Use of Stem Cells to Make Transgenic Animals

Because embryonic stem cells grow in culture, they can be manipulated like many cultured cells. DNA can be transfected into them, and if the proper sequences are present, this DNA can, at low frequency, replace a region of the endogenous chromosome by homologous recombination. If the modified embryonic stem cells are subsequently injected into developing embryos at the blastula stage, they are, with low frequency, able to colonize the cell population that will produce germ cells. When such blastulas grow to adulthood, a proportion of their gametes will carry a chromosome with the modification engineered in the embryonic stem cells. Furthermore, this chromosome will now be inherited by all of their progeny, giving rise to a line of **transgenic** animals. This method is widely used in research to knock out genes by designing the original DNA construct so that when it enters the chromosome by homologous chromosome, a critical region of a particular gene is deleted or disrupted. The use of knockout mice has revolutionized the study of developmental biology by allowing investigators to determine the function of specific genes in intact animals. Another of the many applications of this technology is to use homologous recombination to introduce a human gene of choice into a particular genetic locus that will be expressed only in a specific tissue. This has, for example, allowed the expression of therapeutically important human proteins in animals such as sheep, in which the protein is secreted at high levels into the milk and can be readily purified for clinical use.

Note the distinction between transgenic animals and reproductive cloning. "Cloned" animals are produced by introducing a somatic cell nucleus into an enucleated egg. Experiments first in frogs and later in mammals, such as Dolly the sheep, established that such eggs can support the development of a cloned animal. Transfer of nuclei from lymphocytes and olfactory neurons has been used to derive healthy adult mice. This approach requires the reversal of the epigenetic changes in the nucleus that drove the differentiation of the adult cell. Reprogramming is not well understood and occurs relatively rarely when a nucleus is transferred from a differentiated cell into an egg. Such cloning does not involve the use of stem cells, but embryonic stem cells are produced along the way.

Therapeutic Applications of Stem Cells

In situations in which committed stem cells can be isolated from an adult organ, it is now possible to regenerate damaged tissues by transplanting these stem cells from patients themselves or from donors. The best example is transplantation of bone marrow stem cells to treat patients whose bone marrow has been damaged by cancer, chemotherapy, or other disease. Adverse immunologic reactions are a challenge for transplants from donors other than an identical twin. On one hand, the immune system of the recipient can reject the transplanted cells. On the other hand, lymphocytes contaminating the donor stem cells can mount an immunologic attack on the recipient. Using purified hematopoietic stem cells (ideally, the patient's own stem cells) rather than mixed bone marrow cells avoids this problem. Knowing how to expand hematopoietic stem cells in vitro would be helpful. This approach is already used for treating burns with epidermal stem cells. Normal skin is used as a source of committed skin stem cells, which are multiplied in culture and used to regenerate all of the layers of the skin.

Stem cells might be used to regenerate other damaged tissues, including the insulin-producing cells that are lost in type I diabetes, but appropriate stem cells are not available for many organs, including the pancreas, brain, and heart. Even with appropriate stem cells in hand, much remains to be learned about how to grow them and then direct them to differentiate into mature tissues.

Two approaches are being used to increase the supply of stem cells, either by differentiation of pluripotent stem cells or by converting adult stem cells from bone marrow or another source into the desired type of committed stem cell. Embryonic stem cells have the potential to regenerate any damaged tissue, but sources of human embryonic stem cells are limited, and acquiring them

Continued

from early embryos discarded by fertility clinics is unacceptable to some people. Alternatively, embryos produced by somatic cell nuclear transfer (cloning), ideally from the patient who requires treatment, can give rise to pluripotent embryonic stem cells. However, the production of such "artificial" human embryos is also highly controversial.

Adult stem cells are an alternative to embryonic stem cells. This approach has the advantage that stem cells can be isolated from bone marrow, blood, and skin by using antibodies that recognize specific surface protein "markers"; however, these specialized stem cells do not produce differentiated cells for regeneration of other tissues. In the future, this will require methods to convert a readily available type of stem cell, such as hematopoietic stem cells, into other types of stem cells. Then patients could provide the cells to regenerate their own damaged tissues. Some researchers have claimed success with such "transdifferentiation" of adult stem cells, but scientists remain skeptical about most of these experiments.

G_1 Regulation:
A Matter of Life and Death

To exit from G_1 and commit to a new cycle of proliferation, cells must pass through the restriction point gate controlled by Rb family members. The key to this gate is the phosphorylation of Rb by Cdks, so signals such as growth factors and mitogens that activate Cdks set up a feedback loop that promotes passage of the gate. Of course, in the real world, accidents happen, and the G_1 DNA damage checkpoint provides a way to block cell-cycle progression even in the presence of growth factors and mitogens. The complex G_1 regulatory networks have a potential impact on all of us. If they are disrupted by mutations or damage, the result is cancer. In fact, very few cancers have intact restriction point control networks.

ACKNOWLEDGMENTS

Thanks go to Jiri Bartek and Martin Raff for their suggestions on revisions to this chapter.

SELECTED READINGS

Blais A, Dynlacht BD: Hitting their targets: An emerging picture of E2F and cell cycle control. Curr Opin Genet Dev 14:527-532, 2004.

Blanpain C, Fuchs E: Epidermal stem cells of the skin. Annu Rev Cell Dev Biol 22:339-373, 2006.

Bryder D, Rossi DJ, Weissman IL: Hematopoietic stem cells: The paradigmatic tissue-specific stem cell. Am J Pathol 169:338-346, 2006.

Cardozo T, Pagano M: The SCF ubiquitin ligase: Insights into a molecular machine. Nat Rev Mol Cell Biol 5:739-751, 2004.

DeGregori J: The Rb network. J Cell Sci 117:3411-3413, 2004.

Ekholm SV, Reed SI: Regulation of G(1) cyclin-dependent kinases in the mammalian cell cycle. Curr Opin Cell Biol 12:676-684, 2000.

Fuchs E, Tumbar T, Gausch G: Socializing with the neighbors: Stem cells and their niche. Cell 116:769-778, 2004.

Hochedlinger K, Jaenisch R: Nuclear reprogramming and pluripotency. Nature 441:1061-1067, 2006.

Jackson PK, Eldridge AG: The SCF ubiquitin ligase: An extended look. Mol Cell 9:923-925, 2002.

Jorgensen P, Tyers M: How cells coordinate growth and division. Curr Biol 14:R1014-R1027, 2004.

Kastan MB, Bartek J: Cell-cycle checkpoints and cancer. Nature 432:316-323, 2004.

McGowan CH, Russell P: The DNA damage response: Sensing and signaling. Curr Opin Cell Biol 16:629-633, 2004.

Morrison SJ, Kimble J: Asymmetric and symmetric stem-cell divisions in development and cancer. Nature 441:1068-1074, 2006.

Muotri AR, Gage FH: Generation of neuronal variability and complexity. Nature 441:1087-1093, 2006.

Rando TA: Stem cells, ageing and the quest for immortality. Nature 441:1080-1086, 2006.

Scadden DT: The stem-cell niche as an entity of action. Nature 441:1075-1079, 2006.

Sherr CJ: The INK4a/ARF network in tumour suppression. Nat Rev Mol Cell Biol 2:731-737, 2001.

Shi X, Garry DJ: Muscle stem cells in development, regeneration and disease. Genes Dev 20:1692-1708, 2006.

Veit B: Stem cell signalling networks in plants. Plant Mol Biol 60:793-810, 2006.

Weissman IL, Anderson DJ, Gage F: Stem and progenitor cells: Origins, phenotypes, lineage commitments and transdifferentiation. Annu Rev Cell Dev Biol 17:387-403, 2001.

CHAPTER 42

S Phase and DNA Replication

Accurate replication of DNA, which is crucial for cellular propagation and survival, occurs during the S phase (DNA *s*ynthesis phase) of the cell cycle. This chapter begins with a brief primer on the events of replication and then discusses its regulation. Next, the chapter covers the proteins that bind origins of replication and ensure that each region of DNA is replicated once and only once per cell cycle. It closes by discussing how the structure of the nucleus influences replication.

DNA Replication: A Primer

One of the most exciting predictions of the Watson-Crick model for the structure of DNA was a mechanism for DNA replication. Because DNA strand pairing is determined by complementary base pairing, it was logical to propose the existence of DNA polymerases, enzymes that would move along a single strand of DNA, recognize each base in turn, and insert the proper complementary base at the end of the growing chain. Thus, one *might* have surmised that only a single enzyme was required for DNA synthesis. In fact, DNA replication in eukaryotic cells involves a complex macromolecular machine.

In the basic reaction of DNA replication, the 3′ hydroxyl at the end of the growing DNA strand makes a nucleophilic attack on the α-phosphate of the incoming nucleoside triphosphate to form a phosphodiester bond. This incorporates the nucleotide into the growing chain and releases pyrophosphate (Fig. 42-1). Subsequent hydrolysis of the pyrophosphate provides the driving force for the reaction. This reaction requires the presence of a template strand of DNA that specifies, through base pairing, which of the four nucleoside triphosphates is added to the growing complementary strand.

Before discussing DNA replication and its regulation, an introduction to some terminology describing the geometry of replicating DNA is required. The exact site on the chromosomal DNA where replication begins is termed the **origin of bidirectional replication.** As the term *bidirectional* implies, two sets of DNA replication machinery head off in opposite directions from the origin. Each set of replication machinery, together with the DNA that it is replicating, is called a **replication fork** because at the site of replication, one parental DNA molecule splits into two (Fig. 42-2). It is not known whether replication forks move along the DNA like trains along a track or whether the fork sits at a stationary site (referred to as a replication factory) through which the DNA is "reeled in" as it is replicated.

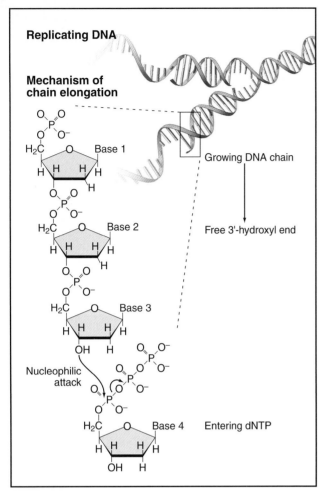

Figure 42-1 MECHANISM OF DNA POLYMERIZATION. A 3′ OH group at the end of a growing DNA chain makes a nucleophilic attack on the ∝-phosphate of a triphosphate precursor in the active site of polymerase (enzyme not shown here). dNTP, nucleoside triphosphate.

The bidirectional nature of DNA replication causes a fundamental problem, as DNA synthesis invariably proceeds in a 5′ to 3′ direction. Replication of the so-called **leading strand** poses no problems. This is the strand along which the fork moves in a 3′ to 5′ direction, so

the newly synthesized DNA is laid down smoothly in a 5′ to 3′ direction (Fig. 42-2). However, the other template strand faces in the opposite direction, apparently requiring DNA polymerase to synthesize DNA in the wrong direction as the replication fork progresses away from the origin (i.e., adding nucleotides in a 3′ to 5′ direction). No DNA polymerase with this polarity has been found. Instead, this **lagging strand** replicates in a series of short segments. Every time the DNA strands have been peeled apart (unwound) by 250 nucleotides or so, a polymerase/primase complex (see Fig. 42-11) initiates DNA synthesis on the lagging strand, with the polymerase running back toward the replication origin in a 5′ to 3′ direction. Locally, synthesis on the lagging strand proceeds in a direction *opposite to the overall direction of fork movement.* Synthesis of each lagging strand fragment stops when DNA polymerase runs into the 5′ end of the previous fragment. Thus, the lagging strand is copied in a highly *discontinuous* fashion into short fragments known as **Okazaki fragments** (named after their discoverer [Fig. 42-2]). Fig. 42-11 describes the enzymes and events at the replication fork in greater detail.

Origins of Replication

Bacteria such as *Escherichia coli* replicate their circular chromosomes using two replication forks starting from a single **origin of replication** (Fig. 42-3A), but eukaryotes must use multiple origins of replication to duplicate their large genomes during a relatively short S phase, which can be limited to as little as a few minutes in some early embryos. These numerous origins are distributed along the chromosome: up to 400 in budding yeast and about 60,000 in human cells. These origins are positioned so that all of the DNA is replicated in the available time, and to be on the safe side, more origins are prepared than are actually needed.

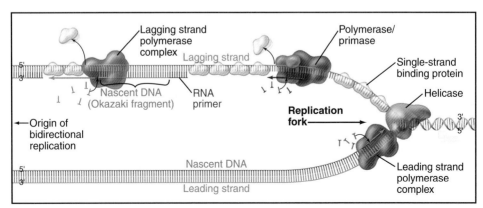

Figure 42-2 KEY COMPONENTS AND EVENTS AT THE REPLICATION FORK.

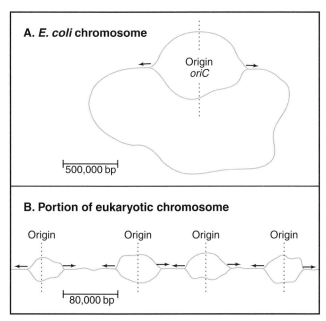

A. *E. coli* chromosome

Origin
oriC

500,000 bp

B. Portion of eukaryotic chromosome

Origin   Origin   Origin   Origin

80,000 bp

Figure 42-3   A, The *E. coli* chromosome is a simple replicon with a single origin of replication. In cells, this chromosome has a complex, highly supercoiled structure. **B,** Eukaryotic chromosomes have multiple origins of replication.

The existence of multiple origins creates a potential hazard: If any origin were used more or less than once per cell cycle, genes would be duplicated or lost. How is the "firing" of all of these origins orchestrated so that each is used once and only once per S phase? Cells manage this problem by a mechanism termed *licensing*, which ensures that each origin is used once and only once per S phase. Each origin is licensed to replicate once and only once per cell cycle. Replication of the origin removes the license, which cannot normally be renewed until the cell has completely traversed the cycle and has passed through mitosis.

A unit of chromosomal DNA whose replication is initiated at a single origin is termed a **replicon.** The origin is defined genetically as a **replicator** element. The classic replicon is the *E. coli* chromosome (which is 4×10^6 base pairs [bp] in size); this has a single replicator site called *oriC* (Fig. 42-3). An **initiator** protein (product of the *E. coli* DnaA gene [Fig. 42-12]) binds to this origin and either directly or indirectly promotes melting of the DNA duplex, giving the replication machinery access to two single strands of DNA. Other factors bind to the initiator, and their concerted action produces a wave of DNA replication proceeding outward in both directions along the DNA (a replication "bubble") at about 750 to 1250 bases per second.

An average human chromosome contains about 150×10^6 bp of DNA. Because the replication machinery in mammals moves only about 20 to 100 bases per second (probably reflecting the fact that the DNA is packaged

into chromatin [see Chapter 13]), it would take up to 2000 hours to replicate this length of DNA from a single origin. In most human cells, the duration of the S phase is about eight hours. This means that at least 25 to 125 origins of replication would be required to replicate an average chromosome in the allotted time. In fact, origins of replication are much more closely spaced than this. It has been estimated that mammalian origins of replication are spaced about 100,000 to 150,000 bp apart. Thus, approximately 60,000 origins of replication participate in replication of the entire human genome.

To explain the events at origins of replication, the budding yeast *Saccharomyces cerevisiae* serves as a good example. Its DNA replication is better understood than that of any other eukaryote.

Replication Origins in *S. Cerevisiae*

About 400 origins of replication participate in replicating the budding yeast genome. A major breakthrough in understanding DNA replication in *S. cerevisiae* was the identification of short (100 to 150 bp) segments of DNA that act as replication origins in vivo when cloned into a yeast plasmid (circular DNA molecule). These **autonomously replicating sequences** (or **ARS elements**) allow yeast plasmids to replicate in parallel with the cellular chromosomes (Fig. 42-4). ARS elements are often, although not always, bona fide replication origins in their native chromosomal context. Replication always initiates within ARS elements, but not all ARS elements act as origins of DNA replication in every cell cycle.

Yeast replication origins are spaced about every 30,000 bp, with a maximum separation of about 130,000 bp. Even this longest interval should replicate easily within the 30 minutes available during the S phase. Because the number of origins exceeds the number required to replicate the genome within the allotted time, some origins need not "fire" every cell cycle. The probability that any given origin will be used in a given cell cycle ranges from less than 0.2 to more than 0.9. It is important to note that replication of an origin by a fork coming from an adjacent origin inactivates it, thereby preventing excess replication during the cell cycle.

The ARS element does two things to establish an origin of replication. First, it has conserved sequences that act as binding sites for a protein complex that marks it as a potential origin. Second, it has nearby sequences that can readily be induced to unwind (become unbase-paired).

Budding yeast ARS elements share a common DNA sequence motif called the **ARS core consensus sequence:** 5'-(A/T)TTTAT(A/G)TTT(A/T)-3' (Fig. 42-5). Single base mutations at several locations within this

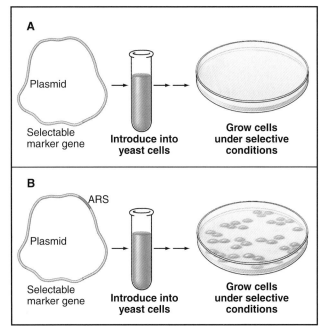

Figure 42-4 THE PLASMID ASSAY FOR IDENTIFICATION OF AN AUTONO-MOUSLY REPLICATING SEQUENCE ELEMENT (ORIGIN OF DNA REPLICATION) IN BUDDING YEAST. The plasmid at *left* has a selectable marker gene (e.g., a gene required for the synthesis of an essential amino acid) plus (in panel **B**) an ARS element. This plasmid is transferred into growing yeast cells that are defective in the marker gene carried by the plasmid, and these cells are then plated out on agar medium that lacks the essential amino acid. Only cells containing a form of the plasmid that can be replicated will grow to make colonies. **A,** A plasmid lacking an ARS fails to replicate and is lost from the cells. These cells cannot grow into colonies on plates that lack the essential amino acid. **B,** If the plasmid contains an ARS element, it replicates along with the chromosomal DNA and is maintained in the population. These cells grow into colonies in the absence of the essential amino acid.

sequence completely inactivate ARS activity. Other, less well-conserved DNA sequences also contribute to the activity of the ARS as a replication origin. One of these, termed B1, together with the ARS core, forms the binding site for a complex of six proteins (five of which are AAA ATPases) termed the **origin recognition**

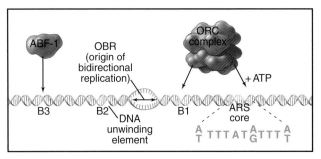

Figure 42-5 THE ORGANIZATION OF THE ARS1 ELEMENT. ORC binds to the ARS core sequence plus element B1. B2 is a sequence that can readily be induced to unwind. The OBR (origin of bidirectional replication) is the site where DNA synthesis actually begins. B3 is a binding site for an auxiliary factor called ABF-1 that is both a transcriptional activator and an activator of the ARS element.

complex (ORC [see later section]). The DNA unwinding element is thought to be another short sequence (B2) located a bit further along the DNA. DNA synthesis begins at an origin of bidirectional replication midway between the ORC binding site and the DNA unwinding element.

ORC was identified by its ability to bind the 11-bp ARS core sequence (Fig. 42-5). This binding has two noteworthy features. First, it requires adenosine triphosphate (ATP), which remains associated with the ORC complex. Second, in yeast, the ORC complex remains bound to the origins of replication across the entire cell cycle. Thus, something other than the presence of ORC must be responsible for regulating the periodic activation of origins in the S phase (see Fig. 42-14). In metazoans, ORC behavior is more complex; the largest subunit, Orc1, cycles on and off the DNA in a cell-cycle-regulated manner.

ARS elements typically contain binding sites for other sequence-specific DNA binding proteins, such as transcription factors. For example, a transcription factor called ARS-binding factor 1 (ABF-1) binds to the B3 sequence within the ARS1 element (Fig. 42-5). Deletion of the ABF-1 binding site only slightly reduces the ability of ARS1 to act as a replication origin in vivo. Furthermore, substitution of DNA binding sequences for other transcription factors within the B3 sequence has little effect on replication efficiency.

In addition to their role in DNA replication, several ORC components also seem to regulate heterochromatin formation and transcription (see Chapters 13 and 15). This cross talk between the machinery used for transcription and DNA replication may explain why regions of chromosomes with actively transcribed genes typically replicate early in the S phase (see the discussion that follows). The Orc6 subunit also functions in mitosis at kinetochores and during cytokinesis. Its detailed role in those processes is not known.

Replication Origins in Mammalian Cells

Far less is known about the structure and function of mammalian origins of DNA replication than about ARS elements in budding yeast. Attempts to develop a mammalian equivalent to the yeast ARS assay have had few successes. It is now accepted that mammalian origins of replication are much more complex than those of their budding yeast counterparts. Mammalian origin activity is affected by DNA sequence, DNA modifications, chromatin structure, and nuclear organization.

At present, two types of mammalian replication origins are known. The first is exemplified by the origin of replication adjacent to the lamin B2 gene (Fig. 42-6A). This origin "fires" within the first several minutes of the S phase, and a variety of methods have succeeded in mapping it to a stretch of less than 500 bp. Within

A. Mapping a simple replication origin

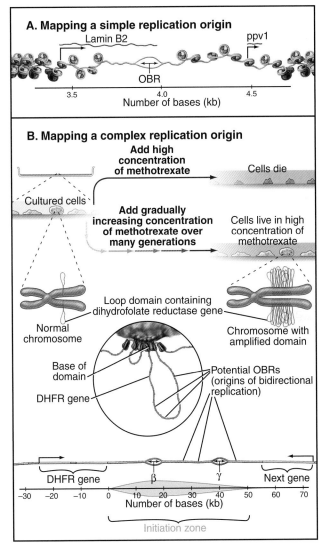

B. Mapping a complex replication origin

Figure 42-6 DNA REPLICATION ORIGINS IN MAMMALS. **A,** A simple DNA replication origin. Replication of the DNA adjacent to the lamin B2 gene appears to initiate entirely from a single origin, as shown. ppv1 is a gene next to the lamin B2 gene. **B,** A complex DNA replication origin near the dihydrofolate reductase (DHFR) gene. Normal cells are killed by exposure to methotrexate, but it is possible to select resistant cell lines by growing them in progressively increasing concentrations of the drug, selecting at each stage for cells that survive. Use of this procedure on hamster cells has resulted in a cell line that contains about 1000 copies of a 230,000-bp domain containing the dihydrofolate reductase gene. This region of DNA is replicated using origins found within a 55,000-bp region adjacent to the dihydrofolate reductase gene. Low levels of initiation of replication occur throughout the entire 55,000-bp region, but most initiation occurs at two specific origins, called β and γ.

this region, a single origin of bidirectional replication appears to be used. Thus, the lamin B2 origin of replication appears to be analogous to the well-characterized budding yeast origins.

The second is exemplified by the widely studied replication origin lying just downstream of the hamster

gene for dihydrofolate reductase, an enzyme that is essential for biosynthesis of thymidine. This origin is accessible to experimental study because it is possible to select for cells with this chromosomal region amplified as hundreds or even thousands of copies (Fig. 42-6B). By looking for the first regions of the amplified DNA to replicate, the origin of replication was initially located within a region of about 55,000 bp. It now appears that DNA replication can initiate with low efficiency at roughly 20 sites distributed throughout this broad zone. Two of these sites are used with relatively higher efficiency, accounting for about 20% of all initiation in the region. These sites, termed Ori-β and Ori-γ (Fig. 42-6), each encompass about 0.5 to 2 kb of DNA.

A third view of vertebrate DNA replication origins came from studies of DNA replication in *Xenopus* eggs. Once activated by fertilization or by various experimental tricks, *Xenopus* eggs divide about an hour later and then undergo a rapid sequence of cell cycles, each of which lasts about 30 minutes. Any DNA that is injected into these eggs is rapidly and efficiently replicated. Prokaryotic DNA and eukaryotic DNA are replicated with similar efficiency, and careful studies demonstrated that this replication initiates randomly with respect to DNA sequence (i.e., does not use defined origins). This promiscuous initiation of DNA replication appears to be a specialized adaptation by early embryos to permit replication of the chromosomes in the very brief temporal window available.

The emerging view is that the replication machinery is highly conserved between budding yeasts and vertebrates but that the location of replication origins is much more flexible in vertebrates. This might in part reflect the diverse range of cell cycles required to make a complex metazoan. The mix of conserved components with divergent uses is a recurring theme in DNA replication.

Assembly of the Prereplication Complex

To preserve the integrity of the genome, each origin of replication must "fire" only once per cell cycle. We now have a reasonable understanding of the various solutions to this problem that have been reached by differing model organisms and vertebrates.

Recall that yeast ORC is stably bound to replication origins throughout the cell cycle. However, ORC is not the trigger for DNA replication. Rather, it acts as a "landing pad" for assembly of a **prereplication complex** of other proteins that initiates DNA replication. During late anaphase or very early G₁ phase, several proteins, including **Cdc6p** and **Cdt1,** bind to the ORC complex at origins of replication (Table 42-1). ORC-Cdc6p-Cdt1

Table 42-1

BIOCHEMICAL ACTIVITIES REQUIRED FOR REPLICATION OF DNA IN EUKARYOTES

Activity	Name of Protein
Origin recognition	ORC (*origin recognition complex*; five of six subunits are AAA ATPases)
Pre-replication complex	Cdc6 (recruits Mcm 2-7) Cdt1 (recruits Mcm 2-7) Mcm 10 (stimulates Cdc45 and polymerase α binding)
Origin activation	Cdk2-cyclin A Cdc7p-Dbf4p Cdc45p (recruits RPA and polymerases. Needed for elongation of growing chain) GINS complex (needed for polymerase binding and elongation of growing chain)
DNA unwinding (helicase)	Mcm 2-7 proteins (precede other fork components) Mcm 8 (controversial, may be elongation helicase)
Stabilization of single-stranded DNA	RPA (binds single-stranded DNA)
Polymerase/primase	DNA polymerase α (no editing function)
Replicative polymerases	DNA polymerase δ DNA polymerase ε (both have 3′–5′ exonuclease editing capability)
Processivity factor	PCNA (ring-shaped clamp that slides along the DNA. Keeps polymerases δ and ε attached to the template strand so that they make longer chains; coordination of cell cycle control and replication; role in repair)
PCNA loader	RF-C (Binds primer: template junction. AAA ATPase. Loading factor for PCNA, important for polymerase switch)
Closing Factors	
Removal of RNA primer	Fen1 5′ ⇒ 3′ exonuclease RNase H
Ligation of discontinuous DNA fragments	DNA ligase I
Releasing superhelical tension	DNA topoisomerase I
Disentangling daughter strands	DNA topoisomerase II

then recruits a complex of Mcm proteins to the origin and loads it onto the DNA. This prereplication complex of ORC, Cdc6p, CDT1, and **minichromosome maintenance (Mcm) proteins** (Fig. 42-7) assembles at each replication origin before the onset of the S phase.

Mcm proteins were identified in a screen for genes of budding yeast that are required for the stability of small artificial chromosomes. Six of these *Mcm* genes encode a structurally related group of proteins, termed Mcm 2-7, that are required for DNA replication. Mcm 2-7 proteins form a hexameric complex that is thought to be shaped like a doughnut. Somehow, Cdc6p–Cdt1 uses ATP hydrolysis to thread DNA through the central hole of the Mcm doughnut. Although the function of the Mcm 2-7 complex is not known for certain, the predominant view is that it is a DNA helicase, an enzyme that uses ATP hydrolysis to separate DNA strands (see Fig. 42-11). It is currently thought that Mcm 2-7 binding to the prereplication complex is the key point of regulation at which origins are "licensed" so that they replicate only once per cell cycle.

In mammals, licensing occurs in several stages, all before passage of the restriction point (see Chapter 41). During telophase, Cdc6, Cdt1, and Mcm 2-7 bind to origins all across the chromosomes. Later, in the early G_1 phase, these licensed origins are somehow processed to select the subset of origins that will fire in the subsequent S phase. A third step establishes the relative temporal order in which origins will fire.

At least three mechanisms regulate licensing. The first involves negative regulation of Cdc6p activity by Cdks, which inhibit Cdc6p–Cdt1 from loading Mcm proteins onto DNA. At the exit from mitosis, destruction of cyclins and synthesis of inhibitory proteins inactivates Cdks, creating a window of time between anaphase and the restriction point for licensing replication origins (see Fig. 40-18). Once mammalian cells pass the restriction point, the levels of Cdk2–cyclin E, and subsequently, Cdk2–cyclin A rise again (see Fig. 41-11) preventing the reassembly of prereplication complexes until after the next mitosis. In yeasts, the single Cdk that is complexed with B-type cyclins inhibits prereplication complex reassembly. Experimental inactivation of Cdk1 during the G_2 phase in the fission yeast *Schizosaccharomyces pombe* demonstrated the importance of kinase activation: Cells lacking Cdk1 activity assembled prereplication complexes on already replicated DNA and then carried out further rounds of "illegal" DNA replication without division.

In vertebrates a protein called **geminin** is a critical regulator of origin "licensing." Geminin binds to Cdt1 and prevents it from loading Mcm proteins onto DNA. The anaphase-promoting complex/cyclosome (APC/C) (see Fig. 40-16) degrades or inactivates geminin, keeping its concentration very low from anaphase through late G_1 when prereplication complexes assemble. Accumulation of geminin starting in the S phase prevents the assembly of new prereplication complexes until after the next mitosis. Yeasts lack geminin, but in vertebrates, regulation of geminin and Cdt1 levels by proteolysis appears to be the primary method of controlling origin licensing.

A third way to regulate origin "licensing" involves sequestering molecules that are required to assemble the prereplication complex in the cytoplasm following the onset of the S phase. This was first suggested by studies of DNA replication in *Xenopus* egg extracts (see Fig. 40-8) in which nuclei replicate their DNA once and only once unless their nuclear envelopes are perforated, in which case the DNA replicates again. In living cells, this regulation by the nuclear envelope appears to be significant only in yeasts, in which factors that are excluded from the nucleus after replication include Mcm proteins.

Components of the prereplication complex are absent from differentiated (G_0) cells. In fact, detection of these proteins with antibodies in cells from cervical smears is currently being developed as a sensitive method for the early detection of cancer cells (Fig. 42-8).

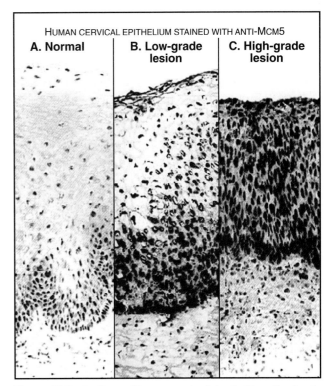

Figure 42-8   Sections of human cervix stained with antibodies to Mcm5. **A,** Normal G_0 cells in this stratified epithelium lack Mcm5 and other replication proteins. **B–C,** Cancer cells express Mcm5 at higher levels as they become more malignant. (Adapted from Williams GH, Romanowski P, Morris L, et al: Improved cervical smear assessment using antibodies against proteins that regulate DNA replication. Proc Natl Acad Sci U S A 95:14932–14937, 1998.)

Signals That Start Replication

A classic experiment (Fig. 42-9) demonstrated that (1) a cytoplasmic inducer triggers the transition into the S phase and (2) this inducer triggers DNA replication in a G_1 nucleus but not in a G_2 nucleus. The inducer is very likely a combination of protein kinases, including Cdk-cyclin pairs, as well as a specialized kinase, Cdc7p-Dbf4p. In mammals, Cdk2–cyclin E, whose activity is maximal at the G_1/S transition (Fig. 42-10), phosphorylates Rb, thereby opening the restriction point "gate" and allowing the E2F/DP dimer to function as a transcription factor and stimulate the transcription of genes involved in DNA replication (see Chapter 41). In addition to cyclin E itself, genes targeted by E2F include cyclin A, Cdc25A, enzymes required for synthesis of DNA precursors (dihydrofolate reductase, thymidine kinase, and thymidylate synthase), origin-binding proteins Cdc6p, Orc1, Cdt1 and its inhibitor geminin, and two components of the replication machinery (DNA polymerase α and proliferating cell nuclear antigen [PCNA]; see Fig. 42-11).

In the S phase, the Cdk inhibitor p27^{Kip1} is a target for the SCF^{Skp2} ubiquitin ligase complex, which marks it

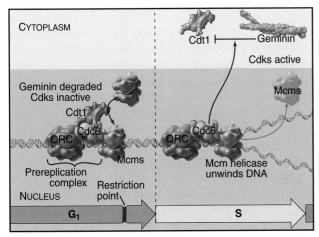

Figure 42-7   COMPONENTS OF THE PREREPLICATION COMPLEX AND THEIR FATE AFTER THE INITIATION OF DNA REPLICATION.

for destruction by proteasomes (see Chapter 40). SCF gets its name from three of its components: Skp2, cullin, and F-box proteins (see Fig. 40-17). Skp2, which is short for "S-phase kinase-associated protein," got its name because it was first identified in a complex with Cdk2–cyclin A. This kinase targets proteins for recognition by SCF, which recognizes and ubiquitinates its substrates only after they have been phosphorylated at certain key positions. E2F/DP and cyclin E are also degraded when cells enter the S phase, and this is apparently triggered by Cdk2–cyclin A (Fig. 42-10).

The second kinase involved with initiation of DNA replication is Cdc7p with its associated subunit Dbf4p. This kinase seems to act at the level of individual DNA replication origins. Careful analysis has revealed that Cdc7p-Dbf4p is required for firing of origins in both early and late S phase. Cdc7p is capable of phosphorylating several Mcm proteins. This phosphorylation may somehow trigger the start of replication fork movement.

Dbf4p, which is responsible for targeting Cdc7p to origins, is very unstable from anaphase through G_1 phase. This period of Dbf4 instability coincides with the cell-cycle period during which prereplication complexes are assembled, and it may provide a mechanism

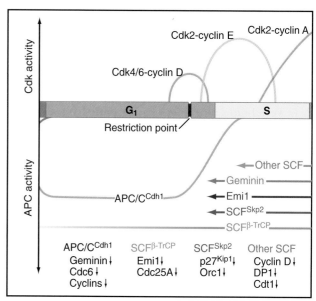

Figure 42-10 PROTEIN DEGRADATION IN THE REGULATION OF DNA REPLICATION. Degradation of geminin, Cdc6, Cdc25A, and cyclins during G_1 keeps Cdk activity low and allows prereplication complex formation. Degradation of p27Kip1 and inactivation of the APC/C^{Cdh1} by Emi1 allows the activation of Cdks to levels sufficient for the initiation of the S phase. Once cells enter the S phase, the G1/S regulatory machinery (cyclins D and E and the E2F cofactor DP1) is degraded. Degradation of Cdt1 and accumulation of geminin block reassembly of prereplication complexes.

to ensure that origins do not fire prematurely until the cell is ready to enter the S phase.

At the onset of DNA replication, each origin of replication has bound to it the ORC complex, Cdc6p-Cdt1, and multiple hexameric Mcm complexes. (See Table 42-1 for a description of the major activities involved in DNA replication. See Box 42-1 for an introduction to DNA replication in *E. coli*.)

Mechanism of DNA Synthesis

For DNA replication to start, the paired strands of the double helix must be separated. This permits the DNA polymerase to bind and begin synthesizing the daughter strand. DNA strand separation is driven by a DNA helicase, an enzyme that uses ATP hydrolysis to peel apart the paired strands of the DNA double helix. Despite exhaustive efforts, the identity of this helicase is not firmly established in eukaryotes, but it is striking that both viral and bacterial helicases are hexameric protein complexes. This, plus limited experimental evidence, has led to the general belief that the hexameric Mcm complex is the eukaryotic DNA helicase. Other helicases may also participate.

Locally, DNA replication appears to start when the Cdk2-cyclin A and Cdc7p-Dbf4p kinases activate the prereplication complex. Key phosphorylated proteins include Mcm 2–7 and Cdc6 (Fig. 42-11A). Phosphoryla-

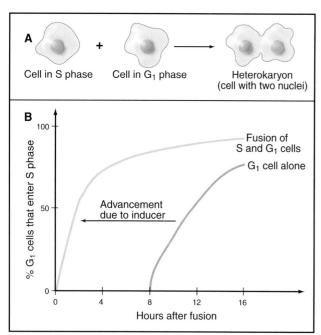

Figure 42-9 CELL FUSION EXPERIMENT SHOWING THE EXISTENCE OF A POSITIVE INDUCER OF THE S PHASE. **A,** Synchronized cells in different stages of the cycle were fused to yield two nuclei in a single cytoplasm. **B,** If the fusion involved nuclei from G_1 and S cells, the G_1 nucleus was induced to enter the S phase sooner than expected. If the fusion involved nuclei from S and G_2 cells, the G_2 nucleus failed to rereplicate its DNA (not shown). (Redrawn from Rao PN, Johnson RT: Mammalian cell fusion: Studies on the regulation of DNA synthesis and mitosis. Nature 225:159–164, 1970.)

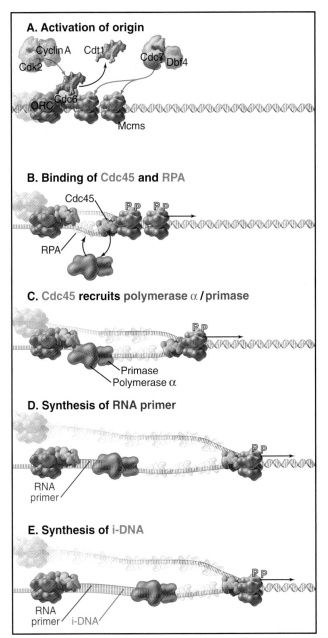

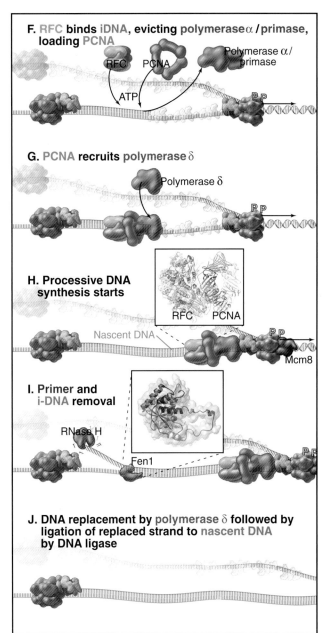

Figure 42-11 THE MAIN EVENTS OF DNA REPLICATION. For a more detailed description, see the text. (PDB file for Fen1: 1A76. PDB file for RFC/PCNA: 1SXJ. PDB file for Cdt1: 1WLQ.)

tion triggers a change in the binding of Cdc6p and Cdt1 to the DNA. Cdc6p remains bound to the chromatin throughout the S phase, while Cdt1 is released and degraded. Activation recruits to the origin a protein called **Cdc45p** together with a single-strand DNA-binding protein, **RPA** (Fig. 42-11B). Several other proteins also bind at this time, but their detailed functions are still being elucidated (Table 42-1).

Cdc45p appears to associate with the Mcm proteins and promote the binding of RPA, forming a complex that somehow activates the Mcm helicase. Cdc45p and RPA then recruit DNA polymerase to the origin (Fig. 42-11C). As the helicase starts to separate the DNA strands,

moving outward in both directions from the origin of bidirectional replication, RPA stabilizes the separated strands, ensuring that they do not base-pair with one another again. Recent results suggest that the Mcm 8 protein may take over as the helicase once the replication fork has moved away from the replication origin (Fig. 42-11H), but this remains under investigation.

The separated DNA strands are ready for replication, but DNA synthesis always involves addition of an incoming nucleoside triphosphate to a free 3′ OH group at the terminus of a *preexisting* nascent polynucleotide (Fig. 42-1). In the absence of a nascent DNA chain, how does DNA polymerase get started? This problem is solved by

BOX 42-1
DNA Replication in Escherichia Coli

The DNA replication system of *Escherichia coli* has been reconstituted entirely from purified components. Analysis of this system reveals many similarities with eukaryotic replication, indicating that this process is highly conserved. *E. coli* DNA replication can be subdivided into three phases: initiation, elongation, and termination. Thus far, at least 28 polypeptides are known to be involved.

Initiation: *E. coli* chromosomal DNA replication initiates within a 245-bp region, termed *oriC*. This region contains four 9-bp binding sites for the *E. coli* initiator protein, DnaA. Nearby are three repeats of a 13-bp A: T-rich sequence. *oriC* also contains specific binding sites for two small histone-like proteins called HU and IHF. Replication is initiated with the cooperative binding of 10 to 20 DnaA monomers to their specific binding sites (Fig. 42-12). To be active, these monomers must each have bound ATP. Binding of DnaA permits unwinding of the DNA at the 13-bp repeats, in a reaction that requires the histone-like proteins. Next, DnaC binds to DnaB and escorts it to the unwound DNA. DnaB is the key helicase that will drive DNA replication by unwinding the double helix, but it binds DNA poorly on its own in the absence of its DnaC escort. Once DnaB has docked onto the DNA, DnaC is released, and the helicase can then start to unwind the DNA, provided that ATP, SSB, and DNA gyrase are present. SSB is a single-stranded DNA binding protein that stabilizes the unwound DNA, and DNA gyrase is a topoisomerase (see Chapter 13) that removes the twist that is generated when the two strands of the double helix are separated.

Elongation: As in eukaryotes, *E. coli* DNA replication involves a leading strand, with the daughter DNA synthesized as a single continuous molecule, as well as a lagging strand, with the DNA synthesized as discontinuous Okazaki fragments. All daughter strands are started by an RNA primase that deposits primers of 11 ± 1 nucleotides. The enzyme that actually synthesizes the DNA is the polymerase III holoenzyme, which has at least 10 subunits. This contains polymerase and proofreading subunits and is held to the DNA by a doughnut-like "sliding clamp" (β). The β is loaded onto the DNA by a pentameric complex in a process that requires ATP. The parallel with PCNA and RFC in eukaryotes is striking. Activities specific for the lagging strand include RNase H, which removes the RNA primers; DNA polymerase I, which fills in the gaps left behind by primer removal; and DNA ligase, which links the Okazaki fragments together. DNA replication in *E. coli* is significantly faster than it is in eukaryotes, with the fork moving at a rate of about 1000 bp per second. This higher speed is presumed to be at least partially attributable to the absence of nucleosomes on the bacterial chromosome.

Termination: A specialized termination zone is found on the circular *E. coli* chromosome opposite *oriC*. This zone contains binding sites called *ter* sites, to which the *ter* binding protein binds. This protein appears to block the movement of DNA helicases, such as DnaB, thereby stalling the DNA replication fork. Following termination of replication, a specialized topoisomerase, the product of the *parC* and *parE* genes, is required to separate the daughter chromosomes from one another.

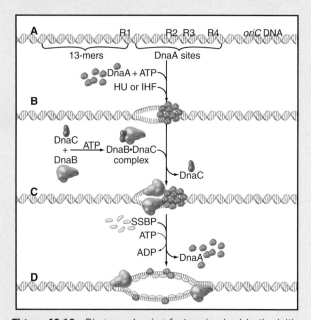

Figure 42-12 Diagram showing factors involved in the initiation of DNA replication in *E. coli*. **A,** DNA sequences at OriC. **B,** Unwinding of the origin. **C,** Binding of helicase. **D,** The template, now ready for binding of DNA polymerase. (Adapted from Baker TA, Wickner SH: Genetics and enzymology of DNA replication in *Escherichia coli*. Annu Rev Genet 26:447–477, 1992.)

a DNA-dependent RNA polymerase called a primase, which, like other RNA polymerases, *can* initiate synthesis de novo without the need for a 3′ OH group. In eukaryotes, all DNA chains are started by a complex of DNA polymerase α and a primase subunit, collectively known as **Pol α/Primase.** Primase synthesizes an RNA chain of about 10 nucleotides to which DNA polymerase α adds another 20 to 30 nucleotides of so-called initiator DNA (iDNA) (Fig. 42-11D–E). These initiating reactions are potentially hazardous, because DNA polymerase α lacks proofreading ability. Any errors in matching up an incoming base would create a mutation. Given the huge number of initiation events that are required to replicate an entire genome, this potential for errors is not acceptable. Therefore, the RNA primer and most or all of the initiator DNA laid down by Pol α/Primase are subsequently replaced.

Once Pol α/Primase has done its job, two further essential factors act. A pentameric protein complex called **replication factor C (RFC)** binds the 3′ end of the initiator DNA. RFC uses energy from ATP hydrolysis to load the trimeric protein **PCNA** onto the DNA (see Fig. 42-11F–G). The PCNA trimer is doughnut-shaped, and when the DNA is inserted into its central hole, it is topologically locked onto the DNA. RFC binding and PCNA loading displace Pol α/Primase from the DNA, and PCNA then recruits **DNA polymerases** δ and ε to the DNA. Moving along with the sliding platform of PCNA, these polymerases then process along the DNA, synthesizing DNA continuously on the leading strand (see Fig. 42-11H). On the lagging strand, they synthesize about 250 bp of DNA until they run into the next Okazaki fragment. Cdc45p may be a scaffolding factor that holds the Mcm hexamer and the replicative DNA polymerases together as the fork moves.

Both polymerases δ and ε have associated exonuclease activities. This enables them to proofread the newly synthesized DNA and correct any mistakes that they have made. This may explain the amazing fidelity of DNA replication, with typically only one error per 10^9 bp polymerized.

The final steps of DNA replication are removal of the RNA primer (and probably initiator DNA) and ligation of adjacent stretches of newly synthesized DNA. Removal of the primer can be accomplished in two ways (Fig. 42-11I). On one hand, an RNA exonuclease called **RNase H** can chew in from the 5′ end of the primer. However, this enzyme cannot remove the last ribonucleotide that is joined to initiator DNA. That requires a second nuclease, called **Fen1.** Alternatively, Fen1 can do the whole job itself if it gets help from a helicase. In this case, the helicase peels the RNA (and possibly the initiator DNA) away from the template, creating a sort of flap. Fen1 then cleaves at the junction where the flap is anchored to the DNA template, removing the oligomer of unwanted nucleotides in one step.

Following removal of initiator RNA, the Pol δ/PCNA complex extends the upstream nascent chain until it runs into the 5′ end created by Fen1. DNA ligase I then joins the two stretches of DNA together (Fig. 42-11J).

Higher-Order Organization of DNA Replication in the Nucleus

A wide variety of experimental evidence revealed that the unit of replication in eukaryotic chromosomes is not the individual replicon but rather a replicon cluster. Evidence for this higher-order organization of DNA replication within the nucleus was first obtained by fiber autoradiography. Cells were fed radioactive precursors for DNA synthesis and then examined by electron microscopy. (For an explanation of this technique, see Fig. 40-3.) The spatial distribution of DNA replication during the S phase is more readily observed by using BrdU, a nucleotide base analog that is incorporated into DNA by the replication machinery in place of thymidine (this is called by its more correct name of Br-dUTP in Fig. 42-13). Incorporation of BrdU into DNA makes the newly synthesized daughter DNA strand heavier, allowing its separation from the parental DNA by centrifugation on a cesium chloride density gradient (see Chapter 6). In addition, specific antibodies that recognize DNA containing either BrdU or the related reagents IdU and CldU can be used to localize the changing patterns of DNA synthesis as cells traverse the S phase. More recently, analogs have been developed in which the Br in Fig. 42-13A has been replaced by a fluorescent group. This allows the newly replicated DNA to be observed directly in living cells.

These methods reveal up to 1000 sites of active replication, called **replication foci,** at any one time during the S phase in a mammalian cell nucleus (Fig. 42-13B–C and E–F). Given that each of these replication foci is active for only about one hour out of the eight- to ten-hour S phase, a cell will replicate DNA at about 10,000 of these foci. Given roughly 60,000 origins in a mammalian cell, each replication focus represents five or six replication origins that are activated coordinately. These replication foci may be associated with the nuclear matrix or nucleoskeleton (see Chapter 13).

Temporal Control of Replication during the S Phase

The term *S phase* gives the impression that all DNA replicates more or less synchronously, but this is far from true. At any given time during the S phase, only 10% to 15% of the replicons actively synthesize DNA. Some replicate earlier, others later. It is important to note that this pattern of replication is not random; some origins consistently replicate early in the S phase, whereas others consistently replicate late in the S phase. Overall, the human genome can be subdivided into at least 1000 "zones," each of which replicates at a characteristic time during the S phase. The organization of replication zones corresponds roughly to the organization of chromosomes into banding patterns: early-replicating regions typically correspond to gene-rich R bands, whereas late-replicating regions typically correspond to gene-poor G-bands (Fig. 42-13D; compare with Fig. 13-14). A similar division of chromosomes into early- and late-replicating regions also holds true for budding yeast, although many fewer replication origins are involved.

BrdU labeling experiments show that the basic unit of chromosomal DNA replication is a cluster of roughly five replication origins that fire coordinately. What must now be superimposed on this view of the replicating chromosome is a second level of regulation: the time at which each replicon cluster fires during the S phase. This can be seen clearly by synchronizing cells at the beginning of the S phase, releasing them from cell-cycle arrest, and then exposing them to BrdU at various times thereafter. This experiment reveals very distinctive patterns of DNA synthesis occurring at different times during the S phase (Fig. 42-13B–C and E–F). Early on, euchromatin replicates throughout the nucleus. Later, replicating regions appear concentrated around nucleoli and other areas of more condensed chromatin. Toward the end of the S phase, replication is largely concentrated in blocks of heterochromatin. These observations show that DNA replication occurs throughout the nucleus, wherever DNA is located. DNA does not move to a small number of discrete sites to be replicated (as was previously thought).

The most striking aspect of these patterns of DNA synthesis is their reproducibility from one cell cycle to the next. For example, regions of DNA labeled early in the S phase overlap little or not at all with DNA labeled three hours later (Fig. 42-13C and E). However, DNA labeled at corresponding points of the S phase in two successive cell cycles superimposes almost entirely. Thus, the chromosomal substructure that gives rise to replication foci is stable from one cell cycle to the next. This strongly suggests that particular regions of chromosomes are organized into reproducible structural domains and that each domain has a particular "window" during the S phase during which it replicates. This is significant. In one study, chromosomal regions that replicated at the wrong time during the S phase as a result of a mutation in an ORC subunit had a defective condensed structure in the next mitosis.

The timing of replication of particular replication origins has been studied most carefully in budding yeast. First, a procedure was developed whereby all cells in a population could be induced to enter the S phase synchronously. Next, the shift in the density of the DNA following BrdU incorporation was used to distinguish between DNA that had replicated and DNA that

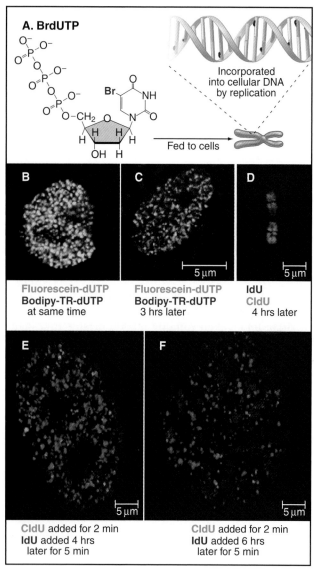

A. BrdUTP

Incorporated into cellular DNA by replication

Fed to cells

B	C	D
Fluorescein-dUTP **Bodipy-TR-dUTP** at same time	Fluorescein-dUTP **Bodipy-TR-dUTP** 3 hrs later	IdU CldU 4 hrs later

5 µm | 5 µm

E | F

5 µm | 5 µm

CldU added for 2 min **IdU** added 4 hrs later for 5 min

CldU added for 2 min **IdU** added 6 hrs later for 5 min

Figure 42-13 VISUALIZATION OF DNA REPLICATION WITHIN THE NUCLEUS. **A,** The protocol for fluorescent labeling of newly replicated DNA. BrdUTP is introduced into DNA in place of dTTP. The incorporated BrdU molecules are detected by fluorescence labeling with labeled antibodies. **B,** In a related technology, *green*-dUTP and *red*-dUTP, when added together, show the many sites of DNA replication in a cell nucleus. Because both UTP analogs are incorporated simultaneously into the DNA, the sites of replication appear *yellow*. **C,** *Green*-dUTP is followed by *red*-dUTP added three hours later. The later sites of DNA replication show very little overlap with the earlier sites. **D,** Mitotic chromosome from a cell that was labeled early in the S phase with IdU *(green)*, and then four hours later with CldU *(red)*. The late-replicating and early-replicating regions of the chromosome are segregated into discrete bands. **E,** CldU *(green)* added early in the S phase and IdU *(red)* added four hours later show little overlap. **F,** CldU *(green)* added early in the S phase and IdU *(red)* added six hours later show no overlap. The *large red blocks* of labeling seen with the IdU are characteristic of the pattern of replicating heterochromatin seen late in the S phase. Bodipy-TR-dUTP, a *red* fluorescent form of dUTP; BrdUTP, Bromo-deoxyuridine triphosphate; CldU, Chlorine-dUTP; Fluorescein-dUTP, a *green* fluorescent form of dUTP; IdU, Iodine-dUTP. All are used in place of dTTP (thymidine triphosphate) in DNA synthesis. (B–C, Courtesy of P. R. Cook, University of Oxford, England; reproduced from Manders EMM, Kimura H, Cook PR: Direct imaging of DNA in living cells reveals the dynamics of chromosome formation. J Cell Biol 144:813–821, 1999. Copyright 1999 The Rockefeller University Press. D, Courtesy of A. I. Lamond, University of Dundee, Scotland; reproduced from Ferreira J, Paolella G, Ramos C, et al: Spatial organization of large-scale chromatin domains in the nucleus: A magnified view of single chromosome territories. J Cell Biol 139:1597–1610, 1997. Copyright 1997 The Rockefeller University Press. E–F, Reproduced from Ma H, Samarabandu J, Devdhar RS, et al: Spatial and temporal dynamics of DNA replication sites in mammalian cells. J Cell Biol 143:1415–1425, 1998. Copyright 1998 The Rockefeller University Press.)

had not (Fig. 42-14). It then became relatively simple to take DNA probes from different regions of the chromosome and determine when each replicated (changed its density) during the S phase. This protocol demonstrated that each ARS element replicates at a characteristic time during the S phase.

There are at least three possible explanations for the sequence of replication patterns seen for different chromosomal regions:

1. Local chromatin structures, established as a result of gene expression, might somehow influence the time of replication. Thus, transcriptionally active loci (where transcription factors are already bound) have a head start over other regions of the chromosomes, permitting them to initiate DNA replication first. This mechanism can explain instances where the timing of replication of a particular locus differs between cell types. For

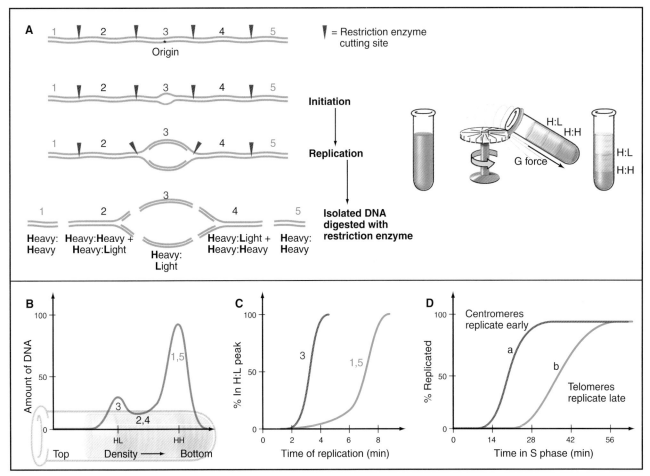

Figure 42-14 Measurement of the time of replication of particular chromosomal regions in *Saccharomyces cerevisiae*. **A–C,** This protocol is based on a classic density shift experiment of Messelson and Stahl that proved that DNA replication is semiconservative. *S. cerevisiae* cells are grown for several generations in a medium containing ^{13}C and ^{15}N heavy isotopes. As a result, their DNA is fully substituted with heavy isotopes. At the beginning of the experiment, the cells are synchronized so that they enter the S phase in a single wave. At the same time, the heavy (H) isotope medium is removed and replaced with "light medium" (L) containing ^{12}C and ^{14}N. At various times after the initiation of the S phase, aliquots of cells are removed, and the DNA is isolated. The DNA is then cleaved with restriction enzymes so that the chromosomes are cut into many fragments. DNA from each time point is then subjected to CsCl density gradient centrifugation. When any local region of DNA is replicated, its density alters from heavy/heavy to heavy/light. After very short incubations with light isotopes, only DNA near the origin of replication will be heavy/light; all other DNA will be heavy/heavy. These two populations of molecules are separated from one another by the density gradient centrifugation. To examine the timing of replication of a specific gene, a cloned segment of DNA corresponding to the region of interest is used to probe (by DNA hybridization) the heavy/heavy and heavy/light peaks from each gradient. The time of replication of each locus is the time at which the restriction fragment being detected by DNA hybridization moves from the heavy/heavy peak to the heavy/light peak. The numbers in panels **B** and **C** refer to the numbered regions of the chromosomes shown in **A. D,** Data from a replication timing experiment show that in budding yeast, centromeres replicate early in the S phase and telomeres replicate late. To generate *curve a,* fractions from a gradient like that shown in panel **B** were hybridized to a cloned centromere region. To generate *curve b,* fractions from the same gradient were hybridized to a cloned telomere region probe. Note that in mammalian cells, centromeres replicate late and telomeres replicate earlier. (This figure is based on the work of the laboratory of B. J. Brewer and W. L. Fangman.

example, in mammalian genomes the region of DNA containing the β-globin gene (encoding a protein subunit of hemoglobin) replicates from a single origin lying just upstream of the gene. This region of more than 200-kb of DNA replicates early in erythroid cells, in which the β-globin gene is expressed, but later in other cells, in which the gene is inactive.

2. The position of origins in the nucleus may influence when they replicate. It has been suggested that replication origins fire in a sequence that is established during G₁ (see earlier). This sequence may reflect the gradual redistribution of chromosomes to their preferred positions as the nuclear organization is gradually reestablished after mitosis.

3. Specific factors may activate various origins of replication in sequential order during the S phase. In yeast, the Cdc7p-Dbf4p kinase must act on later origins of replication for them to fire. This kinase promotes the binding of Cdc45p and RPA, both of which bind to origins only as they are about to fire throughout the S phase. In addition, the Rad53p protein kinase regulates firing of late origins of replication in budding yeast. Rad53p (known as Chk2 in higher eukaryotes) is an important component of DNA damage checkpoints, which have a particularly important role to play during the S phase (see Fig. 40-4).

The Intra-S Checkpoint

A powerful group of three checkpoints, which we here collectively call the intra-S checkpoint, monitors the process of DNA replication and stops it if DNA breaks or stalled replication forks are detected (Fig. 42-15). A third aspect of these checkpoints is to delay the onset of mitosis until the replication of the genome is complete.

These checkpoints have similarities and differences compared to other DNA damage checkpoints. For example, unlike the G₁ DNA damage checkpoint, p53-mediated transcription is not required. However, as is the case in the G₁ and G₂ phases, if DNA breaks are detected, the kinases ATM and ATR and their downstream effectors phosphorylate Cdc25A, triggering its rapid destruction mediated by SCF$^{β\text{-TrCP}}$ (see Fig. 41-12). The resulting inactivation of Cdks during the S phase prevents Cdc45p from loading onto prereplication complexes and blocks the initiation of new replication forks. This prevents replication forks from running across DNA breaks, which could lead to chromosome breaks and the loss of genetic material, with lethal consequences for the cell.

The intra-S checkpoint also detects stalled replication forks. Why would a replication fork stall? This could happen if, for example, the fork encounters a damaged DNA base or bases that it cannot "read." Stopping the fork gives time for the DNA repair machinery to detect and repair the damage (see Box 43-1). Stalled forks activate the ATR kinase, leading to Cdc25A inactivation as described earlier and the cessation of new fork initiation. In addition, through an unknown mechanism, the intra-S checkpoint also has a mechanism to protect existing forks from disassembly. This is important because replication forks contain unwound and nicked DNA molecules that could be turned into breaks if the structure disassembled.

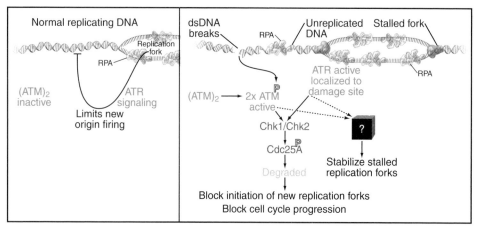

Figure 42-15 THE INTRA-S CHECKPOINT. If DNA breaks are detected, the ATM kinase activates downstream kinases Chk1 and Chk2, leading to phosphorylation of Cdc25A and its subsequent ubiquitin tagging and degradation. This blocks the initiation of new replication forks as well as cell-cycle progression more generally. If DNA persists in unreplicated form or if replication forks stall, the ATR kinase activates a similar downstream response. In addition, an as-yet-unknown mechanism stabilizes stalled replication forks so that they can be repaired and replication completed. p53 is not involved in the intra-S checkpoint.

ATR kinase is activated by binding single-stranded DNA associated with RPA. As this is normally present at every replication fork during DNA replication, ATR signaling appears to be an intrinsic aspect of the replication process. It has been proposed that ATR normally limits excessive firing of replication origins by keeping the concentration of Cdc25A low and coordinates replication with other cell-cycle events. For example, Chk2, a kinase activated by ATM and ATR (Fig. 42-15), is required for the dependence of late origin firing on completion of early replication. This role during the normal S phase could explain why ATR is essential for the life of the cell.

Synthesis of the Histone Proteins

Chromatin contains approximately equal weights of DNA and core histones. Human cells require about 62×10^6 copies of each core histone, assuming a genome size of 6.2×10^9 bp and 200 bp per nucleosome. Because about 90% of histone transcription occurs during the S phase, enormous amounts of these proteins are made during a relatively brief period. Histone synthesis apparently keeps pace, in part, because there are about 40 sets of histone genes.

Synthesis of histones during the S phase is tightly coupled to ongoing DNA replication. If replication is blocked either by addition of drugs or by temperature-sensitive mutants, histone synthesis declines abruptly shortly thereafter. This link between histone synthesis and DNA replication appears to involve at least three components (Fig. 42-16).

First, *transcription of the histone genes rises* three-fold to fivefold as cells enter the S phase. Each histone gene has a cell-cycle-responsive element in its promoter to which a transcription factor binds specifically during the S phase.

Second, the *processing of histone mRNAs increases* sixfold to 10-fold as cells enter the S phase. Histone mRNAs are not polyadenylated, and the primary transcripts are considerably longer than the mature forms.

Processing of the 3′ end of histone pre-mRNAs involves the U7 snRNP (see Chapter 16), a portion of which recognizes histone mRNA and base-pairs with it during processing. Cell-cycle-dependent regulation of processing appears to involve changes in the accessibility of the necessary portion of U7 snRNA. This region is inaccessible in G_0 cells but becomes accessible when cells that have reentered the cycle begin the S phase. The mechanism for this change in RNA conformation is not known.

Third, *changes in the stability of the mRNA* also regulate histone synthesis. Normally, the level of histone mRNA on free polysomes drops rapidly by about 35-fold as cells enter the G_2 phase. If DNA synthesis is interrupted during the S phase, a region at the 3′ end of the mature message somehow targets the mRNA for degradation. If this region is removed from the 3′ terminus of the histone mRNA, the normal link between ongoing replication and mRNA stability is lost. Furthermore, this sequence, transposed onto the 3′ terminus of a globin mRNA, renders that mRNA sensitive to degradation if DNA synthesis is blocked. Degradation of histone mRNA requires ongoing protein synthesis, and it has been speculated that histones themselves participate in the control.

As discussed in Chapter 13, specialized variant forms of histones are synthesized and inserted into the chromatin outside of the S phase. These histones are encoded by mRNAs with introns and normal poly(A) tails and are therefore not processed by the specific S phase–associated pathway (see Chapter 16). Their insertion into chromatin is typically correlated with RNA transcription rather than DNA replication.

Other Events of the S Phase

Although the bulk of attention on the S phase focuses on the duplication of the chromosomes, at least one other essential function required for stability of the genome also occurs at this time. This is duplication of the centrosomes, which will go on at the next mitosis

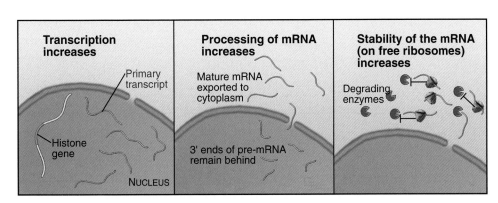

Transcription increases

Primary transcript

Histone gene

NUCLEUS

Processing of mRNA increases

Mature mRNA exported to cytoplasm

3′ ends of pre-mRNA remain behind

Stability of the mRNA (on free ribosomes) increases

Degrading enzymes

Figure 42-16 THREE WAYS IN WHICH HISTONE EXPRESSION IS ELEVATED DURING THE S PHASE.

to set up the poles of the mitotic spindle that are responsible for accurate partitioning of the replicated chromosomes. (See Chapter 34 for a discussion of centrosome duplication.)

With the completion of DNA replication and duplication of the centrosomes, the cell is ready to divide. As the levels of Cdk activity rise toward the threshold that is sufficient to trigger mitotic entry and other factors necessary for mitosis accumulate, the cell continues to screen the integrity of the DNA to ensure that the genome has been replicated correctly and that no harmful DNA damage has occurred in the interim. These checks, together with other ongoing preparations for mitosis, are the principal events of the G_2 phase (see Chapter 43).

ACKNOWLEDGMENT

Thanks go to Julian Blow for suggestions on revisions to this chapter.

SELECTED READINGS

Baker TA, Wickner SH: Genetics and enzymology of DNA replication in Escherichia coli. Annu Rev Genet 26:447-477, 1992.

Bartek J, Lukas C, Lukas J: Checking on DNA damage in S phase. Nat Rev Mol Cell Biol 5:792-804, 2004.

Bell SP, Dutta A: DNA replication in eukaryotic cells. Annu Rev Biochem 71:333-374, 2002.

Diffley JF: Regulation of early events in chromosome replication. Curr Biol 14:R778-R786, 2004.

Gilbert DM: In search of the holy replicator. Nat Rev Mol Cell Biol 5:848-855, 2004.

Hübscher U, Maga G, Spadari S: Eukaryotic DNA polymerases. Annu Rev Biochem 71:133-163, 2002.

Jónsson ZO, Hübscher U: Proliferating cell nuclear antigen: More than a clamp for DNA polymerases. BioEssays 19:967-975, 1997.

Kearsey SE, Cotterill S: Enigmatic variations: Divergent modes of regulating eukaryotic DNA replication. Mol Cell 12:1067-1075, 2003.

Kearsey SE, Maiorano D, Holmes EC, Todorov IT: The role of MCM proteins in the cell cycle control of genome duplication. BioEssays 18:183-190, 1996.

Reed SI: Ratchets and clocks: The cell cycle, ubiquitylation and protein turnover. Nat Rev Mol Cell Biol 4:855-864, 2003.

Stillman B: Cell cycle control of DNA replication. Science 274:1659-1664, 1996.

Waga S, Stillman B: The DNA replication fork in eukaryotic cells. Annu Rev Biochem 67:721-751, 1998.

CHAPTER 43

G_2 Phase and Control of Entry into Mitosis

The G_2 phase was originally defined simply as a gap between the completion of DNA replication and the onset of mitosis. In fact, definition of this phase is not entirely straightforward, as progression from interphase into mitosis is gradual, with early mitotic prophase sharing characteristics of both interphase and mitosis. Here, we define the G_2 phase as the period from the end of the S phase until mid-prophase, that is, until activation of the main mitotic kinase, Cdk1–cyclin B1.

This chapter begins with the biochemical basis for the G_2/mitosis (M) transition and discusses how the G_2 checkpoint delays this transition if DNA damage is detected. Finally, the chapter introduces the major pathways that cells use to attempt to repair damaged DNA.

Enzymology of the G_2/Mitosis Transition

The transition between the G_2 phase and mitosis is the most profound morphologic and physiological change that occurs during the life of a growing cell, matched only by the dramatic changes that occur during death by apoptosis (see Chapter 46). Entry into mitosis is controlled by a network of stimulatory and inhibitory protein kinases and phosphatases, presided over by Cdk1–cyclin B1. (Chapter 40 introduced the components involved in the G_2/M transition.)

Cdk1, the driving force for entry into mitosis, is present at a constant level throughout the cell cycle. Cdk1 regulation is multifaceted (see Fig. 40-14), including binding of cyclin cofactors, inhibition and activation by phosphorylation, binding of inhibitory molecules, and changes in subcellular localization.

Mammalian cells have at least three **B-type cyclins:** B1, B2, and B3. Cyclin B1 is essential for triggering the G_2/M transition, and disruption of its gene has lethal consequences. Cyclin B1, newly synthesized during the latter part of the cell cycle, binds Cdk1 and shuttles it in and out of the nucleus. Importin β carries the Cdk1–cyclin B1 complex into the nucleus, and then Crm1 rapidly exports it back to the cytoplasm (see Chapter 16). Cdk1–cyclin B2 associates with the Golgi apparatus during interphase and might function in Golgi disassembly during mitosis (see Fig. 44-4). Cyclin B3 appears to function only during meiosis in mammals.

As cells approach the G_2/M transition, a combination of one stimulatory and two inhibitory kinases control activation of Cdk1–cyclin B1. The activating kinase, called

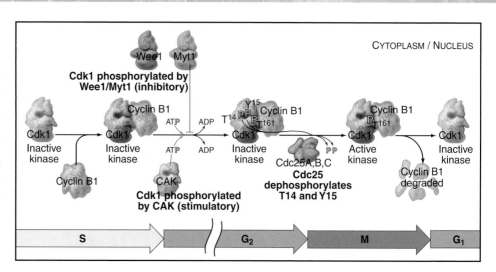

Figure 43-1 Regulation of Cdk1 by cyclin binding and protein phosphorylation from the late S phase through mid-mitosis. (Structure for Wee1 kinase provided by E. N. Baker prior to release to the Protein Data Bank; based on Squire CJ, Dickson JM, Ivanovic I, Baker EN: Structure of human Wee1A kinase: Kinase domain complexed with inhibitor PD0407824. Structure 13:541–550, 2005. PDB file: 1X8B.)

CAK (Cdk-activating kinase; actually Cdk7–cyclin H), is located in the nucleus. CAK phosphorylates Cdk1 on T^{161}, allowing the refolding of the active site cleft that is required for the enzyme to bind substrates (see Chapter 40). Two other kinases, Wee1 and Myt1, counteract the action of CAK (Fig. 43-1). Wee1 is localized to the nucleus, where it inhibits Cdk1 by phosphorylating Y^{15} adjacent to the ATP-binding site. The role of Wee1 as a mitotic inhibitor is clearly demonstrated in *S. pombe*: Overexpression of functional Wee1 delays or prevents the entry of cells into mitosis (Fig. 43-2). Myt1 associated with the Golgi apparatus and endoplasmic reticulum inhibits Cdk1 while it resides in the cytoplasm by phosphorylating T^{14} and Y^{15}. Together, Wee1 and Myt1 ensure that Cdk1 remains inactive as it shuttles into and out of the nucleus (Fig. 43-3). This combination of stimulatory and inhibitory modifications holds Cdk1–cyclin B1 poised for a burst of activation.

The three Cdc25 protein phosphatases remove the inhibitory phosphates from Cdk1–cyclin B1 and trigger the G2/M transition. Cdc25s are dual-specificity protein phosphatases (see Fig. 25-5) that remove phosphates from serine (S), threonine (T), and tyrosine (Y) residues, including the inhibitory phosphates from T^{14} and Y^{15} of Cdk1. Cdc25s are regulated by stimulatory and inhibitory phosphorylation, by alterations in their subcellular localization, and by ubiquitin-mediated proteolysis. Cdc25A, the only one of the three to be indispensable for life, functions at both the G1/S and G2/M transitions, whereas Cdc25B and Cdc25C have roles in the G2/M transition. The preferred targets of the individual Cdc25 isoforms are not known.

Cdc25A and Cdc25C are relatively inactive during interphase for three reasons (Fig. 43-4). First, phosphorylation on a serine residue creates a binding site for a member of the 14-3-3 group of adapter proteins (see Fig. 25-10). These proteins bind sites on target proteins containing serines flanked by several other characteristic amino acids, but only when the critical serine is phosphorylated. This is an example of the general mechanism whereby phosphorylation regu-

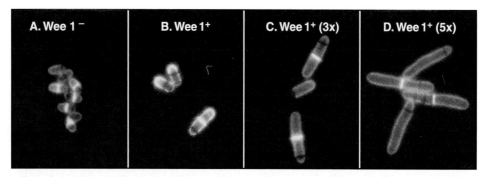

Figure 43-2 The effect of changing cellular levels of Wee1 protein on cell-cycle progression in fission yeast. **A,** Cells that lack functional Wee1 protein enter mitosis too soon in the cell cycle and are smaller than wild-type cells **(B). C–D,** Cells that express excess Wee1 protein are too effective at inactivating Cdk1 and are severely delayed in their ability to enter mitosis (hence their larger size). (From Russell P, Nurse P: Negative regulation of mitosis by Wee1+, a gene encoding a protein kinase homolog. Cell 49:559–567, 1987.)

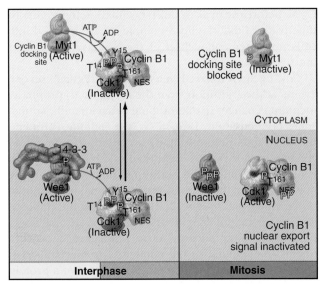

Figure 43-3 Summary of the patterns of Myt1 and Wee1 phosphorylation of Cdk1 in the cytoplasm and nucleus in interphase and mitosis. NES, nuclear export sequence. (Based on an original figure by Helen Piwnica-Worms. 14-3-3 protein, PDB file: 1YWT.)

mitosis. Whether this same mechanism operates in mitotic cells is not known.

Since Cdk1–cyclin B1 is inactive unless activated by a Cdc25 phosphatase, a molecular trigger is required to start the amplification cycle. Members of the **Polo family of protein kinases** are candidates for this role, by activating Cdc25. These kinases and their substrates share amino acid motifs called "polo boxes," which bind to other polo boxes after they have been phosphorylated. Polo kinases recognize certain substrates only after they have been "primed" by phosphorylation by another kinase. This allows for additional levels of control and rapid amplification of the phosphorylation response. Polo family kinases are involved in a variety of mitotic events, including formation of a bipolar spindle, cytokinesis, and passage through certain cell-cycle checkpoints. They reside at the centrosome during interphase and phosphorylate a number of centrosomal proteins in addition to Cdc25.

Changes in Subcellular Localization at the G₂/M Transition

Cyclin B1 (with associated Cdk1) and Cdc25C have both nuclear import and nuclear export signals, so they shuttle in and out of the nucleus throughout interphase (Fig. 43-5). Cdc25A resides in the nucleus. During interphase, Cdk1–cyclin B1 and Cdc25C spend most of their time in the cytoplasm. Inhibitory phosphorylation of Cdk1 and Cdc25C keeps Cdk1 activity low.

Early in prophase, phosphorylation of cyclin B1 inactivates its nuclear export signal and promotes its nuclear import (see Chapter 16), allowing Cdk1–cyclin B1 to accumulate rapidly in the nucleus within five minutes (Figs. 43-3 and 43-6). Cdc25C also stops shuttling at the G₂/M transition, probably as a result of phosphorylation by Polo kinase. The best evidence seems to indicate that the Cdk1–cyclin B that accumulates in the nucleus

lates interactions between proteins in response to physiological signals (see Chapter 25). Association of 14-3-3 with Cdc25A interferes with its binding to Cdk1–cyclin B1 and inhibits its import into the nucleus. Because Cdc25C has an intrinsic nuclear export sequence, the 14-3-3-bound form of Cdc25C is primarily cytoplasmic.

Second, phosphorylation at other sites targets Cdc25A for ubiquitination by SCF^{βTrCP} and destruction by proteasomes. Third, full activation of Cdc25s requires phosphorylation of their amino-terminal region. In meiotic cells, phosphorylation of this site is initiated by a protein kinase called Polo (see next paragraph) and then completed by the Cdc25 substrate, Cdk1–cyclin B1, creating a powerful positive feedback amplification loop that provides a burst of Cdk activity and triggers entry into

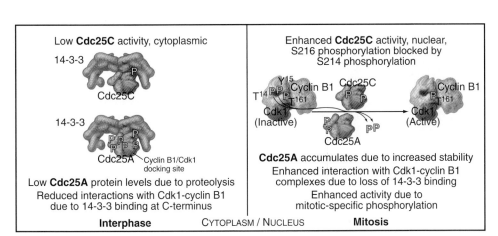

Figure 43-4 Regulation of Cdc25A and Cdc25C activity in interphase and mitosis. (Based on an original figure by Helen Piwnica-Worms.)

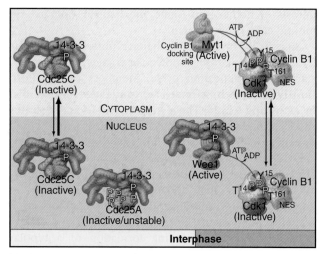

Figure 43-5 Shuttling of components between the nucleus and cytoplasm contributes to the regulation of Cdk1–cyclin B1 during interphase. (Based on an original figure by Helen Piwnica-Worms.)

is already active, but restriction of Cdk–cyclin B complexes to the nucleus together with Cdc25A and Cdc25C significantly increases their local concentration (the volume of the nucleus is much less than the volume of the cytoplasm) and might contribute to the final burst of Cdk1–cyclin B1 activation.

Cdk1–Cyclin A and the Initiation of Prophase

As is noted in Chapter 42, Cdk2–cyclin A plays a critical role during the S phase. Several lines of evidence have revealed that a Cdk–cyclin A complex also helps to trigger the G_2/M transition. First, inactivation of cyclin A, either by mutation in *Drosophila* or by injection of anti–cyclin A antibodies into cultured cells, arrests the cell cycle in G_2. Second, Cdk–cyclin A activity peaks at

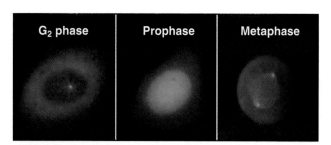

Figure 43-6 Rapid movement of cyclin B1 from the cytoplasm into the nucleus at the onset of prophase and subsequent association with the spindle during mitosis. (Courtesy of Christina Karlsson and Jonathon Pines, Wellcome/CRC Institute, Cambridge, England.)

G_2/M, before the peak of Cdk1–cyclin B1 activity. Finally, if activated Cdk2–cyclin A complexes are injected into cells just after completion of the S phase, cells enter mitosis prematurely.

Cdk–cyclin A kinase is most likely to regulate several events at the transition from the G_2 phase to prophase, including changes in microtubule behavior and chromosome condensation. Late in G_2, the half-life of microtubules drops dramatically from about 10 minutes to about 30 seconds (see Table 44-1). This, coupled with centrosomes' enhanced ability to initiate microtubule polymerization, completely transforms the organization of the microtubule cytoskeleton. Centrosomes take on the appearance of spindle poles and migrate apart over the surface of the nucleus. At the same time, chromatin begins to condense in the nucleus. The mechanism of chromosome condensation is not known, but a protein complex called condensin is required for this condensation to begin during prophase (see Fig. 13-19). Condensin does not associate tightly with chromosomes during interphase; association with chromosomes requires phosphorylation of two of its subunits by a Cdk. This occurs at G_2/M. As chromosomes condense, several mitosis-specific kinetochore proteins also move into the nucleus and associate with kinetochores (see Chapter 13).

These events occur while most Cdk1–cyclin B1 is in the cytoplasm. It is most likely, therefore, that Cdk1–cyclin A triggers at least the nuclear events of prophase (Fig. 43-7). In fact, microinjection of a specific inhibitor of Cdk1–cyclin A causes prophase cells to return rapidly to interphase; chromosomes decondense, rounded prophase cells flatten, and the interphase microtubule network returns. Commitment to mitosis appears to be irreversible only after Cdk1–cyclin B1 enters the nucleus.

Summary of the Main Events of the G_2/M Transition

Synthesis of cyclin B1 in the latter portion of the S and G_2 phases leads to assembly of Cdk1–cyclin B heterodimers that shuttle into and out of the nucleus, spending most of their time in the cytoplasm associated with microtubules. In the late S and G_2 phases, activation of Cdk1–cyclin A initiates mitotic prophase, beginning with changes in microtubule dynamics and chromosome condensation. Several events trigger entry into the active phase of mitosis. Cdc25A becomes stabilized and no longer binds 14-3-3 proteins. This results in the accumulation of Cdc25A and allows more efficient interactions between Cdc25A and Cdk1–cyclin B. The phosphate-binding site for 14-3-3 proteins on Cdc25C becomes dephosphorylated, allowing it to accumulate

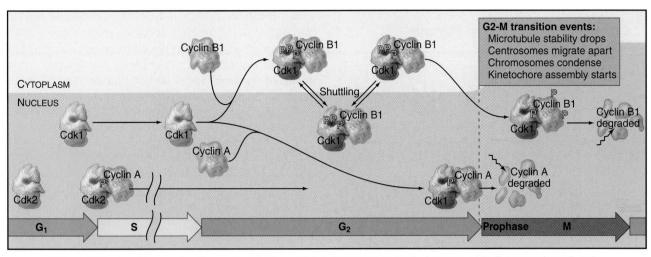

Figure 43-7 Locations and patterns of activation of Cdk1 complexed to cyclin A versus cyclin B across the cell cycle.

in the nucleus. In addition, phosphorylation of cyclin B1 blocks its export from the nucleus and promotes its import, thus causing Cdk1-cyclin B1 to accumulate rapidly in the nucleus. The inhibitory kinase Wee1 is also dephosphorylated, and its activity drops. Cdc25A and Cdc25C activate Cdk1-cyclin B1 by removing inhibitory phosphates on T^{14} and Y^{15}. This starts in the cytoplasm and then may be stimulated as the proteins concentrate in the nucleus. There, the action of Cdk1–cyclin B1 on the nuclear lamina triggers nuclear envelope breakdown and drives the cell into mitosis. Fig. 43-8 summarizes the network regulating Cdk1–cyclin B activation.

Why did such an elaborate system evolve to regulate the G₂/M transition? The answer appears to lie in the

exquisite sensitivity provided by the interlocking network of stimulatory and inhibitory activities. On the one hand, this network ensures a rapid, almost explosive, final transition into mitosis. On the other, it provides a number of ways to delay the G₂/M transition if the cell detects damage to chromosomes. Mitosis with chromosomal damage can lead to cell death or cancer.

The G₂ Checkpoint

Separation of sister chromatids during mitosis is a potential danger point for a cell. If DNA is damaged after it is replicated, the cell can use information present in sister chromatids (which have one good copy and one bad copy) to guide the repair process. However, once sisters separate, such a corrective mechanism is impossible. In addition, if a cell enters mitosis before completing replication of its chromosomes, the attempt to separate sister chromatids causes extensive chromosomal damage. To minimize these hazards, a checkpoint operates in the G₂ phase to block mitotic entry if DNA is damaged or DNA replication is incomplete.

Exposure of cells to agents that damage DNA, including certain chemicals or ionizing radiation, halts the cell cycle temporarily in the G₂ phase. This **G₂ delay** gives cells an opportunity to repair damaged DNA before entering mitosis. Studies of radiation induced G₂ delay in budding yeast identified a major cell-cycle checkpoint in G₂ sensitive to the status of the cellular DNA. Cells that are defective in this checkpoint are much more sensitive to radiation injury than are wild-type cells because they continue to divide, despite the

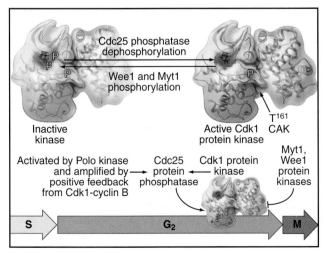

Figure 43-8 Summary of the Cdk1 feedback regulation mechanism at the G₂/M transition.

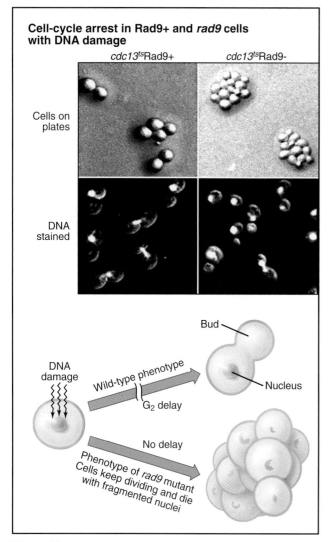

Cell-cycle arrest in Rad9+ and *rad9* cells with DNA damage

cdc13^{ts}Rad9+   cdc13^{ts}Rad9-

Cells on plates

DNA stained

Bud

Nucleus

DNA damage

Wild-type phenotype

G$_2$ delay

No delay

Phenotype of *rad9* mutant
Cells keep dividing and die with fragmented nuclei

Figure 43-9 MUTATION OF GENES REQUIRED FOR THE G$_2$ CHECKPOINT. Cells that are defective in the G$_2$ checkpoint (*Rad9* mutants of budding yeast) cannot delay their entry into mitosis in the presence of damaged DNA and therefore divide themselves to death. Rad-9 is a component of the PCNA-like 9-1-1 damage sensor complex. (Courtesy of Ted Weinert, University of Arizona, Tucson.)

cyclin B kinase, which is high in mitosis and low in interphase. In the absence of nuclei, an inhibitor of DNA polymerases (such as the fungal toxin aphidicolin) has no effect on such extracts, which continue to cycle unabated between the S and M phases. On the other hand, if the extract contains more than 400 nuclei/μL undergoing synchronous cycles of DNA replication and

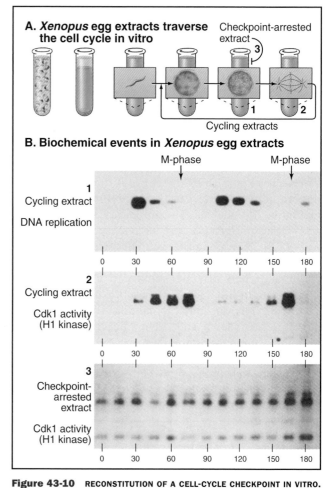

A. *Xenopus* egg extracts traverse the cell cycle in vitro   Checkpoint-arrested extract

Cycling extracts

B. Biochemical events in *Xenopus* egg extracts

M-phase   M-phase

1 Cycling extract DNA replication

0   30   60   90   120   150   180

2 Cycling extract Cdk1 activity (H1 kinase)

0   30   60   90   120   150   180

3 Checkpoint-arrested extract Cdk1 activity (H1 kinase)

0   30   60   90   120   150   180

Figure 43-10 RECONSTITUTION OF A CELL-CYCLE CHECKPOINT IN VITRO. **A,** Cell-cycle transitions in a cell-free extract. **B,** Panel 1: DNA replication was measured by adding ^{32}P-labeled dCTP to the extract and subsequently isolating the DNA, running it in a gel, and detecting incorporation of the radioactive label by autoradiography. *Panel 2:* Cdk1–cyclin B activity was assayed on the basis of the ability of active enzyme to phosphorylate added histone H1 (which was similarly subjected to gel electrophoresis and autoradiography). These panels show that DNA replication and Cdk activity alternate in these in vitro cell cycles. Cdk activity declines precipitously at the end of mitosis. *Panel 3:* If the concentration of nuclei is increased beyond a threshold level and an inhibitor of DNA replication is added, the G$_2$ checkpoint detects the partly replicated DNA and stops the extract from entering mitosis. Cdk activity now remains at about 10% of the level needed to trigger mitosis. (B, Redrawn from Dasso M, Newport JW: Completion of DNA replication is monitored by a feedback system that controls the initiation of mitosis in vitro: Studies in *Xenopus*. Cell 61:811–823, 1990.)

presence of broken or otherwise damaged chromosomes (Fig. 43-9). This continued division in the face of DNA damage leads to cell death, presumably due to accumulated chromosomal defects, as well as chromosome loss.

The G$_2$ checkpoint also monitors the completion of DNA replication. Remarkably, this aspect of the checkpoint even works in vitro in cell-free extracts. As is described in Box 40-3, highly concentrated extracts made from *Xenopus* eggs can be induced to undergo a cyclic alteration in cell-cycle phases, even in the absence of added nuclei. Passage through the different phases can be followed by monitoring the activity of Cdk1–

mitosis, aphidicolin brings the cycling to a halt before M phase. This experiment appears to reconstitute the G₂ checkpoint in vitro (Fig. 43-10). Furthermore, it reveals that partly replicated nuclei release an inhibitory signal that stops the cycle.

The G₂ Checkpoint and Cancer

Defects in the G₂ checkpoint are associated with cancer, since failure to correct damage to tumor suppressor genes can compromise the G₁ checkpoint in subsequent cell cycles. For example, suppose that radiation damages a nucleotide base in the gene for the retinoblastoma susceptibility protein (Rb; see Fig. 41-10). If this happens in the S or G₂ phase, information in the undamaged copy of the gene can be used to repair the damage. Delaying the cell cycle increases the chance of successful repair. On the other hand, if the checkpoint fails and the cell enters mitosis, sister chromatids separate from one another, and the damage is never repaired. As a consequence, one daughter cell from that division has a defective pRb gene, impairing its ability to regulate its growth at the restriction point in the next G₁ phase. Loss of tumor suppressor genes such as pRb and p53 is a major cause of cancer (see Chapter 41).

The G₂ checkpoint minimizes this problem by detecting DNA damage and either delaying entry into mitosis

until the damage is fixed or triggering cell suicide by apoptosis. The checkpoint works by modulating the activities of the components that control the G₂/M transition.

How the G₂ Checkpoint Works

The minimal machinery of a DNA damage checkpoint (see Fig. 40-4) involves **sensors** that detect DNA damage, **transducers** (usually protein kinases) that produce a biochemical signal as a result of the detected damage, and **effectors** (both protein kinases and transcriptional activators) that either directly or indirectly block cell-cycle progression. The sensors are not yet as well characterized as are the transducers and effectors. This section discusses this machinery as a prelude to consideration in Box 43-1 of the mechanisms that repair damaged DNA.

The sensors that detect DNA damage have not yet been entirely characterized (Fig. 43-11). The two apical kinases ATM and ATR (see Fig. 40-4) are mobilized quickly to the sites of DNA damage. However, ATM is activated before it gets to the DNA, and the identity of the earliest sensor of DNA damage remains unclear. The 9-1-1 protein complex (described later) and the enzymes that are involved in processing damaged DNA are also possible sensors of the DNA damage.

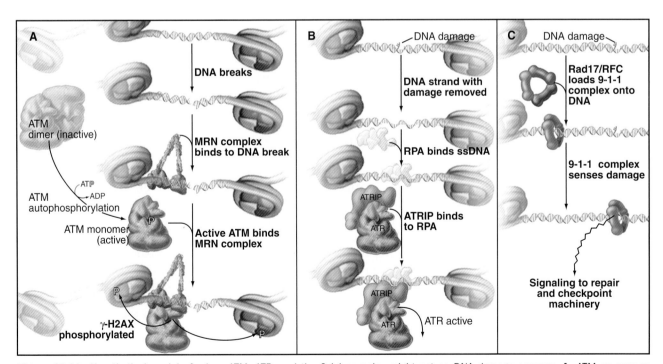

Figure 43-11 Hypothetical models for how ATM, ATR, and the 9-1-1 complex might act as DNA damage sensors. **A,** ATM as sensor. **B,** ATR as sensor. **C,** The 9-1-1 complex as sensor.

Table 43-1

KEY DNA REPAIR GENE DEFECTS ASSOCIATED WITH HUMAN DISEASE

Human Disease	Pathway	Genes Defective*
Ataxia-telangiectasia (AT)	Checkpoint	ATM
Seckel syndrome	Checkpoint	*ATR*
Xeroderma pigmentosum	NER	*XP-A, XP-B, XP-C, XP-D, DDB-2, XP-F, XP-G, POLH*
Cockayne syndrome	NER	*XP-B, XP-D, CSA, CSB*
Trichothiodystrophy	NER	*XP-D*
Hereditary nonpolyposis colon cancer	MMR	*MSH2, PMS2, MLH1*
AT-like disorder	DSB repair	*MRE11*
Nijmegen breakage syndrome	DSB repair	*NBS1*
Breast cancer predisposition	HR	*BRCA1, BRCA2*
LIG4 syndrome	NHEJ	*LIGIV*
Severe combined immune deficiency	NHEJ	*ARTEMIS*

*This list is an outline. For an updated list of the approximately 130 human DNA repair genes known to date, the reader is referred to http://www.cgal.icnet.uk/DNA_Repair_Genes.html#refs.

NER, nucleotide excision repair; MMR, mismatch repair; DSB, double-strand break; HR, homologous recombination; NHEJ, nonhomologous end joining.

Two kinases, ATM and ATR (see Fig. 40-4), are key transducers of the DNA damage response. ATM responds to DNA damage any time during the cell cycle, but ATR appears to respond only if DNA is damaged prior to the completion of replication. Thus, ATM is essential for the G_2 DNA damage checkpoint to arrest the cell cycle when DNA damage occurs after replication is complete.

The activation of ATM involves autophosphorylation, which causes inactive dimers to dissociate into active monomers. Subsequently the Nbs1 subunit of the MRN complex (Fig. 43-11A; see also Fig. 12-13) recruits ATM monomers to the DNA break and initiates the full-blown checkpoint response. The MRN complex has a key role in repair of double-strand breaks in DNA. The Nbs1 gene is mutated in humans with Nijmegen breakage syndrome (Table 43-1).

ATR exists in cells in a constitutive complex with a second subunit, ATR-interacting protein (ATRIP). ATRIP binds to the single-strand DNA binding protein RPA, an essential component of the DNA replication fork (Fig. 43-11B). DNA damage often results directly or indirectly in the presence of single-stranded DNA, which can be produced by the damaging event itself or as a by-product of the DNA repair process. This single-stranded DNA binds RPA and then, through the action of ATRIP, recruits and activates ATR.

Interestingly, the interactions of ATR with ATRIP and ATM with NBS1 both involve short peptide sequences at the very C-terminus of ATRIP and NBS1. These are the only features that NBS1 and ATRIP have in common. Somehow, this binding may alter the structures of the ATM and ATR in a way that turns on the checkpoint response. Since the kinases are already activated prior to recruitment to the sites of DNA damage, activation of the checkpoint response may require additional functions, such as acquiring selectivity for certain key substrates.

ATR depends on two other protein complexes to mount a checkpoint response. One is the trimeric **9-1-1 complex,** which gets its name from its subunits Rad9, Hus1, and Rad1 (Fig. 43-11C). The 9-1-1 complex resembles proliferating cell nuclear antigen (PCNA), the doughnut-shaped processivity factor that is indispensable during DNA replication (see Fig. 42-11). PCNA is loaded onto DNA by the pentameric replication factor C (RFC) ATPase during DNA replication and anchors DNA polymerases and other factors to DNA. A similar enzyme composed of one special subunit, Rad17, plus the four small subunits of RFC is believed to load the 9-1-1 complex onto DNA at or near sites of damage. This speculation is supported by the observation that mutants in four of the RFC subunits are defective in G_2 checkpoint control in yeasts and *Drosophila*.

The role of the 9-1-1 complex is not certain. It could be involved in recognition of damage as it slides along the DNA; it could act as a sliding clamp tethering specialized polymerases that repair the damaged DNA; or it could act as a mobile landing pad for other factors involved in processing damaged DNA.

When DNA damage activates ATM and ATR, they phosphorylate several important substrates, including the **tumor suppressor protein p53,** and two protein **checkpoint kinases** called **Chk1** and **Chk2.** When activated by phosphorylation, Chk1 phosphorylates

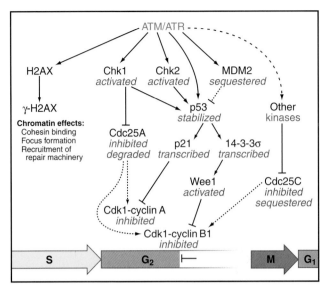

Figure 43-12 HOW THE G₂ CHECKPOINT BLOCKS THE G₂ → M TRANSITION FOLLOWING ACTIVATION OF ATM AND/OR ATR BY DNA DAMAGE. *Dotted lines* show activities that are switched off by the checkpoint. The *dashed line* between ATM/ATR and the kinase that inhibits Cdc25C indicates that this pathway is not yet known. (Based on an original figure by Helen Piwnica-Worms.)

the Cdc25A protein phosphatase (Fig. 43-12). This has at least two consequences. First, it produces binding sites for a 14-3-3 protein, which blocks Cdc25A from activating Cdk1–cyclin B. Second, phosphorylation by Chk1 targets Cdc25A for ubiquitin-mediated proteolysis. This ensures that levels of Cdc25A remain low. In addition, activation of the G₂ checkpoint maintains Cdc25C in a 14-3-3-bound form. This prevents Cdc25C from accumulating in the nucleus and from activating Cdk1–cyclin B as it shuttles in and out of the nucleus.

The transcription factor p53 is phosphorylated and activated by the ATM/ATR kinases following DNA damage. Activated p53 then drives the expression of a number of G₂ checkpoint genes. Although p53 is not required to arrest the cell cycle in G₂ phase in response to DNA damage, it is required to prolong this cell-cycle arrest. p53 stimulates the expression of the **Cdk inhibitor p21,** which inhibits Cdk1–cyclin A 100-fold better than it inhibits Cdk1–cyclin B1. p21 expression thus provides an effective way of blocking the initiation of prophase by Cdk1–cyclin A. p21 also participates in the G₁ DNA damage checkpoint.

p53 also drives the expression of 14-3-3σ, an adapter protein that may interfere with shuttling of Cdk1–cyclin B1 between the nucleus and cytoplasm. Binding of 14-3-3σ maintains the Wee1 inhibitory kinase in a *more* active state, ensuring that the Cdk1–cyclin B1 complex remains inactive. Disruption of the gene for 14-3-3σ is fatal for cells if they sustain DNA damage. Instead of

activating their G₂ checkpoint, they enter an aberrant state with characteristics of both mitosis and apoptosis, and then die.

Another substrate of ATM and ATR is the **specialized histone isoform H2AX.** H2AX phosphorylated by ATM and/or ATR is known as γ-**H2AX.** γ-H2AX spreads rapidly across sites of DNA damage, called "foci." These γ-H2AX foci recruit key proteins for signaling, DNA repair machinery, and the cohesin complex, which holds replicated sister chromatids together (see Fig. 13-19). In the case of double-strand DNA breaks, a particularly dangerous form of DNA damage, the unbroken sister chromatid provides a template to ensure that the break is repaired correctly.

ATM and ATR signaling often involves proteins known as **adapters** (also called mediators). The best-known ATR adapter is a protein called **claspin,** a normal component of replication forks, which is conserved between yeasts and humans. ATR phosphorylates claspin, which recruits Chk1 to stalled replication forks for phosphorylation by ATR. This amplifies the checkpoint response.

Phosphorylation of the ATM adapter, 53BP1, recruits Chk2 to sites of damage where it can be activated by ATM. BRCA1 is another adapter that functions in DNA repair. BRCA1 is of interest because its gene is mutated in 90% of cases of inherited familial breast and ovarian cancer. Both 53BP1 and BRCA1 have protein motifs called BRCT domains that recognize and bind to specific phosphorylated sequences on target proteins. BRCT motifs may recruit proteins to γ-H2AX foci by binding to the phosphorylated histone.

Ideally, checkpoint activation has one of two outcomes. If DNA damage is so extensive that it cannot be repaired, the cell commits suicide by a pathway called apoptosis (see Chapter 46). Less serious damage can be repaired by one of the systems described in Box 43-1.

Transition to Mitosis

The complex web of stimulatory and inhibitory activities that regulates Cdk activity in the G₂ phase enables exquisite control of the G₂/M transition. On the one hand, it poises Cdk1–cyclin B in a state in which it is ready for the explosive burst of activation that triggers the G₂/M transition. At the same time, the complex pathways afford many points where the process may be regulated. These are the basis of the G₂ checkpoint control that prevents cells from segregating their chromosomes if genomic DNA cannot meet stringent quality control standards. Eventually, however, if all goes well, Cdk1–cyclin A and Cdk1–cyclin B1 are activated, and the cell embarks on mitosis, probably the most dramatic event of its life.

BOX 43-1
DNA Repair in Vertebrates

BY CIARAN MORRISON (NATIONAL UNIVERSITY
OF IRELAND, GALWAY)

Every human cell experiences about 10^5 DNA damage events each day. Cell division must not occur with inaccurately replicated or damaged genomes, as this may cause cell death or heritable mutation. A number of systems have evolved to repair damaged DNA (Fig. 43-13). Their activities depend on the particular form of DNA damage sustained by the cell. These repair mechanisms also act in concert with the apoptotic machinery to ensure that if the DNA damage cannot be repaired, the cell will die (see Chapter 46). DNA damage checkpoints are a critical component of the cellular response to DNA damage (see Fig. 40-4), as they impose a delay in the cell cycle during which cells have a chance to repair their genomes.

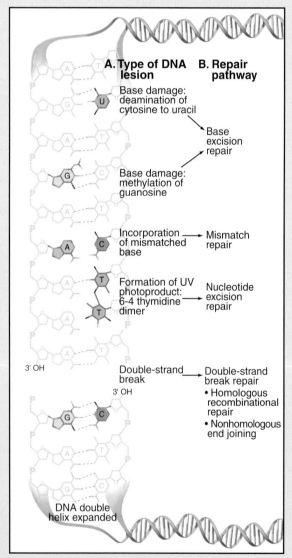

Figure 43-13 EXAMPLES OF DNA DAMAGE AND THE REPAIR PATHWAYS THAT RESPOND TO DIFFERENT TYPES OF LESION.

Base Excision Repair

Bases in DNA can become oxidized, reduced, alkylated, or deaminated owing to endogenous activities or environmental stress. Damaged bases are cut away from the DNA sugar-phosphate backbone by a damage-recognizing **glycosylase,** leaving an abasic site (Fig. 43-14A). **Abasic sites,** which also can be generated directly by DNA damage, are then removed by cleavage of the sugar-phosphate backbone mediated by certain glycosylases and endonucleases. The missing sequence is then reconstructed from its complementary strand by DNA polymerase β, with DNA ligase III-Xrcc1 completing the repair by sealing the gaps in the backbone.

Nucleotide Excision Repair

Bulky DNA adducts caused by chemical agents or environmental stress (particularly ultraviolet radiation from sunlight) are excised by a complex, though well-understood, reaction (Fig. 43-14B). Defects in nucleotide excision repair genes cause the human genetic disease **xeroderma pigmentosum** (XP), which is characterized by hypersensitivity to sunlight and predisposition to skin cancer. Eight proteins encoded by genes mutated in xeroderma pigmentosum (Table 43-1) take part in nucleotide excision repair, providing one of the best examples in which human genetics has helped to unravel a complicated biological process. **Recognition** of the DNA lesion involves the heterotrimeric replication protein RPA, XPA, and XPC and the nine-subunit transcription factor TFIIH, which contains XPB and XPD. ATP-dependent unwinding of the DNA by XPB and XPD forms a **preincision complex.** XPG, which replaces XPC in the complex, makes an **incision** six to nine bases 3′ of the damaged base, and XPF-Ercc1 cuts 20 to 25 bases 5′ of the damage site. This releases a short single-stranded DNA fragment containing the damaged DNA. After excision, DNA polymerases δ or ε fills in the gap by copying the undamaged strand. Prokaryotes have a similar system of adduct recognition, removal, and repair involving the UvrA, UvrB, and UvrC proteins; however, the enzymes that are involved are not conserved between kingdoms, an unusual occurrence for DNA repair systems.

Mismatch Repair

Errors in DNA replication that have not been detected by the proofreading activity of the DNA polymerase are recognized by a dimer consisting of the MSH2/ MSH6 proteins. When a mismatch is detected, this heterodimer undergoes an ATP-dependent transition to a **sliding clamp** and recruits a second heterodimer, consisting of MLH1 and PMS2 (Fig. 43-14C). To distinguish between the original ("correct") sequence and the newly synthesized DNA strand, this sliding clamp complex can then translocate along the DNA until a break is reached, such as that found between Okazaki fragments. The broken strand is there-

BOX 43-1
DNA Repair in Vertebrates—cont'd

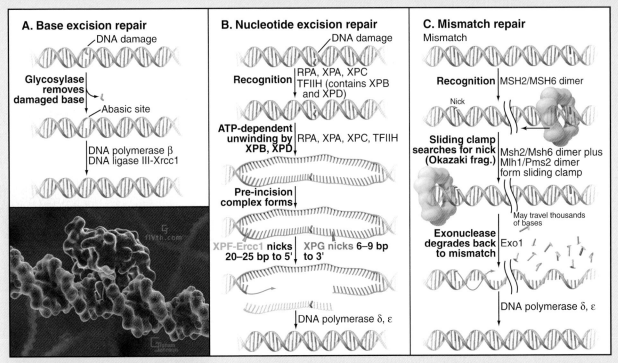

Figure 43-14 PATHWAYS FOR THE REPAIR OF BASE DAMAGE, BULKY ADDUCTS, SUCH AS THYMIDINE DIMERS FORMED BY ULTRAVIOLET LIGHT, OR MISMATCHED BASES. For detailed descriptions, see the text. The *inset* in the panel on base excision repair shows human 3-methyladenine DNA glycosylase complexed to DNA (PDB file: 1BNK). This enzyme scans the DNA for bases that are not strongly H-bonded, uses its "finger" to swing them up into the pocket for scanning, and—if bad—catalyzes excision of that base. (Inset illustration by Graham Johnson (www.fivth.com) for the Howard Hughes Medical Institute, copyright 2004, all rights reserved. Reference: Lau AY, Scharer OD, Samson L, et al: Crystal structure of a human alkylbase-DNA repair enzyme complexed to DNA: Mechanisms for nucleotide flipping and base excision. Cell 95:249–258, 1998.)

fore identified as the newly synthesized DNA strand. The mismatch repair complex then recruits the exonuclease EXO1 and degrades the newly synthesized DNA strand all the way back to the misincorporated base. The resultant long single-stranded region is stabilized by binding of RPA and eventually filled in by the replicative DNA polymerases δ and/or ε.

Double-Strand Break Repair

DNA double-strand breaks are particularly hazardous forms of damage, as they carry the risk of losing chromosomal material or, if misrepaired, causing chromosomal translocations. Two major pathways are responsible for dealing with these lesions, which can be caused by ionizing radiation or radiomimetic drugs or arise spontaneously after replication. Homologous recombinational repair uses undamaged DNA sequence as a template for the accurate repair of double-strand breaks, this sequence usually being derived from the sister chromatid after replication. Nonhomologous end-joining repairs double-strand breaks with no requirement for homology and therefore carries a much higher risk of introducing mutations. Nonhomologous end-joining is the predominant activity that repairs double-strand breaks in the G₁ and early S phase, while homologous

recombination becomes more important in the late S and G₂ phase. Both pathways require the activity of the MRN protein complex (Mre11/RAD50/Nbs1), which localizes to DNA double-strand breaks and is also found at telomeres (see Fig. 12-13). The exonuclease activity of this complex resects (chews back) broken DNA ends to provide single-stranded DNA substrates for the repair systems.

The key protein that is required for homologous recombinational repair in mammalian cells is **Rad51,** the eukaryotic homologue of *E. coli* RecA (Fig. 43-15A). Rad51 forms an extended nucleoprotein filament on single-stranded DNA and catalyses the search for homologous sequences, strand pairing, and strand exchange. Also involved in this process is Rad54, a helicase that is believed to facilitate strand invasion when the single-stranded region forces its way into the complementary DNA duplex on the undamaged sister chromatid. Following invasion of the recombining DNA strands, polymerase activity extends the DNA beyond the site of the double-strand break and forms a **Holliday junction** (Fig. 43-15B). Resolution of the Holliday junction and filling-in of the repaired DNA sequences results in complete repair of the lesion.

Nonhomologous end-joining is initiated at a DNA double-strand break by binding of the Ku70 and Ku80

Continued

BOX 43-1
DNA Repair in Vertebrates—cont'd

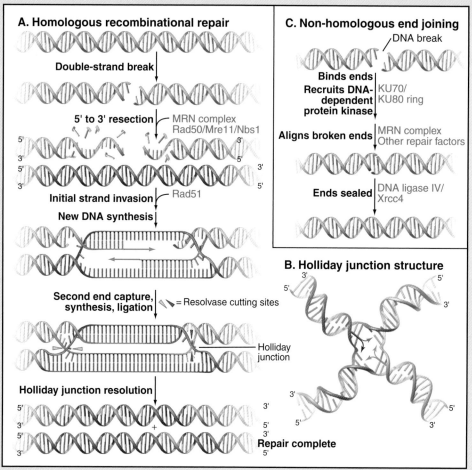

Figure 43-15 PATHWAYS FOR THE REPAIR OF DNA DOUBLE-STRAND BREAKS. A double-strand break is recognized by the PI3-kinase family members ATM or ATR and a cell-cycle delay ensues (see Fig. 40-4). The break is then bound by repair factors in the homologous recombination or the nonhomologous end-joining pathway of DNA repair. It is not known what factors control the "choice" between these pathways. **A,** Homologous recombination pathway of DNA repair. The MRN complex chews back the DNA at a break, leaving a single-stranded overhang that is stabilized by RPA (not shown). It is believed that the MRN complex also plays a role in keeping the broken ends in proximity to one another. Next, RAD51 forms a nucleoprotein filament on the single-stranded DNA, displacing the RPA. The RAD51 nucleoprotein filament then initiates homology searching and repairs the DNA break by inserting the extended single-stranded DNA into homologous sequences (usually on the sister chromatid *[blue]*) and allowing homologous recombination and DNA repair/resynthesis to occur. Capture of the second single-stranded DNA end allows the formation of a joint molecule with a double Holliday junction. Resolution of this Holliday junction structure results in accurate, templated repair of the double-strand break. **B,** A Holliday junction formed by four complementary oligonucleotides complexed to the enzyme Cre (not shown). The Holliday junction is a dynamic structure *(arrows)* that can migrate along the DNA. (PDB file: 3CRX.) **C,** Nonhomologous end-joining pathway of DNA repair. Nonhomologous end-joining is initiated by break recognition by the Ku70/Ku80 heterodimer, which recruits DNA-PK and tethers the broken ends. The breaks are then processed in a reaction involving the MRN complex and other repair factors. DNA-PK's precise role is not yet entirely clear. Next, DNA ligase IV/XRCC4 is recruited to the processed double-strand break, which is ligated back together. (B, Reference: Gopaul DN, Guo F, Van Duyne GD: Structure of the Holliday junction intermediate in Cre-loxP site-specific recombination. EMBO J 17:4175–4187, 1998.)

heterodimer as a ring to which the **DNA-dependent protein kinase** catalytic subunit binds, stimulating other repair factors and aligning the broken ends of the DNA (Fig. 43-15C). The ends are finally sealed by DNA ligase IV, which exists in complex with XRCC4. Nonhomologous end-joining is also necessary for V(D)J recombination and therefore for the development of the immune system (see Fig. 28-10).

Given the importance of accurate transmission of the genetic material, it is not surprising that a number of diseases, key among which is cancer, are associated with deficiencies in DNA repair. Table 43-1 summarizes the impact that mutations in the key DNA repair genes can have in disease. Note that many DNA repair activities are essential for life and therefore have not been described in any human diseases.

ACKNOWLEDGMENTS

Thanks go to Jonathon Pines, Helen Piwnica-Worms, and Carl Smythe for their suggestions on revisions to this chapter. We are especially grateful to Ciaran Morrison, who wrote the new box on DNA repair.

SELECTED READINGS

Abraham RT: Cell cycle checkpoint signaling through the ATM and ATR kinases. Genes Dev 15:2177–2196, 2001.

Melo J, Toczyski D: A unified view of the DNA-damage checkpoint. Curr Opin Cell Biol 14:237–245, 2002.

Morgan DO: Cyclin-dependent kinases: Engines, clocks and micro-processors. Annu Rev Cell Biol 13:261–291, 1997.

Nigg EA: Cell division: Mitotic kinases as regulators of cell division and its checkpoints. Nat Rev Mol Cell Biol 2:21–32, 2001.

O'Connell MJ, Walworth NC, Carr AM: The G2-phase DNA-damage checkpoint. Trends Cell Biol 10:296–303, 2000.

Ohi R, Gould KL: Regulating the onset of mitosis. Curr Opin Cell Biol 11:267–273, 1999.

Petrini JHJ, Stracker TH: The cellular response to DNA double-strand breaks: Defining the sensors and mediators. Trends Cell Biol 13:458–462, 2003.

Pines J: Four-dimensional control of the cell cycle. Nat Cell Biol 1:E73–E79, 1999.

Sancar A, Lindsey-Boltz LA, Ünsal-Kaçmaz K, Linn S: Molecular mechanisms of mammalian DNA repair and the DNA damage checkpoints. Annu Rev Biochem 73:39–85, 2004.

Shiloh Y (ed): Bridge over broken ends: The cellular response to DNA breaks in health and disease. Special issue of DNA Repair 3:779–1251, 2004.

Smits VA, Medema RH: Checking out the G(2)/M transition. Biochim Biophys Acta 1519:1–12, 2001.

Wood RD, Mitchell M, Sgouros J, Lindahl T: Human DNA repair genes. Science 291:1284–1289, 2001.

Mitosis and Cytokinesis

Mitosis is the division of a somatic cell (a vegetative cell in yeast) into two daughter cells. The daughters are usually identical copies of the parent cell, but the process can be asymmetrical. For example, division of stem cells gives rise to one stem cell and another daughter cell that goes on to mature into a differentiated cell. See Box 41-1 for examples.

Traditionally, mitotic events are subdivided into six phases: **prophase, prometaphase, metaphase, anaphase, telophase,** and **cytokinesis** (Fig. 44-1). The dramatic reorganization of both the nucleus and cytoplasm during the mitotic phases is brought about by activation of a number of protein kinases, including Cdk1–cyclin B–p9 (abbreviated here as "Cdk1 kinase"; see Chapter 40). After activation by Cdc25 phosphatase, Cdk1 kinase accumulates in the nucleus, where it joins Cdk1–cyclin A, which was activated somewhat earlier (see Chapter 43). These two Cdk1 kinase complexes operate both as master controllers and as workhorses that directly phosphorylate many proteins whose functional and structural status is altered during mitosis.

Mitosis is an ancient eukaryotic process, and a number of variations emerged during evolution. Many single-celled eukaryotes, including yeast and slime molds, undergo a **closed mitosis,** in which spindle formation and chromosome segregation occur within an intact nuclear envelope to which the spindle poles are anchored. This chapter focuses on **open mitosis,** as used by most plants and animals, in which the nuclear envelope disassembles before the chromosomes segregate. Figure 44-2 summarizes some of the important events during the various mitotic phases.

Prophase

Prophase, the transition from G_2 into mitosis, begins with the first visible condensation of the chromosomes and disassembly of the nucleolus (Fig. 44-3). In the cytoplasm, the interphase network of long microtubules centered on a single centrosome (see Fig. 34-17) is converted into two radial arrays of short microtubules called *asters*. Most types of intermediate filaments disassemble, the Golgi and endoplasmic reticulum fragment, and both endocytosis and exocytosis are curtailed.

Nuclear Changes in Prophase

Chromosome condensation, the landmark event at the onset of prophase, often begins in isolated patches of chromatin at the nuclear periphery. Later, chromosomes condense into two threads, termed **sister chromatids,** which are closely paired along

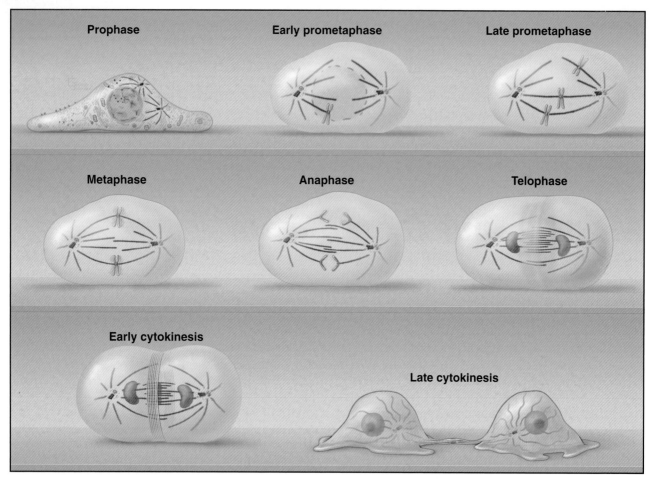

Prophase **Early prometaphase** **Late prometaphase**

Metaphase **Anaphase** **Telophase**

Early cytokinesis

Late cytokinesis

Figure 44-1 OVERVIEW OF THE PHASES OF MITOSIS.

their entire lengths. Although chromosome condensation was first observed more than a century ago, the biochemical mechanism remains a mystery. Protein kinases are thought to drive mitotic chromosome condensation by phosphorylating a number of the hundreds of proteins associated with mitotic chromosomes. The onset of condensation correlates with phosphorylation of histones H1 by Cdk1 kinase and H3 by **Aurora-B** protein kinase, and both are widely used as physiological markers for mitotic cells. However, chromosome condensation still occurs when both of these phosphorylation events are blocked. Possibly, some combination of histone modifications might provide a "code" that promotes chromatin condensation (see Fig. 13-3).

Two pentameric protein complexes, **condensin** I and II, are major constituents of mitotic chromosomes with an essential role in chromosome architecture (see Fig. 13-19). The two complexes share a pair of ABC ATPases, SMC2, and SMC4 (structural *m*aintenance of *c*hromosomes) but have two different sets of three auxiliary proteins. Condensin II enters the cell nucleus during prophase, where it is required for prophase chromosome condensation. However, chromosomes of ver-

tebrate cells that lack condensin condense rapidly once the nuclear envelope breaks down at the onset of prometaphase, so condensin is not directly responsible for mitotic chromosome condensation. Chromosomes that lack condensin separate normally at the beginning of anaphase but appear to fall apart while moving toward the spindle poles. This appears to reflect defects in their underlying structure, and condensin is required for proteins of the chromosome scaffold to assemble properly (see Fig. 13-19). The molecular explanation for these effects is not known. In vitro, condensin complexes can promote coiling and compaction of DNA, but the significance of this is also unknown.

Cytoplasmic Changes in Prophase

Most of the cytoskeleton reorganizes during prophase. Most notably, the microtubule array changes from an extensive network permeating the cytoplasm into two dense, radial arrays of short, dynamic microtubules around the duplicated centrosomes (see Chapter 34). Each of these **asters** eventually becomes one **pole** of the mitotic spindle. During prophase, the two asters

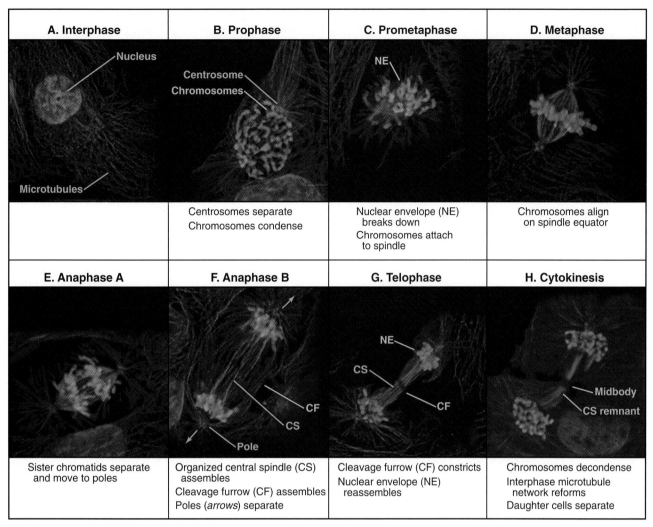

A. Interphase	B. Prophase	C. Prometaphase	D. Metaphase
	Centrosomes separate Chromosomes condense	Nuclear envelope (NE) breaks down Chromosomes attach to spindle	Chromosomes align on spindle equator

E. Anaphase A	F. Anaphase B	G. Telophase	H. Cytokinesis
Sister chromatids separate and move to poles	Organized central spindle (CS) assembles Cleavage furrow (CF) assembles Poles (arrows) separate	Cleavage furrow (CF) constricts Nuclear envelope (NE) reassembles	Chromosomes decondense Interphase microtubule network reforms Daughter cells separate

Figure 44-2 OVERVIEW OF THE PHASES OF MITOSIS AND DEFINITION OF THE MOST IMPORTANT TERMS. **A–C,** *Prophase–prometaphase*: The Cdk1 kinases trigger condensation of replicated sister chromatids, disassembly of the nuclear envelope and Golgi, and a dramatic reorganization of the cytoskeleton. These changes abolish the barrier between the chromosomes and cytoplasm. As cytoplasmic microtubules contact the condensed chromosomes, they attach at the kinetochores (see Fig. 13-20). Interaction of motor proteins on the chromosomes with microtubules produces jostling movements that culminate with the chromosomes aligned at the midplane of a bipolar scaffolding of microtubules (the spindle). **D–F,** *Metaphase–anaphase*: Once all of the chromosomes achieve a bipolar attachment to the spindle, an inhibitory signal is switched off. This leads to activation of a proteolytic network that destroys proteins responsible for holding sister chromatids together and also inactivates Cdk1 by destroying its cyclin B cofactor (see Flg. 40-18). These changes trigger separation of the sister chromatids, which then move toward opposite spindle poles. **G–H,** *Telophase–cytokinesis*: Targeting of nuclear envelope components back to the surface of the chromatids subsequently leads to the re-formation of two daughter nuclei. In most cells, the two daughter nuclei and the surrounding cytoplasm are partitioned by cytokinesis following the contraction of an actin-myosin ring. (Micrographs courtesy of William C. Earnshaw.)

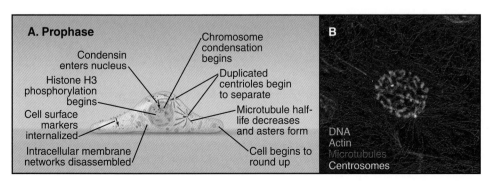

Figure 44-3 INTRODUCTION TO PROPHASE. **A,** Summary of the major events of prophase. **B,** Distribution of DNA *(blue),* microtubules *(red),* actin *(green),* and gamma tubulin (centrosomes *[yellow]*) in a prophase PtK1 (rat kangaroo) cell. (B, Courtesy of Dr. Alexey Khodjakov, Wadsworth Center, Albany, New York.)

Table 44-1

COMPARISON OF MICROTUBULE DYNAMICS IN INTERPHASE AND MITOTIC NEWT LUNG CELLS

Parameter	Interphase	Mitosis
Elongation rate	7 µm/min	14 µm/min
Elongation time before catastrophe	71 s	60 s
Shortening rate	17 µm/min	17 µm/min
Probability of rescue from catastrophe*	0.046/s	0
Length	100 µm	14 µm

*Most cellular microtubules grow constantly by addition of subunits to their free ends but occasionally stop growing and begin shrinking rapidly (a "catastrophe"). Unless shrinking is reversed (a "rescue"), the microtubule completely disappears. (Data from Gliksman NR, Skibbens RV, Salmon ED: How the transition frequencies of microtubule dynamic instability regulate microtubule dynamics in interphase and mitosis. Mol Biol Cell 4:1035–1050, 1993.)

usually migrate apart across the surface of the nuclear envelope, signaling the start of spindle assembly (Fig. 44-3).

Mitotic microtubules behave like interphase microtubules in many ways (see Chapter 34). They are nucleated at their minus ends, they grow by addition of tubulin subunits at their free plus ends, and they undergo random catastrophes during which they rapidly shorten. To a large extent, the prophase changes in microtubule organization can be explained by two simple biochemical changes: (1) increased microtubule-nucleating activity of centrosomes and (2) altered dynamic instability properties of the microtubules (Table 44-1; also see Chapter 34). Interphase microtubules have a high probability of recovering from catastrophes, so they grow quite long. Mitotic microtubules grow more rapidly but exist only transiently. This is because when they undergo a catastrophe, they usually shorten all the way back to the centrosome, with little chance of rescue. These differences in dynamic instability can be reproduced in vitro in mitotic and interphase cellular extracts. They appear to arise, at least in part, from counterbalancing interactions between microtubule-associated proteins, which promote microtubule stability, and kinesin-13 (see Fig. 36-13), which promotes microtubule disassembly.

Other cytoskeletal elements that disassemble during prophase include most, but not all, classes of intermediate filaments (including the nuclear lamins) and specialized actin filament structures, such as stress fibers. However, the junctional complexes between adjoining cells are maintained in epithelial cells. As a result of the cytoskeletal reorganization, most cells round up during prophase. This is particularly evident for animal cells that are cultured on a flat substrate, but cells in tissues also change their shape dramatically during mitosis.

RNA transcription of the chromosomes stops during mitosis. Although a number of mechanisms contribute to this change, phosphorylation of components of the transcriptional machinery by Cdk1 kinase appears to be the predominant mechanism. Cdk1 kinase phosphorylation of ribosomal elongation factor EF2a also stops ongoing protein synthesis and assembly of new ribosomes. Phosphorylation of several nucleolar proteins leads to disassembly of the nucleolus.

The Golgi apparatus and endoplasmic reticulum fragment or vesiculate during prophase (Fig. 44-4). In addition, many membrane-mediated events, including fluid-phase pinocytosis, endocytosis, exocytosis, and intracellular sorting of membrane components (see Chapters 21 and 22), greatly decrease. Golgi disassembly is driven by several kinases, including Cdk1. The first step of the process is fragmentation of the Golgi into smaller mini-stacks. The second step is still being investigated. Some evidence argues that Cdk1 phosphorylation of key components prevents the fusion of transport vesicles back into Golgi stacks (see Chapter 21), the net result being that the Golgi buds apart into small vesicles. Other evidence suggests that an imbalance of vesicle flow between the Golgi and the endoplasmic reticulum results in the Golgi being absorbed

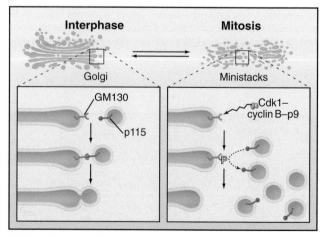

Figure 44-4 GOLGI APPARATUS DYNAMICS IN INTERPHASE AND MITOSIS. Disassembly in mitosis is driven by phosphorylation of components blocking fusion of Golgi membranes.

into the ER during mitosis. Whatever the mechanism of its disassembly, Golgi reassembly begins again during anaphase, following inactivation of Cdk1 kinase. Some Golgi derived vesicles contribute to the plasma membrane during cleavage furrow ingression at the end of mitosis (see later).

Prometaphase

In cells that undergo an open mitosis, prometaphase begins abruptly with disassembly of the nuclear envelope (Fig. 44-5). Microtubules growing outward from the spindle poles penetrate holes in the nuclear envelope, make contact with the chromosomes, and attach to them at specialized structures called **kinetochores** (see Fig. 13-20). Interactions of the two opposing kinetochores of paired sister chromatids with microtubules from opposite poles of the spindle ultimately result in alignment of the chromosomes in a group midway between the poles. An important cell cycle checkpoint (see Chapter 40) known as the **spindle checkpoint** delays the onset of chromosome segregation until any attachment errors have been corrected and all chromosomes have achieved a bipolar attachment.

Nuclear Envelope Disassembly in Prometaphase

Nuclear envelope disassembly involves the removal of two membrane bilayers coupled with disassembly of the nuclear pores and the fibrous **nuclear lamina** meshwork that underlies the inner bilayer (Fig. 44-6). Protein phosphorylation triggers breakdown of the nuclear envelope but the critical targets and mechanisms are not entirely known. Phosphorylation of the nuclear lamins at two sites flanking the central coiled-coil causes the lamina network to disassemble into subunits and might contribute to disassembly of the envelope. Cdk1 kinase can phosphorylate these lamin residues in vitro, but other kinases might participate in vivo. Additionally, phosphorylation of nucleoporins leads to nuclear pore disassembly. This fenestrates the nuclear envelope, dissolving the barrier between nucleus and cytoplasm. Interaction between microtubules and dynein associated with the nuclear envelope may also rip holes in the envelope.

Nuclear envelope components are dispersed in the cytoplasm from prometaphase until telophase (Fig. 44-6), but the mechanism may differ in various cell types. In fertilized amphibian eggs, the nuclear membrane breaks up into small vesicles that disperse in the cytoplasm. In vertebrate somatic cells, the nuclear envelope may be absorbed into the endoplasmic reticulum, which remains as an extensive tubular network throughout mitosis. In both cases, lamin B remains associated with the dispersed nuclear envelope, whereas lamins A and C and many proteins of the nuclear pore complexes disperse as soluble subunits.

During prophase, kinetochores transform from nondescript balls of condensed chromatin into organized plaques on the surface of the chromosomes. By early

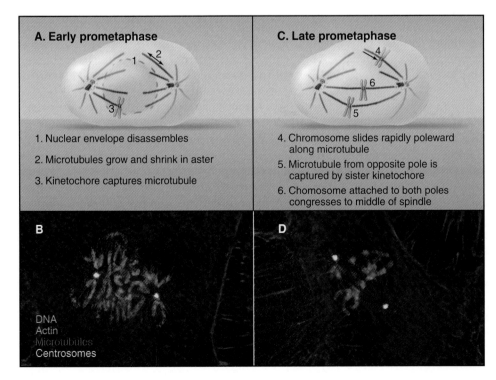

A. Early prometaphase

1. Nuclear envelope disassembles
2. Microtubules grow and shrink in aster
3. Kinetochore captures microtubule

C. Late prometaphase

4. Chromosome slides rapidly poleward along microtubule
5. Microtubule from opposite pole is captured by sister kinetochore
6. Chromosome attached to both poles congresses to middle of spindle

B

D

DNA
Actin
Microtubules
Centrosomes

Figure 44-5 INTRODUCTION TO PROMETAPHASE. **A,** Summary of the major events of early prometaphase. **B,** Distribution of DNA *(blue)*, microtubules *(red)*, actin *(green)*, and gamma tubulin (centrosomes *[yellow]*) in early prometaphase PtK1 (rat kangaroo) cells. **C,** Summary of the major events of late prometaphase. **D,** Distribution of DNA, actin, microtubules, and centrosomes in late prometaphase PtK1 cells. (B and D, Courtesy of Dr. Alexey Khodjakov, Wadsworth Center, Albany, New York.)

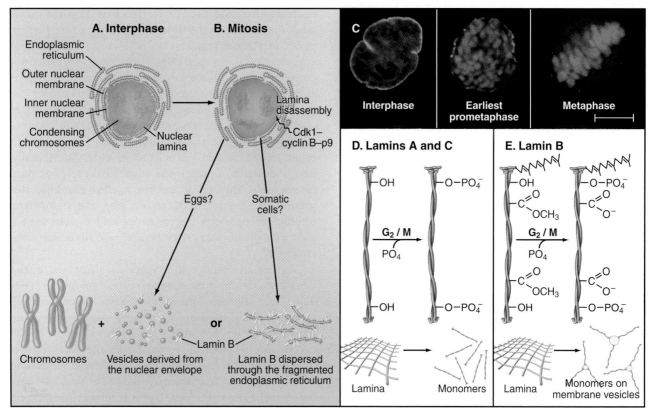

Figure 44-6 **DISASSEMBLY OF THE NUCLEAR ENVELOPE DURING MITOSIS. A–B,** Two contrasting models explaining the fate of the nuclear envelope during the transition from interphase to mitosis in a higher eukaryote. **C,** Micrographs showing solubilization of lamin A fused to GFP during mitosis. Scale bar is 10 μm. **D–E,** Reversible disassembly of lamins A, C, and B is driven by posttranslational modifications of the lamin polypeptides. (C, Courtesy of William C. Earnshaw.)

prometaphase, the characteristic trilaminar disk structure (see Fig. 13-20) can be seen. Each sister chromatid has a kinetochore. Thus, **sister kinetochores** are located on opposite faces of the mitotic chromosome. Only one of the two sister kinetochores faces a given spindle pole at any one time.

Organization of the Mitotic Spindle

The mature metaphase spindle is a bilaterally symmetrical structure with centrally located chromosomes flanked by arrays of microtubules radiating from the poles (Fig. 44-7).

Three predominant classes of microtubules are present in the metaphase spindle (Fig. 44-12). **Kinetochore microtubules** have their plus ends embedded in the kinetochore and their minus ends at or near the spindle pole. They characteristically form bundles, called **kinetochore fibers,** which contain anywhere from 1 microtubule in the budding yeast to more than 200 microtubules in some higher plants. Each human kinetochore binds about 20 microtubules. Up to about 80% of the approximately 2200 spindle microtubules in humans may be present in kinetochore fibers. **Interpo-**

lar microtubules are distributed throughout the body of the spindle and do not attach to kinetochores. Their minus ends may terminate near the pole but are not physically linked to it so that they appear to be free at both ends. Many interpolar microtubules penetrate between and through the chromosomes and extend for some distance beyond them. Thus, the central spindle contains a large number of interdigitated antiparallel microtubules. Tracking these spindle microtubules by electron microscopy has revealed a tendency for the interdigitated microtubules of opposite polarity to pack next to one another. During late anaphase, these antiparallel microtubules bundle to form a structure, called the **central spindle,** that appears to have important roles during cytokinesis. **Astral microtubules** project out from the poles and have a role in orienting the spindle in the cell through interactions with the cell cortex. All of the microtubules within each aster have the same polarity, with their minus ends proximal to the pole. Each unit of a spindle pole, with its associated kinetochore and interpolar and astral microtubules, is referred to as a **half-spindle.**

Spindle structure is largely determined by a combination of microtubule dynamics plus the action of at least

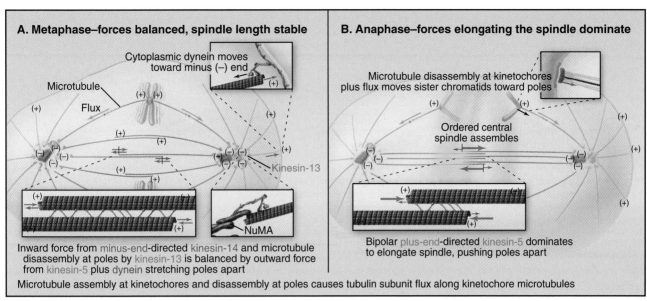

Figure 44-7 ROLE OF MOTORS IN SPINDLE STRUCTURE. The mitotic spindle is a dynamic entity whose structure depends on microtubule assembly/disassembly plus the balance of forces that act to slide microtubules relative to one another and to pull the poles together or apart. **A,** In metaphase, the structure is at steady state. The forces that tend to elongate the spindle, including cytoplasmic dynein (which moves toward microtubule minus ends, pulling the poles out toward the cell cortex) and bipolar kinesin-5 (which moves toward microtubule plus ends, pushing the poles apart), are counterbalanced by kinesin-14, which moves toward microtubule minus ends (and pulls the poles together) and microtubule disassembly at the spindle poles. Dynein and its associated protein, NuMA, also have an important role in organization of the spindle pole. **B,** In anaphase, the balance of kinesin activity shifts, microtubule disassembly at the poles declines, and the spindle undergoes a dramatic elongation. During anaphase, bipolar kinesin-5 and PRC1 also have important roles in organizing the central spindle, which is essential for subsequent assembly and function of the cleavage furrow.

seven different types of kinesins plus cytoplasmic dynein (see Chapter 36). These motors often work in opposition to one another. As a result, the spindle is a highly dynamic structure whose morphology changes as the balance of forces shifts between the various motors. For example, inactivating one or more kinesins with drugs or switching a temperature-sensitive mutant to the nonpermissive temperature can cause the spindle to collapse rapidly on itself. Consequently, chromosomal movements and changes in spindle morphology are complex processes that reflect both the dynamic growth and shrinkage of microtubules plus the net vectorial output of multiple antagonistic and synergistic motors. These various components interact; for example, force exerted by motors can influence the dynamic assembly/disassembly of microtubules.

Spindle Assembly

In metazoans, spindle assembly starts in prophase with the separation of the asters. In most cells, each aster is organized around a centrosome, consisting of a centriole pair and associated pericentriolar material. γ-**Tubulin** ring complexes in the pericentriolar material efficiently nucleate microtubules (see Fig. 34-16), so each aster acts as a **microtubule organizing center.** By the end of prophase, the spindle consists of two asters linked by a

few interpolar microtubules. Cytoplasmic dynein at the cell cortex exerts an outward force separating the asters, whereas kinesin-14 motors (which move toward microtubule minus ends) on the interpolar microtubules exert a counterbalancing force holding the asters together.

This balance of forces changes when the nuclear envelope breaks down. Bipolar kinesin-5 motors are phosphorylated by Cdk1 kinase and concentrate in the central spindle, where they cross-link adjacent antiparallel interpolar microtubules. Kinesin-5 moves toward the plus ends of microtubules. If such a motor attaches to two adjacent antiparallel microtubules and begins to move, it will cause them to slide apart (Fig. 44-7). Thus, the action of kinesin-5 motors pushes the spindle poles apart. The two half-spindles do not separate because they are physically linked via the chromosomes, with sister kinetochores attached to opposite spindle poles.

Also at this time, the asters mature into focused spindle poles. The pericentriolar material efficiently nucleates the assembly of new microtubules with their minus ends at the pole. In addition, cytoplasmic dynein transports free microtubules that are nucleated throughout the cytoplasm to the centrosome along astral microtubules for incorporation into the spindle. The focused microtubule array at the pole forms partly owing to the tethering of microtubules by centrosomes, and partly

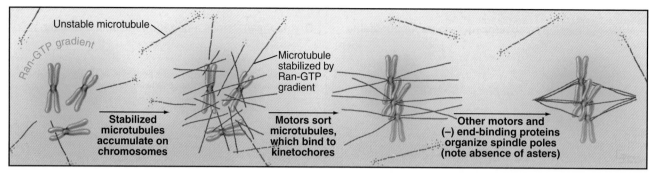

Figure 44-8 ASSEMBLY OF A BIPOLAR SPINDLE IN THE ABSENCE OF CENTROSOMES. A gradient of Ran-GTP stabilizes microtubules around chromosomes, releasing spindle assembly factors. Microtubules that accumulate around the chromosomes are sorted and organized by motor proteins and are subsequently focused to make poles by motors and (–) end-binding proteins such as NuMA. These spindle poles lack prominent astral microtubules.

due to the concerted action of various motors and microtubule cross-linking proteins such as nuclear mitotic apparatus protein **(NuMA).** NuMA is released from the nucleus on nuclear envelope breakdown, and it accumulates near the poles at the minus ends of microtubules.

In large cells that lack centrosomes, such as eggs, spindle formation depends on an alternative pathway that is also active in cells with centrosomes (Fig. 44-8). Chromosomes stabilize nearby microtubules, which are then organized into a bipolar spindle by motor proteins and NuMA. This spindle assembly pathway involves importin α and β, two proteins that direct traffic through nuclear pores during interphase (see Fig. 16-14). Importin α and β inhibit mitotic spindle formation by sequestering several essential proteins, including NuMA. Chromosomes counteract this by releasing spindle assembly factors such as NuMA from importin α and β. The mechanism depends on the association of the GTP exchange factor RCC1 (Ran-GEF in Fig. 14-17) with chromosomes. RCC1 produces a local gradient of the active GTPase Ran-GTP, which dissociates NuMA from importin α and β just as it does during protein import into the nucleus. In this case, however, the net result is microtubule stabilization and assembly of the mitotic spindle.

If centrosomes are removed or destroyed experimentally, somatic cells can also use motor proteins to organize microtubules into bipolar spindles that lack asters but are otherwise remarkably normal. However, only about half of the cells that have lost centrosomes manage to complete mitosis successfully. Thus, centrosomes are not required to form spindles, but they do contribute to successful chromatid separation and cytokinesis by helping to orient the spindle within the dividing cell.

Chromosome Attachment to the Spindle

Dynamic microtubules of prometaphase asters scan the cytoplasm searching for both binding sites that will capture and stabilize their distal plus ends and for other components, including free microtubules. Breakdown of the nuclear envelope makes the condensed chromosomes accessible to the microtubules. Chance encounters with kinetochores during cycles of growth result in the plus ends of microtubules being captured by the kinetochore. **Capture** probably involves the nine-component KMN complex, which contains two components capable of binding weakly to microtubules. One of these, the helical Ndc80 complex (see Fig. 13-21) binds along the sides of microtubules forming fine hairs visible in the electron microscope. Other members of the complex provide an anchoring site for Ncd80 in the kinetochore. Captured microtubules are about five-fold less likely to depolymerize catastrophically than free microtubules. When catastrophes do occur, the microtubules depolymerize back to the pole, recycling tubulin subunits for incorporation into other, growing microtubules.

Initial attachment of a chromosome to a microtubule often involves a lateral interaction between the corona region of the kinetochore (see Fig. 13-20) and the side of a microtubule (Fig. 44-9). Cytoplasmic dynein then slides the chromosome rapidly along the microtubule toward the pole. These steps were first seen in animal cells, and a similar pattern of chromosome attachment and movement also occurs in budding yeast cells.

Capture of the first microtubule by a kinetochore causes the chromosome to move initially toward the spindle pole from which that microtubule originated. Historically, it has been thought that subsequent capture of a microtubule emanating from the opposite spindle pole by the sister kinetochore provides a counterforce that tugs the chromosome in the opposite direction. This **bipolar attachment** produces a balance of opposing forces that, together with the action of kinesin family motor proteins distributed along the chromosome arms, results in the gradual movement of the chromosome toward a point midway between the spindle poles. These movements are accompanied by coordinated shrinkage of the microtubules at the leading kinetochore and growth of microtubules at the

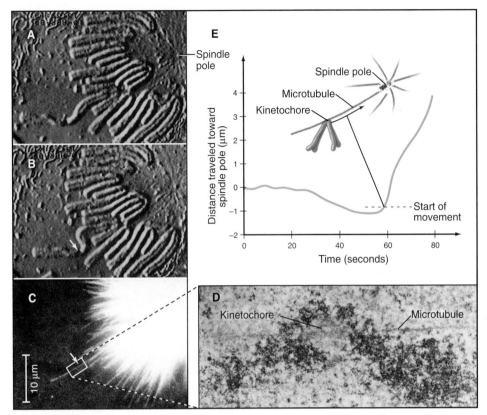

Figure 44-9 INITIAL CHROMOSOMAL MOVEMENTS DURING PROMETAPHASE. **A–B,** Chromosomal movements initiate with the capture of a microtubule by the kinetochore. This results first in movement toward the pole from which that microtubule originated. These images come from a study in which living cells, observed by differential interference microscopy, were subjected to rapid chemical fixation just after a chromosome had attached to the spindle *(arrow).* **C,** Attachment of the chromosome to the spindle was confirmed by indirect immunofluorescence staining for tubulin and, ultimately, by thin-section electron microscopy **(D). E,** The graph shows the movements of the chromosomes before and after attachment. (Reproduced from Rieder CL, Alexander SP, Rupp G: Kinetochores are transported poleward along a single astral microtubule during chromosome attachment to the spindle in newt lung cells. J Cell Biol 110:81–95, 1990. Copyright 1990 The Rockefeller University Press.)

trailing kinetochore. More recently, it has been shown that chromosomes attached to only one spindle pole (mono-oriented) can move toward the spindle equator if the unattached kinetochore associates with the kinetochore fiber of a chromosome that has already become aligned at the spindle equator. In this case, the mono-oriented chromosome glides away from the pole to which it is attached toward the spindle midzone, where it is more likely to capture microtubules emanating from the opposite pole. This motion of one chromosome along the kinetochore fiber of another chromosome requires the kinesin-7 motor CENP-E, which is associated with the kinetochore of the moving chromosome.

The attachment of microtubules to kinetochores can be reproduced and studied in vitro by mixing together chromosomes, isolated centrosomes, and tubulin subunits. Under these circumstances, the plus ends of microtubules growing out from centrosomes attach to the chromosomes. Surprisingly, chromosome-bound microtubules can either lengthen or shorten *at the attached end* without detaching from the chromosome. This tethering of dynamic microtubules is an essential aspect of chromosome movements during mitosis.

Correcting Errors in Chromosome Attachment to the Spindle

The goal of mitosis is to partition the replicated chromosomes accurately to two daughter cells. Therefore, all chromosomes must attach correctly to both spindle poles before being segregated. Three sorts of errors are common: (1) chromosomes with one or both kinetochores lacking attached microtubules, (2) chromosomes with both sister kinetochores attached to the same spindle pole, (3) chromosomes with a single kinetochore attached simultaneously to both spindle poles. Correcting these errors takes time, and the **spindle checkpoint** (see next section) delays mitotic progression to allow the correction process to occur.

Attachment of both sister kinetochores to a single spindle pole is rare, since sister kinetochores are positioned on opposite faces of the chromosome (see Fig. 13-20). When it occurs, one or both kinetochores must detach for the chromosome to achieve a bipolar orientation. Chromosome attachment to opposite spindle poles is more stable than attachment to a single pole, because the *tension* generated by bipolar attachment (where forces pull a chromosome simultaneously toward oppo-

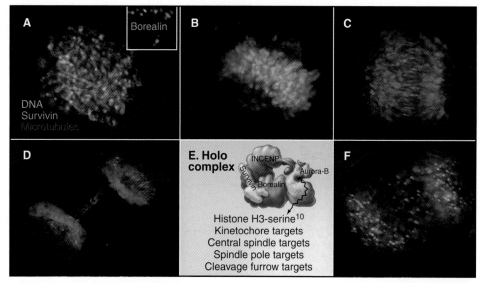

Figure 44-10 CHROMOSOMAL PASSENGER PROTEINS REGULATE MITOTIC EVENTS. These proteins are present at centromeres in prometaphase **(A)** and metaphase **(B)**, but transfer to the spindle midzone at anaphase **(C)** and midbody at anaphase **(D)**. **E,** Components and some targets of the chromosomal passenger complex, showing the Aurora B protein kinase complexed with INCENP, Survivin, and Borealin. **F,** If the complex function is inhibited (in this case by RNAi depletion of Borealin), chromosome attachment errors are common and many chromosomes fail to segregate properly in anaphase. Distribution of DNA *(blue)*, microtubules *(red)*, and survivin-GFP *(green)* in human mitotic cells. **Inset in A,** Distribution of DNA *(blue)*, kinetochores *(red)*, and Borealin *(green)* in a prometaphase cell. (A–D, Micrographs by Sally Wheatley and William C. Earnshaw. F and Inset in A, Micrographs by Ana Carvalho, Reto Gassmann, and William C. Earnshaw. Inset in A and F, Reproduced from Gassmann R, Carvalho A, Henzing AJ, et al: Borealin: A novel chromosomal passenger required for stability of the bipolar mitotic spindle. J Cell Biol 166:179–191, 2004, by copyright permission of The Rockefeller University Press. A–C, From Wheatley SP, McNeish IA: Survivin: A protein with dual roles in mitosis and apoptosis. Int Rev Cytol 247:35–88, 2005.)

site spindle poles) preferentially stabilizes microtubule connections to both kinetochores. It follows that the attachment of a single kinetochore to both spindle poles is more insidious, as that kinetochore is under tension, and the attachments are therefore stable. In fact, attachment of a single kinetochore to both poles seems to be the most common cause of chromosome segregation errors in cultured mammalian cells.

Both of these chromosome attachment errors are corrected through the action of Aurora B protein kinase, a member of the **chromosomal passenger complex,** along with inner centromere protein (INCENP), surviving, and borealin (Fig. 44-10). The other subunits target Aurora B to its various points of action during mitosis and regulate the kinase activity. The complex concentrates in the inner centromeres (the heterochromatin beneath and between the two sister kinetochores) during prometaphase and metaphase. As sister chromatids separate at anaphase, the complex moves to the overlapping interpolar microtubules of the central spindle and to the cell cortex, where the cleavage furrow will form, ultimately winding up in the intercellular bridge during cytokinesis. The chromosomal passenger complex is required to complete cytokinesis but also contributes to the correction of chromosome attachment errors and to the operation of the checkpoint that delays the cell cycle in response to those errors (Fig. 44-10).

Aurora B responds to tension on kinetochores to correct chromosome attachment errors. It phosphorylates both Ndc80 and the Dam1 complex, which are involved in microtubule binding to the kinetochore (see Fig. 13-21). Aurora B phosphorylation strongly inhibits Ndc80 binding to microtubules, and this may signal the kinetochore to let go of the attached microtubule. When a chromosome is correctly attached to both spindle poles, tension may stretch the kinetochore away from the chromosomal passenger complex buried in the chromatin beneath. This might stabilize the chromosome-microtubule interaction by preventing the kinase from phosphorylating the kinetochore.

Finding Time to Fix Chromosome Attachment Errors: The Spindle Checkpoint

Segregation of replicated chromosomes into daughter cells is extremely accurate. For example, budding yeasts lose a chromosome only once in 100,000 cell divisions. Perhaps surprisingly, the frequency of chromosome loss may be 20-fold to 400-fold higher for human cells grown in culture. To achieve even this level of accuracy, most cells must delay entry into anaphase until all chromosomes are attached to both poles of the mitotic spindle. This delay is caused by a cellular quality control pathway

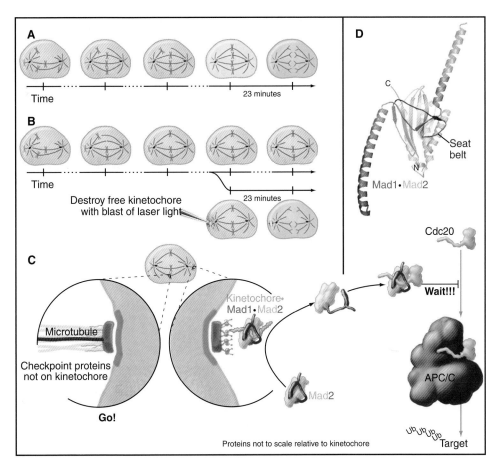

Figure 44-11 THE SPINDLE CHECK-POINT. Signaling by unattached kinetochores stops the cell from entering anaphase until all chromosomes have made a proper bipolar spindle attachment. **A,** As long as there is a chromosome that is not properly attached to the spindle (*beige* cells), the cell does not enter anaphase. The cell enters anaphase about 20 minutes after chromosome attachment is complete (*green* cells). **B,** In a cell with a persistently maloriented chromosome, anaphase entry is delayed (*beige* cells). If the unattached kinetochore is destroyed with a high-powered laser, the cell enters anaphase about 20 minutes later. This proves that the unattached kinetochore sends an inhibitory signal. **C,** The unattached kinetochore sends a signal via the Mad2 protein that ultimately inhibits the APC/C, blocking the degradation of cyclin B and securin and thereby blocking the transition into anaphase. **D,** Mad2 protein shown in its complex with Mad1 protein.

or checkpoint—the **spindle checkpoint**—that senses the completion of chromosome alignment at metaphase (Fig. 44-11). This nomenclature is nearly universal, but it is worth noting that this checkpoint actually monitors kinetochore activity rather than spindle structure. The spindle checkpoint differs from the DNA damage checkpoints in that its default setting is "on" as cells enter mitosis. It shuts off only when every chromosome is properly attached to the spindle.

The spindle checkpoint involves the products of the mitotic arrest–defective genes (MAD) and the budding-uninhibited-by-benzimidazole (BUB) genes. These were originally identified in yeast in genetic screens for cells that continued to try to divide when the spindle was disassembled by drugs. The Mad and Bub proteins are conserved from yeast to human. They accumulate at kinetochores early in mitosis, when the checkpoint is "on" (i.e., during prophase or prometaphase), and most are gradually displaced as microtubules bind and the kinetochores come under tension.

The target of the spindle checkpoint is Cdc20. This protein is thought to be a substrate recognition factor for the APC/C, a ubiquitin-protein ligase (E3 enzyme; see Chapter 23 and Fig. 40-16) that marks target proteins for destruction by proteasomes by decorating them with ubiquitin. Key APC/C substrates include cyclin B and a protein called securin, an inhibitor of the enzyme that triggers separation of sister chromatids at anaphase (see Fig. 44-16). Despite intense study, the mechanistic details are still debated.

Mad1 protein binds to kinetochores that are not properly attached to the spindle (Fig. 44-11). The best guess is that Mad1 then binds **Mad2.** A loop on Mad2 wraps around Mad1 like a safety belt to make a complex that resides stably at kinetochores. This complex can bind additional Mad2 molecules and convert them to a conformation activated for Cdc20 binding. The "primed" Mad2 molecules are then released either on their own or as part of a "mitotic checkpoint complex"; they bind Cdc20, and the APC/C is inhibited. As each chromosome becomes attached to both poles of the spindle, its inhibitory signals are removed. When the last chromosome has achieved a proper attachment, the last source of inhibitory Mad2 complexes is extinguished, and mitosis can proceed.

In metazoans, two of the checkpoint components are protein kinases, and one of these, **BubR1,** may be involved in sensing the quality of kinetochore attachments to the spindle. When the nuclear envelope breaks down at prometaphase, the COOH-terminus of the **CENP-E** kinesin binds to BubR1 located in the outer plate of the kinetochore. This interaction stimulates the

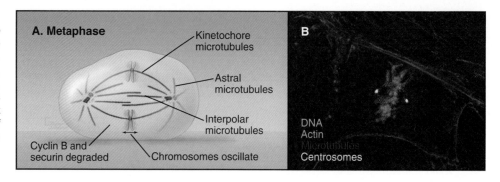

Figure 44-12 INTRODUCTION TO METAPHASE. **A,** Summary of the major events of metaphase. **B,** Distribution of DNA *(blue)*, microtubules *(red)*, actin *(green)*, and gamma tubulin (centrosomes *[yellow]*) in a metaphase PtK1 (rat kangaroo) cell. (B, Courtesy of Dr. Alexey Khodjakov, Wadsworth Center, Albany, New York.)

BubR1 kinase activity, a possible early step in activating the checkpoint. Subsequent microtubule binding by CENP-E then shuts the kinase off again. Thus, CENP-E may function in recognition of microtubule binding by the kinetochore. The yeast homolog of BubR1 is not a kinase; furthermore, yeasts lack CENP-E. Therefore, how they sense microtubule attachment to kinetochores remains mysterious.

Loss of the spindle checkpoint causes a catastrophic, premature entry into anaphase in higher eukaryotes, regardless of the status of chromosome alignment. This leads to an unequal distribution of sister chromatids to daughter cells, causing a genetic imbalance of the daughter cells known as **aneuploidy.** Yeasts can live without the checkpoint genes, but their loss is lethal for mice, which die early during embryogenesis. Humans with mutations in BubR1 have the disorder mosaic variegated aneuploidy, and mice heterozygous for various checkpoint components also show increased aneuploidy. Mosaic variegated aneuploidy is associated with an increased cancer risk, but as yet, no clear link has been established between mutations in other spindle checkpoint genes and cancer.

Metaphase

When all of the chromosomes have attained bipolar orientations (attached to both spindle poles) and moved to positions roughly midway between the two spindle poles, the cell is said to be in metaphase (Fig. 44-12). The compact grouping of chromosomes at the middle of the spindle is referred to as the **metaphase plate.** Destruction of cyclin B and securin (see Fig. 44-16) triggered by the APC/C begins as soon as the last chromosome achieves a bipolar orientation and continues throughout metaphase. Loss of securin is the signal for the separation of sister chromatids, the first sign of anaphase onset. Degradation of cyclin A, which with Cdk1 had an important role in triggering the entry into mitosis, begins earlier, at the entry into prometaphase, and is completed by mid-metaphase.

Microtubule Flux within the Metaphase Spindle

Although the average length of the kinetochore microtubules is roughly constant during metaphase, the microtubules change continuously in three ways. First,

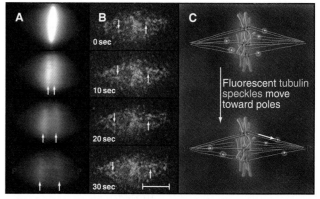

Figure 44-13 MICROTUBULE FLUX IN METAPHASE. **A,** Cells entering mitosis are injected with tubulin subunits modified chemically by attachment of a caged fluorescent dye. This type of dye becomes fluorescent after being irradiated with ultraviolet light. When cells enter metaphase and labeled tubulin is incorporated into the spindle, the central spindle is illuminated with a narrow stripe of ultraviolet light. This activates a narrow band of fluorescent tubulin subunits. With time, these subunits approach the spindle poles (P). Because the length of kinetochore microtubules is constant during this time, the labeled tubulin molecules must migrate along the microtubule toward the pole *(arrows)*. This can occur if new subunits are added to the microtubule at the kinetochore and old subunits are removed at the pole. **B,** Microtubule flux at metaphase in a *Drosophila* embryo visualized by fluorescence speckle microscopy. Embryos were injected with very low levels of fluorescent tubulin, which, instead of decorating the entire spindle, appears as speckles distributed along the microtubules. If a very sensitive camera is used, these speckles can be seen to move toward the poles, reflecting the flux in the underlying microtubules. Scale bar is 5 μm. **C,** Movement of labeled tubulin speckles toward the spindle poles. (A, Courtesy of Arshad Desai and the MBL Cell Division Group, Marine Biology Laboratory, Woods Hole, Massachusetts; reprinted by permission from Macmillan Publishers Ltd. from Mitchison TJ, Salmon ED: Mitosis: A history of division. Nat Cell Biol 3:E17–E21, 2001, copyright 2001. B, Courtesy of Paul Maddox and Arshad Desai, University of California, San Diego.)

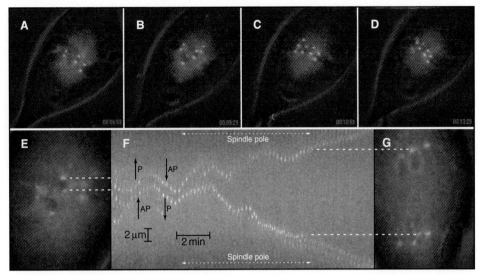

Figure 44-14   Kinetochore oscillations between P (poleward) and AP (away from the pole) movement during late prometaphase and anaphase in PtK1 (rat kangaroo) cells. **A–D,** Images showing the movements of several pairs of sister kinetochores, labeled with GFP-Cdc20 *(green)*, combined with phase-contrast images of the cell *(red)*. **E** and **G,** Higher-magnification views of sister kinetochores (marked with *dashed lines*) in prometaphase and anaphase, respectively. **F,** Kymograph (collage of images of a vertical strip showing the same two kinetochores at various time points during the movie) showing the movements of these two kinetochores. P and AP movements are indicated. Note that oscillations can occur even during anaphase. P movement involves microtubule shrinkage at the leading kinetochore and microtubule growth at the trailing kinetochore (which is undergoing AP movement away from its associated kinetochore). Spindle poles are near the top and bottom of panels E to G. (Micrographs courtesy of E. D. Salmon, University of North Carolina, Chapel Hill.)

there is constant net addition of new tubulin subunits (about 10 subunits per second) to the plus end of the microtubules, where they are attached to the kinetochore. Second, a comparable number of tubulin subunits is continuously lost from the minus end of the kinetochore tubules at the spindle poles. Therefore, tubulin subunits slowly migrate through kinetochore microtubules from the kinetochore to the pole (Fig. 44-13). This **subunit flux** or treadmilling is caused by microtubule depolymerization at the poles driven by kinesin-13 family members. Third, all microtubules attached to each kinetochore change coordinately in length during chromosomal oscillations (see next section).

Chromosome Oscillations during Metaphase

In many cells, even though chromosomes remain, on average, balanced at the middle of the spindle, they jostle one another and undergo numerous small excursions toward one pole or the other throughout metaphase (Fig. 44-14). These oscillations are slow, about 1.5 μm/minute (gain or loss of about 40 tubulin subunits per microtubule per second), perhaps because they require the simultaneous shortening or lengthening of the approximately 20 microtubules attached to each kinetochore in vertebrate cells. The oscillatory movements reverse every few minutes. Both active movements by motor proteins and fluctuations in the length

of kinetochore microtubules contribute to chromosome oscillations during metaphase, but their relative contributions may vary in different cell types. Although the movements of paired sister chromatids are usually coordinated, uncoordinated movements can stretch or compress centromeric chromatin. Thus, although each kinetochore can act independently, some mechanism (perhaps tension sensors in the kinetochore) usually coordinates their actions.

In some cells, microtubules interact with kinesin-4 and kinesin-10 **chromokinesins** associated with the chromosome arms in addition to kinetochores. These secondary interactions contribute to the stable alignment of chromosomes on the central spindle at metaphase.

Anaphase

The separation of sister chromatids at the onset of anaphase is one of the most dramatic events of the entire cell cycle (Fig. 44-15). Sister chromatids move to opposite spindle poles **(anaphase A),** and the poles move apart **(anaphase B).** Anaphase is also the time when the mitotic spindle activates the cell cortex in preparation for cytokinesis.

The dramatic physiological transition of the cytoplasm at anaphase is triggered by the action of two forms of the APC/C and degradation of key proteins. Anaphase A follows activation of APC/C^{Cdc20} (i.e., the

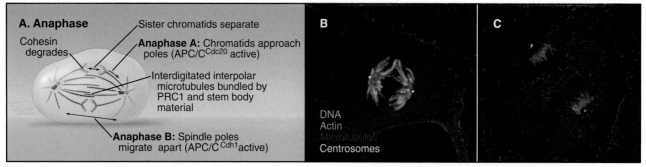

Figure 44-15 INTRODUCTION TO ANAPHASE. **A,** Summary of the major events of anaphase. **B–C,** Distribution of DNA *(blue)*, microtubules *(red)*, actin *(green)*, and gamma tubulin (centrosomes *[yellow]*) in early and late anaphase PtK1 (rat kangaroo) cells. (B–C, Courtesy of Dr. Alexey Khodjakov, Wadsworth Center, Albany, New York.)

APC/C with substrate specificity determined by Cdc20) during metaphase, which targets cyclin B for degradation and causes Cdk activity to fall (see Fig. 40-18). Anaphase B depends on activation of APC/C^{Cdh1}, which forms only when Cdk kinase activity has dropped. This is because Cdh1 phosphorylated by Cdk1 kinase cannot bind to the APC/C. APC/C^{Cdh1} targets polypeptides whose destruction by the proteasome is required for the cell to exit from mitosis and return to interphase.

Biochemical Mechanism of Sister Chromatid Separation

Separation of sister chromatids is regulated by the chromosomes themselves, not by the mitotic spindle. Under certain circumstances, sister chromatids can separate in the absence of microtubules, ruling out forces from the spindle in the process.

Studies of the budding yeast led to a major breakthrough by revealing three factors that regulate sister chromatid separation: a protein complex known as **cohesin,** a protease known as **separase,** and an inhibitor of the protease known as **securin** (Fig. 44-16). This system is conserved from yeast to human.

Cohesin is a complex of four proteins that resembles the condensin complex (see Fig. 13-19). Like condensin, cohesin has two large subunits from the SMC (structural maintenance of chromosomes) family. These proteins, SMC1 and SMC3, are complexed with proteins called Scc1 (which has other names omitted here for simplicity) and Scc3. Additional proteins are required for the stable loading of this complex onto DNA. Cells with mutations in cohesin components separate sister chromatids prematurely in mitosis, resulting in chaotic chromosome missegregation. This system is very ancient; an SMC-related protein is required for orderly chromosome segregation in bacteria.

Exactly how cohesin holds sister chromatids together is unknown, but a variety of evidence suggests that it could form a ring with a diameter of 40 nm, large enough to encircle two sister chromatids like a lasso. In yeast,

the complex functions only if it binds chromosomes during DNA replication, and one factor involved is a specialized form of the RFC complex that loads PCNA rings onto DNA (see Fig. 42-11). Cohesin accumulates at preferred sites on the chromosomes, often near centromeres in budding yeast or in regions of heterochromatin in fission yeast. In vertebrates, most cohesin dissociates from the chromosome arms by late metaphase, owing to the action of protein kinases such as Plk1 and Aurora B, but some remains associated with heterochromatin flanking centromeres until the onset of anaphase.

Cleavage of two key proteins triggers sister chromatid separation at anaphase. The first of these, securin, is an inhibitor of the separase protease. After the last chromosome forms a bipolar attachment to the spindle, the spindle checkpoint is switched off. This allows APC/C^{Cdc20} to tag securin with ubiquitin, leading to its destruction by proteasomes throughout metaphase. When securin levels fall below a critical threshold, separase is unleashed to cleave the Scc1 subunit of cohesin. Cleavage of Scc1 either breaks or disassembles the cohesin ring, allowing the sister chromatids to separate, thereby triggering the onset of anaphase. Phosphorylation of the separase cleavage site on Scc1 by a protein kinase can increase the cleavage of Scc1 by separase. Thus, the proteolysis of Scc1 is integrated and coordinated with the activities of the various mitotic kinases (see Chapter 40).

Human securin is overexpressed in some pituitary tumors, and the protein can act as an oncogene in cultured cells (see Fig. 41-10). Overexpression of securin may disrupt the timing of chromosome segregation, leading to chromosome loss and ultimately contributing to cancer progression.

Mitotic Spindle Dynamics and Chromosome Movement during Anaphase

Anaphase is dominated by the orderly movement of sister chromatids to opposite spindle poles brought

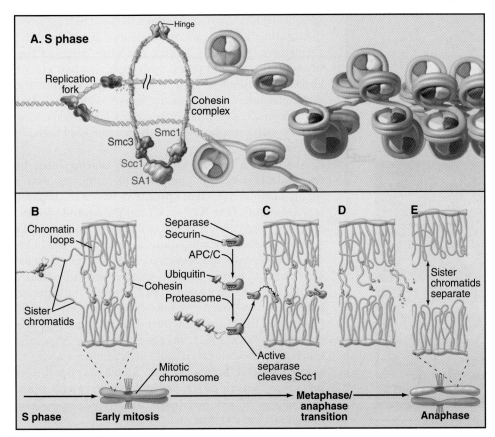

Figure 44-16 REGULATION OF SISTER CHROMATID PAIRING BY THE COHESIN COMPLEX. **A–B,** The cohesin complex forms a ring with a diameter of 35 nm that is loaded onto the chromosomes during DNA replication. The mechanism by which cohesins promote sister chromatid pairing is not known; this is one speculative model. At the onset of anaphase, degradation of its securin inhibitor liberates active separase enzyme. **C–E,** Separase then cleaves cohesin subunit Scc1, and the two sister chromatids are able to separate from one another and move toward opposite spindle poles.

about by the combined action of motor proteins and changes in the length of microtubules. Anaphase chromosome movements occur in two phases (Fig. 44-15). **Anaphase A,** the movement of the sister chromatids to the spindle poles, requires a shortening of the kinetochore fibers. During **anaphase B,** the spindle elongates, pushing the spindle poles apart. The poles separate partially because of interactions between the antiparallel interpolar microtubules of the central spindle and partially because of intrinsic motility of the asters. Most cells use both components of anaphase, but one component may be strongly exaggerated in relation to the other.

Microtubule disassembly on its own can move chromosomes (see Fig. 37-8). Energy for this movement comes from hydrolysis of GTP bound to assembled tubulin, which is stored in the conformation of the tubulin subunits. Chromosomes appear to use motor molecules such as cytoplasmic dynein in the kinetochore corona to hold onto disassembling microtubules. These motors must "run" toward the poles without losing their grip as the microtubules disassemble behind them. In addition, at yeast kinetochores the Dam1 ring (green in Fig. 13-21) can remain associated with disassembling microtubules. Other kinesin "motors" influence the dynamic instability of the spindle microtubules. Members of the kinesin-13 class, which encircle micro-

tubules near kinetochores and at spindle poles, use ATP hydrolysis to promote microtubule disassembly rather than movement.

Anaphase A chromosome movement involves a combination of microtubule shortening and translocation of the microtubule lattice due to flux of tubulin subunits (Fig. 44-13). The contributions of the two mechanisms vary among different cell types. When living vertebrate cells are injected with fluorescently labeled tubulin subunits, the spindle becomes fluorescent (Fig. 44-17). If a laser is used to bleach a narrow zone in the fluorescent tubulin across the spindle between the chromosomes and the pole early in anaphase, the chromosomes approach the bleached zone much faster than the bleached zone approaches the spindle pole. This shows that the chromosomes "eat" their way along the kinetochore microtubules toward the pole. In these cells, subunit flux accounts for only 20% to 30% of chromosome movement during anaphase A, and this flux is dispensable for chromosome movement. In *Drosophila* embryos, in which subunit flux accounts for about 90% of anaphase A chromosome movement, the chromosomes catch up with a marked region of the kinetochore fiber slowly, if at all.

Anaphase B appears to be triggered by the inactivation of the minus end-directed kinesin-14 motors, so that all of the net motor force favors spindle elongation. Three factors contribute to overall lengthening of the

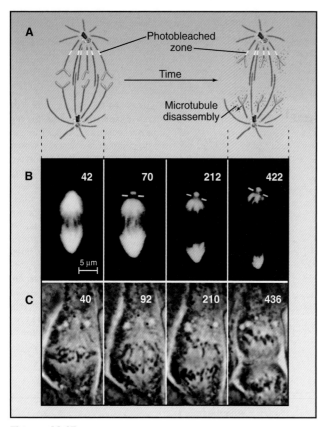

Figure 44-17 CHROMOSOMES MOVE ON SHRINKING MICROTUBULES DURING ANAPHASE. **A,** Mitotic cells are injected with a fluorescently labeled tubulin that rapidly becomes incorporated into the spindle. Just after anaphase onset, a laser is used to photobleach a stripe *(white)* across the spindle near the upper pole. The live cell is monitored over time by fluorescence **(B)** and phase contrast **(C)** microscopy. In this mammalian cell, the chromosomes approach the bleached stripe much faster than the stripe approaches the spindle pole. In other organisms with higher rates of microtubule flux in their spindles, the bleached zone would also move appreciably toward the pole. The numbers are time in seconds. (B–C, Reproduced from Gorbsky GJ, Sammak PJ, Borisy GG: Microtubule dynamics and chromosome motion visualized in living anaphase cells. J Cell Biol 106:1185–1192, 1988. Copyright 1988 The Rockefeller University Press.)

spindle: sliding apart of the interdigitated half-spindles, microtubule growth, and intrinsic motility of the poles themselves (Fig. 44-7). During the latter stages of anaphase B, the spindle poles, with their attached kinetochore microtubules, appear to move away from the interpolar microtubules as the spindle lengthens. This astral movement involves interaction of the astral microtubules with cytoplasmic dynein molecules anchored in the cortical cytoplasm.

Anaphase B spindle elongation is accompanied by reorganization of the interpolar microtubules into a highly organized **central spindle** between the separating chromatids (Fig. 44-15). Within the central spindle, an amorphous dense material called **stem body matrix** stabilizes bundles of antiparallel microtubules and holds together the two interdigitated half-spindles. Proteins concentrated in the central spindle help to regulate cytokinesis. One key factor, PRC1 (*p*rotein *r*egulated in *c*ytokinesis), is inactive when phosphorylated by Cdk kinase and functions only during anaphase when Cdk activity declines. PRC1 directs the binding of several kinesins to the central spindle. Each kinesin appears to target a specific protein kinase, such as Aurora B, to a particular domain of the central spindle, where phosphorylation of key substrates then regulates spindle elongation and cytokinesis.

Telophase

During telophase, the nuclear envelope re-forms on the surface of the separated sister chromatids, which typically cluster in a dense mass near the spindle poles (Fig. 44-18). Some further anaphase B movement may still occur, but the most dramatic change in cellular structure at this time is the constriction of the cleavage furrow and subsequent cytokinesis.

Reassembly of the Nuclear Envelope

Nuclear envelope reassembly begins during anaphase and is completed during telophase (Fig. 44-19). As in

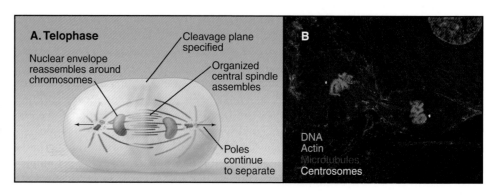

Figure 44-18 INTRODUCTION TO TELOPHASE. **A,** Summary of the major events of telophase. **B,** Distribution of DNA *(blue)*, microtubules *(red)*, actin *(green)*, and gamma tubulin (centrosomes [*yellow*]) in a telophase PtK1 (rat kangaroo) cell. (B, Courtesy of Dr. Alexey Khodjakov, Wadsworth Center, Albany, New York.)

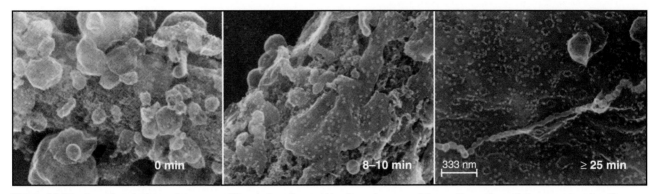

Figure 44-19   Scanning electron microscopy of the stages of assembly of membrane vesicles on the surface of chromosomes in a *Xenopus* egg cytosolic extract. A solution containing membrane vesicles was added to isolated chromatin from *Xenopus* sperm, fixed, and then imaged by field emission scanning electron microscopy. Each panel shows the time of incubation prior to fixation. (Micrographs courtesy of K. L. Wilson, Johns Hopkins Medical School, Baltimore, Maryland. A and C, From Wiese C, Goldberg MW, Allen TD, et al: Nuclear envelope assembly in *Xenopus* extracts visualized by scanning EM reveals a transport-dependent "envelope smoothing" event. J Cell Sci 110:1489–1502, 1997.)

spindle assembly, Ran-GTP promotes early steps of nuclear envelope assembly by releasing near the surface of the chromosomes key components that were sequestered by importin β. Most of these factors are not yet identified, but they include several nuclear pore components.

The mechanism of nuclear envelope reassembly is debated, in part because the fate of the nuclear membrane during mitosis is unclear. If the nuclear envelope disassembles to discrete vesicles as it does in eggs, then envelope reassembly is a classic membrane-sorting problem (see Fig. 21-12) that requires the fusion of membrane vesicles. In eggs, Ran-GTP and unknown factors direct the fusion of at least two or three discrete populations of membrane vesicles to re-form the nuclear envelope. On the other hand, if the nuclear membrane is absorbed into the endoplasmic reticulum during mitosis, as in vertebrate somatic cells, then reassembly involves lateral movements of membrane components within the membrane network and their stabilization at preferred binding sites at the periphery of the chromosomes.

Lamin subunits disassembled in prophase are recycled to re-form the nuclear envelope at the end of mitosis. Reassembly of the nuclear lamina is triggered by removal of mitosis-specific phosphate groups and methyl-esterification of several COOH side chains on lamin B (Fig. 44-6). B-type lamins are among the earliest components of the nuclear envelope to target to the surface of the chromosomes during mid-anaphase. Either at this time or shortly thereafter, other proteins associated with the inner nuclear membrane, including BAF, LAP2, and lamin B receptor (see Fig. 14-8), join the forming envelope. Lamin A enters the re-forming nucleus later during telophase, after the reassembly of nuclear pore complexes and reestablishment of nuclear import pathways. Its assembly into the peripheral lamina occurs

slowly over a period of several hours in the G_1 phase. Transport of lamins through nuclear pores appears to be essential for nuclear reassembly. If lamin transport is prevented, chromosomes remain highly condensed following cytokinesis, and the cells fail to reenter the next S phase.

Cytokinesis

Cytokinesis is the process that divides a mitotic cell into two daughter cells (Fig. 44-20). Cytokinesis involves a number of mechanistically distinct events. These include signaling to specify the cleavage plane (Fig. 44-21), assembly and regulation of the contractile apparatus, specific alterations (including targeted growth) of the cell membrane, and the final separation (abscission) of the two daughter cells.

In animals, protozoa, and most fungi a **contractile ring** of **actin** filaments and **myosin-II** separates daughter cells at the end of mitosis. Myosin-II pulls on the ring of actin filaments, applying tension to the plasma membrane, much like contraction of smooth muscle (see Figs. 39-20 and 39-21). Because the contractile ring is confined to a narrow band of cortex around the equator, it forms a **cleavage furrow,** constricting the plasma membrane locally and pinching the cell in two like a purse string (Fig. 44-20). Signals from the mitotic spindle and cell cycle machinery control the position of this ring and the timing of its constriction.

Protozoa, animals, fungi, and plants use an evolutionarily conserved set of components to implement different strategies to separate daughter cells. For example, both fission yeast and fruit fly cells use signals from polo kinase, a Rho GTPase, and a GTPase-activating protein (GAP) to direct the assembly of a contractile ring of actin, myosin-II, and other conserved components, in

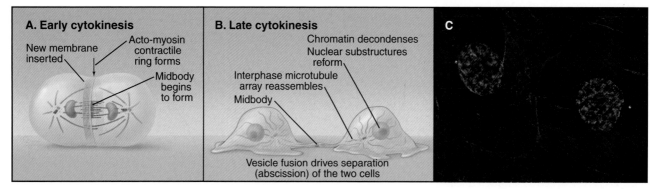

Figure 44-20   INTRODUCTION TO CYTOKINESIS. **A–B,** Summary of the major events of cytokinesis. **C,** Distribution of DNA *(blue)*, microtubules *(red)*, actin *(green)*, and gamma tubulin (centrosomes *[yellow]*) in a PtK1 (rat kangaroo) cell undergoing cytokinesis. (C, Courtesy of Dr. Alexey Khodjakov, Wadsworth Center, Albany, New York.)

spite of the fact that the yeast has a closed mitosis and the flies have an open mitosis. Plants divide by targeted fusion of membrane vesicles to build a new cell wall rather than constricting a cleavage furrow as animals do (Box 44-1 and Fig. 44-22A). However, the final abscission of animal cells also involves targeted fusion of vesicles, and the process is controlled by syntaxins in plants, animal cells, and fungi. Differences between various model organisms may be apparent or real, but they have certainly complicated the quest for a unified model for cytokinesis. Cytokinesis in prokaryotes is genuinely different, since completely different proteins are involved (Fig. 44-22B).

Although cytokinesis has been studied for more than 100 years, it has posed a number of challenges. Cytokinesis research typically employs living cells, because biochemical reconstitution of cleavage furrow assembly and function has yet to be achieved. Because many different essential proteins and other macromolecules are required, genetic analysis in yeasts, *Drosophila,* and *Caenorhabditis elegans* has been particularly informative: In fission yeast, more than 60 different genes are known to contribute to cytokinesis. More recently, this information has been complemented with RNAi analysis in *C. elegans, Drosophila,* and vertebrate tissue culture cells.

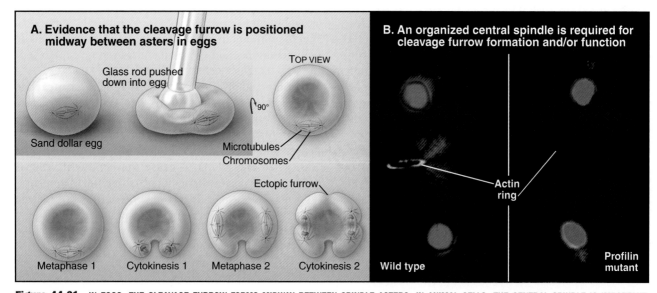

Figure 44-21   IN EGGS, THE CLEAVAGE FURROW FORMS MIDWAY BETWEEN SPINDLE ASTERS. IN ANIMAL CELLS, THE CENTRAL SPINDLE IS IMPORTANT. **A,** A classic experiment in which a sand-dollar egg is caused to adopt a toroid shape. At cytokinesis 2, the egg cleaves into four cells, and a furrow forms between the back sides of the two spindles. (For a description of this and other classic experiments in cytokinesis, see the book by Rappaport in the Selected Readings list.) **B, left,** A wild-type *Drosophila* spermatocyte undergoing cytokinesis, with the contractile ring stained in *yellow.* **Right,** In a profilin mutant, no central spindle forms, and the cell fails to form a contractile ring. (Micrographs courtesy of Professor Maurizio Gatti, University of Rome, Italy. B, From Giansanti MG, Bonaccorsi S, Williams B, et al: Cooperative interactions between the central spindle and the contractile ring during *Drosophila* cytokinesis. Genes Dev 12:396–410, 1998.)

Signals Regulating the Position of the Cleavage Furrow

Elegant experimental data from classic studies on fertilized echinoderm eggs suggest that a **cleavage stimulus,** emitted by the mitotic spindle, specifies the position of the cleavage furrow midway between the poles and perpendicular to the long axis of the spindle, thereby ensuring that the cleavage process separates the daughter nuclei (Fig. 44-21). In fertilized eggs, the poles, with their large astral arrays of microtubules, are regarded as the source of the cleavage stimulus, as furrows can be induced to form midway between two poles, even when no chromosomes are present. In addition, a signal emitted by the bundled microtubules of the central spindle appears to modulate the behavior of the furrow signaled by the poles.

The molecular nature of the cleavage stimulus itself remains a mystery in animals, although several of its features are known:

1. The signal moves from the spindle of echinoderm eggs to the cortex in a straight line at about 7 μm/minute. Microtubules are required, so the signal might be carried toward the cortex along the microtubules. In *Drosophila* spermatocytes, furrowing commences immediately after the cell cortex comes into close proximity with microtubule bundles.

2. Exposure to the cleavage stimulus for only about one minute commits the cortex to assemble a contractile ring. Cortical commitment results in production of a self-propagating furrow that can spread hundreds of micrometers across the surface of very large cells, such as fertilized eggs. If the spindle is removed after commitment, the furrow constricts part way but then regresses.

3. The mitotic apparatus appears to emit the cleavage stimulus throughout anaphase. A mitotic spindle can induce multiple transient furrows if it is experimentally repositioned within the cell.

Although signals from the poles of the mitotic spindle suffice to induce cytokinesis in large invertebrate embryos, other mechanisms contribute information to position the cleavage furrow between the daughter nuclei. In fission yeast, with closed mitosis, the nucleus determines the position of cleavage. In animal somatic cells, the organized central spindle plays a critical role, both early and late in cytokinesis. *Drosophila* mutants that fail to form a central spindle cannot initiate cytokinesis. In contrast, *C. elegans* embryos that lack a central spindle can initiate but not complete the process.

Assembly and Regulation of the Contractile Ring

Exposure of the cell cortex to the cleavage stimulus culminates in the assembly of a **contractile ring** consisting of a very thin (0.1 to 0.2 μm) array of actin filaments attached to the plasma membrane at many sites around the equator (Fig. 44-23). Polymerization of the actin filaments depends on formins (see Fig. 33-12). Small, bipolar filaments of myosin-II are interdigitated with actin filaments. The plasma membrane adjacent to this actin-myosin ring undergoes alterations in its lipid composition that are important for the function of the contractile ring.

Membrane furrowing requires actin and the motor activity of myosin-II (see Fig. 36-5). In animals, the small GTPase RhoA regulates actin polymerization by formins as well as constriction of the ring. Many other proteins are required for cytokinesis to go to completion. In their absence, furrowing begins, but the cleavage furrows ultimately regress, producing binucleated cells. This large class of proteins includes anillin, the chromosomal passenger proteins (Aurora-B kinase and its associated subunits [Fig. 44-10]) and a complex of Rho-GAP with a kinesin-6, among many others. Anillin helps to keep active myosin-II focused into an organized contractile ring throughout cytokinesis.

The chromosomal passengers and the Rho-GAP/kinesin-6 complex are required both for animal cells to assemble the central spindle and for the completion of cytokinesis. Although neither fits all criteria to be the cleavage stimulus, it is worth noting that both RhoA and the chromosomal passenger proteins require microtubules to localize to the site of cleavage furrow formation.

Fission yeast assemble a contractile ring along a well-defined pathway by recruiting proteins from cytoplasmic pools (Fig. 44-24). Polo kinase releases an anillin-like protein from the nucleus to mark the cortex in the middle of the cell and recruit myosin-II and a formin. Profilin activates the formin to polymerize actin filaments. Myosin-II pulls the actin filaments together into a ring around the equator of the cell (Fig. 44-23).

The assembly pathway is not yet understood in animal cells. INCENP and anillin move from the interphase nucleus to the cortex around the cell equator in early anaphase (Fig. 44-23). Some preexisting actin filaments are recruited intact into the contractile ring from adjacent areas of the cortex, whereas other filaments form de novo in the developing ring by assembly from monomers. Formins and profilin are involved, so the pathway resembles that in fission yeast. Myosin-II for the contractile ring is derived from various interphase structures. In cultured vertebrate cells, most of the myosin-II comes from stress fibers (see Fig. 33-1) that break down during prophase. Myosin-II is dispersed throughout the cytoplasm until anaphase, when it concentrates in the

BOX 44-1
Variations on a Theme: Cytokinesis in Plants and Bacteria

Plants

Chromosome segregation is similar in plants and animals, but cytokinesis is very different (Fig. 44-2A). Plants lack centrosomes, and during interphase, microtubules radiate out from the surface of the cell nucleus in all directions. In mitosis, the spindle does not focus to sharp poles at metaphase; instead, it assumes a barrel shape with flat poles. Early in mitosis, a band of microtubules and actin filaments forms around the equator of the cell adjacent to the nucleus. This so-called preprophase band disassembles as cells enter prometaphase. Because the entire cell cortex is covered by a meshwork of actin filaments, disassembly of the preprophase band actually leaves an actin-poor zone in a ring where cytokinesis will ultimately occur. This is called the cortical division site. In late anaphase, two nonoverlapping, antiparallel arrays of microtubules form over the central spindle. This structure, the phragmoplast, gradually expands laterally until it makes a mirror-symmetric double disk of short microtubules with their plus ends abutting the plane of cell cleavage. In addition to microtubules, the phragmoplast contains actin filaments and vesicles derived from the Golgi apparatus and endoplasmic reticulum. The Golgi vesicles, containing cell wall materials (see Fig. 32-12), move along phragmoplast microtubules to the equator, where they fuse, forming a membrane network

that will become the new plasma membrane and laying down the material that will become the new cell wall. As the zone of newly deposited membrane expands radially, the ring of microtubules surrounding it similarly expands. Eventually, the new membrane reaches the lateral cell periphery, and fusion with the plasma membrane separates the two daughter cells. The cortical division site, not the spindle, determines the site of cleavage. This was shown by centrifuging mitotic cells to displace the spindle from the central location where it initially formed. Late in mitosis, the phragmoplast formed at the midzone of the displaced spindle, but this phragmoplast then migrated to the plane of the preprophase band, where cytokinesis occurred.

Bacteria

The strategy for cytokinesis in bacteria is similar to that in animal cells (Fig. 44-22B), but the molecules are completely different. Most bacterial cells cleave as a result of constriction of a ring of the FtsZ protein (*filamentous temperature-sensitive;* mutants in *fts* genes cannot divide and make long filaments on cells). This is called the Z ring. FtsZ is the prokaryotic homolog of eukaryotic tubulins, but it assembles into filaments rather than tubules. As for tubulins (see Fig. 34-4), FtsZ polymerization requires bound GTP and hydrolysis of this GTP destabilizes the polymers.

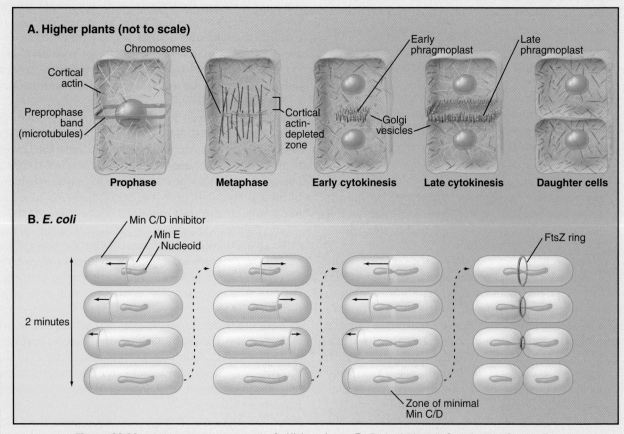

Figure 44-22   REGULATION OF CYTOKINESIS. **A,** Higher plants. **B,** *Escherichia coli.* See the text for details.

BOX 44-1
Variations on a Theme: Cytokinesis in Plants and Bacteria—cont'd

The Z ring is positioned at the cell equator of *Escherichia coli* by the action of three gene products: MinC, MinD, and MinE (*minicell* mutants divide at inappropriate locations and give birth to tiny cells). MinD is an enzyme that recruits MinC to the cell cortex, where it inhibits Z-ring formation. MinE is an antagonist of MinC/MinD action. This system works in a truly remarkable way. MinE forms a ring at the cell equator that migrates along the inner surface of the cell membrane until it reaches the end of the cell, at which point it disassembles. The ring then reforms in the center of the cell and sweeps toward the other end of the cell. As it moves, MinE inactivates the MinC/MinD inhibitory complex on the cell cortex. The inhibi-

tory complex rapidly reestablishes itself on the cell cortex behind the moving MinE ring. It takes about two minutes for each sweep of the MinE ring along half of the cell, and this cycle is repeated continuously until the FtsZ ring assembles at the cell center. No one knows how MinE and FtsZ locate the center of the cell. *Bacillus subtilis* uses an alternative mechanism to position the Z ring for cytokinesis. Interestingly, chloroplasts use a similar system for their division, and FtsZ has been detected in mitochondria of certain primitive eukaryotes. Mitochondria of higher eukaryotes appear to use another GTPase, dynamin, for a similar cleavage mechanism (see Chapter 19, under the section titled "Biogenesis of Mitochondria").

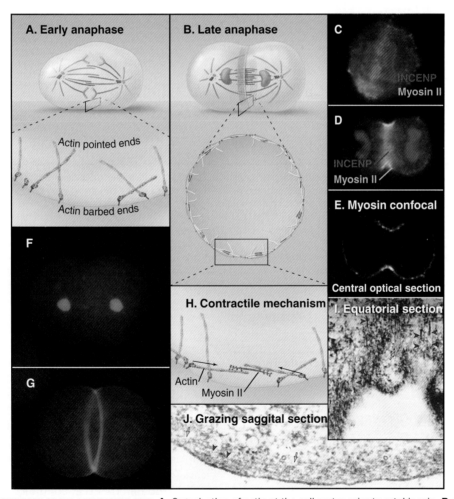

Figure 44-23 **ORGANIZATION OF THE CONTRACTILE RING. A,** Organization of actin at the cell cortex prior to cytokinesis. **B,** Distribution of actin and myosin at the start of ring contraction. **C,** INCENP *(red)* concentrates at the site where the cleavage furrow will form just before myosin *(green)*. **D,** INCENP and myosin concentrate in the contractile ring during contraction. **E,** Confocal micrograph shows the distribution of myosin in a contracting contractile ring. **F–G,** Dividing invertebrate egg with DNA *(blue)* and actin *(red)* in the contractile ring. **H,** Organization of actin and myosin filaments during cytokinesis. **I–J,** Electron micrographs showing actin filaments in the contractile ring. Note the thick filaments that are thought to be myosin-II filaments *(red arrowheads)* and the actin filaments *(yellow arrows)*. (C–D, Courtesy of William C. Earnshaw. E, I, and J, Courtesy of P. Maupin, Johns Hopkins Medical School, Baltimore, Maryland. F–G, Courtesy of Professor Issei Mabuchi, University of Tokyo, Japan. References: Maupin P, Pollard TD: Arrangement of actin filaments and myosin-like filaments in the contractile ring and actin-like filaments in the mitotic spindle of dividing HeLa cells. J Ultrastr Res 94:92–103, 1986; Maupin P, Phillips CL, Adelstein RS, Pollard TD: Differential localization of myosin-II isozymes in human cultured cells and blood cells. J Cell Sci 107:3077–3090, 1994; Eckley DM, Ainsztein AM, MacKay AM, et al: Chromosomal proteins and cytokinesis. J Cell Biol 136:1169–1183, 1997.)

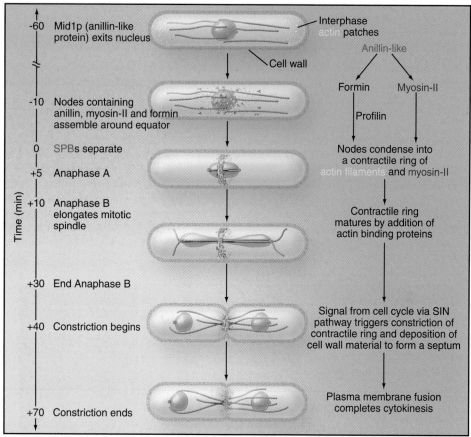

Figure 44-24   Cytokinesis in fission yeast *Schizosaccharomyces pombe*. During interphase, microtubules *(red)* position the nucleus in the middle of the cell. Actin filaments concentrate in small patches *(yellow)* in the cortex at the two growing ends of the cell (see Fig. 33-1). The mitotic spindle is inside the nucleus, as the nuclear membrane does not break down during mitosis. As the cell enters mitosis, an anillin-like protein moves from the nucleus to the equatorial cortex, where it sets up nodes of proteins, including myosin-II and a formin. The formin grows actin filaments *(yellow)*, and myosin-II pulls the nodes together into a continuous contractile ring. At the end of anaphase a signaling system consisting of a GTPase and three protein kinases (the septation initiation network, SIN) triggers constriction of the contractile ring and associated synthesis of new cell wall to form a septum. The septum is a three-layered structure, with the primary septum flanked by two secondary septae. Digestion of the primary septum separates the daughter cells. (Reference: Wu J-Q, Kuhn JR, Kovar DR, Pollard TD: Spatial and temporal pathway for assembly and constriction of the contractile ring in fission yeast cytokinesis. Dev Cell 5:723–734, 2004.)

cortex, especially around the equator where the furrow forms.

Constriction of the Cleavage Furrow

Cleavage furrow ingression is widely believed to be driven by contraction of the contractile ring, though some researchers believe that alterations in the physical characteristics (e.g., tension and stiffness) of the plasma membrane may also have a role to play. Constriction of the ring probably involves a sliding filament mechanism, similar to muscle (see Figs. 39-12 and 39-20). During the early stages of furrowing, the contractile ring maintains a constant volume, but the structure disassembles completely by the end of cleavage. Thus, during the later stages of cytokinesis, contraction is accompanied by disassembly of the ring.

The role of myosin-II as the motor for cytokinesis was established by microinjection of inhibitory antibodies into echinoderm embryos and confirmed by genetic inactivation in the slime mold *Dictyostelium*. Slime mold amoebas that lack the myosin-II heavy chain still extend pseudopodia, round up during mitosis, and complete nuclear division but cannot form a normal cleavage furrow. Mutant cells accumulate many nuclei, because the mitotic cycle continues. The mutants can proliferate if grown on a substratum to which they are tightly adherent by using pseudopods to pull themselves apart into smaller cells.

Constriction of the contractile ring is regulated so that it does not begin until after the onset of anaphase B, when sister chromatids are well separated. Local release of calcium appears to initiate constriction of the contractile ring in some cells. The calcium may activate the enzyme **myosin light chain kinase,** which, in turn, activates myosin-II (see Fig. 39-21). Exposure of dividing cells to agents that stimulate the release of calcium accelerates the appearance and rate of propagation of the cleavage furrow, whereas injection of compounds that bind calcium can inhibit cytokinesis. Other kinases and counterbalancing phosphatases are also involved, so regulation of myosin-II in cytokinesis is actually quite complex.

Membrane Addition and Abscission

As the contractile ring pulls the cell membrane inward, the single cell that entered mitosis is gradually transformed into two daughter cells joined by a thin intercellular bridge (Fig. 44-20). This process requires a significant net increase in the surface area of the cell. New plasma membrane is inserted adjacent to the leading edge of the furrow. The source of the new membrane appears to be secretory vesicles derived from the Golgi apparatus, and addition to the cleavage furrow is a specialized form of exocytosis. Fusion of vesicles providing the new membrane depends on specific syntaxins, t-SNAREs (see Chapter 21) that promote vesicle fusion along the secretory pathway. Targeted endocytosis is also important for cytokinesis, although its role is unclear.

The plasma membrane in the cleavage furrow has a discrete composition. In budding yeast, this compartment is delineated by rings made from polymers of septins, a family of GTP-binding proteins. Septins are essential for cytokinesis in *Saccharomyces cerevisiae* but not fission yeast.

In most animal cells, contraction of the cleavage furrow ultimately reduces the cytoplasm to a thin intercellular bridge between the two daughter cells. The intercellular bridge contains a highly ordered, antiparallel array of microtubules derived from the spindle with a dense knob, the **midbody,** at its center (Fig. 44-20). Isolated midbodies contain over 160 proteins, about one third involved in various aspects of membrane trafficking.

The midbody is encircled by a dense ring of proteins that includes the kinesin-6 that is essential for central spindle assembly (see the earlier section titled "Assembly and Regulation of the Contractile Ring") and a protein known as **centriolin,** which is associated with the centrosome for the rest of the cell cycle. A related yeast protein regulates the exit from mitosis. The conserved domain of centriolin binds the **exocyst,** a multisubunit protein complex that targets secretory vesicles to the plasma membrane (see Chapter 21, under the section titled "Tethering Factors"). These secretory vesicles accumulate near the midbody and fuse with the plasma membrane to separate the two daughter cells from one another. The details of this fusion event are not yet understood. The exocyst complex also contributes to cytokinesis in budding and fission yeasts.

In some tissues, intercellular bridges remain open as **ring canals.** After several rounds of nuclear division with incomplete cytokinesis, the network of cells maintains cytoplasmic continuity as each former contractile ring matures into a larger ring canal. During *Drosophila* oogenesis, four rounds of nuclear division with persistent ring canals creates 15 nurse cells, all in continuity with the oocytes (Fig. 44-25). The cytoplasmic continuity through ring canals allows nurse cells to transfer their cytoplasm into the developing egg, thus greatly increasing its stockpile of proteins and mRNAs available for use in early development. In mammals, incomplete cytokinesis is notable in the testis, where ring canals connect several hundred developing sperm cells.

Exit from Mitosis

To exit from mitosis, cells must inactivate the Cdk1 kinase. This reverses the biochemical and structural changes that are characteristic of mitosis and prepares the cell for proliferation in the next cell cycle. The exit from mitosis is better understood in the yeasts than in animal cells.

In budding yeast, a signaling pathway called the mitotic exit network (MEN) terminates mitosis, promotes contraction of the contractile ring, and initiates septation. The pathway consists of a small GTPase and protein kinases. Cdk kinase activity suppresses the pathway until anaphase, when Cdk activity drops sharply. The MEN GTPase is associated with one spindle pole body (the yeast version of the centrosome), while its key regulator, a GTP exchange factor, is located in the bud. Elongation of the mitotic spindle during ana-

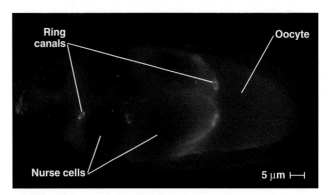

Figure 44-25 Incomplete cytokinesis in a *Drosophila* egg chamber leaves cells joined by ring canals. Colocalization of actin *(red)* and the ring canal protein *kelch (green)* in the ring canals makes them appear *yellow*. In the *Drosophila* egg chamber, ring canals connect nurse cells to each other and to the oocyte. Late in oocyte development, a contraction of the nurse cells forces much of their cytoplasmic contents through the ring canals and into the oocyte. This is one way in which the oocyte gains the stockpile of components that are needed for early development of the fly embryo. (Courtesy of Reed Kelso and Lynn Cooley, Yale University, New Haven, Connecticut.)

phase B moves the GTPase into the bud, where it is activated.

The MEN activates a phosphatase, Cdc14p, by releasing it from sequestration in the nucleolus. Cdc14p inhibits Cdk kinase activity in two ways: First, it inhibits the degradation of a Cdk inhibitor protein, which accumulates and inhibits the Cdk; second, it dephosphorylates Cdh1, which binds the APC/C and triggers the degradation of B-type cyclins and other proteins. Cdc14p also triggers other events during anaphase, including the transfer of chromosomal passenger proteins to the central spindle.

In fission yeast, proteins homologous to the MEN drive the cell out of mitosis. It is not known whether animal cells use a similar program to promote the exit from mitosis. Cdc14 phosphatase is required for cytokinesis in *C. elegans,* but the contributions of other components of the mitotic exit network have not yet been established.

ACKNOWLEDGMENTS

Thanks go to Susan Biggins, Kevin Hardwick, and Bruce Nicklas for their suggestions on revisions to this chapter.

SELECTED READINGS

Albertson R, Riggs B, Sullivan W: Membrane traffic: A driving force in cytokinesis. Trends Cell Biol 15:92-101, 2005.

Balasubramanian MK, Bi E, Glotzer M: Comparative analysis of cytokinesis in budding yeast, fission yeast and animal cells. Curr Biol 14:R806-R818, 2004.

Burgess DR, Chang F: Site selection for the cleavage furrow at cytokinesis. Trends Cell Biol 15:156-162, 2005.

Collas P, Courvalin J-C: Sorting nuclear membrane proteins at mitosis. Trends Cell Biol 10:5-8, 2000.

Hirano T: Chromosome cohesion, condensation, and separation. Annu Rev Biochem 69:115-144, 2000.

Jürgens G: Plant cytokinesis: Fission by fusion. Trends Cell Biol 15:277-283, 2005.

Mitchison TJ, Salmon ED: Mitosis: A history of division. Nat Cell Biol 3:E17-E21, 2001.

Nasmyth K, Peters JM, Uhlmann F: Splitting the chromosome: Cutting the ties that bind sister chromatids. Science 288:1379-1385, 2000.

Piekny A, Werner M, Glozer M: Cytokinesis: Welcome to the Rho zone. Trends Cell Biol 15:651-658, 2005.

Rappaport R: Cytokinesis in Animal Cells: Developmental and Cell Biology Series. Cambridge, England, Cambridge University Press, 1996.

Sharp DJ, Rogers GC, Scholey JM: Microtubule motors in mitosis. Nature 407:41-47, 2000.

Sullivan SM, Maddock JR: Bacterial division: Finding the dividing line. Curr Biol 10:R249-R252, 2000.

Vagnarelli P, Earnshaw WC: Chromosomal passengers: The four dimensional regulation of mitotic events. Chromosoma 113:211-222, 2004.

Von Dassow G, Bement WM: A ring-like template for abscission. Dev Cell 9:578-580, 2005.

Wittmann T, Hyman A, Desai A: The spindle: A dynamic assembly of microtubules and motors. Nat Cell Biol 3:E28-E34, 2001.

CHAPTER 45

Meiosis

Meiosis (from the Greek, meaning "reduction") is a specialized program of two coupled cell divisions used by eukaryotes to maintain the proper chromosome number for the species during sexual reproduction. The number of chromosomes is halved in meiosis; therefore, the subsequent fusion of male and female gametes restores the proper chromosome number for the species. The reduction in chromosome number is achieved by randomly separating **homologous chromosomes,** each pair of which is composed of one chromosome donated by the mother and one donated by the father. This pairing and subsequent separation of homologous chromosomes are typically made possible by genetic recombination, which occurs during the lengthy and complex prophase of the first meiotic division. The random segregation of homologous chromosomes and the genetic recombination that make this possible form the physical basis of the laws of classical genetics, first proposed by Gregor Mendel in 1866.

The unique events of meiosis occur in the first division, termed **meiosis I** (Figs. 45-1 and 45-2). Because the daughter cells have half the number of chromosomes, meiosis I is also known as the **reductional division.** The second division, **meiosis II,** is similar in most respects to mitosis: Sister chromatids segregate from each other, and the number of chromosomes remains the same (Box 45-1; see also Chapter 44). Meiosis II is called the **equational division.** Meiosis is an ancient process that occurs in virtually all higher eukaryotes, including the animal, fungal, and plant kingdoms.

Each human somatic cell has 23 pairs of homologous chromosomes (46 in all). One of each pair is donated by each parent in the egg and sperm, respectively. The number of homologs, 23, is known as the **haploid** chromosome number. In animals, the only haploid cells are gametes (sperm and eggs). At fertilization, haploid gametes fuse to form a zygote, restoring the **diploid** chromosome number of 46. In plants, the haploid phase is represented by gametophytes, which produce ovules and pollen. In most fungi, such as yeasts, haploid and diploid forms are alternate phases of the life cycle.

Much of our knowledge of meiosis is based on studies from the budding yeast, *Saccharomyces cerevisiae.* The use of powerful yeast genetic analysis has enabled an extensive study of the role of particular gene products in meiosis in vivo. Furthermore, because yeast meiosis produces four equivalent spores, it is possible to examine all products of meiosis genetically and biochemically.

Thanks go to Maria del Mar Carmena at the University of Edinburgh for her contributions to this revision of the first-edition chapter.

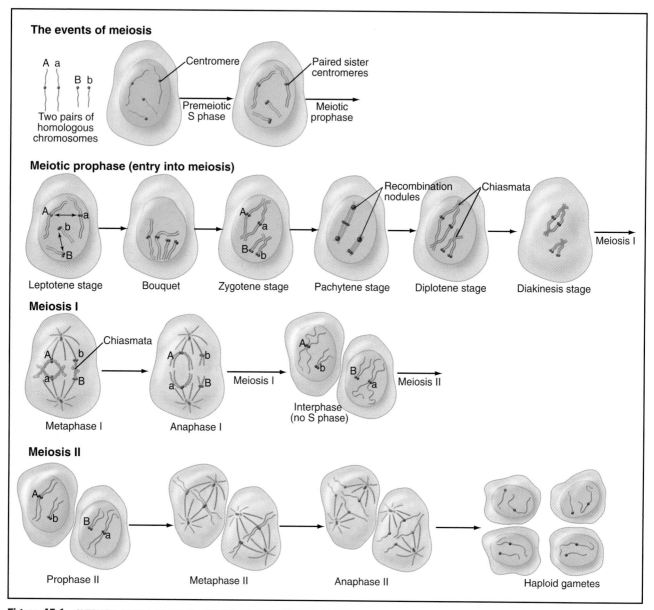

Figure 45-1 OVERVIEW OF THE PHASES OF MEIOSIS, SHOWING IMPORTANT STRUCTURES AND REGULATORY MOLECULES. See the text for a detailed explanation.

Meiosis: An Essential Process for Sexual Reproduction

Without meiosis, there would be no sex because every fusion of gametes would increase the number of chromosomes in the progeny. Sexual reproduction is an important survival strategy that offers organisms a mechanism for altering the genetic makeup of offspring. This strategy has been conserved throughout higher eukaryotes and is inextricably linked with the mechanism of meiosis.

Homologous (maternal and paternal) chromosomes separate from each other in meiosis I. For each pair of

homologs, the choice of spindle orientation in meiosis I is random (i.e., each homolog has two equivalent options for the direction to migrate). Thus, for humans (with 23 pairs of homologous chromosomes), each gamete has 2^{23} (more than 8 million) possible chromosome complements as a result of the independent assortment of subtly different (polymarphic) chromosomes alone. This process does not create new versions of genes, but it guarantees the production of offspring with novel *combinations* of chromosomes.

Meiosis I also produces novel *versions* of chromosomes by exchange of DNA segments between homologs. This occurs because each chromosome must

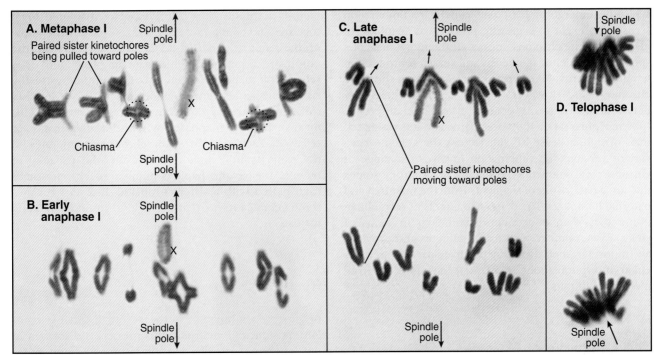

Figure 45-2 First meiotic division stages from the grasshopper *Pyrgomorpha conica* (2n in males = 18 autosomes + 1 X chromosome). **A,** Metaphase I. **B,** Onset of anaphase I. **C,** Anaphase I. **D,** Late anaphase I spermatocytes stained with lactopropionic orcein. All chromosomes are telocentric. Seven bivalents shown in the metaphase I spermatocyte have a single chiasma, while the two bivalents that are observed at the extremes have two chiasmata. The sex chromosome (X) remains unpaired and moves to a single spindle pole. (Images courtesy of José A. Suja and Julio S. Rufas, Universidad Autónoma de Madrid, Spain.)

BOX 45-1
Important Differences between Meiosis and Mitosis

Meiosis involves two cell divisions. The two meiotic divisions are preceded by a round of DNA replication. There is no DNA replication between meiosis I and meiosis II.

The products of meiosis are haploid. The products of mitosis are diploid.

The products of meiosis are genetically different. After recombination and random assortment of homologs in meiosis I, the sister chromatids that segregate in meiosis II are different from each other. In normal mitosis, sister chromatids are identical.

Prophase is longer in meiosis I. Proper orientation and segregation of homologous chromosomes is achieved thanks to the pairing, synapsis (synaptonemal complex formation), and recombination that occur in a lengthened prophase during the first meiotic division. In humans, mitotic prophase lasts well under an hour, while meiotic prophase lasts many days in males and many years in females.

Recombination is increased in meiosis. Recombination occurs in prophase I of meiosis at a rate 100-fold to 1000-fold higher than that in mitosis. The process has two main consequences: the formation of chiasmata and the introduction of genetic variation. Chiasmata are structures that physically link the homologous chromosomes after crossover and play an essential role in meiotic chromosome segregation.

Kinetochore behavior differs in meiosis. During meiosis I, kinetochores of sister chromatids attach to spindle microtubules emanating from the same pole. Homologous kinetochore pairs connect to opposite poles. In mitosis, sister kinetochores attach to spindle microtubules coming from opposite poles.

Chromatid cohesion differs in meiosis. Sister chromatid cohesion is essential for orientation of bivalents (paired homologous chromosomes) on the metaphase I spindle. During anaphase of meiosis I, cohesion is destroyed between sister chromatid arms, and chiasmata are released to allow segregation of homologs. Cohesion at sister centromeres persists until the onset of anaphase II, when it is lost to permit segregation of sisters. In prometaphase of meiosis II, sister chromatids are joined only by the centromeres, whereas at the beginning of mitotic prometaphase, sisters are joined all along the arms.

typically undergo at least one genetic recombination (crossover) event to segregate properly at anaphase of meiosis I. If the chromosomes of all the individuals of a species were identical, meiosis and sexual reproduction would only provide different combinations of the same chromosomes. However, human chromosomes vary between individuals, averaging about one difference (polymorphism) per 1000 base pairs, and it is estimated that, overall, at least 10^6 sites across the genome have variant versions. Recombination involves exchange of chromosomal segments, producing new chromosomes that are a patchwork of segments from the maternal and paternal homologs. The combined effects of recombination and random assortment of homologs in meiosis I yields a vast number of different gametes and provides an important source of genetic diversity that permits eukaryotic populations to adapt to changing environmental conditions.

The Language of Meiosis

Meiosis can be confusing because it has a language of its own, characterized by a number of unusual terms. The best way to understand meiosis is in terms of the essential biological processes that are involved. This reduces the process to only three essential key terms: **pairing, recombination,** and **segregation.** Each is discussed in detail later in this chapter, so they are defined only briefly here.

Pairing is the alignment of homologous chromosomes with one another within the cell nucleus. There are two stages of pairing. In *alignment*, DNA sequences on one chromosome find the corresponding DNA sequences on the homologous chromosome in the presence of the billions of base pairs of DNA in the cell nucleus. Recombination drives the pairing process but is completed later. In the second stage, *synapsis,* the paired homologous chromosomes become intimately associated with one another. A specialized scaffolding structure called the synaptonemal complex mediates this process.

Recombination, the physical exchange of DNA between homologous chromosomes, is the key event governing chromosome behavior during meiotic prophase. Recombination drives the pairing process and can occur without synapsis under specialized circumstances. Specialized chromatin structures called **chiasmata** (from the Greek, meaning "X-shaped cross") form at sites where recombination has been completed. These chiasmata keep homologous chromosomes paired with one another until anaphase of meiosis I.

Meiosis is all about the *segregation* of the paired homologous chromosomes. This process shows some key differences from mitosis (Box 45-1). When the homologs are balanced at the metaphase plate of the

meiosis I spindle, it is the chiasmata that hold them together and counteract the pulling force of the spindle on the kinetochores (Fig. 45-2). Cohesion between the chromatid arms holds chiasmata in place until it is released at anaphase of meiosis I. Centromeres of the sister chromatids remain associated with one another throughout meiosis I until anaphase of meiosis II. This means that at anaphase, when the chiasmata are released, each pair of sister chromatids migrates to the same spindle pole. As a result, the progeny of meiosis I have the haploid number of chromosomes each paired with a sister chromatid. Box 45-2 reviews some genetics terms that are helpful in understanding meiosis.

Recombination

Because recombination is the key to the behavior of chromosomes in meiosis I, this process is discussed in detail herein to provide a mechanistic underpinning for understanding later events. Meiotic recombination is very similar to the process of homologous recombinational repair of double-strand DNA breaks in somatic cells (review Box 43-1 and Fig. 43-15 as a prelude to studying meiotic recombination).

Two key differences distinguish meiotic recombination from the repair process in somatic cells. First, meiotic cells create double-strand DNA breaks on purpose, using a specialized enzyme called Spo11. Second, somatic cells repair DNA breaks using the corresponding DNA sequence on their sister chromatid as a guide. Meiotic cells use the homologous chromosome instead. The mechanism for this switch in selectivity is not known.

Spo11 generates programmed double-strand DNA breaks very early during meiotic prophase (Fig. 45-3). Spo11 is a type II DNA topoisomerase (see Chapter 13, under the section titled "Proteins of the Mitotic Chromosome and Chromosome Scaffold") that cleaves both DNA strands in a reaction that produces a covalent linkage between a tyrosine on the enzyme and the cleaved phosphodiester backbone. Where it has been measured, Spo11 creates about threefold to fivefold more DNA breaks than ultimately complete the recombination pathway to produce reciprocal exchanges of DNA between homologous chromosomes, or **crossovers.** An alternative pathway is thought to process the excess breaks, producing **noncrossover** events (Box 45-2 and Fig. 45-3I-J). Each pair of homologous chromosomes thus undergoes many noncrossover events and a very few crossover events (often only one) during meiosis I prophase.

In both mice and yeast, double-strand breaks generated by Spo11 are required for normal segregation of homologous chromosomes. In *Spo11*-null mice,

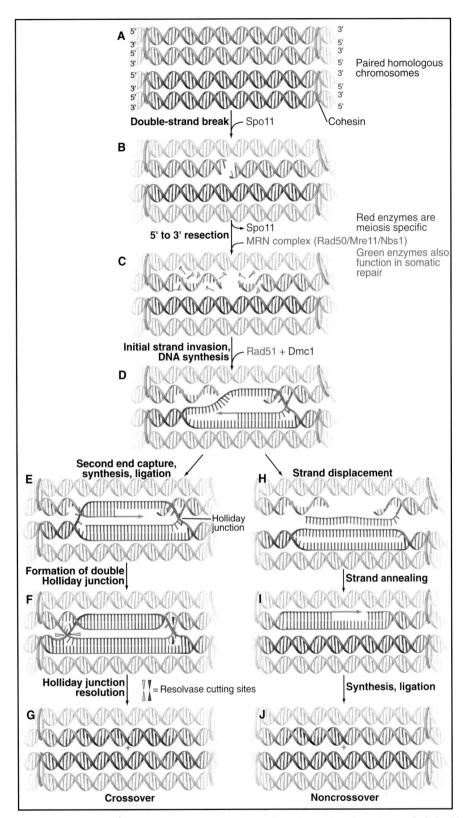

Figure 45-3 THE EVENTS OF RECOMBINATION. Recombination occurs between homologs rather than sisters. **A,** Paired homologous chromosomes. Sister chromatids are held tightly together by cohesin, shown here schematically as hoops. **B,** Spo11 makes a double-strand break. **C,** Resection of the break. **D,** First strand invasion. At this point, the pathway splits in two, one outcome leading to a crossover and the other to a noncrossover. **Crossover pathway: E,** The second resected strand invades its homologous partner. New DNA synthesis fills the gaps. **F,** The resulting molecule contains a double Holliday junction (see Fig. 43-15B). If the resolvase (nuclease) cuts the double Holliday junction asymmetrically as shown (i.e., one vertical and one horizontal cut), the result is a crossover **(G).** If the cuts are symmetrical, a noncrossover molecule is produced. **Noncrossover pathway: H,** In most cases, the invading DNA strand is ejected prior to stabilization and formation of a double Holliday junction. **I,** DNA gap-filling and ligation yield a noncrossover chromosome **(J).**

BOX 45-2
Brief Overview of Genetic Terminology

A comprehensive introduction to the field of genetics is beyond the scope of this text. However, here are a number of terms used by geneticists that will assist in the understanding of the discussion of genetic recombination and its role in meiosis (also see Box 6-2).

The **genotype** of an organism is the combination of genes present on the chromosomes of that organism. The **phenotype** is the physical manifestation of the action of these gene products (i.e., the appearance and macromolecular composition of the organism). In discussing recombination, scientists typically refer to the presence or absence of specific genetic markers. Each **genetic marker** is a particular DNA sequence in or around a gene that can be monitored by examining the phenotypes of the cells that carry it. A genetic marker might be the presence of a functional gene, a mutation with altered activity, or simply a polymorphism of DNA sequence that has no known functional consequence.

A **haploid** organism has one copy of each chromosome. A **diploid** organism has two homologous copies of each chromosome. A diploid organism that is **homozygous** for a particular genetic marker has the same sequence of that particular region of the DNA on both the maternal and paternal homologous chromosomes. A **heterozygous** organism has different forms of the genetic markers on the two homologous chromosomes. Although the physical events of genetic recombination occur in both homozygotes and heterozygotes, they are most readily detected in the latter.

Two genetic markers located on different chromosomes will separate from one another in the anaphase of meiosis I 50% of the time as a result of the random distribution of chromosomes to the two spindle poles. If they are on the same chromosome, they will be *linked* to one another unless the chromosome undergoes a genetic recombination event between them. The greater the separation of two markers on one chromosome, the more likely it is for such an intervening recombination event to occur.

Two types of recombination events occur during meiosis (Fig. 45-3). The first of these—**noncrossover** events (frequently referred to as **gene conversion**)—may involve the *loss* of one or more genetic markers. Noncrossover events are the most common outcome of the programmed double-strand DNA breaks that occur during leptotene. They are thought to involve the invasion of a double helix by a region of single-stranded DNA with complementary sequence but then ejection of this sequence before assembly of a Holliday junction and completion of recombination.

The second type of recombination event—**crossing over**—involves the physical breakage and reunion of DNA strands on two different chromosomes, typically producing a balanced exchange of DNA sequences. This is what most people think of as recombination. In recombination by crossing over, the makeup of genetic markers remains constant; it is the linkage between different markers that changes.

---

recombination is not initiated, and synapsis, if it occurs at all, is aberrant, often involving nonhomologous chromosomes (Fig. 45-4). In these mutant mice, spermatocytes die by apoptosis early in meiotic prophase, and oocytes die somewhat later. In contrast, the nematode *Caenorhabditis elegans* and the fruit fly *Drosophila melanogaster* do not require Spo11-induced double-strand breaks for synapsis of homologous chromosomes.

Once the DNA double-strand breaks have been produced, they are processed by the $5' \rightarrow 3'$ exonuclease MRN (Mre11/Rad50/Nbs1), which chews back one strand of the double helix (a process called resection), leaving single-stranded tails at the $3'$ end of the DNA molecules (Fig. 45-3C; see also Fig. 43-15). The same exonuclease functions in somatic DNA repair and in meiotic recombination.

Next, the single-stranded tails "invade" the other chromosomes, looking for complementary DNA sequences. This process is driven by Rad51 and Dmc1, two proteins that are related to the *E. coli* RecA protein,

which is essential for DNA recombination in bacteria. These proteins polymerize into nucleoprotein filaments on DNA and use ATP hydrolysis to catalyze homologous pairing and strand exchange reactions. The process inserts a single-stranded region of DNA into a double helix, displacing one of the two paired strands. Dmc1 functions only in meiosis, but Rad51 has other essential functions as well. Dmc1 may promote the search for homologous chromosomes, rather than sister chromatids as occurs in somatic DNA repair. Mutants that lack Dmc1 are defective in homologous chromosome pairing. Rad51p and Dmc1p are found in structures called **early recombination nodules** that are distributed along the chromosome axes early in meiosis (Fig. 45-9).

It is now believed that if only one single strand successfully invades the homologous chromosome, the outcome is a noncrossover event, whereas invasion of both single-strand tails leads to crossovers. The double invasion produces branched intermediates known as double **Holliday junctions** (Fig. 45-3F–G; see also Fig.

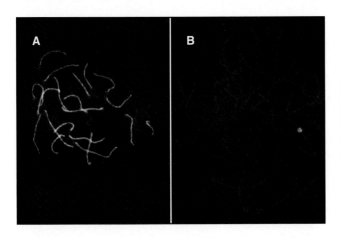

Figure 45-4 Pairing of homologous chromosomes is severely disrupted in the Spo11 mutant. Pachytene chromosomes from wild-type mice **(A)** and mice in which the Spo11 gene has been disrupted **(B)**. (From Baudat F, Manova K, Yuen JP, et al: Chromosome synapsis defects and sexually dimorphic meiotic progression in mice lacking Spo11. Mol Cell 6:989–998, 2000.)

43-15B). These are then cleaved by as yet unknown nucleases and converted to mature crossover recombination products.

A second system for segregating homologs in meiosis I has been found in fruit flies and yeast. This process of **achiasmate segregation** functions on chromosomes that have *not* undergone genetic recombination. Flies have two types of achiasmate segregation, depending on whether homologous or nonhomologous chromosomes are involved. One model for homologous achiasmate segregation proposes that nonrecombined chromosomes remain paired owing to stickiness of heterochromatin at the end of pachytene and, as a result, segregate properly in anaphase I of meiosis. Heterologous achiasmate segregation uses an entirely distinct but unknown mechanism that does not require previous physical pairing of the chromosomes that segregate from one another.

D. melanogaster males do not bother with any of this, do not recombine, and yet still segregate their chromosomes happily in meiosis. So all the complication of meiotic recombination is not the only way to produce haploid gametes. This might be regarded as a cruel joke of evolution by those students who find all the Greek terms of meiotic nomenclature to be daunting.

Tracking the Homologous Chromosomes through the Stages of Meiotic Prophase I

Pairing and recombination of homologous chromosomes take place during **prophase** of meiosis I. In the discussion of these processes, it is necessary to refer to the five stages of meiotic prophase: leptotene, zygotene, pachytene, diplotene, and diakinesis (Fig. 45-1). As the understanding of meiotic prophase advances, the sig-

nificance of these stages is being reassessed. In particular, these morphologic stages do not correspond directly to the steps of meiotic recombination, as was assumed previously.

The start of **leptotene** (from the Greek, meaning "thin ribbon") is defined by the first visible condensation of the chromosomes. Paired sister chromatids begin to condense as arrays of loops flanking a single dense protein-containing axis (Fig. 45-5A–B). This axis consists of proteins that play a role in mitotic chromosome structure as well as proteins that are specialized for meiotic chromosomes. For example, the cohesin complex is a prominent component of this axial structure (see Fig. 13-19), but several of its components are replaced by meiosis-specific forms. According to recent models, recombination begins during leptotene with the formation of double-strand breaks, which are processed and a few selected for crossovers. By the end of leptotene, homologous chromosomes are aligned loosely about 400 nm apart (Fig. 45-6D–G).

During **zygotene** (from the Greek, meaning "yoke ribbon"), the next portion of prophase, homolog pairing, goes to completion in a process known as **synapsis** (Fig. 45-5C–D). This involves the assembly of a protein scaffold, the **synaptonemal complex.** Also in early zygotene, the telomeres cluster in a region of the nuclear envelope, giving rise to the "bouquet" arrangement of chromosomes (see next section). In **pachytene** (from the Greek, meaning "thick ribbon"), synapsis is complete, with the homologs joined together along their lengths by synaptonemal complex (Fig. 45-5E). During pachytene, crossovers are believed to mature into structures called **chiasmata** that will hold homologous chromosomes together through meiosis I metaphase.

Early in **diplotene** (from the Greek, meaning "double ribbon"), the synaptonemal complex disassembles, and chromosomes decondense (Fig. 45-5F). Later on, they start condensing again. Sister chromatids remain closely associated, whereas homologous chromosomes tend to

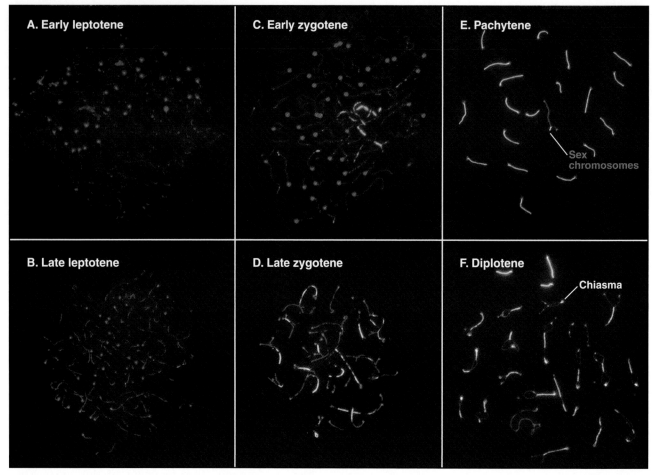

Figure 45-5   IMMUNOFLUORESCENCE IMAGES OF PROPHASE I SUBSTAGES IN MOUSE SPERMATOCYTES. These images demonstrate the pairing and synapsis of homologous chromosomes by localization of the synaptonemal complex proteins SCP3 (a component of the axial elements *[red]*) and SCP1 (a component of the transverse filaments that is present only when homologs are synapsed *[green]*). Centromeres are *blue*. (Images courtesy of Paula Cohen, Cornell University, Ithaca, New York.)

separate from each other, held by the chiasmata. This part of meiotic prophase may last for days or years, depending on the sex and organism (up to 45 years or more in female humans).

In females, the chromosomes are very actively transcribed during diplotene, as the egg busily stores up materials for use during the first few divisions of embryonic development. In animal diplotene cells, the chromosomes have prominent loops and are known as **lampbrush chromosomes** (see Fig. 13-13). These loops are visible because the DNA is massively coated with nascent RNA transcripts and their associated proteins.

Diakinesis (from the Greek, meaning "across movement") is the prometaphase of meiosis I. Following nuclear envelope breakdown, homologous chromosomes become particularly short and condensed. At metaphase I, the bivalents (pairs of homologous chromosomes) are aligned at a metaphase plate (Figs. 45-1 and 45-2). Each homolog (a pair of tightly linked sister chromatids) is attached to a single pole of the meiotic spindle. Chiasmata resist the pulling forces within the spindle.

At anaphase I, the release of cohesion along the chromosome arms (but not between centromeres of sister chromatids) allows chiasmata to be resolved and homologs to move to opposite spindle poles. After telophase I, there is no DNA replication, and cells enter directly in the second meiotic division, which is mechanistically similar to mitosis. In the eggs of most female vertebrates, meiosis is arrested at metaphase II until fertilization.

The normal separation of chromosomes or chromatids is referred to as **disjunction** (disjoining). Mistakes in this separation are referred to as **nondisjunction.** Nondisjunction in meiosis I and II results in the production of gametes with either too many or too few chromosomes, a condition known as **aneuploidy.**

Chromosomal *Ikebana:* The Bouquet Stage

During leptotene, the chromosomal telomeres attach apparently randomly to the surface of the nuclear enve-

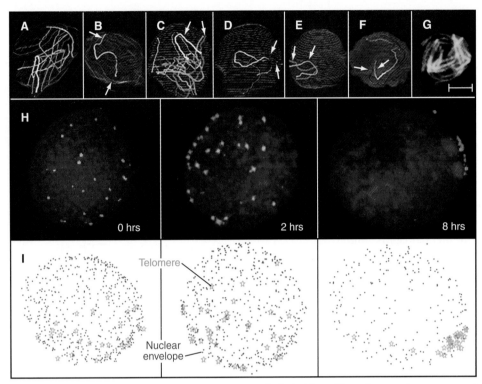

Figure 45-6 CHROMOSOMAL MOVEMENTS DURING EARLY MEIOTIC PROPHASE. **A–G, Pairing of homologous chromosomes during leptotene in the ascomycete *Sordaria*.** Scale bar is 1 μm in **A–F** and 5 μm in **G. A–B,** In early leptotene, homologous chromosomes (visualized in panels **A–F** by electron microscope reconstructions of serial-sectioned nuclei) are not yet aligned with one another. **C–E,** In mid-leptotene, regions of some homologs begin to align. (In panel **D,** only the telomeres have aligned. In panel **E,** the pair of homologs is fully aligned.) **F,** The alignment of homologs is complete by late leptotene. **G,** The alignment of homologs also can be seen by light microscopy using Spo76-GFP, a component of the chromosome axes. **H–I, Stages of formation of the bouquet arrangement in rye. H,** Telomeres *(green)* were detected in nuclei by in situ hybridization (see Fig. 13-15) after 0, 2, and 8 hours in culture. Chromatin is *red.* **I,** Three-dimensional models of the nuclei (nuclear periphery *[red dots]*, telomere position *[green stars]*). (A–G, Adapted from Tesse S, Aurora Storlazzi A, Kleckner N, et al: Localization and roles of Ski8p protein in Sordaria meiosis and delineation of three mechanistically distinct steps of meiotic homolog juxtaposition. Proc Natl Acad Sci U S A 100:12865–12870, 2003. Copyright 2003 National Academy of Sciences, USA. H–I, Adapted from Carlton PM, Cowan CR, Cande WZ: Directed motion of telomeres in the formation of the meiotic bouquet revealed by time course and simulation analysis. Mol Biol Cell 14:2832–2843, 2003. Adapted from *Molecular Biology of the Cell* [Mol Biol Cell 14:2832–2843, 2003; published on-line before print as 10.1091/mbc.E02-11-0760] with the permission of The American Society for Cell Biology.)

lope. As leptotene progresses, in most organisms these telomeres gradually move together to occupy the region of the nuclear envelope closest to the centrosome (spindle pole body in yeasts [Fig. 45-6]). In this region, chromosome axes attach to a dense plaque on the inner surface of the nuclear envelope. This clustering of telomeres in the nucleus requires the presence of microtubules in the cytoplasm. How this process is coordinated across the nuclear envelope is not known. Telomere clustering appears to be maximal at the leptotene-zygotene transition, when the chromosomes radiating into the nuclear interior resemble a bouquet of flowers, hence the name "bouquet stage." The bouquet is a nearly universal feature of this phase of meiosis, although ironically, the popular model organisms *C. elegans* and *D. melanogaster* are exceptions.

The role of this dramatic reorganization of the nuclear interior is still being debated. Homologous chromosome pairing and the initiation of recombination precede and do not absolutely require bouquet formation. However, bouquet formation does make meiotic prophase faster and more efficient; homolog pairing is slow in mutants that are defective in bouquet formation. One attractive proposal is that formation of the bouquet increases the efficiency of strand invasion during recombination. It is possible that this meiosis-specific reorganization of the nucleus is one factor that biases the strand exchange in meiotic recombination toward homologous chromosomes instead of sister chromatids, as occurs in mitotic DNA repair.

Dispersal of the bouquet is linked to the recombination pathway, possibly to completion of the processing of noncrossover events. In any event, the bouquet scatters at pachytene, with dispersal of the telomeres on the membrane, followed by centrosome separation. By diplotene, the telomeres detach from the nuclear membrane.

Pairing and Synapsis in More Detail

Pairing describes the side-by-side alignment of homologous chromosomes at a distance. Homologs are paired in nonmeiotic cells in some organisms, such as the fruit fly *D. melanogaster* and budding yeast *Saccharomyces cerevisiae,* but not in vertebrates. As was mentioned earlier, pairing involves a search of homologous sequences for one another. The entire genome is scanned during this process, because even when a single gene is transposed onto a different chromosome, this gene can still find its homologous partner. In certain organisms, such as *C. elegans,* pairing can involve specialized DNA sequences; however, this does not generally appear to be the case.

The earliest pairing events involve a tendency of homologous chromosome territories to move together in the nucleus even before leptotene chromosome condensation. The mechanism is unknown. Next, programmed double-strand breaks created by Spo11 initiate the recombination pathway during leptotene. In parallel, the condensing homologous chromosomes align with one another at a distance of about 400 nm (Figs. 45-6 and 45-7). Genetic analysis in budding yeast revealed that mutants defective in the earliest stages of recombination are also defective in homolog pairing.

The process of homolog alignment that follows the generation of double-strand breaks almost certainly involves the invasion of neighboring DNA duplexes by single-stranded DNA coated with Rad51 and Dmc1. Thus, the process of recombination has an extremely important role both in the exchange of genetic material and in the mechanics of chromosome behavior during meiotic prophase. There is probably more to homolog pairing than just meiotic recombination, however. Homologous chromosomes still pair in some systems that lack recombination (e.g., certain *D. melanogaster* recombination mutants), synaptonemal complex formation (asynaptic mutants in yeast), or both (e.g., normal *D. melanogaster* males).

Homolog pairing initiated during leptotene becomes much more intimate during **synapsis** as the chromosomes become linked by transverse fibers to form the **synaptonemal complex.** This structure looks roughly like railroad tracks with a third rail running down the center (Figs. 45-7 and 45-8). The two outer rails, 90 to 100 nm apart, traditionally termed *lateral elements,* are the axes of the paired sister chromatids. For the sake of simplicity, this chapter refers to them as *axial* elements throughout meiosis I. Thin transverse filaments lying perpendicular to the axial elements appear to connect them to each other and to the central element (the "third rail"). Synaptonemal complex formation is initiated at a limited number of sites along the paired homologous chromosomes. These often correspond to sites where recombination events will mature into crossovers. Synapsis begins during zygotene, and by pachytene, a continuous synaptonemal complex is observed between homologous chromosomes (Fig. 45-5C–E).

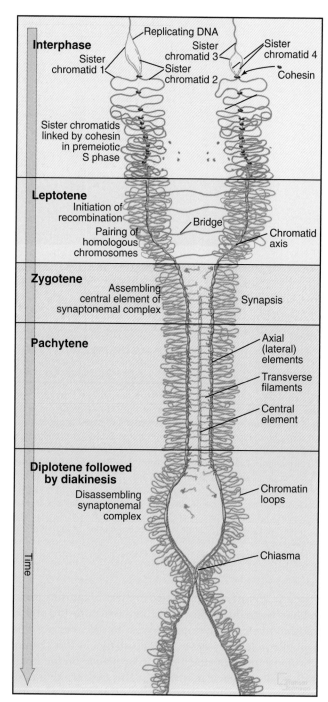

Figure 45-7 STRUCTURAL ORGANIZATION OF THE HOMOLOGOUS CHROMOSOMES AND SYNAPTONEMAL COMPLEX DURING THE VARIOUS STAGES OF MEIOTIC PROPHASE.

It used to be thought that the synaptonemal complex aligns homologous chromosomes in preparation for recombination, but it is now clear that homolog pairing and the initiation of recombination precede synapsis. Furthermore, yeast mutants that affect synaptonemal complex formation do not affect pairing (i.e., homologous chromosomes pair but do not synapse),

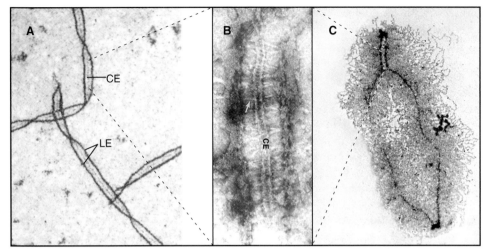

Figure 45-8 SELECTED ELECTRON MICROGRAPHS OF THE SYNAPTONEMAL COMPLEX. **A,** Low-magnification view of maize synaptonemal complexes stained with silver. The lateral (LE) and central elements (CE) are clearly seen. **B,** A negatively stained cricket synaptonemal complex following treatment with deoxyribonuclease (DNase). The central element (CE) and transverse filaments *(arrow)* are visible. **C,** A whole mount of zygotene chromosome of the silk moth. Cells in meiotic prophase were swollen and then lysed under gentle conditions with detergent. The chromosomes were then centrifuged onto thin carbon films so that they could be examined by electron microscopy. The axial elements are easily seen on this chromosome. Chromatin loops radiate outward from both the unpaired axial elements and the paired lateral elements (where synapsis has occurred). (A, Adapted from Gillies CB: Electron microscopy of spread maize pachytene synaptonemal complexes. Chromosoma 83:575–591, 1981. B, Adapted from Solari AJ, Moses MJ: The structure of the central region in the synaptonemal complexes of hamster and cricket spermatocytes. J Cell Biol 56:145–152, 1973, by copyright permission of The Rockefeller University Press. C, From Rattner JB, Goldsmith M, Hamkalo BA: Chromatin organization during meiotic prophase of *Bombyx mori.* Chromosoma 79:215–224, 1980.)

and under certain artificial circumstances, it is possible for nonhomologous chromosomes to undergo synapsis.

It is more likely that synapsis brings recombination to a close and converts recombination sites into chiasmata that hold homologous chromosomes paired until anaphase of meiosis I. Double Holliday junctions produced during recombination persist throughout most of pachytene but are then converted to mature crossover and noncrossover recombination products, presumably within the synaptonemal complex.

Synaptonemal Complex Components

Both genetic and biochemical approaches have identified components of the synaptonemal complex. Perhaps the best studied is the budding yeast protein Zip1p, which is found in mature synaptonemal complex, between the axial elements (Fig. 45-9). Zip1p is predicted to have extensive regions of coiled-coil and is thought to assemble into a rod-shaped dimer. If the length of the Zip1p coiled-coil is altered, then synaptonemal complexes are produced in which the spacing between axial elements is altered. In *zip1* mutants, recombination is initiated but fails to be completed at about 10% of sites. As a result, cells arrest late in prophase (see later discussion of the so-called pachytene checkpoint in the section titled "Cell-Cycle Regulation

of Meiotic Events"). In mammals, a protein called Scp1 is localized in the transverse filaments. Scp1 has no sequence similarity to Zip1p, but both share a common organization: a coiled-coil flanked by two globular domains.

Several protein components of the axial elements (sister chromatid axes) have also been identified. One

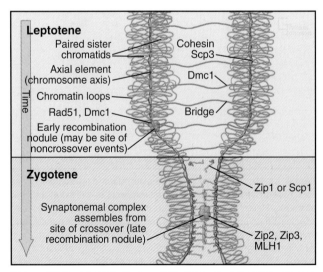

Figure 45-9 DIAGRAM OF THE HOMOLOGOUS CHROMOSOMES AND SYNAPTONEMAL COMPLEX SHOWING THE LOCATIONS OF A NUMBER OF WELL-CHARACTERIZED COMPONENTS.

of these, Scp3, interacts with the cohesin complex (see later) and also with Rad51p and Dmc1p. In Scp3 knockout mice, the axial elements are much less prominent, and the axis of the condensed chromosome is about twofold longer. Other proteins of the synaptonemal complex, including Scp1, can still assemble, but chromosomes in male germ cells lack chiasmata and are unpaired. As a result, the germ cells die in pachytene/diplotene. It thus appears that in the mouse, Scp3 is required for axial condensation of meiotic chromosomes and for normal cohesion between sister chromatids, leading to formation of stable chiasmata. Human males who are mutant in Scp3 lack chiasmata, fail to segregate chromosomes normally in meiosis, and produce no viable sperm.

Chiasmata

The role of recombination in regulating chromosome dynamics during meiosis is most evident during the segregation of homologous chromosomes in meiosis I, mediated by chiasmata. Chiasmata (singular: chiasma) are specialized chromosomal structures that hold the homologous chromosomes together until anaphase I (Figs. 45-1 and 45-10). They are formed at sites where programmed DNA breaks generated by Spo11 undergo the full recombination pathway to generate crossovers.

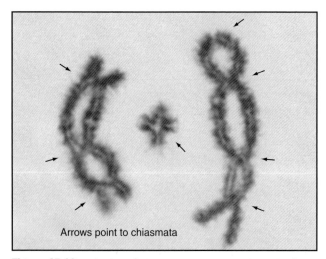

Arrows point to chiasmata

Figure 45-10 BIVALENTS (PAIRED HOMOLOGOUS CHROMOSOMES) ARE HELD TOGETHER BY CHIASMATA AFTER DISASSEMBLY OF THE SYNAPTONEMAL COMPLEX. Here, three diplotene bivalents from the grasshopper species *Chothippus jucundus* are held together by three *(left)*, one *(middle)*, and four *(right)* chiasmata. The *middle* cross-shaped bivalent is telocentric; the other two longer bivalents are submetacentric. (For an explanation of the terminology, see Fig. 12-2.) Lactopropionic orcein staining. (Courtesy of José A. Suja and Julio S. Rufas, Universidad Autónoma de Madrid, Spain.)

It is not known how crossover events, which represent exchanges of DNA sequence information, get turned into chiasmata, the physical structures that link homologous chromosomes during meiosis I. The ultrastructure of chiasmata remains a mystery, but presumably in addition to the intertwined DNA molecules, the protein structures of the chromosome axes are also physically exchanged. Thus, each chiasma consists of two unperturbed sister chromatid arms intertwined with two recombinant arms in which the DNA molecules and their associated protein structures have been spliced. This structure is held in place on the chromosome by cohesion between the sister chromatid arms between the chiasma and the telomeres. One consequence is that chiasmata close to telomeres are unstable, as the length of sister chromatid arms between the chiasmata and the telomeres is insufficient to produce stable cohesion. Thus, crossover formation too close to the telomeres of the homologous chromosomes can lead to failure of chromosome segregation in meiosis.

Only one chiasma per pair of homolog arms is needed to hold homologous chromosomes together during meiosis I. Humans have 39 such arms on the 23 pairs of homologous chromosomes, if one excludes the five acrocentric short arms, which do not normally recombine. Remarkably, there is typically only one chiasma produced for most arms; human males typically have 46 to 53 chiasmata (Fig. 45-11).

Since Spo11 creates many more DNA breaks early in meiosis, a mechanism called **crossover interference** limits the number of breaks that are processed to form crossovers and chiasmata. The designation of a particular DNA break to form a crossover results in a wide zone of surrounding breaks becoming noncrossovers.

The phenomenon of **crossover interference** has been defined genetically for almost 100 years, but its mechanism is unknown. It was thought to be mediated by the synaptonemal complex, since organisms such as the fission yeast *Schizosaccharomyces pombe* and the mold *Aspergillus nidulans* that naturally lack synaptonemal complex also lack interference. However, recent finding show that interference is established and transmitted along the chromosome axes long before the synaptonemal complex forms.

Interestingly, the length of the meiotic chromosome axes (i.e., the length of the synaptonemal complex) is directly proportional to the frequency of meiotic recombination rather than the actual length of DNA in the chromosome. For example, in human females, the synaptonemal complex is roughly 50% longer than it is in males, and females undergo recombination at about twice the frequency of males. This shows yet another link between recombination and the structural dynamics of meiotic chromosomes.

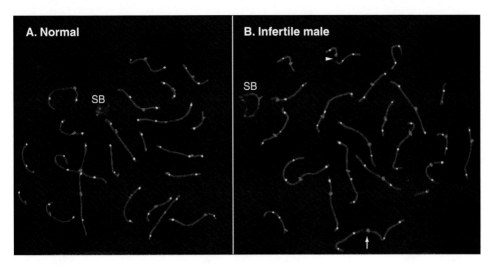

Figure 45-11 **A,** Normal pachytene spread from a testis biopsy showing synaptonemal complexes *(red),* MLH1 foci (recombination sites *[green]*), and centromeres *(blue).* **B,** Abnormal pachytene spread from an infertile patient containing one synaptonemal complex with an area of asynapsis *(arrow)* and one synaptonemal complex with a gap *(arrowhead).* SB, sex body (the paired X and Y chromosomes). (Images courtesy of Renée H. Martin, University of Calgary, Alberta, Canada.)

Cohesion and Chromosomal Movements during Meiosis I

Chromosomes in mitosis achieve a dynamic alignment at metaphase as a result of a balance of forces in the spindle. The two kinetochores of the sister chromatids are attached to opposite spindle poles, and motor proteins located on the chromosomes actively pull each chromatid toward the pole that its kinetochore faces. This force does not produce any net poleward movement during metaphase because the two sister chromatids are held together by cohesion across the centromere until the onset of anaphase (see Fig. 44-16).

In meiosis I, paired homologs (called **bivalents**) are balanced at the metaphase plate. The structure of bivalents has two important differences from that of mitotic chromosomes. First, the kinetochore of each homolog is composed of the two kinetochores of the sister chromatids fused and acting as a single unit. The structure of the meiosis I kinetochore is most easily explained if the two kinetochores are each rotated 90 degrees toward one another relative to their position on mitotic chromosomes (Fig. 45-12A). In yeast, this coorientation of sister kinetochores requires the presence of a meiosis-specific kinetochore protein—monopolin—that associates with sister kinetochores from pachytene until anaphase of meiosis I. Monopolin recruits a protein kinase to kinetochores, but the critical kinase substrates are not known. In some organisms, a strand of material visualized by a specialized silver-staining protocol connects the sister kinetochores. This physical connection is not broken in anaphase I.

A second major difference between bivalents and mitotic chromosomes is in the force that resists the poleward pulling of the kinetochores and restrains the bivalent at the spindle midzone at metaphase. In meiosis

I, this force arises from the adherence of homologs at chiasmata on the chromosome arms (Figs. 45-2 and 45-10). Thus, recombination and chiasma formation are essential parts of the mechanism that guarantees the orderly segregation of homologous chromosomes in meiotic anaphase I. However, recombination alone is not sufficient to ensure the proper segregation of bivalents at meiosis I. This is shown most clearly by the *desynaptic* mutant of maize. In this mutant, homologous chromosomes synapse apparently normally, and normal numbers of recombination events occur, producing chiasmata. However, these chiasmata frequently fall apart as the cells enter the first meiotic M phase. As a result, the homologs tend to segregate randomly in meiosis I. The underlying defect in the *desynaptic* mutation is not known, but the mutation behaves as would be expected for a defect in chromatid arm cohesion.

Work in yeasts, *D. melanogaster,* and *Xenopus laevis,* has identified a protein complex, the **cohesin complex,** that is required to hold sister chromatids together (see Fig. 44-16). Although this has not been proven, cohesin might form a ring that encircles sister chromatids, linking them to one another. In mitosis, cleavage of the cohesin component Scc1 is thought to open the ring, allowing sister chromatids to move apart.

Cohesion is regulated differently in meiosis and mitosis. After premeiotic DNA replication, cohesion keeps sister chromatids together all along the arms, and the cohesin complex makes up a significant portion of the dense axial structure that extends the length of the chromosome. The more robust structure that is seen in meiotic chromosomes may in part be explained by the presence of several meiosis-specific components of the cohesin complex, including Rec8, which fulfills the role played by Scc1 in mitosis.

Tight arm cohesion between sister chromatids causes an interesting problem for the formation of chiasmata.

Figure 45-12 CHROMOSOMAL BEHAVIOR DURING MEIOSIS I AND II. During meiosis I, sister chromatids are tightly paired along their lengths, kinetochore structure is altered, and homologs are held together at the metaphase plate by chiasmata. During anaphase I, loss of cohesion between the arms of sister chromatids releases the chiasmata and allows homologous chromosomes to segregate to opposite spindle poles. During metaphase of meiosis II, sister chromatids are held together at their centromeres. Release of centromeric cohesion at meiosis II allows the sister chromatids to segregate to opposite spindle poles.

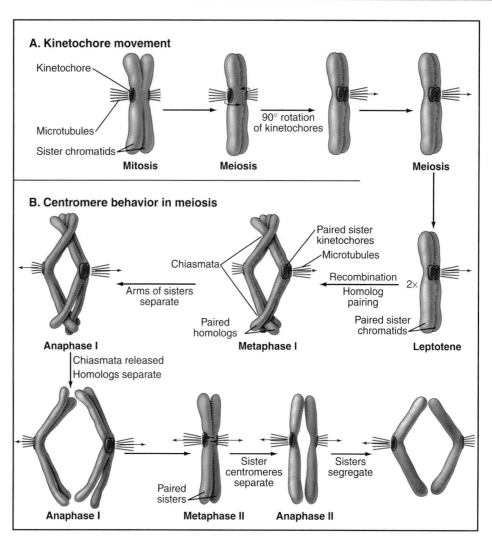

Presumably, when the DNA is exchanged in recombination, the protein backbone of the chromosome axis must also be exchanged. This process apparently occurs within the context of the synaptonemal complex and might involve significant topologic remodeling of the chromosomal axes.

Once chiasmata are assembled, they are held in place by cohesion between the arms of the sister chromatids (Figs. 45-7 and 45-12). This cohesion is retained throughout meiotic prophase and is released only at the onset of anaphase in meiosis I as Rec8 along the chromosome arms is cleaved. Separation of sister chromatid arms "dissolves" the chiasmata, allowing the paired homologous chromosomes to move to opposite spindle poles. In the meantime, the Rec8 at centromeres is protected from cleavage and continues to hold the sister chromatid centromeres tightly paired until anaphase of meiosis II. This protection requires a class of proteins called Shugoshins (from the Japanese, meaning "guardian spirit"), whose mechanism of action is being investigated. Shugoshin requires phosphorylation by Aurora B kinase to associ-

ate stably with centromeres and protect Rec8. This is another job for the chromosomal passenger complex (Fig. 44-10). Centromeric cohesion is released by cleavage of Rec8 at the onset of anaphase II in a process that resembles the release of cohesion during mitosis.

Behavior of the Sex Chromosomes in Meiosis

Of the 46 human chromosomes, the two **sex chromosomes** carry genes that define the sex of the individual. The other 22 pairs of chromosomes are called **autosomes.** Sex chromosomes and autosomes behave differently during meiosis.

Since genetic recombination is required to stabilize homologous chromosomes at the metaphase plate in meiosis I, how is this accomplished for the X and Y chromosomes? The answer in most mammals is that the X and Y chromosomes have a short region of homologous sequence (about 2.6 million base pairs in humans)

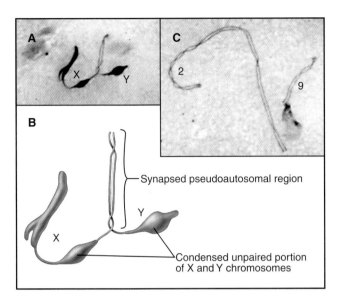

Figure 45-13 THE SEX CHROMOSOMES OF A CHINESE HAMSTER AT PACHYTENE. **A–B,** The X and Y chromosomes are paired at the pseudoautosomal region. Elsewhere, the unpaired chromatin adopts a highly condensed morphology. **C,** Autosomes are completely synapsed and show a lesser degree of condensation. (From Dresser ME, Moses MJ: Synaptonemal complex karyotyping in spermatocytes of the Chinese hamster *(Cricetulus griseus).* IV. Light and electron microscopy of synapsis and nucleolar development by silver staining. Chromosoma 76:1–22, 1980.)

that does pair and undergo genetic recombination during meiosis. This **pseudoautosomal region** must undergo genetic recombination in every meiosis I cell for the X and Y chromosomes to be partitioned correctly. Thus, the X and Y chromosomes act like short homologous chromosomes with large regions of unrelated DNA attached (Fig. 45-13). Unpaired regions of the X and Y chromosomes become highly condensed during late pachytene.

Cell-Cycle Regulation of Meiotic Events

Meiosis employs the full set of functions that regulate the division of somatic cells (see Chapters 40 to 43). However, the peculiarities of the meiotic cell cycle require further mechanisms of regulation. One major difference between meiotic cells and somatic cells is that the meiotic chromosomes must undergo recombination and form chiasmata to segregate properly at the first meiotic division. Yeasts appear to lack a mechanism to detect whether recombination has occurred. Yeast cells that are completely defective in recombination proceed through meiosis with normal timing but disastrous consequences; the chromosomes fail to align properly during meiosis I, and they assort randomly to the daughter cells. On the other hand, yeast cells can

detect the presence of stalled or abnormal recombination intermediates. Such intermediates accumulate if there are problems with the core recombination enzymes or if the assembly of the synaptonemal complex (required for the completion of recombination) is defective. When such problems are detected, cells arrest late in meiotic prophase I. This has been called the pachytene checkpoint, but in fact, the cells arrest late in meiotic prophase by a mechanism that is probably analogous to the G_2 DNA damage checkpoint in somatic cells. Mammalian germ cells that arrest owing to defects in recombination are eliminated by apoptosis.

The same proteins may mediate mitotic and meiotic checkpoints. Proteins such as ataxia telangiectasia-mutated (ATM) kinase, ataxia telangiectasia and Rad3-related (ATR) protein kinase, and their downstream effectors (see Fig. 40-4) are associated with meiotic chromosomes in prophase.

Suppression of DNA Replication between Meiosis I and Meiosis II

One unique aspect of meiosis is that the process involves two M phases with no intervening S phase. On exit from meiosis I, Cdk1 kinase is reactivated immediately. This blocks assembly of prereplication complexes (see Fig. 42-7), thereby blocking DNA replication. At least two pathways contribute to reactivation of Cdk1.

The first involves downregulation of translation of Wee1 protein kinase in meiosis. Wee1 is a mitotic inhibitor (see Fig. 40-14) that inactivates Cdk1 by phosphorylation at Tyr^{15}. The absence of Wee1 in meiosis I was first observed in *X. laevis* but seems to be a universally conserved way of reactivating Cdk1 without an S phase. Ectopic expression of Wee1 in mature *X. laevis* oocytes prevents reactivation of Cdk1 immediately after the meiosis I division. As a result, the oocytes reenter interphase and replicate their DNA. Meiotic cells also express a specialized isoform of Cdc25, the phosphatase that counteracts Wee1 (see Fig. 43-1).

A second mechanism for differentiating meiosis from mitosis involves activation of a specialized mitogen-activated protein (MAP) kinase pathway (see Fig. 27-6) by c-Mos, a meiotic-specific MAP kinase kinase kinase. This pathway activates Cdk1 and other unknown substrates, with profound effects on the meiotic cell cycle (see next section).

The Metaphase II Arrest and the MAP Kinase Pathway

Following their activation and release from the ovary (ovulation), oocytes of many vertebrates arrest in metaphase II of meiosis until they are fertilized. The activity

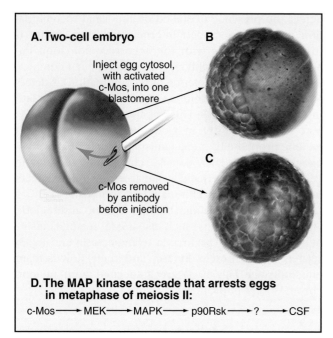

A. Two-cell embryo

Inject egg cytosol, with activated c-Mos, into one blastomere

c-Mos removed by antibody before injection

B

C

D. The MAP kinase cascade that arrests eggs in metaphase of meiosis II:

c-Mos ⟶ MEK ⟶ MAPK ⟶ p90Rsk ⟶ ? ⟶ CSF

Figure 45-14 A, Description of the experiment that identified c-Mos as an essential component of cytostatic factor (CSF) required for arrest of eggs in meiotic metaphase. One blastomere of an *X. laevis* embryo at the two-cell stage was injected with cytoplasm from a metaphase-arrested egg containing CSF activity. **B,** This blastomere (*right half* of the embryo) remained blocked in metaphase while the left blastomere divided many times. **C,** The same experiment was performed, but prior to injection, the c-Mos was removed from the egg cytoplasm by absorption with a specific antibody. Both the injected and uninjected blastomeres continued to divide normally. **D,** The MAP kinase pathway leading to metaphase II arrest in vertebrate eggs. (B–C, Micrographs courtesy of George Vande Woude, NCI, Frederick, Maryland; Adapted from Sagata N, Watanabe N, Vande Woude GF, et al: The c-Mos proto-oncogene product is a cytostatic factor responsible for meiotic arrest in vertebrate eggs. Nature 342:512–518, 1989.)

that is responsible for this arrest was discovered in *X. laevis* eggs arrested in metaphase of meiosis II and is called **cytostatic factor** (CSF). Injection of cytoplasm containing CSF into one blastomere of a two-cell frog embryo blocks the next cell cycle at metaphase, just like the egg (Fig. 45-14). Therefore, CSF can even block somatic cells indefinitely at metaphase in mitosis. CSF activity appears in meiosis II and disappears after fertilization.

One active component of CSF is the *X. laevis* homolog of a well-known viral oncogene, *v-mos,* the transforming gene of the Moloney murine sarcoma virus, which causes solid tumors in mice. DNA hybridization was used to isolate a corresponding cellular gene, ***c-mos,*** from *X. laevis.* The *v-mos* gene is a mutated form of the cellular *c-mos* gene. Vertebrates express *c-mos* exclusively in oocytes and eggs. Injection of either v-Mos or c-Mos proteins into dividing blastomeres of early frog embryos arrests the cells at metaphase (Fig. 45-14). These experiments led to the proposal that c-Mos was CSF.

CSF arrest requires the MAP kinase (MAPK) signal transduction pathway (see Fig. 27-5). Mos activates the pathway by phosphorylating MEK (MAPK-activating kinase), which then activates MAPK. MAPK then activates a downstream kinase called p90Rsk (Fig. 45-14D). Introduction of constitutively active c-Mos or p90Rsk into *X. laevis* eggs is sufficient to induce CSF arrest. However, this is not the whole story, because metaphase arrest is maintained in extracts depleted of p90Rsk. Thus the pathway must include at least one unidentified step beyond p90Rsk.

New research showed that an APC/C inhibitor called Emi2 is a critical component of CSF. A burst of cytoplasmic Ca²⁺ released at fertilization (see Fig. 26-15) activates protein kinase A, which phosphorylates Emi2. This modification creates a binding site for polo kinase, which then also phosphorylates Emi2. Polo phosphorylation marks Emi2 for destruction, resulting in activation of APC/C, termination of the CSF metaphase arrest, and completion of meiosis II.

Timing of Meiosis in Humans

The fate of cells undergoing meiosis, as well as the timing of meiotic events, differs significantly between males and females.

Males produce about 100 million sperm a day in a process called **spermatogenesis.** This process continues throughout adult life. Spermatogenesis starts with the division of stem cells called **spermatogonia** and involves eight divisions prior to meiosis. These divisions are unusual in that cytokinesis is incomplete, and the cells remain connected by intercellular bridges. The process could produce up to 256 cells, but usually, some cells die and others fail to divide, so a more typical number is around 200 cells arising from the initial stem cell division. When these cells pass through meiosis (at which point they are referred to as spermatocytes) the final result is about 800 postmeiotic **spermatids.** Spermatids then undergo a complex program of differentiation, resulting in the production of highly specialized **spermatozoa.** The entire process of spermatogenesis takes about 64 days, the bulk of which is spent in meiosis I. About 16 days are spent in pachytene, the longest stage of the meiosis I prophase. In contrast, only about 8 hours are spent in meiosis II.

In females, each ovary contains a total of about 100,000 primordial follicles, each with an oocyte that is arrested in the diplotene stage of meiosis at about the twelfth to sixteenth week of fetal life. Following puberty, a small number of oocytes become activated and grow each month. One of these activated oocytes matures fully and is shed in response to a surge of luteinizing hormone. The others undergo programmed cell death and degenerate in a process known as atresia. As the oocyte is shed from the ovary, it completes meiosis I and becomes arrested at metaphase of meiosis II by CSF. It remains arrested at this stage until fertilization occurs.

In human females, only one mature egg is produced as a result of meiosis. All of the cell divisions are asymmetrical, the other cells produced by the meiotic cleavages being very small and short-lived. These small cells are referred to as **polar bodies.**

Meiotic Defects and Human Disease

Abnormalities in meiosis are surprisingly common but are not widely observed in human populations because their consequences are extremely severe. In fact, meiotic abnormalities are a leading cause of fetal death, particularly during the first trimester of pregnancy in humans. The two major causes of problems are nondisjunction in the meiotic divisions and the generation of unbalanced chromosomal rearrangements.

When chromosomes fail to segregate properly in one or both meiotic divisions (nondisjunction), the products of meiosis lack the normal haploid complement of chromosomes. Embryos that have gained an entire set of chromosomes are referred to as **polyploid.** In human embryos, polyploidy is a common type of chromosomal abnormality, triploidy (69 chromosomes) being the most common form. It is estimated that 1% to 3% of all conceptions are triploids. Two thirds of these arise from two sperm fertilizing one egg (nothing wrong with meiosis there). In other cases, they come from a diploid gamete, the result of a defective meiotic segregation. The vast majority of triploid embryos do not survive to term.

Most chromosomal abnormalities in human embryos result from the loss or gain of one or more chromosomes during meiosis. This condition is referred to as **aneuploidy.** In most cases, zygotes that arise from aneuploid gametes die during fetal development. (Any fetal death is a spontaneous abortion, commonly called a miscarriage.) It is now thought that at least 50% of all conceptions result in spontaneous abortions. Furthermore, over 60% of those spontaneous abortions are aneuploid. These figures probably underestimate the frequency of meiotic abnormalities and spontaneous abortion during very early pregnancy, as few fetuses that are lost in the first four to six weeks of gestation are sent to a laboratory for karyotyping, and many are never detected at all.

Meiotic errors involving certain autosomes can produce fetuses that survive to birth. Individuals trisomic for chromosome 21 (a condition that is commonly known as **Down syndrome**) have mental retardation and characteristic phenotypic features, including decreased life expectancy. Rare individuals who are trisomic for chromosomes 13 and 18 survive to birth but

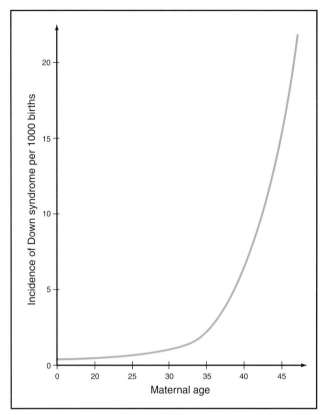

Figure 45-15 THE RELATIONSHIP BETWEEN MATERNAL AGE AND THE INCIDENCE OF DOWN SYNDROME.

typically die shortly thereafter. Why do individuals with Down syndrome survive whereas others affected by aneuploidy do not? Perhaps the very small number (225) of genes on chromosome 21 includes none whose dosage is critical for survival.

The frequency of certain types of aneuploidy, such as trisomy for chromosome 21, increases with the age of the mother. Statistics indicate that only 0.04% of children of mothers who are 20 years old have trisomy 21. This number rises dramatically with maternal age; nearly 5% of the conceptions in mothers 45 years old have trisomy 21 (Fig. 45-15). This maternal age effect is a leading cause of human genetic disease. Some believe that during the many years of arrest of oocytes in meiosis I diplotene, chiasmata joining homologous chromosomes gradually dissociate. A mechanism to explain this is the progressive loss of cohesion between sister chromatids as the mother ages. Mice with a mutation in a key subunit of the cohesin complex (Fig. 45-7; see also Fig. 13-19) exhibit a pattern of chromosome nondisjunction with increasing maternal age that looks much like that seen in aging human mothers. Of course, other factors that are required for accurate chromosome segregation also may be lost or inactivated as oocytes age.

Not all cases of human aneuploidy are the fault of the mother. One of the most common aneuploidies, 45,X

Table 45-1

ANEUPLOIDIES INVOLVING THE SEX CHROMOSOMES IN NEWBORN HUMANS

Karyotype	Frequency	Sex	Comments
47,XXY*	1/1000	M	Klinefelter syndrome. Increased height, sterile, a proportion may have some learning difficulties.
47,XYY	1/1000	M	Increased height, generally fertile, typically with chromosomally normal offspring. A proportion may have some learning difficulties.
Other X or Y aneuploidy	1/1350		
			Total: 1 in 360 male births
47,XXX	1/900	F	Increased height, generally fertile, typically with chromosomally normal offspring. A proportion have serious learning difficulties.
45,X	1/4000	F	Turner syndrome. Reduced height, infertile, normal intelligence. 99% of 45,X embryos terminate as spontaneous abortions.
Other X or Y aneuploidy	1/2700		
			Total: 1 in 580 female births

*This number gives the total number of chromosomes, followed by the complement of sex chromosomes.
Adapted from Nussbaum RL, McInnes RR, Willard HF: Genetics in Medicine, 6th ed. Philadelphia, WB Saunders, 2001, p 150, Table 9-3.

(see Table 45-1 for an explanation of nomenclature), which accounts for nearly 10% of spontaneous abortions, involves the loss of the paternal X or Y chromosome 70% to 80% of the time. In addition, about 7% of instances of trisomy 21 are of paternal origin. Clearly, more than one mechanism is responsible for the generation of aneuploid offspring.

These rather sobering statistics reveal two important facts about human reproduction. First, the production of gametes is error prone. This has been confirmed by direct studies, in which 20% of eggs and 3% to 4% of sperm were found to have chromosomal abnormalities. Second, the much lower rates of chromosomal abnormalities seen in live births (about 0.3% overall [Table 45-1]) reveal that spontaneous abortion is a highly efficient protective mechanism for the elimination of chromosomal imbalances that arise from errors in meiosis.

ACKNOWLEDGMENTS

Thanks go to Paula Cohen, Nancy Kleckner, Gail Stetten, and José Suja for their suggestions on revisions to this chapter.

SELECTED READINGS

Harper L, Golubovskaya I, Cande WZ: A bouquet of chromosomes. J Cell Sci 117:4025–4032, 2004.

Hassold T, Hunt P: To err (meiotically) is human: The genesis of human aneuploidy. Nat Rev Genet 2:280–291, 2001.

Honigberg SM, McCarroll RM, Esposito RE: Regulatory mechanisms in meiosis. Curr Opin Cell Biol 5:219–225, 1993.

Loidl J: Coming to grips with a complex matter. A multidisciplinary approach to the synaptonemal complex. Chromosoma 100:289–292, 1991.

Petronczki M, Siomos MF, Nasmyth K: Un ménage à quatre: The molecular biology of chromosome segregation in meiosis. Cell 112:423–440, 2003.

Rieder CL, Cole R: Chromatid cohesion during mitosis: Lessons from meiosis. J Cell Sci 112:2607–2613, 1999.

Roeder GS: Meiotic chromosomes: It takes two to tango. Genes Dev 11:2600–2621, 1997.

Sagata N: What does Mos do in oocytes and somatic cells? Bioessays 19:13–21, 1997.

Scherthan H: A bouquet makes ends meet. Nat Rev Mol Cell Biol 2:621–627, 2001.

Van Heemst D, Heyting C: Sister chromatid cohesion and recombination in meiosis. Chromosoma 109:10–26, 2000.

Villeneuve A, Hillers KJ: Whence meiosis? Cell 106:647–650, 2001.

Zickler D, Kleckner N: Meiotic chromosomes: Integrating structure and function. Annu Rev Genet 33:603–754, 1999.

CHAPTER 46

Programmed Cell Death

The Necessity for Cell Death in Multicellular Organisms

The ability to undergo **programmed cell death** (Box 46-1) is a built-in latent capacity in virtually all cells of multicellular organisms. Cell death is important for embryonic development, maintenance of tissue homeostasis, establishment of immune self-tolerance, killing by immune effector cells, and regulation of cell viability by hormones and growth factors. It has been proposed that most metazoan cells will die if they fail to receive survival signals from other cells. Abnormalities of the cell death program contribute to a number of diseases, including cancer, Alzheimer's disease, and acquired immune deficiency syndrome (AIDS).

Programmed Cell Death versus Accidental Cell Death: Apoptosis versus Necrosis

Although cells die in many ways, it is useful to focus on the two poles of this spectrum: apoptosis and necrosis. **Apoptosis** is the most commonly described pathway for *programmed* cell death, which is cellular suicide resulting from activation of a dedicated intracellular program (Fig. 46-1). Often, these cells appear completely healthy prior to committing suicide. At the other end of the spectrum is **necrosis,** also called *accidental* cell death, which occurs when cells receive a structural or chemical insult that kills them outright (Fig. 46-2). Examples of such insults include extremes of temperature and physical trauma. The cell itself can also initiate necrosis in response to certain stimuli, particularly when induction of apoptosis is inhibited. In contrast to the orderly biochemical pathways of apoptosis, which involve the action of enzyme cascades and the consumption of ATP, necrosis typically involves a collapse of normal cell physiology as a result of ATP depletion.

Necrosis corresponds to what most of us naively imagine cell death would be like. Owing to lack of cellular homeostasis, water rushes into the dying cell, causing it to swell greatly so that the plasma and organelle membranes burst. As a result, the cell undergoes a generalized process of autodigestion and dissolution, culminating in the spilling of the cytoplasmic contents out into the surroundings (Fig. 46-2). This, in turn, produces local inflammation as phagocytic cells are activated, flock to the site, and ingest the debris (see Chapter 22). Because agents that damage cells act over areas that are large in comparison to the size of a single cell, necrosis often involves large groups of neighboring cells.

BOX 46-1
Key Terms

Programmed Cell Death: An active cellular process that culminates in cell death. This may occur in response to developmental or environmental cues or as a response to physiological damage detected by the cell's internal surveillance networks.

Necrosis (Accidental Cell Death): Cell death that results from irreversible injury to the cell. Cell membranes swell and become permeable. Lytic enzymes destroy the cellular contents, which then leak out into the intercellular space, leading to the mounting of an inflammatory response.

Apoptosis: One type of programmed cell death that initially was characterized by a particular pattern of morphologic changes but now is defined by the action of molecular pathways involving cell surface receptors or mitochondria and resulting in the activation of specialized proteases. The name comes from the ancient Greek, referring to shedding of the petals from flowers or leaves from trees. Apoptosis is observed in all metazoans, including both plants and animals.

Apoptotic death occurs in two phases. During the *latent phase,* the cell looks morphologically normal but is actively making preparations for death. The *execution phase* is characterized by a series of dramatic structural and biochemical changes that culminate in the fragmentation of the cell into membrane-enclosed *apoptotic bodies.* Activities that cause cells to undergo apoptosis are said to be *pro-apoptotic.* Activities that protect cells from apoptosis are said to be *anti-apoptotic.*

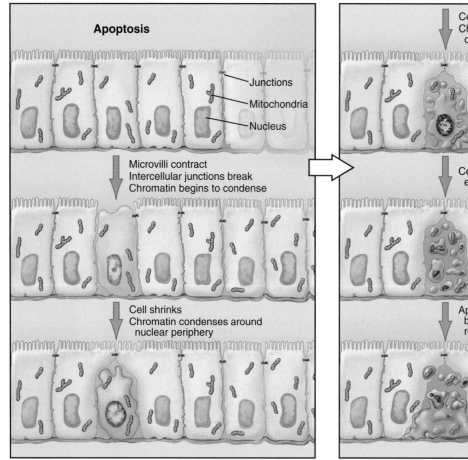
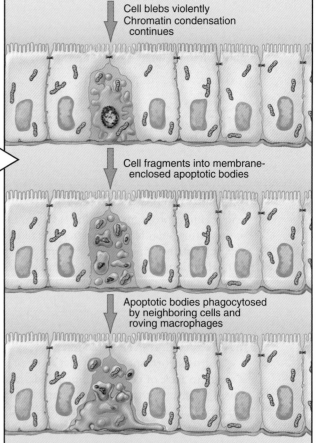

Figure 46-1 **APOPTOSIS—ACTIVE CELLULAR SUICIDE—TYPICALLY AFFECTS SINGLE CELLS.** Neighboring cells remain healthy. Apoptotic cell death usually does not lead to an inflammatory response.

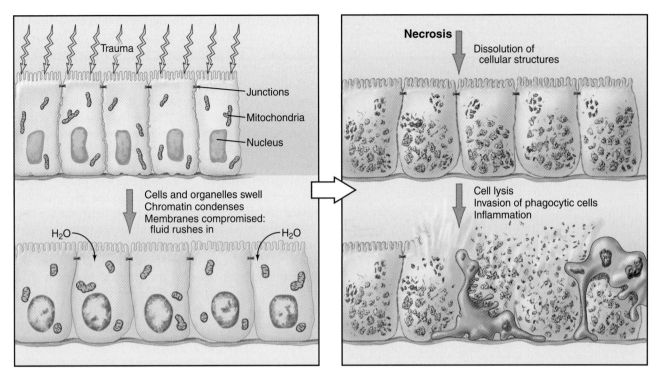

Figure 46-2 NECROSIS IS A RESULT OF INJURY TO CELLS. Typically, groups of cells are affected. In most cases, necrotic cell death leads to an inflammatory response (*red* "angry" macrophages).

In contrast to necrosis, apoptotic cells shrink rather than swelling, as part of a reproducible pattern of structural alterations of both the nucleus and cytoplasm (Fig. 46-1). Apoptosis is a two-stage process. On receipt of the **pro-apoptotic** signal that triggers the pathway to death, cells enter a **latent phase** of apoptosis (Fig. 46-3). Although committed to a pathway that leads to their inevitable demise at some later time, cells in the latent phase look as healthy as their neighbors. The duration of the latent phase of apoptosis is extremely variable, ranging from a few hours to several days. The reason for this variability is not known.

Ultimately, the cells enter the **execution phase** of apoptosis, lasting about an hour, during which they undergo dramatic morphologic and physiological changes. These include (1) loss of microvilli and intercellular junctions (Fig. 46-4); (2) shrinkage of the cytoplasm; (3) dramatic changes in cytoplasmic motility with activation of violent blebbing (Fig. 46-5); (4) loss of plasma membrane asymmetry, with the distribution

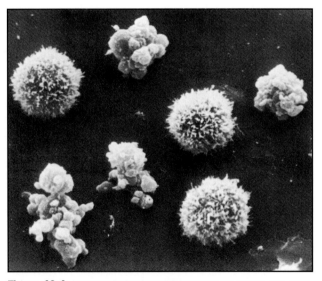

Figure 46-4 SCANNING ELECTRON MICROGRAPH OF INTACT AND APOPTOTIC MOUSE SARCOMA CELLS. Intact cells are covered with microvilli, whereas apoptotic cells have numerous smooth blebs. These cells were stimulated to undergo apoptosis as a result of interference with RNA metabolism. (From Wyllie AH, Kerr JFR, Currie AR: Cell death: The significance of apoptosis. Int Rev Cytol 68:251–305, 1980.)

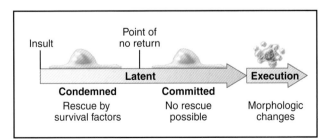

Figure 46-3 THE TWO PHASES OF APOPTOSIS. Note that the latent phase can be subdivided into two stages: a *condemned* stage, during which the cell is proceeding on a pathway toward death but can still be rescued if it is exposed to anti-apoptotic activities, and a *committed* stage, beyond which rescue is impossible.

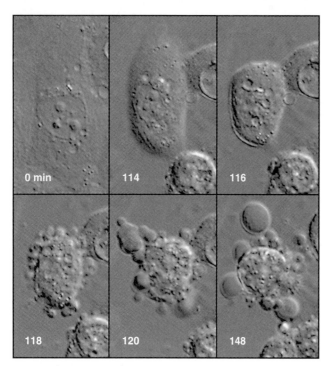

Figure 46-5 APOPTOSIS OF A TRANSFORMED PIG KIDNEY CELL FOLLOW-ING EXPOSURE TO ETOPOSIDE, A DRUG USED IN CANCER CHEMOTHERAPY. The dramatic cytoplasmic blebbing results in the disassembly of the cell into membrane-enclosed vesicles. (Courtesy of L. M. Martins and K. Samejima, Wellcome Trust Institute for Cell Biology, University of Edinburgh, Scotland.)

of phosphatidylserine being randomized so that it appears in the outer membrane leaflet; (5) hypercondensation of the chromatin and its collapse against the nuclear periphery; and (6) the "explosive" fragmentation of the cell into membrane-enclosed **apoptotic bodies** that contain remnants of the nucleus, mitochondria, and other organelles. The plasma membrane retains its integrity throughout the entire process. All of these changes are instigated by the action of a specific set of death-inducing proteases, discussed at length later.

In tissues, apoptotic bodies are rapidly phagocytosed by surrounding cells that recognize the phosphatidylserine and other markers exposed on their surface (Fig. 46-6). Apoptosis can thus be considered to be the disassembly of the cell into "bite-sized" vesicles. Because these vesicles remain membrane bound, the cellular contents are not released into the environment. It is important to note that surface markers on apoptotic bodies cause cells that ingest them to secrete anti-inflammatory cytokines. As a result, apoptotic death does not lead to an inflammatory response.

Nonapoptotic Programmed Cell Death

The terms *apoptosis* and *programmed cell death* are sometimes viewed as synonymous. However, in a number of well-documented systems, cells undergo programmed cell death without the dramatic structural changes that classically define apoptosis. Thus, all apop-

Figure 46-6 PHAGOCYTOSIS OF APOPTOTIC CELLS. **A–C,** Phagocytosis that occurs when cells express "eat me" signals results in the production of anti-inflammatory cytokines. **D,** Electron micrograph of a phagocytosed apoptotic body containing a nuclear fragment. The nucleus of the epithelial cell that engulfed this apoptotic body is shown at *left*. In this case, apoptosis occurred during allograft rejection in a pig. (A, Based on Lauber K, Blumenthal SG, Waibel M, Wesselborg S: Clearance of apoptotic cells: Getting rid of the corpses. Mol Cell 12: 277–287, 2004. B, From Wyllie AH, Kerr JFR, Currie AR: Cell death: The significance of apoptosis. Int Rev Cytol 68:251–305, 1980.)

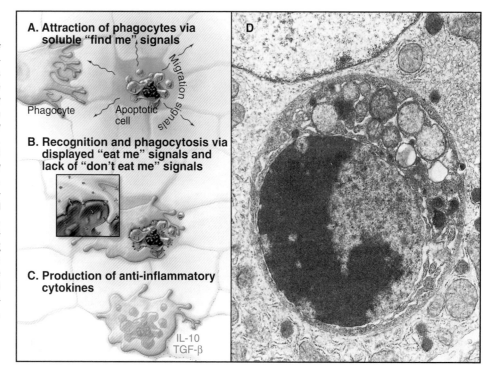

A. Attraction of phagocytes via soluble "find me" signals

Phagocyte   Apoptotic cell

Migration signals

B. Recognition and phagocytosis via displayed "eat me" signals and lack of "don't eat me" signals

C. Production of anti-inflammatory cytokines

IL-10
TGF-β

D

tosis is programmed cell death, but the converse is not necessarily true.

When the adult tobacco hawkmoth emerges from its cocoon, its intersegmental muscles undergo programmed cell death that differs in several ways from apoptosis as described earlier. The chromatin does not condense; DNA is not digested; and cytoplasm does not "boil." Instead, a polyubiquitin gene is induced and plays an important role in intracellular protein degradation (see Chapter 23). Thus, although these muscle cells unquestionably undergo programmed cell death, they apparently do not use the apoptosis pathway.

Classes of Cells That Undergo Programmed Cell Death

At least six distinct classes of cells undergo programmed cell death (examples are given in Fig. 46-7).

Developmentally Defective Cells

During molecular maturation of T-lymphocyte antigen receptors (see Figs. 27-8 and 28-8), immature T cells in the thymus (known as thymocytes) rearrange the genes encoding the receptor α and β chains. Many newly created receptors bind to foreign antigens, but others interact with self-antigens. Cells with receptors recognizing self-antigens are potentially harmful and are eliminated through apoptosis in a process known as **negative selection** (Fig. 46-8). The drug cyclosporin A, which inhibits apoptosis in thymocytes, can cause autoimmune disease.

To function properly, the T-cell receptor must recognize major histocompatibility complex (MHC) glycoproteins on other cells during antigen presentation (see Fig. 27-8). T lymphocytes whose T-cell receptors cannot interact with the spectrum of MHC glycoproteins expressed in a given individual are ineffective in the immune response. These cells die by apoptosis in a process known as **positive selection** (Fig. 46-8). Overall, defects in T-cell receptor assembly are extremely common, and up to 95% of immature T cells die by apoptosis without leaving the thymus.

Similar positive and negative selection steps occur during the maturation of B lymphocytes (see Fig. 28-8), which is accomplished by a combination of gene rearrangements and facilitated mutagenesis. B lymphocytes expressing antibodies directed against self-antigens or producing antibodies whose affinity for antigen is below a critical threshold are eliminated through apoptosis.

Excess Cells

The use of programmed cell death for quality control during development is not limited to the immune system but is also extremely important during brain development. Embryonic ganglia often have many more neurons than are required to enervate their target muscles. Production of excess cells is part of a Darwinian strategy to ensure that a sufficient number of axons reach their targets. Excess neurons that fail to

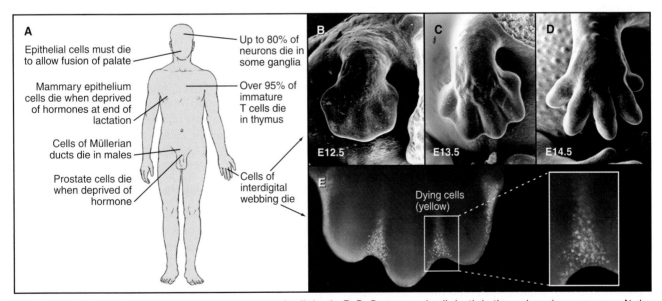

Figure 46-7 A, Types of cells that undergo programmed cell death. **B–D,** Programmed cell death in the embryonic mouse paw. At day 12.5 of development, the digits are fully connected by webbing. By day 13.5, the webbing has started to die, and by day 14.5, all of the webbing cells are gone. **E,** Nuclei of cells undergoing programmed cell death take up acridine *orange,* whereas cells of the surrounding healthy tissue do not. (Micrographs courtesy of William Wood and Paul Martin, Department of Anatomy and Developmental Biology, University College of London, England.)

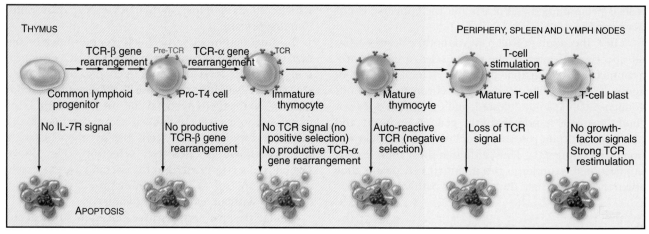

Figure 46-8 EXAMPLES OF SIGNALS THAT PROMOTE DIFFERENTIATION OR PROGRAMMED CELL DEATH OF IMMATURE THYMOCYTES IN THE THYMUS AND MATURE T CELLS IN THE PERIPHERY. Thymocytes that make functional T-cell receptors and do not recognize self-antigens mature, provided that they receive survival signals, such as interleukin-7. Thymocytes undergo apoptosis if they produce defective T-cell receptor, recognize self-antigens, suffer DNA damage, or receive a death stimulus (glucocorticoid hormone). More than 95% of immature thymocytes die without leaving the thymus. (Based on Strasser A: The role of BH3-only proteins in the immune system. Nat Rev Immunol 5:189–200, 2005.)

make appropriate connections have no function and are eliminated by programmed cell death. Up to 80% of neurons in certain developing ganglia die in this way. Because of the importance of apoptosis during its development, the brain is often seriously affected in mice that are engineered to lack components of the apoptotic pathway.

Cells That Serve No Function

The elimination of obsolete cells whose function has been completed is most evident in organisms, such as insects and amphibians, that undergo metamorphosis during development. For example, programmed cell death initiated by a burst of thyroid hormone is responsible for resorption of the tadpole tail.

Mammals also use programmed cell death to eliminate obsolete tissues during development. For example, in humans, the digits of hands and feet are connected by a tissue webbing during embryogenesis. Cells in this webbing serve no purpose in the adult and are eliminated by programmed cell death (Fig. 46-7).

During craniofacial development, the hard palate develops from two lateral precursors, each covered in a protective layer of epithelial cells. As the two halves grow together at the midline of the nasopharynx, they remain separated by this covering of epithelium until, in response to a developmental cue, the epithelial cells at the midline undergo programmed cell death. Then the two halves of the palate can fuse. Failure of the epithelial cells to die at the appropriate time can interfere with the fusion of the bone, causing cleft palate.

Populations of cells that are fully functional may become obsolete as a result of physiological changes in the status of an organism. For example, in male mammals, certain accessory glands of the reproductive system are regulated by the levels of circulating male hormone. If hormone levels fall below a critical threshold, these organs, including the prostate, virtually disappear in a very brief time as their constituent cells undergo massive apoptotic death. Should levels of circulating androgens rise again, the remaining prostatic stem cells proliferate and reconstruct the gland. A similar cycle of growth and involution is seen in the mammary gland of female mammals, which exhibits substantial differences in size and cellular composition in the lactating and nonlactating states. Interference with survival signaling by sex hormones is one important strategy that is commonly used in the treatment of breast and prostate cancer.

Programmed cell death is also used to eliminate certain populations of cells that never served any function to begin with. The Müllerian ducts develop into the female oviduct. In male embryos, progenitors of the Müllerian ducts develop, even though they have no function. Programmed cell death eliminates the constituent cells of these embryonic ducts.

Cells Whose Cell Cycle Is Perturbed

Chapters 40 to 43 describe how biochemical circuits called checkpoints regulate the cell cycle. If DNA is damaged, checkpoint activation blocks cell-cycle progression while repair processes operate. An important downstream effector of checkpoints, the p53 transcription factor, induces the expression of genes encoding proteins that arrest the cell cycle as well as genes encoding proteins that induce cell death. It is generally thought that if the damage cannot be repaired quickly, the pro-death factors win out, and the outcome is apoptosis.

Types of DNA damage that commonly trigger cell death are double-strand breaks induced by ionizing radiation and DNA breaks or other damage induced by chemotherapeutic agents.

A second important cell-cycle checkpoint regulates the transition from the G1 phase to the S phase. Passage of the restriction point (see Fig. 41-7) represents the commitment of the cell to undergo another cycle of DNA replication and division. Restriction point control centers on the regulation of the E2F family of transcription factors. However, E2F not only regulates genes that promote cell-cycle progression; it also induces the expression of genes that promote apoptosis. It is now thought that if E2F is activated too strongly, as, for example, where restriction point control has broken down (see Fig. 41-10), its function as a death inducer takes over, and the cells undergo apoptosis. Cells that die in response to inappropriate signals to proliferate include those that are infected by certain viruses or overexpress genes involved in cell proliferation (such as *c-myc* and *c-fos* [Fig. 46-14]). This ability to recognize an inappropriate stimulus to proliferate and respond to it by undergoing apoptosis may be an important defense against cancer.

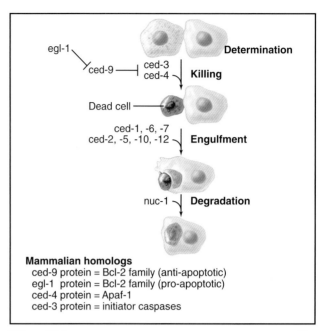

Figure 46-9 GENETIC DISSECTION OF PROGRAMMED CELL DEATH. The *ced* (cell death abnormal) mutants of the nematode worm *C. elegans* affect the killing, engulfment, and degradation stages of programmed cell death.

Virus-Infected Cells

Cells that harbor infectious agents, such as viruses, are harmful to the organism. Cytotoxic T lymphocytes eliminate virus-infected cells by causing them to undergo programmed cell death either by apoptosis or by a second related pathway.

At least part of the loss of mature CD4$^+$ T helper cells (see Fig. 28-8) in people who are infected with HIV-1 results from programmed cell death. When exposed to agents that normally stimulate cell proliferation, these cells instead undergo apoptosis. Paradoxically, it appears that many of these dying cells are not themselves infected with HIV.

Chemotherapeutic Killing of Cells

Exposure of cancer cells to many of the agents that are used in chemotherapy does not kill the cells outright. Instead, they die because the drugs cause intracellular damage that acts as a signal for the induction of apoptotic cell death.

Genetic Analysis of Programmed Cell Death

Several key components that are involved in the apoptotic execution of mammalian cells were first identified by a genetic analysis of the nematode worm *Caenorhabditis elegans*. Because *C. elegans* is optically clear, it is

possible to see every cell in a developing worm by using differential interference contrast optics (see Fig. 6-2). This enabled investigators to develop a complete fate map for *C. elegans* that traces the lineage of each cell in an adult worm back to the fertilized egg. These studies led to the surprising discovery that programmed cell death is one of the most common fates for newborn *C. elegans* cells. Of the 1090 somatic cells that are produced during embryogenesis of the *C. elegans* hermaphrodite, 131 undergo programmed cell death at reproducible locations and times.

Mutations in at least 14 *C. elegans* genes affect programmed cell death (Fig. 46-9). These may be divided into three classes: (1) genes that mark cells for subsequent programmed death, (2) genes that are involved in cell killing and its regulation, and (3) genes that are involved in the phagocytosis and subsequent processing of the cell corpses. These mutants are collectively known as "cell death abnormal" (ced) **mutants.**

The three best-known cell death genes are ***ced-3,*** ***ced-4,*** and ***ced-9.*** *Ced-3* and *ced-4* are required for cells to undergo apoptotic programmed cell death. If either gene is inactivated, all cells throughout the organism that should die by apoptosis are reprieved. These cells remain alive and are apparently functional. Interestingly, these worms have normal life spans. This suggests that programmed cell death is not involved in the normal aging process, at least not in *C. elegans.* *Ced-9* regulates *ced-3* and *ced-4.* In *ced-9* loss-of-function mutants, many cells die that should normally stay alive. This is deleterious for the organism, and *ced-9* mutants die.

These genes all have mammalian counterparts (discussed more fully later). Ced-3 is a member of a specialized family of cell death proteases called caspases. Ced-4 is a scaffolding/adapter protein that plays an essential role in the activation of Ced-3 from its zymogen precursor. Its mammalian counterpart is apoptotic protease-activating factor-1 **(Apaf-1).** Ced-9 is a member of the **Bcl-2** family of cell death regulators. In mammals, some Bcl-2 family members protect against cell death, whereas others actively promote cell death.

Eight *C. elegans* genes encode proteins that are involved in the phagocytosis and processing of cell corpses. Several are signaling proteins with roles in reorganizing the cytoskeleton to permit the cell to move toward and engulf its target. Another, the *nuc-1* gene, encodes one of several nucleases that digest the DNA of the dead cell. In the worm, digestion of the DNA occurs in lysosomes of cells that ingest the corpse. In mammals, this digestion typically is initiated within the dying cell itself. The process of phagocytosis turned out to be surprisingly complex, probably involving both ligand-receptor interactions and directed cell motility.

Signals and Pathways of Apoptosis

Two principal pathways lead to cell death by apoptosis. These are introduced only briefly here. The **intrinsic pathway** (Fig. 46-16) is activated by internal surveillance mechanisms or signals sent (or not sent) by other cells. Signals that induce this pathway include DNA damage, exposure to chemicals that interfere with a variety of cellular pathways, excessive activation of factors that promote cell-cycle progression, and receipt of certain pro-apoptotic stimuli from the surrounding medium. Withdrawal of nutrients or of nurturing signals from the environment also activates the intrinsic pathway. Survival signals include lymphokines, such as interleukin-2 and interleukin-3, which are essential for survival of thymocytes; nerve growth factor, which is required for survival of many neurons; and extracellular matrix, which is required for survival of epithelial cells. Signals that activate the intrinsic pathway converge on mitochondria, which release key factors that drive the apoptotic response.

Signals from other cells are the primary triggers of the **extrinsic pathway** (Fig. 46-17). Direct contact with the target cell activates specific receptors that initiate this pathway, starting on the inner surface of the plasma membrane. Activation of the extrinsic pathway is one strategy that cytotoxic T lymphocytes use to kill cells

that are recognized as foreign (or as harboring foreign pathogens). This pathway is also widely used to control cell populations in the immune system.

Protein Regulators and Effectors of Apoptosis

Since the penalty for misregulation of apoptosis is inappropriate cell death, it is not surprising that the process is carefully regulated. This is essential for cells but complicates matters for students. This section first lays out the overall strategy in generic terms and then fills in some important details.

A cascade of proteases called caspases drives apoptosis. Each caspase is harmless until activated (usually by proteolytic cleavage). The cascade starts with the activation of a small number of initiator caspases, which activate numerous effector caspases. The ability of effector caspases to activate further initiators and effectors further amplifies the cascade.

This strategy of employing amplification and positive feedback has two powerful advantages. First, it can provide a very rapid change in the state of the cytoplasm, from pro-life to pro-death within seconds. Second, because a relatively small number of initiator caspases initiate the cascade, these enzymes are feasible targets for negative regulators that can rapidly quell responses that are initiated under borderline conditions or by mistake. This is beneficial but also complicates the overall system. If initiator caspases start apoptosis and are then inactivated by suppressers, how does the response ever take hold? The answer is at least one more level of regulation: inhibitors of the inhibitors.

The following sections discuss the workhorses of apoptosis—the caspases—followed by regulation of the response.

Caspases

Caspases (cysteine aspartases) are specialized proteases with a cysteine in their active site that cleave on the C-terminal side of aspartate residues. Caspases inactivate cellular survival pathways and specifically activate other factors that promote cell death.

C. elegans has three caspases, one of which (Ced-3) is essential for cell death. In contrast, mammals have at least 13 caspase genes (Fig. 46-10A). Analysis based on sequence comparisons divides caspases into two major subfamilies. The caspase 1 subfamily encodes enzymes that process pro-interleukin-1β to yield mature interleukin-1β. Macrophages secrete this cytokine, which is involved in causing inflammation. In contrast, the caspase 3 subfamily of enzymes participates almost exclusively in apoptotic cell death.

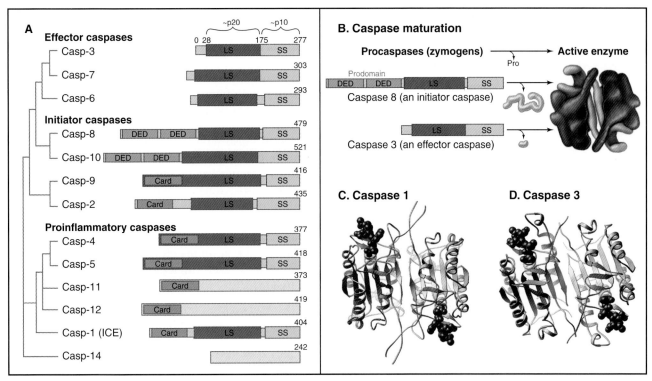

Figure 46-10 INTRODUCTION TO CASPASES. A, The 13 mammalian caspases fall into three groups. Where it has been determined, the portions of the zymogens that give rise to the large *(blue)* and small *(yellow)* subunits are shown. **B,** Initiator caspases have large prodomains that participate in subcellular targeting. Two procaspases come together to form the active enzyme. **C–D,** Crystal structure of caspases 1 and 3. The catalytic residues come primarily from the large subunit *(blue)*. In the pro-inflammatory caspase 1–like enzymes, the catalytic site is relatively open. In the caspase 3–like enzymes (involved in apoptosis), the small subunit *(yellow)* forms a "hood" that limits access to the active site. The space-filling structure *(red)* represents a peptide inhibitor covalently bound in the active site of the enzyme.

Like many proteases, caspases are synthesized as inactive zymogens. All living vertebrate cells apparently synthesize these zymogens constitutively. The caspase zymogen consists of three domains and an N-terminal prodomain followed by the large and small subunits of the mature enzyme (Fig. 46-10A–B). These three domains are separated by aspartate residues, the cleavage target for caspases. Caspase zymogens are usually activated by zymogen cleavage and release of the prodomains. Following cleavage, the two large and two small subunits associate in a compact, block-like heterotetrameric molecule (Fig. 46-10B–D). Cleavage of the zymogens permits a major conformational change in the polypeptide, creating two stable active site pockets between the large and small subunits.

Two classes of caspases are involved in cell death. **Initiator caspases** have long prodomains (Fig. 46-10A). These zymogens exist as monomers in cells and become autoactivated when scaffolding cofactors promote their aggregation. Activation is thought to involve dimerization of the zymogens and might not necessarily require zymogen cleavage. Sequences within the extended prodomains are involved in targeting the initiator caspase zymogens to the appropriate cellular locations and in interactions with scaffolding factors.

Effector caspase zymogens are monomers with short prodomains in healthy cells. These inactive enzymes are incapable of autoactivation under normal circumstances. Instead, they are activated through cleavage by initiator caspases.

Scaffolding proteins and **adapters** play an essential role in the activation of initiator caspases. For the *intrinsic pathway* of cell death, factors released from mitochondria (discussed later) activate the scaffold protein **apoptotic protease activating factor 1 (Apaf-1).** Active Apaf-1 forms a seven-spoked ring-like structure called the **apoptosome** (Fig. 46-16). Binding of the procaspase 9 zymogen to this structure promotes dimerization and activation of the enzyme, which appears to achieve full activity without the necessity of zymogen cleavage. The scaffold proteins for the *extrinsic death pathway* are cytoplasmic domains of cell surface receptors. When these receptors bind their ligands on the surface of other cells, they form stable trimeric complexes that recruit **adapter proteins,** which have multiple protein-protein interaction motifs and link the

There are so many different proteins involved in apoptosis that even experts have a difficult time keeping them all straight. However, an understanding of the general principles is much simplified if the following principle is kept in mind. Most proteins that are involved in apoptosis regulation are built from a relatively limited number of modules, many of which act as sites for protein-protein interactions. The following are the most important modules for apoptosis.

Bcl-2 family members are defined by the presence of short regions of conserved sequence, referred to as *BH domains* (Bcl-2 homology). One of these, the approximately 20-residue BH3 domain, found in all Bcl-2 family members, is thought to promote complex formation between Bcl-2 family members.

The process of caspase targeting and activation is regulated by three domains that, although they are not significantly related to one another at the level of amino acid sequence, all adopt a similar structure in solution. All are regions of approximately 80 to 90 residues that form a characteristic arrangement of six α-helix bundles.

1. The *death domain* (DD) is found in many proteins that are involved in signaling pathways related to cell death. These include cell death receptors, such as Fas (and others), and adapter molecules, such as FADD.

2. The *death effector domain* (DED) is found in adapters such as FADD, the prodomains of caspases 8 and 10, and certain inhibitors of apoptosis.

3. The *caspase recruitment domain* (CARD) is found both in a number of adapter proteins involved in cell death, including CED-4 and Apaf-1, and in caspases 1, 2, and 9.

In general, these domains prefer to interact with themselves (i.e., DD-DD, DED-DED, and CARD-CARD). Such interactions are said to be homophilic. As a result, when a new apoptosis effector protein is cloned, it is possible to predict from an analysis of the sequence which of the known proteins it is most likely to interact with.

procaspase 8 zymogen to the receptor complex (Box 46-2). This leads to the dimerization, activation, self-cleavage, and release of active caspase 8, thereby starting the apoptotic cascade.

Caspases are selective enzymes that cleave a relatively limited subset of cellular proteins (Fig. 46-11). Some targets are structural proteins, but many are involved in cellular signaling. For example, caspases cleave several protein kinases. Many kinases have autoregulatory domains that enable them to be switched on and off in response to physiological stimuli (see Fig. 25-4). Caspase cleavage often neatly removes these regulatory domains, thereby producing constitutively active enzymes. Presumably, these unregulated kinases then activate factors that promote cell death. Caspases also cleave and inactivate a number of proteins that normally function in the detection and repair of DNA damage.

Caspases also act on a number of targets that directly promote cell death. The most obvious example of this is caspase activation of other caspases on the death cascade. Caspases also act indirectly to cause the release from mitochondria of factors that promote cell death through the intrinsic pathway. Caspase cleavage of an inhibitory chaperone is responsible for activation of the nuclease that ultimately destroys the chromosomal DNA of most cells undergoing apoptosis (see later discussion).

Natural Caspase Inhibitors

Because most healthy cells express initiator procaspases with the potential to oligomerize by mistake and kill the cell, it is important to have a mechanism that dampens this "noise" in the pro-apoptotic pathway. The inhibitor of apoptosis protein (IAP) family is defined by the presence of a motif of approximately 80 amino acids known as a baculovirus IAP repeat domain. This is a type of Zn^{2+} finger (Fig. 15-17) that mediates protein-protein interactions. IAP proteins inhibit caspases in two ways. First, they bind the caspase and invade the active site, thereby blocking its access to substrates. Second, several IAPs are also E3 ubiquitin ligases (see Fig. 23-8). When they bind caspases, they ubiquitinate them, thereby tagging them for destruction by proteasomes.

If IAP proteins inactivate caspases, then how is the apoptotic response ever initiated? Cells also express an antidote for the IAPs. This protein, known as second mitochondrial activator of caspases (Smac or DIABLO), is normally sequestered in mitochondria. It is released when the intrinsic pathway of apoptosis is initiated.

IAPs were discovered in studies of the mechanisms viruses use to avoid being eliminated by cell death. When viruses infect cells and disassemble their capsids, they become vulnerable to suicide defense mechanisms: If cells can kill themselves before the virus has had time to complete its life cycle, they will take the virus with them, and the organism will survive. To defend against this, viruses pilfer cellular proteins and adapt them for their own means. For example, insect baculoviruses make two proteins that inhibit apoptosis, keeping the cell alive long enough for the virus to reproduce. One of these, IAP, was derived from a cellular gene. The origin of the second, p35, is less clear. p35 is a broad-spectrum caspase inhibitor that is thought to work by

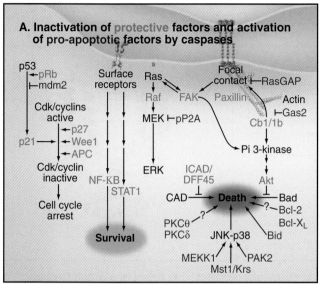

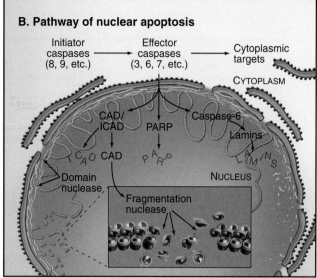

Figure 46-11 SOME WAYS THAT CASPASES PROMOTE CELL DEATH. **A,** Some of the many proteins cleaved by caspases in apoptotic cell death. Proteins shown in *green* normally have a role in keeping the cell alive and are inactivated by caspases. Proteins shown in *red* are turned into active death-promoting factors as a result of caspase cleavage. Proteins shown in *black* are not cleaved and are included to show the pathways that are affected by cleavage. Caspases inactivate a number of pathways that promote cell survival, thereby strongly reinforcing the decision of the cell to die. **B,** Some of the roles of caspases in disassembly of the nucleus.

a serpin-like mechanism. Serpins are special protease substrates that, on cleavage, form a tight complex with the enzyme, thereby inactivating it. Several mammalian pox viruses also make a serpin-like inhibitor of certain caspases called CrmA.

CAD Nuclease and Its Chaperone ICAD

During apoptosis, the chromosomal DNA is destroyed. The many nucleases involved in cleaving the cellular DNA during (and after) apoptotic cell death fall into two classes. **Cell autonomous nucleases** degrade the DNA from within the dying cell (Fig. 46-12A). The best known is the caspase-activated DNase (CAD; see later discussion). In some cell types, a mitochondrial nuclease known as endonuclease G may also be involved. Cell autonomous nucleases are dispensable for cell death and for the life of the organism. They might have evolved to eliminate viral DNA as part of the suicide defense response described in the previous section.

Waste management nucleases clean up the debris after cells die. They either function within lysosomes of cells that have phagocytosed apoptotic cell fragments or are secreted and function in the extracellular space. DNase II, one of the most important waste management nucleases, is essential for life. Mouse embryos that lack DNase II become overwhelmed with undegraded DNA and die.

Cell autonomous nucleases act in two stages. After an initial cleavage of the chromosomes into fragments of roughly 50,000 base pairs, DNA is usually (but not always) cleaved between nucleosomes, producing a characteristic "ladder" of DNA fragments with a periodicity of about 200 base pairs. This ladder is seen when DNA isolated from apoptotic cells is subjected to gel electrophoresis. The responsible nuclease is **CAD.** CAD is normally present in a complex with **ICAD** (inhibitor of CAD [Fig. 46-12C]). The complex of CAD and ICAD is also known as DNA fragmentation factor (DFF). ICAD is a chaperone that must be present for CAD to fold into an active conformation as it is being translated on the ribosome. However, ICAD also inhibits the nuclease activity of CAD. This dual function of ICAD guarantees that only inactive CAD can be synthesized in healthy cells. During apoptosis, caspase 3 cleaves ICAD and releases active CAD nuclease.

Bcl-2 Proteins and the Intrinsic Pathway of Apoptotic Cell Death

As was mentioned previously, mitochondria are key players in a pathway to cell death that is triggered by a variety of toxic insults (Fig. 46-16). These mitochondrial events are regulated by the Bcl-2 family of proteins. The following sections describe this important protein family and their regulation of the intrinsic pathway of apoptosis.

Bcl-2 Proteins

Bcl-2 proteins can be grouped into three subfamilies (Fig. 46-13). Bcl-2 *protectors* protect cells against apoptosis. Bcl-2 *killers* (e.g., Bax and Bak) are pro-apoptotic proteins that actively kill cells. Bcl-2 *regulators*

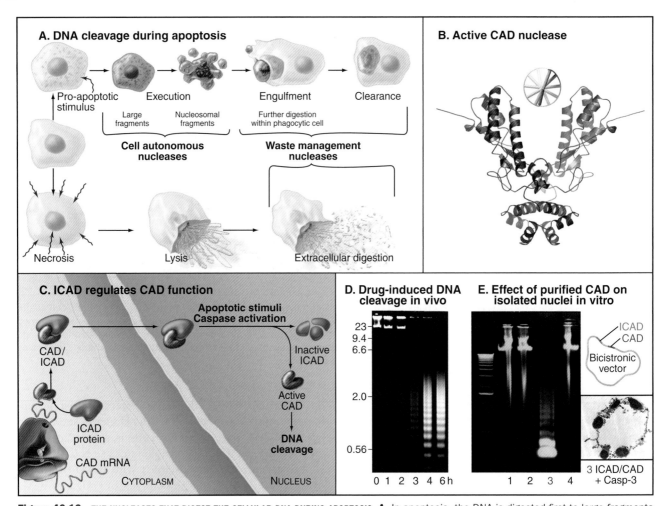

Figure 46-12 THE NUCLEASES THAT DIGEST THE CELLULAR DNA DURING APOPTOSIS. **A,** In apoptosis, the DNA is digested first to large fragments and later to nucleosome-sized pieces (see Fig. 13-1) by cell autonomous nucleases expressed within the dying cell. Waste management nucleases made by other cells also have an essential role in cleaning up apoptotic and necrotic debris. **B,** The predominant cell autonomous nuclease (CAD) has a scissors-like structure. **C,** ICAD is an inhibitory chaperone for CAD, promoting its folding on the ribosome and continuing as an inhibitor when CAD is stored in the nucleus. ICAD cleavage leads to CAD activation. **D,** Cleavage of the chromosomal DNA by CAD during chemotherapy-induced apoptosis of a leukemia cell line. DNA separated according to size by electrophoresis on an agarose gel was stained with ethidium bromide.

E, Activated CAD causes chromatin condensation and appearance of an apoptotic morphology in isolated cell nuclei. Cloned CAD and ICAD were expressed together in *E. coli* (the expression vector is diagrammed at *right*) and incubated with nuclei. ICAD cleavage with caspase 3 released active CAD, which degrades the nuclear DNA *(Lane 3)*. Other lanes: DNA gel size markers *(left)*; nuclei incubated with buffer or caspase 3 alone *(Lanes 1 and 2,* respectively); same experiment as in *Lane 3* but performed by using a mutant ICAD that could not be cleaved by caspase 3 *(Lane 4)*. To the *right* is an electron micrograph of a thin section of one nucleus with condensed chromatin at the nuclear periphery.

(A, Based on Samejima K, Earnshaw WC: Trashing the genome: The role of nucleases during apoptosis. Nat Rev Mol Cell Biol 6:677–688, 2005. B, PDB file: 1VOD. Structure described in Woo EJ, Kim YG, Kim MS, et al: Structural mechanism for inactivation and activation of CAD/DFF40 in the apoptotic pathway. Mol Cell 14:531–539, 2004. D, From Kaufmann SH: Induction of endonucleolytic DNA cleavage in human acute myelogenous leukemia cells by etoposide, camptothecin, and other cytotoxic anticancer drugs: A cautionary note. Cancer Res 49:5870–5878, 1989. E, Courtesy of K. Samejima, Wellcome Trust Institute for Cell Biology, University of Edinburgh, Scotland.)

promote cell killing by either interfering with the protectors or activating the killers. These proteins primarily regulate the release of death-promoting factors from mitochondria when cells receive signals that activate the intrinsic pathway.

C. elegans genetics identified a gene, *ced-9*, that protects cells against apoptosis. In *ced-9* mutants, many cells that normally survive into the adulthood of the organism die during development. This kills the worm.

Human Bcl-2 is functionally and structurally homologous to *C. elegans* Ced-9 and can substitute for it in living worms. This ability of a human gene to protect nematode cells is just one of many examples showing that the fundamental mechanisms that are involved in apoptotic cell death have been conserved over great evolutionary distances.

Bcl-2 family members are defined by the presence of one to four short blocks of conserved protein sequence

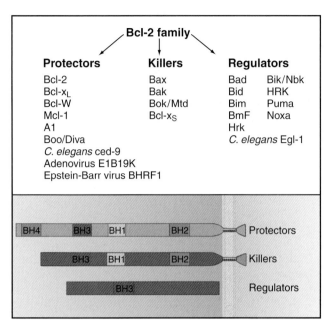

Figure 46-13 Introduction to the Bcl-2 family of proteins.

lymphoma. These particular lymphomas arise when a chromosome translocation, involving chromosomes 14 and 18, moves the *Bcl-2* gene into the immunoglobulin heavy-chain gene cluster, a site of very active gene transcription in B lymphocytes. Elevated transcription of Bcl-2 is thought to be directly responsible for the cancerous phenotype in these patients, making Bcl-2 a cancer-promoting oncogene (see Chapter 41).

Unlike many other oncogenes, *Bcl-2* overexpression does not cause cell proliferation. Instead, it disrupts the balance of regulation between life and death of the affected cells. Cells that overexpress Bcl-2 protein actually grow, if anything, more slowly than do their normal counterparts. However, Bcl-2 overexpressers are highly resistant to many stimuli that normally promote cell death. The net result is an accumulation of B cells: a lymphoma. Figure 46-14 shows an example of Bcl-2 conferring resistance to death when the cell cycle is perturbed by expression of an oncogene.

The Intrinsic Pathway of Apoptotic Death

In addition to their role in energy production, mitochondria have an essential role as sensors of the health of the

called **BH** (Bcl-2 homology) **domains.** Anti-apoptotic Bcl-2 protectors typically have four of the domains. Pro-apoptotic Bcl-2 killers typically have three of these domains, while the Bcl-2 pro-apoptotic regulators have only the BH3 domain. The BH3 domain is a short segment of helix that fits into a groove on the surface of both Bcl-2 protectors and killers, forming a complex that regulates their activity. It is now believed that the Bcl-2 protectors regulate the behavior of Bcl-2 killers by a similar interaction. For example, Bcl-2 protein forms a complex with a pro-apoptotic Bcl-2 killer called Bax, thereby interfering with the ability of Bax to kill cells.

Genetic experiments in mice revealed several different functions for Bcl-2 family members. Mice that are born without Bcl-2 have deficiencies of the immune system that are best understood if one role of this protein in vivo is to render lymphocytes resistant to pro-apoptotic signals during immune system maturation. In contrast, loss of another pro-life family member, Bcl-x$_L$, is lethal. Embryos die, apparently as a result of widespread death of neurons in the central and peripheral nervous systems and hematopoietic cells of the liver. In contrast, loss of the killers Bax plus Bak makes cells highly resistant to apoptosis by a wide variety of intrinsic pathway stimuli.

Bcl-2 Family Members and Cancer

A gene that prevents cells from dying poses a potential danger in multicellular organisms, in which rates of cell proliferation and death must be balanced carefully. In fact, the name *Bcl-2* comes from the discovery that this gene is the culprit responsible for certain types of B-cell

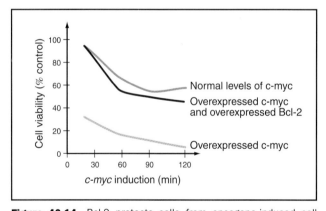

Figure 46-14 Bcl-2 protects cells from oncogene-induced cell death. Chinese hamster ovary cells die when they are induced to express abnormally high levels of the c-myc protein, but simultaneous expression of the Bcl-2 protein rescues them from this effect. These cells contain many copies of the *c-myc* gene under control of a promoter that is activated when the cells are briefly exposed to high temperature (43°C for 90 minutes). The curves show the percentage of viable cells remaining at various times following the induction of c-myc expression. The *Bcl-2* gene was introduced into these cells on a plasmid molecule under the control of a viral promoter, which is always active. The *blue line* represents the parental cell line lacking either the cloned *c-myc* or *Bcl-2* genes. (Note that about 40% of these cells die following the heat treatment used to induce *c-myc* expression.) The *yellow line* shows that the cells that produce high levels of *c-myc* protein alone rapidly die by apoptosis. The *red line* shows that cells expressing both the c-myc and Bcl-2 proteins survive the treatment almost as well as the parental cells. (From Bissonnette RP, Echeverri F, Mahboubi A, et al: Apoptotic cell death induced by c-myc is inhibited by *bcl-2*. Nature 359:552–556, 1992.)

cell. If cells sense insults from which they cannot recover, mitochondria trigger the **intrinsic pathway** of cell death (Fig. 46-16). This pathway is regulated by Bcl-2 family members. The regulation seems straightforward in *C. elegans,* in which the protector CED-9 (Bcl-2–like) binds to the CED-4 scaffolding protein (Apaf-1-like) and interferes with its activation of the CED-3 caspase. Apoptosis is induced when the regulator BH3-only protein EGL-1 binds to CED-9 and blocks it from inactivating CED-4.

In mammals, the situation is more complex, partly because Bcl-2 family members are more numerous and partly because they do not interact in such a straightforward fashion. In mammals, two of the killer proteins, Bax and Bak, are essential for activation of the intrinsic pathway. In healthy cells, Bak is loosely associated with the mitochondrial outer membrane, and Bax is in the cytoplasm (Fig. 46-16). On receipt of a pro-apoptotic stimulus, Bax and Bak insert deeply into the mitochondrial outer membrane, form oligomers, and somehow (not yet known but possibly involving the formation of membrane pores) cause the release of pro-apoptotic factors from the mitochondrial intermembrane space. Binding of anti-apoptotic Bcl-2 family members to Bax/ Bak somehow prevents the release of pro-apoptotic factors from mitochondria. Various BH3-only family members either facilitate Bax/Bak oligomerization or bind and neutralize anti-apoptotic Bcl-2 family members.

The pro-apoptotic factors that are released from the mitochondrial intermembrane space by Bax and Bak include the electron transport protein **cytochrome c** (see Fig. 19-5), Smac, and endonuclease G (Fig. 46-15). These mitochondrial proteins actively promote apoptotic cell death. In the cytoplasm, cytochrome c binds to the scaffolding protein **Apaf-1,** a mammalian homologue of *C. elegans* CED-4 protein, causing it to form a seven-spoked wheel-like structure called the apoptosome (Fig. 46-16). Apaf-1 in the apoptosome binds caspase 9 through an N-terminal **caspase recruitment domain.**

The C-terminal portion of Apaf-1 acts as an autoinhibitor of Apaf-1 function. Binding of cytochrome c and deoxyadenosine triphosphate induces a conformational change that turns off the autoinhibition, thereby permitting binding and autoactivation of seven procaspase 9 monomers. Binding to the apoptosome elevates the catalytic activity of the procaspase 9 zymogen approximately 2000-fold without the need for its cleavage. Thus, the active form of caspase 9 is an oligomeric complex of the zymogen with the apoptosome. Activated caspase 9 then cleaves multiple procaspase 3 zymogens, amplifying the cell death cascade. This cascade can be further amplified in at least two ways. First, caspase 3 cleaves other effector caspases, directly amplifying the cascade. In addition, active caspases cleave the BH3-

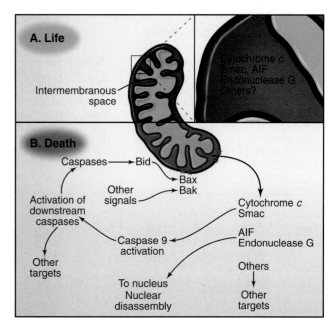

Figure 46-15 MITOCHONDRIA AS INTEGRATORS OF A CELL'S LIFE AND DEATH DECISIONS. **A,** In healthy cells, a number of factors that promote apoptosis are stored in the intermembrane space of the mitochondria. **B,** In cells undergoing apoptosis, caspases trigger the pro-apoptotic Bcl-2 family members to induce the release of these death-promoting factors; this initiates an amplifying cycle that ultimately leads to cell death. AIF, apoptosis-inducing factor.

only protein Bid, which then activates more Bax and Bak in a feedback loop, thereby promoting the release of more cytochrome c and Smac, and enhancing caspase 9 activation.

It was extremely surprising to find that an essential metabolic protein such as cytochrome c has a second function that is essential for death. Among the studies supporting the Jekyll-and-Hyde-like nature of this protein in life and death was the engineering of mice whose cytochrome c can function in electron transport but cannot bind Apaf-1. These mice die as a result of brain abnormalities caused by insufficient cell death.

The Extrinsic Pathway of Apoptotic Death

Cells express at least six different cell surface molecules, collectively termed *death receptors,* that can trigger apoptotic death. These receptors generally bind protein ligands that are expressed on the surface of other cells. This binding activates the receptor, turning on a pathway that leads to apoptotic death.

One well-characterized death receptor is called Fas (also known as Apo1 or CD95), a member of the tumor necrosis factor receptor family (see Fig. 24-10). Fas is a

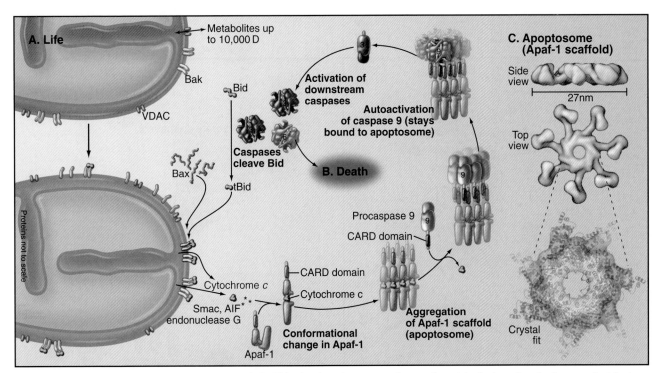

Figure 46-16 THE INTRINSIC CELL DEATH PATHWAY. **A–B,** This drawing shows one of several models for how the death-promoting factors, such as cytochrome c, are released by mitochondria. In this model, Bax and Bak form a pore that releases cytochrome c. Released cytochrome c binds to Apaf-1, inducing formation of the apoptosome, which binds and activates procaspase 9 via scaffold-induced oligomerization. Activated caspase 9 subsequently activates downstream effector caspases, leading to the death of the cell. **C,** Reconstruction of the apoptosome from cryoelectron microscopy *(top)* with crystal structure of Apaf-1 superimposed *(bottom)*. (C, top, Reprinted from Acehan D, Jiang X, Morgan DG, et al: Three-dimensional structure of the apoptosome: Implications for assembly, procaspase-9 binding, and activation. Mol Cell 9:423–432, 2002. Copyright 2002, with permission from Elsevier. C, bottom, Based on Riedl SJ, Li W, Chao Y, et al: Structure of the apoptotic protease-activating factor 1 bound to ADP. Nature 434:926–933, 2005. PDB file: 1Z6T.)

type I membrane protein whose extracellular domain consists of three cysteine-rich domains (see Fig. 24-11, which shows the atomic structure of the related trimeric tumor necrosis factor receptor with bound ligand). The cytoplasmic domain of Fas contains a **death domain** of about 80 residues, which is shared by all of the death receptors (Box 46-2).

The **Fas ligand** is a trimeric 40-kD intrinsic membrane protein found on the surface of cells. Cytotoxic T lymphocytes use Fas ligand to rid the body of virally infected cells. When a cytotoxic T lymphocyte contacts a target cell, the Fas ligand on the lymphocyte surface binds to Fas on the target cell and initiates the extrinsic pathway of apoptotic death (Fig. 46-17). Ligand binding activates signaling from the intracellular death domain of Fas, possibly by stabilizing Fas trimers or by altering their conformation. Activated Fas binds an adapter protein called **FADD** (Fas-associated protein with a death domain). The Fas-FADD complex binds procaspase 8 through interactions involving another type of motif called the **death effector domain,** which is present on both FADD and the prodomain of procaspase 8. On this molecular scaffold, procaspase 8 monomers dimerize and acquire catalytic activity. These dimers

can cleave neighboring dimers, creating and releasing heterotetrameric active caspase 8, which initiates the caspase cascade by activating downstream effector caspases.

This pathway poses considerable risk for the cell. Fas is constitutively present in the cell membrane and appears to have the ability to form at least transient trimers in the absence of binding by its ligand. How do cells avoid the accidental activation of apoptosis caused by chance binding of procaspase 8 zymogens to naturally occurring transient Fas trimers?

Cells express a protein called FLIP (FLICE-like inhibitory protein; FLICE is another name for caspase 8) that looks very much like a catalytically dead version of procaspase 8. When expressed at high levels, FLIP competes with procaspase 8 monomer for binding to FADD, thereby inhibiting the autoactivation of the caspase. This role of FLIP may be to dampen the Fas response locally to ensure that the cascade does not get activated by mistake. When expressed at low levels, FLIP can have the opposite function, facilitating caspase 8 activation by forming a heterodimer with procaspase 8 monomers and causing a conformational change that activates the protease.

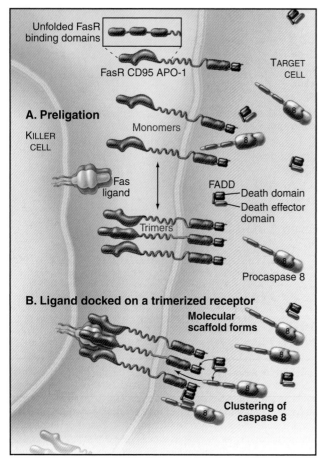

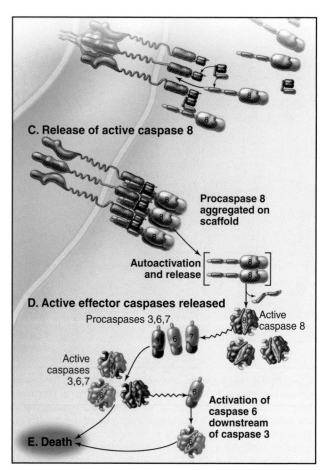

Figure 46-17   THE EXTRINSIC CELL DEATH PATHWAY. The pathways shown here are downstream of the Fas cell death receptor. **A,** Preligation. **B,** Ligand docked on a trimerized receptor. **C,** Release of active caspase. **D,** Release of effector caspases. **E,** Death. (See the text for a detailed description.)

Role of the Fas Death Receptor in Normal and Diseased Cells

Mouse mutants provide clear evidence for an important role of Fas in regulation of the immune system. Mice with mutated *Fas* (the *lpr* mutation) or Fas ligand (the *gld* mutation) accumulate excessive lymphocytes. In the appropriate genetic background, these mice tend to develop autoimmune disorders that, in some cases, resemble the human disease systemic lupus erythematosus. Evidence that Fas is involved in human systemic lupus erythematosus is still scant.

Fas is important in regulating the life span of activated tissue T and B lymphocytes. Normally, T cells die within a few days of their activation during an immune response. Activation initiates the expression of Fas ligand on the T cells themselves. This interacts by an unknown mechanism with Fas already on the cell surface, causing the cell to commit apoptotic suicide. T-cell activation also downregulates the expression of FLIP, thus permitting the more efficient activation of

procaspase 8 by trimerized Fas. A similar mechanism (export of Fas and Fas ligand to the surface of the same cell) is responsible for some examples of p53-induced cell death and some instances of cell death following exposure to chemotherapeutic agents.

Expression of Fas ligand can protect tissues against immune system cells that express Fas. Some tissues, like the lens of the eye and the testis, avoid immune and inflammatory responses by expressing Fas ligand. Immune effector cells that enter these tissues encounter Fas ligand and die by apoptosis. These tissues are known as *immune-privileged*. Not surprisingly, certain tumor cells subvert this strategy as protection against the immune system. Melanoma cells expressing Fas ligand establish tumors particularly efficiently. Some tumor cells, especially colon and lung cancer cells, also defend themselves against immune surveillance with so-called **decoy receptors.** A secreted Fas decoy receptor blocks Fas ligand on cytotoxic cells. Other decoy receptors remain membrane bound but do not signal cell death when they bind ligand because their intracellular domains lack functional death domains.

Linking Apoptosis to the Cell Cycle by p53

No obligate link exists between particular cell-cycle phases and apoptosis. Noncycling G_0 cells can undergo apoptosis, and cycling cells appear able to do so from any cell-cycle phase. However, one link between apoptosis and the cell-cycle machinery has now been firmly established. This involves the p53 tumor suppresser and DNA damage.

The p53 transcription factor is one of the downstream effectors of the DNA damage response pathway (see Fig. 40-4). When cells sense DNA damage induced by agents such as ionizing radiation, levels of p53 rise dramatically (Fig. 46-18). When stabilized and activated by phosphorylation (see Fig. 41-13) p53 upregulates the expression of a number of genes, including the Cdk inhibitor p21, which blocks the entry into the S and M phases. p53 also can trigger an apoptotic response in instances in which the DNA damage is too severe to repair. This tumor suppressor protein is very important in the body's defense against cancer. Mutations in the p53 gene/protein are found in about 50% of all human cancers.

A direct connection between p53 and apoptosis was revealed by overexpression of the cloned p53 gene in different cell types. In most cells, overexpression of p53 arrests the cell cycle at the G_1/S boundary. However, ectopic expression of cloned p53 in certain cancer-derived cell lines causes the cells to undergo apoptosis.

The role of p53 in apoptosis was confirmed in transgenic mice lacking a functional p53 gene (p53 knockout mice). These mice develop normally but are extremely prone to cancer at a very young age. Thus, although mice do not require p53 for programmed cell death during embryogenesis, p53 is critical for apoptosis of certain cells. Thymocytes isolated from p53 knockout mice are extremely resistant to the induction of apoptosis by ionizing radiation and other agents that cause DNA breaks (Fig. 46-18B). However, p53 is not involved in all types of apoptosis. For example, even thymocytes isolated from p53 knockout mice show normal induction of apoptosis following exposure to glucocorticoid hormone (Fig. 46-18).

p53 promotes apoptosis by functioning as a transcriptional activator. It controls, among others, the well-studied death-promoting genes *Bax, Fas (CD95/APO-1)*, and *APAF-1*. However it now appears that the key target gene is *PUMA* (p53 modulated upregulator of apoptosis), a BH3-only protein that promotes apoptotic cell death by activating Bax and Bak. *PUMA* knockout mice show defects in cell death pathways that are essentially identical to those seen in p53 knockout mice and not seen in mice that lack *Bax, Fas, or Apaf-1.*

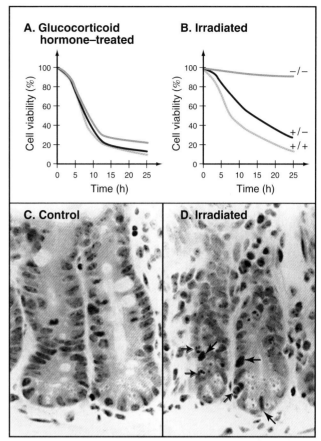

Figure 46-18   **A–B, Survival of thymocytes from three strains of mice after exposure to glucocorticoids or irradiation.** Cell death was due to apoptosis. The strains were as follows: wild-type mice *(yellow)*, heterozygous mice having one good copy of the *p53* gene and one defective copy *(red)*, and mice lacking a functional copy of the *p53* gene *(blue)*. Thymocytes that lack p53 are resistant to radiation-induced apoptosis but show normal induction of apoptosis following exposure to glucocorticoid hormone. **C–D, Induction of p53 accumulation following radiation of the small intestine.** *Black arrows* indicate cells with increased levels of p53. *Red arrows* indicate apoptotic cells. (A–B, From Lowe SW, Schmitt EM, Smith SW, et al: p53 is required for radiation-induced apoptosis in mouse thymocytes. Nature 362:847–849, 1993. C–D, Courtesy of John Hickman, Molecular and Cellular Pharmacology Group, University of Manchester, England.)

Importance of Apoptosis in Human Disease

Studies of apoptosis now account for a substantial fraction of cell biology research. Why has this field so caught the scientific eye? The most likely answer is that apoptosis is a point of intersection between cell signaling pathways, cell structure, the cell cycle, and, of course, human disease. This chapter has mentioned the roles that aberrations in apoptosis play in the etiology of autoimmunity, AIDS, and cancer. Apoptosis is also emerging as a key factor in neurodegenerative diseases, such as Huntington's disease and Alzheimer's disease,

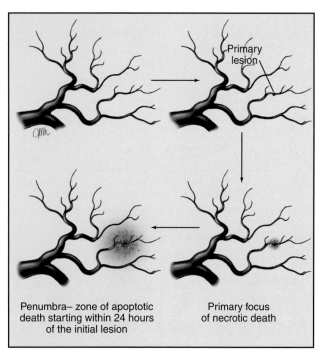

Primary lesion

Penumbra– zone of apoptotic
death starting within 24 hours
of the initial lesion

Primary focus
of necrotic death

Figure 46-19 SECONDARY APOPTOTIC DEATH CAUSED BY OXYGEN DEPRI-
VATION IN THE PENUMBRA GREATLY INCREASES THE SIZE OF THE AFFECTED
AREA OF THE BRAIN IN STROKE.

as well as in myocardial infarction and stroke (Fig.
46-19). At a practical level, the realization that many
successful chemotherapeutic agents act by inducing
cancer cells to undergo apoptosis has motivated searches
for newer and better drugs that elicit this response. One
promising approach is to combine reagents that either
directly promote apoptosis or weaken cellular resistance to apoptosis with cancer chemotherapy. The goal
is to find combinations that increase cell killing synergistically. It is hoped that this strategy will improve
outcomes in cases where tumors are resistant to current
chemotherapy. Conversely, the realization that a large
fraction of the cell deaths in stroke are attributable to a
wave of apoptosis that radiates outward from the original focus of ischemic death has led to the hunt for molecules that will prevent apoptosis during the critical
period following the stroke or infarct. With such important practical problems to be solved, apoptosis will continue to occupy a prominent position in cell biology
research over the coming years.

ACKNOWLEDGMENTS

Thanks go to Scott Kaufmann and Yuri Lazebnik for their
suggestions on revisions to this chapter.

SELECTED READINGS

Abraham MC, Shaham S: Death without caspases, caspases without
death. Trends Cell Biol 14:184-193, 2004.

Breckenridge DG, Xue D: Regulation of mitochondrial membrane
permeabilization by BCL-2 family proteins and caspases. Curr Opin
Cell Biol 16:647-652, 2004.

Cory S, Adams JM: The BCL2 family: Regulators of the cellular life-
or-death switch. Nat Rev Cancer 2:647-656, 2002.

Earnshaw WC, Martins LM, Kaufmann SH: Mammalian caspases:
Structure, activation, substrates and functions during apoptosis.
Annu Rev Biochem 68:383-424, 1999.

Green DR, Kroemer G: The pathophysiology of mitochondrial cell
death. Science 305:626-629, 2004.

Lauber K, Blumenthal SG, Waibel M, Wesselborg S: Clearance of
apoptotic cells: Getting rid of the corpses. Mol Cell 14:277-287,
2004.

Lockshin RA, Zakeri Z: Programmed cell death and apoptosis: Origins
of the theory. Nat Rev Mol Cell Biol 2:545-550, 2001.

Meier P, Finch A, Evan G: Apoptosis in development. Nature 407:796-
801, 2000.

Metzstein MM, Stanfield GM, Horvitz HR: Genetics of programmed
cell death in C. elegans: Past, present and future. Trends Genet
14:410-416, 1998.

Nagata S: Apoptosis by death factor. Cell 88:355-365, 1997.

Raff MC: Social control on cell survival and cell death. Nature
356:397-400, 1992.

Reddien PW, Horvitz HR: The engulfment process of programmed
cell death in Caenorhabditis elegans. Annu Rev Cell Dev Biol
20:193-221, 2004.

Riedl SJ, Shi Y: Molecular mechanisms of caspase regulation during
apoptosis. Nat Rev Mol Cell Biol 5:897-907, 2004.

Savill J, Fadok V: Corpse clearance defines the meaning of cell death.
Nature 407:784-788, 2000.

Shi Y: Caspase activation: Revisiting the induced proximity model.
Cell 117:855-858, 2004.

Strasser A: The role of BH3-only proteins in the immune system. Nat
Rev Immunol 3:189-200, 2005.

Vaux DL: Apoptosis timeline. Cell Death Differ 9:349-354, 2002.

Wyllie AH, Kerr JFR, Currie AR: Cell death: The significance of apoptosis. Int Rev Cytol 68:251-305, 1980.

Glossary

5′ cap. Modified guanosine residue on the 5′ end of mRNAs that protects against degradation

5′ exonuclease. Enzyme that degrades RNA or DNA from the 5′ end

5S RNA. Smallest RNA component of the ribosome, transcribed by RNA polymerase III

14-3-3 domain. Adapter domain that binds serine-phosphate ligands

30-nm fiber. Compacted filament of chromosomal DNA made up of closely packed nucleosomes

AAA ATPase. Family of multimeric enzymes that use ATP hydrolysis to do work in DNA replication, membrane trafficking, and microtubule-dependent motility

A-band. Region of striated muscle sarcomere with myosin thick filaments

ABC transporter. Family of enzymes that pumps diverse solutes and flips lipids across membranes

Acetylcholine. Neurotransmitter for the neuromuscular junction and other synapses

Acetylcholine esterase. Enzyme that degrades acetylcholine

Acrosomal process. Projection of the sperm plasma membrane supported by actin filaments

Actin. Subunit protein of cytoplasmic microfilaments and muscle thin filaments

Actin-related protein (Arp). Family of proteins sharing a common origin and fold with actin

Action potential. Self-propagating, transient change in the membrane potential

Activation loop. Region of protein kinases that must be phosphorylated for the kinase to be fully activated

Acyl-CoA-cholesterol transferase (ACAT). Enzyme of ER membranes that catalyzes the formation of cholesterol esters

ADAR (adenosine deaminase acting on RNA). Enzyme that converts adenine (which base-pairs with uracil) to inosine (which base-pairs with cytosine) by deamination, thereby potentially altering the protein encoded by the mRNA

Adenine. Purine base found in ATP, DNA, and RNA; H-bonds with thymine or uracil

Adenylylcyclase. Enzyme that converts ATP into 3′ to 5′ cyclic AMP

ADF/cofilin. Protein that severs actin filaments and promotes depolymerization

Adherens junction. Intercellular junction that uses cadherins for adhesion and is anchored to actin filaments

Adipocyte. Fat cell

Affinity chromatography. Use of an immobilized ligand to purify interacting macromolecules

Aggrecan. Core protein for a proteoglycan that associates with hyaluronan in cartilage

Agonist. Ligand molecule that activates a receptor

Alpha-actinin. Actin filament cross-linking protein, found in striated muscle Z-disks

Alpha and beta tubulin. Isoforms of tubulin that form the heterodimeric building blocks of microtubules

Alpha-catenin. Adapter protein between cadherins, beta-catenin, and actin filaments

Alpha-helix. Common element of protein secondary structure, right-handed helix with 3.6 amino acid residues per turn

Alpha-satellite. Family of repeated DNA sequences found in human centromeres, composed of monomers ~171 base pairs long, some with binding sites for centromeric protein CENP-B

Alternative splicing. Production of more than one mRNA, and therefore more than one protein product, from a gene by alternative exclusion of exons or inclusion of introns from the mRNA

Alzheimer's disease. Most common dementia of older people, characterized by loss of neurons and formation of intracellular paired helical filaments of tau that aggregate in neurofibrillary tangles

Amide nitrogen. Nitrogen contributed by an amino acid to the peptide bonds of proteins

Amino acid. Building block of proteins, including an amino group, a central α-carbon with a side chain (or R group), and a carboxyl group

Aminoacyl-tRNA synthetases. Enzymes that catalyze covalent coupling of an amino acid to its cognate tRNA

Amino terminus. End of a polypeptide with a free amino group

Anaphase A. The stage of mitosis when sister chromatids separate from each other by moving to the poles of the mitotic spindle, initiated by degradation of proteins that regulate sister chromatid cohesion

Anaphase B. The stage of mitosis when the poles of the mitotic spindle move apart

Anaphase-promoting complex/cyclosome. A ubiquitin-conjugating (E3) enzyme complex that targets proteins, including cyclins and securin, for degradation during mitosis and G_1

Aneuploidy. Excess or missing chromosomes caused by errors in mitosis or meiosis

Antagonist. Ligand molecule that inhibits receptor

Anterograde traffic. Movement of cargo and lipid forward through the secretory system toward the plasma membrane

Anterograde transport. Microtubule-based movements away from the cell center, generally powered by dynein

Antigen-presenting compartment. Phagolysosome specialized for loading MHC Class II molecules with peptides

Antiporter. Carrier proteins that catalyze movements of solutes across membranes up concentration gradients at the expense of transport of a second solute down its concentration gradient in the opposite direction

AP1 complex. Protein complex that directs clathrin coat assembly at the TGN

Apaf-1 (apoptotic protease activating factor 1). Protein activated by cytochrome c that binds procaspase 9 to form the apoptosome, initiating the intrinsic pathway of apoptotic cell death

APC. Product of the adenomatous polyposis coli gene; mutations predispose to colon polyps and cancer

APC/C. *See* Anaphase-promoting complex/cyclosome.

Apical plasma membrane. Region of plasma membrane on the free surface of epithelial cells separated from the basolateral membrane by a ring of tight junctions

Apoptosis. A type of programmed cell death triggered by internal signals or external stimuli and accompanied by characteristic morphologic and biochemical changes

Apoptosome. Seven-spoked ring-like structure containing Apaf-1 and procaspase 9 that starts the proteolytic cascade in the intrinsic (mitochondrial) pathway of apoptosis

Apoptotic bodies. Membrane-enclosed remnants of apoptotic cells

Aquaporins. Family of membrane channels selective for water

Arabidopsis thaliana. Mustard weed; popular genetic model organism favored by plant biologists

Arachidonic acid. A 20-carbon fatty acid with four double bonds; common constituent of membrane lipids and precursor of eicosanoids

Archaea. One of the three domains of life, along with Bacteria and Eukaryotes

Arf. Family of small GTPases, including Sar1 and Arf1-6, that mediate membrane traffic by associations of protein effectors with specific membranes; Arf1 recruits either COPI coat complexes or clathrin to Golgi-like membranes

Arp2/3 complex. Protein complex including Arp2 and Arp3 that nucleates branched actin filaments

Arrestin. Protein that binds and inhibits phosphorylated seven-helix receptors

Assembly proteins (AP1, AP2). Clathrin coat constituents that regulate clathrin coat assembly

Aster. Radial array of dynamic microtubules emanating from the duplicated centrosomes at the poles of the mitotic spindle; has a role in orienting the spindle in the cell through interactions with the cell cortex

ATM (ataxia telangiectasia mutated). Large protein kinase that can initiate the response to DNA damage by activating the downstream kinases Chk1 and Chk2

ATP. Adenosine triphosphate; the common energy-carrying molecule for cellular metabolism; enzymes use the energy released from the hydrolysis of its γ-phosphate for many cellular processes

ATP synthase. Reversible, rotary mitochondrial transmembrane protein that can either hydrolyze ATP to pump protons or use the passage of protons down a gradient across the membrane to synthesize ATP (*see* F-type ATPase)

ATR (ATM and Rad3 related). Large protein kinase that responds to abnormal accumulation of single-stranded DNA by activating downstream kinases Chk1 and Chk2

Aurora-B. Protein kinase in the chromosomal passenger complex that regulates chromosome attachment and cytokinesis during mitosis

Autolysosome. Compartment containing acid hydrolases for intracellular degradation formed by fusion of a nascent autophagic vacuole with a late endosome or lysosome

Autonomic nerve. Nerves of the sympathetic and parasympathetic peripheral nervous systems

Autonomously replicating sequences (ARS). Short (100 to 150 bp) DNA segments that can act as replication origins in yeast

Autophagic vacuole. Compartment for intracellular degradation formed when a flattened membrane cisterna encloses a region of cytoplasm in a vesicle with two membranes

Autophagy. Degradation of intracellular substrates in membrane-bounded compartments

Autosomes. Chromosomes that do not carry genes that define the sex of the individual

Axon. Process of a neuron capable of propagating an action potential and forming synapses with other neurons or muscles

Axoneme. Microtubule-based structural framework of eukaryotic cilia and flagella

Barbed end. Fast-growing end of an actin filament

Barr body. Inactivated X chromosome forming a discrete patch of heterochromatin at the nuclear periphery

Basal body (axonemal). Cylindrical microtubule organizing center composed of nine triplet microtubules located at the base of cilia and flagella

Basal body (bacterial). A transmembrane complex of proteins forming the rotary motor for bacterial flagella

Basal lamina. A thin, planar specialization of extracellular matrix beneath epithelia and around muscle cells and peripheral nerve cells

Base excision repair. Process that replaces oxidized, reduced, alkylated, or deaminated DNA bases

Basolateral plasma membrane. Domain of the cell membrane of epithelial cells facing neighboring cells and the basal lamina, separated from the apical domain by a ring of tight junctions

Bax and Bak. Bcl-2 family proteins that activate the intrinsic pathway of apoptosis by inserting into mitochondrial outer membranes and releasing pro-apoptotic factors

Bcl-2 proteins. Three subfamilies of proteins with BH domains that regulate the release of death-promoting factors from mitochondria: Bcl-2 *protectors* inhibit apoptosis; Bcl-2 *killers* promote apoptosis; Bcl-2 *regulators* interfere with protectors or activate killers

Beta-catenin. Adapter protein between the cytoplasmic domain of cadherins, α-catenin, and actin filaments; also a transcription factor regulated by Wnt signaling pathways

Beta-sheet. Common element of protein secondary structure consisting of parallel or antiparallel strands of polypeptides linked by backbone hydrogen bonds

BH domains (Bcl-2 homology). Conserved sequences of ~20 residues that define Bcl-2 family members; BH3 domain, found in all Bcl-2 family members, promotes interactions of Bcl-2 family members

Bilayer. Planar assembly of lipids with hydrophobic fatty acid chains inside and hydrophilic head groups on both surfaces

BiP. HSP70 family chaperone protein that promotes folding of proteins in the ER lumen

Bipolar attachment. Attachment of the kinetochores of two sister chromatids to microtubules emanating from opposite poles of the mitotic spindle

Bivalents. Paired homologous chromosomes consisting of four sister chromatids held together by chiasmata during meiosis I

Branch point. Site of attachment of the 5′ end of an intron to an adenosine in the lariat intermediate during RNA splicing

Brefeldin A (BFA). Fungal metabolite used experimentally to disassemble the Golgi apparatus by preventing activation of Arf1 by GTP binding

Bright field. Light microscopic imaging system without optical elements to vary the phase or polarity of the light

Bromodomain. Protein motif that binds acetylated N-terminal histone tails

Brown fat. Fat cells with numerous mitochondria specialized for heat production

BUB (budding uninhibited by benzimidazole). Conserved genes encoding proteins essential for the spindle checkpoint

Ca-ATPase pump. P-type membrane pump that uses ATP hydrolysis to transport Ca^{2+} into the endoplasmic reticulum or out of the cell

CAD (caspase-activated DNase). Principal nuclease within apoptotic cells that degrades chromatin into DNA nucleosomal fragments of about 200 base pairs

CAD domain. Extracellular domains of the cadherin family of adhesion proteins

Cadherin. Adhesion proteins that typically bind to like cadherins on other cells

Caenorhabditis elegans. Small nematode worm; genetic model organism favored by developmental biologists

Cajal bodies (coiled bodies). Nuclear structures that accumulate many factors involved in mRNA processing and within which specific nucleotides in snRNAs are modified.

CAK (Cdk-activating kinase). Complex of Cdk7 and cyclin H that phosphorylates Cdk1 on T^{161}, the final step in its activation

Calcium-sensitive dye. Dye that changes its fluorescence on Ca^{2+} binding

Calmodulin. Small calcium ion binding protein that activates numerous effector proteins

Calnexin. Sugar-binding, lectin-like protein in ER lumen

Calnexin cycle. Cycle of modifications that help glycoproteins fold in the ER

Calsequestrin. Ca^{2+} binding protein in the ER lumen of striated muscle

cAMP. Nucleotide with an adenine base and a cyclic phosphodiester bond linking the 3′ and 5′ hydroxyls; an important signaling second messenger

cAMP-gated channel. Family of cation ion channels activated by cAMP binding to a cytoplasmic domain

Cap recognition complex. Proteins that recognize 5′ caps on mRNAs, targeting them for export from the nucleus and to preinitiation complexes on ribosomes

Cap Z. Isoform of heterodimeric capping protein that binds barbed ends of thin filaments in the Z-disk of striated muscles

Capping protein. Heterodimeric protein that caps the barbed ends of actin filaments

Carbohydrate. Sugar molecules with the chemical composition $(CH_2O)_n$

Carbonyl oxygen. The oxygen atom on the carbon atom of peptide bonds

Carboxyl terminus. The end of a polypeptide with a free carboxyl group

Carboxyl-terminal domain (CTD). Region of RNA polymerase II that participates in initiation and coordinates RNA splicing reactions

Cardiac muscle. The striated muscle of the heart

Cardiomyopathy. Genetic diseases of heart muscle leading to heart failure or abnormal rhythms

Cargo selection. Mechanism for cargo sorting into membrane-bound transport carriers

Carrier vesicles. Tubules or larger membrane-enclosed structures that mediate transport among intracellular compartments

Cartilage. Specialized connective tissue consisting largely of collagen fibrils, proteoglycans, and water found in joints, respiratory tract, and developing bones

CAS. Nuclear export receptor that works with RanGTP to displace cargo from importin α

Caspase recruitment domain (CARD). Protein interaction domain found in cell death adapter proteins and certain caspases

Caspases (cysteine aspartases). Proteases with an active site cysteine that cleave at aspartate residues and whose activation triggers apoptotic cell death

Catastrophe. Random change of state whereby an end of a microtubule stops growing and rapidly depolymerizes

Cathepsin K. Proteolytic enzyme secreted by osteoclasts to digest organic components of bone

Caveolae. Small (~50 nm) flask-shaped invaginations of plasma membrane enriched in caveolin, cholesterol, and signaling molecules

Caveolin. Major protein component of caveolae

CDC mutants (cell division cycle mutants). Mutations in genes essential for cell cycle progression that cause yeast to accumulate at a single point in the cell cycle

Cdc20. Target of the spindle checkpoint; thought to be a substrate recognition factor for the APC/C

Cdc25. Three protein phosphatases that remove inhibitory phosphates from T^{14} and Y^{15} of Cdk-cyclin complexes, thereby triggering kinase activation

Cdc42. Small GTPase of the Rho family that regulates actin assembly

Cdc45p. Protein recruited to active origins of replication to activate Mcm proteins, promote RPA binding, and recruit DNA polymerase

Cdk (cyclin-dependent kinase). Kinase that requires association of a cyclin subunit to regulate cell cycle progression

Cdk1–cyclin B. Cell cycle kinase with critical roles in the G_2/M transition and mitosis

Cdk2-cyclin A. Cell cycle kinase with critical roles in S phase and G_2/M transition

cDNA. A DNA copy of a messenger RNA

Ced (cell death abnormal) mutants. Mutations in *C. elegans* genes that affect programmed cell death

Cell cortex. Region of cytoplasm beneath the plasma membrane, typically rich in actin filaments

Cell wall. Extracellular matrix of plants and fungi

Cellulose. Long, unbranched polymer of glucose in plant cell walls; most abundant biopolymer on earth

Cellulose synthases. Plasma membrane enzymes that synthesize cellulose

CEN sequences. Short DNA sequences in budding yeast chromosomes that specify protein-binding sites for assembly of kinetochores

CENP-A. Histone H3 variant, an integral component of kinetochores in species ranging from yeast to man

CENP-B. Protein that binds a 17-bp sequence in α-satellite DNA and establishes an epigenetic state favoring kinetochore assembly on α-satellite DNA arrays

CENP-C. Protein that appears to bridge between the inner and outer kinetochore

Central pair. Two microtubules located in the middle of nine outer doublet microtubules in axonemes

Central spindle. Antiparallel bundle of microtubules that appears late in anaphase and has an important role during cytokinesis

Centrifuge. Machine that spins a sample holder to generate force to sediment particles in liquid samples

Centrin. Family of EF-hand, Ca^{2+} binding proteins similar to calmodulin that are essential for the biogenesis of centrioles (and spindle pole bodies of yeast)

Centrioles. Barrel-shaped structures composed of nine microtubule triplets that organize the centrosome (*see* Basal body)

Centromere. Chromosomal locus, defined by specific DNA sequences and associated proteins that regulates chromosomal movements during mitosis and meiosis

Centrosome. Pair of centrioles and surrounding matrix containing proteins including γ-tubulin that nucleate microtubules and serve as the microtubule-organizing center in most animal cells

Ceramide. Backbone of all sphingolipids that is converted to glucosylceramide and sphingomyelin in the Golgi apparatus

Ceramide transport protein (CERT). Removes newly synthesized ceramide from the ER for transport to the Golgi apparatus

cGMP. Nucleotide with a guanine base and a cyclic phosphodiester bond linking the 3′ and 5′ hydroxyls

Chaperone. Protein that assists the folding of other proteins

Checkpoint. Biochemical circuit that, when active, blocks progression through the cell cycle, either temporarily or, in some cases, permanently

Chemiosmotic cycle. A series of reactions across a lipid bilayer that couples the creation of an ion gradient by an energy-consuming transmembrane pump to energy-requiring transport or ATP synthesis by a second transmembrane protein

Chemotaxis. Process by which a cell moves up a concentration gradient of a chemical attractant

Chiasmata. Chromatin structures at sites where recombination has been completed; keep homologous chromosomes paired until anaphase of meiosis I

Chk1/Chk2 (checkpoint kinases 1/2). Protein kinases activated by ATM and ATR that phosphorylate Cdc25A protein phosphatase and other substrates, thereby blocking cell cycle progression

Chloride channel. Transmembrane ion channel selective for chloride ions

Chlorophyll. Organic molecule that absorbs photons and uses the energy to boost electrons to an excited state

Chloroplast. Eukaryotic organelle derived from a symbiotic cyanobacterium specialized for photosynthesis

Chloroplast stroma. Compartment inside the inner chloroplast membrane devoted to synthesis of three-carbon sugar phosphates, chloroplast proteins, and fatty acids

Cholesterol. Polycyclic lipid with one polar atom found in biological membranes; also the precursor for steroid hormones and bile acids

Chondrocyte. Cell that synthesizes and secretes the extracellular matrix of cartilage

Chromatid. A single chromosomal DNA molecule plus its attendant proteins

Chromatin. DNA plus the proteins that package it within the cell nucleus

Chromatography. Method to separate chemicals based on interactions with an immobile matrix such as a gel or paper; implemented with the matrix in a tubular column or on a plate

Chromodomain (chromatin modification organizer). Motif of 50 amino acids that binds to histone H3 trimethylated on lysine

Chromonema fiber. A chromatin fiber, 100 to 300 nm in diameter, thought to be an element of higher-order packing of chromatin within chromosomes

Chromosomal passenger complex. A complex of Aurora B kinase, inner centromere protein (INCENP), survivin, and borealin that is required to correct chromosome attachment errors, for the spindle checkpoint, and to complete cytokinesis

Chromosome. DNA molecule with its attendant proteins that behaves as an independent unit during mitosis and meiosis

Chromosome cycle. Replication and partitioning of chromosomes into two daughter cells

Chromosome scaffold. Structural proteins left behind after chromosomes are treated with nucleases to remove the DNA and extracted to remove most chromosomal proteins

Chromosome territories. Discrete regions of the interphase nucleus occupied by particular chromosomes

Cilium. Cell surface organelle of eukaryotes based on a microtubule axoneme, usually capable of generating waves or other motions but sometimes immotile sensory structures

Citric acid cycle. Biochemical reactions in the mitochondrial matrix that derives energy by breaking down acetyl-CoA

CKI (cyclin-dependent kinase inhibitor). Class of proteins that negatively regulate Cdks to block cell cycle progression

Clathrin. Protein that forms a three-legged triskelion and a lattice on the cytoplasmic surface of membranes during the formation of buds

Clathrin-coated pit. Invaginated patch of membrane formed by a lattice of clathrin triskelions and adapter molecules on the cytoplasmic surface

Clathrin-mediated endocytosis. Selective uptake of ligands bound to receptors that concentrate in clathrin-coated pits

Claudins. Transmembrane proteins that link plasma membranes together at tight junctions

Cleavage furrow. Constriction of the plasma membrane that pinches a cell in two during cytokinesis as a result of action of a contractile ring of actin filaments and myosin-II

Cleavage stimulus. Signal emitted by the mitotic spindle that specifies the position of the cleavage furrow midway between the poles and perpendicular to the long axis of the spindle

CLIP-170. Protein that concentrates on plus ends of growing microtubules; involved in transport of membranes and behavior of microtubules at kinetochores

Closed mitosis. Form of mitosis in single-celled eukaryotes, including yeast and slime molds in which the mitotic spindle forms and chromosomes segregate within an intact nuclear envelope to which the spindle poles are anchored

Coactivator. Protein complex that facilitates loading of the transcriptional apparatus onto a gene, often by modifying N-terminal histone tails to "open" the chromatin

Codon. Three successive nucleic acid bases in mRNA that specify the position of a particular amino acid in a polypeptide during synthesis on a ribosome

Cohesin. Complex of four proteins that holds sister chromatids together from their replication during the S phase until their separation at the onset of anaphase

Coiled-coil. Left-handed helix of two α-helical polypeptides; either parallel or antiparallel

Colchicine. Drug isolated from the autumn crocus that inhibits microtubule assembly by binding dissociated tubulin dimers

Collagen. Chief fibrous protein of connective tissues, composed of three rod-shaped polypeptides, each folded in type II polyproline helix; many isoforms specialized for cartilage, basal lamina and other connective tissues

Complex I (NADH:ubiquinone oxidoreductase). Complex of proteins in mitochondrial inner membranes and bacterial plasma membranes, which takes electrons from NADH and transfers protons out of the mitochondrial matrix and bacterial cytoplasm

Complex II (succinate:ubiquinone reductase). A transmembrane enzyme complex from mitochondria and Bacteria that takes part in the citric acid cycle, by coupling oxidation of succinate to reduction of flavin adenine dinucleotide (FAD) to $FADH_2$

Complex III (cytochrome bc_1). Transmembrane protein complex from mitochondria and Bacteria that couples oxidation and reduction of ubiquinone to the transfer of protons out of the matrix

Complex IV (cytochrome oxidase). Transmembrane protein complex of mitochondria and Bacteria that takes electrons from four cytochrome c molecules to reduce molecular oxygen to two waters, as well as to pump four protons out of the mitochondrial matrix or bacterial cytoplasm

Condenser. Lenses in microscopes that focus the illuminating beam on the specimen

Condensin I and II. Two pentameric protein complexes with an essential role in chromosome architecture

Conditional mutation. A mutation that gives an abnormal phenotype only under certain conditions such as high temperature

Confocal microscope. Imaging system using pinholes to restrict the illumination to a thin plane in the specimen

Conformational change. Change in the shape of a macromolecule

Connexin. Protein subunit of gap junction channels

Connexon. Hexamer of connexin subunits making up gap junction channels connecting the cytoplasm of adjacent cells

Constitutive heterochromatin. Inactive form of chromatin that remains condensed throughout the cell cycle owing to the presence of special proteins and modifications of the histone proteins

Constitutive secretion. Exocytosis without special stimuli being received by the cell

Contact inhibition. Arrest of cell-cycle progression in G1 when cells growing in culture become surrounded by other cells on all sides, mediated by interactions of cadherins

Contractile ring. Band of actin filaments, myosin-II, and other proteins attached to the plasma membrane around the cortex midway between spindle poles that pinches daughter cells in two like a purse string during cytokinesis

COPI coat complex. Assembly of Arf1 GTPase, coatomer, and a GAP on the cytoplasmic face of VTCs and Golgi membranes to mediate protein sorting, budding, and retrograde transport back to the ER

COPII coat complex. Assembly of Sar1p GTPase, Sec23p•Sec24p, and Sec13p•Sec31p on the cytoplasmic face of the ER to mediate sorting and trafficking of secretory cargo out of the ER

Core histones. Histones H2A, H2B, H3, and H4, which form the disk-like octameric core of nucleosomes

Core mannose oligosaccharide. Branched oligosaccharide rich in mannose that is transferred from dolichol phosphate to the side chain of an asparagine of a newly synthesized protein in the ER lumen

Core protein. Protein modified with glycosaminoglycans to make a proteoglycan

Cotranslational translocation. Movement of a protein across the ER membrane concurrent with its synthesis by a membrane-bound ribosome

CpG islands. Regions of DNA rich in CpG found in and around gene promoters

Crinophagy. Fusion of lysosomes directly with secretory vesicles resulting in the degradation of secretory proteins

Cristae. Folds of the inner mitochondrial membrane

Critical concentration. The concentration of unpolymerized subunits giving equal rates assembly and disassembly at an end of a polymer

Crossbridge. Force-producing connection of a motor protein between its cytoskeletal track and its cargo

Crossover. Physical breakage and reunion of DNA strands on two different chromosomes, typically producing a balanced exchange of DNA sequences

Crossover interference. Uncharacterized mechanism that locally limits the number of DNA breaks that are processed to form crossovers and chiasmata during meiosis

c-Src. Nonreceptor tyrosine kinase important in signaling

Cyanobacteria. Photosynthetic Bacteria (formerly called blue-green algae) with both types of photosystems as well as a manganese enzyme that splits water

Cyclic nucleotide–dependent protein kinases. Kinases regulated by binding of cyclic nucleotides to part of the enzyme or to a separate regulatory subunit

Cyclic nucleotide–gated channels. Cation channels regulated by binding of cyclic nucleotides to cytoplasmic domains

Cyclic-ADP-ribose. Derivative of NAD that sets the sensitivity of ryanodine receptor calcium release channels to the cytoplasmic Ca^{2+} concentration

Cyclin. Class of subunits required for activity of cyclin-dependent kinases that undergo cyclic patterns of accumulation and destruction during the cell cycle

Cyclin-dependent kinase. *See* Cdk.

Cyclooxygenase. Enzymes that convert arachidonic acid into prostaglandin H2

Cytochalasin. Fungal product used experimentally to depolymerize actin filaments in cells

Cytochrome c. Small heme protein, part of electron transport pathway of oxidative phosphorylation and, when released from mitochondria, a trigger for apoptosis

Cytochrome P450. Enzymes of the smooth ER that detoxify endogenous steroids, carcinogenic compounds, and lipid-soluble molecules from the environment

Cytokine. Diverse family of protein hormones and growth factors

Cytokine receptor. Transmembrane receptors for cytokines linked to JAK kinases in the cell

Cytokinesis. Division of the cytoplasm into two daughter cells at the end of mitosis

Cytoplasmic streaming. Bulk movement of organelles and cytoplasm

Cytosine. Pyrimidine base present in DNA and RNA; H-bonds with guanine

Cytoskeleton. The ensemble of protein polymers (including actin filaments, intermediate filaments, and microtubules) forming the mechanical scaffold for the cytoplasm

Cytostatic factor (CSF). A biochemical activity, including the APC/C inhibitor Emi2, that arrests vertebrate oocytes in metaphase II of meiosis until they are fertilized

Dark reactions. Biochemical reactions in chloroplasts that convert carbon dioxide into three-carbon sugar phosphates

Deadenylases. Enzymes that catalyze the stepwise removal of the poly(A) tail of mRNAs, signaling their degradation by removing binding sites for the poly(A)-binding protein (PABP), which when present inhibits cap removal at the other end of the RNA

Death domain (DD). Protein interaction domain in proteins from cell death signaling pathways, including Fas cell death receptors and FADD adapter molecules

Death effector domain (DED). Protein interaction domain in adapters such as FADD, the prodomains of caspases 8 and 10, and in certain inhibitors of apoptosis

Debranching enzyme. Linearizes the lariat mRNA splicing intermediate for degradation by exonucleases

Decapping complex. Removes the 5′ cap from mRNAs, triggering their rapid degradation

Dendrite. Nerve cell process specialized for receiving synapses from other neurons

Dense body. Attachment sites for actin filaments and intermediate filaments in the cytoplasm of smooth muscle cells

Dense fibrillar component. Regions of nucleoli surrounding fibrillar centers

Dephosphorylation. Reaction that removes a phosphate from a protein side chain

Desmin. Intermediate filament isoform expressed by muscle cells

Desmoplakin. Protein link between desmosomal cadherins and intermediate filaments

Desmosome. Intercellular junction mediated by cadherins and anchored to cytoplasmic intermediate filaments

Diacylglycerol (DAG). Diglyceride with two fatty acids and no head group; activates PKC isoforms

Diakinesis. Prometaphase of meiosis I

Dicer. Double-strand-specific RNA endonuclease in the RNAi pathway that generates short RNA duplexes that are incorporated into the RISC complex

Dictyostelium discoideum. A cellular slime mold; popular model organism for studying chemotaxis, motility, and differentiation

Differential interference contrast (DIC). Light microscopy optics generating contrast from local differences in refractive index

Diploid chromosome number (2n). Total number of chromosomes in a diploid organism, comprising pairs of homologous chromosomes, one donated by the mother and the other by the father

Diplotene. Fourth stage of meiotic prophase with decondensed chromosomes held together by chiasmata (can last for decades in female humans)

Dis1/TOG family (called XMAP215 in frogs). Proteins that associate with microtubule plus ends to regulate microtubule assembly and dynamics; required for organization of mitotic spindle poles in animals and cortical arrays of microtubules in plants

Disjunction (disjoining). Normal separation of chromosomes or chromatids in meiosis or mitosis

Disks. Membrane compartments in photoreceptor cells rich in rhodopsin

Disulfide bond. S-S bond formed by oxidation between two cysteine residues

DNA. Polymer of phosphate-linked sugars (deoxyribose) linked to purine and pyrimidine bases that constitutes the genetic information for most organisms

DNA damage checkpoints. Biochemical pathways that detect damaged DNA and then either block cell cycle progression or trigger cell death by apoptosis

DNA polymerases δ and ε. Enzymes that use PCNA to help them process along the DNA, synthesizing DNA continuously on the leading strand. On the lagging strand, they synthesize Okazaki fragments of about 250 bp

DNA replication. Synthesis of two complementary strands from a DNA double helix; duplication of the genome

DNA replication checkpoint. Biochemical mechanism that detects unreplicated DNA or stalled DNA replication forks, stabilizing the latter so that they can be repaired

DNA topoisomerase IIα. An enzyme found in the mitotic chromosome scaffold that alters DNA topology by passing one double-helix strand through another

Dolichol phosphate. Long-chained, unsaturated isoprenoid alcohol with pyrophosphate at one end that is the substrate for the synthesis of oligosaccharide precursors in the cytoplasm and subsequent transfer to asparagines of proteins in the ER lumen

Dominant negative mutation. Mutation giving rise to a deleterious phenotype even in the presence of a wild-type allele

Double-strand break repair. Two processes that repair double-strand breaks in DNA either without a template (nonhomologous end-joining) or using undamaged DNA as a template (homologous recombinational repair) for accurate repair

Down syndrome. Common human aneuploidy with three copies of chromosome 21

Drosophila melanogaster. Fruit fly, genetic model organism popular for studying development

Dynactin complex. Protein complex linking dynein to membrane cargo

Dynamic instability. Behavior of microtubules with growing and shrinking microtubules coexisting at steady state

Dynamin. GTPase that coordinates the invagination, fission, and internalization of clathrin-coated vesicles

Dynein. Motor proteins that use ATP hydrolysis to move toward the minus ends of microtubules, members of AAA ATPase family

Dystroglycan/sarcoglycan complex. Transmembrane complex that stabilizes muscle plasma membranes through interactions with the cytoskeleton and the basal lamina

Dystrophin. Giant protein that links the dystroglycan/sarcoglycan complex to cytoplasmic actin filaments; mutations cause the most common form of muscular dystrophy

E1 enzyme (ubiquitin-activating enzyme). Activates the small protein ubiquitin by forming a thioester bond between the C-terminus of ubiquitin and a cysteine on the enzyme

E2 enzyme (ubiquitin-conjugating enzyme). Either transfers ubiquitin directly to the ε amino group of a lysine of a target protein or combines with a third component (an E3 or ubiquitin-protein ligase) to do so

E2F. Family of 10 transcription factors in mammals that regulate genes promoting cell cycle progression at the restriction point and can trigger cell death by apoptosis

E3 enzyme (ubiquitin-protein ligase). Transfers ubiquitin to the ε amino group of a lysine of a target protein

Early recombination nodules. Sites along chromosomes where DNA strand breaks have occurred and recombination is initiated early in meiosis

EB1. Protein that binds growing microtubule plus ends and associates with APC

E-cadherin. Isoform of cadherin adhesion protein expressed by epithelial cells

EEA1. Tethering factor in the early endosomal membranes

Effector caspases. "Downstream" caspases activated through cleavage by initiator caspases and responsible for most intracellular proteolysis during apoptosis

Ehlers-Danlos syndrome. Human genetic disease with thin skin and lax joints owing to mutations in the genes for fibrillar collagens type III or type IV

Eicosanoids. Diverse class of lipid second messengers derived from arachidonic acid

Elastin. Protein subunit of elastic fibers

Electrical potential. Voltage difference across a membrane

Electrical synapse. Site of rapid transmission of action potentials between neurons through gap junctions

Electron transport pathway. Sequence of reactions in the inner mitochondrial membrane and bacterial plasma membrane that uses energy from the passage of electrons to generate a proton gradient across the membrane to power a chemiosmotic cycle to synthesize ATP

Electrostatic interaction. Attraction of oppositely charged atoms

Elongation factor Tu (eEF-1 in animals). GTPase that delivers tRNAs charged with amino acids to ribosomes and is the timer for the proofreading reaction

Elongation factors. Proteins that facilitate the synthesis of polypeptides on ribosomes

Embryonic stem cells. Precursors of the entire embryo, produced by the first embryonic cell divisions

Emi2. An inhibitor of the APC/C and a key component of cytostatic factor

Endocytosis. Process by which extracellular materials are captured and enclosed within membrane-bound carriers that invaginate and pinch off into the cytoplasm from the plasma membrane

Endoplasmic reticulum (ER). Large, membrane-delineated, intracellular compartment that collects proteins synthesized in the cytoplasm for modification and delivery into the secretory pathway

Endosome. A membrane-bounded compartment for processing materials taken in by endocytosis

Enhancer. Complex cluster of transcriptional regulator binding sites on DNA that increases the rate of initiation from a basal promoter; can function even if located up to 10 kb upstream or downstream from the promoter or in either orientation relative to it

Enthalpy. The internal energy of a system plus the product of its volume times its pressure; the pressure-volume term rarely applies to biological systems, so the internal energy corresponds to the heat contained in the chemical bonds

Entropy. Measure of the disorder in a system

Eosinophil. A type of white blood cell with large granules that stain with eosin; active against parasites

Epidermal growth factor. Protein hormone that activates a receptor tyrosine kinase and promotes growth of epithelial cells

Epidermolysis bullosa. Genetic disease with mutations in keratins resulting in fragility and blistering of skin

Epigenetic trait. Inheritable property of chromosomes carried by enzymatic modification of DNA or proteins associated with DNA rather than being encoded in the nucleotide sequence

Epiphyseal plate. Disk of cartilage whose expansion is responsible for the growth of long bones

Epithelial sodium channel. Channel protein formed by four subunits with two transmembrane segments

Equilibrium constant. Thermodynamic parameter describing the extent of a reaction at equilibrium; related to the change in free energy and to the ratio of the rate constants for the forward and reverse reactions

ER export domain. Site of secretory cargo export from the ER

ERAD (ER-associated protein degradation). Process to move misfolded proteins out of the ER into the cytoplasm for degradation by proteasomes

Erythropoietin. Cytokine driving red blood cell production, produced by the kidney

Escherichia coli. Gram-negative colon bacterium; popular genetic model organism

ESCRT complex. Protein complex that sorts ubiquitinated receptors in early endosomes and drives them into the membrane invaginations of multivesicular bodies

Euchromatin. Transcriptionally active or potentially active chromatin, containing most of the genes

Eukaryote. Organism in which the genome is packaged within a nucleus

Excitable membrane. Plasma membrane with voltage-gated Na- and K-channels, capable of propagating action potentials

Excited state. High-energy state of an electron achieved by absorption of a photon or a chemical reaction, used to generate proton gradients across membranes in photosynthesis and oxidative phosphorylation or to emit a photon during fluorescence

Exonic splicing enhancers (ESEs). RNA sequences that bind SR-proteins and stimulate the use of the flanking 5′ and 3′ splice sites, promoting exon definition by preventing the exon in which they are located from being included in an intron

Exon-junction complex (EJC). Protein complex deposited on mRNA during splicing in the nucleus and retained following export to the cytoplasm, where it is used to identify mRNAs on which translation has terminated prematurely

Exons. Regions of genes that appear in mature RNA molecules

Exosome (endocytosis). Vesicles of invaginated membrane inside multivesicular bodies that are released from cells when MVBs fuse with the plasma membrane

Exosome (RNA processing). Complex of multiple different 3′ to 5′ exonucleases that degrade nuclear RNAs and turnover mRNAs in the cytoplasm

Expansins. Plant proteins that break noncovalent links between cellulose polymers transiently, allowing turgor pressure to expand the volume of the cell

Expressed sequence tag (EST). DNA sequences collected by sequencing random cDNAs

Extracellular matrix. Fibrous proteins, polysaccharides, proteoglycans, and adhesive glycoproteins providing the mechanical support for tissues in animals and plants

Extrinsic pathway of cell death. Process initiated when cell surface ligands activate receptors on target cells, triggering the apoptotic pathway in the target cells

Facultative heterochromatin. DNA sequences located in heterochromatin in some cells and in euchromatin in others; X chromosome inactivation is a classic example of facultative heterochromatin in mammals.

FADD (Fas-associated protein with a death domain). Adapter protein that promotes association of activated Fas receptor with procaspase 8, triggering the extrinsic cell death pathway

Farnesyl. A 15 carbon isoprenyl group used to anchor peripheral proteins to membrane bilayers; conjugated to a cysteine side chain near the C-terminus of the protein

Fas (also known as Apo1 or CD95). A death receptor of the tumor necrosis factor (TNF) receptor family with a death domain (DD) in the cytoplasmic tail

Fas ligand. Trimeric cell surface protein that initiates the extrinsic pathway of apoptotic death when it binds Fas on a target cell

Fast axonal transport. Bidirectional transport of membrane-bound vesicles and organelles on microtubules in nerve axons; anterograde movements powered by kinesin; retrograde movements powered by dynein

Fatty acid oxidation. Biochemical reactions that produce acetyl-CoA from the breakdown of fatty acids

Fen1 (flap nuclease). Nuclease that removes the RNA primer (and probably initiator DNA) during DNA replication

Fibrillar centers. Regions of nucleoli containing rRNA genes, RNA polymerase I, and its associated transcription factors

Fibrillin microfibril. A polymer of the protein fibrillin, the scaffold for laying down elastin in elastic fibers

Fibrin. Blood protein that polymerizes to clot blood

Fibrinogen. Blood protein precursor of fibrin and also an adhesion protein for platelets

Fibroblast. Cell that synthesizes most of the extracellular matrix in connective tissues

Fibronectin. Adhesive glycoprotein that connects fibers and cells in the extracellular matrix; multiple isoforms, one circulating in blood forms a provisional matrix in wounds

Filopodium (also microspike). Finger-like extension of plasma membrane supported by a bundle of actin filaments

First-order reaction. A reaction with one reactant

Flagellum (bacterial). Helical protein polymer forming the propeller for bacterial motility

Flagellum (eukaryotic). Motile cell surface organelle powered by an axoneme; plural = flagella

Fluid-phase endocytosis. Ingestion of extracellular fluid in a vesicle formed by the plasma membrane

Fluorescence. Emission of light from a molecule after excitation by a shorter-wavelength, more energetic photon

F-met-leu-phe. A chemotactic tripeptide released by Bacteria that attracts white blood cells

Focal adhesion kinase. A nonreceptor tyrosine kinase active in focal contacts

Focal contact. Plasma membrane specialization with integrins to adhere to the extracellular matrix; associated with cytoplasmic signaling proteins

Formin. Dimeric protein that stimulates actin filament nucleation and remains attached to the growing barbed end during assembly of contractile rings, filopodia, and other bundles of actin filaments

Free energy. Thermodynamic energy in a system available to do work

Freeze fracture. A method to prepare specimens for electron microscopy involving freezing, fracturing, etching (sublimation) of water from the fractured surface, and rotary shadowing with metal

FtsZ. Protein with the same fold as tubulin that participates in cytokinesis in Bacteria and Archaea

F-type ATPase. Reversible, rotary membrane pumps that use transport of protons down a concentration gradient to drive the synthesis of ATP or use ATP hydrolysis to pump protons

Fusion protein (membrane traffic). Protein that mediates fusion of a carrier with an acceptor membrane

Fusion protein (molecular biology). Fusion of coding sequences from two proteins to produce a hybrid protein

G-protein. GTPase subunit of trimeric GTPases

G-protein-coupled receptor kinase. Serine/threonine kinases activated by G-protein beta-subunits, which phosphorylate and inactivate seven helix receptors

G_0 phase. Cell cycle state of nondividing (often terminally differentiated) cells

G_1 phase (first gap phase). Interval in cell cycle between mitosis and DNA replication

G_2 checkpoint. Cell cycle checkpoint operating in the G_2 phase to block mitotic entry if DNA is damaged or DNA replication is incomplete

G_2 delay. Temporary halt in cell cycle progression observed in cells with damaged DNA as a result of function of the G_2 checkpoint

G_2 phase (second gap phase). Interval between the completion of DNA replication and mitosis

G_α. Membrane-anchored GTP-binding subunit of trimeric G-proteins

G_β. Subunit of trimeric G-proteins

G_γ. Membrane-anchored subunit of trimeric G-proteins

Gamma-tubulin. Tubulin isoform crucial for microtubule nucleation found in ring complexes in pericentriolar material

Gamma-tubulin ring complex (γTuRC). Complex of 10 to 13 γ-tubulin molecules and 8 associated polypeptides that nucleates microtubule assembly

GAP (GTPase activating protein). Proteins that stimulate GTP hydrolysis by small GTPases, reversing the association of the GTPase with effector proteins

Gap junction. Intercellular junction composed of connexons, channels that conduct molecules smaller than 1 kD between cells

GEF (guanine nucleotide exchange factors). Proteins that bind small GTPases and stimulate the dissociation of GDP, allowing GTP binding to activate the GTPase

Gel electrophoresis. Use of an electric field to separate molecules according to their size and charge in a gel matrix

Gel filtration chromatography. Method to separate molecules based on their size (hydrodynamic radius)

Gelsolin. Calcium-sensitive actin filament severing and capping protein

Geminin. Cell cycle–regulated protein that regulates "licensing" of origins of DNA replication in metazoans by binding Cdt1 and preventing preinitiation complex assembly

Gene. Segment of DNA encoding a functional RNA or protein product

Genetic code. The correspondence between nucleotide triplets in mRNAs to amino acids in a polypeptide; one to six different triplet codons encode each amino acid

Genetic marker. Particular DNA sequence that can be monitored by examining the phenotypes of the cells that carry it

Genome. The entire DNA complement of an organism

Genomics. The study of genomes by cloning and sequencing the DNA and by analyzing and comparing the sequences

Genotype. Combination of genes present on the chromosomes of an organism

Glutamate. Amino acid and neurotransmitter

Glutamate receptor. Cation channel activated by binding glutamate

Glycerol. Three-carbon molecule with a hydroxyl group on each carbon

Glycerolphospholipid. *See* Phosphoglyceride.

Glycoconjugate. Protein modified with one or more sugars

Glycolipid. Lipid modified with one or more sugars

Glycolysis. Biochemical reactions that derive energy from the breakdown of glucose to form ATP and other energy-carrying metabolites

Glycoprotein. Protein modified with one or more sugars

Glycosaminoglycan. Polysaccharide polymers, generally composed of a repeated pair of sugars

Glycosidases. Enzymes that remove sugars from glycoproteins

Glycosidic bond. Ether bond between sugar residues

Glycosphingolipid. Sphingolipid modified with one or more sugars

Glycosylation. Process that conjugates sugars with proteins and lipids

Glycosylphosphatidylinositol tail. Phosphoglyceride that is linked to the C-terminus of a protein by a short oligosaccharide and a phosphatidylinositol head group

Glycosyltransferases. Enzymes that add sugar residues to proteins

Golgi apparatus. Major compartment of the secretory membrane system for processing glycoproteins and sorting molecules in the lumen and lipid bilayer

Granular component. Region of the nucleolus for ribosome subunit assembly

Grb2. Adapter protein consisting of two SH3 domains and one SH2 domain

Green fluorescent protein. Jellyfish protein that absorbs blue light and emits green light; often fused to other proteins for observing their distribution in live cells

GroEL. Barrel-shaped chaperonins that use ATP hydrolysis to assist the folding of nascent polypeptides

Growth cone. Motile tip of a growing nerve cell process

Growth cycle. Increase in cellular mass

Growth factors. Proteins that promote the growth of cell mass

Growth hormone. Pituitary hormone that controls body size

GST fusion protein. Hybrid protein consisting of a protein of interest fused to glutathione-S-transferase, which allows purification by binding to glutathione immobilized on beads

GTP exchange factor. *See* GEF.

GTPase. Family of proteins activated by GTP binding (allowing interactions with effector proteins) and inactivated by GTP hydrolysis and γ-phosphate dissociation

GTPase-activating protein. *See* GAP.

Guanine. Purine base present in DNA and RNA; H-bonds with cytosine

Guanine nucleotide dissociation inhibitor (GDI). Protein that prevents exchange of GDP for GTP on Rabs and other small GTPases

Guanylylcyclase. Transmembrane and cytoplasmic enzymes that synthesize cGMP from GTP

Half-spindle. Portion of mitotic spindle consisting of a spindle pole with its associated kinetochore and interpolar and astral microtubules

Haploid chromosome number (n). Number of chromosomes donated by the mother or the father in a diploid organism; only haploid cells in animals are gametes (sperm and eggs)

Hedgehog. Signaling protein that helps to establish boundaries between cells of different fates during embryogenesis

Helicase. Enzyme that uses ATP hydrolysis to dissociate complementary strands of nucleic acids or remove secondary structure or bound proteins from nucleic acids

Helix-loop-helix proteins. Transcription factors with a basic region to recognize specific DNA sequences plus two helical dimerization domains separated by a loop region

Helix-turn-helix proteins. Transcription factors composed of two helices, one of which binds a recognition sequence of 6 bp in the major groove of DNA

Hemicellulose. Branched polysaccharide associated with cellulose in microfibrils in plant cell walls

Hemidesmosome. Plasma membrane specialization with integrins to bind the basal lamina and anchored to intermediate filaments in the cytoplasm

Heterochromatin. Transcriptionally inert, condensed chromatin rich in histone H3 trimethylated on lysine 9

Heterochromatin protein 1 (HP1). Protein that binds nucleosomes containing histone H3 trimethylated on lysine 9 and recruits other components of heterochromatin

Heterogeneous nuclear RNA. Incompletely processed precursors of mRNA

Heterozygous. In a diploid organism, the condition in which a particular genetic marker has different forms on the two homologous chromosomes

Hexose. A six-carbon sugar

Histone code hypothesis. Proposal that posttranslational modifications of histones determine the level of functional activity of particular regions of chromatin

HMG-CoA reductase. ER membrane enzyme that catalyzes a step in cholesterol biosynthesis

Holliday junctions. Intermediates in the recombination process consisting of branched DNA structures formed between two recombining DNA molecules

Holocentric chromosomes. Chromosomes with centromere activity distributed along the whole surface of the chromosome during mitosis

Homeodomain. DNA-binding domains of 60 amino acids found in transcription factors that specify body segments during development

Homogenize. Grind up or physically disrupt cells or tissues

Homologous chromosomes. Pairs of chromosomes (in diploid organisms) one of which is donated by the mother and the other by the father

Homozygous. In a diploid organism, the condition in which a particular genetic marker has the same sequence on both the maternal and paternal homologous chromosomes

HOX (homeobox) gene. Class of genes for transcription factors that specify the development of embryonic segments

Hsp70. Protein chaperones that use ATP hydrolysis to drive a cycle of binding and release of short hydrophobic segments to promote polypeptide folding

Hsp90. Protein chaperones that maintain steroid receptors in an "open" state, ready to bind their ligands

hTERT. The reverse transcriptase subunit of telomerase

Hyaluronan. Very large glycosaminoglycans consisting of alternating D-glucuronic acid and D-N-acetylglucosamine

Hydrogen bond. Weak bonds between an H atom with a partial positive charge and an oxygen or nitrogen atom with a partial negative charge; contribute to stabilizing macromolecule secondary structure and interactions

Hydrophilic. Molecules or groups of atoms in molecules with favorable interactions with water

Hydrophobic. Molecules or groups of atoms in molecules with unfavorable interactions with water

Hydrophobic effect. Phenomenon whereby exclusion of water from complementary surfaces favors macromolecular associations; driven by increases in the entropy of the water

Hydroxyapatite. Crystals of $[Ca_{10}(PO_4)_6(OH)_2]$ in bone matrix

IAP (inhibitor of apoptosis protein). Family of proteins that inhibit caspases characterized by a motif of ~80 amino acids known as a baculovirus IAP repeat (BIR)

I-band. Region of a striated muscle sarcomere with thin filaments but no thick filaments

ICAD (inhibitor of CAD). Chaperone required to fold caspase-activated DNase (CAD) that then inhibits the nuclease until cleaved by a caspase, releasing active CAD

Icosahedron. Closed polyhedron with 12 fivefold vertices

Ig-CAM. Family of cell adhesion proteins with extracellular immunoglobulin-fold domains

Image processing. Optical and computation methods to remove noise, average or make 3D reconstructions of micrographs

Immediate early genes. Genes expressed soon after stimulation of cultured fibroblasts in G_0 with serum

Immunoprecipitation. Method using antibodies to isolate specific proteins from cell extracts

Immunoproteasome. Specialized proteasomes that participate in ubiquitin-independent cleavage of intracellular antigens, such as viral proteins, into peptides of uniform length for presentation by MHC class I on the surface of antigen-presenting cells

Importin α. Adapter protein that recognizes small basic nuclear localization sequences and works with the transport receptor importin β in nuclear import

Importin β (karyopherin β). One class of receptor for proteins with nuclear localization sequences, regulated by Ran GTPase; also functions as a chaperone regulating the assembly of subcellular structures, including the mitotic spindle and nuclear envelope

Import receptor. Proteins that bind cargo proteins with nuclear localization sequences directly or in combination with adapter molecules and facilitate their transport into the nucleus (*see* Importin β)

Imprinting. Epigenetic mechanism that turns a gene off during formation of the egg or sperm and keeps the gene off in all cells that develop from that gamete

Inactivation peptide. A segment of polypeptide that blocks an open ion channel

Initiation codon. Nucleotide triplet AUG in mRNA that specifies methionine, which begins polypeptide chains

Initiation factors. Proteins that coordinate assembly of mRNA and ribosomal subunits to begin the synthesis of a polypeptide

Initiator. DNA sequences in promoters near transcription start sites of many genes

Initiator caspases. Caspases that are autoactivated by association with scaffolding cofactors and propagate apoptosis by cleaving and activating effector caspase zymogens

Inner nuclear membrane. The internal lipid bilayer surrounding the nucleus; associated with nuclear lamina

Inner segment. Part of photoreceptor cells between the cell body and light-absorbing outer segment

Inositol triphosphate (IP$_3$). Cyclohexanol with the 1, 4, and 5 hydroxyls phosphorylated

Insulators. DNA sequences that protect regions of a chromosome from the effects of neighboring regions

Insulin receptor. Receptor tyrosine kinase activated by insulin binding

Integral membrane protein. Protein embedded, at least in part, in a membrane lipid bilayer

Integrin. Family of heterodimeric plasma membrane adhesion proteins that generally bind extracellular matrix molecules and other cells

Intercalated disk. Adhesive junction linking the ends of cardiac muscle cells, anchored to cytoplasmic actin and intermediate filaments

Intercellular bridge. Thin connection between daughter cells at the end of cytokinesis containing an antiparallel array of microtubules derived from the mitotic spindle

Interchromatin granules. Intranuclear concentrations of factors for RNA processing

Interchromosomal domain. Region of nucleoplasm between adjacent chromosome territories

Intermediate filaments. Family of 10-nm filaments composed of α-helical subunits related to keratin

Interphase (or "resting stage"). Part of the cell cycle in which cells are not engaged in division

Interpolar microtubules. Microtubules distributed through the mitotic spindle, apparently free at both ends, that bundle to form the central spindle during anaphase and telophase

Intraflagellar transport. Bidirectional transport of proteins along the axonemes of cilia and flagella

Intrinsic pathway of cell death. Apoptotic pathway triggered by release of pro-apoptotic factors from mitochondria and regulated by Bcl-2 family members

Introns. Regions of genes that are removed from immature RNA molecules by splicing

Inward rectifying channel. Channels with higher conductivity into than out of cells

Ion exchange chromatography. Separation of molecules based on their affinity for charged beads

IP$_3$ receptor. Channels activated by IP$_3$ to release calcium from the ER

Isoforms. Related proteins encoded by different genes or alternatively spliced mRNAs

Isoprenoid tail. Lipids consisting of three to six isoprenyl units (*see* Farnesyl)

JAK. Family of tyrosine kinases associated with cytokine receptors, playfully named "just another kinase"

K$^+$ leak channel. Potassium channel that helps to maintain the resting potential of excitable cell membranes

Kartagener's syndrome. Genetic disease with immobile cilia owing to a defect in dynein

Katanin. AAA ATPase that uses energy from ATP hydrolysis to sever microtubules

KcsA. Bacterial K-channel; first crystal structure of an ion channel

KDEL. C-terminal tetrapeptide sequence used to retain soluble proteins in the ER

Keratin. Family of intermediate filament proteins expressed in epithelial cells

Kinesin. Family of motor proteins using ATP hydrolysis to walk along microtubules, generally toward their plus end

Kinesin-13/kinesin-8. Kinesins that remove subunits from the ends of microtubules

Kinetochore. Structure at the surface of centromeric chromatin that binds microtubules and directs the movements of chromosomes in mitosis

Kinetochore fibers. Bundles of microtubules attached to kinetochores consisting of one microtubule in budding yeast to more than 200 microtubules in higher plants

Kinetochore microtubules. Class of mitotic spindle microtubules with their plus ends embedded in the kinetochore and their minus ends at or near the spindle pole

Lactacystin. Antibiotic that reacts covalently with threonine residues to inactivate proteasomes

Lagging strand. During DNA replication, the DNA strand along which replication occurs in a direction opposite to that of the replication fork, so that the newly synthesized DNA is laid down as a series of short discontinuous segments known as Okazaki fragments

Lamin A. Nuclear lamin encoded by a gene that is subject to many mutations that cause at least 16 human genetic diseases, including Emery-Dreifuss muscular dystrophy

Laminin. Adhesive glycoprotein of the basal lamina

Lampbrush chromosomes. Actively transcribed chromosomes with prominent loops visible during the diplotene stage of meiosis in animals

Lariat. Circular RNA molecule with a tail created early in mRNA splicing

Late endosomes. Mature multivesicular bodies that have not yet fused with lysosomes

Leading edge. Advancing pseudopod of motile cells driven by actin polymerization

Leading strand. During DNA replication, the DNA strand along which replication moves in the same direction as the replication fork, so that newly synthesized DNA is laid down continuously

Lectin. Protein that binds particular sugar molecules

Leptin. Satiety hormone secreted by fat cells and acting on neurons of the hypothalamus in the brain that regulate appetite and bone metabolism

Leptotene. First stage of meiotic prophase, defined by the first visible condensation of chromosomes, during which homologous chromosome pairing and alignment occur

Leucine zipper protein. Dimeric transcription factors with basic regions that recognize specific DNA sequences held together by a coiled-coil stabilized by leucine residues

Leukocyte. White blood cell

Ligand. Molecule that binds to a receptor

Light reactions. Steps in photosynthesis that depend on the continuous absorption of light, including production of high-energy electrons, electron transport to make NADPH, creation of a proton gradient for synthesis of ATP, and generation of oxygen

Light-harvesting complexes. Small, transmembrane proteins that absorb light and transfer energy to a photosynthetic reaction center

Lignins. Polymers of phenylpropanoid alcohols and acids in "secondary" cell walls of plants

LINES (long interspersed nuclear elements). Common class of human retrotransposons with a consensus sequence of 6 to 8 kb that make up about 20% of the human genome

Linker DNA. DNA that links adjacent nucleosomes

Linker histone (H1). Binds to linker DNA, participates in formation of 30-nm fibers and chromatin compaction

Lipid raft. Microdomain in a lipid bilayer enriched in sphingolipids and cholesterol

Lipid-transfer protein (LTP). Protein that catalyzes exchange but not net transfer of lipids between membranes

Listeria. Gram-negative intracellular pathogenic Bacterium that uses actin polymerization for motility

Locus control regions (LCRs). Short regions of DNA rich in binding sites for transcriptional regulators, that create "open" chromatin promoting the expression of nearby genes

Low-density lipoproteins (LDLs). Particles containing dietary and de novo–synthesized cholesterol, which are secreted into the blood for transport to other tissues

Lymphocyte. White blood cell of the adaptive immune system

Lysobisphosphatidic acid. Lipid that promotes bilayer curvature during invagination and formation of intralumenal vesicles in multivesicular bodies

Lysosomal hydrolase. Enzymes concentrated in lysosomes that catalyze degradation of macromolecules by breaking covalent bonds by the addition of water

Lysosomal storage disease. Genetic diseases arising from absence of or defects in lysosomal hydrolases

Lysosome. Membrane-bound organelle containing acid hydrolases, including proteases; provides an acidic environment for digestion of contents

Lysyl oxidase. Extracellular enzyme that catalyzes the cross-linking of collagen and elastin

Macroautophagy. Engulfment into an autophagic vacuole of large volumes of cytoplasm that can include glycogen granules, ribosomes, and organelles

Macropinocytosis. Ingestion of extracellular fluid into a large endocytic structure

MAD (mitotic arrest-defective) genes. Encode proteins that execute the spindle checkpoint, delaying anaphase until all kinetochores are attached correctly to the spindle

Mannose-6-phosphate receptors. Integral membrane proteins that bind lysosomal hydrolases modified with mannose-6-phosphate in the *trans*-Golgi network for delivery to endosomes and lysosomes

MAP-2. High-molecular-weight microtubule associated protein in the tau family

MAP kinase. Serine/threonine kinases activated by phosphorylation in the cytoplasm that move to the nucleus to activate transcription factors required for cell growth and division

MAP kinase kinase. Kinases that activate MAP kinases by phosphorylation of serine and tyrosine

MAP kinase kinase kinase. Serine kinases that activate MAP kinase kinases

Mass spectrometry. Analytical method to measure the mass of molecules with high accuracy

Mast cell. Connective tissue cell activated by binding of antigens to cell surface immunoglobulins causing it to secrete granules containing histamine

Matrix metalloproteinase. Zinc proteases that digest the extracellular matrix of connective tissues

Matrix (mitochondrial). Innermost compartment of mitochondria with enzymes for the citric acid cycle and fatty acid oxidation

Mcm proteins (minichromosome maintenance). Six AAA ATPases that form a hexameric complex thought to have helicase activity to separate DNA strands during replication

Mediator. Complex of over 20 polypeptides that interacts reversibly with RNA polymerase II and other factors to form a "holoenzyme," which requires additional factors to be competent for initiation of transcription

Megacomplex. Complex of many aggrecan proteoglycans with hyaluronan in cartilage

Megakaryocyte. Polyploid bone marrow cell that produces platelets by a budding process

Meiosis. Specialized program of two coupled cell divisions used by eukaryotes to maintain the proper chromosome number for the species during sexual reproduction

Meiosis I. First division of meiosis, in which homologous chromosomes separate, also known as the reductional division because the number of chromosomes is halved

Meiosis II. Second division of meiosis (also called the equational division); resembles mitosis as sister chromatids segregate from each other and the number of chromosomes remains the same

Membrane carriers. Enzyme-like proteins that catalyze movements of solutes across membranes

Membrane channels. Protein pores for rapid movement of specific ions and solutes across membranes

Membrane peroxisomal targeting sequence (mPTS). Amino acid sequences that target proteins to peroxisomal membranes

Membrane potential. Voltage difference across a lipid bilayer

Membrane pumps. Transmembrane enzymes that use ATP hydrolysis or another energy source to move solutes across membranes up concentration gradients

Membrane skeleton. Network of actin filaments and accessory proteins associated with the cytoplasmic face of cellular membranes

Messenger RNA (mRNA). RNA molecules transcribed by RNA polymerase II and containing the sequence of bases that specify the sequences of amino acids in polypeptide chains

Metaphase. Third phase of mitosis with all chromosomes attached to both spindle poles and aligned near the equator of the mitotic spindle

Metaphase plate. Compact grouping of chromosomes at the middle of the mitotic spindle with all pairs of sister chromatids attached to both spindle poles

Microarray. Ordered pattern of spots of nucleic acids or proteins on a glass slide used for large-scale automated binding reactions such as measuring levels of mRNAs

Microelectrode. Glass capillary with a micrometer tip used to record the membrane potential of a single cell

Micro-RNA (miRNA). Small RNAs of about 22 nucleotides excised from larger precursors and associated with the RISC complex that represses translation of target mRNAs or directs their cleavage by the slicer endonuclease

Microtubule. Stiff cylindrical polymers of α- and β-tubulin that support a variety of cellular structures and serve as tracks for movements powered by motor proteins called kinesins and dyneins

Microtubule-associated proteins (MAPs). Proteins that regulate microtubule properties by binding tubulin dimers, by stabilizing or severing polymers, or by associating with microtubule ends

Microtubule-organizing center (MTOC). Structures containing γ-tubulin that nucleate microtubule assembly and usually anchor microtubule minus ends

Microvillus. Finger-like extension of plasma membrane supported by a bundle of actin filaments

Midbody. Dense knob surrounding antiparallel microtubules in the thin intercellular bridge between daughter cells following constriction of the cleavage furrow

Minus end. Slower-growing end of a microtubule terminating with α-tubulin

Mismatch repair. DNA repair process that removes errors that occur during DNA replication

Mitochondria. Eukaryotic organelle derived from a symbiotic proteobacterium specialized for oxidative phosphorylation to form ATP, fatty acid oxidation, and the citric acid cycle

Mitochondrial matrix. Innermost compartment of mitochondria with enzymes for citric acid cycle and fatty acid oxidation

Mitogen/mitogenic signals. Factors or signals coming from other cells and from the extracellular matrix that promote cell cycle progression

Mitosis (M phase). Cell cycle phase when chromosomes and other cellular components are partitioned to two daughter cells

Mitotic spindle. Framework of microtubules (between two centrosomes in animal cells or two spindle pole bodies in fungi) that segregates chromosomes during mitosis

M-line. Connections between the centers of thick filaments in striated muscles

Monocyte. White blood cell, precursor of tissue macrophages and osteoclasts

Motor end plate. *See* Neuromuscular junction.

Motor nerve. Axon of a neuron in the brain stem or spinal cord that controls muscle contraction

Motor proteins. Enzymes that used energy from ATP hydrolysis to produce force and motion on actin filaments or microtubules

Motor unit. All of the skeletal muscle cells controlled by one motor neuron

MPF (maturation-promoting factor, M phase–promoting factor). Activity discovered by developmental biologists that causes interphase cells to enter mitosis; later shown to be an active Cdk with a cyclin partner

mRNA. *See* Messenger RNA.

Mucin. Heavily glycosylated cell surface proteins, ligands for selectins

Multiple drug resistance proteins. ABC transporters that pump drugs and other hydrophobic molecules out of cells

Multivesicular body (MVB). Endocytic compartment derived from early endosomes by the inward invagination of vesicles forming sites for degradation of lipids and membrane proteins

Mus musculus. The mouse; commonly studied as a representative mammal with highly developed genetics

Mutation. Any alternation of genomic DNA sequences

Myc. Transcriptional factor that promotes expression of genes for cell cycle progression (cyclins E and D2) and represses expression of Cdk inhibitors (CKI and INK)

Myofibril. Contractile unit of striated muscle composed of many sarcomeres in series

Myosin. Family of motor proteins using ATP hydrolysis to apply tension to actin filaments

Myosin light chain kinase. Serine/threonine kinase activated by calcium-calmodulin that phosphorylates the regulatory light chain of myosin-II to trigger contraction of smooth muscle and constriction of the contractile ring during cytokinesis

Myosin-II. Principal myosin of muscles and contractile rings of dividing cells

Myristoyl tail. Fourteen-carbon fatty acid added to the N-terminus of peripheral membrane proteins including c-Src tyrosine kinase

Myt1. Cytoplasmic kinase that phosphorylates at T^{14} and Y^{15} in the active site of Cdk1 inhibiting its activity until it is activated by dephosphorylation during M phase

NADH. Reduced form of nicotinamide adenine dinucleotide; an energy carrier in cells

Na⁺K⁺-ATPase. P-type pump using ATP hydrolysis to pump Na^+ out of and K^+ into animal cells

Nebulin. Giant protein that extents from end to end of striated muscle thin filaments

Necrosis. Cell death resulting from irreversible injury involving leaking cell membranes, destruction of cellular contents lysosomal enzymes, and local inflammation

Negative selection. Apoptotic cell death of potentially harmful lymphocytes with T-cell receptors that recognize self-antigens

Negative staining. Method to prepare specimens for electron microscopy by drying them in a puddle of heavy metal salts

N-end rule. Presence of certain amino acids at the N-terminus of a protein causes it to be ubiquitinated by a specific E3 enzyme and subsequently destroyed

Neocentromere. Functional centromeres that form rarely on noncentromeric DNA

Nernst equation. Relation between the concentrations of an ion on the two sides of a selectively permeable membrane and the equilibrium membrane potential

Nerve ending. *See* Synapse.

Netrin. Diffusible protein that signals attraction or repulsion of growth cones and capillaries

Neural crest cell. Embryonic cells that form sympathetic nervous system, pigment cells of skin, adrenal medullary cells, and many other cells

Neurofilament. Intermediate filaments of neurons

Neuromuscular junction. Synapse between a motor nerve and a skeletal muscle cell

Neurotransmitter. Small organic ions used for chemical communication between nerves and between nerves and other cells

Neutrophil. White blood cell specialized for phagocytosis and destruction of bacteria

Nicotinic acetylcholine receptor. Cation channel activated by binding acetylcholine

Nitric oxide. Gas that serves as a second messenger, by activating guanylylcyclase

Nitric oxide synthase. Enzyme that liberates nitric oxide from arginine

N-linked oligosaccharide. Sugar polymer conjugated to side chain of a protein asparagine residue

Nocodazole. Synthetic chemical that inhibits microtubule assembly by binding dissociated tubulin dimers

Noncrossover (gene conversion). Most common outcome of programmed double-strand DNA breaks during meiotic prophase; may involve loss of one or more genetic markers

Nondisjunction. Mistakes in the separation of chromosomes or chromatids in meiosis or mitosis resulting in aneuploidy, daughter cells with too many or too few chromosomes

Nonhistone proteins. Proteins of chromatin and chromosomes that are not histones

Nonsense mediated decay (NMD). Process by which the presence of a premature translation termination signal (or nonsense codon) strongly destabilizes mRNA

NSF (*N*-ethyl maleimide [NEM]-sensitive factor). AAA ATPase that uses the energy from ATP hydrolysis to dissociate cis-SNARE complexes and recycles the SNAREs for another round of membrane fusion

N-terminal tails. About 30 amino acids at the N-terminus of core histones that regulate chromatin compaction

Nuclear envelope. Double lipid bilayer that encloses the nucleus; outer membrane contiguous with the ER

Nuclear export sequence (NES). Short peptide sequence recognized by carrier proteins that direct a protein for transport out of the nucleus

Nuclear lamina. Meshwork of intermediate filaments (nuclear lamins) that stabilizes the inner nuclear envelope

Nuclear lamins. Type V intermediate filament proteins that make up the nuclear lamina

Nuclear localization sequence (NLS). Short peptide sequence recognized by carrier proteins (transport receptors) that direct the protein for transport into the nucleus

Nuclear matrix or nucleoskeleton. Residual structures that remain when isolated nuclei are subjected to digestion with nucleases and extraction of the bulk of the histones

Nuclear pore complexes. Channels bridging both the inner and outer nuclear membranes that provide the sole route for communication between the nucleus and cytoplasm during interphase

Nuclear receptor. Family of transcription factors activated by lipid soluble ligands, including steroid hormones; active receptors enter the nucleus to regulate gene expression

Nucleation. Initial steps in the assembly of polymeric macromolecular structures

Nucleic acid. Polymers of nucleotides linked by phosphodiester bonds, RNA, and DNA

Nucleolus. Nuclear subdomain specialized for ribosome biogenesis

Nucleolus-organizing regions (NORs). Remnants of nucleolar fibrillar centers that remain associated with rRNA genes in condensed mitotic chromosomes

Nucleoplasm. The cellular region enclosed within the nuclear envelope

Nucleoporins. Family of about 30 structural proteins that regulate access through the nuclear pore

Nucleoside. Five-carbon sugar (ribose or deoxyribose) with a base on C1

Nucleosome. Complex of 165 base pairs of DNA wrapped twice around a protein core consisting of two copies each of the histones H2A, H2B, H3, and H4

Nucleosome core particle. 146 base pairs of DNA wrapped around a core consisting of a histone octamer

Nucleosome remodeling complex. Enzyme using energy from ATP hydrolysis to alter the location of nucleosomes on DNA

Nucleotide. Five-carbon sugar (ribose or deoxyribose) with a base on C1 and one to three phosphates on C5

Nucleotide excision repair. Process that replaces chemically modified bases in DNA

Nucleus. Membrane-bounded compartment in eukaryotes containing genomic DNA and machinery for RNA synthesis and processing

Objective. Microscope lens that collects light scattered by specimens

Occludin. Transmembrane protein subunit of tight junctions

Odorant. Vast array of volatile organic molecules that activate olfactory receptors to detect smells

Okazaki fragment. Short segments of newly synthesized DNA formed during DNA replication

Olfactory sensory neuron. Cells in the nose that detect and signal the presence of odorant molecules by sending action potentials into the central nervous system

Oligosaccharyl transferase. ER enzyme associated with translocons that transfers core oligosaccharides from dolichol to an asparagine in an appropriate sequence of a growing polypeptide

O-linked oligosaccharide. Glycosaminoglycans conjugated to a serine or threonine side chain

Oncogene. Gene that predisposes to oncogenic (cancerous) transformation of cells when the protein product is activated inappropriately; generally components of signal transduction pathways that regulate cellular growth and proliferation

Op18/stathmin. Protein that binds two tubulin dimers and inhibits their assembly

Open mitosis. Mitosis in which the nuclear envelope disassembles before chromosomes segregate, as in most plants and animals

Open probability. Fraction of the time that an ion channel is open

Operon. Prokaryotic transcription units containing more than one gene, often encoding physiologically related proteins

ORC (origin recognition complex). Complex of six proteins that marks origins of replication for the association with other proteins essential for replication

Origin of replication (defined genetically as a replicator element). Positions on the chromosome where DNA replication initiates

Osteoblast. Cell that secretes organic components of bone matrix

Osteoclast. Multinucleated cell formed by fusion of monocytes, specialized for bone resorption

Osteocyte. Cell surrounded by the bone matrix; can lay down or resorb matrix locally

Osteogenesis imperfecta. A variety of congenital fragile bone syndromes often caused by mutations in collagen

Osteon (Haversian system). Rod-shaped element of long bones formed by concentric layers of bone laid down on the inner surface of a resorption canal

Osteopetrosis. Disease with overgrown, dense bones owing to a failure of bone resorption due to lack of osteoclasts

Osteoporosis. Disease characterized by loss of bone tissue

Outer doublet. Pair of one complete and one incomplete microtubule in a ring of nine in axonemes

Outer nuclear membrane. Lipid bilayer continuous with the ER and sharing its functions

Outer segment. Part of photoreceptor cells with light-absorbing membranes; a modified cilium

Oxidative phosphorylation. Biochemical reactions in mitochondria and certain bacteria that utilize energy from the breakdown of nutrients to synthesize ATP from ADP

P4-type ATPase. Variant P-type ATPase pump that flips lipids between the leaflets of bilayers

p21. Protein that blocks cell cycle progression by inhibiting Cdk1-cyclin A; its expression is turned on by p53 in response to DNA damage

p53. Transcription factor activated in response to DNA damage, which turns on expression of proteins that block cell-cycle progression or induce apoptosis

Pacemaker. Heart muscle cells that spontaneously generate action potentials and drive rhythmic contractions

Pachytene. Third stage of meiotic prophase, during which synapsis is complete and crossovers mature into chiasmata

Pairing. Side-by-side alignment of homologous chromosomes at a distance during meiotic prophase

Parathyroid hormone. Stimulates osteocytes to mobilize calcium from bone matrix

Patch clamp. Glass micropipette that is applied to the surface of a cell or a piece of membrane to record electrical events in single ion channels

PAX (paired box) genes. Class of genes that specify the development of embryonic segments

PCNA (proliferating cell nuclear antigen). Doughnut-shaped trimer topologically locked onto the DNA by RFC that acts as a molecular "tool belt" to which numerous proteins involved with DNA replication and repair bind to achieve a stable association with the DNA

PDZ domain. Family of adapter domains that recognize C-terminal sequences of target proteins

Pectin. Branched polysaccharide associated with cellulose in microfibrils in plant cell walls

Pentose. Five-carbon sugar

Peptide bond. Amide bond between the amino group of one amino acid and the carboxyl group of another amino acid

Peptidyl prolyl isomerase. ER enzyme that catalyzes the interconversion of cis and trans peptide bonds involving proline

Pericentriolar material (PCM). Matrix surrounding pairs of centrioles that links them together and contains gamma-tubulin ring complexes, which nucleate microtubules

Perichondrium. Capsule of connective tissue that covers the surface of cartilage

Perichromatin fibrils. Nucleoplasmic structures on the surface of condensed chromatin that contain splicing factors and RNA packaging proteins

Perinuclear space. Compartment continuous with the lumen of the ER that separates the inner and outer nuclear membranes

Periosteum. Connective tissue capsule on the surface of bones

Peripheral membrane protein. Protein associated with either surface of a biological membrane by a covalently attached lipid, electrostatic interactions, or partial insertion into the bilayer; can be extracted by a basic solution

Peroxins. Proteins that recognize and deliver proteins to peroxisomes

Peroxisomal biogenesis disorders. Diseases arising from defects in peroxisome formation

Peroxisomal targeting signal type 1 (PTS1). Three C-terminal amino acids that target enzymes to the lumen of peroxisomes

Peroxisomal targeting signal type 2 (PTS2). N-terminal sequences that target proteins to the lumen of peroxisomes

Peroxisomes. Membrane-bounded organelles containing oxidative enzymes

Phagocytosis. Process by which cells ingest large particles such as bacteria, foreign bodies, and remnants of dead cells

Phagolysosome. Organelle formed on fusion of a phagosome with a lysosome

Phalloidin. Cyclic peptide produced by poisonous mushrooms that has a high affinity for and stabilizes actin filaments; when conjugated with fluorescent dye, it is used to label actin filaments in cells

Phase contrast. Microscopic optical system generating contrast from differences in refractive index between a specimen and a reference beam

Phenotype. Physical manifestation of the action of the genotype of an organism (refers to both the appearance and macromolecular composition of the organism)

Phosphatidylcholine. Glycerolphospholipid with a choline head group

Phosphatidylinositol. Glycerolphospholipid with an inositol (cyclohexanol) head group that can be phosphorylated on carbons 3, 4, and 5 either singly or in combination to produce polyphosphoinositides

Phosphatidylinositol 3-kinase. Lipid kinase that phosphorylates the 3 hydroxyl of phosphatidylinositol

Phosphatidylinositol 4,5-bisphosphate (PIP$_2$). Phosphatidylinositol with phosphate esterified to the hydroxyls of inositol C4 and C5

Phosphatidylserine. Glycerolphospholipid with a serine head group

Phosphodiester bond. Phosphate esterified to two hydroxyls (can link either different molecules or within the same molecule in cyclic phosphodiesters)

Phosphodiesterase. Enzyme that catalyzes the conversion of 3′ 5′ cyclic nucleotides to the corresponding nucleoside monophosphate

Phosphoglyceride (glycerolphospholipid). Lipid with fatty acids esterified to the C1 and C2 hydroxyls of glycerol and phosphate on C3

Phospholipase A2. Enzyme that catalyzes cleavage of the ester bond between glycerol C2 and the fatty acid of a phosphoglyceride

Phospholipase C. Enzyme that catalyzes cleavage of the ester bond between glycerol C3 and the phosphate link to the head group of a phosphoglyceride

Phospholipase D. Enzyme that catalyzes cleavage of the ester bond between the phosphate and the head group of a phosphoglyceride

Phosphorylation. Formation of an ester bond between a phosphate and a hydroxyl of an amino acid, sugar, lipid, or other molecule

Photoreceptor cells. Sensory cells that express rhodopsin or other photoreceptor molecules and respond to absorption of photons

Photosynthesis. Biochemical reactions in chloroplasts and certain bacteria that utilize energy from absorption of photons to synthesize ATP

Photosystem I. Light-absorbing and electron carrier proteins in the membranes of purple bacteria, green filamentous bacteria, cyanobacteria, and chloroplasts that use energy from the absorption of photons to produce a proton gradient across the membrane to drive the synthesis of ATP

Photosystem II. Light-absorbing and electron carrier proteins in the membranes of green sulfur bacteria, heliobacteria, cyanobacteria, and chloroplasts that use energy from the absorption of photons to produce a proton gradient across the membrane to drive the synthesis of ATP

Phragmoplast. Arrays of microtubules formed by plant cells to deliver vesicles from the Golgi apparatus and ER to form new plasma membrane for cytokinesis

Pinocytosis. Ingestion of extracellular fluids by vesicles formed from the plasma membrane

Plakoglobin. Adapter protein linking cadherins and intermediate filaments in desmosomes

Plasma membrane. Membrane forming the boundary of the cell

Plasmadesmata. Intercellular junction between plant cells providing continuity between their cytoplasms

Plasmid. Circular DNA molecule that can replicate and propagate through generations in cells

Plasmid cloning. Isolation of a piece of DNA by propagation in a plasmid from a single founder cell

Platelet. Small cellular fragments in blood responsible for patching defects in small blood vessels and promoting clotting

Platelet-derived growth factor. Protein growth factor released by activated platelets that stimulates proliferation of cells expressing the appropriate receptor tyrosine kinase

Pleckstrin homology (PH) domain. Adapter domains that bind phosphorylated inosities; found in multiple proteins

Plectin. Protein that links intermediate filaments to integrins, microtubules and actin filaments

P-loop. Polypeptide segments of cation ion channels that form selectivity pores

Pluripotent stem cells. Stem cells whose progeny can form multiple specialized cells; embryonic stem cells form all adult cells; bone marrow pluripotent stem cells form all blood cells

Plus end. Faster-growing end of a microtubule terminating with β-tubulin

PML bodies (promyelocytic leukemia bodies). Nuclear structures of unknown function containing an E3 ubiquitin ligase called PML

Pointed end. Slower-growing end of actin filaments

Polar bodies. Small cells produced by asymmetrical cell divisions during female meiosis

Polarized cell. Cell with functionally distinct apical and basolateral plasma membrane domains separated by tight junctions; internal contents are also polarized

Polo. Protein kinases regulating several aspects of cell cycle control; active on substrates that have been "primed" by prior phosphorylation by another kinase

Poly-A tail. Fifty to 200 adenine residues added posttranscriptionally to the 3′ end of most eukaryotic mRNAs

Polymerase chain reaction (PCR). Method using heat-stable DNA polymerases to amplify DNA sequences by cycles of replication, strand dissociation, and further replication in the presence of excess primer sequences

Polymerase α/primase. Enzyme that initiates DNA replication by synthesizing an RNA chain of about 10 nucleotides to which DNA polymerase α adds another 20 to 30 nucleotides of "initiator DNA," all subsequently replaced by more accurate polymerases

Polypeptide. Polymer of amino acids linked by peptide bonds

Polyploidy. Common chromosomal abnormality with an entire extra set of chromosomes

Polysomes. Complex of a mRNA with multiple ribosomes, each synthesizing the same polypeptide

Polytene chromosomes. Giant chromosomes in some tissues of insect larvae, consisting of more than 1000 identical DNA molecules packed side by side in register

Polytopic protein. Protein that spans a membrane multiple times

Porins. Transmembrane proteins of the outer membrane of gram-negative bacteria and mitochondria forming channels for passage of molecules of less than 5000 D

Position effect. Repression of an actively transcribed gene that has been translocated into close proximity to constitutive heterochromatin, due to spreading of heterochromatin across the gene

Positive selection. Pathway of apoptotic death of lymphocytes that will be ineffective in immune responses because they express T-cell receptors that fail to interact with any of the MHC glycoproteins expressed by the individual

Postsynaptic. On the receiving side of a synapse

Posttranslational targeting. Mechanisms that move completed polypeptides across membrane bilayers into mitochondria, chloroplasts, and peroxisomes and out of Bacteria

Posttranslational translocation. Translocation of a protein across the ER membrane after it is fully synthesized in the cytoplasm

pRb. Family of transcriptional regulators (three in mammals) that control the activity of E2F family transcription factors and control cell cycle progression at the restriction point

Preinitiation complex (transcription). Complexes of TATA box–binding protein and associated factors that promote the initiation of transcription

Preinitiation complex (translation). Assembly of mRNA and proteins on a small ribosomal subunit

Prenucleolar bodies. Particles containing nucleolar components that associate with NORs during nucleolar reassembly after mitosis

Prenylation. Lipid modification that anchors proteins on cytoplasmic surfaces of membranes (see Isoprenoid tail)

Preprocollagen. Precursor to collagen with a signal sequence and assembly domains at both ends

Prereplication complex. Protein complex of ORC, Cdc6p, CDT1, and Mcm proteins that assembles at each replication origin once per cell cycle before the onset of S phase

Presequences. Amino acid sequences that target polypeptides to mitochondria

Presynaptic. On the sending side of a synapse

Primary cilium. Nonmotile cilium that serves as a sensory organelle; found on most animal cells

Primary constriction. Waist-like stricture at the centromere of mitotic chromosomes where the two sister chromatids are most intimately paired

Primitive mesenchymal cell. Stem cell for connective tissue cells

Proapoptotic. Signal or protein that triggers the apoptotic pathway of cell death

Processed pseudogenes. DNA sequences created by reverse transcription of mature mRNAs by a LINE reverse transcriptase and insertion back into the genome

Procollagen. Trimeric precursor of collagen held together by C-terminal assembly domains

Profilin. Protein that binds polyproline and actin monomers, catalyzes actin nucleotide exchange

Programmed cell death. Active cellular process that culminates in cell death in response to developmental signals, environmental cues, or physiological damage

Proliferation. Expansion of cell numbers by division

Prometaphase. Phase of mitosis beginning with nuclear envelope breakdown (in higher eukaryotes) and attachment of chromosomes to microtubules from the two poles of the forming mitotic spindle

Promoter. Assembly of DNA sequences required to form a preinitiation complex and initiate transcription

Prophase. First phase of mitosis, defined by chromosome condensation inside an intact nuclear envelope accompanied by changes in the dynamics of cytoplasmic microtubules

Prostaglandins. Family of lipid second messengers derived from arachidonic acid

Proteasome. Barrel-shaped multienzyme complex that degrades target proteins (typically tagged with chains of ubiquitin) into short peptides with recycling of intact ubiquitin monomers

Protein. One or more polypeptides folded into a functional three-dimensional structure

Protein coats. Polymeric structures that assemble on the cytoplasmic surface of membranes, causing them to bud off coated vesicles

Protein disulfide isomerase (PDI). Enzyme that catalyzes exchange of protein of disulfide (S-S) bonds in the ER lumen

Protein domain. Independently folded part of a protein

Protein folding. Conversion a linear polypeptide into a particular three-dimensional structure

Protein kinase. Enzyme that catalyzes formation of phosphate esters on hydroxyl groups of proteins

Protein kinase A (PKA). Protein kinase regulated by cAMP binding to a regulatory subunit

Protein kinase C (PKC). Protein kinase regulated by binding of diacylglycerol or other lipids and calcium to its regulatory domains

Protein phosphatase. Enzyme that catalyzes the hydrolysis (removal) of phosphate esters from hydroxyl groups of proteins

Protein targeting. Mechanisms that deliver a protein to a particular location in a cell

Proteoglycans. Proteins modified with O-linked glycosaminoglycans, found in secretory granules and extracellular matrix

Protofilaments. Longitudinally oriented filaments of tubulin dimers, 13 of which make up the cylindrical wall of most microtubules

Pseudoautosomal region. Region of sequence homology between male and female sex chromosomes that must undergo genetic recombination in meiosis I for sex chromosomes to partition correctly

Pseudogene. Nonfunctional DNA sequences derived from gene transcripts that have been reverse transcribed and inserted back into the chromosome

Pseudopod. Cellular protrusion responsible for cellular locomotion

Pseudosubstrate. Region of polypeptide similar to a substrate contained in a kinase or a kinase regulatory subunit that inhibits access of substrates to the kinase by binding to the active site

PTB domain. Adapter domain that binds particular peptides with a phosphotyrosine, found in multiple proteins

R (regulatory) subunits. Proteins that inhibit PKA but dissociate when they bind cAMP

Rab. Family of small GTPases that control protein-protein interactions between transport carriers and docking complexes on target membranes

Rac. Family of small GTPases related to Rho that regulate actin assembly

RAD51. Eukaryotic homolog of *E. coli* RecA, associates with single-stranded DNA and catalyzes the search for homologous sequences, strand pairing, and strand exchange during DNA recombination and repair

Radial spoke. Multiprotein connection between the central pair and outer doublets of axonemes

Raf. MAP kinase kinase kinase activated by Ras

Ran. Small GTPase that provides direction to nuclear transport; within the nucleus, Ran-GTP dissociates imported proteins from their carriers and binds proteins for export to their carriers; also functions in spindle assembly in eggs

Ran GAP1. Cytoplasmic GTPase-activating protein that stimulates GTP hydrolysis by Ran

Ras. Small GTPase that couples activation of growth factor receptor tyrosine kinases to Raf at the start of the MAP kinase pathway

Ras-GEF. Nucleotide exchange factor called SOS that activates Ras

Rate constant. Proportionality constant between the concentration(s) of reactant(s) and the rate of a reaction

RCC1 (regulator of chromosome condensation). Ran guanine nucleotide exchange factor (GEF) that associates tightly with chromatin throughout the cell cycle and maintains a high concentration of RanGTP in the nucleus

Reaction center. Complex of proteins with light-absorbing chromophores and electron transfer cofactors that absorb light and initiate an electron transport pathway that pumps protons out of Bacteria and thylakoids of chloroplasts

Receptor. Macromolecule that selectively binds particular partner molecules (ligands), initiating a cellular response

Receptor serine/threonine kinase. Family of receptors that bind ligands related to transforming growth factor beta and initiate signaling through cytoplasmic serine/threonine kinase domains

Receptor tyrosine kinase. Family of receptors that bind growth factors and initiate signaling through cytoplasmic tyrosine kinase domains

Receptor-mediated endocytosis. Facilitated uptake of an extracellular ligand due to its binding to a receptor that undergoes endocytosis

Recombination. Physical exchange of DNA strands between homologous chromosomes, during meiosis 1 drives chromosomal pairing and formation of chiasmata that are critical for segregation of homologous chromosomes

Recycling endosome. Endosome located in the perinuclear Golgi region where receptors returning to the cell surface accumulate

Reductional division. First division of meiosis when homologous chromosomes separate and the chromosome number halves

Reductionism. Experimental strategy relying on characterization and reconstitution of isolated molecular components of complex biological systems

Regulated secretory pathway. Route for concentrating and packaging proteins in storage granules for discharge from the cell in response to hormonal or neural stimulation

Repetitive DNA. Sequences present in many copies (thousands, in some cases) in eukaryotic genomes

Replication foci. Up to 1000 or more sites of replication observed in eukaryotic nuclei during S phase, each representing five or six coordinately activated replication origins

Replication fork. Site of DNA replication consisting of a parental DNA molecule unwound into two strands along with the replication machinery on both strands

Replicon. Region of chromosomal DNA replicated from a single origin of replication

Rescue (in dynamic instability). Random transition of a microtubule from a phase of rapid shortening to regrowth

Residual body. Mature lysosome containing a large amount of undegraded material

Restriction point. Checkpoint in late G_1 phase that blocks cells from committing to a proliferation cycle unless nutrients and mitogens are present and the cell senses appropriate interactions with the surrounding extracellular matrix

Retina. Epithelium at the back of the vertebrate eye with an array of photoreceptor cells

Retinal. Vitamin A derivative that serves as the chromophore for rhodopsin, the photon receptor in the eye

Retrieval pathway. Recycling of proteins and lipids from the Golgi back to the ER

Retrograde traffic. Flow of cargo and lipids back toward the ER

Retrograde transport. Movement of membrane-bound particles toward the cell body of neurons

Retromer. Protein complex involved in transport from late endosomes to *trans*-Golgi network

Retrotranslocon. Channel proposed to export proteins from the ER lumen or membrane into the cytoplasm for degradation

Retrotransposons. Transposable elements of DNA that move via RNA intermediates

Reverse genetics. Study of gene function by engineering desired mutations into cloned coding regions of genes

Reverse transcriptase. Specialized DNA polymerase that copies RNA into DNA

RFC (replication factor C). Protein complex that binds the $3'$ end of initiator DNA and uses energy from ATP hydrolysis to load the trimeric protein PCNA onto the DNA

RGD motif. Tripeptide (arginine-glycine-aspartic acid) used by several extracellular ligands to bind integrins

RGS proteins. Proteins that stimulate GTP hydrolysis by α-subunits of trimeric G-proteins

Rho. Family of small GTPases that regulate contraction mediated by myosin-II and other aspects of the actin cytoskeleton; essential for cytokinesis

Rhodopsin. Seven-helix receptor protein with covalently bound retinal that absorbs photons in the retina

Rho-GDI. Protein that binds Rho-GDP and blocks activation by GEFs

Ribose. Five-carbon sugar, component of RNA

Ribosomal RNA (rRNA). Three of the four RNA molecules forming the bulk of ribosomes including the catalytic site; precursor RNA cotranscribed by RNA polymerase and processed into 18S, 5.8S, and 25S/28S rRNAs

Ribosome. Complex of ribosomal RNAs with multiple proteins that catalyzes the synthesis of polypeptides

Ribozymes. RNAs with catalytic activity independent of proteins, including group I and group II self-splicing introns and ribosomal RNA

Ribulose phosphate carboxylase (called RUBISCO). Most abundant protein on earth, catalyzes the combination of a five-carbon sugar with carbon dioxide to form two molecules of the three-carbon sugar 3-phosphoglycerate in the stroma of chloroplasts

Rickettsia. Alpha proteobacteria closely related to mitochondria; cause of typhus and other diseases

Ring canals. Intercellular bridges that remain open following incomplete cytokinesis to maintain cytoplasmic continuity between daughter cells in specialized tissues

RISC. *See* RNA-induced silencing complex.

RNA. Polymer of phosphate-linked sugars (ribose) linked to purine and pyrimidine bases used to carry genetic information, catalyze reactions, bind ligands, or assemble with proteins in macromolecular complexes

RNA editing. Covalent modifications of individual nucleotides, which alter their base-pairing potential and thereby change the amino acid that is incorporated during protein synthesis; increasing the diversity of protein products that can be coded by the genome

RNA interference (RNAi). Experimental use of double-stranded RNAs complementary to a target mRNA to trigger its cleavage by RISC complex

RNA polymerase. Enzyme that transcribes (synthesizes) RNA complementary to a DNA template

RNA-induced silencing complex (RISC). Multienzyme complex that promotes the maturation of miRNAs and can cleave target RNAs, repress translation of mRNAs, or inhibit transcription of target genes via formation of heterochromatin

RNase H. Exonuclease that removes the RNA primer used to start DNA replication by chewing in from the 5′ end

Rod. Photoreceptor cell for sensitive detection of a broad range of wavelengths

Rough endoplasmic reticulum. Subdomain of ER with associated ribosomes synthesizing proteins for secretion and insertion into membranes and specialized for protein folding

RPA. Single-strand DNA-binding protein recruited by Cdc45 and Mcm proteins to stabilize separated strands of DNA during replication and repair

Ryanodine receptor. Calcium release channel of the endoplasmic reticulum

S phase (synthetic phase). Portion of the cell cycle when DNA is replicated

Saccharomyces cerevisiae. Budding yeast; popular genetic model organism for studying basic cell biology

SAM complex (sorting and assembly machinery of the outer membrane). Protein complex for translocation of proteins into chloroplasts

Sar1. Small GTPase that recruits COPII coat complexes to the ER membrane

Sarcomere. Contractile unit of striated muscle consisting of a bipolar array of overlapping actin and myosin filaments

Sarcoplasmic reticulum. Smooth ER of striated muscles specialized for rapid release and reuptake of the calcium ions that regulate contraction

Satellite DNAs. Repeated DNAs clustered in discrete areas of chromosomes, e.g., flanking centromeres

Scanning electron microscope. Optical system to scan a fine electron beam over a metal-coated specimen and create an image from secondary electrons emitted from the surface

SCF. Class of E3 ubiquitin ligase containing Skp1/Skp2, a cullin, and an F-box protein; important for cell cycle control by proteolysis

Schizosaccharomyces pombe. Fission yeast; popular genetic model organism for studying the cell cycle

SDS. Sodium dodecylsulfate; ionic detergent used to solubilize proteins for separation on the basis of size by gel electrophoresis

Sec61 complex. *See* Translocon.

SecA. Bacterial enzyme that uses ATP hydrolysis to promote the translocation of proteins through SecYE translocons

SecB. Bacterial chaperone for newly synthesized proteins to prevent folding and maintain a state competent for translocation

Second messengers. Calcium ions and small molecules including cyclic nucleotides and lipids that carry biochemical signals inside cells

Secondary constriction. Region of a chromosome associated with the nucleolus-organizing region

Secondary structure. Regular structures formed by polypeptides, especially α-helices and beta-sheets

Second-order reaction. Chemical reaction with two reactants

Secretory cargo. Transmembrane and lumenal proteins transported through the secretory system

Secretory granule. Membrane-bounded packets of concentrated secretory proteins prepared for secretion

Secretory membrane system. Distributes proteins and lipids synthesized in the ER to other sites using vesicular intermediates for transport between the ER, Golgi apparatus, and plasma membrane

Securin. Inhibitor of the separase protease that cleaves proteins to trigger the onset of sister anaphase chromatid separation

Segmental duplications. Regions of DNA ≥ 1000 base pairs with ≥ 90% sequence identity that are present in more than one copy but are not transposons

Selectin. Plasma membrane adhesion receptor for mucins on other cells

Self-assembly. Capacity of macromolecules to form large structures without guidance by templates

Self-cleaving ribozymes. RNAs with the capacity to cleave themselves in the absence of proteins

Senescence. Terminal G_0 state with viable but nondividing cells

Separase. Protease that cleaves a component of cohesin, triggering the onset of anaphase sister chromatid separation

Seven-helix receptor. A large class of receptor proteins composed of seven transmembrane α-helices, coupled to cytoplasmic trimeric G-proteins

Sex chromosomes. Chromosomes that carry genes that define the sex of an organism

SH2 domain. Family of adapter domains that bind peptides including a phosphorylated tyrosine, found in many signaling proteins

SH3 domain. Family of adapter domains that bind proline-rich peptides, found in many signaling proteins

Side chain. Chemical group on the α-carbon of an amino acid

Signal peptidases. Enzymes that cleave signal peptides from proteins after translocation of proteins across membranes

Signal recognition particle (SRP). RNA-protein complex that serves as an adapter between signal sequences and the translocon of endoplasmic reticulum

Signal sequence. N-terminal hydrophobic polypeptide signal that directs proteins to the ER

Signal transduction. Reactions that convert a stimulus into a change in the behavior of a cell

SINES (short interspersed nuclear elements). Retrotransposons of about 300 bp that make up about 13% of the human genome

Sinoatrial node. Cluster of heart muscle cells that generate the action potentials that produce rhythmic contractions

siRNA. Exogenus 22–nucleotide RNAs introduced into cells to trigger the destruction of target complementary RNAs by the RISC complex

Sister chromatids. Products of DNA replication, two identical DNA molecules, each packaged by chromatin proteins

Skeletal muscle. Striated muscle cells controlled by motor neurons in the spinal cord and brain stem

Slicer (Ago2). Component of the RISC complex that cleaves target RNA sequences that are perfectly complementary to miRNAs associated with RISC

Slow axonal transport. Transport of structural proteins and cytoplasmic enzymes from their site of synthesis near the nucleus along nerve cells process; some of these components move by rare short bursts of fast transport along microtubules

Smad. Family of cytoplasmic transcription factors activated to enter the nucleus after phosphorylation by receptor serine/threonine kinases following binding of ligands

Small heterochromatic RNAs (shRNAs). RNAs generated by transcription of both strands of DNA that associate with a nuclear complex called RITS (RNA-induced transcriptional silencing), which is related to the cytoplasmic RISC complex and induce heterochromatin formation and silencing of the transcribed locus

Small interfering RNAs. *See* siRNA.

Small nuclear RNAs (snRNAs). RNAs that function in complexes with proteins in small nuclear ribonucleoprotein (snRNP) particles to recognize signals in the pre-mRNA that identify introns and exons during splicing

Small nucleolar RNAs (snoRNA). Small RNAs, mostly excised from introns of RNAs transcribed by RNA polymerase II, that are involved in selection of the sites of modification of RNA bases during the maturation of functional RNAs

S/MARs (scaffold/matrix attachment regions). Regions of DNA that associate with the nuclear matrix and chromosome scaffold in biochemical fractionation experiments

SMC proteins (structural maintenance of chromosomes). ATPases that form part of the condensin and cohesin complexes that are essential for mitotic chromosome structure, regulation of sister chromatid pairing, DNA repair and replication, and regulation of gene expression

SMN protein (survival of motor neurons). Subunit of a large protein complex that promotes the assembly of Sm-proteins on snRNA, gene mutated in spinal muscular atrophy

Smooth endoplasmic reticulum. Subdomain of ER lacking ribosomes and dedicated to drug metabolism, steroid synthesis, and calcium homeostasis

Smooth muscle. Muscle cells without highly organized sarcomeres found in the walls of blood vessels and internal organs

Sm-proteins. Seven closely related proteins that assemble into a heptameric ring structure on snRNAs

SNAP receptor (SNARE). Family of proteins that participates in the fusion of carriers with their appropriate acceptor compartment

Speckles. Clusters of nucleoplasmic interchromatin granules containing factors involved in RNA processing

Spectrin. Actin-binding protein of the membrane skeleton of the plasma membrane and some cytoplasmic organelles; identified in red blood cell ghosts

Spermatids. Male germ cells that have completed meiosis but not yet differentiated into mature sperm

Spermatogenesis. Process that produces sperm

Spermatogonia. Stem cells that give rise to sperm

Spermatozoa. Mature sperm

Sphingomyelin. Sphingolipid with a choline or ethanolamine head group

Spindle checkpoint (metaphase checkpoint). Process that delays the onset of anaphase until every chromosome is properly attached to the mitotic spindle

Spindle pole. One of the duplicated centrosomes plus its associated pericentriolar material that nucleate microtubules during mitosis

Spindle pole body. Plaque-like structure embedded in the nuclear envelope of fungi that contains γ-tubulin and acts as the microtubule organizing center for mitosis

Splicing. RNA maturation reactions that cut out specific regions (introns) and rejoin the remaining RNA (exons)

sRNAs. Small RNAs of around 22 nucleotides that associate with the RNA-induced silencing complex (RISC) can lead to cleavage of target RNAs, repress translational of mRNAs, or inhibit transcription of target genes via formation of heterochromatin

SRP-receptor. Transmembrane receptor in ER that binds the complex of ribosome, nascent polypeptide chain, and SRP prior to cotranslational translocation

SR-proteins. Protein factors important for alternative splicing that contain domains rich in serine-arginine dipeptides

START. Point in the G_1 phase of budding yeast after which cells are committed to complete the cell cycle

STAT. Family of cytoplasmic transcription factors activated to enter nucleus after phosphorylation by JAK kinases

Stathmin. *See* Op18/stathmin.

Stem body matrix. Amorphous dense material within the central spindle that stabilizes bundles of antiparallel microtubules and holds together the two interdigitated half-spindles

Stem cell niche. Special environments created by tissue cells and the extracellular matrix that help stem cells maintain their status as stem cells

Stem cells. Cells with the capacity to produce, through intermittent asymmetrical cell division, both a self-renewing stem cell and a second cell with the capacity to differentiate into more specialized cells

Stem loop. RNA sequence that forms an antiparallel double helix with a loop at the end

Step size. Distance moved by a motor protein during one cycle of ATP hydrolysis

Stratified epithelium. Form of epithelium with multiple layers of cells on a basal lamina

Stress fiber. Bundle of actin filaments, myosin-II, and other proteins linking focal adhesions in nonmuscle cells

Striated muscle. Skeletal and cardiac muscles that have a striped appearance owing to alignment of the sarcomeres

Subunit. Macromolecular building block for a larger structure

Subunit flux (treadmilling). Flow of actin or tubulin subunits through their polymers as a result of net addition of subunits to one end and loss of subunits from the other end, observed for microtubules in mitotic spindles

Switch I/II. Regions of GTPases that change conformation depending on binding of GTP or GDP

Symporter. Carrier proteins that catalyze movements of solutes across membranes up concentration gradients at the expense of transport of a second solute down its concentration gradient in the same direction

Synapse. Specializations of nerve cells for rapid communication with other nerve and muscle cells in which the sending cell concentrates vesicles with a neurotransmitter prepared for secretion and the receiving cell concentrates receptors for that neurotransmitter

Synapsis. Intimate pairing of homologous chromosomes during zygotene of meiosis-I

Synaptic vesicle. Small vesicles filled with neurotransmitter concentrated in presynaptic endings

Synaptonemal complex. Protein scaffold assembled between homologous chromosomes during synapsis in meiotic prophase; looks like railroad tracks with a third rail running down the center

T tubule. Invaginations of plasma membrane in striated muscles that communicate action potentials deep into the cytoplasm

Tail-anchored protein. Protein inserted into membranes posttranslationally using a hydrophobic C-terminal anchor

Talin. Adapter protein between integrins and actin filaments in focal contacts

Targeting signals. Amino acid sequences that are both necessary and sufficient to guide proteins to their final destinations

TATA box. Promoter element for many genes transcribed by RNA polymerase II, consisting of the consensus sequence TATAAAA, recognized by TATA box–binding protein (TBP)

TATA box–binding protein (TBP). Protein that binds the TATA box, bending the DNA and promoting the assembly of the RNA polymerase preinitiation complex

Tau. Family of microtubule-associated proteins, including tau, MAP2, and MAP4, characterized by conserved microtubule-binding motifs that stabilize microtubules

Taxol. Cancer chemotherapeutic drug isolated from the bark of the Western yew that binds β-tubulin and stabilizes microtubules

Telomerase. Specialized form of reverse transcriptase, containing both RNA and protein subunits that is responsible for maintaining DNA sequences at telomeres

Telomere. Structure at both ends of chromosomal DNA molecules that protects the ends and ensures their complete replication

Telophase. Fifth phase of mitosis, initiated by reformation of the nuclear envelope on the surface of the chromatin

Temperature-sensitive (ts) mutants. Conditional mutants, functional at a low *permissive* temperature but not at a higher *restrictive* temperature

Termination. Reactions specified by a termination codon (UAA, UAG, or UGA) at the 3′ end of the coding sequence that complete the synthesis of a polypeptide and release the polypeptide and mRNA from a ribosome

Termination codons. The nucleotide triplets (UAA, UGA, UAG) that stop peptide synthesis

Terminator. Sequences in bacterial RNAs that trigger dissociation of a transcript and RNA polymerase when RNA polymerase reaches the end of a gene or operon

Tetanus. Maximal contraction of skeletal muscle achieved by repetitive stimulation by the motor neurons

Tethering factors. Rod-shaped proteins that tether membrane carriers to the cytoskeleton and target organelles prior to fusion

TGF-β. *See* Transforming growth factor–β.

Thick filament. Large bipolar filaments of myosin-II in striated muscles; interleaved with thin filaments

Thin filament. Actin-based filaments in muscle cells; interleaved with thick filaments

Thin section. Slice of plastic-embedded tissue for viewing by transmission electron microscopy

Threshold. Membrane potential required to activate voltage-gated Na-channels and initiate an action potential

Thrombin. Blood enzyme that cleaves the plasma protein fibrinogen into fibrin during clotting

Thylakoid membranes. Chloroplast membranes containing proteins for photosynthesis

Thymine. Pyrimidine base found in DNA; H-bonds with adenine

Thymosin β-4. Small protein that sequesters actin monomers

Tic (translocon at the inner membrane of chloroplasts). Integral membrane proteins specialized to transport proteins across the inner chloroplast membrane

Tight junction. Intercellular junction that occludes the extracellular space and regulates the passage of solutes between epithelial cells

Tim complexes (translocase of the inner mitochondrial membrane). Integral and peripheral membrane of the inner mitochondrial membrane that transport proteins into the matrix or inner membrane

Tissue stem cells. Stem cells with the capacity to renew themselves and to produce daughter cells that differentiate into a limited range of specialized cells

Titin. Giant striated muscle protein that extends between Z-disks and M-lines

Toc (translocon at the outer membrane of chloroplasts). Integral membrane proteins that transport proteins across the outer chloroplast membrane

Tom complex (translocase of the outer mitochondrial membrane) Integral and peripheral membrane protein complex of the outer mitochondrial membrane that translocates polypeptides into mitochondria

Transcription. Synthesis of RNA complementary to a DNA template strand

Transcription elongation. Phase of transcription in which RNA polymerase synthesizes an RNA strand complimentary to the sequence of the template DNA

Transcription factor. Proteins that associate with promoter sequences and are necessary for specific transcription by purified RNA polymerases in vitro

Transcription initiation. First phase of transcription including formation of a preinitiation complex leading to an open complex with unwound DNA and formation of the first phosphodiester bond between the first two complementary ribonucleotides

Transcription termination. Final phase of transcription when RNA polymerase reaches a signal on DNA that causes an extended pause in elongation, release of the nascent transcript, and base pairing of the DNA

Transcription unit. Gene-coding and regulatory (*cis*-acting) DNA sequences that direct transcription initiation, elongation, and termination

Transcytosis. Vesicular transport of extracellular ligands through the cytoplasm across a cell

Transducin. Trimeric G-protein coupled to rhodopsin in photoreceptor cells

Transesterification. Reactions during RNA splicing when new phosphodiester bond formation is coupled with breaking of old bonds, so, in principal, input of energy is not required

Transfer RNA (tRNA). Adapters between amino acids and mRNA codons during protein synthesis; these small RNAs carry a particular amino acid on one end and have on the other end the sequence of bases (anticodon) complementary for one of the mRNA codons that specifies that amino acid

Transformed cell. A cell lacking normal growth control that keeps proliferating as long as nutrient and mitogen supplies last regardless of whether it is touching neighboring cells or not

Transforming growth factor–β (TGF-β). Activates a serine/threonine kinase receptor and pathways that promote the differentiation of mesenchymal cells

Transgenic. Organism with a genome containing foreign genes

Trans-Golgi network (TGN). Exit face of the Golgi apparatus specialized for sorting cargo to various destinations

Transit sequences. Amino acid sequences that target polypeptides to chloroplasts

Translation. Protein synthesis catalyzed by ribosomes and guided by the sequence of nucleotides in mRNA that specifies the sequence of amino acids in a polypeptide

Translocon. Protein-conducting channel composed of Sec61 complex in the ER and SecYE complex in Bacteria

Transmembrane segment. Part of a polypeptide that extends into or through a lipid bilayer

Transmission electron microscope. Optical system that uses a beam of electrons focused by electromagnetic lenses to produce an image

Transposable elements (transposons). DNA segments dispersed throughout a genome, that either are now or were formerly capable of moving from place to place in the DNA

Transposons. *See* Transposable elements.

Treadmilling. *See* Subunit flux.

Trigger factor. Protein chaperone associated with bacterial ribosomes

Trimeric G-protein. Signal transduction complex consisting of a GTPase (alpha subunit), beta subunit and gamma subunit; GTP binding to the alpha subunit dissociates it from beta/gamma; both alpha and beta-gamma subunits can activate target molecules

tRNA. *See* Transfer RNA.

Tropomodulin. Protein that blocks the pointed end of actin filaments and binds tropomyosin

Tropomyosin. Alpha-helical coiled-coil protein that binds end to end along actin filaments

Troponin. Trimeric protein that binds calcium and cooperates with tropomyosin to regulate contraction of striated muscles

TRP channels. Family of cation channels that serve as temperature sensors among other functions

t-SNARE. *See* SNAP receptor.

Tumor necrosis factor. Inflammatory protein that activates trimeric receptors

Tumor suppressor. Gene that predisposes to cancer when inactivated; protein products are typically negative regulators of cell proliferation

Tunicamycin. Drug that inhibits the glycosylation of dolichol phosphate and therefore the formation of N-linked glycoproteins

Two-hybrid assay. Bioassay for protein interactions based on interacting proteins reconstituting a split transcription factor and activating a reporter gene

Type 1 transmembrane protein. Protein with its N-terminus facing the ER lumen or cell exterior, C-terminus in the cytoplasm and transmembrane segment spanning the membrane

Type 2 transmembrane protein. Protein with its N-terminus in the cytoplasm, C-terminus facing the ER lumen or cell exterior and transmembrane segment acting as an internal signal sequence

Ubiquitin. Small protein that when attached to the ε amino group of a lysine of a target protein, either signals the target protein for destruction or marks it for other interactions

Ubiquitin-activating enzyme. *See* E1 enzyme.

Ubiquitin-conjugating enzyme. *See* E2 enzyme.

Unfolded protein response (UPR). Response pathway triggered by excess misfolded proteins in the ER that leads to activation of genes controlling ER function

Uniporter. Carrier proteins that catalyze movements of solutes across membranes down concentration gradients

Unique-sequence DNA. DNA sequences typically present in a single copy per haploid genome, often coding regions of genes

Unprocessed pseudogenes. DNA sequences created either by reverse transcription of unspliced precursor mRNAs or by local duplications of the chromosome that generally occur as a result of recombination between transposable elements

Uracil. Pyrimidine base found in RNA; H-bonds with adenine

Vacuolar ATPase. V-type H$^+$ transporting ATPase pump that progressively acidifies the compartments along the endocytic pathway

van der Waals interaction. Distance-dependent attraction or repulsion of closely spaced atoms

Vesicle-tubule carrier (VTC). Pleomorphic transport intermediates that ferry secretory cargo from the ER to the Golgi apparatus

Vesicular transport. Mechanism to deliver cargo between donor and acceptor membrane-bound compartments involving small vesicles or tubular-vesicular carriers

Vimentin. Subunit of intermediate filaments in mesenchymal cells

Vinblastine. Drug isolated from periwinkle that interferes with microtubule dynamics by binding between tubulin dimers at the ends of microtubules; useful in cancer treatment

Vinculin. Actin-binding adapter protein concentrated in focal contacts

Voltage-gated channel. Ion channels with a domain that senses the electrical potential across the membrane and opens the channel gate above a certain threshold

v-SNARE. *See* SNAP receptor.

WASp. Protein that activates Arp2/3 complex to form branched actin filaments; product of the gene mutated in Wiskott-Aldrich syndrome, an X-linked immunodeficiency and bleeding disorder

Wee1. Nuclear protein kinase that phosphorylates Y^{15} in the active site of Cdk1, thereby inhibiting its function as part of a mechanism that holds Cdk1-cyclin B1 poised for a burst of activation

Wortmannin. Inhibitor of phosphatidylinositol 3-kinase

WW domain. Adapter domains that bind certain phosphoserine and phosphothreonine peptides; found in many proteins

Xeroderma pigmentosum (XP). Human genetic disease characterized by hypersensitivity to sunlight and predisposition to skin cancer caused by defects in nucleotide excision repair genes

Z-disk. Anchoring site for the barbed ends of striated muscle actin filaments

Zonula adherens. Ring-shaped adhesive junction around the apex of epithelial cells based on cadherins and anchored to cytoplasmic actin filaments

Zygotene. Second stage of meiotic prophase, defined by pairing of homologous chromosomes and clustering of telomeres giving rise to a "bouquet" arrangement of chromosomes

Index

Page numbers followed by f indicate figures; page numbers followed by t indicate tables; page numbers followed by b indicate boxes.